3RD EDITION

HEALTH ASSESSMENT IN NURSING

DISCLAIMER

This work is provided 'as is', and the publisher disclaims any and all warranties, express or implied, including any warranties as to accuracy, comprehensiveness, or currency of the content of this work.

This work is no substitute for individual patient assessment based upon healthcare professionals' examination of each patient and consideration of, among other things, age, weight, gender, current or prior medical conditions, medication history, laboratory data and other factors unique to the patient. The publisher does not provide medical advice or guidance and this work is merely a reference tool. Healthcare professionals, and not the publisher, are solely responsible for the use of this work including all medical judgments and for any resulting diagnosis and treatments.

Given continuous, rapid advances in medical science and health information, independent professional verification of medical diagnoses, indications, appropriate pharmaceutical selections and dosages, and treatment options should be made and healthcare professionals should consult a variety of sources. When prescribing medication, healthcare professionals are advised to consult the product information sheet (the manufacturer's package insert) accompanying each drug to verify, among other things, conditions of use, warnings and side effects and identify any changes in dosage schedule or contraindications, particularly if the medication to be administered is new, infrequently used or has a narrow therapeutic range. To the maximum extent permitted under applicable law, no responsibility is assumed by the publisher for any injury and/or damage to persons or property, as a matter of products liability, negligence law or otherwise, or from any reference to or use by any person of this work.

HEALTH ASSESSMENT IN NURSING

3RD EDITION

Peter Lewis BN, CertCC, MNEd, PhD
Associate Professor, School of Nursing, Midwifery and Social Work
University of Queensland, Brisbane, Queensland

David Foley BSc, RN, A&ECert, MN, PhD
Lecturer, Adelaide Nursing School,
The University of Adelaide, Adelaide, South Australia

Original US edition by

Janet R. Weber, RN, EdD
Professor Emeritus, Department of Nursing
Southeast Missouri State University
Cape Girardeau, Missouri, USA

Jane H. Kelley, RN, PhD
Retired Professor, School of Nursing
Indiana Wesleyan University
Louisville, Kentucky, USA

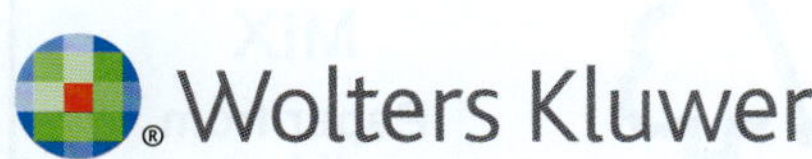

Philadelphia • Baltimore • New York • London
Buenos Aires • Hong Kong • Sydney • Tokyo

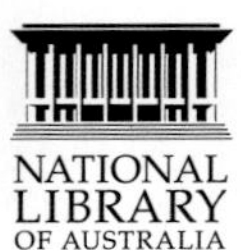

A catalogue record for this work is available from the National Library of Australia

Publishing Director – Asia Pacific: Vaughn Curtis
Senior Project & Program Manager: Helena Klijn
Project Coordinator: Elizabeth Ryan
Editor: New Best-set Typesetters Ltd
Proofreader: Marnie Firipis
Indexer: Max McMaster
Cover and internal design: Lisa Petroff Design
Rights and picture research: Karen Forsyth, Copper Leife
Typesetter: New Best-set Typesetters Ltd
Printer: C&C Offset Printing Co., Ltd, China

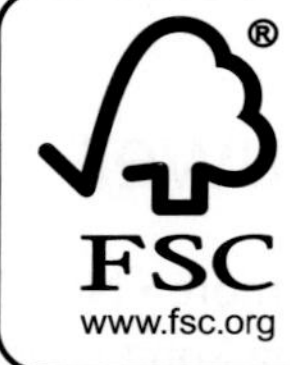

MIX
Paper from responsible sources
FSC® C008047

CCS0620

Contents

CONTRIBUTORS

AUSTRALIA AND NEW ZEALAND

Christopher AITKEN
AdvDipHlthSc, BHlthScN, RN, MClinSc, MACN
Clinical and Simulated Learning Environments Coordinator, Technical Services, Queensland University of Technology, Brisbane, Queensland
Chapter 39 The value of simulation-based learning

Julie BOWEN-WITHINGTON
Family Planning Cert, Women's Health Cert, Dip Tchg (Tertiary), GCert (Fam & CommHlth), BAppSci (Nursing), RN, RM, PGDipED, MA HlthSci (Nursing)
Principal Lecturer (Simulation), Te Hoe Ora ki Manawa, Department of Health Practice, Ara Institute of Canterbury, Christchurch, New Zealand
Chapter 21 Breasts and the lymphatic system

Kate CAMERON
OncNursCert, CertIV TAE, RN, GDip NSc, MNSc, PhD
Senior Lecturer, Adelaide Nursing School, University of Adelaide, Adelaide, South Australia
Clinical Practice Director, Cancer/Heart and Lung, Central Adelaide Local Health Network, Adelaide, South Australia
Chapter 35 Assessing families
Chapter 38 Assessing communities

Ryan CLARKE
RN, GDip (Online Learning), MTeaching (Secondary)
Clinical Nurse Educator, GAMA Healthcare Ltd., Melbourne, Victoria
Sessional Lecturer, University of South Australia, Adelaide, South Australia
Chapter 19 Mouth, throat, nose and sinuses

Tiffany CONROY
DipBusFLM, BN, RN, GCert (UnivTeach&Learn), MNSc, PhD, FACN
Senior Research Fellow, College of Nursing and Health Sciences, Flinders University, Adelaide, South Australia
Chapter 24 Abdomen

Jenny DAVIS
BAppSci (Nursing), RN, RM, BHIM (Hons), GCHE, GDip (Crit Care), GDip (Periop), MMid, PhD
Senior Lecturer, School of Nursing and Midwifery, La Trobe University, Melbourne, Victoria
Chapter 10 Assessing culture

Charlotte de CRESPIGNY AM
DipAppSc (Nursing), BN, RN, GDipPHC (Addiction), PhD
Adjunct Professor of Drug and Alcohol Nursing, School of Nursing, The University of Adelaide, South Australia
Chapter 11 Assessment in Aboriginal and Torres Strait Islander communities

Amye EDEN
BMid, GradCertMid, MMid
Lecturer in Midwifery, School of Nursing and Midwifery, University of South Australia, Adelaide, South Australia
Chapter 31 Assessing childbearing women

Iain EVERETT
BN, RN, GCert (Emerg Nurs), MPH, MNP
Lecturer/Nurse Practitioner, School of Nursing, The University of Adelaide/Queen Elizabeth Hospital, Adelaide, South Australia
Chapter 2 Collecting subjective data

Robyn FAIRHALL
BAppSci (Adv Nsg), RN, RM, MNSt, PhD
Senior Lecturer, Monash Nursing & Midwifery, Monash University, Victoria
Chapter 4 Validating and documenting data

David FOLEY
BSc, RN, A&ECert, MN, PhD
Lecturer, Adelaide Nursing School, The University of Adelaide, Adelaide, South Australia
Chapter 7 Assessing general status and vital signs
Chapter 8 Assessing pain: The fifth vital sign
Chapter 34 Assessing older people
Chapter 37 Assessing people with intellectual disabilities
Chapter 39 The value of simulation-based learning

Amanda FOX
RN, GDip HP, PhD
Senior Lecturer, School of Nursing, Queensland University of Technology, Brisbane, Queensland
Chapter 17 Eyes

Andrew GARDNER
DIP MEDICAL HYPNOSIS, BN, RN, MMHN, MBUSADMIN, PHD
Member of the Australian College of Mental Health Nurses
Senior Lecturer (Mental Health Nursing), School of Nursing, Midwifery and Social Work, The University of Queensland, Brisbane, Queensland
Chapter 36 Assessing alcohol, tobacco and other drug-related issues

Aaron GROGAN
A&E CERT, BN, RN, NP, MNP, MBA
Senior Lecturer, School of Nursing, Midwifery and Social Work, The University of Queensland, Brisbane, Queensland
Chapter 26 Male genitalia
Chapter 27 Anus, rectum and prostate
Chapter 29 Nervous system

Glenda HAWLEY
DIPAPPSCI (Nursing Management), RN (1st prize), RM, GDIP (Health Promotion), PHD
Lecturer, School of Nursing Midwifery & Social Work, University of Queensland, Brisbane, Queensland
Chapter 32 Assessing newborns and infants

Kat HITE
CERTIV T&A, RN, GCERT (Online Learning), GDIP (ICU), LLN
Nurse Educator, CALHN Nursing Education, Adelaide, South Australia
Chapter 3 Collecting objective data

Ainsley JAMES
BN, RN, MN, GRADCERT.HED, GRADCERT.PAEDS, PHD, MACN
Lecturer/Program Coordinator (Gippsland), School of Nursing and Healthcare Professions, Federation University Australia (Gippsland campus), Victoria
Chapter 10 Assessing culture

Jacqueline JAUNCEY-COOKE
RN, GRAD CERT HEALTH PROF EDUC, GRAD DIP CRIT CARE, MNRS, PHD
School of Nursing, Midwifery & Social Work, The University of Queensland, Queensland
Chapter 15 Skin, hair and nails

Sandra JOHNSTON
BHLTHSC, RN, GCERT (Management), GDIP (Sexual Health), MBA, PHD
Lecturer, School of Nursing, Queensland University of Technology, Brisbane, Queensland
Chapter 17 Eyes

Elyce KENNY
BN, RN, GRAD CERT (Nurs Ed), GRAD DIP PAED CHILD & YTH HLTH NURSING
Associate Lecturer, School of Nursing, The University of Adelaide, Adelaide, South Australia
Chapter 33 Assessing children and adolescents

Peter LEWIS
CERTCC, BN, MNED, PHD
Associate Professor, School of Nursing, Midwifery and Social Work, University of Queensland, Brisbane, Queensland
Chapter 4 Validating and documenting data
Chapter 5 Analysing data using critical thinking skills
Chapter 20 Thorax and lungs
Chapter 22 Heart and neck vessels
Chapter 28 Musculoskeletal system
Chapter 30 Pulling it all together

Patricia MEAD
BN, GDIP Health Counselling, MPHC
Acting Nursing Director, Acting Manager Acute & State-wide Services, Division of Child & Adolescent Mental Health, Women's & Children's Health Network, South Australia
Chapter 6 Assessing mental status and psychosocial developmental level

Andrew ORMSBY
BN, RN, MN, PHD
Group Captain, Director Air Force Health, Department of Defence, Canberra
Chapter 13 Assessing spirituality and religious practices

Joanne RAMSBOTHAM
CERT ADULT ED, EM, RN, MN CHILD HEALTH, PHD
Senior Lecturer, School of Nursing, Queensland University of Technology, Brisbane, Queensland
Chapter 18 Ears

Philippa RASMUSSEN
BN, RN, GCERT (CAMHN), GDIP (Psych St), MHN, MN, PHD
Associate Professor, Adelaide Nursing School, The University of Adelaide, Adelaide, South Australia
Deputy Dean International, Faculty of Health and Medical Sciences, The University of Adelaide, Adelaide, South Australia
Chapter 6 Assessing mental status and psychosocial developmental level

Charrlotte SEIB
RN, PHD
Senior Lecturer, School of Nursing and Midwifery, Griffith University, Gold Coast, Queensland
Co-lead, Women's Wellness Research Group, Menzies Health Institute Queensland, Griffith University, Gold Coast, Queensland
Chapter 25 Female genitalia

Linda A. STARR
DIPAPPSCI (Nursing), BN (Nursing), RN, GDIPED (Dist Ed), MHN, GCLP, LLB, LLM, PHD
Associate Professor, School of Nursing and Midwifery, Flinders University, Bedford Park, South Australia
Chapter 9 Assessing victims of violence

Snez STOLIC
RN, GCertEd, MAppSc, PhD
Lecturer, School of Nursing, Midwifery and Indigenous Health, Charles Sturt University, New South Wales
Chapter 1 The nurse's role in health assessment: Collecting and analysing data
Chapter 14 Assessing nutrition
Chapter 16 Head and neck
Chapter 23 Peripheral vascular system

Helen TOPIA
CT Nursing, BN, RN, MW, MAs APN, NP
Lecturer/Nurse Practitioner, Health Care Practice Nursing, Auckland University of Technology, Auckland, New Zealand
Chapter 12 Assessment in Māori communities

UNITED STATES

(Chapter numbers refer to *Health Assessment in Nursing* by Janet R Weber and Jane H Kelley; 5th edition)

Shirley ASHBURN
RN, BSN, MS
Professor of Nursing, Cypress College
Cypress, California
Chapter 7

Jill CASH
MSN, APN
Family Nurse Practitioner, Southern Illinois Rheumatology
Herrin, Illinois
Chapters 29, 30, 31

Kathy CASTEEL
APRN, MSN, FNP-BC
Family Nurse Practitioner
Columbia, Missouri
Chapter 14

Brenda JOHNSON
RN, PhD
Professor, Southeast Missouri State University
Cape Girardeau, Missouri
Chapter 32

Bobbi PALMER
APRN, MSN, FNP-BC
FNP Program Director, Southeast Missouri State University
Cape Girardeau, Missouri
Case Studies

Ann D. SPRENGEL
RN, EdD
Professor, Director of Undergraduate Studies
Department of Nursing, Southeast Missouri State University
Cape Girardeau, Missouri
Chapters 13, 22

Michelle TANZ
DNP, APRN, FNP-BC
Assistant Professor, Southeast Missouri State University
Cape Girardeau, Missouri
Chapter 8

Lisa WAGGONER
DNP, APN, FNP-BC
Assistant Professor, Arkansas State University
Jonesboro, Arkansas
Chapters 26, 27

Madonna WEISS
APRN, MSN, FNP-BC
Instructor, Southeast Missouri State University
Cape Girardeau, Missouri
Case studies and consultant for photo shoot

Cathy YOUNG
DNSc, RN, FNP-BC
Coordinator of FNP Track, Arkansas State University
Jonesboro, Arkansas
Chapter 10

REVIEWERS

AUSTRALIA AND NEW ZEALAND

Jann FIELDEN
RCPN, TCERT, PGCERT(Nsg), MA(Nsg)
Lecturer / Teaching Scholar, School of Health & Human Sciences, Southern Cross University, Gold Coast, Queensland

Ann FRAMP
RN, M ADV NURS PRAC, PHD
Lecturer in Nursing and Discipline Leader, School of Nursing and Midwifery, University of the Sunshine Coast, Maroochydore, Queensland

Sandra GOETZ
RN, MHLTHSC, GRAD CERT HIGHERED, SFHEA, MACN
Lecturer, School of Nursing and Midwifery, Griffith University, Brisbane, Queensland

Roslyn HALEY
RN, BNSC, MED
Lecturer in Nursing, School of Nursing and Midwifery, University of South Australia, Adelaide, South Australia

Geoffrey HARVEY
RN, CEN, BA, BHSC, MN (Adv Prac), CATA
Programme Leader Competence Assessment Programme for Registered Nurses, School of Nursing, Otago Polytechnic, Otago, New Zealand
Senior Lecturer, School of Nursing, Otago Polytechnic, Otago, New Zealand

Jennifer HOSKING
BN, GCERTHIGHERED, GRADDIPNURS(Crit Care), MNURSPRAC
Lecturer, School of Nursing and Midwifery, Deakin University, Geelong, Victoria

Victoria KAIN
RN, MN, PHD
Senior Lecturer, School of Nursing and Midwifery, Griffith University, Brisbane, Queensland

Annabel MATHESON
RN, BNURS, DIPHLTHSCI (Nursing), PHD
Senior Lecturer, School of Nursing, Midwifery and Indigenous Health, Charles Sturt University, Bathurst, New South Wales

Joy PERTILE
RN, MN, APN IN PRIMARY CARE AND EMERGENCY MEDICINE IN THE USA.
Lecturer, University of Tasmania, Sydney campus

Maryanne PODHAM
DIP APSCI, BHSC (Nursing), GCERT (Rural and Remote Nursing), GCERT (Clinical Education), MN
Lecturer, School of Nursing, Midwifery and Indigenous Health, Charles Sturt University, Dubbo, New South Wales

Mereana RAPATA-HANNING
RN, MN, GCLTT
Principal Lecturer, Te Kura Tapuhi | School of Nursing, Otago Polytechnic, Dunedin, New Zealand

Rebecca SCHULTZ
BA, BNG, RN, GRADCERTDIAB, MRP
Lecturer, School of Nursing, Edith Cowan University, Perth, Western Australia

Bronwyn SMITH
RN, BA, MPASR
Lecturer, School of Nursing and Midwifery, Western Sydney University, Sydney, New South Wales

Kiriaki STEWART
BN, RN, GDN (High Dependency), MNSC, MR (HLTH) CANDIDATE
Lecturer, School of Nursing & Midwifery, University of South Australia, Adelaide, South Australia

PREFACE

As nurses provide more care in acute care settings, clinics, family homes, rehabilitation centres and long-term care facilities, they need to be better prepared to perform accurate and timely health assessments. No matter where a nurse practises, two components are essential for accurate collection of patient data: a comprehensive knowledge base and expert nursing assessment skills.

With this third Australian and New Zealand edition of *Health Assessment in Nursing*, our goal is to help students to acquire the skills they need to perform nursing assessments in an ever-changing healthcare environment. This edition offers students in-depth, accurate information, illustrations and learning tools to help them develop skills in collecting both subjective and objective data.

In addition to nursing assessment skills, today's nurses need expert critical thinking skills to analyse the data they collect and to detect patient problems—whether they are nursing problems that can be treated independently by nurses, collective problems that can be treated in conjunction with other healthcare practitioners, or medical problems that require referral to appropriate professionals. This text encourages students to use critical thinking skills to analyse the data they collect.

FEATURES OF THE TEXT

Case studies in each chapter highlight the focus for that chapter. Each case study is presented sequentially throughout the chapter and in full at the end with corresponding critical thinking questions. The critical thinking questions have been structured to guide your progress through the chapter content, to help link the theoretical content with clinical practice and to ensure deep level learning.

> **CASE STUDIES**
>
> *In order for you to apply the theory discussed in the chapter, the following short case studies have been included so that you think about what you are reading and apply it.*
>
> - Emma is beginning her graduate rotation on an endocrine ward that adopts a team nursing approach to care. Although Emma intends to start her shift with a brief head-to-toe assessment of her ... seem more concerned

Focus on simulation Links to Laerdal simulation-based scenarios and to sim cases. Chapter 39 highlights the value of interactive, simulation-based learning, which is a vital component in healthcare education today. It empowers students to develop their knowledge and skills and to integrate theory with practice in realistic clinical settings, offering a rich, content-based immersive learning experience in a risk-free environment.

Links to Laerdal simulation-based scenarios Wolters Kluwer Health's partnership with healthcare simulation experts Laerdal enables this edition of *Health Assessment in Nursing* to provide references to the Australian and New Zealand Nursing education scenarios developed by Laerdal Australia, The Council of Deans of Nursing and Midwifery (Australia & New Zealand) and the National League for Nursing. These simulation scenarios address major learning objectives and different levels of complexity, and are pedagogically designed to facilitate acquisition of knowledge and skills in all key aspects of nursing care, from health assessment to patient management. The scenarios form the basis of the extensive learning experience that case-based learning in a simulated environment provides, enabling students to prepare for clinical placement and to acquire the knowledge and skills essential for professional registration and practice in today's complex healthcare environment. These scenarios are available to subscribers.

Links to sims cases In addition to the Laerdal simulation-based scenarios, five scenarios designed to be used in a simulation setting have been specifically written for this text and are available on thePoint. These scenarios have been developed so that teachers can deliver more immersive simulation experiences to teach assessment of the following topics: mental status, pain, victims of violence, elderly patients and patients with intellectual disabilities.

> **SIMULATED LEARNING**
>
> 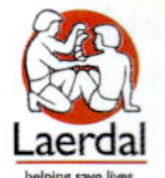
>
>
> **Having completed this chapter, explore the scenarios of Doris Bowman Parts 1 and 2. Doris is a 39-year-old female who is postoperative following a total abdominal hysterectomy. Incorporating the health assessment content in this chapter with your existing theoretical knowledge and clinical experience, progress through the simulation scenarios (this is best done in a small group). How would you manage Doris's care? When reflecting on your management of Doris, what do you think you did well and what do you think you can improve? Consider why you think this and also how you ... manage a similar problem in the future.**
>
> **... you have considered**

Older adult considerations boxes throughout the text include tips and information on adapting the assessment process to older adults, emphasising the person-centred approach and describing how some physical changes are normal adaptations to ageing rather than abnormal health findings. *Older adult considerations* boxes are in addition to Chapter 34, 'Assessing older adults', which provides an in-depth assessment of functional health in older adults, a demographic group that is growing in size in both Australia and New Zealand.

> **OLDER ADULT CONSIDERATIONS**
> Patients older than 80 years should recall two to four words after 5 minutes and possibly after 10 and 30 minutes with hints that prompt recall.

Paediatric considerations highlight considerations for babies and young children.

> **PAEDIATRIC CONSIDERATIONS**
> A normal temperature range for a child is usually 37°C and up to 38°C. Unless you are using a tympanic thermometer specifically designed for children less than 3 years old, a digital or electronic thermometer under the arm is the safest way to take an infant's or toddler's temperature.

Cultural considerations are included where relevant to highlight important considerations for particular cultural groups and to emphasise the need for cultural competency in healthcare practice.

> **CULTURAL CONSIDERATIONS**
> Eye contact and facial expressions such as smiling differ in some cultures. Eye contact is often related to status or gender (who initiates eye contact with whom), and smiling often does not imply agreement with the speaker, or friendliness. See Chapter 10 for more details.

Clinical tips are included throughout to help highlight critical content necessary for a thorough assessment, and to scaffold this upon existing knowledge.

> **CLINICAL TIP**
> When assessing the level of consciousness, always begin with the least noxious stimulus: verbal, tactile, to painful.

Safety tips alert the student to key information to ensure safe assessment practice.

> **SAFETY TIP**
> Use the rectal route only if other routes are not practical (e.g. patient cannot cooperate, is comatose, or cannot close mouth, or a tympanic thermometer is unavailable). Never force the thermometer into the rectum and never use a rectal thermometer for patients with severe coagulation disorders, recent rectal, anal, vaginal or prostate surgeries, diarrhoea, haemorrhoids, colitis or faecal impaction.

Watch and learn and **Concepts in action** icons highlight online videos and animations ancillaries that help explain key concepts. Online ancillary resources are available for both students and lecturers who have purchased the text.

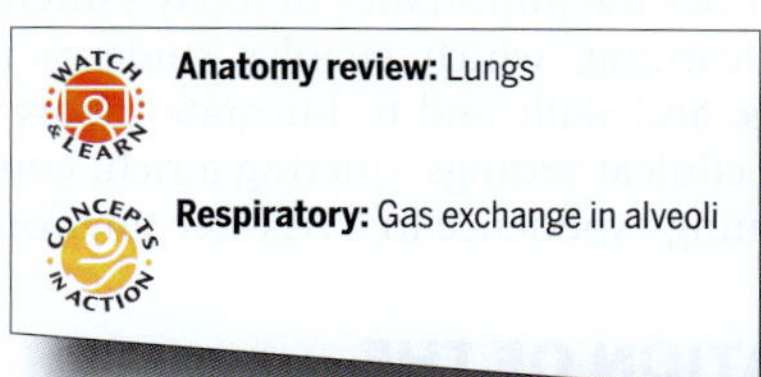

ORGANISATION OF THE TEXT

This third Australian and New Zealand edition of *Health Assessment in Nursing* has five units:

- Unit 1 Nursing data collection, documentation and analysis
- Unit 2 Integrative holistic nursing assessment
- Unit 3 Nursing assessment of physical systems
- Unit 4 Nursing assessment of special groups
- Unit 5 Health assessment and simulation-based learning.

Unit 1 describes the nurse's role in health assessment. It introduces the student to data collection and analysis as part of the nursing process. Separate chapters provide in-depth information about each step of the assessment process: collecting subjective data, collecting objective data, validating and documenting data, and analysing the data. The process of using critical thinking skills to assess patients is also discussed.

Unit 2 introduces the student to the concept that the patient should never be viewed as an isolated individual. Content covered in this unit is applicable throughout the entire patient assessment. The unit begins by explaining how to obtain an overall view or general impression of the patient. Assessment techniques to determine the patient's mental status and comfort level are described, as are ways to determine if the patient is a victim of violence; and ways to assess how culture, spirituality, religion and nutrition affect the patient's holistic health. Considerations in health assessment in Aboriginal and Torres Strait Islander and Māori cultures are also described.

Unit 3 immerses the student in actual assessment techniques for all body systems. Separate chapters cover techniques for each body system. Techniques to adapt for both the younger and the older patient are highlighted. The unit concludes with a chapter titled 'Pulling it all together', which shows the student how to integrate and individualise the assessment of all body systems. Students can use the examples provided to model their own data collections, analyses and formulation of diagnoses, collaborative problems or referrals.

Unit 4 reinforces the need to adapt assessment to the context of the patient. Chapters provide specific information about ways to assess childbearing women, newborns and infants, children and adolescents, people with intellectual disabilities, alcohol or drug-impaired patients, older adults, families and communities. Separate chapters for each of these groups allow students easy access to the information they need when taking another course, such as paediatric nursing or community health nursing. For example, rather than looking for toddler considerations in each body system chapter, the student need only look to Chapter 33 to find head-to-toe information about the toddler. The chapter on assessing older adults provides an in-depth assessment of functional health of the elderly population.

Unit 5 describes the importance of today's interactive, simulation-based learning, which enables students to develop their knowledge and skills and to integrate theory with practice in realistic clinical settings, offering a rich, content-based immersive learning experience in a risk-free environment.

ORGANISATION OF THE ASSESSMENT CHAPTERS

Assessment chapters walk students through the entire assessment process from an anatomy and physiology review, to data collection and analysis. Integration of a case study and corresponding critical thinking questions is designed to engage the student with the chapter content as well as to ground this content through real-life application. The assessment chapters include the following organisation:

- Integrated case study
- Structure and function
- Health assessment
- Collecting subjective data: The nursing health history
- Collecting objective data: Physical examination
- Validating and documenting findings
- Analysis of data
- Diagnostic reasoning: Possible conclusions
- Complete case study (combines the integrated case study with a COLDSPA table and concept map).

The **integrated case study** is presented sequentially throughout the chapter. Individual components of the case study are aligned with corresponding content. Critical thinking questions are posed to focus the student's thoughts: they reflect the content just covered and also require the application of this content using a problem-solving approach to determine what content may subsequently follow in the chapter and why. The ability to answer these questions will also provide immediate feedback as to how well past content has been absorbed.

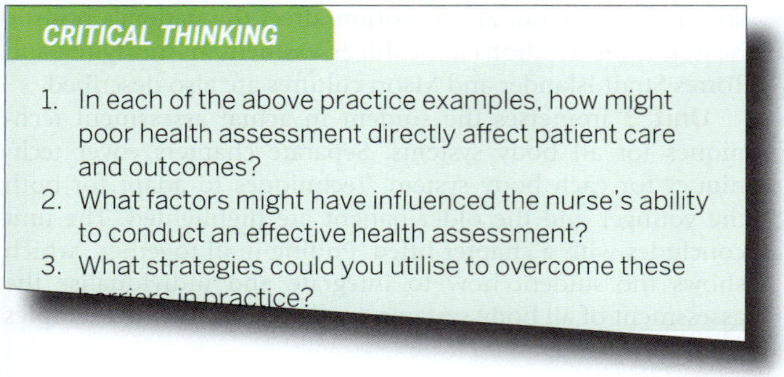

CRITICAL THINKING

1. In each of the above practice examples, how might poor health assessment directly affect patient care and outcomes?
2. What factors might have influenced the nurse's ability to conduct an effective health assessment?
3. What strategies could you utilise to overcome these barriers in practice?

Structure and function sections review key anatomy and physiology, which provide the knowledge base the nurse draws on to complete assessment. Health assessment sections give in-depth assessment parameters, including nursing health history, physical assessment, and validation and documentation of the data.

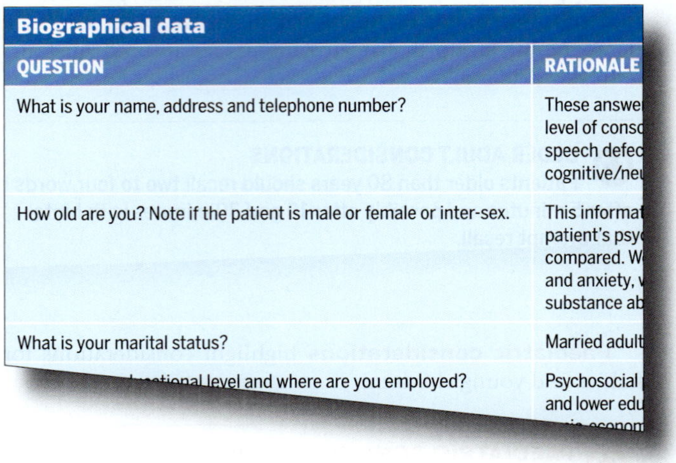

Biographical data

QUESTION	RATIONALE
What is your name, address and telephone number?	These answe level of consc speech defec cognitive/neu
How old are you? Note if the patient is male or female or inter-sex.	This informat patient's psyc compared. W and anxiety, v substance ab
What is your marital status?	Married adult
...ucational level and where are you employed?	Psychosocial and lower edu ...ic econom

Nursing health history information is presented in two columns: column one gives examples of questions to ask the patient and column two gives the rationale for asking each question. This approach is designed to help students to understand the 'whys' behind the 'whats', promoting critical thinking.

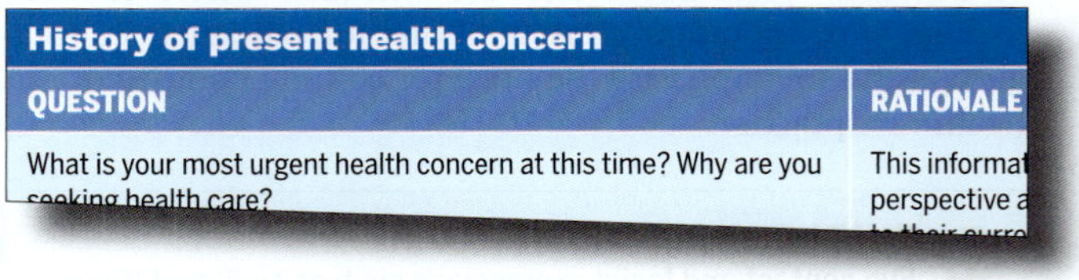

History of present health concern

QUESTION	RATIONALE
What is your most urgent health concern at this time? Why are you seeking health care?	This informat perspective a ...

Next, **physical examination procedures** are illustrated in a step-by-step fashion across three columns. Column one describes how to perform specific aspects of the examination; column two presents normal findings and normal variations; and column three presents a variety of abnormal findings. In addition, abnormal findings depict common abnormal findings, helping students to identify their findings. Sample documentation is also included.

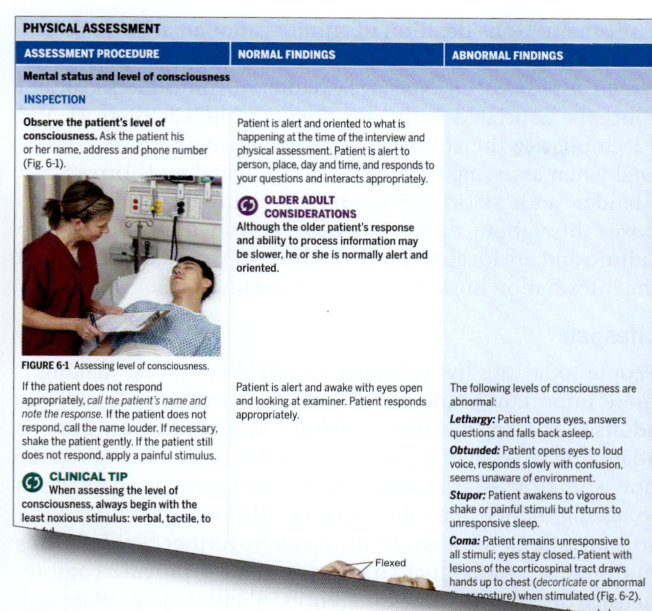

PHYSICAL ASSESSMENT		
ASSESSMENT PROCEDURE	NORMAL FINDINGS	ABNORMAL FINDINGS
Mental status and level of consciousness		
INSPECTION		
Observe the patient's level of consciousness. Ask the patient his or her name, address and phone number (Fig. 6-1). FIGURE 6-1 Assessing level of consciousness.	Patient is alert and oriented to what is happening at the time of the interview and physical assessment. Patient is alert to person, place, day and time, and responds to your questions and interacts appropriately. OLDER ADULT CONSIDERATIONS Although the older patient's response and ability to process information may be slower, he or she is normally alert and oriented.	
If the patient does not respond appropriately, *call the patient's name and note the response.* If the patient does not respond, call the name louder. If necessary, shake the patient gently. If the patient still does not respond, apply a painful stimulus. CLINICAL TIP When assessing the level of consciousness, always begin with the least noxious stimulus: verbal, tactile, to	Patient is alert and awake with eyes open and looking at examiner. Patient responds appropriately.	The following levels of consciousness are abnormal: *Lethargy:* Patient opens eyes, answers questions and falls back asleep. *Obtunded:* Patient opens eyes to loud voice, responds slowly with confusion, seems unaware of environment. *Stupor:* Patient awakens to vigorous shake or painful stimuli but returns to unresponsive sleep. *Coma:* Patient remains unresponsive to all stimuli; eyes stay closed. Patient with lesions of the corticospinal tract draws hands up to chest (*decorticate* or abnormal flexor posture) when stimulated (Fig. 6-2).

Sample of subjective data

Mr X is concerned about forgetting students' names in his class over the past semester. Also misplaces objects more frequently than in the past. Concerned this will impair his abilities as a teacher. Memory loss and misplacing things increase as the day progresses. No history of stroke, meningitis or head injury. No family history of Alzheimer disease. Brother had bipolar disorder. Is able to perform normal activities of daily living but

Sample of objective data

Mental status: Alert and oriented to person, place, day and time. Provided correct biographical information regarding: age (54 years), address and marital status (married). Holds a master's degree in education. Teaches Year 6 mathematics. Clean and well-groomed appearance. Good eye contact, with pleasant, cooperative disposition. Speech clear with moderate tone. Appears anxious over forgetting names and location of objects. Looking

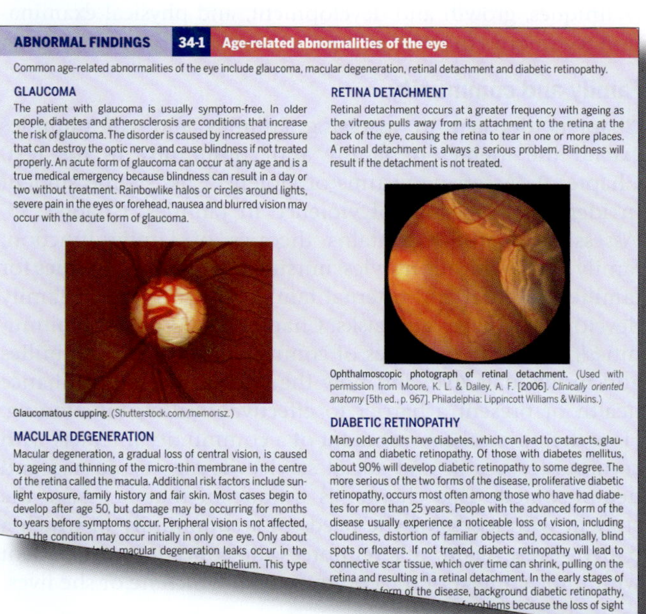

ABNORMAL FINDINGS 34-1 Age-related abnormalities of the eye

Common age-related abnormalities of the eye include glaucoma, macular degeneration, retinal detachment and diabetic retinopathy.

GLAUCOMA

The patient with glaucoma is usually symptom-free. In older people, diabetes and atherosclerosis are conditions that increase the risk of glaucoma. The disorder is caused by increased pressure that can destroy the optic nerve and cause blindness if not treated properly. An acute form of glaucoma can occur at any age and is a true medical emergency because blindness can result in a day or two without treatment. Rainbowlike halos or circles around lights, severe pain in the eyes or forehead, nausea and blurred vision may occur with the acute form of glaucoma.

Glaucomatous cupping. (Shutterstock.com/memorisz.)

MACULAR DEGENERATION

Macular degeneration, a gradual loss of central vision, is caused by ageing and thinning of the micro-thin membrane in the centre of the retina called the macula. Additional risk factors include sunlight exposure, family history and fair skin. Most cases begin to develop after age 50, but damage may be occurring for months to years before symptoms occur. Peripheral vision is not affected, and the condition may occur initially in only one eye. Only about

RETINA DETACHMENT

Retinal detachment occurs at a greater frequency with ageing as the vitreous pulls away from its attachment to the retina at the back of the eye, causing the retina to tear in one or more places. A retinal detachment is always a serious problem. Blindness will result if the detachment is not treated.

Ophthalmoscopic photograph of retinal detachment. (Used with permission from Moore, K. L. & Dailey, A. F. [2006]. *Clinically oriented anatomy* [5th ed., p. 967]. Philadelphia: Lippincott Williams & Wilkins.)

DIABETIC RETINOPATHY

Many older adults have diabetes, which can lead to cataracts, glaucoma and diabetic retinopathy. Of those with diabetes mellitus, about 90% will develop diabetic retinopathy to some degree. The more serious of the two forms of the disease, proliferative diabetic retinopathy, occurs most often among those who have had diabetes for more than 25 years. People with the advanced form of the disease usually experience a noticeable loss of vision, including cloudiness, distortion of familiar objects and, occasionally, blind spots or floaters. If not treated, diabetic retinopathy will lead to connective scar tissue, which over time can shrink, pulling on the retina and resulting in a retinal detachment. In the early stages of the milder form of the disease, background diabetic retinopathy,

Finally, the integrated case study is presented with a COLDSPA table and concept map to assist the student with a complete review of chapter content, data analysis and the diagnostic reasoning process.

COLDSPA

Example for memory loss

Use the COLDSPA mnemonic as a guideline to collect needed addition, the following questions help elicit important inform

Mnemonic	Question
Character	Describe the sign or symptom (feeling, appearance, sound, sme or taste, if applicable).
Onset	When did it begin?
	Where is it? Does it radiate? Doe anywhere else?

Sections on **validating and documenting findings, analysis of data, diagnostic reasoning** and **possible conclusions** assist students in their collation and analysis of data.

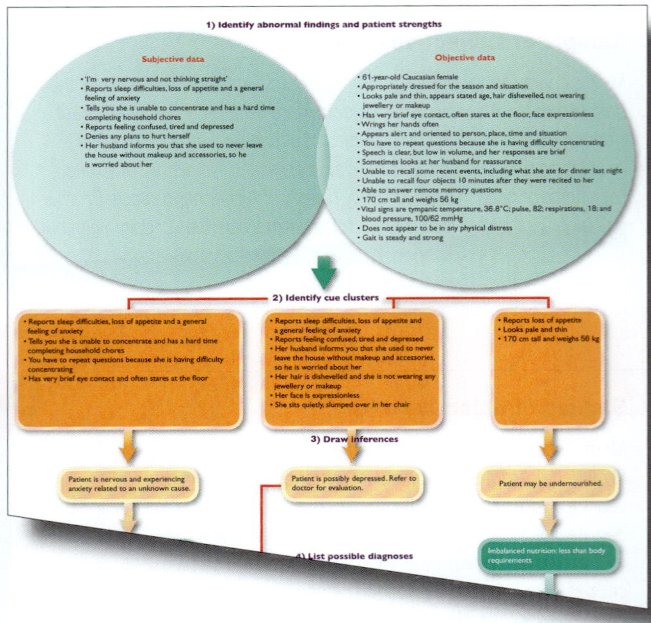

THEMES OF THE TEXT

Health promotion

Health promotion and patient wellness are important baseline concepts in *Health Assessment in Nursing*. Asking the types of questions exemplified in the *Nursing history* sections of the chapters provides the nurse with an opportunity to promote health—particularly in regard to nutrition, activity and exercise, sleep and rest, medication use and abuse, self-care responsibilities, social activities, family relationships, education and careers, stress levels and coping strategies, and adaptation to the environment and community. The Promote health displays detail risks and describe risk reduction tips, providing an excellent resource for students to use to teach patients ways to reduce risk factors.

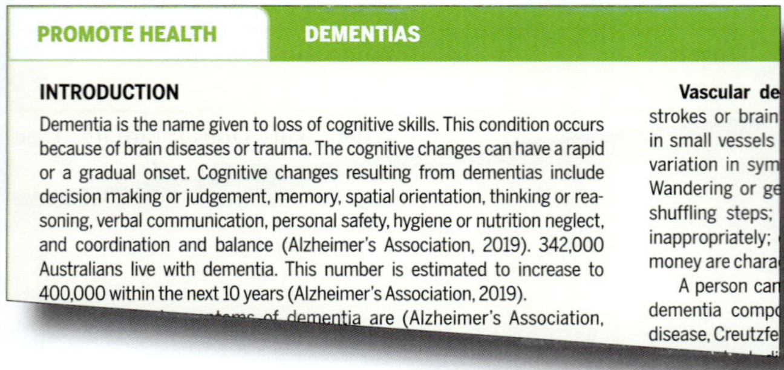

PROMOTE HEALTH DEMENTIAS

INTRODUCTION

Dementia is the name given to loss of cognitive skills. This condition occurs because of brain diseases or trauma. The cognitive changes can have a rapid or a gradual onset. Cognitive changes resulting from dementias include decision making or judgement, memory, spatial orientation, thinking or reasoning, verbal communication, personal safety, hygiene or nutrition neglect, and coordination and balance (Alzheimer's Association, 2019). 342,000 Australians live with dementia. This number is estimated to increase to 400,000 within the next 10 years (Alzheimer's Association, 2019).

strokes or brain
in small vessels
variation in sym
shuffling steps;
inappropriately;
money are chara
A person ca
dementia comp
disease, Creutzfe

Culture

In today's health care environment, both healthcare providers and healthcare recipients present with a vast cultural diversity. This poses new ideas, practices and challenges for nursing assessment. Consideration of culture is not an aside to assessment: it is an integral component and has a high priority in *Health Assessment in Nursing*. Chapter 10 introduces cultural concepts associated with assessment, while Chapters 11 and 12 emphasise the culturally important aspects to be considered when assessing the health of Aboriginal and Torres Strait Islander and Māori communities. Cultural considerations boxes throughout further highlight considerations related to culture and are located where the student would expect to find the information during an actual assessment.

Lifespan

People today are living longer and healthier lives, making it more important than ever to meet the health needs of older adults. Chapters in Unit 3 include information on how to adapt the assessment process to older adults and describe how some physical changes are actually normal adaptations to ageing, rather than abnormal health findings. Older adult considerations throughout the chapters further highlight this information. Individual chapters in Unit 4 provide comprehensive discussion of the differences inherent in assessing very young and elderly patients, as well as childbearing women. These chapters explain and illustrate the uniqueness of differences in regard to body structures and functions, interview techniques, growth and development, and physical examination techniques in these groups.

Family and community

Chapters devoted to assessing families and communities extend the themes of family and community in the text. Chapter 9, 'Assessing victims of violence', assists the student in identifying the use of violence in families. Chapter 35, 'Assessing families', contains theories of family function, family communication styles, nursing interview techniques for families, internal and external family structuring, and family development stages and tasks. Chapter 38, 'Assessing communities', addresses the types of communities in which families and individuals live, and how the community may enhance health or present a barrier to effective, healthy functioning. How the physical environment of a community interacts with community health and social services is also explained and demonstrated. This chapter is unique in that it assists the student with assessing the needs of a community in which a patient lives. Again, this reinforces the concept of the patient within the context of the community in which he or she lives.

A COMPREHENSIVE PACKAGE FOR LEARNING AND TEACHING

Ancillary resources available on thePoint* for instructors and students

To further facilitate learning and teaching, an extensive suite of online resources is available for lecturers and students whose institutions have adopted this text. These may be accessed at the text's accompanying website located on thePoint (http://thePoint.lww.com).

ONLINE RESOURCES

An extensive range of additional resources to enhance teaching and learning and to facilitate understanding may be found online at the text's accompanying website, located on thePoint at http://thepoint.lww.com. These include Watch and Learn videos, Concepts in Action animations, journal articles, case studies, discussion topics and quizzes.

... may also access Lippincott Procedures,

Student resources

- Journal articles
- Concepts in action animations
- Watch and learn videos

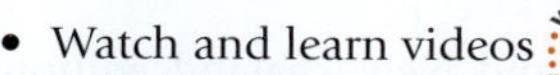

- Learning objectives

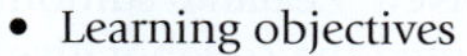

Instructor resources

- Five clinical scenarios on mental status, pain, victims of violence, elderly patients and patients with intellectual disabilities
- Question testbanks
- Discussion topics and answers
- Image bank
- PowerPoint presentations
- Case studies and answers
- Assignments and answers
- Pre-lecture quizzes and answers

A POWERFUL RESOURCE FOR STUDENTS AND LECTURERS

The third edition of *Health Assessment in Nursing* enables students and lecturers alike to rely on a dynamic teaching and learning resource—a unique combination of authoritative text, complemented by an extensive suite of resources in every format, all designed to extend the student's understanding and to assist the lecturer in teaching preparation.

Peter Lewis
David Foley

ACKNOWLEDGEMENTS

Christine and Joseph for love and patience; Dad, Mum, Peter and Patricia for guidance; God for my countless blessings.
Peter Lewis

My thanks for the support of my wife, Suzanne, and the encouragement of my children, Ted, John, Rosie and Michael. Teaching my nursing students health assessment has been a privilege that inspires me to cultivate their compassion.
David Foley

Preparing the third Australian and New Zealand edition of *Health Assessment in Nursing* has required the collaborative effort of academics, specialist clinicians and publishing staff. We gratefully acknowledge the expert knowledge and hard work these individuals have shared through their contribution of adapted content, review and comment. Special thanks to Liz Ryan for her tireless work in coordinating the review of this third edition.

Peter Lewis and David Foley; Brisbane 2020

UNIT 1 NURSING DATA COLLECTION, DOCUMENTATION AND ANALYSIS

CHAPTER 1

The nurse's role in health assessment: Collecting and analysing data

HOW TO USE THIS TEXTBOOK

Unlike most other health assessment textbooks, this text has an acute care focus. It presents content in a way that promotes student mastery of core assessment techniques relevant to actual nursing practice in acute care settings. In our experience, nursing students often feel overwhelmed when learning health assessment because of the large volume of information presented. It is important that you approach learning this material with some key points in mind.

First, it is not realistic to expect that new nursing graduates will possess every assessment skill necessary for all areas of nursing practice. Graduates with a strong foundation in health assessment and clinical reasoning skills should be capable of learning and applying additional assessment skills relevant to specialty areas. This is supported by research on the use of physical assessment skills in nursing practice. Birks et al. (2013) found from 1,220 surveys that students were taught to perform 121 physical assessment skills, yet only 34% of the skills were actually used on a daily or weekly basis by practising Registered Nurses (RN) in Australia. Birks et al. (2014), however, stated that 80% of the 53 Australian educators surveyed reported providing only 50% of 121 physical assessment skills. Taken together, these findings suggest a disconnection between what is taught and what is practised. The authors of the abovementioned studies argue, consistent with the approach taken in this textbook, that educators should focus on skills that are likely to be used in actual practice to inform nursing care. The Nursing Council of New Zealand Competencies for Registered Nurse (NCNZ/Te Kaunihera Tapuhi o Aotearoa, 2016) requires that nurses use scientific evidence, professional knowledge and clinical judgement to be able to meet Competency 2.2, which is the ability to undertake a comprehensive and accurate nursing assessment in a variety of settings. The Nursing and Midwifery Board of Australia (2017) requires that RNs are able to conduct comprehensive and systematic health assessment and assessment techniques to collect relevant and accurate information as incorporated into the Registered Nurse Standards for Practice.

Seminal research of physical assessment content taught in undergraduate nursing programs in the U.S. found that, of the 122 skills included on the survey, 81% were reportedly being taught in most programs; however, less than 25% of these skills were regularly used in clinical practice (Giddens & Eddy, 2009). Although there is evidence that only a subset of physical assessment skills is routinely used by RNs in practice, the authors suggest that nursing health assessment textbooks may be contributing to this finding, given that the volume of information included has continually expanded to meet a perceived market need. Nursing educators may feel obligated to cover all of the physical assessment techniques described in the textbooks. Moreover, because of their inexperience, students often have difficulty differentiating between the techniques that are important to learn and those that have little relevance for entry-level practice (Osborne et al., 2015)

Second, this textbook should be used as a tool to develop clinical judgement skills. Working through clinical scenarios and related critical thinking questions in each chapter allows you to practise 'thinking like a nurse' and helps prepare you for clinical placement.

Third, this health assessment textbook focuses on providing a solid foundation for interpreting physical assessment findings gathered in a health history and physical assessment. Tables and figures are used throughout the book to help emphasise normal and abnormal assessment findings. Assessment should be supported by knowledge in anatomy and physiology, pathophysiology and medical-surgical nursing. In this textbook, we can provide only a review of the key concepts of these subjects.

WHY LEARN HEALTH ASSESSMENT?

Acquiring health assessment skills is one of the most important and challenging aspects of becoming an RN. It includes the systematic collection of subjective and objective data so the nurse can make clinical judgements about a patient's health status. In doing so, the nurse may collect physiological, psychological, socio-cultural and developmental patient data.

Picture yourself in the following clinical situations:

- You walk into Mrs Tam's room for the first time. She is sitting on the edge of the bed crying and has not changed into a hospital gown. You introduce yourself and say, 'You seem very upset.' Mrs Tam tells you she is concerned about her ailing mother being left at home alone while she is in the hospital for breast cancer surgery.
- You arrive for work in the residential care home and take handover of your patient, Mr Stevanovic. He has been found unresponsive. You need to perform a primary and secondary survey on Mr Stevanovic to assess his sudden deterioration and to determine the appropriate immediate interventions.
- You work in the emergency department and need to check on Mr Nguyen, who has just come in complaining of dull pain near the navel, nausea and vomiting and a fever. When you enter the room you see the patient splinting his abdomen and a very anxious wife, already asking you a lot of questions.

Although often invisible to others, assessment comprises a major part of what expert RNs do. As a nurse, you will constantly observe situations and collect information to make clinical judgements. This occurs no matter what the setting: hospital, clinic, home, community or long-term care. Each of the above situations requires the collection of additional data before making a clinical judgement. For example, is Mrs Tam capable of caring for herself? Is Mr Stevanovic haemodynamically stable? What is Mr Nguyen's gastrointestinal status? What are the concerns and information needs of Mrs Nguyen? Additional information may be gathered from further direct observations of the patient and surroundings. In addition, you may also collect data by talking with the patient.

Learning to assess patients systematically and comprehensively is important because your assessment drives all components of the nursing process. Incomplete or inaccurate assessment leads to errors in identifying problems or results in poor judgements, which put your patients at risk of ineffective, inefficient or unsafe nursing care (Alfaro-LeFevre, 2014). Assessment data provide the foundation on which nurses base their decisions, interventions and evaluations. In the acute care setting, nurses are usually the first health care professional to identify and act on changes in a patient's condition at the bedside. Nurses draw on their health assessment skills to identify life-threatening complications and recognise subtle and overt changes that reflect deterioration of the patient's condition. Through early detection and intervention for patient problems, nurses save lives and improve patient outcomes every day.

Without an adequate knowledge base of health assessment skills and associated clinical terminology, nurses are unable to communicate with other members of the multidisciplinary team in a meaningful way about a patient's condition or clinical management. In order to be respected and valued members of the health care team, nurses also need to be able to use the same language as their colleagues.

Although health assessment is an essential competency of nursing education and it has been taught in undergraduate nursing programs for several decades. Reliance on others and technology, lack of time, ward culture, lack of confidence, lack of role models and lack of influence on patient care are all factors that affect nurses' ability to perform health assessment (Douglas et al., 2014). Effective strategies in performing an effective health assessment include a logical structured approach (Smith & Rushton, 2015) and avoiding distractions.

CASE STUDIES

In order for you to apply the theory discussed in the chapter, the following short case studies have been included so that you think about what you are reading and apply it.

- Emma is beginning her graduate rotation on an endocrine ward that adopts a team nursing approach to care. Although Emma intends to start her shift with a brief head-to-toe assessment of her patients, all the other nurses seem more concerned about completing patient showering and bed making. They don't seem comfortable with physical assessment and see it as 'something the doctor does'. After a while, Emma starts to prioritise completing these tasks over the clinical assessment of her patient load.
- Akari is working in a medical ward and is allocated to a patient after surgery who has had a chest drain inserted after a pneumothorax. Akari reads the medical officer orders, which state 'hourly checks for oscillation and bubbling', but she has no idea what this means. She contacts the medical officer, who says that she needs to assess for 'check for water swings in the seal chamber and look for any bubbles'. However, she does not understand what the instruction means or how to do them.
- Muhammad has just finished a clinical placement in a coronary care unit where he learned to auscultate patients' heart sounds with a stethoscope. During his next clinical placement on a surgical ward he continued to do this during patient assessment. There was no reason why he should not. However, the nurses on the new ward did not follow this practice. They gave him strange looks and made such offhand remarks as, 'What's with the stethoscope? Are you pretending to be a doctor or something?' or sarcastic comments whenever he performed the skill such as, 'Hear anything good?' In response, Muhammad stopped including heart sounds in his cardiac assessments.

CRITICAL THINKING

1. In each of the above practice examples, how might poor health assessment directly affect patient care and outcomes?
2. What factors might have influenced the nurse's ability to conduct an effective health assessment?
3. What strategies could you utilise to overcome these barriers in practice?

Table 1-1 Phases of the nursing process

Phase	Title	Descripting
I	Relationship	Establishing rapport with patient
II	Assessment	Collecting subjective and objective data
III	Diagnosis	Analysing subjective and objective data to make a professional nursing judgement (nursing diagnosis, collaborative problem or referral)
IV	Planning	Determining outcome criteria and developing a plan
V	Implementation	Carrying out the plan
VI	Evaluation	Assessing whether outcome criteria have been met and revising the plan as necessary

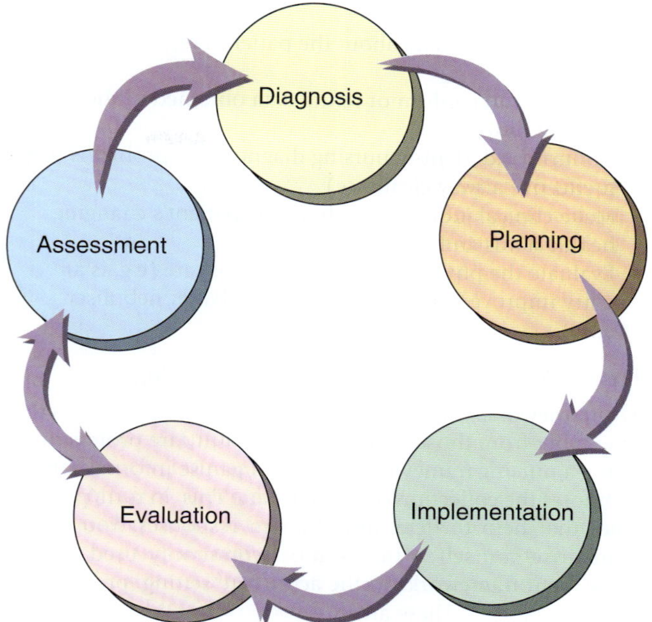

FIGURE 1-1 Each step of the nursing process depends on the accuracy of the preceding step. The steps are also overlapping because you might have to move more quickly on some problems than others. While evaluation involves examining all the previous steps, it especially focuses on achieving desired outcomes. The arrow between assessment and evaluation goes in both directions because assessment and evaluation are ongoing processes as well as separate phases. When the outcomes are not as anticipated, the nurse needs to revisit (reassess) all the steps, collect new data and formulate adjustments to the plan of care. (Alfaro, R. (2014). *Applying nursing process: A tool for critical thinking* (8th ed.). Philadelphia: Lippincott Williams & Wilkins.) Nursing health history and physical examination differs greatly from that of a medical or other type of health care examination (e.g. dietary assessment or examination for physiotherapy

HEALTH ASSESSMENT: A NURSING FOCUS

Interaction with a patient begins by establishing rapport through active listening and an empathic approach, which enables the nursing process that begins with assessment. Assessment is the first and most critical phase of the nursing process. If data collection is inadequate or inaccurate, incorrect nursing judgements may be made that adversely affect the remaining phases of the process: problem identification, planning, implementation and evaluation (Table 1-1). Although the assessment phase of the nursing process precedes the other phases in the formal nursing process, nurses are always aware that assessment is ongoing and continuous throughout all the phases of the nursing process. The nursing process should be thought of as circular, not linear (Fig. 1-1). Every health care professional performs assessments to make professional judgements related to patients.

The purpose of a nursing health assessment is to collect subjective and objective data to determine a patient's overall level of functioning in order to make a professional clinical judgement. The nurse collects physiological, psychological, socio-cultural, developmental and spiritual data about the patient. Thus, the nurse performs holistic data collection.

The mind, body and spirit are considered to be interdependent factors that affect a person's level of health. Nurses focus on how patients' health status affects their activities of daily living and how patients' activities of daily living affect their health. For example, in a patient with a medical diagnosis of chronic heart failure, the patient's response to illness may be anxiety or a lack of energy to carry out normal daily activities. These are human responses to heart failure that can be identified and treated by nurses.

In addition, the nurse assesses how the patient interacts within their family, culture and community and how the patient's health status affects the family and community. In contrast, the doctor performing a medical examination focuses primarily on the patient's physiological status; less focus may be placed on psychological, socio-cultural or spiritual well-being. Similarly, a physiotherapist would focus more on the patient's musculoskeletal system and ability to perform activities of daily living.

Thus, although nursing, medicine and allied health share common knowledge and skills for health assessment, the *purposes* for which the knowledge and skills are used differ:

- A medical assessment is used to evaluate the aetiology of disease and make a medical diagnosis.
- A nursing assessment is used to evaluate the *response* of the whole person to actual or potential health problems, which then inform nursing priorities and interventions.

For example, abnormal findings from a neurological assessment may be used:

- By a medical practitioner to make a clinical diagnosis of a brain lesion
- By an RN to consider nursing diagnoses related to functional ability and capacity for self-care (e.g. risk of falls), to determine the influence of disability on the patient's and family's lifestyles, and to gain insight into what these findings mean to the patient: all potential foci for independent nursing intervention
- By a physiotherapist to plan therapy involving exercise, splints or ambulatory aids.

Both the doctor and the RN auscultate a patient's lung sounds and determine that they are diminished and a wheeze is present. How will they use this assessment data differently?

The doctor listens to:

- Diagnose the cause of the abnormal sounds (e.g. asthma)
- Determine appropriate medical intervention (e.g. a prescription for salbutamol).

The RN listens to:

- Gather baseline data about the patient's respiratory function
- Supplement, confirm or refute data obtained in the nursing history
- Confirm and identify nursing diagnoses or problems (e.g. ineffective airway clearance)
- Make clinical judgements about the patient's changing health status and management
- Evaluate the physiological outcomes of care (e.g. is air entry improved and wheeze decreased after nebuliser use?).

Frameworks for health assessment in nursing

The frameworks used to collect nursing health assessment data may differ from those used by other health care professionals. Using a nursing framework helps to organise information and promotes the collection of holistic data. This, in turn, provides clues that help to determine human responses. You should familiarise yourself with the most commonly used nursing assessment frameworks in the acute care setting, presented in Tables 1-2 to 1-5. These are:

- Gordon's 11 Functional Health Patterns (Table 1-2)
- The Emergency Care Cycle (Table 1-3)
- The Body Systems Framework (Table 1-4)
- The Head-To-Toe Framework (Table 1-5).

Because there are so many nursing health assessment frameworks available for organising data, using one assessment framework would limit the use of this text and ignore many other valid nursing assessment framework methods. Therefore, the objective of this textbook is to provide you with the essential raw material necessary to perform a thorough health assessment without locking into one particular framework. You can take the information in this book and adapt it to the nursing assessment framework of your choice, relevant to the patient and context of care. The book is organised around a head-to-toe assessment of body parts and systems. In each chapter, the nursing health history is organised according to a 'generic' nursing history framework, which is an abbreviated version of the complete nursing health history detailed in Chapter 3. The questions asked in each chapter concentrate on that particular body part or system and are broken down into four sections:

- History of present health concern
- Past health history
- Family history
- Lifestyle and health practices.

After the health history, the physical assessment section provides the procedure, normal findings and abnormal findings

Table 1-2 Physical assessment frameworks: Gordon's 11 Functional Health Patterns

1. Health Perception—Health Management Pattern
   Subjective data: Perception of health status and health practices used by patient to maintain health
   Objective data: Appearance, grooming, posture, expression, vital signs, height, weight
2. Nutritional–Metabolic Pattern
   Subjective data: Dietary habits, including food and fluid intake
   Objective data: General physical survey, including examination of skin, mouth, abdomen and cranial nerves (CN) V, IX, X and XII
3. Elimination Pattern
   Subjective data: Regularity and control of bowel and bladder habits
   Objective data: Skin examination, rectal examination
4. Activity–Exercise Pattern
   Subjective data: Activities of daily living that require energy expenditure
   Objective data: Examination of musculoskeletal system, including gait, posture, range of motion (ROM) of joints, muscle tone and strength; cardiovascular examination; peripheral vascular examination; thoracic examination
5. Sexuality–Reproduction Pattern
   Subjective data: Sexual identity, activities and relationships; expression of sexuality and level of satisfaction with sexual patterns; reproduction patterns
   Objective data: Genitalia examination, breast examination
6. Sleep–Rest Pattern
   Subjective data: Perception of effectiveness of sleep and rest habits
   Objective data: Appearance and attention span
7. Cognitive–Perceptual Pattern
   For the purposes of this handbook, the cognitive pattern has been divided into two parts: (a) the sensory-perceptual pattern, to include the senses of hearing, vision, smell, taste and touch; and (b) the cognitive pattern, to include knowledge, thought perception and language.
   a. Sensory–Perceptual Pattern
      Subjective data: Perception of ability to hear, see, smell, taste and feel (including light touch, pain and vibratory sensation)
      Objective data: Visual and hearing examinations, pain perception, cranial nerve examination; testing for taste, smell and touch
   b. Cognitive Pattern
      Subjective data: Perception of messages, decision making, thought processes
      Objective data: Mental status examination
8. Role–Relationship Pattern
   Subjective data: Perception of and level of satisfaction with family, work and social roles
   Objective data: Communication with significant others, visits from significant others and family, family genogram
9. Self-Perception–Self-Concept Pattern
   Subjective data: Perception of self-worth, personal identity, feelings
   Objective data: Body posture, movement, eye contact, voice and speech patterns, emotions, moods and thought content
10. Coping–Stress Tolerance Pattern
    Subjective data: Perception of stressful life events and ability to cope
    Objective data: Behaviour, thought processes
11. Value–Belief Pattern
    Subjective data: Perception of what is good, correct, proper and meaningful; philosophical beliefs; values and beliefs that guide choices
    Objective data: Presence of religious articles, religious actions and routines, and visits from clergy

From Weber, J. R. (2017). *Nurses' handbook of health assessment* (9th ed.). Philadelphia: Wolters Kluwer Health.

Table 1-3 Physical assessment frameworks: The Emergency Care Cycle

The Emergency Care Cycle: Primary survey	The Emergency Care Cycle: Secondary survey
A = Airway • Clear and open airway • Assess for airway obstruction or respiratory distress B = Breathing • Assess respirations, air entry, colour C = Circulation • Check central pulse for quality and rate, skin colour, capillary refill D = Disability • Brief neurological assessment including level of consciousness (e.g. Alert, Responds to verbal stimulation, to Pain, Unconscious [mnemonic: AVPU]) • Assess pupils for size, shape, equality and response to light • Limb assessment for strength and sensation	E = Exposure/environmental control • Remove clothing for further physical assessment • Maintain temperature within normal limits F = Full set of vital signs/further investigations • TPR, BP, other investigations G = Give comfort measures • Pain/anxiety assessment H = History and Head-to-toe assessment • Allergies, Medication history, Past health history, Last meal, Events/Environment prior to illness (mnemonic: AMPLE) • Systematic head-to-toe assessment

Table 1-4 Physical assessment frameworks: The Body Systems Framework

- Integumentary
- Head, Eyes, Ears, Nose and Throat (mnemonic: HEENT)
- Cardiovascular
- Respiratory
- Gastrointestinal
- Genitourinary
- Musculoskeletal
- Neurological
- Endocrine
- Psychosocial

Table 1-5 Physical assessment frameworks: The Head-To-Toe Framework

- General survey
- Vital signs
- Head and neck
- Upper extremities
- Posterior chest
- Anterior chest
- Abdomen
- Lower extremities
- General neurological

for each step of examination of a particular body part or system. The collected data based on the patient's answers to the types of questions asked in the nursing history, along with the objective data gathered during the hands-on physical assessment, enable the nurse to make judgements concerning nursing and collaborative problems, and the need for patient teaching.

The end result of a nursing assessment is the formulation of nursing problems (or diagnoses) that require nursing care, the identification of collaborative problems that require interdisciplinary care and the identification of medical problems that require immediate referral.

Types of health assessment

The four basic types of assessment are:

- Initial comprehensive assessment
- Ongoing or partial assessment
- Focused or problem-oriented assessment
- Emergency assessment.

Each varies in the amount and type of data collected.

Initial comprehensive assessment

An initial comprehensive assessment involves collecting subjective data about the patient's perception of the health of all body parts or systems, health history, family history, and lifestyle and health practices (which include information related to the patient's overall function), as well as objective data gathered during a step-by-step physical examination.

The nurse typically collects the subjective data, especially those related to the patient's overall function. However, depending on the setting (hospital, community, clinic or home), other members of the health care team may participate in various parts of the objective data collection. For example, in a hospital setting the doctor usually performs a total physical examination when the patient is admitted (if this was not previously done in the general practitioner's office). A physiotherapist may perform a musculoskeletal examination, as in the case of a patient with a stroke, and a dietitian may take anthropometric measurements in addition to a subjective nutritional assessment. In some rural settings, a nurse practitioner may perform the entire physical examination. In the home setting, the nurse is usually responsible for performing most of the physical examination.

Regardless of who collects the data, a total health assessment (subjective and objective data regarding functional health and body systems) is needed when the patient first enters the health care system and periodically thereafter to establish baseline data against which future health status changes can be measured and compared. The frequency of comprehensive assessments depends on the patient's age, risk factors, health status, health promotion practices and lifestyle.

Ongoing or partial assessment

An ongoing or partial assessment of the patient consists of data collection that occurs after the comprehensive database is established. This gathering of data consists of an overview of the patient's body systems and health patterns as a follow-up on his or her health status. Any problems that were initially detected in the patient's body system or health patterns are reassessed in less depth to determine any major changes (deterioration or improvement) from the baseline data (Fig. 1-2). In addition, a brief reassessment of the patient's normal body system or health patterns is performed to detect any

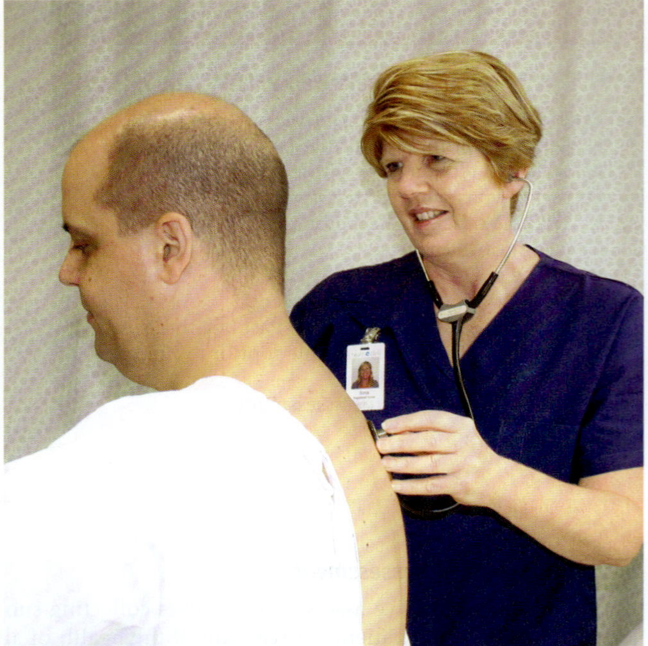

FIGURE 1-2 The nurse listens to the patient's lung sounds to determine any changes from the baseline data.

new problems. This type of assessment is usually performed whenever the nurse or another health care professional has an encounter with the patient. This type of assessment may be performed in the hospital, community or home setting. For example, a patient admitted to the hospital with lung cancer requires frequent assessment of lung sounds. A total assessment of skin would be performed less frequently, with the nurse focusing on the colour and temperature of the extremities to determine the level of oxygenation.

Focused or problem-oriented assessment

A focused or problem-oriented assessment does not take the place of the comprehensive health assessment. It is performed when a comprehensive database exists for a patient who comes to the health care agency with a specific health concern. A focused assessment consists of a thorough assessment of a particular patient problem and does not cover areas unrelated to the problem. For example, if your patient tells you he has ear pain, you would ask him questions about the pain, possible hearing loss, dizziness, ringing in his ears and personal ear care. Asking questions about his sexual functioning or normal bowel habits would be unnecessary and inappropriate. The physical examination should focus on his ears, nose, mouth and throat. At this time, it would not be appropriate to repeat all system examinations such as the heart and neck vessels or abdominal assessment.

Emergency assessment

An emergency assessment is a very rapid assessment performed in life-threatening situations (Fig 1-3). In such situations (choking, cardiac arrest, drowning), an immediate diagnosis is needed to provide prompt treatment. An example of an emergency assessment is the evaluation of the patient's airway, breathing and circulation when cardiac arrest is suspected. The only concern during this type of assessment is to determine the status of the patient's life-sustaining physical functions.

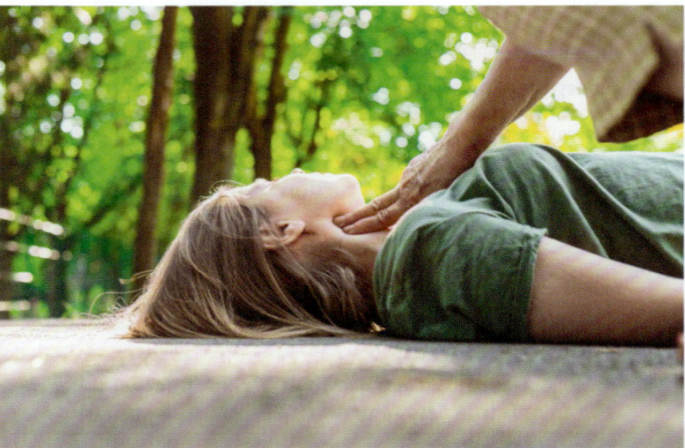

FIGURE 1-3 Assessment of the carotid pulse is vital in an emergency assessment. (iStockphoto.com/Madrolly.)

OVERVIEW OF THE STEPS OF HEALTH ASSESSMENT

The assessment phase of the nursing process has four major steps:

1. Collection of subjective data
2. Collection of objective data
3. Validation of the data
4. Documentation of the data.

Although there are four steps, they tend to overlap, and you may perform two or three steps concurrently. For example, you may ask your patient if she has dry skin while you are inspecting the condition of the skin. If she answers 'no', but you notice that the skin on her hands is very dry, validation with the patient may be performed at this point.

Each part of the assessment is discussed briefly in the following sections. However, Chapters 2, 3 and 4 provide an in-depth explanation of each of the four steps. In addition, these steps are covered throughout this text. All nursing assessment chapters contain the following sections: collecting subjective data, collecting objective data, and a combined validation and documentation section.

Preparing for the assessment

Before actually meeting the patient and beginning the nursing health assessment, there are several things you should do to prepare. It is helpful to review the patient's chart, if available. Knowing the patient's basic biographical data (age, sex, religion and occupation) is useful. These details provide background about chronic diseases and gives clues to how a present illness may impact the patient's activities of daily living. Also useful is documented information regarding the patient's medical diagnoses and progress notes. These give you an opportunity to verify what you read with what the patient tells you and to ask further questions as needed. Reviewing the patient's status with other health care team members who have taken care of or interacted with the patient is also helpful. Often a patient may reveal and share important data with some team members and not others.

After reviewing the patient chart or discussing the patient's status with others, remember to keep an open mind and to avoid premature judgements that may alter your ability to collect accurate data. For example, do not assume that a 30-year-old female patient who happens to be a nurse knows everything regarding hospital routine and nursing care, or that a 60-year-old male patient with diabetes mellitus needs teaching regarding nutrition. Keep an open mind. Validate information with the patient and be prepared to collect additional data.

Also use this time to educate yourself about the patient's diagnoses or tests performed. The patient may have a medical diagnosis you have never heard of or have not dealt with in the past. You may review the chart and find that the patient had a special blood test and the results were abnormal and that you are not familiar with this test. If this is the case, you should consult the necessary resources (e.g. textbooks, journal articles, hospital policy) to learn about the test and the implications of its findings.

Once you have gathered some basic data about the patient, take a minute to reflect on your own feelings regarding your initial encounter with the patient. For example, the patient may be a 20-year-old with a drug overdose. If you are 20 years old and are a very health-conscious person who does not drink, smoke, take illegal drugs or drink caffeine, you need to take time to examine your own feelings to avoid biases, judgements and the tendency to project your own feelings onto the patient. You must be as objective and open as possible. Other patient situations that may require more reflection time include those involving sexually transmitted infections, terminal illnesses, amputation, paralysis, early teenage pregnancies, human immunodeficiency virus (HIV) infection or acquired immunodeficiency syndrome (AIDS), and termination of pregnancy.

Finally, remember to obtain and organise materials that you will need for the assessment. The materials may be assessment tools such as a guide to interview questions, or forms on which to record data collected during the health history interview and physical examination. Also gather any equipment (e.g. stethoscope, thermometer) necessary to perform a nursing health assessment.

Collecting subjective data

The collection of subjective data is usually performed by a health history interview. The subjective data can be collected from the primary source (the patient) or secondary sources (the patient's family or friends or other health care professionals such as paramedics).

Subjective data are generally what patients communicate or perceive regarding their health status. Subjective data are sensations or symptoms (e.g. pain, hunger), feelings (e.g. happiness, sadness), perceptions, desires, preferences, beliefs, ideas, values and personal information that can be elicited and verified only by the patient. To elicit accurate subjective data, learn to use effective interviewing skills with a variety of patients in different settings. The major areas of subjective data include:

- Biographical information (e.g. name, age, religion, occupation)
- Physical symptoms related to each body part or system (e.g. eyes and ears, abdomen)
- Past health history
- Family history
- Health and lifestyle practices (e.g. health practices that put the patient at risk, nutrition, activity, relationships, cultural beliefs and practices, family structure and function, community environment).

The skills of interviewing and the components of a health history are discussed in Chapter 3.

Collecting objective data

Objective data are directly observed or measured by the nurse. They are also known as signs or overt data. The combination of subjective and objective data provides an overall picture of the patient's health status. Objective data include:

- Physical characteristics (e.g. skin colour, posture)
- Body functions (e.g. heart rate, respiratory rate)
- Appearance (e.g. dress and hygiene)
- Behaviour (e.g. mood, affect)
- Measurements (e.g. blood pressure, temperature, height, weight)
- Results of laboratory testing (e.g. platelet count, X-ray findings).

Objective data are obtained by general observation and by using the four physical examination techniques: inspection, palpation, percussion and auscultation. Another source of objective data is the patient's health record, which is the document that contains information about what other health care professionals (i.e. nurses, doctors, physiotherapists, dietitians, social workers) observed about the patient. Objective data may also be observations noted by the family or significant others about the patient. See Table 1-6 for a comparison of objective and subjective data.

Validating the data

Validation of assessment data is a crucial part of assessment that often occurs along with the collection of subjective and objective data. It serves to ensure that the assessment process is not terminated before all relevant data have been collected, and it helps to prevent the documentation of inaccurate data. What types of assessment data should be validated, the different ways to validate data and identifying areas where data are missing are all parts of the process. Validation of data is discussed in detail in Chapter 4.

Documenting the data

Documentation of assessment data is an important component of assessment because it forms the database for the entire nursing process and provides data for all other members of the health care team. The documentation of data from health histories, physical assessment forms and patient records creates a legal document used to plan care and communicate information from one health care provider to another. The documentation of data is a vital tool to monitor the progress of patients and elicit the quality of care provided. In order for the documentation to be useful and effective, nurses must adhere to strict guidelines. Information must be accurate, confidential, complete and detailed. When documenting data, the nurse must use appropriate abbreviations, symbols and clinical terminology that reflect standard and professional practices. Chapter 4 discusses the types of documentation, the purpose of documentation, what to document, guidelines for documentation and different types of documentation forms.

Table 1-6 Comparing subjective and objective data

	Subjective	Objective
Description	Data elicited from and verified by the patient	Data directly or indirectly observed through measurement
Sources	Patient Family and significant others Patient record Other health care professionals	Observations and physical assessment findings of the nurse or other health care professionals Documentation of assessments made in patient record Observations made by the patient's family or significant others
Methods used to obtain data	Patient interview	Observation and physical examination
Skills needed to obtain data	Interview and therapeutic communication skills Caring ability and empathy Listening skills	Inspection Palpation Percussion Auscultation
Examples	'I have a headache.' 'It frightens me.' 'I'm not hungry.'	Respirations 16 per minute Blood pressure 180/100 mmHg, apical pulse 80 and irregular X-ray film reveals fractured pelvis

ANALYSIS OF ASSESSMENT DATA

Analysis of data is the second phase of the nursing process. Analysis of the collected data goes hand-in-hand with the rationale for performing a nursing assessment. The purpose of assessment is to arrive at conclusions about the patient's health. To arrive at conclusions, the nurse must analyse the assessment data. Indeed, nurses often begin to analyse the data in their mind while performing assessment. To achieve the goal or anticipated outcome of the assessment, the nurse makes sure the data collected are as accurate and thorough as possible.

During this phase, the nurse analyses and synthesises data to determine whether the data reveal a nursing problem (sometimes expressed formally as a nursing diagnosis), a collaborative problem or a problem that needs to be referred to another discipline (referral).

The North American Nursing Diagnosis Association International (NANDA International, 2018–2020) has defined a nursing diagnosis as 'a clinical judgment about individual, family or community responses to actual or potential health problems or life processes. Nursing diagnosis provides the basis for selection of nursing interventions to achieve outcomes for which the nurse has accountability' (Herdman & Kanitsuru, 2018, p. 155).

Collaborative problems are defined by Carpenito (2017) as certain physiological complications that nurses monitor to detect their onset or changes in status. Nurses manage collaborative problems by implementing both doctor- and nurse-prescribed interventions to reduce further complications. Referrals occur because nurses assess the 'whole' physical, psychological, social, cultural and spiritual patient and, therefore, often identify problems that require the assistance of other health care professionals. Chapter 5 provides information about data analysis and problem identification.

The process of data analysis

To arrive at a nursing diagnosis, collaborative problem or referral, you must go through the steps of data analysis. This process requires diagnostic reasoning skills, often called critical thinking. The process can be divided into four major steps:

1. Suspend judgement (don't jump to a conclusion immediately).
2. Consider all possibilities regarding what might be going on for this patient and, if needed, collect more data (ask questions and consult with members of the intradisciplinary team).
3. Balance all information collected; ask: 'How does this relate to this patient now?' (Consider wider contexts for this patient, including determinants of health, lifestyle, values, health beliefs and practices of the patient).
4. Make a clinical decision holistically (view the person both as whole and within the context of his or her life, not just individual signs and symptoms) with accompanying clear rationale.

Each of these steps is explained in detail in Chapter 5. In addition, each assessment chapter in this text contains a section called 'Analysis of data', which uses these steps to analyse the assessment data presented in a specific patient case study related to the chapter content.

SUMMARY

Nursing health assessment differs in purpose, framework and end result from all other types of professional health care assessment. Assessment is the first and most critical step of the nursing process, and accuracy of assessment data affects all other phases of the nursing process. There are four types of nursing assessment: initial comprehensive, ongoing or partial, focused or problem-oriented and emergency. Health assessment can be divided into four steps: collection of subjective data, collection of objective data, validation of the data and documentation of the data.

It is difficult to discuss nursing assessment without taking the process one step further. Data analysis is the second step of the nursing process and the end result of nursing assessment. The purpose of data analysis is to reach conclusions concerning the patient's health. These conclusions are in the form of patient's problems, activating interventions or a need for referral. To arrive at conclusions, the nurse must go through eight steps of critical thinking or clinical reasoning.

These are:

1. Consider the patient's situation—includes listing the facts or describing the person, object or context
2. Collect cues or information—involves collecting or gathering information, for example handover report, patient history and chart, results and subject and objective data
3. Process information—requires analysis of the data, interpretation, discrimination and making deductions or opinions, and considering actions
4. Identify problems or issues—making inferences to diagnose the patient's problem
5. Establish goals—identifying what you would like to see occur, what the desired outcome is in a selected realistic time frame
6. Take action—selecting a course of action, choosing the most appropriate from those available
7. Evaluate outcomes—identifying the outcome of the intervention, whether the situation has improved or deteriorated
8. Reflect on process and new learning—critiquing or contemplating what you have learnt from the situation, considering if you would have done anything differently (Levett-Jones, 2017).

ONLINE RESOURCES

An extensive range of additional resources to enhance teaching and learning and to facilitate understanding may be found online at the text's accompanying website, located on thePoint at http://thepoint.lww.com. These include Watch and Learn videos, Concepts in Action animations, journal articles, case studies, discussion topics and quizzes.

Subscribers may also access Lippincott Procedures, an extensive online point-of-care procedure guide that provides reliable step-by-step instructions for more than 1700 procedures, including 450 evidence-based Australian procedures, and skills in a variety of speciality settings, together with a wealth of supporting information.

References

Alfaro-LeFevre, R. (2014). *Applying nursing process: The foundation for clinical reasoning* (8th ed.). Philadelphia: Wolters Kluwer Health/Lippincott Williams & Wilkins.

Birks, M., Cant, R., James, A., et al. (2013). The physical assessment skills by registered nurses in Australia: Issues for nursing education. *Collegian (Royal College of Nursing, Australia), 20*(1), 27–33.

Birks, M., Jones, A., Chung, C., et al. (2014). The teaching of physical assessments skills in pre-registration nursing programmes in Australian. *Collegian (Royal College of Nursing, Australia), 21*(3), 245–253.

Carpenito, L. J. (2017). *Handbook of nursing diagnosis* (15th ed.). Philadelphia: Lippincott Williams & Wilkins.

Douglas, C., Osbourne, S., Reid, C., et al. (2014). What factors influence nurses assessment practices? Development of the Barriers to nurse use of physical assessment scale. *Journal of Advanced Nursing, 70*(11), 2683–2694.

Giddens, J. F. & Eddy, L. (2009). A survey of physical examination techniques taught in undergraduate nursing programs: Are we teaching too much? *The Journal of Nursing Education, 48*(1), 24–29.

Herdman, T. H. & Kanitsuru, S. (Eds). (2018). *NANDA International Inc Nursing diagnoses: Definitions and classification 20184–2020* (11th ed.). New York: Thieme/NANDA International.

Levett-Jones, T. (2017). *Clinical reasoning: Learning to think like a nurse* (2nd ed.). Frenchs Forest NSW: Pearson.

Nursing and Midwifery Board of Australia. (2017). Registered nurse standards for practice. Viewed December 2018 at https://www.nursingmidwiferyboard.gov.au/Codes-Guidelines-Statements/Professional-standards/registered-nurse-standards-for-practice.aspx.

Nursing Council of New Zealand/Te Kaunihera Tapuhi o Aotearoa. (2016 Amendment). Nursing Council of New Zealand. Viewed December 2018 at http://www.nursingcouncil.org.nz/Nurses.

Osborne, S., Douglas, C., Reid, C., et al. (2015). The primacy of vital signs – acute care nurses and midwives' use of physical assessment skills: A cross sectional study. *International Journal of Nursing Studies, 52*(5), 915–962.

Smith, J. & Rushton, M. (2015). How to perform respiratory assessment. *Nursing Standard, 30*(7), 34–36. doi:10.7748/ns.30.7.34.s45.

Weber, J. R. (2017). *Nurses' handbook of health assessment* (9th ed.). Philadelphia: Wolters Kluwer Health.

Selected readings

MacDonald, E. W., Boulton, J. L. & Davis, J. L. (2018). E-Learning and nursing assessment skills and knowledge – an integrative review. *Nurse Education Today, 66*, 166–174.

Martin, C. T. (2016). The value of physical examination in mental health nursing. *Nurse Education in Practice, 17*, 91–96.

CHAPTER 2

Collecting subjective data

Collecting subjective data is an integral part of nursing health assessment. Subjective data consist of:

- Sensations or symptoms
- Feelings
- Perceptions
- Desires
- Preferences
- Beliefs
- Ideas
- Values
- Personal information.

These types of data can be elicited and verified only by the patient. Subjective data provide clues to possible physiological, psychological and sociological problems. They also provide the nurse with information that may reveal a patient's risk for a problem as well as areas of strengths for the patient.

The information is obtained through interviewing. Therefore, effective interviewing skills are vital to accurate and thorough collection of subjective data.

CRITICAL THINKING

1. If you are not confident interviewing patients, what steps could you take to improve your interviewing technique and gain confidence?

INTERVIEWING

Obtaining a valid nursing health history requires professional, interpersonal and interviewing skills. The nursing interview is a communication process that has two focuses:

1. Establishing rapport and a trusting relationship with the patient to elicit accurate and meaningful information
2. Gathering information on the patient's developmental, psychological, physiological, socio-cultural and spiritual statuses to identify deviations that can be treated with nursing and collaborative interventions or strengths that can be enhanced through nurse–patient collaboration.

Phases of the interview

The nursing interview has four basic phases: introductory, working, and summary and closing. These phases are briefly explained by describing the roles of the nurse and the patient during each one.

Introductory phase

After introducing himself or herself to the patient, the nurse explains the purpose of the interview, discusses the types of questions that will be asked, explains the reason for taking notes and assures the patient that confidential information will *remain* confidential. The nurse also makes sure that the patient is comfortable (physically and emotionally) and has privacy. It is essential for the nurse to develop trust and rapport at this point in the interview. This can begin by conveying a sense of priority and interest in the patient. Developing rapport depends heavily on verbal and non-verbal communication on the part of the nurse. In addition, you may also collect data by talking to the patient or their significant other. These types of communication are discussed later in the chapter.

Working phase

During this phase, the nurse elicits the patient's comments about major biographical data, reasons for seeking care, history of the present health concern, past health history, family history, review of body systems for current health problems, lifestyle and health practices, and developmental level. The nurse then listens, observes cues and uses critical thinking skills to interpret and validate information received from the patient. The nurse and patient collaborate to identify the patient's problems and goals. The facilitating approach may be free-flowing or more structured with specific questions, depending on the time available and the type of data needed.

Summary and closing phase

During the summary and closing, the nurse summarises information obtained during the working phase and validates problems and goals with the patient (see Chap. 4), then identifies and discusses possible plans to resolve the problem (potential problems and complications or risks; see Chap. 5). Finally, the nurse asks whether anything else concerns the patient and if there are any further questions.

CRITICAL THINKING

2. How would you know whether you have managed to establish rapport with a patient during the interview?
3. Describe the critical thinking skills that you would use to interpret and validate the information that patients supply. How can you confirm what patients tell you about themselves?

Communication during the interview

The patient interview involves two types of communication: non-verbal and verbal. Several special techniques and certain general considerations will improve both types of communication and promote an effective and productive interview.

Non-verbal communication

Non-verbal communication is as important as verbal communication. Your appearance, demeanour, posture, facial expressions and attitude strongly influence how the patient perceives the questions you ask. Never overlook this type of communication or take it for granted.

Appearance

First take care to ensure that your appearance is professional. The patient is expecting to see a health professional; therefore, you should look the part. Wear comfortable, neat professional attire or a uniform. Be sure your nametag, including credentials, is clearly visible. Your hair should be neat and not in any extreme style; some nurses like to wear long hair pulled back. Fingernails should be short and neat; jewellery should be minimal. In some hospital, the policies are bare below the elbows—so no watches, bracelets or too many rings.

Demeanour

Your demeanour should also be professional. When you enter a room to interview a patient, display poise. Focus on the patient and the upcoming interview and assessment. Do not enter the room laughing loudly, yelling to a colleague or muttering under your breath. This appears unprofessional to the patient and will have an effect on the entire interview process. Greet the patient calmly and focus your full attention on him or her. Do not be overwhelmingly friendly or 'touchy'; many patients are uncomfortable with this type of behaviour. It is best to maintain a professional distance.

Facial expression

Facial expressions are often an overlooked aspect of communication. Because your facial expression often shows what you are truly thinking (regardless of what you are actually saying), keep a close check on your facial expression. No matter what you think about a patient or what kind of day you are having, keep your expression neutral and friendly. If your face shows anger or anxiety, the patient will sense it and may think it is directed towards him or her. If you cannot effectively hide your emotions, you may want to explain that you are angry or upset about a personal situation, but admitting this to the patient to develop a trusting relationship and genuine rapport is not advised according to the Registered Nurse standards for practice (Nursing and Midwifery Board [NMBA], 2018) and the International Council of Nurses code of ethics for nurses (ICN, 2012). You may need to have another nurse continue with the interview.

Portraying a neutral expression does not mean that your face lacks expression. It means using the right expression at the right time. If the patient looks upset, you should appear, and be, understanding and concerned. Conversely, smiling when the patient is on the verge of tears will cause the patient to believe you do not care about his or her problem.

Attitude

One of the most important non-verbal skills to develop as a health care professional is a non-judgemental attitude. You should practise the concepts of cultural safety towards all patients who should be accepted, regardless of beliefs whether secular or religious, nationality, political beliefs, ethnicity and culture, gender, lifestyle and health care practices. Do not act superior to the patient or appear shocked, disgusted or surprised at what you are told. These attitudes will cause the patient to feel uncomfortable opening up to you and important data concerning his or her health status could be withheld.

Being non-judgemental involves not 'preaching' to the patient or imposing your own sense of ethics or morality. Focus on health care and how you can best help the patient to achieve the highest possible level of health. For example, if you are interviewing a female patient who smokes, avoid lecturing condescendingly about the dangers of smoking. Also avoid telling her that she is foolish or portraying an attitude of disgust. This will only harm the nurse–patient relationship and will do nothing to improve the patient's health. The patient is, no doubt, already aware of the dangers of smoking. Forcing guilt on her is unhelpful. Accept the patient, be understanding of the habit and work together to improve the patient's health. This does not mean you should not encourage the patient to quit; it means that how you approach the situation makes a difference. Let the patient know you understand that it is hard to quit smoking, support her efforts to quit and offer suggestions on the latest methods available to help kick the smoking habit.

Silence

Another non-verbal technique to use during the interview process is silence. Periods of silence allow you and the patient to reflect and organise your thoughts, which facilitates more accurate reporting and data collection.

CRITICAL THINKING

4. Do you think that beginning a question with 'Why . . .' is a reasonable way to ask someone about their health practices and beliefs? For example, are there any problems asking a patient, 'Why do you smoke?' Could you ask this question another way?
5. During an interview it is good practice to allow periods of silence, but how long should these periods be allowed to last?

Listening

Listening is the most important skill to learn and develop fully in order to collect complete and valid data from your patient. To listen effectively, you need to maintain good eye contact in the majority of contexts, smile or display an open, appropriate facial expression, maintain an open body position (open arms and hands, and leaning forwards). Some people do not like or avoid direct eye contact, and some people are very silent for a variety of reasons be they cultural or part of their personality or character. It is important to build rapport and communication. One practical tip could be asking the patient what they may be interested in and then finding a common link with that interest while you are undertaking another task during the interview or assessment. This can be done with minimal eye contact.

Avoid preconceived ideas or biases about your patient. To listen effectively, you must keep an open mind. Avoid crossing your arms, sitting back, tilting your head away from the patient, thinking about other things, or looking blank or inattentive. Becoming an effective listener takes concentration and practice.

In addition, several non-verbal affects or attitudes may hinder effective communication. They may promote discomfort or distrust. Display 2-1 describes communication styles to avoid.

Verbal communication

Effective verbal communication is essential to a patient interview. The goal of the interview process is to elicit as much data about the patient's health status as possible. Several types of questions and techniques to use during the interview are discussed in the following sections.

Open-ended questions

Open-ended questions are used to elicit the patient's feelings and perceptions. They typically begin with the words 'how' or 'what'. An example of this type of question is 'How have you been feeling lately?' These types of questions are important because they require more than a one-word response from the patient and therefore encourage description. Asking open-ended questions may help to reveal significant data about the patient's health status.

Closed-ended questions

Use closed-ended questions to obtain facts and to focus on specific information. The patient can respond with one or two words. The questions typically begin with the words 'when' or 'did'. An example of this type of question is 'When did your headache start?' Closed-ended questions are useful in keeping the interview on course. They can also be used to clarify or obtain more accurate information about issues disclosed in response to open-ended questions. For example, in response to the open-ended question 'How have you been feeling lately?' the patient says, 'Well, I've been feeling really sick in my stomach and I don't feel like eating because of it.' You may be able to follow up and learn more about the patient's symptom with a closed-ended question such as 'When did the nausea start?'

Word list

Another way to ask questions is to provide the patient with a choice of words to choose from in describing symptoms, conditions or feelings. This list approach helps you to obtain specific answers and reduces the likelihood of the patient's perceiving or providing an expected answer. For example, 'Is the pain severe, dull, sharp, mild, cutting or piercing?' 'Does the pain occur once every year, day, month or hour?' Repeat choices as necessary.

DISPLAY 2-1 COMMUNICATION STYLES TO AVOID

Non-verbal communication styles to avoid

Excessive or insufficient eye contact

Avoid extremes in eye contact. Some patients feel very uncomfortable with too much eye contact; others believe that you are hiding something from them if you do not look them in the eye. Therefore, it is best to use a moderate amount of eye contact. For example, establish eye contact when the patient is speaking to you but look down at your notes from time to time. A patient's cultural background often determines how he or she feels about eye contact (see the section on cultural variations in communication for more information).

Distraction and distance

Avoid being occupied with something else while you are asking questions during the interview. This behaviour makes the patient believe that the interview may be unimportant to you. Avoid appearing mentally distant as well. The patient will sense your distance and will be less likely to answer your questions thoroughly. Also try to avoid physical distance exceeding 1 m during the interview. Rapport and trust are established when the patient senses your focus and concern are solely on the patient and the patient's health. Physical distance may portray a non-caring attitude or a desire to avoid close contact with the patient.

Standing

Avoid standing while the patient is seated during the interview. Standing puts you and the patient at different levels. You may be perceived as the superior, making the patient feel inferior. Care of the patient's health should be an equal partnership between the health care provider and the patient. If the patient is made to feel inferior, he or she will not feel empowered to be an equal partner and the potential for optimal health may be lost. In addition, vital information may not be revealed if the patient believes that the interviewer is untrustworthy, judgemental or disinterested.

Verbal communication styles to avoid

Biased or leading questions

Avoid using biased or leading questions. These cause the patient to provide answers that may or may not be true. The way you phrase a question may actually lead the patient to think you want him or her to answer in a certain way. For example, if you ask 'You don't feel bad, do you?' the patient may conclude that you do not think she should feel bad and will answer 'no' even if this is not true.

Rushing through the interview

Avoid rushing the patient. If you ask the patient questions on top of questions, several things may occur. First, the patient may answer 'no' to a series of closed-ended questions when he or she would have answered 'yes' to one of the questions if it was asked individually. This may occur because the patient did not hear the individual question clearly or because the answers to most were 'no' and the patient forgot about the 'yes' answer in the midst of the others. With this type of interview technique, the patient may believe that his or her individual situation is of little concern to the nurse. Taking time with patients shows that you are concerned about their health and helps them to open up. Finally, rushing someone through the interview process undoubtedly causes important information to be left out of the health history. A patient will usually sense that you are rushed and may try to help hurry the interview by providing abbreviated or incomplete answers to questions.

Reading the questions

Avoid reading questions from the history form. This deflects attention from the patient and results in an impersonal interview process. As a result, the patient may feel ill at ease opening up to formatted questions.

Paraphrasing

Rephrasing information the patient has provided is an effective way to communicate during the interview. This technique helps you to clarify information the patient has stated; it also enables you and the patient to reflect on what was said. For example, your patient, Mr G, tells you that he has been really tired and nauseated for 2 months and that he is scared because he fears he has some horrible disease. You might rephrase the information by saying, 'You're thinking that you have a serious illness?'

Well-placed phrases

Patient verbalisation can be encouraged by well-placed phrases from the nurse. If the patient is in the middle of explaining a symptom or feeling and believes that you are not paying attention, you may fail to get all the necessary information. Listen closely to the patient and use phrases such as 'yes' or 'I agree' to encourage the patient to continue.

Inferring

Inferring information from what the patient tells you and what you observe in the patient's behaviour may elicit more data or verify existing data. Be careful not to lead the patient to answers that are not true (see verbal communication styles to avoid in Display 2-1 for more information). An example of inferring information is as follows: Your patient, Mrs J, tells you that she has bad pain. You ask where the pain is and she says, 'My stomach.' You notice that she has her hand on the right side of her lower abdomen and seems to favour her entire right side. You say, 'It seems you have more difficulty with the right side of your stomach' (use the word 'stomach' because that is the term the patient used to describe the abdomen). This technique, if used properly, helps to elicit the most accurate data possible from the patient.

Providing information

Another important thing to consider throughout the interview is to provide the patient with information as questions and concerns arise. Make sure you answer every question as well as you can. If you do not know the answer, explain that you will find out for the patient. The more patients know about their own health, the more likely they are to become equal participants in caring for their health.

As with non-verbal communication, several verbal communication techniques may hinder effective communication (see Display 2-1).

Special considerations during the interview

Three variations in communication must be considered as you interview patients: older adult, cultural and emotional. These variations affect the non-verbal and verbal techniques you use during the interview. Imagine, for example, that you are interviewing an 82-year-old woman and you ask her to describe how she has been feeling. She does not answer you and she looks confused. This older patient may have some hearing loss. In such a case, you may need to modify the verbal technique of asking open-ended questions.

CRITICAL THINKING

6. How would you obtain descriptions of symptoms from a child, or a person with an intellectual disability?

Older adult variations in communication

Age affects and commonly slows all body systems to varying degrees. However, normal aspects of ageing do not necessarily equate with a health problem, so it is important not to approach an interview with an elderly patient assuming that there is a health problem. Older patients have the potential to be as healthy as younger patients.

When interviewing an elderly patient, you must first assess hearing acuity. Hearing loss occurs normally with age, and undetected hearing loss is often misinterpreted as mental slowness or confusion. If you detect hearing loss, speak slowly, face the patient at all times during the interview and position yourself so that you are speaking on the side of the patient that has the ear with better acuity. Do not assume that all elderly persons are hard of hearing so do not yell at the patient.

Older patients may have more health concerns than younger patients and may seek health care more often. Many times, older patients with health problems feel vulnerable and scared. They need to believe that they can trust you before they will open up to you about what is bothering them. Thus, establishing and maintaining trust, privacy and partnership with the older patient is particularly important (Fig. 2-1). It is not unusual for elderly patients to be taken for granted and their health complaints ignored, causing them to become fearful of complaining. It is often disturbing to the older patient that his or her health problems may be discussed openly among many health care providers and family members. Assure your elderly patients that you are concerned, that you see them as equal partners in health care and that what is discussed will be between you, their health care provider and them.

Speak clearly and use straightforward language during the interview with the elderly patient. Avoid medical jargon and modern slang. Ask questions in simple terms, but do not talk down to the patient. It is important to not be overly familiar and use condescending language such as 'dear' or 'love'. Being older physically does not mean the patient is slower mentally. Showing respect is important. However, if the patient is mentally confused or forgetful, it is important to have a significant other (e.g. spouse, child, close friend) present during the interview to provide or clarify the data.

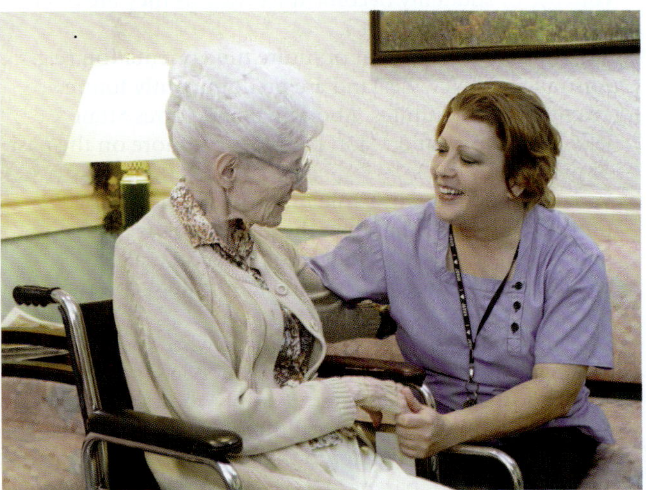

FIGURE 2-1 Establishing and maintaining trust, privacy, and partnership with older adults' sets the tone for effectively collecting data and sharing concerns.

Cultural variations in communication

Ethnic and cultural variations in communication and self-disclosure styles may significantly affect the information obtained (Andrews & Boyle, 2011; Giger, 2012; Maier-Lorentz, 2008). Be aware of possible variations in the communication styles of yourself and the patient. If misunderstanding or difficulty in communicating is evident, seek help from an expert—what some professionals call a 'culture advisor' employed by the health care facility or a support person of your choice. This person should be thoroughly familiar not only with the patient's language, culture and related health care practices but also with the health care setting and system of the dominant culture.

Frequently noted variations in communication styles include:

- Reluctance to reveal personal information to strangers for various cultural reasons
- Variation in willingness to openly express emotional distress or pain
- Variation in ability to receive information (listen)
- Variation in meaning conveyed by language. For example, a patient who does not speak the predominant language may not know what a certain medical term or phrase means and therefore will not know how to answer your question. Use of slang with non-English speakers is discouraged as well. Keep in mind that it is hard enough to learn proper language, let alone the idiom vernacular. The non-English speaker will likely have no idea what you are trying to convey.
- Variation in use and meaning of non-verbal communication: eye contact, stance, gestures and demeanour. For example, direct eye contact may be perceived as rude, aggressive or immodest by some cultures, whereas lack of eye contact may be perceived as evasive, insecure or inattentive by other cultures; a slightly bowed stance may indicate respect in some groups; size of personal space affects one's comfortable interpersonal distance; touch may be perceived as comforting or threatening.
- Variation in disease or illness perception: culture-specific syndromes or disorders are accepted by some groups (e.g. in Central Australian traditional culture when people collapse or suddenly become unconscious they are often described as 'having a fit').
- Variation in past, present or future time orientation (e.g. Australia and New Zealand are predominantly future oriented; other cultures, Aboriginal and Torres Strait Islander peoples and Māori people focus more on the past or present).
- Variation in the family's role in the decision-making process: a person other than the patient or the patient's parent may be the major decision maker regarding appointments, treatment or follow-up care for the patient.

You may have to interview a patient who does not speak your language. To perform the best interview possible, it is necessary to use an interpreter. Possibly the best interpreter would be a culture expert (or culture advisor). Consider the relationship of the interpreter to the patient. If the interpreter is the patient's child, parent or a person of a different sex, age or social status, interpretation may be impaired. Also keep in mind that communication through use of pictures may be helpful when working with some patients.

Emotional variations in communication

Not every patient you encounter will be calm, friendly and eager to participate in the interview process. Patients' emotions vary for a number of reasons. They may be scared or anxious about their health or about disclosing personal information, angry that they are sick or about having to have an examination, or depressed about their health or other life events—or they may have an ulterior motive for having an assessment performed. Patients may also have some sensitive issues with which they are grappling and may turn to you for help. Often people can become annoyed when they are asked the same question again and again. It is important that nurses do their 'homework' to build on the story the person has given, to inform the safe and timely nursing care. Some helpful ways to deal with patients with various emotions are discussed in Display 2-2.

DISPLAY 2-2 INTERACTING WITH PATIENTS WITH VARIOUS EMOTIONAL STATES

When interacting with an anxious patient

- Provide the patient with simple, organised information in a structured format.
- Explain who you are and your role and purpose.
- Ask simple, concise questions.
- Avoid becoming anxious like the patient.
- Decrease any external stimuli and do not hurry.

When interacting with an angry patient

- Approach this patient in a calm, reassuring, in-control manner.
- Allow him or her to ventilate feelings. However, if the patient is out of control, do not argue with or touch the patient.
- Obtain help from other health care professionals as needed.
- Avoid arguing and facilitate personal space so the patient does not feel threatened or cornered.

When interacting with a depressed patient

- Express interest in and understanding of the patient and respond in a neutral manner.
- Do not try to communicate in an upbeat, encouraging manner. This will not help the depressed patient.

When interacting with a manipulative patient

- Provide structure and set limits.
- Differentiate between manipulation and a reasonable request.
- If you are not sure whether you are being manipulated, obtain an objective opinion from other nursing colleagues.

When interacting with a seductive patient

- Set firm limits on overt sexual patient behaviour and avoid responding to subtle seductive behaviours.
- Encourage the patient to use more appropriate methods of coping in relating to others.

When discussing sensitive issues (for example, sexuality, dying, spirituality)

- First be aware of your own thoughts and feelings regarding dying, spirituality and sexuality; then recognise that these factors may affect the patient's health and may need to be discussed with someone.
- Ask simple questions in a non-judgemental manner.
- Allow time for ventilation of the patient's feelings as needed.
- If you do not feel comfortable or competent discussing personal, sensitive topics, you may make referrals as appropriate, for example, to a pastoral counsellor for spiritual concerns or to other specialists as needed.

The information gathered from the interview should inform the nursing actions or interventions that need to be taken.

COMPLETE HEALTH HISTORY

The health history is an excellent way to begin the assessment process because it lays the groundwork for identifying nursing problems and provides a focus for the physical examination.

The importance of the health history lies in its ability to provide information that will assist the examiner in identifying areas of strength and limitation in the individual's lifestyle and current health status. It is critical that the patient's health literacy is taken into account when conducting the interview and completing a health history. Data from the health history also provide the examiner with specific cues to health problems that are most apparent to the patient. Then these areas may be more intensely examined during the physical assessment. When a patient is having a complete, head-to-toe physical assessment, collection of subjective data usually requires that the nurse take a complete health history. The complete health history is modified or shortened when necessary. For example, if the physical assessment will focus on the heart and neck vessels, the subjective data collection would be limited to the data relevant to the heart and neck vessels.

When taking a health history, begin by explaining to the patient why the information is being requested; for example, 'so that I will be able to plan individualised nursing care with you'. This section of the chapter explains the rationale for collecting the data, discusses each part of the health history and provides sample questions. The health history has eight sections:

- Biographical data
- Reasons for seeking health care
- History of present health concern
- Past health history
- Family health history
- Review of systems (ROS) for current health problems
- Lifestyle and health practices
- Developmental level (this is a judgement that the nurse makes based on the interview—it is not something that the patient 'reports'; see also Chaps 33 and 37 for more on assessing children and patients with intellectual disabilities).

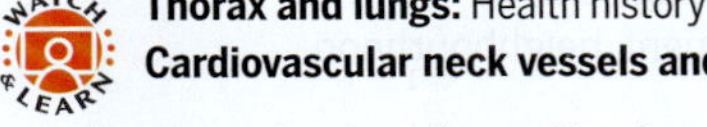

Thorax and lungs: Health history taking
Cardiovascular neck vessels and heart: Health history taking

The organisation for collecting data in this text is a generic nursing framework that you can use as is or adapt to use with any nursing framework. See Assessment tool 2-1 for a summary of the components of a complete patient health history. This can be used as a guide for collecting subjective data from the patient.

Biographical data

Biographical data usually include information that identifies the patient, such as name, address, phone number, gender and who provided the information—the patient or significant others. The patient's date of birth, medical record number or similar identifying data may also be included.

When students are collecting the information and sharing it with instructors, addresses and phone numbers should be deleted and initials used to protect the patient's privacy. However, the name of the person providing the information needs to be included to assist in determining its accuracy. The patient is considered the primary source and all others (including the patient's medical record) are secondary sources. In some cases, the patient's immediate family or carer may be a more accurate source of information than the patient. An example would be an elderly patient's wife who has kept the patient's medical records for years or the legal guardian of a patient with mental disabilities. In any event, validation of the information by a secondary source may be helpful. It may be appropriate to use a qualified interpreter during the interview process to ensure that the information obtained is accurate and that the patient and any significant others are able to ask questions and receive clear answers. It is important to be aware of the patient's and significant other's health literacy during the interviewing and assessment.

The patient's culture, ethnicity and subculture may be determined by collecting data about the patient's date and place of birth, nationality or ethnicity, marital status, religious or spiritual practices, and primary and secondary languages spoken, written and read. This information helps you to examine special needs and beliefs that may affect the patient or family's health care. A primary language is usually the one spoken in the family during early childhood and the one in which the person thinks. However, if the patient was educated in another language from kindergarten onwards, that may be the primary language and the birth language would be secondary.

Gathering information about the patient's educational level, occupation and working status at this point in the health history assists you in tailoring questions to the patient's level of understanding. In addition, this information can help to identify possible patient strengths and limitations affecting health status. For example, if the patient was recently downsized from a high-power, high-salary position, the effects of overwhelming stress may play a large part in his or her health status.

Finally, asking who lives with the patient and identifying significant others indicates the availability of potential carers and support people for the patient. Absence of support people would alert you to the (possible) need for finding external sources of support.

Reasons for seeking health care

This category includes two questions: 'What is your major health problem or concern at this time?' and 'How do you feel about having to seek health care?' The first question assists the patient in focusing on the most significant health concern and answers the nurse's question, 'Why are you here?' or 'How can I help you?' Doctors call this the patient's chief complaint or presenting complaint, but a more holistic approach for phrasing the question may draw out concerns that reach beyond just a physical complaint and may address stress or lifestyle changes.

The second question encourages the patient to discuss fears or other feelings about having to see a health care provider. For example, a woman visiting a nurse practitioner may state her major health concern as 'I found a lump in my breast.' She may be able to respond to the second question by voicing fears that she has been reluctant to share with her significant others. This question may also draw out descriptions of her previous experiences—both positive and negative—with other health care providers.

ASSESSMENT TOOL 2-1 Nursing Health History Format (Used for Patient Care Plan)

Biographical data

- Name
- Address
- Phone
- Gender
- Provider of history (patient or other)
- Date of birth
- Place of birth
- Race or ethnic background
- Educational level
- Occupation
- Significant others or support persons

Reasons for seeking health care

- Reason for seeking health care
- Feelings about seeking health care

History of present health concern

- Character (How does it feel, look, smell, sound, etc.?)
- Onset (When did it begin; is it better, worse or the same since it began?)
- Location (Where is it? Does it radiate?)
- Duration (How long does it last? Does it recur?)
- Severity (How bad is it on a scale of 0 [barely noticeable] to 10 [e.g. worst pain ever experienced]?)
- Pattern (What makes it better? What makes it worse?)
- Associated factors (What other symptoms do you have with it? Will you be able to continue doing your work or other activities [leisure or exercise]?)

Past health history

- Problems at birth
- Childhood illnesses
- Immunisations to date
- Adult illnesses (physical, emotional, mental)
- Surgeries
- Accidents
- Prolonged pain or pain patterns
- Allergies

Family health history

- Age of parents (Living? Deceased date?)
- Parents' illnesses
- Grandparents' illnesses
- Aunts' and uncles' age and illnesses
- Children's ages and illnesses or disabilities

Review of systems for current health problems

- Skin, hair and nails
- Head and neck
- Ears
- Eyes
- Mouth, throat, nose and sinuses
- Thorax and lungs
- Breasts and regional lymphatics
- Heart and neck vessels
- Peripheral vascular
- Abdomen
- Male genitalia
- Female genitalia
- Anus, rectum and prostate
- Musculoskeletal system
- Neurological status
- Cognitive and mental health status
- Urinary and bowel function
- Nutritional status

Lifestyle and health practices

- Description of a typical day (a.m. to p.m.)
- 24-hour dietary intake (foods and fluids)
- Who purchases and prepares meals
- Activities on a typical day
- Exercise habits and patterns
- Sleep and rest habits and patterns
- Use of medications and other substances (caffeine, nicotine, alcohol, over-the-counter medications recreational drugs)
- Self-concept
- Self-care responsibilities
- Social activities for fun and relaxation
- Social activities contributing to society
- Relationships with family, significant others and pets
- Values, religious affiliation, spirituality
- Past, current and future plans for education
- Type of work, level of job satisfaction, work stressors
- Finances
- Stressors in life, coping strategies used
- Residency, type of environment, neighbourhood, environmental risks

History of present health concern

This section of the health history takes into account several aspects of the health problem and asks questions whose answers can provide a detailed description of the concern. First, encourage the patient to explain the health problem or symptom in as much detail as possible by focusing on the onset, progression and duration of the problem; signs and symptoms, and related problems; and what the patient perceives as causing the problem. You may also ask the patient to evaluate what makes the problem worse, what makes it better, which treatments have been tried, what effect the problem has had on daily life or lifestyle, what expectations are held about recovery and the ability to provide self-care.

Because there are many characteristics to be explored for each symptom, a memory helper—known as a mnemonic—can help you to complete the assessment of the sign, symptom or health concern. Many mnemonics have been developed for this purpose (e.g. PQRST, COLDSPA, OLDCART, COLDSTER, LOCSTAAM). The mnemonic used in this text is COLDSPA, which is designed to help you explore symptoms, signs or health concerns (see Display 2-3). The COLDSPA example below provides a sample application of the COLDSPA mnemonic adapted to analyse back pain.

The patient's answers provide a great deal of information about the problem, especially how it affects the patient's lifestyle and activities of daily living. This helps you to evaluate the patient's insight into the problem and plans for managing it. You can also begin to postulate potential problems from this initial information.

Problems or symptoms particular to body parts or systems are covered in the nursing history section under 'History of present health concern' in the physical assessment chapters. Each identified symptom must be described for clear understanding of probable cause and significance. This will inform the nursing actions or interventions that need to be taken followed by evaluating their effectiveness.

DISPLAY 2-3 COMPONENTS OF THE COLDSPA SYMPTOM ANALYSIS MNEMONIC

Mnemonic	Question
Character	Describe the sign or symptom (feeling, appearance, sound, smell or taste if applicable).
Onset	When did it begin?
Location	Where is it? Does it radiate? Does it occur anywhere else?
Duration	How long does it last? Does it recur?
Severity	How bad is it? How much does it bother you?
Pattern	What makes it better or worse?
Associated factors/How it **A**ffects the patient	What other symptoms occur with it? How does it affect you?

Past health history

This portion of the health history focuses on questions related to the patient's past, from the earliest beginnings to the present. These questions elicit data related to the patient's strengths and weaknesses in his or her health history. The patient's strengths may be physical (e.g. optimal body weight), social (e.g. active in community services), emotional (e.g. expresses feeling openly) or spiritual (often turns to faith for support). The data may also point to trends of unhealthy behaviours such as smoking or lack of physical activity. The information gained from these questions assists you in identifying risk factors that stem from previous health problems. Risk factors may be to the patient or to his or her significant others.

Information covered in this section includes questions about birth, growth, development, childhood illnesses, immunisations, allergies, previous health problems, hospitalisations, surgeries, pregnancies, births, previous accidents, injuries, pain experiences, and emotional or psychiatric problems. Sample questions include:

- 'Can you tell me how your mother described your birth? Were there any problems? As far as you know, did you progress normally as you grew to adulthood? Were there any problems that your family told you about or that you experienced?'
- 'What illnesses did you have as a child, such as measles or mumps? What immunisations did you get and are you up to date now?' (See Display 2-4 for recommended immunisations.)
- 'Do you have any chronic illness? If so, when was it diagnosed? How is it treated? How satisfied have you been with the treatment?'
- 'What illnesses have you had? How were the illnesses treated?'

COLDSPA

Sample application of COLDSPA: Exploring the symptoms of back pain

Mnemonic	Question	Patient response example
Character	Describe the sign or symptom (feeling, appearance, sound, smell or taste, if applicable).	'What does the pain feel like?'
Onset	When did it begin?	'When did this pain start?'
Location	Where is it? Does it radiate? Does it occur anywhere else?	'Where does it hurt the most? Does it radiate or go to any other part of your body?'
Duration	How long does it last? Does it recur?	'How long does the pain last? Does it come and go or is it constant?'
Severity	How bad is it? How much does it bother you?	'How intense is the pain? Rate it on a scale of 1 to 10.'
Pattern	What makes it better or worse?	'What makes your back pain worse or better? Are there any treatments you've tried that relieve the pain?'
Associated factors/How it Affects the patient	What other symptoms occur with it? How does it affect you?	'What do you think caused it to start? Do you have any other problems that seem related to your back pain? How does this pain affect your life and daily activities?'

DISPLAY 2-4 RECOMMENDED ADULT IMMUNISATION SCHEDULE: AUSTRALIA AND NEW ZEALAND

Australia

National Immunisation Program Schedule

From 1 April 2019

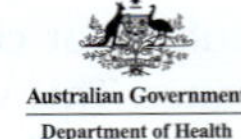

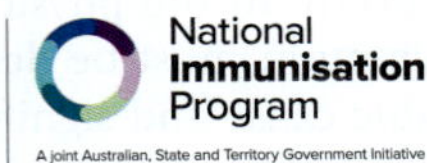

Age	Disease	Vaccine Brand
Childhood vaccination (also see influenza vaccine)		
Birth	• Hepatitis B (usually offered in hospital)[a]	H-B-Vax® II Paediatric or Engerix B® Paediatric
2 months Can be given from 6 weeks of age	• Diphtheria, tetanus, pertussis (whooping cough), hepatitis B, polio, *Haemophilus influenzae* type b (Hib) • Pneumococcal • Rotavirus[b]	Infanrix® hexa Prevenar 13® Rotarix®
4 months	• Diphtheria, tetanus, pertussis (whooping cough), hepatitis B, polio, *Haemophilus influenzae* type b (Hib) • Pneumococcal • Rotavirus[b]	Infanrix® hexa Prevenar 13® Rotarix®
6 months	• Diphtheria, tetanus, pertussis (whooping cough), hepatitis B, polio, *Haemophilus influenzae* type b (Hib)	Infanrix® hexa
Additional vaccines for Aboriginal and Torres Strait Islander children (QLD, NT, WA and SA) and medically at-risk children	• Pneumococcal	Prevenar 13®
12 months	• Meningococcal ACWY • Measles, mumps, rubella • Pneumococcal	Nimenrix® M-M-R® II or Priorix® Prevenar 13®
Additional vaccines for Aboriginal and Torres Strait Islander children (QLD, NT, WA and SA)	• Hepatitis A	Vaqta® Paediatric
18 months	• *Haemophilus influenzae* type b (Hib) • Measles, mumps, rubella, varicella (chickenpox) • Diphtheria, tetanus, pertussis (whooping cough)	ActHIB® Priorix-Tetra® or ProQuad® Infanrix® or Tripacel®
Additional vaccines for Aboriginal and Torres Strait Islander children (QLD, NT, WA and SA)	• Hepatitis A	Vaqta® Paediatric
4 years	• Diphtheria, tetanus, pertussis (whooping cough), polio	Infanrix® IPV or Quadracel®
Additional vaccines for medically at-risk children[c]	• Pneumococcal	Pneumovax 23®

DISPLAY 2-4 RECOMMENDED ADULT IMMUNISATION SCHEDULE: AUSTRALIA AND NEW ZEALAND (continued)

Australia (continued)

National Immunisation Program Schedule

From 1 April 2019

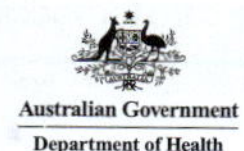

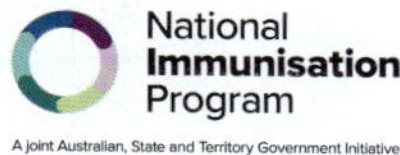

Age	Disease	Vaccine brand
Adolescent vaccination (also see influenza vaccine)		
12–<13 years (School programs[d])	• Human papillomavirus (HPV)[e] • Diphtheria, tetanus, pertussis (whooping cough)	Gardasil®9 Boostrix®
14–<16 years (School programs[d])	• Meningococcal ACWY	Nimenrix®
Adult vaccination (also see influenza vaccine)		
15–49 years Aboriginal and Torres Strait Islander people with medical risk factors[c]	• Pneumococcal	Pneumovax 23®
50 years and over Aboriginal and Torres Strait Islander people	• Pneumococcal	Pneumovax 23®
65 years and over	• Pneumococcal	Pneumovax 23®
70–79 years[f]	• Shingles (herpes zoster)	Zostavax®
Pregnant women	• Pertussis (whooping cough)[g] • Influenza[h]	Boostrix® or Adacel®

Funded annual influenza vaccination[h]

6 months and over with certain medical risk factors[c]

All Aboriginal and Torres Strait Islander people 6 months and over

65 years and over

Pregnant women

a Hepatitis B vaccine: Should be given to all infants as soon as practicable after birth. The greatest benefit is if given within 24 hours, and must be given within 7 days.
b Rotavirus vaccine: First dose must be given by 14 weeks of age, the second dose by 24 weeks of age.
c Refer to the current edition of *The Australian Immunisation Handbook* for all medical risk factors.
d Contact your state or territory health service for school grades eligible for vaccination.
e Observe Gardasil®9 dosing schedules by age and at-risk conditions. 2 doses: 9 to <15 years—6 months mininimum interval. 3 doses: ≥15 years and/or have certain medical conditions—0, 2 and 6 month schedule. Only 2 doses funded on the NIP unless 12-13 year old has certain medical risk factors.
f All people aged 70 years old, with a five year catch-up program for people aged 71–79 years old until 31 October 2021.
g Single dose recommended each pregnancy, ideally between 20–32 weeks, but may be given up until delivery.
h Refer to annual influenza information for recommended vaccine brand for age.

- Contact your State and Territory Health Department for further information on any additional immunisation programs specific to your State or Territory.
- All people aged less than 20 years are eligible for free catch up vaccines.
- Adult refugees and humanitarian entrants are eligible for free catch up vaccines.

For more information

health.gov.au/immunisation

State/Territory	Contact Number
Australian Capital Territory	(02) 6205 2300
New South Wales	1300 066 055
Northern Territory	(08) 8922 8044
Queensland	13 HEALTH (13 4325 84)
South Australia	1300 232 272
Tasmania	1800 671 738
Victoria	1300 882 008
Western Australia	(08) 9321 1312

As the NIP Schedule is subject to regular amendments, this figure is an example only. Access the online and most up-to-date version of the NIP Schedule at https://www.health.gov.au/health-topics/immunisation/immunisation-throughout-life/national-immunisation-program-schedule. (© Commonwealth of Australia.)

Continued on following page

DISPLAY 2-4 RECOMMENDED ADULT IMMUNISATION SCHEDULE: AUSTRALIA AND NEW ZEALAND (continued)

New Zealand

Vaccines for the National Immunisation Schedule

A reference card for vaccinators and other health professionals

immunise
our best protection

Age	Vaccines
Pregnancy	Tdap injection (Boostrix®) + Influenza 1 injection. Brand varies.
6 Weeks	RV1 oral vaccine (Rotarix®) + DTaP-IPV-Hep B/Hib injection (Infanrix® hexa) + PCV10 injection (Synflorix®)
3 Months	RV1 oral vaccine (Rotarix®) + DTaP-IPV-Hep B/Hib injection (Infanrix® hexa) + PCV10 injection (Synflorix®)
5 Months	DTaP-IPV-Hep B/Hib injection (Infanrix® hexa) + PCV10 injection (Synflorix®)
15 Months	Hib injection (Hiberix®) + MMR injection (Priorix®) + PCV10 injection (Synflorix®) + Varicella injection (Varilrix®)
4 Years	DTaP-IPV injection (Infanrix® IPV) + MMR injection (Priorix®)
11–12 Years	Tdap injection (Boostrix®) + HPV injection (Gardasil® 9) (2 doses, 6 months apart)
45 Years	Td injection (ADT® Booster)
65 Years	Td injection (ADT® Booster) + Influenza 1 injection (annually). Brand varies. + Shingles injection (Zostavax®)

(New Zealand Ministry of Health (NZMOH). National Immunisation Schedule. Available via https://www.healthed.govt.nz/system/files/resource-files/HE1308_National%20Immunisation%20schedule_0.pdf, CC BY 4.0 International License, Jan 2017, revised May 2019.)

- Do you have any allergies and if you have had an allergic reaction what happened?
- 'Have you ever delivered a baby? If so how many?'
- 'Have you ever been hospitalised or had surgery? If so, when? What were you hospitalised for or what type of surgery did you have? Were there any complications?'
- 'Have you experienced any accidents or injuries? Please describe them.'
- 'Have you experienced pain in any part of your body? Please describe the pain.'
- 'Have you ever been diagnosed with or treated for emotional or mental problems? If so, please describe their nature and any treatment received. Describe your level of satisfaction with the treatment.'

How patients frame their previous health concerns suggests how they feel about themselves and is an indication of their sense of responsibility for their own health. For example, a male patient who has been obese for years may blame himself for developing diabetes and fail to comply with his diet, whereas another patient may be very willing to share the treatment of her diabetes and her success with an insulin pump in a support group. Some patients are very forthcoming about their past health status; others are not. It is helpful to have a series of alternative questions for less responsive patients and for those who may not understand what is being asked.

Family health history

As researchers discover more and more health problems that seem to run in families and that are genetically based, the family health history assumes greater importance. In addition to genetic predisposition, it is also helpful to see other health problems that may have affected the patient by virtue of having grown up in the family and being exposed to these problems. For example, family members who smoke can affect other

DISPLAY 2-4 RECOMMENDED ADULT IMMUNISATION SCHEDULE: AUSTRALIA AND NEW ZEALAND (continued)

New Zealand (continued)

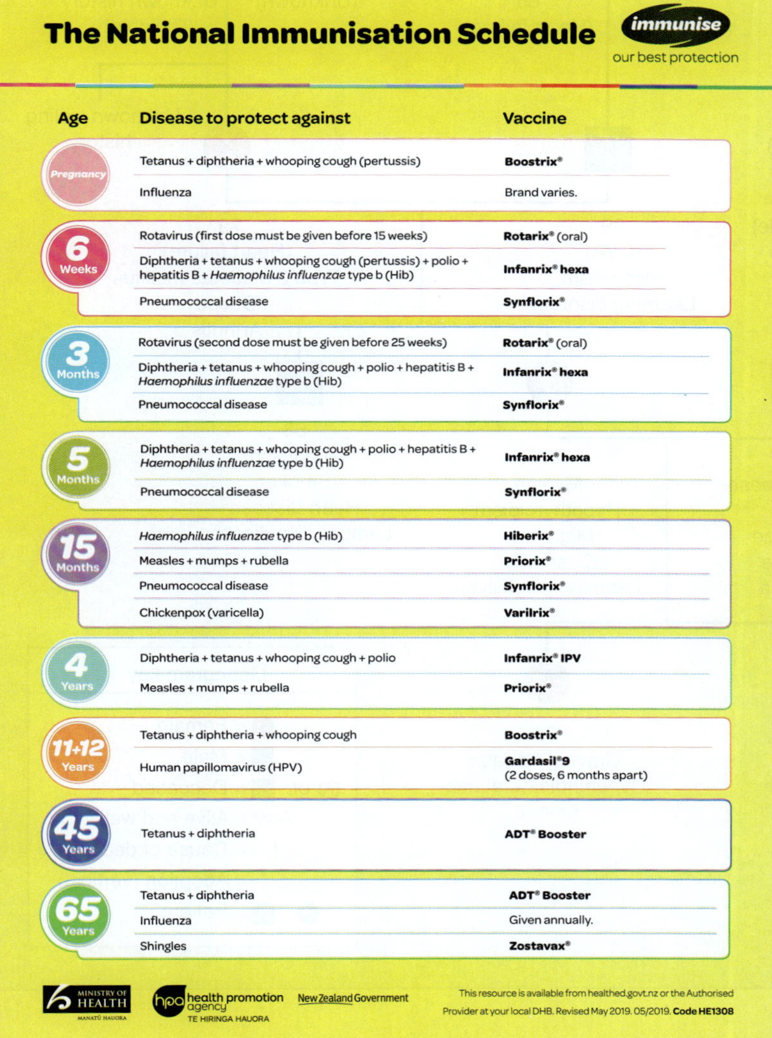

The National Immunisation Schedule

immunise
our best protection

Age	Disease to protect against	Vaccine
Pregnancy	Tetanus + diphtheria + whooping cough (pertussis)	Boostrix®
	Influenza	Brand varies.
6 Weeks	Rotavirus (first dose must be given before 15 weeks)	Rotarix® (oral)
	Diphtheria + tetanus + whooping cough (pertussis) + polio + hepatitis B + *Haemophilus influenzae* type b (Hib)	Infanrix® hexa
	Pneumococcal disease	Synflorix®
3 Months	Rotavirus (second dose must be given before 25 weeks)	Rotarix® (oral)
	Diphtheria + tetanus + whooping cough + polio + hepatitis B + *Haemophilus influenzae* type b (Hib)	Infanrix® hexa
	Pneumococcal disease	Synflorix®
5 Months	Diphtheria + tetanus + whooping cough + polio + hepatitis B + *Haemophilus influenzae* type b (Hib)	Infanrix® hexa
	Pneumococcal disease	Synflorix®
15 Months	*Haemophilus influenzae* type b (Hib)	Hiberix®
	Measles + mumps + rubella	Priorix®
	Pneumococcal disease	Synflorix®
	Chickenpox (varicella)	Varilrix®
4 Years	Diphtheria + tetanus + whooping cough + polio	Infanrix® IPV
	Measles + mumps + rubella	Priorix®
11+12 Years	Tetanus + diphtheria + whooping cough	Boostrix®
	Human papillomavirus (HPV)	Gardasil®9 (2 doses, 6 months apart)
45 Years	Tetanus + diphtheria	ADT® Booster
65 Years	Tetanus + diphtheria	ADT® Booster
	Influenza	Given annually.
	Shingles	Zostavax®

Ministry of Health Manatū Hauora · health promotion agency Te Hiringa Hauora · New Zealand Government

This resource is available from healthed.govt.nz or the Authorised Provider at your local DHB. Revised May 2019. 05/2019. **Code HE1308**

(New Zealand Ministry of Health (NZMOH). National Immunisation Schedule. Available via https://www.healthed.govt.nz/system/files/resource-files/HE1308_National%20Immunisation%20schedule_0.pdf, CC BY 4.0 International License, Jan 2017, revised May 2019.)

family members in at least two ways. First, the second-hand smoke can compromise the physical health of non-smoking family members; second, the smoker may serve as a negative role model for children, inducing them to take up the habit as well. Another example is obesity; recognising it in the family history can alert you to a potential risk factor.

The family history should include as many genetic relatives as the patient can recall. Include maternal and paternal grandparents, aunts and uncles on both sides, parents, siblings and the patient's children. Such thoroughness usually identifies those diseases that may skip a generation such as autosomal recessive disorders. Include the patient's spouse but indicate that there is no genetic link. Identifying the spouse's health problems could explain disorders in the patient's children not indicated in the patient's family history.

Drawing a genogram helps to organise and illustrate the patient's family history. Use a standard format so others can easily understand the information. Also provide a key to the symbols used. Female relatives are usually indicated by a circle and male relatives are identified by a square. Marking an X in the circle or square and listing the age at death and the cause of death note a deceased relative. Identify all relatives, living or dead, by age and provide a brief list of diseases or conditions. If the relative has no problems, the letters 'A/W' (alive and well) should be placed next to the age. Straight vertical and horizontal lines are used to show relationships. A horizontal dotted line can be used to indicate the patient's spouse; a vertical dotted line can be used to indicate adoption. A sample genogram is illustrated in Figure 2-2.

After the diagrammatic family history, prepare a brief summary of the types of health problems present in the family. For example, the patient in the genogram depicted in Figure 2-2 has longevity, obesity, heart disease, hypertension (HTN), arthritis, thyroid disorders, type 2 diabetes mellitus (formerly

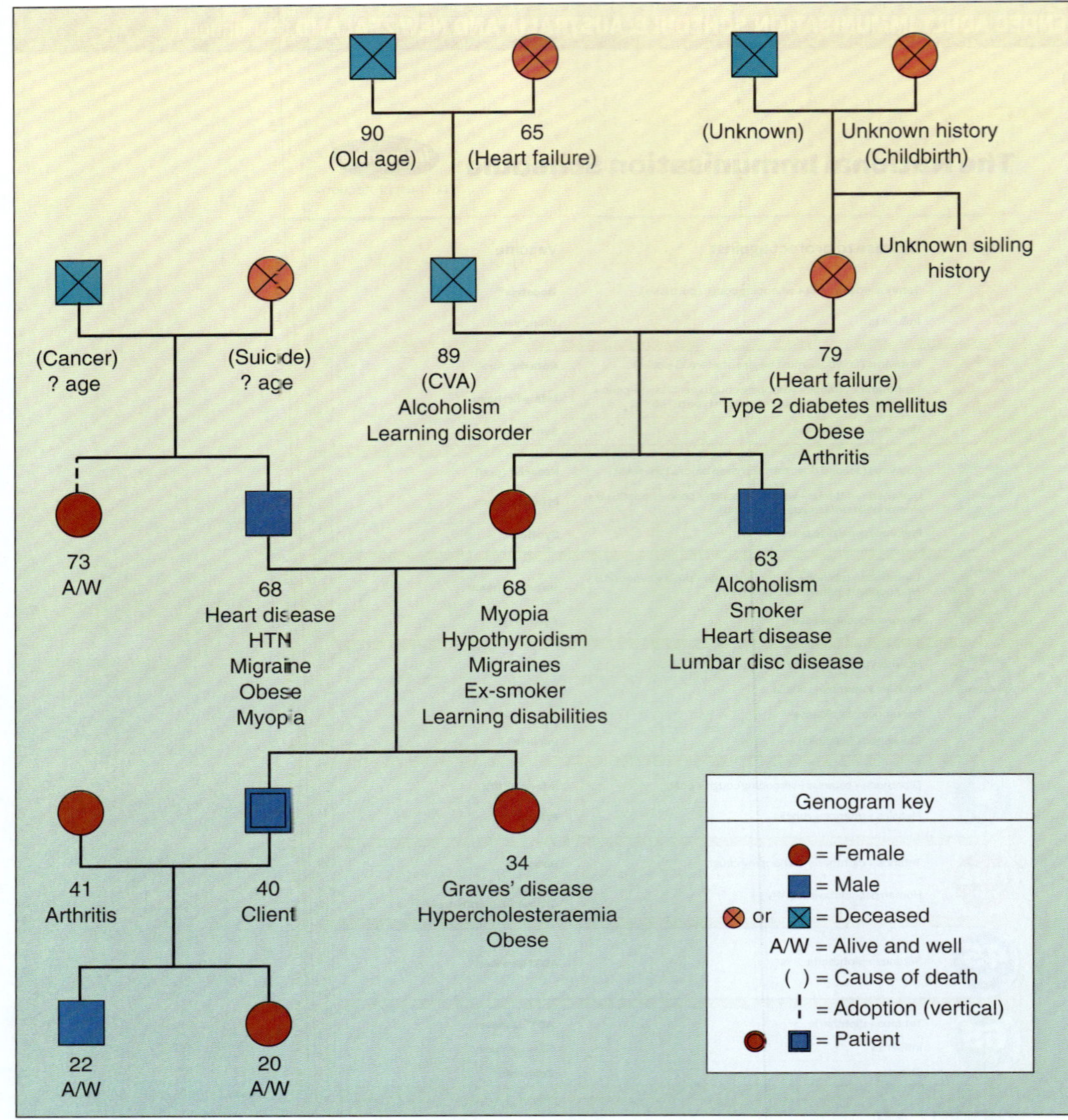

FIGURE 2-2 Genogram of a 40-year-old male patient.

known as non-insulin-dependent diabetes mellitus), alcoholism, smoking, myopia, learning disabilities, hyperactivity disorder and cancer (one relative) on his maternal side. On his paternal side are obesity, heart disease, hypercholesterolaemia, back problems, arthritis, myopia and cancer. His paternal history is not as extensive as his maternal history because his father was adopted. In addition, his sister is obese and has Graves' disease and hypercholesterolaemia. His wife has arthritis; his children are both A/W.

Review of systems for current health problems

In the review of systems (or review of body systems), each body system is addressed and the patient is asked specific questions to draw out current health problems or problems from the recent past that may still affect the patient or that are recurring. Care must be taken in this section to include only the patient's subjective information and not your observations.

During the review of body systems, document the patient's descriptions of his or her health status for each body system and note the patient's denial of signs, symptoms, diseases or problems that you ask about but are not experienced by the patient. For example, under the area 'Head and neck', the patient may answer that there are no problems but in response to your questioning about headaches, stiffness, pain or cracking in the neck with motion, swelling in the neck, difficulty swallowing, sore throat, enlarged lymph nodes and so on, the patient may suddenly remember that he or she did have a sore throat a week ago that was self-treated with zinc lozenges. This information might not have emerged without specific questioning.

The questions about problems and the clinical manifestations of disorders should be asked in terms that the patient understands, but findings may be recorded in standard medical terminology. If the patient appears to have a limited vocabulary or health literacy, you may need to ask questions in several different ways and use very basic lay terminology. If the patient is well educated and seems familiar with medical terminology, do not insult him or her by talking at a much lower level. The most obvious information to collect for each body part or system is listed below. See the physical assessment chapters for in-depth questions and rationales for each particular body part or system:

- *Skin, hair and nails:* Skin colour, temperature, condition, excessive sweating, rashes, lesions, balding, dandruff, condition of nails
- *Head and neck:* Headache, swelling, stiffness of neck, difficulty swallowing, sore throat, enlarged lymph nodes
- *Ears:* Hearing, ringing or buzzing, earaches, drainage from ears, dizziness and exposure to loud noises
- *Eyes:* Vision, eye infections, redness, excessive tearing, halos around lights, blurring, loss of side vision, moving black spots or specks in visual fields, flashing lights, double vision, eye pain
- *Mouth, throat, nose and sinuses:* Condition of teeth, tongue and gums; lumps, sore throat; mouth lesions; hoarseness; rhinorrhoea; nasal obstruction; frequent colds; sneezing or itching of eyes, ears, nose or throat; nose bleeds; snoring
- *Thorax and lungs:* Difficulty breathing, wheezing, pain, shortness of breath during routine activity, orthopnoea, cough or sputum, haemoptysis, respiratory infections
- *Breasts and regional lymphatics:* Lumps or discharge from nipples, dimpling or changes in breast size or appearance of the nipples, swollen or tender lymph nodes in axilla
- *Heart and neck vessels:* Last blood pressure, ECG tracing or findings, chest pain or pressure, palpitations, oedema
- *Peripheral vascular:* Swelling, or oedema, of legs and feet; pain at rest or only on walking; cramping; sores on legs; colour or texture changes on the legs or feet
- *Abdomen:* Indigestion, difficulty swallowing, nausea, vomiting, abdominal pain, gas, jaundice, hernias and or lumps
- *Male genitalia:* Excessive or painful, burning sensation during urination, frequency or difficulty starting and maintaining urinary stream, leaking of urine, blood noted in urine, sexual problems, perineal lesions, penile drainage or discharge, pain, swelling or redness of the scrotum, difficulty achieving an erection or difficulty ejaculating, exposure to sexually transmitted infections
- *Female genitalia:* Sexual problems; sexually transmitted infections; voiding problems (e.g. dribbling, hesitancy, incontinence, pain and burning and offensive discharge on urination); reproductive data such as age at menarche, menstruation (length and regularity of cycle), pregnancies and type of problems with delivery, abortions, pelvic pain, birth control, menopause (date or year of last menstrual period) and use of hormone replacement therapy. Painful lumps of the labia. Pain and discomfort during sexual intercourse.
- *Anus, rectum and prostate:* Bowel habits, pain with defecation, haemorrhoids, blood in stool, constipation, diarrhoea
- *Musculoskeletal:* Swelling, redness, pain and stiffness of joints, ability to perform activities of daily living, muscle strength and change in balance
- *Neurological:* General mood, behaviour, depression, anger, concussions, headaches, loss of strength or sensation, coordination and balance, difficulty speaking, memory problems, strange thoughts or actions, difficulty learning.

Lifestyle and health practices profile

This is a very important section of the health history because it deals with the patient's human responses, which include nutritional habits, activity and exercise patterns, sleep and rest patterns, use of medications and substances, self-concept and self-care activities, social and community activities, relationships, values and beliefs systems, education and work, stress level and coping style, and environment.

Here patients describe how they are managing their lives, their awareness of healthy versus toxic living patterns, and the strengths and supports they have or use. When assessing this area, use open-ended questions to promote a dialogue with the patient. Follow up with specific questions to guide the discussion and clarify the information as necessary. Be sure to pay special attention to the cues the patient may provide that point to possibly more significant content and the non-verbal communication displayed by the patient. Take brief notes so that pertinent data are not lost and so there can be follow-up if some information needs clarification or expansion.

In this section, each area is discussed briefly then followed by a few sample questions.

Description of a typical day

This information is necessary to elicit an overview of how the patient sees his or her usual pattern of daily activity. The questions you ask should be vague enough to allow the patient to provide the orientation from which the day is viewed, for example, 'Please tell me what an average or typical day is for you. Start with when you wake in the morning and continue until bedtime.' Encourage the patient to discuss a usual day, which, for most people, includes work or school. If the patient gives minimal information, you may ask additional specific questions to draw out more details.

Nutrition and weight management

Ask the patient to recall what consists of an average 24-hour intake for him or her with emphasis on what foods are eaten and in what amounts. Also ask about snacks, fluid intake and other substances consumed. Depending on the patient, you may want to ask who buys and prepares the food and when and where meals are eaten. These questions uncover food habits that are health promoting as well as those that are less desirable. The patient's answers about food intake should be compared with current national guidelines (see Online resources and Chap. 14). Resources are available from the Australian Department of Health and the New Zealand Ministry of Health. They are designed to teach people what types and amounts of food to eat to ensure a balanced diet, promote health and prevent disease. Consider reviewing posters with the patient and explaining what a serving size is. The patient's fluid intake should be compared with the general recommendation of 6 to 8 glasses of water or non-caffeinated fluids daily. It is also important to ask about the patient's bowel and bladder habits at this time (included in the review of symptoms). Sample questions include:

- 'What do you usually eat during a typical day? Please tell me the kinds of foods you prefer, how often you eat throughout the day and how much you eat.'
- 'Do you eat out at restaurants frequently?'
- 'Do you eat only when hungry? Do you eat because of boredom, habit, anxiety, depression?'
- 'Who buys and prepares the food you eat?'
- 'Where do you eat your meals?'
- 'How much and what types of fluids do you drink?'

Activity level and exercise

Assess how active the patient is during an average week either at work or at home. Inquire about regular exercise. Some patients believe that if they do heavy physical work at their job, they do not need additional exercise. Make it a point to distinguish between activities done when working, which may be stressful and fatiguing, and exercise, which is designed to reduce stress and strengthen the individual. Compare the patient's answers with the recommended exercise regimen of regular aerobic exercise for 20 to 30 minutes at least three times a week. Explain to the patient that regular exercise reduces the risk of heart disease, strengthens the heart and lungs, reduces stress and helps with weight management.

Sample questions include:

- 'What is your daily pattern of activity?'
- 'Do you follow a regular exercise plan? What types of exercise do you do?'
- 'Are there any reasons why you cannot follow a moderately strenuous exercise program?'
- 'What do you do for leisure and recreation?'
- 'Do your leisure and recreational activities include exercise?'

Sleep and rest

Inquire whether the patient feels he or she is getting enough sleep and rest. Questions should focus on specific sleep patterns such as how many hours a night the person sleeps, interruptions, whether the patient feels rested, problems sleeping (e.g. insomnia), rituals the patient uses to promote sleep and concerns the patient may have regarding sleep habits. The patient may have expressed some of this information already, but it is useful to gather data in a more systematic and thorough manner at this time. Inquiries about sleep can bring out problems, such as anxiety, which manifest as sleeplessness, or inadequate sleep time, which can predispose the patient to accidents. Compare the patient's answers with the normal sleep requirement for adults, which is usually between 5 and 8 hours per night. Keep in mind that sleep requirements vary depending on age, health and stress levels.

Sample questions include:

- 'Tell me about your sleeping patterns.'
- 'Do you have trouble falling asleep or staying asleep?'
- 'How much sleep do you get each night?'
- 'Do you feel rested when you awaken?'
- 'Do you nap during the day? How often and for how long?'
- 'What do you do to help you fall asleep?'

See Promote health—Sleep disorders: Insomnia and Display 2-5. For more detailed discussions of sleep and insomnia, see the work edited by Mansfield and McEvoy (2013), *Sleep disorders: A practical guide for Australian health care practitioners.*

Further information

Understanding sleep and sleep-related health problems

- Australasian Sleep Association
- Sleep Health Foundation
- https://www.health.govt.nz/your-health/healthy-living/food-activity-and-sleep/sleeping/sleep-tips-adultsYes
- Harvard University Sleep & Health
- Sleep disorders: A practical guide for Australian health care practitioners (ed. Mansfield, D. R. & McEvoy, R. D.) (2013). *MJA, 199*(8), Supplement.

DISPLAY 2-5 STANFORD SLEEPINESS SCALE

This is a quick way to assess how alert you are feeling. During the day when you go about your business, ideally you would want a rating of '1'. Take into account that most people have two peak times of alertness daily, at about 9 a.m. and 9 p.m. Alertness wanes to its lowest point at around 3 p.m. and after that it begins to build again. Rate your alertness at different times during the day. If your score is greater than '3' during a time when you should feel alert, you may have a serious sleep debt and require more sleep.

Degree of sleepiness	Scale rating
Feeling active, vital, alert or wide awake	1
Functioning at high levels, but not at peak; able to concentrate	2
Awake, but relaxed; responsive but not fully alert	3
Somewhat foggy, let down	4
Foggy; losing interest in remaining awake; slowed down	5
Sleepy, woozy, fighting sleep; prefer to lie down	6
No longer fighting sleep, sleep onset soon; having dream-like thoughts	7
Asleep	X

Hoddes, E., Zarcone, V., Smythe, H., Phillips, R., Dement, W. C. (July 1973). Quantification of Sleepiness: A New Approach. *Psychophysiology 10*(4), 431–436. John Wiley & Sons, Inc. All Rights Reserved.

- The relationship between functional health literacy and obstructive sleep apnea and its related risk factors and comorbidities in a population cohort of men. Li, J. J., Appleton S. L., Wittert G. A., et al., (2014).
- Impact of five nights of sleep restriction on glucose metabolism, leptin and testosterone in young adult men. Reynolds A. C., Dorrian J., Liu P. Y., et al., (2012).

Medication and substance use

The information gathered about medication and substance use provides you with information concerning the patient's lifestyle and self-care ability. Medication and substance use can affect the patient's health and cause loss of function or impaired senses. In addition, certain medications (over-the-counter) and substances can increase the patient's risk of disease. Because many people use alternative and naturopathy therapies, which may include vitamins and a variety of herbal supplements, it is important to ask which are used and how often. Prescription medications may interact with these supplements (e.g. garlic decreases coagulation and interacts with warfarin). Sample questions include:

- 'What medications have you used in the recent past and what do you use currently, both those that your doctor prescribed and those that you can buy over the counter at a pharmacy? For what purpose did /do you take the medication? How much (dose) and how often did/do you take the medication?'
- 'How much beer, wine or other alcohol do you drink, on average?'
- 'Do you drink coffee or other beverages containing caffeine (e.g. cola)?' If so, 'How much and how often?'
- 'Do you now or have you ever smoked cigarettes or used any other form of nicotine? How long have you been smoking/did you smoke? How many packs per week? Tell me about any efforts to quit.'

PROMOTE HEALTH **SLEEP DISORDERS: INSOMNIA**

A person who reaches the average life expectancy of approximately 80 years or so could have spent at least 28 of those years asleep, 'the perceptual disengagement from the environment', as expressed by Mansfield and McEvoy (2013, p. 5). This activity accounts for a major portion of our lives but is often taken for granted. The consequences of sleep loss remain under-recognised across the community. The link between healthy sleep and healthier individuals warrants further investigation and understanding. Some common disorders are obstructive sleep apnoea (OSA), shift-work disorder, insomnia, delayed sleep-phase disorder and sleep disorders in children.

INSOMNIA

Insomnia is defined according to the *Diagnostic and statistical manual of mental disorders, fifth edition* 'as difficulty getting to sleep, staying asleep or having restorative sleep despite having adequate opportunity for sleep, together with associated impairment of daytime functioning with symptoms being persistent for at least 4 weeks' (Cunnington et al., 2013, in Mansfield & McEvoy, p. 36).

Insomnia is a common disorder affecting 13% to 33% of the Australian population who have problems either getting to sleep or staying asleep. According to Cunnington et al. (in Mansfield & McEvoy, 2013), insomnia can be comorbid with other physical and mental health disorders with, for example, approximately 50% of people with depression having comorbid insomnia. It also leads to an increased risk of further depression and is associated with hypertension.

Acute insomnia is insomnia with symptoms occurring for less than 4 weeks. On the other hand, once people have had sleep problems past the 4-week point, their thought processes and behaviour towards sleep change and become maladaptive, propagating the problem. Here insomnia needs to be viewed as a chronic illness by health clinicians so there is emphasis on strategies to prevent relapses rather than focus on treating acute episodes. Acute and chronic insomnia require different management approaches.

Risk factors

Regarding insomnia:

- Most common sleep disorder
- 25% males and 10% adult females are affected
- Obstructive sleep apnoea is strongly associated with increased mortality and cardiovascular disease in middle-aged populations

Regarding chronic insomnia:

- Unlikely to resolve spontaneously
- Characterised with cycles of relapse and remission or persistency
- Best managed using non-pharmacological strategies such as cognitive–behavioural therapy
- For sufferers of insomnia with ongoing symptoms, medication has a role

Teach risk reduction tips

Cognitive-behavioural therapy interventions for insomnia include:

- Stimulus control:
  - BED = SLEEP
  - No reading, watching TV, talking on the phone or using social media before sleep or while in bed
  - Aim for positive association with the bedroom environment and sleeping
- Sleep-restriction therapy:
  - Strict bedtime and rising schedule and fixed wake time
- Relaxation techniques:
  - Breathing
  - Visual imagery
  - Meditation
- Cognitive therapy:
  - Identify beliefs that might conflict with adhering to the various interventions
  - Use of mindfulness in relation to sleep
- Sleep hygiene education such as environmental, physiological and behavioural habits that promote good sleep:
  - Avoid long daytime naps, keep a regular sleep–wake schedule, avoid stimulants (e.g. caffeine), limit alcohol intake before bed, and have a quiet, dark bedroom

Summarised from Mansfield, D. R. & McEvoy, R. D. (Eds) for the Australian Sleep Association and the Sleep Health Foundation. (2013). *Sleep disorders: A practical guide for Australian health care practitioners.* Supplement to *Medical Journal of Australia, 99*(8). See also the Sleep Well Clinic of New Zealand at www.sleepwellclinic.co.nz.

- 'Have you ever taken any medication not prescribed by your health care provider? If so, when, what type, how much and why?'
- 'Have you ever used, or do you now use, recreational drugs—amphetamines, marijuana and other party/designer drugs? Describe any usage oral, inhaled or in through your veins.'
- 'Do you take vitamins or herbal supplements, naturopathic or traditional medicines? If so, what?'

Self-concept and self-care responsibilities

This includes assessment of how the patient views himself or herself and investigation of all behaviours that the person does to promote health while ensuring cultural safety of patients from culturally and linguistically diverse backgrounds. Examples of subjects to be addressed include sexual responsibility; basic hygiene practices; regularity of health care checkups (i.e. dental, visual, medical); breast or testicular self-examination; and accident prevention and hazard protection (e.g. using smoke alarms, wearing seat belts and sunscreen).

You can correlate answers to questions in this area with health-promotion activities discussed previously and with risk factors from the family history. This will help to point out patient strengths and needs for health maintenance. Questions to the patient can be open-ended, but the patient may need prompting to cover all areas. Sample questions include:

- 'What do you see as your talents or special abilities?'
- 'How do you feel about yourself? About your appearance?'
- 'Can you tell me what activities you do to keep yourself safe and healthy or to prevent disease?'
- 'Do you practise safe sex?'
- 'How do you keep your home safe?'
- 'Do you drive safely?'
- 'In the last 3–5 years what health check-ups and screenings have you had?
- 'How often do you see the dentist or have your eyes (vision) examined?'

Social activities

Questions about social activities help you to discover what outlets the patient has for support and relaxation and whether the patient is involved in the community beyond family and work. Information in this area also helps to determine the patient's current level of social development. Sample questions include:

- 'What do you do for fun and relaxation?'
- 'With whom do you socialise most frequently?'
- 'Are you involved in any community activities?'
- 'How do you feel about your community?'
- 'Do you think that you have enough time to socialise?'
- 'What do you see as your contribution to society?'

Relationships

Ask patients to describe the composition of the family into which they were born and about past and current relationships with these family members. In this way, you can assess problems and potential support from the patient's family of origin. In addition, similar information should be sought about the patient's current family (Fig. 2-3). If the patient does not have any family by blood or marriage, then information should be gathered about any significant others (including pets) who may constitute the patient's 'family'. Sample questions include:

- 'Who is (are) the most important person(s) in your life? Describe your relationship with that person (those people).'
- 'What was it like growing up in your family?'
- 'What is your relationship like with your spouse or partner?'
- 'What is your relationship like with your children?'
- 'Describe any relationships you have with significant others.'
- 'Do you get along with your in-laws?'
- 'Are you close to your extended family?'
- 'Do you have any pets?'
- 'What is your role in your family? Is it an important role?'
- 'Are you satisfied with your current sexual relationship? Have there been any recent changes in this relationship?'

Values and belief systems

Assess the patient's values. In addition, discuss the patient's philosophical, religious and spiritual beliefs. Some patients may not be comfortable discussing values or beliefs. Their feelings should be respected. However, the data can help to identify important problems or strengths. Sample questions include:

- 'What is most important to you in life?'
- 'What do you hope to accomplish in your life?'
- 'Do you have a religious affiliation? Is this important to you?'
- 'Is a relationship with God, a God (or another higher power) an important part of your life?'
- 'What gives you strength and hope?'

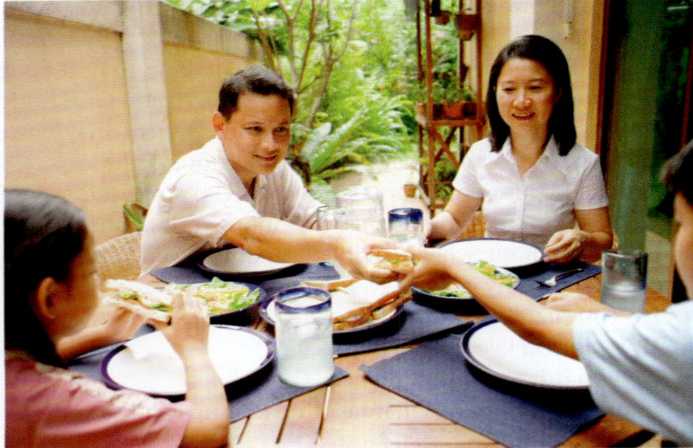

FIGURE 2-3 Discussing family relationships is a key way to assess support systems. (Shutterstock.com/Asia Images Group.)

Education and work

Questions about education and work help to identify areas of stress and satisfaction in the patient's life. If the patient does not perceive that he or she has sufficient education or does not enjoy work, assistance or support may be needed to make changes. Sometimes discussing this area will help patients to feel good about what they have accomplished and promote their sense of life satisfaction. Questions should bring out data about the kind and amount of education the patient has, whether the patient enjoyed school, whether the patient perceives his or her education as satisfactory or whether there were problems and what plans the patient may have for further education, either formal or informal. Similar questions should be asked about work history. Sample questions include:

- 'Tell me about your experiences in school or about your education.'
- 'Are you satisfied with the level of education you have? Do you have future educational plans?'
- 'What can you tell me about your work? What are your responsibilities at work?'
- 'Do you enjoy your work?'
- 'How do you feel about your colleagues?'
- 'What kind of stress do you have that is work related? Any major problems?'
- 'Who is the main provider of financial support in your family?'
- 'Does your current income meet your needs?'

Stress levels and coping styles

To investigate the amount of stress that patients perceive they are under and how they cope with it, ask questions that address what events cause stress for the patient and how he or she usually responds. In addition, find out what the patient does to relieve stress and whether these behaviours or activities can be construed as adaptive or maladaptive. To avoid denial responses, non-directive questions or observations regarding previous information provided by the patient may be an easy way to get the patient to discuss this subject. Sample questions include:

- 'What types of things make you angry?'
- 'How would you describe your stress level?'
- 'How do you manage anger or stress?'
- 'What do you see as the greatest stressors in your life?'
- 'Where do you usually turn for help in times of crisis?'

Environment

Ask questions regarding the patient's environment to assess health hazards unique to the patient's living situation and lifestyle. Look for physical, chemical or psychological situations that may put the patient at risk. These may be found in the patient's neighbourhood, home, work or recreational environment. They may be controllable or uncontrollable. Sample questions include:

- 'What risks are you aware of in your environment such as in your home or neighbourhood, on the job or in any activities in which you participate?'
- 'What types of precautions do you take, if any, when playing contact sports, using harsh chemicals or paint, or operating machinery?'
- 'Do you believe you are ever in danger of becoming a victim of violence? Explain.'

SUMMARY

Collecting subjective data is a key step of the nursing health assessment. Subjective data consist of information elicited and verified only by the patient. Interviewing is the means by which subjective data are gathered. Two types of communication are useful for interviewing: non-verbal and verbal. Three variations in communication—Older persons, cultural and emotional—may be encountered during the patient interview.

The complete health history is performed to collect as much subjective data about a patient as possible. It consists of eight sections: biographical data, reasons for seeking health care, history of present health concern, past health history, family health history, review of body systems for current health problems, lifestyle and health practices profile, and developmental level. The information gathered will inform the nursing actions or interventions that need to be taken followed by evaluating the effectiveness of those interventions.

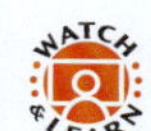

Beginning the physical assessment

ONLINE RESOURCES

An extensive range of additional resources to enhance teaching and learning and to facilitate understanding may be found online at the text's accompanying website, located on thePoint at http://thepoint.lww.com. These include Watch and Learn videos, Concepts in Action animations, journal articles, case studies, discussion topics and quizzes.

Subscribers may also access Lippincott Procedures, an extensive online point-of-care procedure guide that provides reliable step-by-step instructions for more than 1700 procedures, including 450 evidence-based Australian procedures, and skills in a variety of speciality settings, together with a wealth of supporting information.

References

Andrews, M. & Boyle, J. (2011). *Transcultural concepts in nursing care* (6th ed.). Philadelphia: Lippincott Williams & Wilkins.

Giger, J. (2012). *Transcultural nursing: Assessment and intervention* (6th ed.). St Louis: Mosby/Elsevier.

International Council of Nurses. (2012). The ICN code of ethics for nurses. Viewed October 2019 at https://www.icn.ch/sites/default/files/inline-files/2012_ICN_Codeofethicsfornurses_%20eng.pdf

Li, J. J., Appleton, S. L., Wittert, G. A., et al. (2014). *Sleep*, *37*(3), 571–578.

Maier-Lorentz, M. M. (2008). Transcultural nursing: Its importance in nursing practice. *Journal of Cultural Diversity*, *15*(1), 37–43.

Mansfield, D. R. & the Australasian Sleep Association and the Sleep Health Foundation (Eds). (McEvoy, R. D., 2013). *Sleep disorders: A practical guide for Australian health care practitioners*. Supplement to Medical Journal of Australia, 199(8). Available at www.mja.com.au/journal/2013/199/8/supplement.

Nursing and Midwifery Board of Australia (NMBA). (2018). Code of conduct for nurses. Viewed October 2019 at www.nursingmidwiferyboard.gov.au/documents/default.aspx?record=WD17%2f23849&dbid=AP&chksum=ki92NMPa9thp9f9ZhTQNJg%3d%3d

Reynolds, A. C., Dorrian, J., Liu, P. Y., et al. (2012). *PLoS ONE*, *7*(7), e41218.

Selected readings

Department of Health. (2019). Australia's physical activity and sedentary behaviour guidelines and the Australian 24-hour movement guidelines. Viewed October 2019 at https://www1.health.gov.au/internet/main/publishing.nsf/Content/health-pubhlth-strateg-phys-act-guidelines.

National Health and Medical Research Council and the Australian Department of Health and Ageing. (2013). *Australian dietary guidelines* and *Australian guide to healthy eating* (posters). Viewed November 2013 at www.healthyactive.gov.au/internet/healthyactive/Publishing.nsf/Content/eating.

Online resources

Australasian Sleep Association: https://www.sleep.org.au/

Australian Government's Eat for Health program (dietary guidelines) and Guide to Healthy Eating posters: www.eatforhealth.gov.au

Department of Health, physical activity guidelines: www.healthyactive.gov.au/internet/healthyactive/publishing.nsf/Content/recommendations-guidelines

New Zealand Ministry of Health, food and nutrition guidelines: www.health.govt.nz/our-work/preventative-health-wellness/nutrition/food-and-nutrition-guidelines

Sleep Health Foundation: www.sleephealthfoundation.org.au

Sleep Well Clinic, New Zealand: www.sleepwellclinic.co.nz

Transcultural nursing: Basic concepts and case studies: www.culturaldiversity.org

Transcultural Nursing Society, theories and models: www.tcns.org

CHAPTER 3

Collecting objective data

A complete nursing assessment includes both the collection of subjective data (discussed in Chap. 2) and the collection of objective data. Objective data include information about the patient that the nurse directly observes during interaction with the patient and information elicited through physical assessment (examination) techniques and diagnostic values. Objective data encompass definitive patient information available through vital signs (discussed in Chap. 7), assessment of mental status and psychosocial development (discussed in Chap. 6), and interpretation of laboratory results and medical information from the interdisciplinary team, such as ultrasound, X-ray, nutritional status and other focused investigations. Collecting objective data also involves the analysis of findings using critical thinking skills (discussed in Chap. 5). In addition, succinct and accurate communication and documentation of findings (discussed in Chap. 4) is essential to enable ongoing assessment, diagnosis, planning, intervention and evaluation of nursing care.

CRITICAL THINKING

1. From the description above, what particular observations would be classified as objective data?
2. Do you think that the scoring of pain is objective data?
3. Is your observation about patient skin colour objective data?

There are instances, such as unexpected patient deterioration, when a more focused assessment is required in order to prioritise and implement appropriate care to align with the terminology of the nursing process. In these instances, it is acceptable to wait until the patient has stabilised before a more holistic and comprehensive nursing assessment is performed (Nelson, 2018).

To become proficient in physical assessment, you must have knowledge and interpretative skills in the following areas:

- Types of and operation of equipment needed for the particular examination (e.g. touch, speech, thermometer, penlight, sphygmomanometer, otoscope, tuning fork, stethoscope)
- Preparation of the setting, yourself, the patient and any other members of the interdisciplinary team or significant others who should be present for the physical assessment
- Performance of the four assessment techniques: inspection, palpation, percussion and auscultation
- Ability to interpret and contextualise data using critical thinking skills and a decision-making framework in order to develop an evicence-based plan of care to achieve best patient outcomes (see Chap. 5) (Toney-Butler & Unison-Pace, 2018).

CRITICAL THINKING

Many medical and allied health professionals are comfortable with using physical assessment skills as part of their role—for example, physiotherapists measure range of movement in joints and doctors listen to heart sounds with a stethoscope. However, nurses can be reluctant to use the skills of palpation, percussion and auscultation. They may feel intimidated by instruments such as otoscopes and ophthalmoscopes.

4. Why do you think that nurses are content to measure vital signs but less confident assessing breath sounds?
5. List the reasons why you think it is important that nurses use the skills of inspection, palpation, percussion and auscultation.

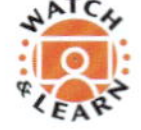

Beginning the physical assessment

EQUIPMENT

Each part of the physical examination requires specific equipment. Table 3-1 lists the equipment necessary for the examination and describes the general purpose of each item. More detailed descriptions of these items of equipment and the procedures for using them are provided in the chapters on the body systems where each item is used. The stethoscope is used as an assessment tool to examine many body systems: as such, this chapter includes a description and guidelines on how to use it.

Table 3-1 Equipment needed for physical examinations

Equipment needed	Purpose
For all examinations	
Gloves	To protect examiner in any part of the examination when the examiner may have contact with blood, body fluids, secretions, excretions and contaminated items or when disease-causing agents could be transmitted to or from the patient
For vital signs	
Sphygmomanometer	To measure diastolic and systolic blood pressure
Stethoscope	To auscultate blood sounds when measuring blood pressure
Thermometer (oral, rectal, tympanic, electronic)	To measure body temperature
Watch with second hand	To time heart rate, pulse rate
Pain rating scale	To determine perceived pain level
For anthropometric measurements	
Skinfold callipers	To measure skinfold thickness of subcutaneous tissue
Flexible tape measure	To measure mid-arm circumference
Platform scale with height attachment	To measure height and weight
For skin, hair and nail examination	
Ruler with centimetre markings	To measure size of skin lesions
Magnifying glass	To enlarge visibility of lesion
Wood light	To test for fungus
For head and neck examination	
Small cup of water	To help patient swallow during examination of the thyroid gland
For eye examination	
Penlight	To test pupillary constriction
Snellen chart	To test distant vision
Ophthalmoscope	To view the red reflex and to examine the retina of the eye
Cover card	To test for strabismus
Newspaper or Rosenbaum Pocket Screener	To test near vision
For ear examination	
Otoscope	To view the ear canal and tympanic membrane
Tuning fork	To test for bone and air conduction of sound
For mouth, throat, nose and sinus examination	
Penlight	To provide light to view the mouth and throat and to transilluminate the sinuses
Tongue depressor	To depress tongue to view throat, check looseness of teeth, view cheeks and check strength of tongue
Piece of small gauze	To grasp tongue to examine mouth
Otoscope with wide-tip attachment	To view the internal nose
For thoracic and lung examination	
Stethoscope (diaphragm)	To auscultate breath sounds
Marking pencil and centimetre ruler	To measure diaphragmatic excursion
For heart and neck vessel examination	
Stethoscope (bell and diaphragm)	To auscultate heart sounds
Two centimetre rulers	To measure jugular venous pressure
For abdominal examination	
Stethoscope	To detect bowel sounds
Marking pencil and tape measure with centimetre markings	To mark area of percussion of organs to measure size
Two small pillows	To place under the patient's knees and head to promote relaxation of abdomen

Continued on following page

Table 3-1 Equipment needed for physical examinations (continued)

Equipment needed	Purpose
For female genitalia examination	
Vaginal speculum and lubricant	To inspect cervix through dilation of the vaginal canal
Slides or specimen container, bifid spatula and cottonwool bud	To obtain endocervical swab and cervical scrape and vaginal pool sample
For anus, rectum, prostate examination	
Lubricating jelly	To promote comfort for patient
Specimen container	To test for occult blood
For peripheral vascular examination	
Stethoscope and sphygmomanometer	To auscultate vascular sounds and measure blood pressure
Flexible tape measure	To measure size of extremities for oedema
Cotton ball and paper clip	To detect light, blunt and sharp touch
Tuning fork	To detect vibratory sensation
Doppler ultrasound probe blood	To detect pressure and weak pulses not easily heard with a stethoscope
For musculoskeletal examination	
Tape measure	To measure size of extremities
Goniometer	To measure degree of flexion and extension of joints
For neurological examination	
Tuning fork	To test for vibratory sensation
Cotton ball, paper clip	To test for light, sharp and dull touch and two-point discrimination
Soap, coffee	To test for smelling perception
Salt, sugar, lemon, gherkin juice	To test for taste perception
Tongue depressor	To test for rise of uvula and gag reflex
Reflex hammer	To test deep tendon reflexes
Coin or key	To test for stereognosis (ability to recognise objects by touch)

Prior to any examination, collect the necessary equipment and place it in the area where the examination will be performed. This promotes organisation and prevents you from leaving the patient in the middle of your assessment to search for a piece of equipment.

PREPARING FOR THE EXAMINATION

How well you prepare the environment, yourself and the patient can affect the quality of the data you collect. As an examiner, you must make sure you have prepared for all aspects of the assessment prior to commencement.

Preparing the environment

The physical examination may take place in a variety of environments such as a hospital room, outpatient clinic, doctor's office, school health office, employee health office or a patient's home. It is important that you strive to ensure that the examination setting meets the following conditions:

- Comfortable, warm room temperature—provide a warm blanket if the room temperature cannot be adjusted
- Private area free of interruptions from others—close the door or pull the curtains if possible
- Quiet area free of distractions—turn off mobile phones, radio, television or other noisy equipment where appropriate
- Adequate lighting—it is best to use sunlight (when available); however, good overhead lighting is sufficient. A portable lamp is helpful for illuminating the skin and for viewing shadows or contours
- Firm examination table or bed at a height that prevents stooping—a fold-up stool may be useful when it is necessary for the examiner to sit for parts of the assessment
- A bedside table and tray to hold the equipment needed for the examination.
- Any specific infection control precautions relevant to the clinical procedure.

CRITICAL THINKING

6. How possible is it to create the right environment for the examination?
7. What strategies could be employed where the environment is less than optimal (e.g. in a busy, noisy and crowded emergency department)?

Preparing yourself

With increasing imperatives to focus on person and family-centred care, the therapeutic relationship between the nurse and patient is essential to enriching the patient experience. This relationship can be maintained by promoting mutual trust and respect (Kornhaber et al., 2016). To promote this as a beginning examiner, it is helpful for you to assess your own feelings and anxieties before examining the patient because anxiety is easily conveyed to the patient, who may already feel uneasy and self-conscious about the examination. Developing confidence in performing a physical assessment can be achieved by practising the techniques on a classmate, friend or relative. The 'pretend patient' should be encouraged to simulate the patient role as closely as possible. It is also beneficial to perform some of the practice assessments with an experienced supervisor or clinician who can provide helpful hints and feedback on technique.

Another essential element of preparing for the physical assessment examination is preventing the transmission of infectious agents (Anderson et al., 2018). In 2007 the Ministry of Health New Zealand (MoHNZ) published its *Guidelines for the control of multidrug-resistant organisms in New Zealand* to be followed by all health care workers caring for patients (MoHNZ, 2007). In 2019, the Australian Commission on Safety and Quality in Health Care (ACSQHC) and the National Health and Medical Research Council (NHMRC) released the publication *Australian guidelines for the prevention and control of infection in healthcare* (NHMRC, 2019). In 2017, the ACSQHC released their second edition of the *National safety and quality in health service (NSQHS) standards* focusing on areas that are considered essential to improving patient safety and quality of care. The combined infection control guidelines for Australia and New Zealand are in Display 3-1.

In addition, the ACSQHC has developed a series of educational interactive online modules focused on infection prevention and control; these modules are based on the Australian guidelines and are aimed to facilitate the identification of risk management strategies to help reduce healthcare-associated infections. There is also the Health Quality & Safety Commission New Zealand (HQSCNZ), which maintains an active online recource, *Infection prevention and control*, to support initiatives aimed at preventing and monitoring health care–associated infections (HQSCNZ, 2019). Links to helpful online resources are provided at the end of this chapter.

The specific precaution or combination of precautions varies contingent on the care to be provided. In conjunction with the national guidelines, the nurse is responsible for adhering to the policies and procedures of the organisation in which he or she is practising. For example, performing venipuncture requires gloves and protective eyewear, but intubation requires gloves, gown or plastic apron, face shield or surgical mask and

DISPLAY 3-1 DOHA* AND MOHNZ† INFECTION CONTROL GUIDELINES

Standard precautions

Assume that every person is potentially infected or colonised with an organism that could be transmitted in the health care setting, and apply the following infection control practices during the delivery of health care.

Hand hygiene

- During the delivery of health care, avoid unnecessary touching of surfaces in close proximity to the patient to prevent both contamination of clean hands from environmental surfaces and transmission of pathogens from contaminated hands to surfaces.
- When hands are visibly dirty, contaminated with proteinaceous material or visibly soiled with blood or body fluids, wash hands with either a non-antimicrobial soap and water or an antimicrobial soap and water.
- If hands are not visibly soiled, or after removing visible material with non-antimicrobial soap and water, decontaminate hands in the clinical situations described later. The preferred method of hand decontamination is with an alcohol-based hand rub (ABHR). Alternatively, hands may be washed with an antimicrobial soap and water. Frequent use of ABHR immediately following hand washing with non-antimicrobial soap may increase the frequency of dermatitis (HHA, n.d.). Perform hand hygiene:
  - Before having direct contact with patients
  - After contact with blood, body fluids or excretions, mucous membranes, non-intact skin or wound dressings
  - After contact with a patient's intact skin (e.g. when taking a pulse or blood pressure or lifting a patient)
  - If hands will be moving from a contaminated body site to a clean body site during patient care
  - After contact with inanimate objects (including medical equipment) in the immediate vicinity of the patient
  - After removing gloves.
- Wash hands with non-antimicrobial soap and water or with antimicrobial soap and water if contact with spores (e.g. *Clostridium difficile* or *Bacillus anthracis*) is likely to have occurred. The physical action of washing and rinsing hands under such circumstances is recommended because alcohols, chlorhexidine, iodophors and other antiseptic agents have poor activity against spores.
- Do not wear artificial fingernails, nail varnish or extenders if duties include direct contact with patients at high risk of infection and associated adverse outcomes (e.g. those in intensive care units [ICUs] or operating rooms).
- Develop an organisational policy on the wearing of non-natural nails by health care personnel who have direct contact with patients outside of the groups specified in the preceding text.

Personal protective equipment

- Observe the following principles of use:
  - Wear personal protective equipment (PPE) (e.g. gloves, gown, plastic aprons, eye or facial protection) when the nature of the anticipated patient interaction indicates that contact with blood or body fluids may occur.
  - Prevent contamination of clothing and skin during the process of removing PPE.
  - Before leaving the patient's room or cubicle, remove and discard PPE.
- **Gloves**
  - Wear gloves when it can be reasonably anticipated that contact with blood or other potentially infectious materials, mucous membranes, non-intact skin or potentially contaminated intact skin (e.g. of a patient incontinent of stool or urine) could occur.
  - Wear gloves with fit and durability appropriate to the task.
    - Wear disposable examination gloves for providing direct patient care.

*DoHA: Department of Health Australia (2004); †MoHNZ: Ministry of Health New Zealand (2007);
‡HSCT: haematopoietic stem cell transplant; **SARS: severe acute respiratory syndrome; ††RSV: respiratory syncytial virus; ‡‡HAI: health care–associated infections.

Continued on following page

DISPLAY 3-1 DOHA* AND MOHNZ† INFECTION CONTROL GUIDELINES (continued)

- Wear disposable examination gloves or reusable utility gloves for cleaning the environment or medical equipment.
- Remove gloves after contact with a patient or the surrounding environment (including medical equipment) using proper technique to prevent hand contamination. Do not wear the same pair of gloves for the care of more than one patient. Do not wash gloves for the purpose of reuse because this practice has been associated with transmission of pathogens.
- Discard single-use gloves as soon as they are damaged.
- Change gloves during patient care if the hands will move from a contaminated body site (e.g. perineal area) to a clean body site (e.g. face).

- **Gowns/plastic apron**
  - Wear a gown or plastic apron that is appropriate to the task, to protect skin and prevent soiling or contamination of clothing during procedures and patient care activities when contact with blood, body fluids, secretions or excretions is anticipated.
    - Wear a gown or plastic apron for direct patient contact if the patient has uncontained secretions or excretions.
    - Remove gown or plastic apron and perform hand hygiene before leaving the patient's environment.
  - Do not reuse gowns or plastic aprons, even for repeated contacts with the same patient.
  - Routine donning of gown or plastic apron upon entrance into a high-risk unit (e.g. ICU, neonatal ICU or HSCT‡ unit) is not indicated.
- **Mouth, nose, eye protection**
  - Use PPE to protect the mucous membranes of the eyes, nose and mouth during procedures and patient care activities that are likely to generate splashes or sprays of blood, body fluids, secretions and excretions. Select masks, surgical face masks, respirators, goggles, face shields and combinations of each according to the need anticipated by the task performed.
  - During aerosol-generating procedures (e.g. bronchoscopy, suctioning of the respiratory tract [if not using in-line suction catheters], endotracheal intubation) in patients who are not suspected of being infected with an agent for which respiratory protection is otherwise recommended (e.g. *Mycobacterium tuberculosis,* SARS**, or haemorrhagic fever viruses), wear one of the following: a face shield that fully covers the front and sides of the face, a mask with attached shield, or a mask and goggles (in addition to gloves and gown).
- **Respiratory hygiene and cough etiquette**
  - Educate healthcare personnel on the importance of source control measures to contain respiratory secretions to prevent droplet and fomite transmission of respiratory pathogens, especially during seasonal outbreaks of viral respiratory tract infections (e.g. influenza, RSV††, adenovirus, parainfluenza virus) in communities.
  - Implement the following measures to contain respiratory secretions in patients and accompanying individuals who have signs and symptoms of a respiratory infection, beginning at the point of initial encounter in a healthcare setting (e.g. triage, reception and waiting areas in emergency departments, outpatient clinics and doctors' offices).
    - Post signs at entrances and in strategic places (e.g. lifts, cafeterias) within ambulatory and inpatient settings with instructions to patients and other persons with symptoms of a respiratory infection to cover their mouth/nose when coughing or sneezing, to use and dispose of tissues, and to perform hand hygiene after hands have been in contact with respiratory secretions.
    - Provide tissues and no-touch receptacles (e.g. pedal-operated lid or open, plastic-lined waste basket) for disposal of tissues.
    - Provide resources and instructions for performing hand hygiene in or near waiting areas in ambulatory and inpatient settings; provide conveniently located dispensers of ABHR and, where sinks are available, supplies for hand washing.
    - During periods of increased prevalence of respiratory infections in the community (e.g. as indicated by increased school absenteeism or increased number of patients seeking care for a respiratory infection), offer masks to coughing patients and other symptomatic persons (e.g. persons who accompany ill patients) upon entry into the facility or medical office and encourage them to maintain special separation, ideally a distance of at least 1 m, from others in common waiting areas. Some facilities may find it logistically easier to institute this recommendation year-round as a standard of practice.

Patient, clinician and environmental safety

- **Patient placement**
  - Include the potential for transmission of infectious agents in patient placement decisions. Place patients who pose a risk of transmission to others (e.g. uncontained secretions, excretions or wound drainage; infants with suspected viral respiratory or gastrointestinal infections) in a single-patient room when available.
  - Determine patient placement based on the following principles:
    - Routes of transmission of the known or suspected infectious agent
    - Risk factors for transmission in the infected patient
    - Risk factors for adverse outcomes resulting from an HAI‡‡ in other patients in the area or room being considered for patient placement
    - Availability of single-patient rooms
    - Patient options for room sharing (e.g. cohorting patients with the same infection).
- **Patient care equipment and instruments or devices**
  - Establish policies and procedures for containing, transporting and handling patient care equipment and instruments or devices that may be contaminated with blood or body fluids.
  - Remove organic material from critical and semicritical instrument or devices using recommended cleaning agents before high-level disinfection and sterilisation to enable effective disinfection and sterilisation processes.
  - Wear PPE (e.g. gloves, gown), according to the level of anticipated contamination, when handling patient care equipment and instruments or devices that are visibly soiled or may have been in contact with blood or body fluids.
- **Care of the environment**
  - Establish policies and procedures for routine and targeted cleaning of environmental surfaces as indicated by the level of patient contact and degree of soiling.
  - Clean and disinfect surfaces that are likely to be contaminated with pathogens, including those that are in close proximity to the patient (e.g. bed rails, overbed tables) and frequently touched surfaces in the patient care environment (e.g. door knobs, surfaces in and surrounding toilets in patients' rooms), on a more frequent schedule compared with that for other surfaces (e.g. horizontal surfaces in waiting rooms).
  - Use hospital-grade disinfectants that have microbiocidal (i.e. killing) activity against the pathogens most likely to contaminate the patient care environment, in accordance with the manufacturer's instructions.
    - Review the efficacy of in-use disinfectants when evidence of continuing transmission of an infectious agent (e.g. rotavirus, *C. difficile,* norovirus) may indicate resistance to the in-use product and change to a more effective disinfectant as indicated.
  - In facilities that provide health care to paediatric patients or have waiting areas with child's play toys (e.g. obstetric and gynaecological rooms and clinics), establish policies and procedures for cleaning

*DoHA: Department of Health Australia (2004); †MoHNZ: Ministry of Health New Zealand (2007);
‡HSCT: haematopoietic stem cell transplant; **SARS: severe acute respiratory syndrome; ††RSV: respiratory syncytial virus; ‡‡HAI: health care–associated infections.

DISPLAY 3-1 DOHA* AND MOHNZ† INFECTION CONTROL GUIDELINES (continued)

and disinfecting toys at regular intervals. Use the following principles in developing this policy and procedures:
  - Select toys that can be easily cleaned and disinfected
  - Do not permit use of stuffed furry toys if they will be shared
  - Clean and disinfect large stationary toys (e.g. climbing equipment) at least weekly and whenever visibly soiled
  - If toys are likely to be mouthed, rinse with water after disinfection; alternatively, wash in a dishwasher
  - When a toy requires cleaning and disinfection, do so immediately or store in a designated labelled container separate from toys that are clean and ready for use.
- Include multiuse electronic equipment in policies and procedures for preventing contamination and for cleaning and disinfecting, especially those items that are used by patients, those used during delivery of patient care and mobile devices that are moved in and out of patient rooms frequently (e.g. daily).
- Protective covers and washable keyboards must be included in cleaning and disinfecting protocols (Doll et al., 2018).

- **Textiles and laundry**
  - Handle used textiles and fabrics with minimum agitation to avoid contamination of air, surfaces and persons.
  - If laundry chutes are used, ensure that they are properly designed, maintained and used in a manner to minimise dispersion of aerosols from contaminated laundry.
- **Safe injection practices**
  The following recommendations apply to the use of needles, cannulas that replace needles and, where applicable, intravenous delivery systems.
  - Use aseptic technique to avoid contamination of sterile injection equipment.
  - Do not administer medications from a syringe to multiple patients, even if the needle or cannula on the syringe is changed. Needles, cannulas and syringes are sterile, single-use items; they should not be reused for another patient or used to access a medication or solution that might be intended for a subsequent patient.
  - Use fluid infusion and administration sets (i.e. intravenous bags, tubing and connectors) for one patient only, and dispose appropriately after use. Consider a syringe or needle and cannula contaminated once they have been used to enter or connect to a patient's intravenous infusion bag or administration set.
  - Use single-dose vials for parenteral medications whenever possible.
  - Do not administer medications from single-dose vials or ampules to multiple patients or combine leftover contents for later use.
  - If multidose vials must be used, both the needle or cannula and syringe used to access the multidose vial must be sterile.
  - Do not keep multidose vials in the immediate patient treatment area and store in accordance with the manufacturer's recommendations; discard if sterility is compromised or questionable.
  - Do not use bags or bottles of intravenous solution as a common source of supply for multiple patients.
- **Infection control practices for special lumbar puncture procedures**
  Wear a surgical mask when placing a catheter or injecting material into the spinal canal or subdural space (i.e. during myelograms, lumbar puncture and spinal or epidural anaesthesia).
- **Worker safety**
  Adhere to federal and state requirements for protection of health care personnel from exposure to bloodborne pathogens.

*DoHA: Department of Health Australia (2004); †MoHNZ: Ministry of Health New Zealand (2007);
‡HSCT: haematopoietic stem cell transplant; **SARS: severe acute respiratory syndrome; ††RSV: respiratory syncytial virus; ‡‡HAI: health care–associated infections.

protective eyewear. General principles to keep in mind while performing a physical assessment include the following:

- Wash your hands before beginning the examination, before a procedure, immediately after accidental direct contact with blood or other body fluids (gloves should be worn if there is a chance of direct contact with blood or other body fluids), after completing the physical examination or after removing gloves and also after touching the patient's surroundings (Zimmerman, 2013). If possible, wash your hands in the examining room in front of the patient to demonstrate and promote safe practice. This assures the patient that you are concerned about his or her safety (Doyle et al., 2017).
- Wear gloves if you have an open cut or skin abrasion, if the patient has an open or weeping cut, if body fluids are being collected (e.g. blood, sputum, wound drainage, urine or stools) for a specimen, if handling contaminated surfaces (e.g. linen, tongue blades, vaginal speculum), and when performing an examination of the mouth, an open wound, genitalia, vagina or rectum. Change gloves, remembering to wash your hands before putting on new gloves, if moving from contaminated to clean body sites, and between patients. You may need to explain the rationale for the use of gloves to the patient in order to reassure him or her, while educating the patient on the importance of protection from infection for all concerned (NHMRC, 2019).
- If a pin or other sharp object is used to assess sensory perception, discard the pin in an appropriate container that has been identified for disposal of sharp items, and use a new one for the next patient.
- Wear a surgical mask, gloves and protective eye wear if performing an examination in which you are likely to be splashed with blood or other body fluid droplets (e.g. if performing an oral examination on a patient who has a chronic productive cough).

Approaching and preparing the patient

The nurse–patient relationship should be established during the patient interview before the physical examination takes place. This is important because it helps to alleviate any tension or anxiety that the patient is experiencing. At the end of the interview, it is important you explain to the patient that the physical assessment will follow and describe what the examination will involve. For example, you might say to a patient, 'Mr Nadal, based on the information you have given me, I believe that a complete physical examination should be performed so I can better assess your health. This will require you to remove your clothing and to put on this hospital gown. You may leave on your underwear until it is time to perform the genital examination.' It is important to ensure that the patient consents to the examination before proceeding.

Respect the patient's desires and requests related to the physical examination. Some patient requests may be simple, such as asking to have a family member or friend present during the examination. It is important to consider that there may be environmental or contextual factors that can hinder a physical assessment—for example, patients may not understand instructions if English is their second language, and some patients may not wish to expose parts of their body because of gender, sexuality or other cultural issues and associated barriers (see Chap. 10 onwards). These factors, and others, can provide a significant barrier to the collection of objective data. If faced with this situation, explain to the patient the importance of the examination and the risk of missing important information if any part of the examination is omitted. Ultimately, however, whether to have the examination is the patient's decision.

CRITICAL THINKING

8. What problems might occur when a family member is present to interpret for a patient who does not speak English?

Within health care, consent involves the principle that a patient gives permission prior to receving any form of treatment, examination or test. Informed consent is the gold standard and is a legal obligation across all health care environments. Informed consent requires clear explanation of the intended intervention, followed by evidence that the patient has clear understanding of what to expect, including possible outcomes (NHS, 2016: OAIC, 2014; NZNO, 2016). In this way, patients are able to make sound decisions about, and contributions to their care. Some health care providers ask the patient to sign a consent form before a physical examination, especially in situations where a vaginal or rectal examination is to be performed. It may be beneficial or even organisation policy to have a witness present for invasive procedures, such as examination of the patient's breasts and genitalia, particularly if the patient is of the opposite gender to the examiner or if there are any concerns that the patient may misconstrue the nature and intent of the assessment. The witness is often another health care professional but can also include someone whom the patient elects (NCNZ, 2012; Nelson, 2018; NMBA, 2018).

Consent is interwoven with ethical, professional and medico-legal implications, and during the process of collecting objective data, the nurse should be mindful of this in all instances of invasive data collection.

If a urine specimen is necessary, explain to the patient the purpose of a urine sample and the procedure for giving a sample, and provide a specimen container to collect the sample. If a urine sample is not necessary, ask the patient to urinate before the examination to promote an easier and more comfortable examination of the abdomen and genital areas. Ask the patient to undress and put on a hospital gown and explain that his or her underwear can be worn until just before the genital examination to promote comfort and privacy. Leave the room while the patient changes into the hospital gown and knock before re-entering the room to ensure the patient's privacy.

Begin the examination with the less-intrusive procedures such as measuring the patient's temperature, pulse, blood pressure, height and weight. These procedures allow the patient to feel more comfortable with the nurse and help to ease patient anxiety about the examination (Nelson, 2018). Some jurisdictions provide uniform data collection charts, such as South Australia's Adult Observation Chart (Fig. 3-1), that are designed according to human factor principles and incorporate track and trigger systems to ensure clinical deterioration is recognised and care escalated according to local guidelines and resources (ACSQHC, 2017). Throughout the examination, continue to explain what procedure is being performed and why. This helps to ease the patient's anxiety. It is usually helpful to integrate health teaching and health promotion during the examination (e.g. breast self-examination techniques during the breast examination).

Approach the patient from the right-hand side of the examination table or bed because most examination techniques are performed with the examiner's right hand (even if the examiner is left-handed). You may ask the patient to change positions frequently, depending on the part of the examination being performed. Prepare the patient for these changes at the beginning of the examination by explaining that these position changes are necessary to ensure a thorough examination of each body part and system. Many patients need assistance getting into the required position. Display 3-2 illustrates various positions and provides guidelines for using them during the examination. Display 3-3 provides considerations for older adult patients.

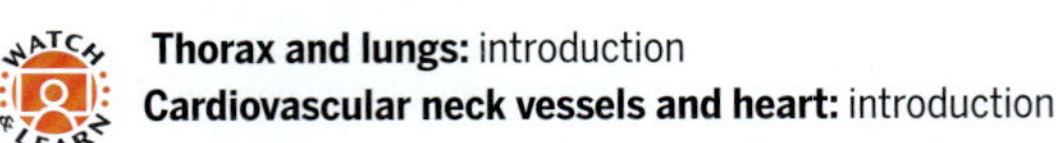

Thorax and lungs: introduction
Cardiovascular neck vessels and heart: introduction

PHYSICAL EXAMINATION TECHNIQUES

Four basic techniques must be mastered before you can competently perform a thorough and complete assessment of the patient. These techniques are inspection, palpation, percussion and auscultation and, when used in conjunction with systematic and continuous collection of patient data extending beyond physical assessment, will help the nurse plan and deliver care that is appropriate and individualised to the patient (Toney-Butler & Unison-Pace, 2018). This chapter provides descriptions of each of the techniques identified above, along with guidelines on how they are performed. These techniques are performed usually in the order identified above, except when the abdomen is being examined the order changes so that auscultation takes place after inspection.

Using each technique for the assessment of specific body systems is described in the appropriate chapter. After performing each of the four assessment techniques, you should ask yourself questions that will facilitate analysis of the data and determine areas in which more data may be needed. These questions include:

- Did the inspection, palpation, percussion or auscultation reveal any deviations from the normal findings? (Normal findings are listed in the second column of the physical assessment sections in the body systems chapters.)
- If there is a deviation, is it a normal physical, gerontological or cultural finding; an abnormal adult finding; or an abnormal physical, gerontological or cultural finding? (Normal gerontological and cultural findings are in the second column of the physical assessment sections in the body systems chapters. Abnormal adult, gerontological and cultural findings can be found in the third column of the physical assessment sections.)
- Based on the findings, is it relevant to ask the patient more questions to validate or obtain more information about the inspection, palpation, percussion or auscultation findings?

Rapid Detection and Response Adult Observation Chart

(MR59A)

Hospital: ....

Affix patient identification label in this box

UR Number: ....

Surname: ....

Given name: ....

Second given name: ....

D.O.B: __ __ / __ __ / __ __ __ __ Sex: ....

Chart Number:

General Instructions

You must record appropriate observations:

- On admission
- At a frequency appropriate for the patient's clinical state but not less than once/shift for acute inpatients
- As per local procedures with a minimum of once daily for patients awaiting discharge placement.

You must record a set of observations including a minimum of respiratory rate, blood pressure, pulse rate, temperature, oxygen saturation and level of consciousness/sedation:

- If the patient is deteriorating or an observation is in a shaded area
- Whenever you are worried about the patient.

Review is required for unrelieved and unexpected pain that continues to trigger escalation for 2 consecutive values despite medication administration.

When graphing observations, place a dot (•) in the centre of the box which includes the current observation in its range of values and connect it to the previous dot with a straight line. If observations fall above or below graphic parameters, write the value in relevant box. For systolic blood pressure, use the symbol indicated on the graphic chart.

Whenever an observation falls within a shaded area, you must initiate the actions required for that colour, unless a modification has been made.

Modifications

If abnormal observations are to be tolerated for the patient's clinical condition, write the acceptable ranges and rationale (where a response will not be triggered) below. Duration of modification must be specified.

	Modification 1	Modification 2	Modification 3	Modification 4
Date	/ /	/ /	/ /	/ /
Time	:	:	:	:
Duration				
Observation(s) and acceptable range				
Brief Rationale *(Full description in medical record)*				
Doctor's Signature				
Doctor's Name *(print)*				
Doctor's Designation				
Nurse Signature				
Nurse Name *(print)*				
Nurse Designation				

Resuscitation Orders as Per Medical Records:

Full Resus: ☐ Modified Resus*: ☐ NFR*: ☐

Transcribed from Medical Records by: Signature .... Name...

**If modified or NFR, look in patient's medical records.*

RDR Adult Observation Chart

MR59A

Page 1 of 4

FIGURE 3-1 Adult observation chart. (Department for Health and Ageing, Government of South Australia, 2013. While current at the time of press, this chart is undergoing a review process and is slated for update in 2020. For the most current information, please see https://www.sahealth.sa.gov.au.)

Continued on following page

Date		
Time		
Respiratory Rate *(breaths/min)*	Write ≥ 36	Write ≥ 36
	31 - 35	31 - 35
	26 - 30	26 - 30
	21 - 25	21 - 25
	16 - 20	16 -20
	11 - 15	11 - 15
	8 - 10	8 - 10
	Write ≤ 7	Write ≤ 7
O_2 Saturation *(%)*	≥ 98	≥ 98
	95 - 97	95 - 97
	90 - 94	90 - 94
	Write ≤ 89	Write ≤ 89
O_2 Flow Rate *(L/min)* Write value:	≥ 7	≥ 7
	6	6
	1 - 4	1 - 4
Delivery Method/Air		
Blood Pressure *(mmHg)* Use systolic blood pressure as trigger for response	Write ≥ 220	Write ≥ 220
	210s	210s
	200s	200s
	190s	190s
	180s	180s
	170s	170s
	160s	160s
	150s	150s
	140s	140s
	130s	130s
	120s	120s
	110s	110s
	100s	100s
	90s	90s
	80s	80s
	70s	70s
	60s	60s
	50s	50s
	Write ≤ 40	Write ≤ 40
Pulse Rate *(beats/min)*	Write ≥ 140	Write ≥ 140
	130s	130s
	120s	120s
	110s	110s
	100s	100s
	90s	90s
	80s	80s
	70s	70s
	60s	60s
	50s	50s
	40s	40s
	Write ≤ 30	Write ≤ 30
Temperature *(°C)*	Write ≥ 39.1	Write ≥ 39.1
	38.6 - 39.0	38.6 - 39.0
	38.1 - 38.5	38.1 - 38.5
	37.6 - 38.0	37.6 - 38.0
	37.1 - 37.5	37.1 - 37.5
	36.6 - 37.0	36.6 - 37.0
	36.1 - 36.5	36.1 - 36.5
	35.6 - 36.0	35.6 - 36.0
	35.1 - 35.5	35.1 - 35.5
	Write ≤ 35	Write ≤ 35
Consciousness/ Sedation Wake patient before scoring	3	3
	2	2
	1	1
	0	0
Pain Score At Rest *(2 consecutive)*	8 - 10	8 - 10
	5 - 7	5 - 7
	0 - 4	0 - 4
Intervention	*See chart overleaf*	*See chart overleaf*

Page 2 of 4

FIGURE 3-1 Adult observation chart. (Department for Health and Ageing, Government of South Australia, 2013. While current at the time of press, this chart is undergoing a review process and is slated for update in 2020. For the most current information, please see https://www.sahealth.sa.gov.au.) **(continued)**

Rapid Detection and Response Adult Observation Chart **(MR59A)** Hospital:	Affix patient identification label in this box UR Number: .... Surname: .... Given name: .... Second given name: .... D.O.B: __ __ / __ __ / __ __ __ __ Sex: ....

Medical Emergency Response (MER) Call

Response Criteria
- Respiratory or cardiac arrest
- Threatened airway
- Significant bleeding
- Any observations in a purple zone
- Unexpected or uncontrolled seizure
- Unattended MDT review
- You are worried about the patient

Actions Required ASAP
- Place emergency call and specify location
- Initiate basic/advanced life support
- Notify senior doctor responsible for patient
- Increase frequency of observations post intervention

Multi Disciplinary Team (MDT) Review

(minimum of registered nurse and medical doctor - check for modifications)

Response Criteria
- Unrelieved chest pain
- Any observations in a red zone
- Urine output <30mL/hr over 4 hours from patient with IDC or patient has not voided for over 12 hours
- You are worried about the patient

Actions Required
- MDT to review patient within 30 minutes (Country Hospitals refer to local guidelines)
- Increase frequency of observations
- If MDT not attended within 30 minutes escalate to MER

*** 3 or more observations in the red zone, escalate to MER**

RN Review and Notify Shift Coordinator

Response Criteria
- Any observations in a yellow zone
- New or unexplained behavioural change
- You are worried about the patient

Actions Required
- Registered nurse must review the patient
- Increase frequency of observations
- Manage anxiety, pain and review O_2 requirements

*** 3 or more observations in the yellow zone, escalate to MDT Review**

Level of Consciousness / Sedation

Score	Descriptor	Stimulus	Response	Duration
3	Difficult to rouse (severe respiratory depression)	Pain, shoulder squeeze, jaw thrust	Brief eye opening OR any movement OR no response	N/A
2	Easy to rouse, difficulty staying awake	Voice, light touch	Eye opening and eye contact	<10 seconds
1	Easy to rouse	Voice, light touch	Eye opening and eye contact	>10 seconds
0	Awake, alert	N/A	N/A	N/A

Page 3 of 4

FIGURE 3-1 Adult observation chart. (Department for Health and Ageing, Government of South Australia, 2013. While current at the time of press, this chart is undergoing a review process and is slated for update in 2020. For the most current information, please see https://www.sahealth.sa.gov.au.) **(continued)**

Continued on following page

Rapid Detection and Response Adult Observation Chart (MR59A) Hospital:	Affix patient identification label in this box UR Number: .... Surname: .... Given name: .... Second given name: .... D.O.B: __ __ / __ __ / __ __ __ __ Sex: ....

Additional Observations

Date																		
Time																		
Initials																		
Designation																		

Interventions or Review

If you administer an intervention or review, record here and note letter in intervention row over page in appropriate time column.		Initial *Please print*	Designation
a			
b			
c			
d			
e			
f			
g			
h			

Page 4 of 4

FIGURE 3-1 Adult observation chart. (Department for Health and Ageing, Government of South Australia, 2013. While current at the time of press, this chart is undergoing a review process and is slated for update in 2020. For the most current information, please see https://www.sahealth.sa.gov.au.) **(continued)**

DISPLAY 3-2 POSITIONING THE PATIENT

Sitting position
The patient should sit upright on the side of the examination table. In the home or office setting, the patient can sit on the edge of a chair or bed. This position is good for evaluating the head, neck, lungs, chest, back, breasts, axillae, heart, vital signs and upper extremities. This position is also useful because it permits full expansion of the lungs and allows the examiner to assess symmetry of upper body parts. Some patients may be too weak to sit up for the entire examination. They may need to lie down (supine position) and rest throughout the examination. Other patients may be unable to tolerate the position for any length of time. An alternative position is for the patient to lie down with his or her head elevated.

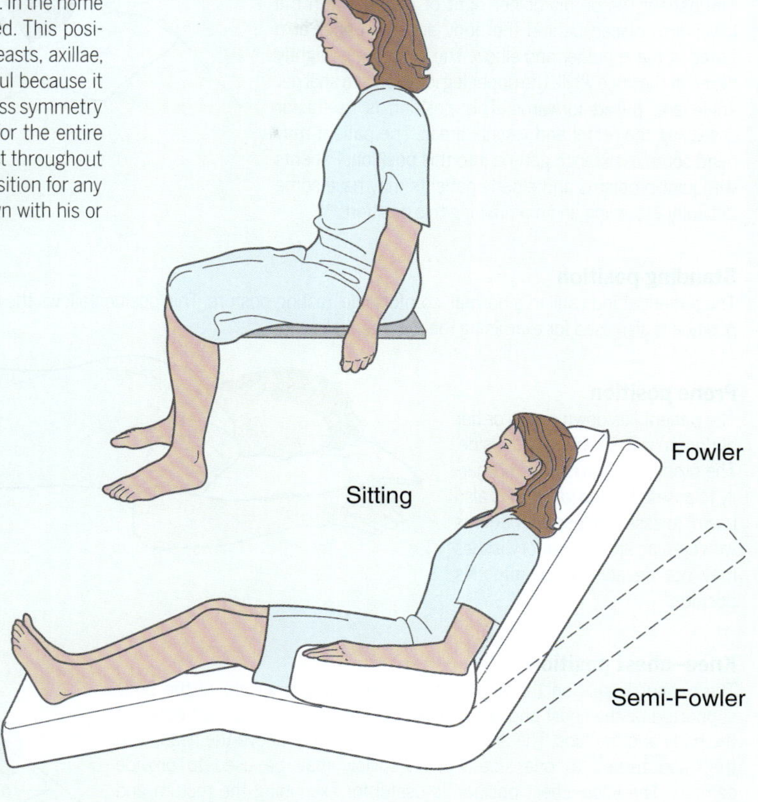

Fowler position
When the patient is lying on their back with the head of the bed or examination table elevated at a 15–90-degree angle the patient is in a Fowler position. A 15–30-degree angle classifies as low-Fowler; 30–45-degree angle as semi-Fowler; and 60–90-degree angle as a high-Fowler position. This position allows for abdominal muscle relaxation and is more comfortable for patients suffering respiratory or cardiac issues (Anchala, 2016).

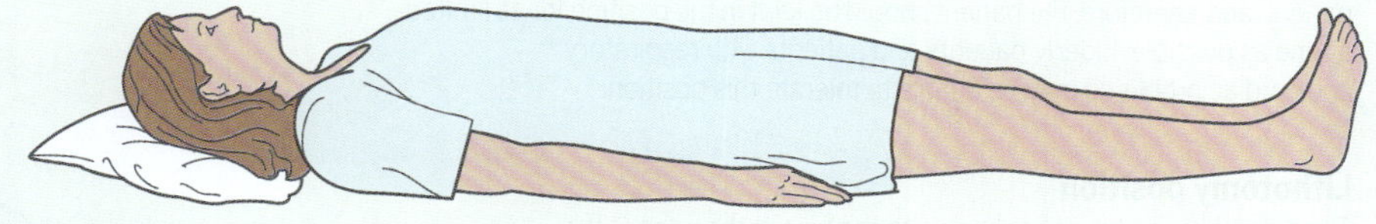

Supine position
Ask the patient to lie down with the legs together on the examination table (or bed if in a home setting). A small pillow may be placed under the head to promote comfort. If the patient has trouble breathing, the head of the bed may need to be raised. This position allows the abdominal muscles to relax and provides easy access to peripheral pulse sites. Areas assessed with the patient in this position may include head, neck, chest, breasts, axillae, abdomen, heart, lungs, pelvic area and extremities.

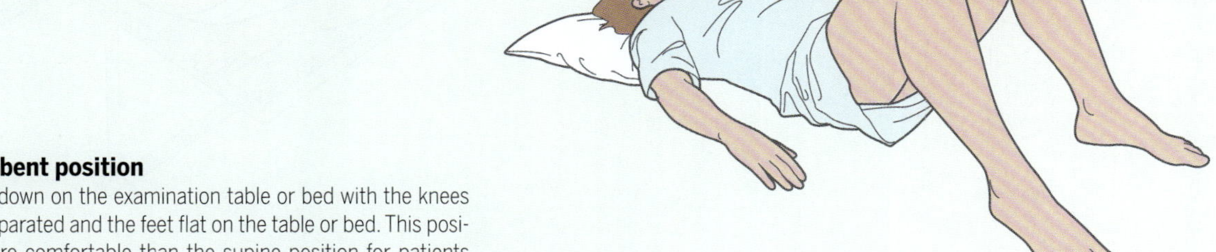

Dorsal recumbent position
The patient lies down on the examination table or bed with the knees bent, the legs separated and the feet flat on the table or bed. This position may be more comfortable than the supine position for patients with pain in the back or abdomen. Areas that may be assessed with the patient in this position include head, neck, chest, axillae, lungs, heart, extremities, breasts and peripheral pulses. It is also used for digital vaginal or rectal examination. The abdomen should not be assessed because the abdominal muscles are contracted in this position.

Continued on following page

DISPLAY 3-2 POSITIONING THE PATIENT (continued)

Left lateral position with upper thigh flexed

The patient lies on his or her right or left side with the lower arm placed behind the body and the upper arm flexed at the shoulder and elbow. The lower leg is slightly flexed at the knee while the upper leg is flexed at a sharper angle and pulled forwards. This position is useful for assessing the rectal and vaginal areas. The patient may need some assistance getting into this position. Patients with joint problems and elderly patients may have some difficulty assuming and maintaining this position.

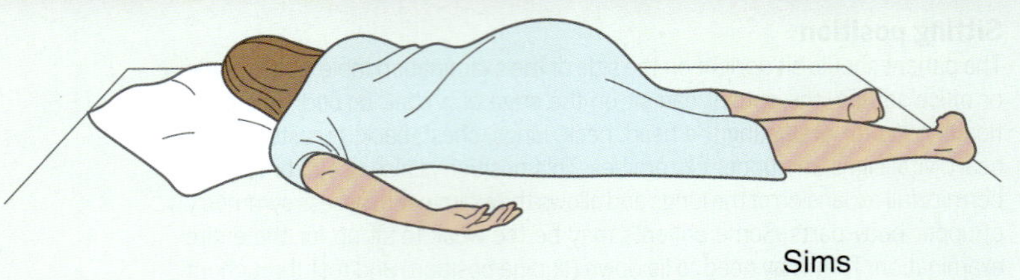

Standing position

The patient stands still in a normal, comfortable, resting posture. This position allows the examiner to assess posture, balance, body habitus and gait. This position is also used for examining the male genitalia.

Prone position

The patient lies down on his or her abdomen with the head to the side. The prone position is used primarily to assess the hip joint but is also useful to assess the spine. Patients with cardiac and respiratory issues may not be able to tolerate this position.

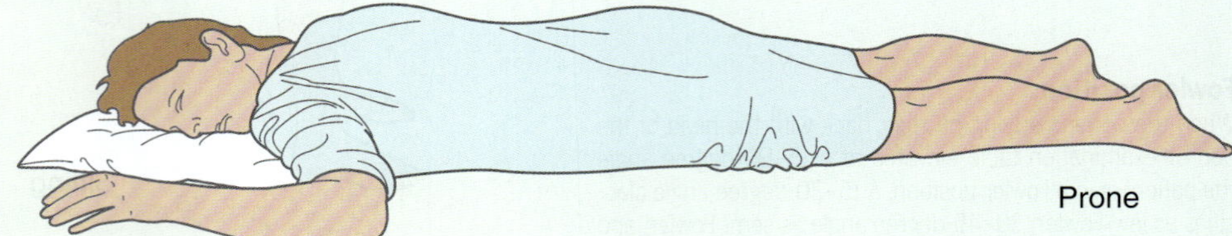

Knee–chest position

The patient kneels on the examination table with the weight of the body supported by the chest and knees. A 90-degree angle should exist between the body and the hips. The arms are placed next to or above the head, with the head turned to one side. A small pillow may be used to provide comfort. The knee–chest position is useful for examining the rectum and prostate. This position may be embarrassing and uncomfortable for the patient, and, therefore, the patient should be kept in the position for as limited a time as possible. Elderly patients and patients with respiratory and cardiac problems may be unable to tolerate this position.

Knee–chest

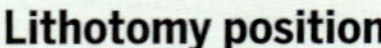

Lithotomy position

The patient lies on his or her back with the hips at the edge of the examination table and the feet supported by stirrups. The lithotomy position is used to examine the female genitalia, reproductive tracts and the rectum. The patient may require assistance getting into this position. It is an exposed position, and patients may feel embarrassed. In addition, elderly patients may not be able to assume this position for very long or at all. Therefore, it is best to keep the patient well draped during the examination and to perform the examination as quickly as possible.

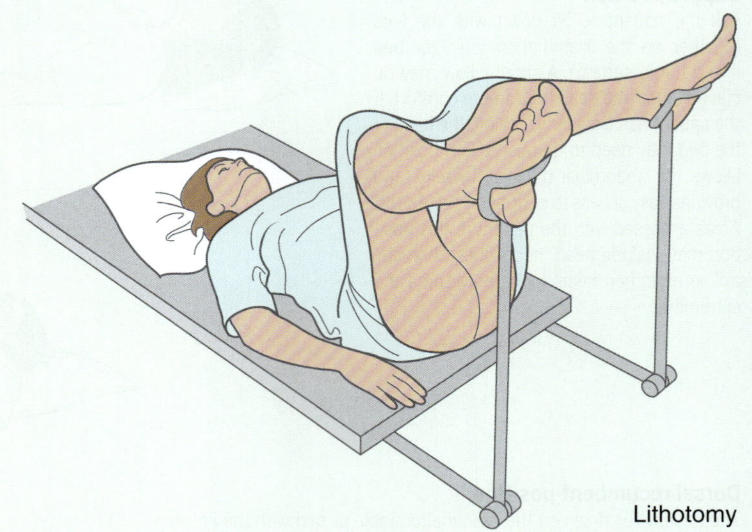

- Based on the observations and data, does the physical assessment need to focus on other related body systems?
- Is validation of the inspection, palpation, percussion or auscultation findings required by your supervisor or another clinician?
- Should the patient and data findings be referred to a primary care provider such as the patient's original referring medical practitioner?
- Are there environmental or contextual factors that are hindering the physical assessment, such as those already discussed?

DISPLAY 3-3 GENERAL CONSIDERATIONS FOR EXAMINING OLDER ADULTS

- Some positions may be very difficult or impossible for the older patient to assume or maintain because of decreased joint mobility and flexibility (see Display 3-2). Therefore, try to perform the examination in a manner that minimises position changes.
- It is a good idea to allow rest periods for the older adult, as required.
- Some older patients may process information at a slower rate, so it is important to explain the procedure and integrate teaching in a clear and slow manner.
- See Chapter 34 for assessing the older patient.

These questions help ensure that data are complete and accurate and facilitate analysis (Toney-Butler & Unison-Pace, 2018).

Inspection

Inspection involves using the senses of vision, smell and hearing to consciously observe and detect any normal or abnormal findings. This technique is used from the moment you meet the patient and continues throughout the examination. Inspection precedes palpation, percussion and auscultation because the latter techniques can potentially alter the appearance of what is being inspected. Although most of the inspection involves the use of the senses only, a few body systems require the use of special equipment (e.g. ophthalmoscope for the eye inspection, otoscope for the ear inspection).

The following guidelines should be used to practise the technique of inspection:

- Make sure the room is a comfortable temperature. A room that is too cold or too hot can alter the normal behaviour of the patient and the appearance of the patient's skin.
- Use good lighting, preferably sunlight. Fluorescent lights can alter the true colour of the skin. In addition, abnormalities may be overlooked with dim lighting.
- Look, listen, smell and observe before touching. Touch can alter appearance and distract you from a complete, focused observation.
- Completely expose the body part being inspected while draping the rest of the patient as appropriate.
- Note the following characteristics while inspecting the patient: colour, patterns, size, location, consistency, symmetry, movement, behaviour, odours and sounds.
- Compare the appearance of symmetrical body parts (e.g. eyes, ears, arms, hands) or both sides of any individual body part (Thomas, 2017).

Palpation

Palpation consists of using parts of the hand to touch and feel for the following characteristics: texture (rough or smooth), temperature (warm or cold), moisture (dry or wet), mobility (fixed or movable, still or vibrating), consistency (soft, hard or fluid-filled), strength and rhythm of pulses (strong or weak, thready or bounding, regular or irregular), size (small, medium or large), shape (well defined or irregular) and degree of tenderness.

Three different parts of the hand—the fingerpads, ulnar or palmar surface and dorsal surface—are used during palpation.

Table 3-2 Parts of hand to use when palpating

Hand part	Sensitive to
Fingerpads	Fine discriminations: pulses, texture, size, consistency, shape, crepitus
Ulnar or palmar surface	Vibrations, thrills, fremitus
Dorsal (back) surface	Temperature

Each part of the hand is particularly sensitive to certain characteristics. You should determine which characteristic you are trying to palpate and refer to Table 3-2 to find which part of the hand is best to use. Several types of palpation can be used to perform an assessment; they include light, moderate, deep and bimanual palpation. The depth of the structure being palpated and the thickness of the tissue overlying that structure determine whether you should use light (surface less than 1 cm), or deep palpation (2 to 5 cm). Bimanual palpation is the use of both hands to hold and feel a body structure.

In general, your fingernails should be short and your hands should be a comfortable temperature. Standard precautions should be followed if applicable. Proceed from light palpation, which is safest and the most comfortable for the patient, to moderate palpation and finally to deep palpation. Specific instructions on how to perform the four types of palpation follow:

- *Light palpation:* To perform light palpation (Fig. 3-2), place your dominant hand lightly on the surface of the structure. There should be very little or no depression (less than 1 cm). Feel the surface structure using a circular motion. Use this technique to feel for pulses, tenderness, surface skin texture, temperature and moisture.

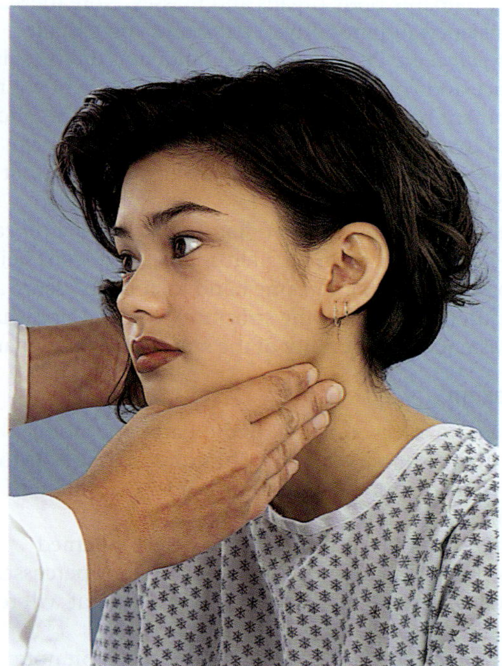

FIGURE 3-2 Light palpation. (© B. Proud.)

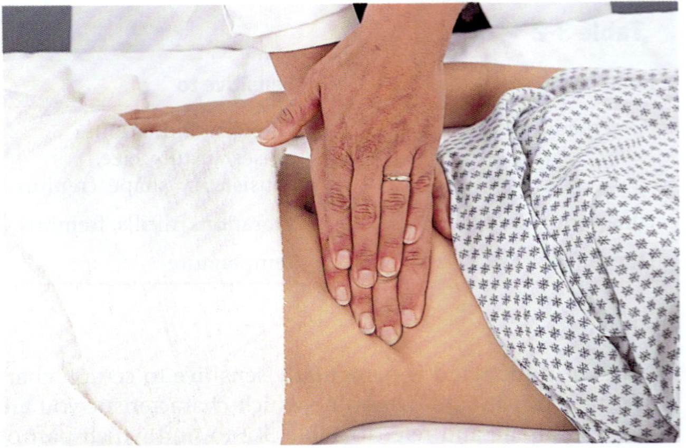

FIGURE 3-3 Deep palpation. (© B. Proud.)

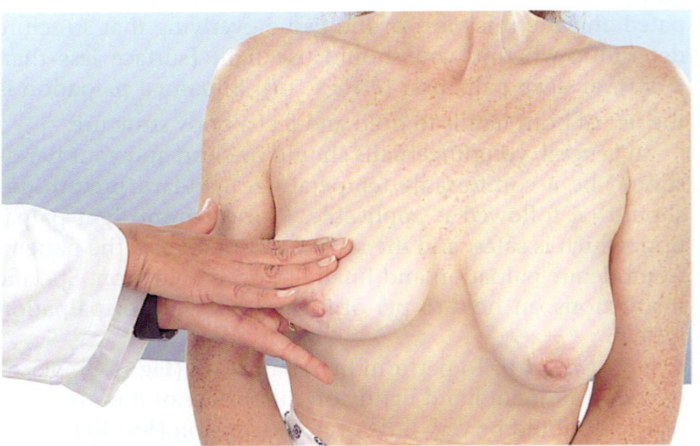

FIGURE 3-4 Bimanual palpation of the breast. (© B. Proud.)

- *Moderate palpation:* Depress the skin surface 1 to 2 cm with your dominant hand and use a circular motion to feel for easily palpable body organs and masses. Note the size, consistency and mobility of structures you palpate.
- *Deep palpation:* Place your dominant hand on the skin surface and your non-dominant hand on top of your dominant hand to apply pressure (Fig. 3-3). This should result in a surface depression between 2.5 and 5 cm. This allows you to feel very deep organs or structures that are covered by thick muscle.
- *Bimanual palpation:* Use two hands, placing one on each side of the body part (e.g. uterus, breasts, spleen) being palpated (Fig. 3-4). Use one hand to apply pressure and the other hand to feel the structure. Note the size, shape, consistency and mobility of the structures you palpate.

Percussion

Percussion involves tapping body parts to produce sound waves. These sound waves or vibrations enable you to assess underlying structures. Percussion has several different assessment uses, including:

- *Eliciting pain:* Percussion helps to detect inflamed underlying structures. If an inflamed area is percussed, the patient's response may indicate, or the patient will report, that the area feels tender, sore or painful.
- *Determining location, size and shape:* Percussion note changes between borders of an organ and its neighbouring organ can elicit information about location, size and shape.

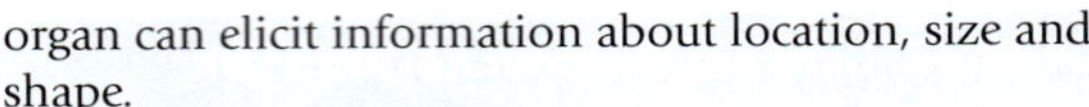

- *Determining density:* Percussion helps to determine whether an underlying structure is filled with air or fluid or is a solid structure.
- *Detecting abnormal masses:* Percussion can detect superficial abnormal structures or masses. Percussion vibrations penetrate approximately 5 cm deep. Deep masses do not produce any change in the normal percussion vibrations.
- *Eliciting reflexes:* Deep tendon reflexes are elicited using the percussion hammer.

The three types of percussion are direct, blunt and indirect. Direct percussion (Fig. 3-5) is the direct tapping of a body part with one or two fingertips to elicit possible tenderness (e.g. tenderness over the sinuses). Blunt percussion (Fig. 3-6) is

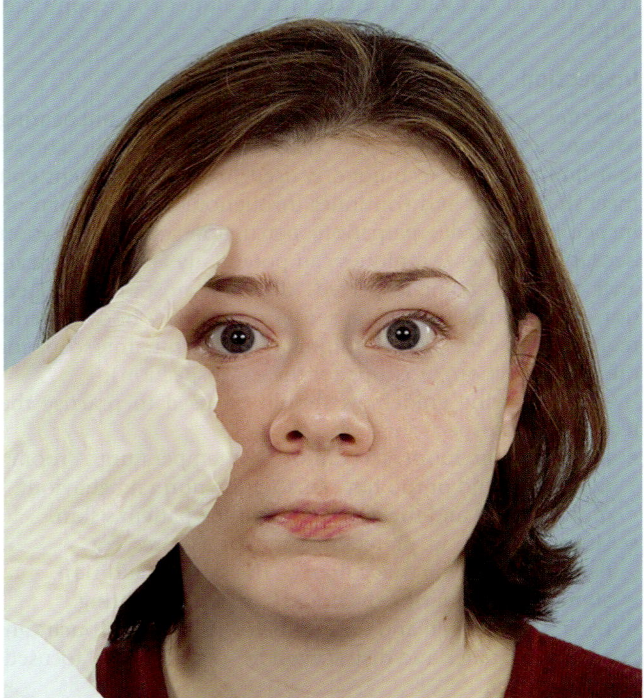

FIGURE 3-5 Direct percussion of sinuses.

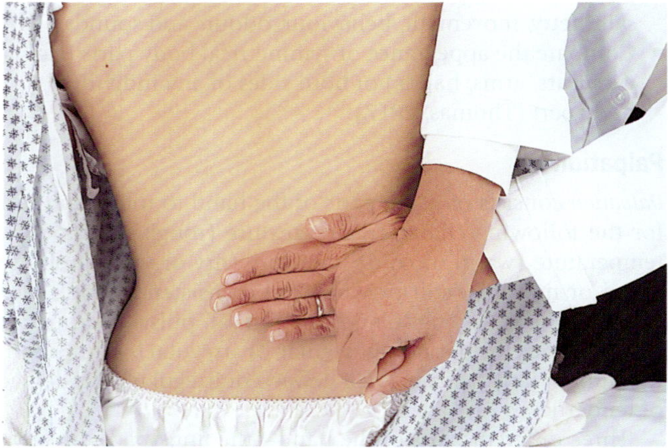

FIGURE 3-6 Blunt percussion of kidneys. (© B. Proud.)

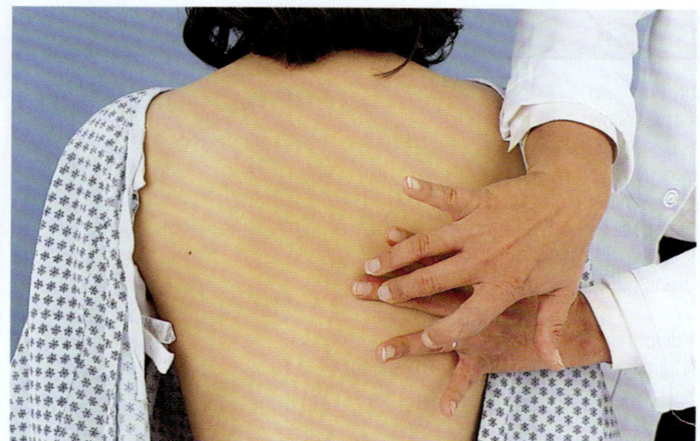

FIGURE 3-7 Indirect or mediate percussion of lungs. (© B. Proud.)

used to detect tenderness over organs (e.g. kidneys) by placing one hand flat on the body surface and using the fist of the other hand to strike the back of the hand flat on the body surface. Indirect or mediate percussion (Fig. 3-7) is the most commonly used method of percussion. The tapping done with this type of percussion produces a sound or tone that varies with the density of the underlying structures. As density increases, the sound of the tone becomes quieter. Solid tissue produces a soft tone, fluid produces a louder tone and air produces an even louder tone. These tones are referred to as percussion notes and are classified according to origin, quality, intensity and pitch (Table 3-3).

The following techniques help to develop proficiency in the technique of indirect percussion:

- Place the middle finger of your non-dominant hand on the body part intended for percussion.
- Keep your other fingers off the body part being percussed because they will damp the tone elicited.
- Use the pad of the middle finger of your other hand (ensure that this fingernail is short) to strike the middle finger of your non-dominant hand that is placed on the body part.
- Withdraw your dominant middle finger immediately to avoid damping the tone.
- Deliver two quick taps and listen carefully to the tone.
- Use quick, sharp taps by quickly flexing your wrist, not your forearm.

You can practise percussing by tapping your thigh to elicit a flat tone and your puffed-out cheek to elicit a tympanic tone. A good way to detect changes in tone is to fill a carton halfway with fluid and practise percussing on it. The tone will change from resonance over air to a duller tone over the fluid.

Auscultation

Auscultation is a type of assessment technique that requires the use of a stethoscope to listen for heart sounds, movement of blood through the cardiovascular system, movement of the bowel and movement of air through the respiratory tract. A stethoscope is used because these body sounds are not audible to the human ear. The sounds detected using auscultation are classified according to the intensity (loud or soft), pitch (high or low), duration (length) and quality (musical, crackling, raspy) of the sound (see Equipment spotlight 3-1).

The following guidelines should be followed as you practise the technique of auscultation:

- Eliminate distracting or competing noises from the environment (e.g. radio, television, machinery).
- Expose the body part intended for auscultation. Do not auscultate through the patient's clothing or gown. Rubbing against the clothing obscures the body sounds.
- Use the diaphragm of the stethoscope to listen for high-pitched sounds, such as normal heart sounds, breath sounds and bowel sounds, and press the diaphragm firmly on the body part being auscultated.
- Use the bell of the stethoscope to listen for low-pitched sounds such as abnormal heart sounds and bruits (abnormal loud, blowing or murmuring sounds heard during auscultation). Hold the bell lightly on the body part being auscultated.

SUMMARY

Collecting objective data is essential for a complete nursing assessment. You must have knowledge and interpretative skills to become proficient in collecting objective data: necessary equipment and how to use it; preparing the environment, yourself and the patient or relevant others for the examination; how to perform the four basic assessment techniques; and how to interpret the data and apply critical thinking skills to ensure appropriate and timely intervention to avoid preventable adverse patient outcomes (covered in Chap. 5). Collecting objective data requires a great deal of practise to become proficient. Proficiency is needed because how the data are collected can affect the accuracy of the information elicited.

Table 3-3 Sounds (tones) elicited by percussion

Sound	Intensity	Pitch	Length	Quality	Example of origin
Resonance (heard over part air and part solid)	Loud	Low	Long	Hollow	Normal lung
Hyper-resonance (heard over mostly air)	Very loud	Low	Long	Booming	Lung with emphysema
Tympany (heard over air)	Loud	High	Moderate	Drumlike	Puffed-out cheek, gastric bubble
Dullness (heard over more solid tissue)	Medium	Medium	Moderate	Thudlike	Diaphragm, pleural effusion, liver
Flatness (heard over very dense tissue)	Soft	High	Short	Flat	Muscle, bone, sternum, thigh

EQUIPMENT SPOTLIGHT 3-1 HOW TO USE THE STETHOSCOPE

The stethoscope is used to listen for (auscultate) body sounds that cannot ordinarily be heard without amplification (e.g. lung sounds, bruits, bowel sounds). To use a stethoscope, follow these guidelines:

1. Place the earpieces into the outer ear canal. They should fit snugly but comfortably to promote effective sound transmission. The earpieces are connected to binaurals (metal tubing), which connect to rubber or plastic tubing. The rubber or plastic tubing should be flexible and no more than 25 cm long to prevent the sound from diminishing.
2. Angle the binaurals down towards your nose. This will ensure that sounds are transmitted to your eardrums.
3. Use the diaphragm of the stethoscope to detect high-pitched sounds. The diaphragm should be at least 3.8 cm wide for adults and smaller for children. Hold the diaphragm firmly against the body part being auscultated.
4. Use the bell of the stethoscope to detect low-pitched sounds. The bell should be at least 2.5 cm wide. Hold the bell lightly against the body part being auscultated.

Some do's and don'ts

- Warm the diaphragm or bell of the stethoscope before placing it on the patient's skin.
- Explain what you are listening for and answer any questions the patient has. This will help to alleviate anxiety.
- Do not apply too much pressure when using the bell—too much pressure will cause the bell to work like the diaphragm.
- Avoid listening through clothing, which may obscure or alter sounds.

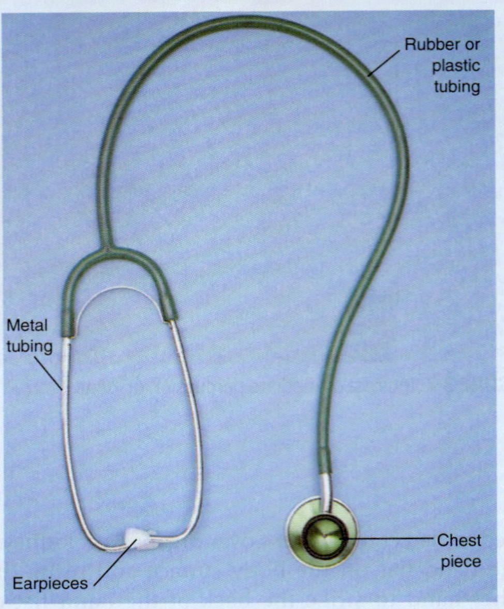

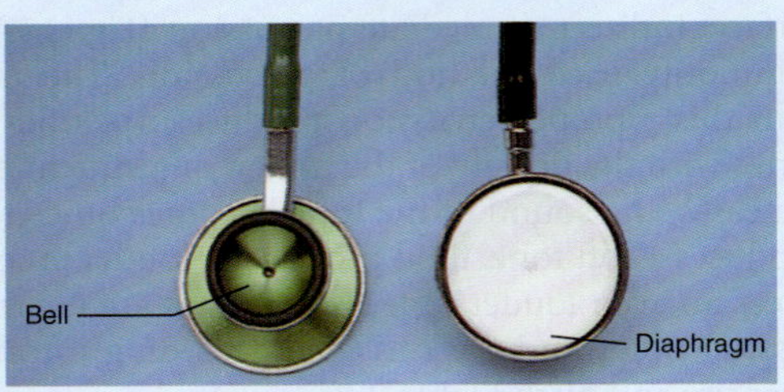

ONLINE RESOURCES

An extensive range of additional resources to enhance teaching and learning and to facilitate understanding may be found online at the text's accompanying website, located on thePoint at http://thepoint.lww.com. These include Watch and Learn videos, Concepts in Action animations, journal articles, case studies, discussion topics and quizzes.

Subscribers may also access Lippincott Procedures, an extensive online point-of-care procedure guide that provides reliable step-by-step instructions for more than 1700 procedures, including 450 evidence-based Australian procedures, and skills in a variety of speciality settings, together with a wealth of supporting information.

References

Anchala, J. (2016). A study to assess the effect of therapeutic positions on haemodynamic parameters among critically ill patients in the intensive care unit at Sri Ramachandra Medical Centre. *Journal of Nursing & Care, 5*(3), Viewed February 2019 at https://pdfs.semanticscholar.org/0b93/45b58e463a98dec95471f3a96644dd03f116.pdf.

Anderson, D. J., Harris, A. & Baron, E. L. (2018). Infection prevention: Precautions for preventing transmission of infection. UpToDate. Viewed February 2019 at https://www.uptodate.com/contents/infection-prevention-precautions-for-preventing-transmission-of-infection/print. Wolters Kluwer.

Australian Commission on Safety and Quality in Health Care (ACSQHC). (2017). *National safety and quality health service standards* (2nd ed.). Sydney: ACSQHC.

Australian Commission on Safety and Quality in Healthcare (ACSQHC) & National Health and Medical Research Council (NHMRC). (2019). *Australian guidelines for the prevention and control of infection in healthcare*. Canberra: Australian Government. Viewed August 2019 at https://www.nhmrc.gov.au/file/14289/download?token=QNDTcrjY.

Department of Health Australia (DoHA). (2004). *Infection control guidelines for the prevention of transmission of infectious diseases in the healthcare setting 2004. Part 1: 7.2. Chemical disinfectants and sterilants. Part 3:13.1–13.5. Protective personal equipment*. Canberra: Department of Health and Ageing.

Doll, M., Stevens, M. & Bearman, G. (2018). Environmental cleaning and disinfection of patient areas. *International Journal of Infectious Diseases, 67*, 52–57.

Doyle, G. A., Xiang, J., Zaman, H., et al. (2017). Patient attitudes and participation in hand co-washing in an outpatient clinic before and after a prompt. *Annals of Family Medicine, 15*(2), Viewed February 2019 at https://www.ncbi.nlm.nih.gov/pmc/articles/PMC5348233/pdf/0150155.pdf.

Health Quality & Safety Commission New Zealand. (2019). Infection Prevention & Control. Viewed February 2020 at https://www.hqsc.govt.nz/our-programmes/infection-prevention-and-control/.

Kornhaber, R., Walsh, K., Duff, J., et al. (2016). Enhancing adult therapeutic interpersonal relationships in the acute health setting: An integrative reivew. *Journal of Multidisciplinary Healthcare, 9*, 537–546.

Ministry of Health New Zealand (MoHNZ). (2007). *Guidelines for the control of multidrug-resistant organisms in New Zealand*. Wellington: Ministry of Health. Viewed February 2019 at www.health.govt.nz/publications.

Nelson, L. (2018). How to conduct a head-to-toe assessment. Nurse.Org, Viewed February 2019 at https://nurse.org/articles/how-to-conduct-head-to-toe-assessment/.

New Zealand Nurses Organisation (NZNO). (2016). Guidelines: privacy, confidentiality and consent in the use of exemplars of practice, case studies, and journaling. Viewed August 2019 at https://www.nzno.org.nz/LinkClick.aspx?fileticket=SXS5iY5CdGk%3D&portalid=0.

NHS. (2016). Overview: Consent to treatment. NHS England. Viewed February 2019 at https://www.nhs.uk/conditions/consent-to-treatment/.

Nursing and Midwifery Board of Australia (NMBA). (2018). Code of conduct for nurses. Professional standards. Viewed August 2019 at https://www.nursingmidwiferyboard.gov.au/Codes-Guidelines-Statements/Professional-standards.aspx.

Nursing Council of New Zealand (NCNZ). (2012). *Code of conduct for nurses*. Viewed August 2019 at https://www.nursingcouncil.org.nz/Public/Nursing/Code_of_Conduct/NCNZ/nursing-section/Code_of_Conduct.aspx?hkey=7fe9d496-9c08-4004-8397-d98bd774ef1b.

Office of the Australian Information Commissioner (OAIC). (2014). *Australian privacy principles*. Viewed August 2019 at https://www.oaic.gov.au/privacy/australian-privacy-principles/.

Thomas, M. (2017). Nursing assessment. The Royal Children's Hospital Melbourne. Viewed February 2019 at https://www.rch.org.au/rchcpg/hospital_clinical_guideline_index/nursing_assessment/.

Toney-Butler, T. J. & Unison-Pace, W. J. (2018). Nursing admission assessment and examination. [[Updated 19 January 2019]. In *StatPearls*. [Internet]. Treasure Island, FL: StatPearls Publishing. Viewed February 2019 at https://www.ncbi.nlm.nih.gov/books/NBK493211/.

Zimmerman, P. (2013). Asepsis and infection prevention and control. Chap. 33. In J. Dempsey, S. Hillege, & R. Hill (Eds). *Fundamentals of nursing: A person-centred approach to care*. Sydney: Lippincott Williams & Wilkins.

Selected reading

Hand Hygiene Australia (HHA). (n.d.). Hand care issues. Viewed February 2019 at https://www.hha.org.au/hand-hygiene/what-is-hand-hygiene/hand-care-issues.

Online resources

Australian Commission on Safety and Quality in Health Care (ACSQHC): www.safetyandquality.gov.au

Centre for Cultural Competence Australia: www.ccca.com.au

Hand Hygiene Australia: www.hha.org.au

Hand Hygiene New Zealand: https://www.hqsc.govt.nz/our-programmes/infection-prevention-and-control/projects/hand-hygiene/

Joanna Briggs Institute Library: www.joannabriggslibrary.org/jbilibrary

New Zealand Ministry of Health: www.health.govt.nz

Preventing and Controlling Healthcare-Associated Infection Standard: https://www.safetyandquality.gov.au/sites/default/files/migrated/National-Safety-and-Quality-Health-Service-Standards-second-edition.pdf

Guidelines for the Control of Multidrug-resistant organisms in New Zealand: https://www.health.govt.nz/system/files/documents/publications/guidelines-for-control-of-multidrug-resistant-organisms-dec07.pdf

Infection Prevention and Control—New Zealand https://www.hqsc.govt.nz/our-programmes/infection-prevention-and-control/

Royal Australasian College of Surgeons: www.surgeons.org

World Health Organization, hand hygiene: www.who.int/gpsc/5may/en

CHAPTER 4

Validating and documenting data

Validation and documentation of data often occur concurrently with the collection of subjective and objective assessment data, but looking at each step separately can help to emphasise the importance of each step in nursing assessment.

VALIDATING DATA

Purpose of validation

Validation of data is the process of confirming or verifying that the subjective and objective data you have collected are reliable and accurate. The steps of validation include deciding whether the data require validation, determining ways to validate the data and identifying areas where data are missing. Failure to validate data may result in the premature closure of the assessment or the collection of inaccurate data. Errors during assessment cause judgements to be made on unreliable data, which result in diagnostic errors during the second part of the nursing process—the analysis of data (determining patient diagnoses). Thus, validation of the data collected during assessment of the patient is crucial to the first step of the nursing process.

Data requiring validation

Not every piece of data you collect must be verified. For example, you would not need to verify or repeat the patient's pulse, temperature or blood pressure unless certain conditions exist. Conditions that require data to be rechecked and validated include:

- *Discrepancies or gaps between the subjective and objective data.* For example, a male patient tells you that he has no pain, yet you find he has a high blood pressure, a high heart rate and dilated pupils. The patient is also grimacing and cannot lie still in bed.
- *Discrepancies or gaps between what the patient says at one time then at another time.* For example, your female patient says she has never had surgery, but later in the interview she mentions that her appendix was removed when she was 12 years old.
- *Findings that are very abnormal or inconsistent with other findings.* For example, the following are inconsistent with each other: the patient has a temperature of 40 °C, is resting comfortably and has skin that is warm to the touch but is not flushed or diaphoretic.

Methods of validation

There are several ways to validate your data:

- Recheck your own data through a repeat assessment. For example, take the patient's temperature again with a different thermometer.
- Clarify data with the patient by asking additional questions. For example, if a patient is holding his abdomen, the nurse may assume he is having abdominal pain, when actually the patient is very upset about his diagnosis and is feeling nauseated.
- Verify the data with another health care professional. For example, ask a more experienced nurse to listen to the abnormal heart sounds you think you have just heard.
- Compare your objective findings with your subjective findings to uncover discrepancies. For example, if the patient states that she 'never gets any time in the sun', yet she has dark, wrinkled and suntanned skin, you need to validate the patient's perception of never getting any time in the sun and the possible use of sun beds and so on.

Identification of areas where data are missing

Once you establish an initial database, you can identify areas where more data are needed. You may have overlooked certain questions. In addition, because data are examined in a grouped format, you may realise that additional information is required. For example, if an adult patient weighs only 44.5 kg, you would explore further to see if the patient recently lost weight or this has been his or her usual weight for an extended time. If a patient tells you he or she lives alone, you may need to identify the existence of a support system, his or her degree of social involvement with others and the ability to function independently.

DOCUMENTING DATA

In addition to validation, the documentation of assessment data is crucial to the first step in the nursing process. The significance of this aspect of assessment is addressed specifically by various national nursing and midwifery practice Acts, accreditation and funding agencies (e.g. Australian Nursing & Midwifery Accreditation Council, The Joint Commission, the Australian Council on Healthcare Standards and the Nursing Council of New Zealand), professional organisations (local, state and national) and institutional agencies (acute, transitional, long-term and home care). Assessment and documentation policies and procedures exist in health care institutions that provide not only documentation criteria but also assistance for form completion. The categories of information on the forms are designed to ensure that the nurse gathers pertinent information needed to meet the standards and guidelines of the specific institutions mentioned previously and to develop a plan of care for the patient.

Purpose of documentation

The primary reason for documenting the initial assessment is to provide the health care team with a database that becomes the foundation for care of the patient. Documentation helps to identify health problems, formulate diagnoses and plan immediate and ongoing interventions. If the diagnosis or problem is made without supporting assessment data, incorrect conclusions and interventions may result.

The initial and ongoing assessment documentation database also establishes a way of communicating with multidisciplinary team members. With the advent of computer-based documentation systems, this database can link to other documents and health care departments, eliminating the repetition of similar data collection by other health team members. Display 4-1 describes the many other purposes that assessment documentation serves.

Nurses use comprehensive and systematic nursing databases that streamline data collection and organisation yet maintain a concise record that satisfies legal standards. These databases may be paper based or electronic; for example, the eHealth patient record system (My Health Record) announced by the Australian Government in 2010 (Department of Health and Ageing, 2011) and the Health Identity Program in the New Zealand Ministry of Health. A number of electronic data systems are used in Australian and New Zealand hospitals. Data systems and electronic patient records allow a more efficient integration of information within, and between, health care providers. Clinical information systems also provide a single location (as opposed to multiple patient charts in a single institution or different charts on the same patient across multiple institutions) for the entry, storage and utilisation of all patient information such as admission and assessment documentation, medication histories and diagnostic test results. Benefits include improved patient safety due to a reduction in errors, caused by illegible writing or incomplete patient data sets, enhanced research capabilities and more efficient management practices. Concerns about patient confidentiality, risks of patient data being hacked, difficulties in the integration of legacy systems of patient information storage, the number of different clinical information systems in use across health sectors and cost implications have meant that the uptake of electronic data systems has varied within, and between, states and regions (Allen-Graham et al., 2018; Burridge et al., 2018).

Information requiring documentation

Every institution is unique when it comes to documenting assessments. However, two key elements need to be included in all documentation: *nursing history* and *physical assessment*, also known as *subjective* and *objective data*. Most data collection starts with subjective data and ends with objective data. The reason for this is that information gained from collecting a subjective history will generally guide the physical assessment that is required.

As discussed in previous chapters, subjective data consist of the information that the patient or significant others tell the nurse, and objective data are what the nurse observes through inspection, palpation, percussion and auscultation. It is important to remember to document only what the patient tells you and what you observe—not what you interpret or infer from the data. Interpretation or inference is performed during the analysis phase of the nursing process (see Chap. 5).

It should also be remembered that 'pertinent negatives' can also be documented. A pertinent negative is a finding that you might expect in a patient but which is absent (e.g. if the patient suffered a blunt trauma to the head but does not have a headache). The inclusion of pertinent negatives indicates to others your assessment was thorough. It also indicates that additional assessments have been conducted, even if the findings were negative.

Subjective data

Subjective data typically consist of biographical data, current health concerns and symptoms (or the patient's chief complaint), past health history, family history, and lifestyle and health practices information:

DISPLAY 4-1 PURPOSES OF ASSESSMENT DOCUMENTATION

- Provides a chronological source of patient assessment data and a progressive record of assessment findings that outline the patient's course of care.
- Ensures that information about the patient and family is easily accessible to members of the health care team; provides a vehicle for communication; and prevents fragmentation, repetition and delays in carrying out the plan of care.
- Establishes a basis for screening or validating proposed diagnoses.
- Acts as a source of information to help diagnose new problems.
- Offers a basis for determining the educational needs of the patient, family and significant others.
- Provides a basis for determining eligibility for care and funding. Careful recording of data can support funding or gain additional funding for transitional or skilled care needed by the patient.
- Constitutes a permanent legal record of the care that was, or was not, given to the patient.
- Forms a component of patient acuity system or patient classification systems (Meleis, 2017). Numeric values may be assigned to various levels of care to help determine the staffing mix for the unit.
- Provides access to significant epidemiological data for future investigations and research and educational endeavours.
- Promotes compliance with legal, accreditation, funding and professional standard requirements.

- *Biographical* data typically consist of the patient's name, age, occupation, ethnicity, religion and support systems or resources.
- The present *health concern review* is recorded in statements that reflect the patient's *current symptoms.* Statements should begin with the phrase, 'Patient (or significant other) states …' Describe items as accurately and descriptively as possible. For example, if a patient complains of difficulty breathing, report how the patient describes the problem, when the problem started, what started it, how long it occurred and what makes their breathing better or worse. Use a memory tool, such as a COLDSPA mnemonic, described in Chapter 2, to explore further every symptom reported by the patient. This information provides the health care team members with details that help in diagnosis and clinical problem solving. Sometimes you may need to record the absence of specific signs and symptoms (e.g. no vomiting, diarrhoea or constipation).
- *Past health history* data tell the nurse about events that happened before the patient's admission to the health care facility, or the current encounter with the patient. The data may be about previous hospitalisations, surgeries, treatment programs, acute illness, chronic illnesses and injuries. Be sure to include all pertinent information, for example, the dates of hospitalisation. Also, be sure to include all data, even negative history (e.g. 'Patient denies prior surgeries').
- *Family history* data include information about the patient's biological family (e.g. family history of diseases or behaviours that may be genetic or familial). A genogram may be helpful in recording the family history (see Chap. 2).
- *Lifestyle and health practices* information typically details risk behaviours such as past or present smoking; alcohol use; medication use (prescribed, over-the-counter or illicit); environmental factors that may affect health; social and psychological factors that may affect the patient's health; patient and family health education needs; family and other relationships; and treatment and disease data. Be sure to be comprehensive yet succinct.

Objective data

After you complete the nursing history, the physical examination begins. This examination includes inspection, palpation, percussion and auscultation. Data from the physical examination help further define the patient's problems, establish baseline data for ongoing assessments and validate the subjective data obtained during the nursing history interview. A variety of systematic approaches may be used, for example, head-to-toe, major body systems, functional health patterns or human response patterns.

No matter which approach is used, these general rules apply:

- Make notes as you perform the assessments, and document them as concisely as possible.
- Avoid documenting general non-descriptive or non-measurable terms such as normal, abnormal, good, fair, satisfactory or poor.
- Instead, use specific descriptive and measurable terms about what you inspected, palpated, percussed and auscultated (i.e. 7.5 cm in diameter, red excoriated edges, with purulent yellow drainage).

Guidelines for documentation

The way that the nursing assessments are recorded varies among practice settings. However, the following guidelines apply to all settings.

- *Document legibly or print neatly in non-erasable ink.* Errors in documentation are usually corrected by drawing one line through the entry, writing 'error' and initialling the entry.
- *Never obliterate the error* with white correction fluid or tape, an eraser or a marking pen. Keep in mind that the health record is a legal document.
- *Use correct grammar and spelling. Use only abbreviations that are acceptable and approved by the institution.* Avoid slang, jargon or labels, unless they are direct quotes.
- *Avoid wordiness that creates redundancy.* For example, do not record: 'Auscultated gurgly bowel sounds in right upper, right lower, left upper and left lower abdominal quadrants. Heard 36 gurgles per minute.' Instead record: 'Bowel sounds present in all quadrants at 36 per minute.'
- *Use phrases instead of sentences to record data.* For example, avoid recording: 'The patient's lung sounds were clear both in the right and left lungs.' Instead record: 'Bilateral lung sounds clear.'
- *Record data findings, not how they were obtained.* For example, do not record: 'Patient was interviewed for past history of high blood pressure, and blood pressure was taken.' Instead record: 'Has 3-year history of hypertension treated with medication. BP sitting right arm 140/86 mmHg; left arm 136/86 mmHg.'
- *Write entries objectively without making premature judgements or diagnoses.* Use quotation marks to identify clearly the patient's responses. For example, record: 'Patient crying in room, refuses to talk, husband has gone home' instead of 'Patient depressed due to fear of breast biopsy report and not getting along well with husband.' Avoid making inferences and diagnostic statements until you have collected and validated all data with the patient and his or her family.
- *Record the patient's understanding and perception of problems.* For example, record: 'Patient expresses concern regarding being discharged soon after gallbladder surgery because of inability to rest at home with six children.'
- *Avoid recording the word 'normal' for normal findings.* For example, do not record: 'Liver palpation normal.' Instead record: 'Liver span 10 cm in right MCL and 4 cm in MSL. No tenderness on palpation.' However, in some health care settings, only abnormal findings are documented if the policy is to chart only by exception. In that case, no normal findings would be documented in any format.
- *Record complete information and details for all patient symptoms or experiences.* For example, do not record: 'Patient has pain in lower back.' Instead record: 'Patient reports aching–burning pain in lower back for 2 weeks. Pain worsens after standing for several hours. Rest and ibuprofen used to reduce pain. No radiation of pain. Rates pain as 7 on scale of 0 to 10.'
- *Include additional assessment content when applicable.* For example, include information about the carer or last medical contact.
- *Support objective data with specific observations obtained during the physical examination.* For example, when describing the emotional status of the patient as depressed, follow it with a description of the ways depression is demonstrated such

as 'dressed in dirty clothing, avoids eye contact, unkempt appearance and slumped shoulders.'

Assessment forms used for documentation

Standardised assessment forms have been developed to ensure that content in documentation and assessment data meets regulatory requirements and provides a thorough database. The type of assessment form used for documentation varies by health care institution. In fact, a variety of assessment forms may even be used within an institution. Typically, however, three types of assessment forms are used to document data: an initial assessment form, frequent or ongoing assessment forms, and focused or specialised assessment forms.

Initial assessment form

An initial assessment form is called a *nursing admission* or *admission database*. Four types of frequently used initial assessment documentation forms are known as open-ended, cued or checklist, integrated cued checklist, and nursing minimum data set forms. Display 4-2 describes each type of initial assessment form. In addition, Figure 4-1 provides an example of documentation where vital signs are required to be recorded in a graphic format that promotes easy visualisation of abnormalities and the rapid comparison of recorded assessment data between different time periods. This graphic representation is also important as it clearly presents clinical trends and should facilitate earlier clinical intervention if required. The NSW Health Standard Adult General Observation (SAGO) Chart is predominantly used in the acute care setting.

Frequent or ongoing assessment forms

Various institutions have created flow charts to help staff record and retrieve data for frequent reassessments. As noted earlier, an example of a flow chart used in the clinical setting is the NSW Health Standard Adult General Observation (SAGO) Chart. This chart was included in this chapter because it clearly demonstrates the importance of being aware of a patient's baseline observations, recognising the importance of not only observing and recording patient data but also contextualising observations and observing for any immediate or progressive change from one period to the next for individual patients rather than standard expectations (Fig. 4-1).

Progress notes (Fig. 4-2) may be used to document unusual events, responses, significant observations or interactions because the data are inappropriate for flow records. *Clinical pathways* streamline the documentation process and prevent needless repetition of data. Emphasis is placed on the quality, not quantity, of documentation.

Focused or specialised assessment forms

Some institutions may use assessment forms that are focused on one major area of the body or require a specific history for patients who have a particular problem. Examples include cardiovascular or neurological assessment documentation forms, which focus on a major area of the body, whereas short-stay areas within the hospital such as day surgery or medical imaging focus on a specific history (Fig. 4-3). Forms may be also be customised and used as a screening tool to assess specific concerns or risks such as falling or skin problems. These forms are usually abbreviated versions of admission data sheets, with specific assessment data related to the purpose of the assessment.

24/10/2019 Patient short of breath with laboured respirations of 32/minute. Chest barrel shaped. Skin reddish. Decreased tactile fremitus percussed bilaterally. Bilateral hyperresonance. Respiratory and diaphragmatic excursion decreased. Has nonproductive cough, decreased breath sounds with wheezing and prolonged expirations. Patient states,'I'm so short of breath.'

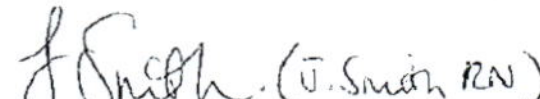

FIGURE 4-2 Documentation of assessment findings on a narrative progress note.

DISPLAY 4-2 FEATURES OF TYPES OF INITIAL ASSESSMENT FORMS

Open-ended forms (traditional form)
- Calls for narrative description of problem and listing of topics
- Provides lines for comments
- Individualises information
- Provides 'total picture', including specific complaints and symptoms in the patient's own words
- Increases risk of failing to ask a pertinent question because questions are not standardised
- Requires a lot of time to complete the database

Cued or checklist forms
- Standardises data collection
- Lists (categorises) information that alerts the nurse to specific problems or symptoms assessed for each patient (see Fig. 4-1)
- Usually includes a comment section after each category to allow for individualisation
- Prevents missed questions
- Promotes easy, rapid documentation
- Makes documentation somewhat like data entry because it requires nurse to place checkmarks in boxes instead of writing narrative
- Poses chance that a significant piece of data may be missed because the checklist does not include the area of concern

Integrated cued checklist
- Combines assessment data with identified diagnoses
- Helps cluster data, focuses on diagnoses, assists in validating diagnosis labels and combines assessment with problem listing in one form
- Promotes use by different levels of carers, resulting in enhanced communication among the disciplines

Nursing minimum data set
- Comprises format commonly used in long-term care facilities
- Has a cued format that prompts nurse for specific criteria; usually computerised
- Includes specialised information, such as cognitive patterns, communication (hearing and vision) patterns, physical function and structural patterns, activity patterns and restorative care
- Meets the needs of multiple data users in the health care system
- Establishes comparability of nursing data across clinical populations, settings, geographical areas and time

NSW GOVERNMENT | Health

STANDARD ADULT GENERAL OBSERVATION CHART

FAMILY NAME	MRN
GIVEN NAME	☐ MALE ☐ FEMALE
D.O.B. ____/____/____	M.O.
ADDRESS	
LOCATION	
COMPLETE ALL DETAILS OR AFFIX PATIENT LABEL HERE	

☐ Altered Calling Criteria

ALL OBSERVATIONS MUST BE GRAPHED

OTHER CHARTS IN USE

☐ Neurological Observation ☐ Insulin Infusion ☐ Alcohol Withdrawal
☐ Fluid Balance ☐ Pain / Epidural / Patient Control Analgesia ☐ Resuscitation Plan
☐ Anticoagulant ☐ Neurovascular ☐ Other __________

PRESCRIBED FREQUENCY OF OBSERVATIONS

Observations must be performed routinely at least 8th hourly, unless advised below

	EXAMPLE				
DATE:	dd/MM/yy				
Time:	hh:mm				
Frequency Required	Twice daily				
Medical Officer Name (BLOCK letters)	P. SMITH				
Medical Officer Signature	P. SMITH				
Attending Medical Officer Signature	R. Bloggs				

ALTERATIONS TO CALLING CRITERIA
MUST BE REVIEWED WITHIN 72 HOURS OR EARLIER IF CLINICALLY INDICATED
Any alterations MUST be signed by a Medical Officer and confirmed by Attending Medical Officer
Document rationale for altering CALLING CRITERIA in the patient's health care record

		EXAMPLE				
DATE:		dd/MM/yy				
TIME:		hh:mm				
Next review due Date & Time		dd/MM/yy hh:mm				
Respiratory Rate	Yellow Zone	30-34				
	Red Zone	≥ 35				
SpO_2	Yellow Zone					
	Red Zone					
Heart Rate	Yellow Zone					
	Red Zone					
Blood Pressure	Yellow Zone					
	Red Zone					
Other	Yellow Zone					
	Red Zone					
Medical Officer Name (BLOCK letters)		P. SMITH				
Medical Officer Signature		P. SMITH				
Attending Medical Officer Signature		R. Bloggs				

INTERVENTIONS / COMMENTS / ACTIONS

	Date	Time	
1.			
2.			
3.			
4.			

STANDARD ADULT GENERAL OBSERVATION CHART SMR110.010

Page 1 of 4

FIGURE 4-1 The NSW Health Standard Adult General Observation (SAGO) Chart. (© Clinical Excellence Commission. 2020.)

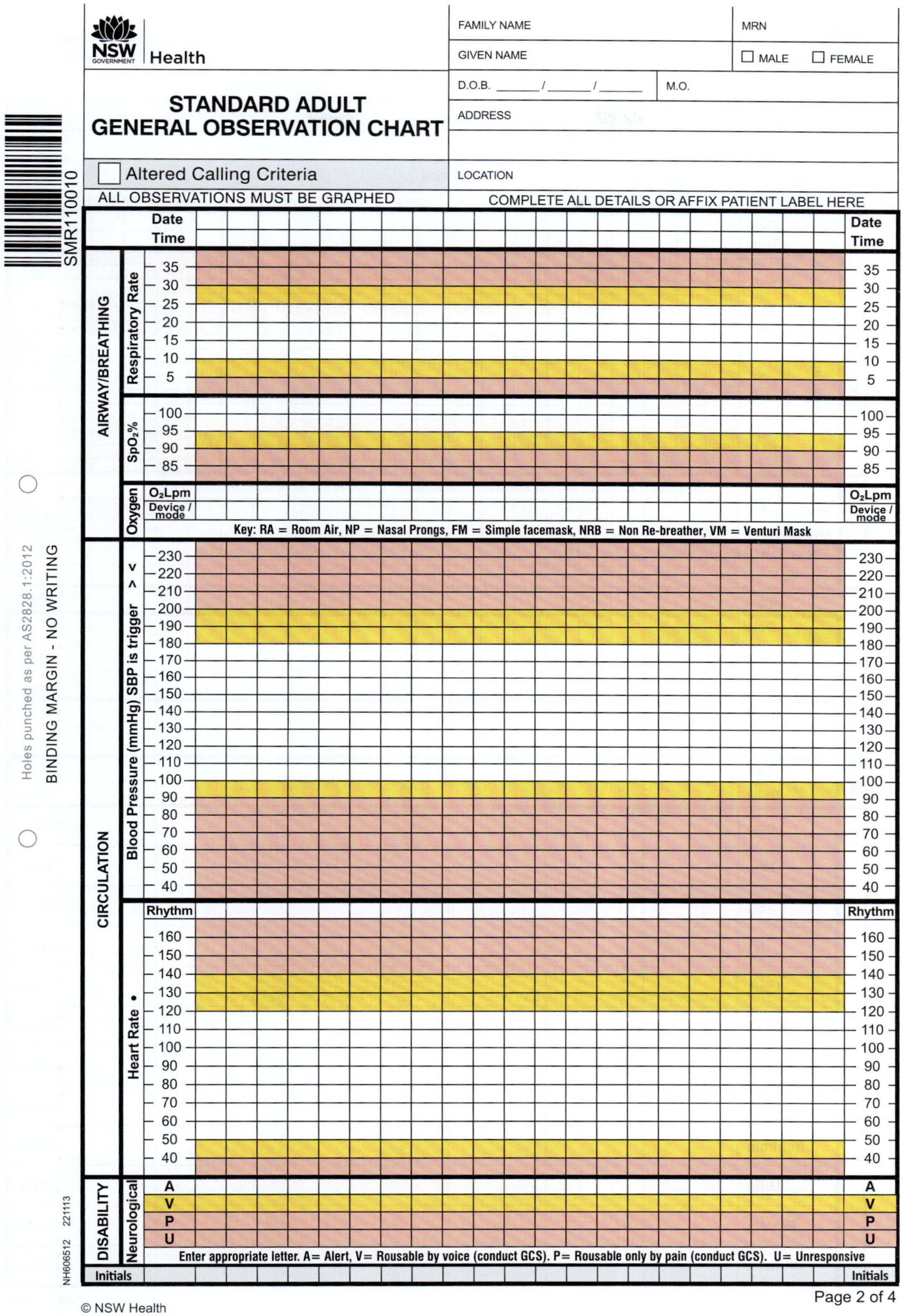

NSW GOVERNMENT Health

STANDARD ADULT GENERAL OBSERVATION CHART

FAMILY NAME | MRN
GIVEN NAME | ☐ MALE ☐ FEMALE
D.O.B. _____/_____/_____ | M.O.
ADDRESS
LOCATION

☐ Altered Calling Criteria

ALL OBSERVATIONS MUST BE GRAPHED

COMPLETE ALL DETAILS OR AFFIX PATIENT LABEL HERE

SMR110010

Holes punched as per AS2828.1:2012

BINDING MARGIN - NO WRITING

		Date / Time		Date / Time
AIRWAY/BREATHING	Respiratory Rate	35, 30, 25, 20, 15, 10, 5		35, 30, 25, 20, 15, 10, 5
	SpO2%	100, 95, 90, 85		100, 95, 90, 85
	Oxygen	O2Lpm		O2Lpm
		Device / mode		Device / mode
		Key: RA = Room Air, NP = Nasal Prongs, FM = Simple facemask, NRB = Non Re-breather, VM = Venturi Mask		
CIRCULATION	Blood Pressure (mmHg) SBP is trigger ˅ ˄	230, 220, 210, 200, 190, 180, 170, 160, 150, 140, 130, 120, 110, 100, 90, 80, 70, 60, 50, 40		230, 220, 210, 200, 190, 180, 170, 160, 150, 140, 130, 120, 110, 100, 90, 80, 70, 60, 50, 40
		Rhythm		Rhythm
	Heart Rate •	160, 150, 140, 130, 120, 110, 100, 90, 80, 70, 60, 50, 40		160, 150, 140, 130, 120, 110, 100, 90, 80, 70, 60, 50, 40
DISABILITY	Neurological	A, V, P, U		A, V, P, U
		Enter appropriate letter. A= Alert, V= Rousable by voice (conduct GCS). P= Rousable only by pain (conduct GCS). U= Unresponsive		
Initials				Initials

NH606512 221113

FIGURE 4-1 The NSW Health Standard Adult General Observation (SAGO) Chart. (© Clinical Excellence Commission. 2020.) *(continued)*

Continued on following page

NSW GOVERNMENT | Health

	FAMILY NAME
	MRN
	GIVEN NAME
	☐ MALE ☐ FEMALE
STANDARD ADULT GENERAL OBSERVATION CHART	D.O.B. _____/_____/_____
	M.O.
	ADDRESS
☐ Altered Calling Criteria	LOCATION
ALL OBSERVATIONS MUST BE GRAPHED	COMPLETE ALL DETAILS OR AFFIX PATIENT LABEL HERE

		Date		Date
		Time		Time
EXPOSURE	Temperature (°C) ●	41		41
		40.5		40.5
		40		40
		39.5		39.5
		39		39
		38.5		38.5
		38		38
		37.5		37.5
		37		37
		36.5		36.5
		36		36
		35.5		35.5
		35		35
		34.5		34.5
		34		34
Pain		Assess pain level at rest and with movement. Enter R for at rest, M for movement		
		Severe (7-10)		Severe (7-10)
		Moderate (4-6)		Moderate (4-6)
		Mild (1-3)		Mild (1-3)
		Nil		No pain
		Initials		Initials
Blood Glucose		Date		Date
		Time		Time
		BGL		BGL
Bowels		Date		Date
Weight		Date		Date
		☐ Daily		Daily
Urinalysis		Date		Date
		Time		Time
		SG		SG
		pH		pH
		Leuk		Leuk
		Blood		Blood
		Nitrite		Nitrite
		Ketones		Ketones
		Bilirubin		Bilirubin
		U/Bil		U/Bil
		Protein		Protein
		Glucose		Glucose

Page 3 of 4

FIGURE 4-1 The NSW Health Standard Adult General Observation (SAGO) Chart. (© Clinical Excellence Commission. 2020.) *(continued)*

REFER TO YOUR LOCAL CLINICAL EMERGENCY RESPONSE SYSTEM (CERS) PROTOCOL FOR INSTRUCTIONS ON HOW TO MAKE A CALL TO ESCALATE CARE FOR YOUR PATIENT

CHECK THE HEALTH CARE RECORD FOR AN END OF LIFE CARE PLAN WHICH MAY ALTER THE MANAGEMENT OF YOUR PATIENT

Yellow Zone Response

IF YOUR PATIENT HAS ANY YELLOW ZONE OBSERVATIONS OR ADDITIONAL CRITERIA* YOU MUST

1. Initiate appropriate clinical care
2. Repeat and increase the frequency of observations, as indicated by your patient's condition
3. Consult promptly with the **NURSE IN CHARGE** to decide whether a **CLINICAL REVIEW** (or other CERS) call should be made

Consider the following:

- What is usual for your patient and are there documented 'ALTERATIONS TO CALLING CRITERIA'?
- Does the trend in observations suggest deterioration?
- Is there more than one Yellow Zone observation or additional criterion?
- Are you concerned about your patient?

IF A CLINICAL REVIEW IS CALLED:

1. Reassess your patient and escalate according to your local CERS if the call is not attended within 30 minutes or you are becoming more concerned
2. Document an A-G assessment, reason for escalation, treatment and outcome in your patient's health care record
3. Inform the Attending Medical Officer that a call was made as soon as it is practicable

***Additional YELLOW ZONE Criteria**

- Increasing oxygen requirement
- Poor peripheral circulation
- Excess or increasing blood loss
- Decrease in Level of Consciousness or new onset of confusion
- Low urine output persistent for 4 hours (< 100mLs over 4 hours or < 0.5mL/kg/hr via an IDC)
- Polyuria, in the absence of diuretics (urine output > 200mL/hr for 2 hours)
- Greater than expected fluid loss from a drain
- New, increasing or uncontrolled pain (including chest pain)
- Blood Glucose Level < 4mmol/L or > 20mmol/L with no decrease in Level of Consciousness
- Ketonaemia > 1.5mmol/L or Ketonuria 2 + or more
- **Concern by patient or family member**
- **Concern by you or any staff member**

CONSIDER IF YOUR PATIENT'S DETERIORATION COULD BE DUE TO SEPSIS, A NEW ARRHYTHMIA, HYPOVOLAEMIA/HAEMORRHAGE, PULMONARY EMBOLUS/DVT, PNEUMONIA/ATELECTASIS, AN AMI, STROKE, OR AN OVERDOSE/OVER SEDATION

Red Zone Response

IF YOUR PATIENT HAS ANY RED ZONE OBSERVATIONS OR ADDITIONAL CRITERIA# YOU MUST CALL FOR A RAPID RESPONSE (as per local CERS) AND

1. Initiate appropriate clinical care
2. Inform the **NURSE IN CHARGE** that you have called for a **RAPID RESPONSE**
3. Repeat and increase the frequency of observations, as indicated by your patient's condition
4. Document an A-G assessment, reason for escalation, treatment and outcome in your patient's health care record
5. Inform the Attending Medical Officer that a call was made as soon as it is practicable

#Additional RED ZONE Criteria

- **Cardiac or respiratory arrest**
- **Airway obstruction or stridor**
- **Patient unresponsive**
- Deterioration not reversed within 1 hour of Clinical Review
- Increasing oxygen requirements to maintain oxygen saturation > 90%
- Arterial Blood Gas: PaO_2 < 60 or $PaCO_2$ > 60 or pH < 7.2 or BE < -5
- Venous Blood Gas: $PvCO_2$ > 65 or pH < 7.2
- Only responds to Pain (P) on the AVPU scale
- Sudden decrease in Level of Consciousness (a drop of 2 or more points on the GCS)
- Seizures
- Low urine output persistent for 8 hours (< 200mLs over 8 hours or < 0.5mL/kg/hr via an IDC)
- Blood Glucose Level < 4mmol/L or > 20mmol/L with a decreased Level of Consciousness
- Lactate ≥ 4mmol/L
- **Serious concern by any patient or family member**
- **Serious concern by you or any staff member**

Holes punched as per AS2828.1:2012

BINDING MARGIN - NO WRITING

Page 4 of 4

FIGURE 4-1 The NSW Health Standard Adult General Observation (SAGO) Chart. (© Clinical Excellence Commission. 2020.) *(continued)*

NSW GOVERNMENT | Health
South Eastern Sydney Local Health District
Illawarra Shoalhaven Local Health District

Facility:

FAMILY NAME | MRN
GIVEN NAME | ☐ MALE ☐ FEMALE
D.O.B. _______ / _______ / _______ | M.O.
ADDRESS

LOCATION / WARD

COMPLETE ALL DETAILS OR AFFIX PATIENT LABEL HERE

CLINICAL PROCEDURE SAFETY CHECKLIST LEVEL 2

If this checklist is not completed or check is incorrect, IIMs notification to be entered

SEI090032

Time Out is to be completed immediately before the surgery or procedure starts.

Name of Proceduralist who led checklist ______________________________

Name of Procedure ______________________________

☐ Confirm all Team Members have introduced themselves by name and role

Patient Identification Confirmed	☐ Yes	
Procedure Verified and Matches Consent	☐ Yes	
Allergy/Adverse Reaction Check	☐ Yes	☐ No
Anticipated Critical Events	☐ Yes	☐ No
Correct Site / Side / Level Verified and Matches Consent	☐ Yes	
Site Marked	☐ Yes	☐ No ☐ N/A
Imaging data confirmed	☐ Yes	☐ N/A
Correct implants / prostheses (types / size / side) are available	☐ Yes	☐ N/A
Any special equipment needed is available	☐ Yes	☐ N/A
Patient position confirmed	☐ Yes	☐ N/A
Does the patient need antibiotic prophylaxis	☐ Yes	☐ No
If yes, has it been given according to the guidelines	☐ Yes	☐ No
Has the patient received thromboprophylaxis		
Anticoagulant	☐ Yes	☐ Not Required
Mechanical	☐ Yes	☐ Not Required
Does the patient need any special pre-operative medications	☐ Yes	☐ N/A
If yes, have they been given	☐ Yes	

Form completed by: ______________________________

Designation: ______________________ Date: __________ Time: __________

Post Procedure

Document the procedure and advice for clinical handover in the patient's Healthcare record. Ensure patient is aware of post-procedure health advice. Label any specimens/images correctly. Document any post-procedure tests where clinically relevant. Equipment problems/issues documented and advised to relevant staff.

Holes Punched as per AS2828.1: 2012
BINDING MARGIN - NO WRITING

S0140SESIS 300519

CLINICAL PROCEDURE SAFETY CHECKLIST LEVEL 2

SEI090.032

NO WRITING

Page 1 of 2

FIGURE 4-3 Clinical Procedure Safety Checklist. (© South Eastern Sydney Local Health District. 2019.)

Health NSW Government — South Eastern Sydney Local Health District, Illawarra Shoalhaven Local Health District	FAMILY NAME	MRN
Facility:	GIVEN NAME	☐ MALE ☐ FEMALE
	D.O.B. ____/____/____	M.O.
CLINICAL PROCEDURE SAFETY CHECKLIST LEVEL 2	ADDRESS	
	LOCATION / WARD	
	COMPLETE ALL DETAILS OR AFFIX PATIENT LABEL HERE	

LEVEL 2 PROCEDURES

		Requirements	
Definition	**Examples**	**Pre-procedure (including Team Time Out)**	**Post procedure**
- Proceduralist often supported by an assisting proceduralist/s - Usually requires written consent - Does not involve procedural sedation or general/regional anaesthesia - Usually performed in wards, emergency departments, clinics, imaging departments, interventional suites	- Lumbar puncture - Insertion of chest tube - Ascitic tap - Stress test - Diagnostic interventional procedures - Nuclear Medicine therapies - Non-superficial Biopsies - IV or IT administration of chemotherapy - Centrally inserted central venous access device[8]	**STOP and confirm the following before commencing the procedure** - Proceduralist/assisting proceduralist/s introductions, where appropriate - Patient identification - Procedure verification - procedure + site/side/level, where appropriate, matches consent - Patient position - Essential imaging reviewed - Allergy/adverse reaction check - Special medication/s administered - Antibiotics - Implants and special equipment - Anticipated critical events	- Document procedure in patient's health care record or Radiology Information System - Advice for clinical handover - Equipment problems/ issues - Specimens/images labelled correctly - Post procedure tests where clinically relevant eg. CXR post insertion of chest tube

Document Number PD2017_032

Holes Punched as per AS2828.1: 2012

BINDING MARGIN - NO WRITING

SEI090032

Page 2 of 2 NO WRITING

FIGURE 4-3 Clinical Procedure Safety Checklist. (© South Eastern Sydney Local Health District. 2019.) *(continued)*

SUMMARY

Validation and documentation are two crucial aspects of the nursing health assessment. Nurses need to perform these two steps of assessment thoroughly and accurately.

Validation of data verifies the assessment data gathered from the patient. It consists of determining which data require validation, implementing techniques to validate them and identifying areas that require further assessment data.

Documentation of data is the act of recording the patient assessment findings. Nurses first need to understand the purpose of documentation, then learn which information to document, be aware of and follow the individual documentation guidelines of their particular health care facility. In addition, it is important for nurses to be familiar with the different documentation forms used in other health care institutions.

ONLINE RESOURCES

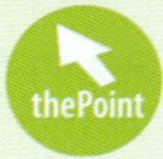

An extensive range of additional resources to enhance teaching and learning and to facilitate understanding may be found online at the text's accompanying website, located on thePoint at http://thepoint.lww.com. These include Watch and Learn videos, Concepts in Action animations, journal articles, case studies, discussion topics and quizzes.

Subscribers may also access Lippincott Procedures, an extensive online point-of-care procedure guide that provides reliable step-by-step instructions for more than 1700 procedures, including 450 evidence-based Australian procedures, and skills in a variety of speciality settings, together with a wealth of supporting information.

References

Allen-Graham, J., Mitchell, L., Heriot, N., et al. (2018). Electronic health records and online medical records: An asset or a liability under current conditions? *Australian Health Review, 42*, 59–65. http://dx.dio.org/10.1071/AH16095.

Burridge, L., Foster, M., Geraghty, T., et al. (2018). Person-centred care in a digital hospital: Observations and perspectives from a specialist rehabilitation setting. *Australian Health Review, 42*, 529–535. https://dio.org/10.1071/AH17156.

Department of Health and Ageing (Australian Government). (2011). eHealth: National E-Health Strategy. Available at www.health.gov.au/internet/main/publishing.nsf/content/national+Ehealth+strategy.

Meleis, A. I. (2017). *Theoretical nursing: Development and progress* (6th ed.). Philadelphia: Lippincott Williams & Wilkins.

Okaisu, E. M., Kaikwani, F., Wanyana, G., et al. (2014). Improving the quality of nursing documentation: An action research project. *Curationis, 38*(1), Art.#1251. doi:10.4102/curationis.v3171.1251.

Selected readings

Akhu-Zaheya, L., Al-Maaitah, R. & Bani Hani, S. (2018). Quality of nursing documentation: Paper-based health records versus electronic-based health records. *Journal of Clinical Nursing, 27*, e578–e589. doi:10.1111/jocn.14097.

Burnie, J., Heist, C., Donoghue, K., et al. (2018). Successful implementation of electronic trauma documentation in a level 111 trauma center—It can be done. *Online Journal of Nursing Informatics*, Available at http://www.himss.org/ojni.

Carpenito, L. J. (2017). *Nursing care plans and documentation: Transitional patient & family-centred care* (7th ed.). Philadelphia: Lippincott Williams & Wilkins.

Ding, S., Lin, F. & Gillespie, B. M. (2016). Surgical wound assessment and documentation of nurses: An integrative review. *Journal of Wound Care, 25*(3), 232–240.

Heidarizadeh, K., Rassouli, M., Manoochehri, H., et al. (2017). Nurses' perception of challenges in the use of an electronic nursing documentation system. *Computers, Informatics, Nursing: CIN, 35*(11), 599–605. doi:10.1097/CIN.00000000000358.

Islam, M., Poly, T. N. & Li, Y. C. (2018). Recent advances of clinical information systems: Opportunities and challenges. *Yearbook of Medical Informatics*, doi: 10.1055/s-0038-1667075.

Johnson, L., Edward, K. L. & Giandinota, J. (2018). A systematic literature review of accuracy in nursing car plans and using standardised nursing language. *Collegian (Royal College of Nursing, Australia), 25*, 355–361. Available at www.elsevier.com/locate/coll.

Pagulayan, J., Eltair, S. & Faber, K. (2018). Nurse documentation and the electronic health record. *American Nurse Today, 13*(9), 48. Available at www.AmericanNurseToday.com.

Penoyer, D. A., Cortelou-Ward, K. H., Noblin, A. M., et al. (2014). Use of electronic health record documentation by healthcare workers in an acute care hospital system. *Journal of Healthcare Management, 59*(2), 130–144.

Petkovšek-Gregorin, R. & Skela-Savič, B. (2015). Nurses' perceptions and attitudes towards documentation in nursing. *Obzornik zdravstvene nege, 49*(2), 106–125. http://dx.doi.org/10.14528/snr.2015.49.2.50.

Staunton, P. & Chiarella, M. (2017). *Law for nurses and midwives* (8th ed.). Sydney: Elsevier.

Tubaishat, A. (2018). Perceived usefulness and perceived ease of use of electronic health records among nurses: Application of technology acceptance modelled. *Informatics for Health & Social Care, 43*(4), 379–389. doi:10.1080/17538157.2017.1363761.

Vowden, L. & Vowden, P. (2015). Documentation in pressure ulcer prevention and management. *Wounds UK, 11*(3), 6–9.

Online resources

Aged Care Quality and Safety Commission: https://www.agedcarequality.gov.au/

Australian Council on Healthcare Standards (ACHS): https://www.achs.org.au/

Australian Health Practitioner Regulation Agency: https://www.ahpra.gov.au/

Australian Nursing & Midwifery Accreditation Council (ANMAC): https://www.anmac.org.au/

Midwifery Council of New Zealand/Te Tatau o te Whare Kahu: https://www.midwiferycouncil.health.nz/

New Zealand Ministry of Health: https://www.health.govt.nz/

Nursing and Midwifery Board of Australia (NMBA): https://www.nursingmidwiferyboard.gov.au/

Nursing Council of New Zealand/Te Kaunihera Tapuhi o Aotearoa: http://www.nursingcouncil.org.nz/

CHAPTER 5

Analysing data using critical thinking skills

ANALYSIS OF DATA AND CRITICAL THINKING

A primary responsibility of any nurse is to undertake health assessments and collect patient data. However, the nurse's role goes beyond documenting data in the chart or passing on to members of the multidisciplinary team. The critical thinking skills that underpin nursing assessment include: determining which data should be collected in each situation; which data indicate the need for additional assessment; and which data should be passed on to others (as well as the speed of data transition). Although nurses are not in a position to provide a medical diagnosis for a patient, it is unrealistic to think that after completing relevant tertiary studies and acquiring clinical experience, they have no idea of what is happening with a patient. Therefore, what is expected of a nurse is an understanding of why specific assessments are made and what specific findings will indicate. The nurse is also expected to be aware that specific findings will often pose new questions requiring additional patient assessment. This chapter addresses the analysis of data nurses collect and the use of critical thinking skills to determine what it is that nurses should do with this information (see Display 5-1). This chapter addresses the development of clinical judgement.

DISPLAY 5-1 ESSENTIAL ELEMENTS OF CRITICAL THINKING

- Keep an open mind.
- Generate a rationale to support opinions or decisions.
- Reflect on thoughts before reaching a conclusion.
- Use past clinical experiences to build knowledge.
- Acquire an adequate knowledge base that continues to build.
- Be aware of the interactions of others.
- Be aware of the environment.

Alfaro-LeFevre (2009, p. 99; 2011) explains the concept of clinical judgement well. She states:

> Developing clinical judgement—clinical reasoning skills—is one of the most important and challenging aspects of becoming a nurse. It's important because people's lives depend on it. It's challenging because thinking in the clinical setting is often fraught with more anxiety and risks than any other situation … [it] entails things like knowing what to look for, how to recognise when a patient's status is changing, and what to do about it. For beginners, this is particularly taxing because it requires an ability to recall facts, put them together into a meaningful whole, and apply the information to a current clinical situation (a situation which is often fluid and changing).

Clinical judgement is a skill that must be built over time. Student or graduate nurses are expected to demonstrate emerging clinical judgement skills that are in a constant state of growth. Consequently, students or graduates are expected to think about what it is they are doing, and to be able to justify their practice within its expected scope. It should be remembered that all knowledge starts with nothing. As a nursing student, knowledge is scaffolded over a three-year program. Lifelong learning skills are also embedded into nursing curricula because it is recognised that nurses do not graduate knowing everything; they are required to continue to improve their knowledge over the course of their career. Given this, nursing students should consider the following three points:

1. Know what is normal.
2. Subjective data are important: ask the patient questions.
3. Always validate data and findings.

Knowing what is normal allows the nurse to recognise what is abnormal. Although student nurses or new practitioners might not at first be able to interpret what an 'abnormality' is (or what it means for the patient), they can seek clarification and support from other members of the health care team. This facilitates recognition of 'abnormality' so the student then knows what is normal *and* this one new 'abnormality'. The list of 'abnormalities' the student is familiar with will increase with experience and exposure and contribute to the advancement of his or her clinical judgement skills.

Asking the patient questions is worthwhile. Patients will frequently know what is wrong with them if the problem is an existing one. Alternatively, the answers patients provide to the questions asked will often direct the future assessments that will be undertaken and help exclude some potential assessments that might have been considered.

Validation of findings is important because interventions are based on assessments. If the assessment data are not accurate, the intervention may not be warranted. Furthermore, consider not just a verification of the assessment findings, but also supplementary assessments that might provide additional data to support earlier findings and assist in determining patient interventions. No single finding should be considered in isolation: it should always be validated with supporting data to ensure optimal patient care.

THE DIAGNOSTIC REASONING PROCESS

If you are confident of your work during the *assessment phase*, you are ready to analyse your data—the *diagnostic phase* of the nursing process. This phase consists of the following essential components: grouping and organising data, validating data and comparing data with norms, clustering data to make inferences, generating possible hypotheses regarding the patient's problems, formulating a professional clinical judgement, and validating the judgement with the patient. These basic components have been organised in various ways to break the process of diagnostic reasoning into easily understood steps. Regardless of how the information is organised or the title of the steps, diagnostic reasoning always consists of these components.

This text presents *seven distinct steps* (outlined below) used to provide a clear, concise explanation of how to perform data analysis. Each step is described in detail. In addition, these seven steps are described throughout the textbook in the 'Analysis of data' sections towards the end of the assessment chapters in Units 2 and 3. We will use the following case study as an example of diagnostic reasoning.

CASE STUDY

You are working on a surgical ward during a clinical placement and are asked by your buddy Registered Nurse (RN) to take routine postoperative observations on a patient who is 24 hours post-laparoscopic appendicectomy and is to be discharged later in your shift. When you take his body temperature, you find it is 38 °C.

CRITICAL THINKING

Alfaro-LeFevre (2009, 2011) states that using 'sound clinical judgement' means drawing valid conclusions and acting appropriately, based on those conclusions (e.g. monitor more closely, begin independent treatment or contact a more experienced clinician to activate the chain of command). Based on the case study above:

1. Do you consider this body temperature significant or abnormal?
2. What would you do about it?
3. How did you come to these conclusions?

Step one: Identify abnormal data

Carpenito-Moyet (2005) states that interpreting data involves two key activities: recognising data as significant (or abnormal) and assigning meaning to (or being able to explain) significant data. As a student, determining the clinical significance of assessment data takes practice. You may use a number of strategies, such as:

- Asking the patient if the finding is normal for them.
- Comparing data with healthy norms and reference ranges.
- Using the patient as their own control (e.g. compare findings with baseline data; always look for symmetry and bilateral equality).
- Considering variations of 'normal' based on the patient's history (e.g. consider how pre-existing health problems or treatments might affect assessment findings).

CLINICAL TIP
As a student nurse, remember to report anything you suspect to be abnormal.

Identifying abnormal findings requires nurses to apply their knowledge of normal human anatomy, physiology and psychosocial development. Collected assessment data should be compared with reference texts and literature that provide standards and values for physical and psychological norms (i.e. height, nutritional requirements, growth and development).

As discussed in Chapter 4, it is important that you verify or validate abnormal assessment findings to prevent errors in clinical decisions and practice. Checking the accuracy of measurements and findings during data collection is an important example; there have been many clinical examples of patients who were identified as confused when in fact the assessment of their mental status was confounded by sensory deficits such as visual or hearing impairments. Having a more experienced colleague validate abnormal findings is also a useful strategy.

CASE STUDY

As the temperature was taken tympanically, you are satisfied the correct technique was followed. The probe with protective sheath was placed inside the external ear canal with gentle pressure, coming in contact with all sides of the ear canal, while the pinna was pulled in an upwards direction, to help straighten the external auditory canal to ensure measurement accuracy. You take a reading in the opposite ear, which shows 38.1 °C.

CRITICAL THINKING

4. How would you validate the accuracy of the body temperature you obtained?

CLINICAL TIP
Seek opportunities to practise physical assessment skills when on clinical placement and compare your findings with your buddy RN or other available clinicians.

Step two: Cluster data

One piece of assessment data rarely provides enough information to make a clinical judgement; nurses cluster together relevant data to identify actual or potential health problems and develop a plan of care. For example, in the case study, an elevated body temperature in a postoperative patient could have many causes and, without further assessment, a sound clinical judgement cannot be made. Abnormal data identified in the case study should trigger a focused nursing assessment in order to interpret the finding.

CLINICAL TIP

Vital signs are never interpreted in isolation; they form part of the overall clinical assessment of a patient. When interpreting vital signs, always compare them with established norms, patient baselines and trends.

CASE STUDY

You discuss the finding with your buddy RN, who explains that a low-grade fever appearing soon after surgery (24 to 48 hours) is often part of the body's inflammatory response. Other common causes of postoperative fever include atelectasis, pneumonia, wound infection, urinary tract infections or infected IV sites. Also, because your patient has had an appendicectomy, he should be observed for evidence of peritonitis. With this information in mind, you return to the patient to complete a focused assessment in order to confirm or rule out these potential causes.

On assessment:

- General survey: The patient looks well and appears to be in no acute discomfort or distress. On the observation chart, the temperature pattern shows a low-grade fever since admission. Other vital signs are within normal limits (heart rate 70, respiratory rate 14, blood pressure 120/70 mmHg, SpO_2 98% on room air).
- Chest: Lungs are clear to auscultation.
- Abdomen: Soft, slight tenderness at wound sites. Bowel sounds active. No guarding.
- Wounds: Port sites are dry and intact.
- Extremities: intravenous cannula in right hand without redness, oedema or tenderness.

CRITICAL THINKING

5. What problems might an elevated temperature suggest in a postoperative patient?
6. What specific complications after an appendicectomy might cause a fever?
7. Based on your answers, what other focused nursing assessments would you undertake?

During step two, the nurse is to group together abnormal data that seem to be related, looking for relationships, patterns or trends among data. Identifying meaningful data clusters is a difficult skill for student nurses until they have developed enough knowledge and clinical experience to draw on. For example, in the case study, the buddy RN with postoperative care experience was immediately able to consider the most likely possible causes of this patient's elevated temperature: respiratory complication (atelectasis), surgical complication (peritonitis) or a normal variation in response to appendicitis and surgery. In order to confirm or refute these inferences, the experienced RN is quickly able to focus their assessment and gather additional data.

As a student, sorting data into categories of an assessment framework (e.g. functional health patterns or body systems) may help you to cluster relevant data together to identify patterns (e.g. all data about elimination are considered together, or all the cardiovascular data are considered together). However, clustering data usually involves a process of inductive reasoning by grouping all significant data that are related, regardless of the pattern or system in which individual cues are found. *Concept mapping* can be a useful strategy to analyse relationships among data. Working through the case study examples in each chapter of this text will also improve your ability to identify data clusters.

Step three: Draw inferences

Step three requires the nurse to determine the meaning of data clusters and formulate reasoned conclusions about the patient's actual or potential health problems.

CRITICAL THINKING

8. Do case study data support any of the possible causes of elevated temperature identified by the buddy RN?
9. What reasoned conclusion can you make about this patient's postoperative recovery?

CASE STUDY

Based on the focused assessment data, you rule out any of the possible complications identified earlier. Although the patient's temperature is elevated, there are no data that suggest a problem at this time. In collaboration with your buddy RN, you decide the appropriate course of action is to monitor the patient's temperature more frequently before discharge.

CRITICAL THINKING

When discussing your decision with another student nurse on placement, she asks why you didn't reduce the patient's temperature with antipyretics such as paracetamol.

10. Why is it unnecessary to reduce the patient's temperature?

Health problems that are identified by the nurse fall into two categories: *nursing diagnoses* and *collaborative problems*. Nursing diagnoses are health-related problems that are managed primarily by nursing care. In the case study, for example, you may collect data that suggest the patient has deficient knowledge about postoperative care before discharge. This is something for which the nurse would intervene and manage independently (e.g. patient education about managing surgical wounds and signs of infection). Therefore, the nurse would move to step four: stating the problem using a nursing diagnosis.

However, if the inference you draw from a data cluster requires both medical and nursing interventions to resolve the problem, then this suggests a collaborative problem. Collaborative problems are defined as 'certain physiological complications that nurses monitor to detect onset or changes in status. Nurses manage collaborative problems using doctor-prescribed and nurse-prescribed interventions to minimise the complications of events' (Carpenito, 2012). Because nurses spend the most time with patients, they play a critical role in detecting and reporting signs and symptoms that may suggest a medical diagnosis or complication. For example, nurses caring for a patient after surgery are accountable for monitoring for signs of potential complications, such as bleeding.

In the case study, for example, had you clustered further abnormal data along with the patient's temperature of 38 °C, such as increasing abdominal tenderness with guarding, nausea and absent bowel sounds, this would have suggested the potential complication of peritonitis. In this situation you would notify the medical team and initiate collaborative interventions to manage the complication. Collaborative problems are equivalent in importance to nursing diagnoses but represent the interdependent or collaborative role of nursing.

Step four: Propose possible diagnoses

When writing a formal statement, nurses often use a common language to describe and conceptualise the problems they assess and treat. Nursing diagnoses reflect nursing's unique focus on the patient's *human responses* to actual or potential health problems (compared with medical diagnoses, which focus on the disease process or pathology). The North American Nursing Diagnosis Association International (NANDA-I) taxonomy is an accepted framework in Australia and New Zealand. However, it is not used consistently by nurses in practice throughout Australian health care settings. Nurses often adapt the NANDA-I terminology to meet their own contexts and specific patient needs. Although there are criticisms of the NANDA taxonomy, nursing diagnoses are discussed in this text because they offer a framework for students to conceptualise and identify problems that may be treated independently by the nurse. For the most part, however, rather than use the term 'nursing diagnoses' this text will use the more general term 'diagnosis'. A diagnosis, whether medical, nursing or otherwise, will directly affect the patient and require resolution by any or all members of the health care team. Although nurses may identify particular diagnoses, and medical or other allied health professionals identify others, it should be a collaborative approach that resolves the diagnosis, regardless of which specific health profession leads the intervention.

A 'risk' diagnosis indicates the patient does not currently have the problem but is at high risk of developing it (e.g. risk of impaired skin integrity related to immobility, poor nutrition and incontinence). Nurses frequently identify potential health problems or undertake risk assessments, for example, to identify patients at risk of falls or pressure ulcers.

An actual diagnosis indicates the patient is currently experiencing the stated problem or has a dysfunctional pattern (e.g. impaired skin integrity: reddened area on right buttocks). Table 5-1 provides a comparison of risk and actual diagnoses.

Step five: Check for defining characteristics

At this point in analysing the data, the nurse must check whether the defining characteristics of the chosen diagnoses are represented in the data clusters in order to choose the most accurate diagnoses and delete those diagnoses that are not valid or accurate for the patient. This step is often difficult because diagnostic labels overlap, making it hard to identify the most appropriate diagnosis. For example, the diagnostic categories of impaired gas exchange, ineffective airway clearance and ineffective breathing patterns all reflect respiratory problems, but each is used to describe a very different human response pattern and set of defining characteristics. Reference texts such as Carpenito's (2012) *Handbook of nursing diagnosis* can assist the student to determine the appropriateness of the diagnostic statement.

Step six: Confirm or rule out diagnoses

If the data cluster does not meet the defining characteristics, you can rule out that particular diagnosis. If the data cluster does meet the defining characteristics, the diagnosis should be verified with the patient.

Validation is also important with the patient who has a collaborative problem. If the patient has a collaborative problem, you need to inform him or her about which signs you are monitoring. For example, in the laparoscopic appendicectomy case study, you would be taking the patient's vital signs every 30 minutes immediately postoperatively (and then 60 minutes) for the next several hours to monitor for any signs of postoperative complications. As the patient is 24 hours post surgery at this point, you would likely be monitoring his or her observations fourth hourly; although you have established the low-grade fever is a normal physiological response to postoperative inflammation, it is still something that you would want to monitor.

Step seven: Document and act on conclusions

Be sure to document all of your professional judgements and the data that support those judgements in the progress notes

Table 5-1 Comparison of risk and actual diagnoses

	Risk diagnoses	Actual diagnoses
Patient status	State of risk for identified problem	State of health problems
Format for stating	'Risk of …'	Nursing diagnoses and 'related to' clause
Examples	Risk of altered body image Risk of altered family processes Risk of ineffective breastfeeding Risk of impaired skin integrity	Disturbed body image related to hand wound that is not healing Interrupted family processes related to hospitalisation of patient Ineffective breastfeeding related to poor mother–infant attachment Impaired skin integrity related to immobility

or clinical pathway. The documentation of data collection before analysis is described in Chapter 4. Guidelines for correctly documenting nursing diagnoses, collaborative problems and referrals are described in the sections that follow.

Nursing diagnoses are often documented and worded in different formats. The most useful formats for actual and at-risk nursing diagnoses are described below. In addition, the major conclusions of a nursing assessment are compared in Table 5-2. Frequently in Australian and New Zealand hospitals, however, rather than list nursing diagnoses, nurses simply chart the patients' progress, problems, interventions and plan for the shift they have just managed. It is important to record your cares and concerns carefully and not simply provide this information in a verbal handover or on the care plan. This information should also be documented in the patient chart.

Risk diagnoses

A risk diagnosis describes a situation in which an actual diagnosis will most likely occur if the nurse does not intervene. In this case, the patient does not have any symptoms or defining characteristics that are manifested, and thus a shorter statement is sufficient:

'Risk of' *diagnostic label* related to (r/t) + *aetiology*

Example: Risk of *infection* r/t *surgical incision*

Actual diagnoses

The most useful format for an actual nursing diagnosis is:

NANDA label (for problem) + r/t + *aetiology* + as manifested by (AMB) + *defining characteristics*

Example: Acute pain r/t *surgical incision* AMB *patient's report of abdominal pain, tense and guarded abdomen, facial grimacing and tachycardia*

Shorter formats are often used to describe patient problems. However, the above format provides all of the necessary information and provides the reader with the clearest and most accurate description of the patient's problem.

Collaborative problems and referrals

Collaborative problems should be documented as risk of complications (RC) of: _________ (specify, e.g. paralytic ileus). In a shortened form, this is written as 'RC of: _______'. Nursing goals for the collaborative problem should be documented, as well as which parameters the nurse must monitor (e.g. bowel sounds) and how often they should be monitored. The nurse also needs to indicate when the doctor or nurse practitioner should be notified, and to identify nursing interventions to help prevent the complication from occurring and nursing interventions to be initiated if a change occurs.

LEARNING TO THINK LIKE A NURSE

Developing the confidence to make clinical judgements comes with accumulating both knowledge and experience. It is a process that develops with time and practice. A beginning nurse attempts to make accurate diagnoses but, because of a lack of knowledge and experience, often finds that he or she has made diagnostic errors. Experts have an advantage because they know when exceptions can be applied to the rules that the novice is accustomed to using and applying. Beginning nurses

Table 5-2 Major conclusions of assessment

	Actual problem diagnosis	Potential problem diagnosis	Collaborative problem	Problem for referral
Who identifies the concern?	Nurse	Nurse	Nurse or other provider	Nurse or other provider
Who deals with the concern?	Nurse (independent practice)	Nurse (independent practice)	Nurse (interdependent practice)	Other provider
What content knowledge is needed?	Nursing science Sciences Basic studies	Nursing science Sciences Basic studies	Nursing science Sciences Basic studies Domain of other providers	Nursing science Sciences Basic studies Domain of other providers
What minimum work experience is needed?	Average	Better than average	Average	Average
What does first part of conclusion statement look like?	Taxonomy label or other descriptive label	Usually taxonomy label of 'Risk of …'	Risk of complication (RC)	N/A
Are related factors included?	Yes, unless unknown	Yes (mandatory)	Sometimes	N/A
What might complete statement look like?	Disturbed self-esteem related to knowledge deficit, ineffective coping as new mother and loss of job	Risk of impaired skin integrity related to immobility, incontinence and fragile skin	RC: Rejection of kidney transplant	Unsafe housing (referral is necessary)

tend to see things as right or wrong, whereas experts realise there are shades of grey or areas between right and wrong. Novices also tend to focus on details and may miss the big picture, whereas experts have a broader perspective in examining situations. Although a lack of experience may be seen as problematic, if the novice sees each clinical experience as an opportunity to learn and improve through engaging with other members of the multidisciplinary team, his or her experience will develop quickly. Experience combined with exposure to new situations will, over time, serve only to help the novice move towards being the nurse he or she aspires to be.

One of the best models to explain how experienced nurses make clinical judgements in practice was developed by Tanner (2006). The overall process of clinical judgement includes four key aspects:

- Using a perceptual recognition of the situation at hand, termed 'noticing'. Experienced RNs immediately recognise abnormal data and possible problems based on: their expectations of each clinical encounter, which stem from their knowledge of the particular patient and his or her patterns of responses; their clinical or practical knowledge of similar patients, drawn from experience; and their textbook knowledge.
- Developing a sufficient understanding of the situation to respond, termed 'interpreting'—Noticing triggers reasoning patterns that allow the nurse to interpret the situation and respond with interventions. For example, in order to confirm or refute their initial grasp of the situation, experienced RNs must quickly be able to focus their assessment and gather additional data.
- Deciding on a course of action deemed appropriate for the situation, which may include no immediate action, termed 'responding'.
- Attending to the patient's responses to intervention, and reviewing the outcomes of the action, focusing on the appropriateness of all of the preceding aspects (i.e. what was noticed, how it was interpreted and how the nurse responded), termed 'reflecting'. Thus, reflection completes the cycle, contributing to the RNs ongoing clinical knowledge development and his or her capacity for clinical judgement in future situations.

The challenge for you as a student nurse is to move beyond mastering the skills of data collection to develop your confidence in analysing and interpreting findings, identifying and clustering abnormal data and determining nursing priorities. Although beginning nurses lack the depth of knowledge and expertise that experienced nurses have, they can still learn to improve their clinical judgement skills. Ethridge (2007) found that new nurse graduates learned to 'think like a nurse' and develop confidence in making clinical judgements through multiple clinical experiences with a wide variety of patients, support from educators and experienced nurses, and sharing experiences with their peers. Making the most of clinical placements by seeking opportunities to develop these skills is essential in the transition from student nurse to beginning practitioner.

CLINICAL TIP

Use every opportunity on clinical placement to ask RNs how they make clinical judgements. What assessments did they perform to make decisions about patient care? What was the reasoning behind their decision?

Pitfalls during assessment and analysis

Students can also improve their diagnostic accuracy by becoming aware of, and avoiding, the several pitfalls of diagnosing. These pitfalls decrease the reliability of cues and decrease diagnostic accuracy. There are two sets of pitfalls: those that occur during the assessment phase, and those that occur during the analysis of data phase.

The first set of pitfalls (specific to the validation of data—this includes the occasional requirement to collect additional data) is discussed in detail in Chapter 4. The importance of making assessments systematically and comprehensively cannot be overstated. Student nurses often include too few unreliable or invalid data, and have an insufficient number of assessment findings available to support the diagnoses.

The second set of pitfalls occurs during the analysis phase. Cues may be clustered yet unrelated to each other. For example, the patient may be very quiet and appear depressed. A nurse may assume the patient is grieving because her husband died a year ago, but the patient may just be fatigued because of all the diagnostic tests she has just undergone.

Another common error is quickly diagnosing a patient without hypothesising several diagnoses. For example, a nurse may assume that a patient with type 1 diabetes who has been re-admitted with hyperglycaemia has a knowledge deficit concerning self-management. However, further exploration of data reveals that the patient has low self-esteem and feelings of powerlessness and hopelessness in controlling a labile, fluctuating blood glucose level. The nurse's goal is to avoid making diagnoses without taking sufficient time to process the data and explore the situation carefully.

Finally, do not overlook consideration of the patient's *cultural background* when analysing data. Patients from other cultures may be misdiagnosed because the defining characteristics and labels for specific diagnoses do not accurately describe the human responses in their culture. Therefore, it is essential to look closely at cultural norms and responses for various patients (these are discussed further in Chaps 10 to 13).

ANALYSIS OF DATA THROUGHOUT HEALTH ASSESSMENT IN NURSING

The purpose of assessing a patient is to analyse the *subjective* and *objective* data collected. The steps of data collection and analysis overlap in health assessment. In the clinical assessment chapters in Units 2 and 3, the 'Analysis of data' sections have been developed to help new nurses visualise, understand and practise analysing data (diagnostic reasoning). Breaking the assessment skills into individual chapters should serve to remind novice practitioners that not all assessments need to be completed, depending on the patient's presenting symptoms. For example, it might be decided a patient presenting with a cough will require only a respiratory assessment. However, after asking the patient questions, it might be determined that the cough is related to a recently prescribed angiotensin-converting-enzyme inhibitor for the management of cardiac failure. It would then be decided that a cardiac assessment (and a vascular assessment, depending on the degree of heart failure) will also be completed.

The 'Analysis of data' sections consist of two parts. The first part, called 'Diagnostic reasoning: Possible conclusions', may contain such subheadings as 'Potential patient risks', 'Potential patient problems', 'Selected collaborative problems' and 'Medical problems'. These headings are used so that students become familiar with common possible conclusions related to a particular body part or system.

The second part is entitled 'Case study'. Here either the case study that has been interspersed throughout the chapter is reassembled as one piece or another case study is introduced. Following this case study are the key steps of clinical reasoning and the accompanying data for each step based on the case study. This part illustrates exactly how to analyse data and which information to include in each of the key steps of diagnostic reasoning. It helps the student grasp the concepts of critical thinking and data analysis.

SUMMARY

Analysis of data is the second step of the nursing process. It is the purpose and end result of assessment. It is often called the diagnostic phase because the purpose of this phase is identification of actual or potential patient problems or need for referral to another member of the multidisciplinary team. The thought process required for data analysis is called diagnostic reasoning—a form of critical thinking.

The key steps developed for this text that explain how nurses should analyse assessment data are as follows:

1. Identify abnormal data.
2. Cluster data.
3. Draw inferences.
4. Propose possible diagnoses.
5. Check for defining characteristics.
6. Confirm or rule out diagnoses.
7. Document and act on conclusions.

Keep in mind that developing sound clinical judgement requires a commitment to developing your knowledge base and making the most of learning opportunities while on clinical placement.

ONLINE RESOURCES

An extensive range of additional resources to enhance teaching and learning and to facilitate understanding may be found online at the text's accompanying website, located on thePoint at http://thepoint.lww.com. These include Watch and Learn videos, Concepts in Action animations, journal articles, case studies, discussion topics and quizzes.

Subscribers may also access Lippincott Procedures, an extensive online point-of-care procedure guide that provides reliable step-by-step instructions for more than 1700 procedures, including 450 evidence-based Australian procedures, and skills in a variety of speciality settings, together with a wealth of supporting information.

References

Alfaro-LeFevre, R. (2009). *Critical thinking and clinical judgment: A practical approach to outcome-focused thinking* (4th ed.). St Louis: Saunders/Elsevier.

Alfaro-LeFevre, R. (2011). *Critical thinking and clinical judgement: A practical approach* (5th ed.). Philadelphia: W.B. Saunders.

Carpenito, L. J. (2012). *Handbook of nursing diagnosis* (14th ed.). Philadelphia: Lippincott Williams & Wilkins.

Carpenito-Moyet, L. J. (2005). *Understanding the nursing process: Concept mapping and care planning for students*. Philadelphia: Lippincott Williams & Wilkins.

Ethridge, S. A. (2007). Learning to think like a nurse: Stories from new nurse graduates. *The Journal of Continuing Education in Nursing, 38*(1), 24–30.

NANDA International. (2011). *Nursing diagnoses: Definitions and classification 2012–2014* (9th ed.). Kaukauna, WI: North American Nursing Diagnosis Association/Hoboken, NJ: Wiley-Blackwell.

Tanner, C. A. (2006). Thinking like a nurse: A research-based model of clinical judgment in nursing. *The Journal of Nursing Education, 45*(6), 204–211.

Selected readings

Carvalho, D. P. S. R. P., Azevedo, I. C., Cruz, G. K. P., et al. (2017). Strategies used for the promotion of critical thinking in nursing undergraduate education: A systematic review. *Nurse Education Today, 57*(10), 103–107.

Siles-González, J. & Solano-Ruiz, C. (2016). Self-assessment, reflection on practice and critical thinking in nursing students. *Nurse Education Today, 45*(10), 132–137.

Tutticci, N., Lewis, P. A., Coyer, F., et al. (2016). Measuring third year undergraduate nursing students' reflective thinking skills and critical reflection self-efficacy following high fidelity simulation: A pilot study. *Nurse Education in Practice, 18*(1), 52–59.

Tutticci, N., Ryan, M., Coyer, F., et al. (2018). Collaborative facilitation of debrief after high fidelity simulation and its implications for reflective thinking: Student experiences. *Studies in Higher Education, 43*(9), 1654–1667.

Zuriguel Pérez, E., Lluch Canut, M. T., Falcó Pegueroles, A., et al. (2015). Critical thinking in nursing: Scoping review of the literature. *International Journal of Nursing Practice, 21*(4), 820–830.

CHAPTER 6

Assessing mental status and psychosocial developmental level

CASE STUDY

Jenny Wilson, a 61-year-old female, has come to the local family clinic where you work. She is accompanied by her husband Steve. When you ask her the reason for her visit she states, 'I am very nervous and not thinking straight.' She sits quietly, slumped over in her chair and often wrings her hands. Her face is expressionless, with minimal eye contact given. You notice that her hair appears unwashed and clothing ill fitting. Steve says he is worried about her because she doesn't leave the house much anymore.

Conceptual foundations

Mental status refers to a patient's level of cognitive and emotional functioning and stability. Mental status is reflected in one's speech, appearance and thought patterns. The ability to think clearly and respond appropriately to daily stressors is necessary to function effectively in the activities of daily living. The World Health Organization (WHO) defines mental health as 'a state of well being in which every individual realizes his or her own potential, can cope with the normal stresses of life, can work productively and fruitfully, and is able to make a contribution to his or her community's condition in which mental functions are successfully performed and there is no mental illness.' Sources of mental health are prevalent in Western societies today, which may affect other body systems when prompt assessment and intervention is delayed. Mental health is one of the eight National Health Priority Areas developed by the Australian government. For more information on mental health in Australia, see www.aihw.gov.au/mental-health. Mental health and addictions are also a New Zealand government health priority: For more information see https://www.health.govt.nz/system/files/documents/publications/ministry_of_health_output_plan_2018_19.pdf

Recent records estimate that more than 450 million people worldwide are suffering with a mental disorder (APA, 2013). The *Diagnostic and statistical manual of mental disorders* (DSM) is published by the American Psychiatric Association (APA) and is widely used for defining mental disorders and identifying symptoms. The fifth edition of the DSM, or DSM-5, was published in May 2013.

The DSM-5 definition for a mental disorder is a disorder that has the following features:

A. A behavioural or psychological syndrome or pattern that occurs in an individual
B. That reflects an underlying psychobiological dysfunction
C. The consequences of which are clinically significant distress (e.g. a painful symptom) or disability (i.e. impairment in one or more important areas of functioning)
D. Must not be merely an expectable response to common stressors and losses (e.g. the loss of a loved one) or a culturally sanctioned response to a particular event (e.g. trance states in religious rituals)
E. That is not primarily a result of social deviance or conflicts with society.

Mental disorders may affect other body systems when prompt assessment and intervention are delayed. For example, people with depression may lose their appetite and over time may develop nutritional deficiencies that affect their gastrointestinal system as well as other body systems.

The term 'psychosocial development' is frequently used in nursing and refers to patients' history and adaptation to their experiences, as seen in their current mental and emotional health, in addition to their self-concept, role development, relationship stress and coping patterns, and spiritual beliefs. In this chapter you will learn to assess both the mental status and psychosocial developmental level of patients. The structure and function of the neurological system can affect one's mental and psychosocial status. Cerebral abnormalities can disturb the patient's intellectual ability, communication ability or emotional responses. Refer to Chapter 16 for a review of the structure and function of the cerebral cortex.

Erik H. Erikson's (1963) theory of psychosocial development will be used in this text to determine the patient's psychosocial developmental level (see also David, 2014).

CASE STUDY

Jenny's mental health

Jenny reports sleep difficulties, a loss of appetite and a general feeling of anxiety. When asked about her daily routine she tells you she is unable to concentrate and has a hard time completing activities. She reports feeling confused, tired and depressed. She denies any plans to hurt herself.

CRITICAL THINKING

1. What further information would you gather from Jenny and/or her partner Steve at this point?

Health assessment

COLLECTING SUBJECTIVE DATA: THE NURSING HEALTH HISTORY

Be alert for all clues that reflect the patient's mental and psychosocial status from the very first interaction you have with the patient. Before asking questions to determine the patient's mental and psychosocial status, explain the purpose of this part of the examination. Explain that some questions you ask may seem irrelevant, but they will help to determine how certain thought processes and activities of daily living are affecting the patient's current health status. For example, it is only through in-depth questioning that the examiner may be able to tell that the patient is having difficulty with concentration, which may be due to excessively stressful life situations or a neurological problem. Tell patients they may decline to answer any questions with which they are uncomfortable. Ensure confidentiality and respect for all that the patient shares with you within the limits of the multidisciplinary team. Ensure the patient knows you will have to report your findings to fellow team members. An important component of this part of the assessment is observing the patient's general behaviour, as well as his or her reaction to the questions.

Problems with other body systems may affect mental status. For example, a patient with low blood sugar may report anxiety, irritability, poor concentration and other mental status changes. Regardless of the source of the problem, the patient's lifestyle and overall level of functioning may be affected. Because of the subjective nature of their mental status and psychosocial development, an in-depth nursing history is necessary to detect problems in areas affecting the patient's daily living activities. For example, the nurse will be able to find out that the patient is having difficulty with concentration or memory only through precise questioning during the interview.

Patients who are experiencing symptoms such as memory loss or confusion may fear they have a serious condition, such as a brain tumour or Alzheimer disease. They may also fear a loss of control, of independence and of role performance. Be sensitive to these fears and concerns because the patient may decline to share important information with you if these concerns are not addressed. Patients would often rather have a physiological problem than a mental disorder because of social stigma, or cultural beliefs that mental health problems may signify weakness such as a lack of self-control or that they are a risk to others. Mental health problems often affect a patient's self-image and self-concept in a negative manner.

While interviewing the patient you may witness them expressing a variety of emotions. For example, the patient may be very anxious about their health problem, or angry they are having a problem with their health. In addition, you may need to discuss sensitive issues such as sexuality, dying or spirituality with your patient. Therefore, there are many interviewing skills you will need to develop to complete a psychosocial history effectively. For expanded guidelines, see Chapter 2, Display 2-2, 'Interacting with patients with various emotional states'.

Biographical data

QUESTION	RATIONALE
What is your name, address and telephone number?	These answers will provide baseline data about the patient's level of consciousness, memory, speech patterns, articulation or speech defects. Inability to answer these questions may indicate a cognitive/neurological defect.
How old are you? Note if the patient is male or female or inter-sex.	This information helps determine a reference point for which the patient's psychosocial developmental level and appearance can be compared. Women tend to have a higher incidence of depression and anxiety, whereas men tend to have a higher incidence of substance abuse and psychosocial disorders.
What is your marital status?	Married adults often report less stress than single or divorced adults.
What is your educational level and where are you employed?	Psychosocial problems appear more often in those with lower incomes and lower educational levels. Patients from higher educational and socio-economic levels tend to participate in more healthy lifestyles.

History of present health concern

QUESTION	RATIONALE
What is your most urgent health concern at this time? Why are you seeking health care?	This information will help the examiner determine the patient's perspective and ability to prioritise the reality of symptoms related to their current health status.

COLDSPA

Example for memory loss

Use the COLDSPA mnemonic as a guideline to collect needed information for each symptom the patient shares. In addition, the following questions help elicit important information.

Mnemonic	Question	Patient response example
Character	Describe the sign or symptom (feeling, appearance, sound, smell or taste, if applicable).	'Cannot remember names of friends I should know and sometimes cannot remember where I put things or where I am going next.'
Onset	When did it begin?	'Three months ago—I thought it was stress, but it is getting worse.'
Location	Where is it? Does it radiate? Does it occur anywhere else?	'I forget people's names at work and at church. I misplace things at work and home all the time.'
Duration	How long does it last? Does it recur?	'I often have to ask people their name because I just cannot recall it. Sometimes it takes me 5 to 10 minutes to remember what I started out to do next.'
Severity	How bad is it? How much does it bother you?	'I cannot get things done as fast as I used to because I am always forgetting what I intended to do and where I put things.'
Pattern	What makes it better or worse?	'Sometimes it is better in the morning after a good night's sleep but gets worse as the day goes on.'
Associated factors/How it Affects the patient	What other symptoms occur with it? How does it affect you?	'I have trouble getting my secretarial work done on time and I am afraid I am going to overlook or lose something important and lose my job.'

Past health history

QUESTION	RATIONALE
Have you ever received medical treatment for a mental health problem or received any type of counselling services? Explain.	Some patients may have had a negative past experience with mental health care services.
Have you ever had any type of head injury, meningitis, encephalitis or a stroke? What changes in your health did you notice as a result of these?	These conditions can affect the developmental level and the mental status of the patient.
Do you have headaches? Describe.	Tension headaches may be seen in patients experiencing stressful situations.
Have you ever served in active duty in the armed forces? Explain.	Post-traumatic syndrome may be seen in veterans who experienced traumatic conditions in military combat.
Do you ever have trouble breathing or have heart palpitations?	Patients with anxiety disorders may hyperventilate or have palpitations.

Continued on following page

Family history

QUESTION	RATIONALE
Is there a history of mental health problems or Alzheimer disease in your family?	Some psychiatric disorders may have a genetic or familial connection such as anxiety, depression, bipolar disorder and/or schizophrenia, or Alzheimer disease.

Lifestyle and health practices

QUESTION	RATIONALE
Can you perform your normal activities of daily living (ADLs)? Describe a typical day. Describe your energy level.	Neurological and mental illnesses can alter one's responses to activities of daily living. Depression may be seen in those with sedentary lifestyles. Anxious patients may be restless, whereas depressed patients may feel fatigued. Patients with eating disorders may exercise excessively.
Describe your normal eating habits.	Poor appetite may be seen with depression, eating disorders and substance abuse.
Describe your daily bowel elimination patterns.	Irritable bowel syndrome or peptic ulcer disease may be associated with psychological disorders.
Describe your sleep patterns.	Insomnia is often seen in depression, anxiety disorders, bipolar disorder and substance abuse.
Do you take any prescribed or over-the-counter medications? How much alcohol do you drink? Do you use recreational drugs such as marijuana, tranquilisers, barbiturates or cocaine?	Use of these substances may alter one's level of consciousness, decrease response times and cause changes in moods and temperament. Inappropriate use of any of these substances may indicate alcoholism or drug abuse problems.
Have you been exposed to any environmental toxins?	Cognition may be altered with toxin exposure.
What religious/spiritual beliefs do you have?	Certain religious or spiritual beliefs can affect the patient's ability to cope in a positive or negative manner.
How do you feel about yourself and your relationship with others?	Patients with a low self-concept may be depressed or suffer from eating disorders or have substance abuse problems. Patients with psychological problems often have difficulty maintaining effective meaningful relationships.
What do you perceive as your role in your family or relationship with your significant other?	Mental health problems often interfere with one's role in families and relationships. In turn, stressful relationships or roles may interfere with one's mental health.

CASE STUDY

Jenny's physical health

Jenny Wilson is 170 cm tall and weighs 56 kg. Her vital signs are temperature 36.8 °C, pulse 82, respirations 18 and blood pressure 100/62 mmHg. She does not appear to be in any physical distress. Her gait is steady and strong.

CRITICAL THINKING

2. Consider some of the physical health issues you think might be affecting Jenny.

COLLECTING OBJECTIVE DATA: PHYSICAL EXAMINATION

Sometimes the *mental status examination* (MSE) may be performed with a complete neurological assessment, which also includes assessment of cranial nerves, motor and cerebellar function, sensory function and reflexes. Among all of these neurological assessments, the MSE assesses the highest level of cerebral integration. The advantage of assessing mental status at the very beginning of the head-to-toe examination is that it provides clues regarding the validity of the subjective information provided by the patient throughout the examination.

CLINICAL TIP

It is best to determine the validity of the patient's responses instead of completing the entire physical examination only to learn that the patient's answers to questions may have been inaccurate. If the nurse finds out that the patient's thought processes are

impaired, another means of obtaining necessary subjective data must be identified, for example, collateral information from carers, relatives and friends, or from medical records.

A comprehensive MSE is quite lengthy and involves great care on the part of the examiner to put the patient at ease. The examination has several parts, including assessment of the patient's level of consciousness, posture, gait, body movements, dress, grooming, hygiene, facial expressions, behaviour and affect, speech, mood, feelings, expressions, thought processes, perceptions and cognitive abilities. Cognitive abilities include orientation, concentration, recent and remote memory, abstract reasoning, judgement, visual perception and constructional ability. The comprehensive mental status examinations (see Assessment tool 6-1) must be administered by a health professional.

ASSESSMENT TOOL 6-1 Mental status examinations

Mental State Examination

A key mental health assessment tool is the Mental State Examination (MSE), which comprises the following major aspects:

Appearance

- For example, posture, body appearance and condition, grooming

Behaviour

- Features; for example, mannerisms, tics
- Descriptors; for example, impassive, restless, agitated, aggressive

Cooperation

- For example, friendly, cooperative, uncooperative, suspicious, hostile, evasive, seductive, perplexed

Affect and mood

Affect: Clinician's observation of the range and appropriateness of the patient's emotions.
- Range; for example, flat, blunted, restricted, normal, labile
- Appropriateness; appropriate or inappropriate in the context of the patient's speech or ideation

Mood: If possible, describe how the patient perceives his or her own mood, preferably using the patient's own words. Clinical descriptors include depressed, anxious, euthymic (normal), irritable, angry and euphoric.

Speech

- Rate: slow, normal, rapid or pressured
- Volume: soft, normal, loud or shouting
- Quantity: nil, spontaneous, normal, talkative or garrulous
- Quality: accent, rhythm, impediments

Thought form and content (judged by listening to the patient's speech)

Thought form
- Quantity—for example, thought blocking, poverty of content, or racing thoughts
- Logical connection or sense of thought— for example, normal, circumstantial, tangential, flight of ideas, loosening of association or incoherence
- Other—for example, clang associations, punning, neologisms, perseveration

Thought content

Any pathological features such as:
- Preoccupations
- Overvalued ideas
- Delusions
- Ideas of reference
- Obsessions
- Compulsions.

What is the subject matter of the patient's thoughts or preoccupations? Are there any suicidal or homicidal ideas?
Note: If there are thoughts of harm to specific persons, consult with a senior colleague regarding duty to warn.

Perception

Any unusual sensory phenomena such as:
- Hallucinations (especially auditory)
- Illusions

Continued on following page

ASSESSMENT TOOL 6-1 Mental status examinations (continued)

- Heightened perception
- Derealisation/depersonalisation.

Note: In older patients with visual or hearing deficits, misinterpretations may occur. These are not necessarily indicative of a mental health problem.

Cognition

Level of consciousness

- Alert
- Hypervigilant
- Drowsy: easily aroused
- Stupor: aroused only by vigorous stimuli
- Coma: unable to be aroused.

Memory

- Immediate, short term (recent) and long term (remote)

Orientation

- Time, place and person

Attention and concentration

- Ability to follow conversation and focus on immediate matters

Insight

An individual's awareness of his or her illness, its effects and implications assessed as good, partial or poor.

Judgement

Ability to accurately assess a situation and act appropriately in response, assessed as intact or impaired. The Mini–Mental State Examination or the Modified Mini–Mental State Examination are useful instruments for screening cognitive functioning.

Risk assessment

A risk assessment is an essential part of all stages of a patient's management. A risk assessment should be conducted as part of the formal assessment. Common risks to consider include:

- Risk of absconding
- Risk of self-harm
- Risk of underlying organic/physical illness being undetected *(e.g. Many physical health conditions have similar symptoms to mental health illnesses, e.g. chest pain [cardiovascular event] and chest pain in anxiety. The treatment trajectories for these conditions are clearly different.)*
- Risk of suicide
- Risk of harm to others.

Mental Health and Drug and Alcohol Office, NSW Department of Health, Sydney (2009). *Mental health for emergency departments—A reference guide* (pp. 17–19).

Folstein Mini–Mental State Examination

Patient's name ___________
Assessor's name ___________ Date ___________
(Maximum 30; <26 = Concern; <24 = Further assessment)

Orientation	Score (max 10)
What is today's date?	_______
What is the year?	_______
What is the month?	_______
What day is today?	_______
What season is it?	_______
What building are we in?	_______
What floor are we on?	_______
What town are we in?	_______
What state are we in?	_______
What country are we in?	_______

ASSESSMENT TOOL 6-1 Mental status examinations (continued)

Registration	Score (max 3)
Ask to repeat: 'ball', 'flag', 'tree'. First repetition is score. Repeat until get right or six times	______
Attention and calculation	Score (max 5)
100 – 7, for 5 subtractions OR Spell 'world' backwards, with 1 for each letter in exactly the right place	______
Recall	Score (max 3)
3 previous words (from Registration, above)	______
Language	Score (max 9)
Name a watch and a pencil (2 points)	______
Repeat the following: 'no ifs, ands, or buts' (1 point) ______	
Follow a three-stage command: 'Take the paper in your right hand, fold it in half and put it on the floor' (3 points)	______
Repeat and obey the following: 'CLOSE YOUR EYES' (1 point)	______
Write a sentence. It must have noun, verb and be sensible (1 point)	______
Draw 2 intersecting pentagons. Must have 10 angles and intersect (1 point)	______
Total score	______/30

Mental Health and Drug and Alcohol Office, *Mental health for Emergency Departments - A Refreence Guide*. NSW Ministry of Health. Amended March 2015.

Another assessment tool for the assessment of mental health and risk, which is validated and used in Australia and New Zealand, is the Health of the Nation Outcome Scales (HoNOS) (Wing et al., 1998). The HoNOS is available in three versions: one for children and adolescents, one for middle-aged adults and another for those over 65 years old. There are 12 scales covering the following four domains: behaviour, impairment, symptom and social. This assessment tool needs to be administered by a health professional trained in its application. You are encouraged to seek the opportunity to be present while the MSE and HoNOS examinations are administered, to augment your learning.

If time is limited and a quick standard measure is needed to evaluate or re-evaluate the patient's mental state, the mental status examinations found in Assessment tool 6-1 may be used to obtain a patient score. If depression is suspected, the depression questionnaire (Self-assessment 6-1) or the Kessler Psychological Distress Scale (K10) (Assessment tool 6-2) may be completed by the patient. The K10 is a widely used tool in Australia and New Zealand for depression. In addition, the

SELF-ASSESSMENT 6-1 DEPRESSION QUESTIONNAIRE

The following DEPRESSION QUESTIONNAIRE has 16 simple questions that may help identify common symptoms of depression. The results can be a helpful way to discuss your condition with your health care provider and actually help him/her diagnose your condition. After answering the questions provided on the following pages, print the completed questionnaire and discuss any concerns with your doctor.

As with any medical illness or condition, only your doctor or other qualified health care professional can provide a diagnosis of depression. The following questionnaire is intended to help you discuss symptoms with a qualified health care professional. This questionnaire is not intended to serve as a substitute for a diagnosis of depression by a qualified health care professional. If you think you may have depression, you should visit your doctor or other qualified health care professional as soon as possible.

Complete the questionnaire below and take the results to your doctor. Choose the items that best describe you over the last 7 days.

1 Falling asleep

0 I never take longer than 30 minutes to fall asleep.
1 I take at least 30 minutes to fall asleep, less than half the time.
2 I take at least 30 minutes to fall asleep, more than half the time.
3 I take more than 60 minutes to fall asleep, more than half the time.

2 Sleep during the night

0 I do not wake up at night.
1 I have a restless, light sleep with a few brief awakenings each night.
2 I wake up at least once a night, but I go back to sleep easily.
3 I awaken more than once a night and stay awake for 20 minutes or more, more than half the time.

3 Waking up too early

0 Most of the time, I awaken no more than 30 minutes before I need to get up.
1 More than half the time I awaken more than 30 minutes before I need to get up.
2 I almost always awaken at least one hour or so before I need to, but I go back to sleep eventually.
3 I awaken at least one hour before I need to, and can't go back to sleep.

4 Sleeping too much

0 I sleep no longer than 7–8 hours/night, without napping during the day.
1 I sleep no longer than 10 hours in a 24-hour period including naps.
2 I sleep no longer than 12 hours in a 24-hour period including naps.
3 I sleep longer than 12 hours in a 24-hour period including naps.

Continued on following page

SELF-ASSESSMENT 6-1 DEPRESSION QUESTIONNAIRE (continued)

5 Feeling sad

0 I do not feel sad.
1 I feel sad less than half the time.
2 I feel sad more than half the time.
3 I feel sad nearly all of the time.

(Please complete either 6 or 7)

6 Decreased appetite

0 There is no change in my usual appetite.
1 I eat somewhat less often or lesser amounts of food than usual.
2 I eat much less than usual and only with personal effort.
3 I rarely eat within a 24-hour period, and only with extreme personal effort or when others persuade me to eat.

7 Increased appetite

0 There is no change from my usual appetite.
1 I feel a need to eat more frequently than usual.
2 I regularly eat more often and/or greater amounts of food than usual.
3 I feel driven to overeat both at mealtime and between meals.

(Please complete either 8 or 9)

8 Decreased weight (within the last two weeks)

0 I have not had a change in my weight.
1 I feel as if I've had a slight weight loss.
2 I have lost 1 kilogram or more.
3 I have lost 4 kilograms or more.

9 Increased weight (within the last two weeks)

0 I have not had a change in my weight.
1 I feel as if I've had a slight weight gain.
2 I have gained 1 kilogram or more.
3 I have gained 4 kilograms or more.

10 Concentration/decision making

0 There is no change in my usual capacity to concentrate or make decisions.
1 I occasionally feel indecisive or find that my attention wanders.
2 Most of the time, I struggle to focus my attention or to make decisions.
3 I cannot concentrate well enough to read or cannot make even minor decisions.

11 View of myself

0 I see myself as equally worthwhile and deserving as other people.
1 I am more self-blaming than usual.
2 I largely believe that I cause problems for others.
3 I think almost constantly about major and minor defects in myself.

12 Thoughts of death or suicide

0 I do not think of suicide or death.
1 I feel that life is empty or wonder if it's worth living.
2 I think of suicide or death several times a week for several minutes.
3 I think of suicide or death several times a day in some detail, or I have made specific plans for suicide or have actually tried to take my life.

13 General interest

0 There is no change from usual in how interested I am in other people or activities.
1 I notice that I am less interested in people or activities.
2 I find I have interest in only one or two of my formerly pursued activities.
3 I have virtually no interest in formerly pursued activities.

14 Energy level

0 There is no change in my usual level of energy.
1 I get tired more easily than usual.
2 I have to make a big effort to start or finish my usual daily activities (for example, shopping, homework, cooking or going to work).
3 I really cannot carry out most of my usual daily activities because I just don't have the energy.

15 Feeling slowed down

0 I think, speak and move at my usual rate of speed.
1 I find that my thinking is slowed down or my voice sounds dull or flat.
2 It takes me several seconds to respond to most questions and I'm sure my thinking is slowed.
3 I am often unable to respond to questions without extreme effort.

16 Feeling restless

0 I do not feel restless.
1 I'm often fidgety, wringing my hands, or need to shift how I am sitting.
2 I have impulses to move about and am quite restless.
3 At times, I am unable to stay seated and need to pace around.

Depression questionnaire scoring

Each of the four possible answers to each quiz question is given an ascending numerical value from 0 to 3, and the total test score is calculated by using the following formula:

Enter the highest score on any 1 of the 4 sleep items, questions 1–4 ______
Enter the score from question 5 ______
Enter the highest score on any 1 appetite/weight item, questions 6–9 ______
Enter the score from question 10 ______
Enter the score from question 11 ______
Enter the score from question 12 ______
Enter the score from question 13 ______
Enter the score from question 14 ______
Enter the highest score on either of the 2 psychomotor items, questions 15 and 16 ______

TOTAL SCORE (Range 0–27)

Interpreting the scores

0–5	None
6–10	Mild
11–15	Moderate
16–20	Severe
21–27	Very severe

Rush, A. J., et al. (2003). The 16-item Quick Inventory of Depressive Symptomatology (QIDS) Clinician Rating (QIDS-C) and Self-Report (QIDS-SR): A psychometric evaluation in patients with chronic major depression. *Biological Psychiatry, 54*, 573–583. Retrieved March 2019 from www.ids-qids.org.

ASSESSMENT TOOL 6-2 Kessler Psychological Distress Scale (K10) questions

All of the time (score 5)	Most of the time (score 4)	Some of the time (score 3)	A little of the time (score 2)	None of the time (score 1)	
Answer each question below with a score (from 1 to 5) that best describes you.					**Score 1, 2, 3, 4, 5**
1. In the past 4 weeks, about how often did you feel tired out for no good reason?					
2. In the past 4 weeks, about how often did you feel nervous?					
3. In the past 4 weeks, about how often did you feel so nervous that nothing could calm you down?					
4. In the past 4 weeks, about how often did you feel hopeless?					
5. In the past 4 weeks, about how often did you feel restless or fidgety?					
6. In the past 4 weeks, about how often did you feel so restless you could not sit still?					
7. In the past 4 weeks, about how often did you feel depressed?					
8. In the past 4 weeks, about how often did you feel that everything was an effort?					
9. In the past 4 weeks, about how often did you feel so sad that nothing could cheer you up?					
10. In the past 4 weeks, about how often did you feel worthless?					

Kessler, R. C., Barker, P. R., Colpe, L. J., Epstein, J. F., Gfroerer, J. C., Hiripi, E., Howes, M. J, Normand, S-L. T., Manderscheid, R. W., Walters, E. E. & Zaslavsky, A. M. (2003). Screening for serious mental illness in the general population. *Archives of General Psychiatry, 60*(2), 184–189.

ASSESSMENT TOOL 6-3 Symptoms of Alzheimer disease

Symptoms

While there are some common symptoms of Alzheimer's disease, everyone is unique. No two cases of Alzheimer's are likely to be the same. People in the early stages of Alzheimer's disease experience lapses of short-term memory. As the disease progresses they may:

- have increasing difficulty managing complex or new tasks
- frequently forget the names of people, places, appointments and recent events
- show a lack of initiative or withdrawal from usual activities
- experience emotional and personality changes, such as frustration, anxiety or sadness
- become more irritable, suspicious or emotionally unresponsive in the face of their increasing disability
- have problems finding the right words or understanding what is said to them.

This information sheet was Alzheimer's New Zealand material from www.alzheimers.org.nz. (Accessed 18 Nov. 2019).

CASE STUDY

Jenny appears to be alert and oriented to person, place, time and situation. However, you find you have to repeat questions because she is having difficulty concentrating. Her responses are brief and low in volume. She sometimes looks to her husband for reassurance. She is unable to recall recent events, including what she ate for dinner last night.

CRITICAL THINKING

3. What subjective and objective data would you need to collect to complete your assessment?

Alzheimer guide (Assessment tool 6-3) may be used by the examiner to determine if the patient has any early warning signs of Alzheimer disease.

Preparing the patient

Questions are intended to collect both subjective and objective data. For example, one question may be to name the day of the week. Another example would be asking the patient to explain where he or she is at the time of the examination. Simply alerting patients to the unusual nature of some of your questions, and your purpose for asking them, is likely to put them at ease. With practice you will learn how to obtain this information without direct questioning, just by observing the patient's responses to other questions during the examination. In preparing the patient it is important to be mindful of cultural and spiritual considerations. These topics are covered in depth in other chapters of this text, for example Chapters 10 and 13.

Equipment

- Pen and paper
- Health of the Nation Outcome Scales (HoNOS) tool (Wing et al., 1998)
- Mini–Mental State Examination (MMSE) (Assessment tool 6-1)
- Kessler Psychological Distress Scale (K10) (Assessment tool 6-2)
- Symptoms of Alzheimer disease (Assessment tool 6-3)

The purpose of the following form is to provide an example framework for a comprehensive physical assessment.

PHYSICAL ASSESSMENT

ASSESSMENT PROCEDURE	NORMAL FINDINGS	ABNORMAL FINDINGS
Mental status and level of consciousness		
INSPECTION		
Observe the patient's level of consciousness. Ask the patient his or her name, address and phone number (Fig. 6-1). 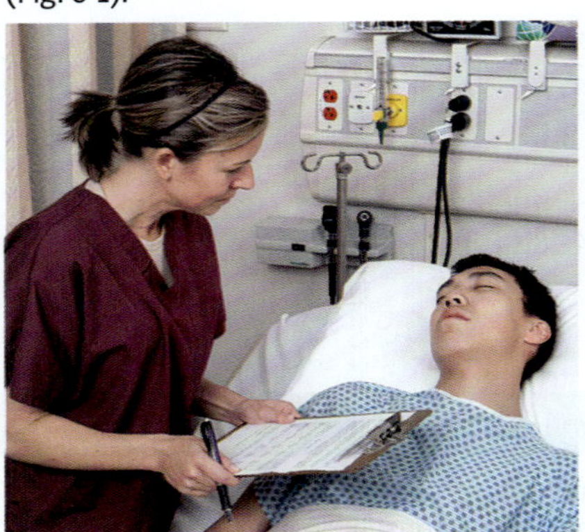 **FIGURE 6-1** Assessing level of consciousness.	Patient is alert and oriented to what is happening at the time of the interview and physical assessment. Patient is alert to person, place, day and time, and responds to your questions and interacts appropriately.  **OLDER ADULT CONSIDERATIONS** **Although the older patient's response and ability to process information may be slower, he or she is normally alert and oriented.**	
If the patient does not respond appropriately, *call the patient's name and note the response.* If the patient does not respond, call the name louder. If necessary, shake the patient gently. If the patient still does not respond, apply a painful stimulus. **CLINICAL TIP** **When assessing the level of consciousness, always begin with the least noxious stimulus: verbal, tactile, to painful.**	Patient is alert and awake with eyes open and looking at examiner. Patient responds appropriately.	The following levels of consciousness are abnormal: ***Lethargy:*** Patient opens eyes, answers questions and falls back asleep. ***Obtunded:*** Patient opens eyes to loud voice, responds slowly with confusion, seems unaware of environment. ***Stupor:*** Patient awakens to vigorous shake or painful stimuli but returns to unresponsive sleep. ***Coma:*** Patient remains unresponsive to all stimuli; eyes stay closed. Patient with lesions of the corticospinal tract draws hands up to chest (*decorticate* or abnormal flexor posture) when stimulated (Fig. 6-2). Patient with lesions of the diencephalon, midbrain or pons extends arms and legs, arches neck and rotates hands and arms internally (*decerebrate* or abnormal extensor posture) when stimulated (Fig. 6-3).

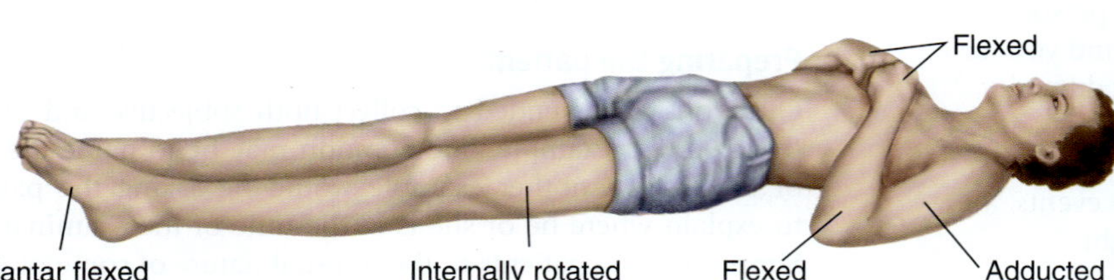

FIGURE 6-2 Decorticate posture. (Fuller, J. & Schaller-Ayers, J. (1994). *Health assessment: A nursing approach*. (2nd ed.) Philadelphia: Wolters Kluwer Health, Inc.)

PHYSICAL ASSESSMENT (continued)

ASSESSMENT PROCEDURE	NORMAL FINDINGS	ABNORMAL FINDINGS

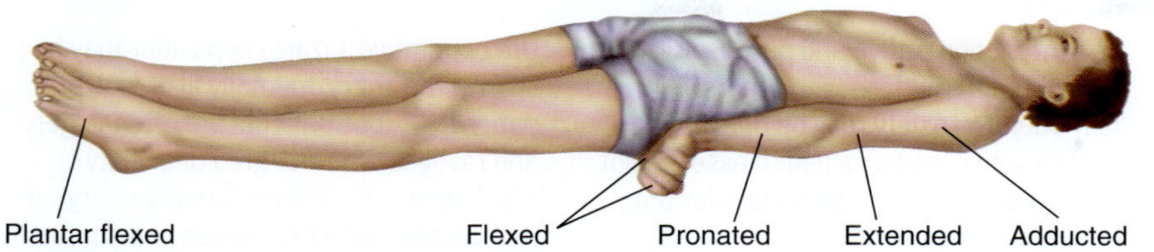

FIGURE 6-3 Decerebrate posture. (Fuller, J. & Schaller-Ayers, J. (1994). *Health assessment: A nursing approach*. (2nd ed.) Philadelphia: Wolters Kluwer Health, Inc.)

ASSESSMENT PROCEDURE	NORMAL FINDINGS	ABNORMAL FINDINGS
Use the Glasgow Coma Scale (GCS) for patients who are at high risk of rapid deterioration of the nervous system (Assessment tool 6-4).	GCS score of 14 indicates an optimal level of consciousness.	GCS score of less than 14 indicates some impairment in the level of consciousness. A score of 3, the lowest possible score, indicates deep coma.
Observe posture, gait and body movements. Be alert for tense, nervous, fidgety and restless behaviour, which may be seen in anxiety or may simply reflect the patient's apprehension during a physical examination.	The patient appears to be relaxed with shoulders and back erect when standing or sitting. Gait is rhythmic and coordinated with arms swinging at sides.	Slumped posture may reflect feelings of powerlessness or hopelessness characteristic of depression or organic brain disease. Bizarre body movements and behaviour may be noted in schizophrenia or may be a side effect of drug therapy or other activity. Tense or anxious patients may elevate their shoulders towards their ears and hold the entire body stiffly.

Continued on following page

ASSESSMENT TOOL 6-4 Using the Glasgow Coma Scale

The Glasgow Coma Scale is useful for rating a patient's response to stimuli. The patient who scores 10 or lower needs emergency attention. The patient with a score of 7 or lower is generally considered to be in a coma.

	Score	
Eye opening response	Spontaneous opening	4
	To verbal command	3
	To pain	2
	No response	1
Most appropriate verbal response	Oriented	5
	Confused	4
	Inappropriate words	3
	Incoherent	2
	No response	1
Most integral motor response (arm)	Obeys verbal commands	6
	Localises pain	5
	Withdraws from pain	4
	Flexion (decorticate rigidity)	3
	Extension (decerebrate rigidity)	2
	No response	1
Total score		3 to 15

PHYSICAL ASSESSMENT (continued)

ASSESSMENT PROCEDURE	NORMAL FINDINGS	ABNORMAL FINDINGS
Mental status and level of consciousness (continued)		
Observe behaviour and affect.	Patient is cooperative and purposeful in his or her interactions with others. Mild to moderate anxiety may be normal in a patient who is having a health assessment performed. Affect is appropriate for the patient's situation.	Uncooperative, bizarre behaviour may be seen in the angry, mentally ill or violent patient. Anxious patients are often fidgety and restless. Some degree of anxiety is often seen in ill patients. Apathy or crying may be seen with depression. Incongruent behaviour may be seen in patients who are in denial of problems or illness. Prolonged, euphoric laughing is typical of mania. **OLDER ADULT CONSIDERATIONS** **In the older adult, purposeless movements, wandering, aggressiveness or withdrawal may indicate neurological deficits.**
Observe dress and grooming. Keep the examination setting and the reason for the assessment in mind as you note the patient's degree of cleanliness and attire. For example, if the patient arrives directly from home, he or she may be neater than if he or she comes to the assessment from the workplace. **CLINICAL TIP** **Be careful not to make premature judgements regarding the patient's dress. Styles and clothing fads (e.g. torn jeans, oversized clothing, baggy pants), developmental level, socio-economic level and culture all influence a person's dress.**	Dress is appropriate for occasion and weather. Dress varies considerably from person to person, depending on individual preference. There may be several normal dress variations depending on the patient's developmental level, age, socio-economic level, and culture or subculture. **OLDER ADULT CONSIDERATIONS** **Some older adults may wear excess clothing because of slowed metabolism and loss of subcutaneous fat, resulting in cold intolerance.**	Unusually meticulous grooming and finicky mannerisms may be seen in obsessive-compulsive disorder. Poor hygiene and inappropriate dress may be seen in depression, schizophrenia, dementia and Alzheimer disease. One-sided neglect may result from lesion in the opposite parietal cortex, usually the non-dominant side. Uncoordinated clothing, extremely light clothing or extremely warm clothing for the weather conditions may be seen on mentally ill, grieving, depressed or poor patients. This may also be noted in patients with heat or cold intolerances. Extremely loose clothing held up by pins or a belt may suggest recent weight loss. Patients wearing long sleeves in warm weather may be protecting themselves from the sun or covering up needle marks secondary to drug abuse. Soiled clothing may indicate homelessness, elderly vision deficits or mental illness.
Observe hygiene. Determine what the normal level of hygiene is for the patient's developmental and socio-economic level and cultural background.	The patient is clean and groomed appropriately for occasion. Stains on hands and dirty nails may reflect certain occupations such as mechanic or gardener.	A dirty, unshaven, unkempt appearance with a foul body odour may reflect depression, drug abuse or low socio-economic level (i.e. homeless patient). Poor hygiene may be seen in dementia or other conditions that indicate a self-care deficit. If the patient is cared for by others, poor hygiene may reflect neglect by carer or carer role strain. Breath odours from smoking or from drinking alcoholic beverages may be noted, as may diet-related odours such as garlic or soy products.

PHYSICAL ASSESSMENT (continued)

ASSESSMENT PROCEDURE	NORMAL FINDINGS	ABNORMAL FINDINGS
Observe facial expressions. Note particularly eye contact and affect. **CULTURAL CONSIDERATIONS** **Eye contact and facial expressions such as smiling differ in some cultures. Eye contact is often related to status or gender (who initiates eye contact with whom), and smiling often does not imply agreement with the speaker, or friendliness. See Chapter 10 for more details.**	Patient maintains good eye contact, smiles and frowns appropriately.	Poor eye contact is seen in depression or apathy. Extreme facial expressions of happiness, anger or fright may be seen in anxious patients. Patients with Parkinson disease may have a masklike, expressionless face. Staring watchfulness appears in metabolic disorders and anxiety. Inappropriate facial expressions (e.g. smiling when expressing sad thoughts) may indicate mental illness. Drooping or gross asymmetry occurs with neurological disorder or injury (e.g. Bell palsy or stroke).
Observe speech. Observe and listen to tone, clarity and pace of speech.	Speech is in a moderate tone, clear, with moderate pace, and culturally appropriate. **OLDER ADULT CONSIDERATIONS** **Normally in older adults, responses may be slowed but speech should be clear and moderately paced.**	Slow, repetitive speech is characteristic of depression or Parkinson disease. Loud, rapid speech may occur in manic phases of bipolar disorder. Disorganised speech, consistent (non-stop) speech, or long periods of silence may indicate mental illness or a neurological disorder (e.g. dysarthria, dysphasia, speech defect, garbled speech). Table 6-1 provides further information about voice and speech problems.
If the patient has difficulty with speech, perform additional tests: • Ask the patient to name objects in the room. • Ask the patient to read from printed material appropriate for his or her educational level. • Ask the patient to write a sentence. **CLINICAL TIP** **Speech is largely influenced by experience, level of education and culture.**	Patient names familiar objects without difficulty. Reads age-appropriate written print. Writes a coherent sentence with correct spelling and grammar.	Patient cannot name objects correctly, read print correctly or write a basic correct sentence. Deficits in this area require further neurological assessment to identify any dysfunction of higher cortical levels.

Continued on following page

Table 6-1 Sources of voice and speech problems

Problem	Description	Source
Dysphonia	Voice volume disorder	Laryngeal disorders or impairment of cranial nerve X (vagus nerve)
Cerebellar dysarthria	Irregular, uncoordinated speech	Multiple sclerosis
Dysarthria	Defect in muscular control of speech (e.g. slurring)	Lesions of the nervous system, Parkinson disease or cerebellar disease
Aphasia	Difficulty producing or understanding language	Motor lesions in the dominant cerebral hemisphere
Wernicke's aphasia	Rapid speech that lacks meaning	Lesion in the posterior superior temporal lobe
Broca's aphasia	Slowed speech with difficult articulation, but fairly clear meaning	Lesion in the posterior inferior frontal lobe

PHYSICAL ASSESSMENT (continued)

ASSESSMENT PROCEDURE	NORMAL FINDINGS	ABNORMAL FINDINGS
Mental status and level of consciousness (continued)		
Observe mood, feelings and expressions. Ask patient 'How are you feeling today?' and 'What are your plans for the future?' **CLINICAL TIP** **Moods and feelings often vary from sadness to joy to anger, depending on the situation and circumstance.**	Cooperative or friendly, expresses feelings appropriate to situation, verbalises positive feelings regarding others and the future, expresses positive coping mechanisms (support groups, exercise, sports, hobbies, counselling).	Expression of prolonged negative, gloomy, despairing feelings is noted in depression (see Self-assessment 6-1). Expression of elation and grandiosity, high energy level, and engagement in high-risk but pleasurable activities is seen in manic phases. Excessive worry may be seen in anxiety or obsessive-compulsive disorders. Eccentric moods not appropriate to the situation are seen in schizophrenia.
Observe thought processes and perceptions. Observe thought processes for clarity, content and perception by inquiring about patient's thoughts and perceptions expressed. Use statements such as 'Tell me more about what you just said' or 'Tell me what your understanding is of the current situation or your health.' **CLINICAL TIP** **When assessing the mental status of an older patient, be sure first to check vision and hearing before assuming the patient has a mental problem.**	Patient expresses full, free-flowing thoughts; follows directions accurately; expresses realistic perceptions; is easy to understand and makes sense; does not voice suicidal thoughts.	Abnormal processes include persistent repetition of ideas, illogical thoughts, interruption of ideas, invention of words or repetition of phrases as in schizophrenia; rapid flight of ideas, repetition of ideas and use of rhymes and punning as in manic phases of bipolar disorder; continuous, irrational fears and avoidance of an object or situation as in phobias; delusion, extreme apprehension; compulsions; obsessions; and illusions are also abnormal (see the glossary for definitions).
Identify possibly destructive or suicidal tendencies in patient's thought processes and perceptions by asking, 'How do you feel about the future?' or 'Have you ever had thoughts of hurting yourself or doing away with yourself?' or 'How do others feel about you?'	Verbalises positive, healthy thoughts about the future and self.	Patients who are suicidal may share past attempts of suicide, give plan for suicide, verbalise worthlessness about self, joke about death frequently. Patients who are depressed or feel hopeless are at higher risk of suicide.
OLDER ADULT CONSIDERATIONS **Use the Geriatric Depression Scale if depression is suspected in the older patient (see Chapter 34). Read the questions to the patient if the patient cannot read.**	Scores 10 or less.	Scores between 10 and 30 may indicate depression.
Observe cognitive abilities. ***Orientation:*** Ask for the patient's name and names of family members (Fig. 6-4) (person); the time such as hour, day, date or season (time); and where the patient lives or is now (place). **CLINICAL TIP** **When assessing orientation to time, place and person, remember that orientation to time is usually lost first and orientation to person is usually lost last.**	Patient is aware of self, others, time, home address and current location. 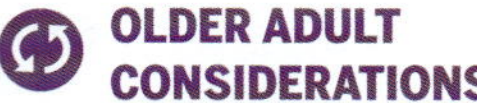 **Some older patients may seem confused, especially in a new or acute care setting, but most know who and where they are and the current month and year.**	Reduced degree of orientation may be seen with organic brain disorders or psychiatric illness such as withdrawal from chronic alcohol use or schizophrenia. (*Note:* Schizophrenia may be marked by hallucinations—sensory perceptions that occur without external stimuli—as well as disorientation.)

PHYSICAL ASSESSMENT (continued)

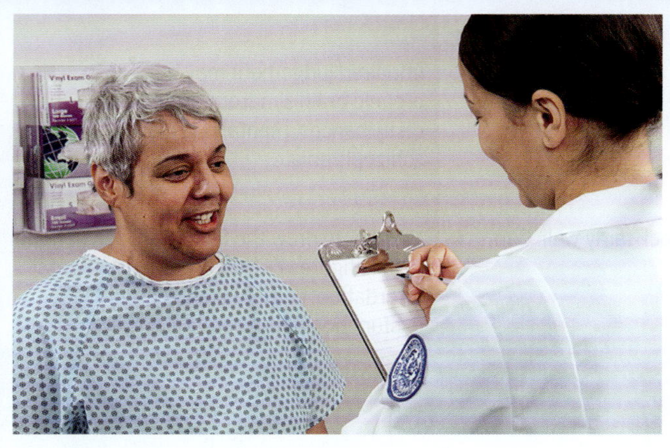

FIGURE 6-4 Assessing orientation by asking the client to identify a family member. (Weber, J.R. & Kelley, J.H. [2017]. Health Assessment in Nursing, 6e, © Wolters Kluwer Health.)

ASSESSMENT PROCEDURE	NORMAL FINDINGS	ABNORMAL FINDINGS
Concentration: Note the patient's ability to focus and stay attentive to you during the interview and examination. Give the patient directions such as 'Please pick up the pencil with your left hand, place it in your right hand, then hand it to me.'	Patient listens and can follow directions without difficulty.  **OLDER ADULT CONSIDERATIONS** **Some older patients may like to reminisce and tend to wander somewhat from the topic at hand.**	Distraction and inability to focus on task at hand are noted in anxiety, fatigue, attention deficit disorders and impaired states due to alcohol or drug intoxication.
Recent memory: Ask the patient 'What did you have to eat today?' or 'What is the weather like today?'	Recalls recent events without difficulty. **OLDER ADULT CONSIDERATIONS** **Some older patients may exhibit hesitation with short-term memory.**	Inability to recall recent events is seen in delirium, dementia, depression and anxiety.
Remote memory: Ask the patient: 'When did you get your first job?' or 'When is your birthday?' Information on past health history also gives clues to the patient's ability to recall remote events.	Patient correctly recalls past events.	Inability to recall past events is seen in cerebral cortex disorders.
Use of memory to learn new information: Ask the patient to repeat four unrelated words. The words should not rhyme and they cannot have the same meaning (e.g. rose, hammer, vehicle, brown). Have the patient repeat these words in 5 minutes, again in 10 minutes and again in 30 minutes.	Patient is able to recall words correctly after a 5-, a 10- and a 30-minute period.  **OLDER ADULT CONSIDERATIONS** **Patients older than 80 years should recall two to four words after 5 minutes and possibly after 10 and 30 minutes with hints that prompt recall.**	Inability to recall words after a delayed period is seen in anxiety, depression or Alzheimer disease. If Alzheimer disease is a concern, use Assessment tool 6-3 to determine with the patient and family if early warning signs are present. Refer to Promote Health—Dementias for more information about Alzheimer disease and other forms of dementia.
Abstract reasoning: Ask the patient to compare objects. For example, 'How are an apple and orange the same? How are they different?' Also ask the patient to explain a proverb. For example, 'A rolling stone gathers no moss' or 'A stitch in time saves nine.' **CLINICAL TIP** **If patients have limited education, note their ability to joke or use puns, which also requires abstract reasoning.**	Patient explains similarities and differences between objects and proverbs correctly. The patient with limited education can joke and use puns correctly.	Inability to compare and contrast objects correctly or interpret proverbs correctly is seen in schizophrenia, mental retardation, delirium and dementia.

Continued on following page

PHYSICAL ASSESSMENT (continued)

ASSESSMENT PROCEDURE	NORMAL FINDINGS	ABNORMAL FINDINGS
Mental status and level of consciousness (continued)		
Judgement: Ask the patient, 'What do you do if you have pain?' or 'What would you do if you were driving and a police car was behind you with its lights and siren turned on?'	Answers to questions are based on sound rationale.	Impaired judgement may be seen in organic brain syndrome, emotional disturbances, mental retardation and schizophrenia.
Visual perceptual and constructional ability: Ask the patient to draw the face of a clock or copy simple figures (Fig. 6-5).	Draws the face of a clock fairly well. Can copy simple figures.	Inability to draw the face of a clock or copy simple figures correctly is seen in mental retardation, dementia and parietal lobe dysfunction of the cerebral cortex.

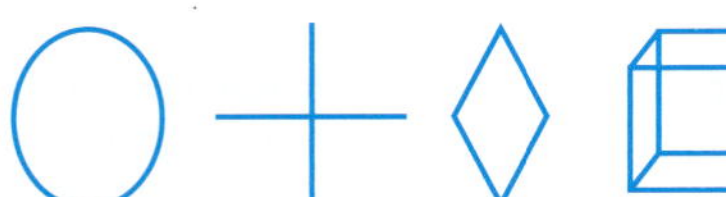
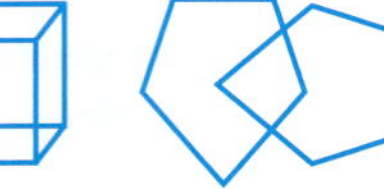

FIGURE 6-5 Figures to be drawn by patient.

ASSESSMENT PROCEDURE	NORMAL FINDINGS	ABNORMAL FINDINGS
Use the Mini–Mental Examination if time is limited and a quick measure is needed to evaluate cognitive function. **CLINICAL TIP** **This examination tests level of orientation, memory, speech and cognitive functions but not mood, feelings, expressions, thought processes or perceptions.**	A score greater than 28 for patients with a high school education and a score of 20 to 30 for patients with less than a high school education is considered normal.	For patients with a high school education, a score less than 26 = concern, and less than 24 = further assessment. ***Caution:*** Note that potential harm from labelling or identifying patients with possible dementia must be weighed against benefits of assessment (Stephan, 2014).

PROMOTE HEALTH **DEMENTIAS**

INTRODUCTION

Dementia is the name given to loss of cognitive skills. This condition occurs because of brain diseases or trauma. The cognitive changes can have a rapid or a gradual onset. Cognitive changes resulting from dementias include decision making or judgement, memory, spatial orientation, thinking or reasoning, verbal communication, personal safety, hygiene or nutrition neglect, and coordination and balance (Alzheimer's Association, 2019). 342,000 Australians live with dementia. This number is estimated to increase to 400,000 within the next 10 years (Alzheimer's Association, 2019).

The general symptoms of dementia are (Alzheimer's Association, 2019):

- Repeatedly asking the same questions
- Becoming lost or disoriented in familiar places
- Being unable to follow directions
- Getting disoriented as to the date or time of day
- Not recognising and being confused about familiar people
- Having difficulty with routine tasks such as paying the bills
- Neglecting personal safety, hygiene and nutrition. Dementia is one of the nine National Health Priority.

Areas identified by the Australian government. For more information on dementia in Australia, see www.aihw.gov.au/dementia.

Alzheimer disease, the most common dementia of the elderly, results from gradual destruction of brain nerve cells and a shrinking brain. Symptoms resemble general dementia symptoms but include loss of recent memory, depression, anxiety, personality changes, unpredictable quirks or behaviours, and problems with language, calculation and abstract thinking. Late in the disease, delusions and hallucinations can occur.

Vascular dementia (multi-infarct dementia) results from small strokes or brain blood supply changes usually caused by blood clots in small vessels (Alzheimer's Association, 2019). Brain location causes variation in symptoms and the symptoms may have a sudden onset. Wandering or getting lost in familiar surroundings; moving with rapid, shuffling steps; loss of bladder or bowel control; laughing or crying inappropriately; difficulty following instructions; and problems handling money are characteristic. This dementia has no cure and is not reversible.

A person can have mixed dementia. Other diseases that may have a dementia component or symptoms similar to dementia include Pick disease, Creutzfeldt–Jakob disease, Huntington disease, Parkinson disease and Lewy body disease, as well as other central nervous system conditions, systemic conditions (nutrition, fever, hormone, poisoning-related), substance abuse, and psychological stress and psychosis.

Ageing has common forms of decline that are often *mistaken* for dementia or resemble dementia. These include slower thinking, problem solving, learning and recall; decreased attention and concentration; more distractedness; and need for hints to jog memory.

Risk factors

- Vascular, cerebrovascular or cardiovascular disease including the development of cerbro vascular accident
- Type 2 diabetes mellitus cardiac disease and hypertension, especially with metabolic syndrome factors: abdominal obesity, hyperchylomicromaemia, low levels of high-density lipoproteins (HDL), hypertension and hyperglycaemia
- Physical, intellectual, social and nutritional habits
- Age; slightly higher in females over 80 years old
- Obesity (especially abdominal) and for obese cigarette smokers

- Genetics, but it is not well understood how diet and environment interact with genetics
- Gait disturbances may correlate with early dementia
- Diet, especially high cholesterol
- Environment, especially heavy metals
- Cigarette smoking
- Alcohol consumption

Teach risk reduction tips

- Consult primary care provider to control vascular, cerebrovascular, cardiovascular diseases, especially including hypertension, diabetes mellitus type 2 and cardiac disease
- Maintain active engagement in mental, physical and social activities
- Eat a healthy diet avoiding high cholesterol and including a variety of fruits and vegetables

DEVELOPMENTAL LEVEL: PSYCHOSOCIAL STATUS

Determining the patient's developmental level is essential to complete the patient's portrait. You do not need to ask the patient additional questions unless major gaps in the data are found or clarification is needed. Instead, group and analyse the data obtained during the health history and compare them with normal developmental parameters (e.g. height, weight, Erikson's psychosocial developmental stages (David, 2014)). This requires integrating all that has been learned about the patient from their health history and using critical thinking to determine any developmental impairment. Standard growth charts can be used to determine physical development.

However, when assessing adults, the area most likely to yield delays or unresolved problems occurs in the psychosocial domain of development. Erikson developed a psychosocial theory that identifies opposing concepts for each developmental stage to describe growth from birth to death (Table 6-2). Although there are implied age ranges attached to these stages and it is hoped that a person might move through them in an orderly fashion, this does not always occur. Thus, it is important to look at the patient's behaviour rather than age to identify the stage of development relative to their age.

Strong indicators that the patient is functioning much below the usual behaviour for their age range may specify areas for possible diagnoses (e.g. developmental delay) and nursing intervention. Sometimes a person skips one or more developmental levels and, at a later stage of maturity, goes back and successfully works through the missed levels. A thorough knowledge of the behaviours and approximate age levels provides the nurse with a powerful tool for assessing and helping a patient grow to his or her full potential. Although the accomplishment of all of the tasks in the stage before moving on is ideal, it is believed that partial resolution is adequate for health, growth and development.

CASE STUDY

Psychosocial assessment

Jenny and Steve have been retired for 2 years. They have one daughter who is living overseas with her partner and their 6-month-old grandson.

CRITICAL THINKING

4. Where do you think Jenny is placed in Erikson's psychosocial developmental stages, and why?

The psychosocial developmental stages of the young adult, middle-aged adult and older adult are discussed in detail in the following section. Each section includes important questions to ask yourself about the patient to determine if he or she has accomplished all of the required tasks in a particular psychosocial developmental stage. If the adult patient does not seem even to have advanced psychologically to the intimacy versus isolation stage, refer to the earlier stages seen in children and adolescents, which are discussed in Chapter 33.

Table 6-2 Erik H. Erikson's psychosocial developmental levels

Developmental level	Basic task	Negative counterpart	Basic virtues
1. Infant	Basic trust	Basic mistrust	Drive and hope
2. Toddler	Autonomy	Shame and doubt	Self-control and will power
3. Preschooler	Initiative	Guilt	Direction and purpose
4. Schoolager	Industry	Inferiority	Method and competence
5. Adolescent	Identity	Role confusion	Devotion and fidelity
6. Young adult	Intimacy	Isolation	Affiliation and love
7. Middlescent	Generativity	Stagnation	Production and care
8. Older adult	Ego-integrity	Despair	Renunciation and wisdom

Adapted from Erikson's Stages of Personality Development, from *Childhood and society* by Erik H. Erikson. Copyright 1950, © 1963 by W.W. Norton & Company, Inc., renewed © 1978, 1991, by Erik H. Erikson.

ASSESSMENT OF ERIKSON'S STAGES (1991) OF PSYCHOSOCIAL DEVELOPMENT

ASSESSMENT PROCEDURE	NORMAL FINDINGS	ABNORMAL FINDINGS
Determine the patient's psychosocial developmental level by answering the following questions. If you do not have enough data to answer these questions, you may need to ask the patient additional questions or make further observations.		
Does the young adult • Accept self—physically, cognitively and emotionally? • Have independence from the parental home? • Express love responsibly, emotionally and sexually? • Have close or intimate relationships with a partner? • Have a social group of friends? • Have a philosophy of living and life? • Have a profession or a life's work that provides a means of contribution? • Solve problems of life that accompany independence from the parental home?	**Intimacy** The young adult should have achieved self-efficacy during adolescence and is now ready to open up and become intimate with others. Although this stage focuses on the desire for a special and permanent love relationship, it also includes the ability to have close, caring relationships with friends of both sexes and a variety of ages. Spiritual love also develops during this stage. Having established an identity apart from the childhood family, the young adult is now able to form adult friendships with his or her parents and siblings. However, the young adult will always be a son or daughter.	**Isolation** If the young adult cannot express emotion and trust enough to open up to others, social and emotional isolation may occur. Loneliness may cause the young adult to turn to addictive behaviours such as alcoholism, drug abuse or sexual promiscuity. Some people try to cope with this developmental stage by becoming very spiritual or social, playing an acceptable role, but never fully sharing who they are or becoming emotionally involved with others. When adults successfully navigate this stage, they have stable and satisfying relationships with important others.
Does the middle-aged adult • Have healthful life patterns? • Derive satisfaction from contributing to the growth and development of others? • Have an abiding intimacy and long-term relationship with a partner? • Maintain a stable home? • Find pleasure in an established work or profession? • Take pride in self and family accomplishments and contributions? • Contribute to the community to support its growth and development?	**Generativity** During this stage, the middle-aged adult is able to share self with others and establish nurturing relationships. The adult will be able to extend self and possessions to others. Although traditionalists tend to think of generativity in terms of raising one's children and guiding their lives, generativity can be realised in several ways even without having children. Generativity implies mentoring and giving to future generations. This can be accomplished by producing ideas, products, inventions, paintings, writings, books, films or any other creative endeavours that are then given to the world for the unrestricted use of its people. Generativity also includes teaching others, children or adults, mentoring young workers or providing experience and wisdom to assist a new business to survive and grow. Also implied in this stage is the ability to guide, then let go of one's creations. Successful movement through this stage results in a fuller and more satisfying life and prepares the mature adult for the next stage.	**Stagnation** Without this important step, the gift is not given and the stage does not come to successful completion. Stagnation occurs when the middle-aged person has not accomplished one or more of the previous developmental tasks and is unable to give to future generations. Sometimes severe losses may result in withdrawal and stagnation. In these cases, the person may have total dependency on work, a favourite child or even a pet, and be incapable of giving to others. A project may never be finished or schooling completed because the person cannot let go and move on. Without a creative outlet, a paralysing stagnation sets in.
Does the older adult • Adjust to the changing physical self? • Recognise changes present as a result of ageing, in relationships and activities? • Maintain relationships with children, grandchildren and other relatives? • Continue interests outside of self and home?	**Integrity** According to Erikson (1950), a person in this stage looks back and either finds that life was good or despairs because goals were not accomplished. This stage can extend over a long time and include excursions into previous stages to complete unfinished business. Successful movement through this stage does not mean that one day a person wakes up and says, 'My life has been good'; rather,	**Despair** If the older person cannot feel grateful for his or her life, cannot accept those less desirable aspects as merely part of living or cannot integrate all of the experiences of life, then the person will spend his or her last days in bitterness and regret and will ultimately die in despair.

ASSESSMENT OF ERIKSON'S STAGES (1991) OF PSYCHOSOCIAL DEVELOPMENT (continued)

ASSESSMENT PROCEDURE	NORMAL FINDINGS	ABNORMAL FINDINGS
• Complete transition from retirement at work to satisfying alternative activities? • Establish relationships with others who are his or her own age? • Adjust to deaths of relatives, spouse and friends? • Maintain a maximum level of physical functioning through diet, exercise and personal care? • Find meaning in past life and face inevitable mortality of self and significant others? • Integrate philosophical or religious values into self-understanding to promote comfort? • Review accomplishments and recognise meaningful contributions he or she has made to community and relatives?	it encompasses a series of reminiscences in which the person may be able to see past events in a new and more positive light. This can be a very rich and rewarding time in a person's life, especially if there are others with whom to share memories and who can assist with reframing life experiences (Fig. 6-6). For some people, resolution and acceptance do not come until the final weeks of life, but this still allows for a peaceful death.	

CLINICAL TIP
Erikson's Psychosocial Developmental Stages are based on ego development with distinct conflicts (indicated as 'Normal findings' and 'Abnormal findings' in this section) across the lifespan. These stages are a lifelong process and may overlap each other.

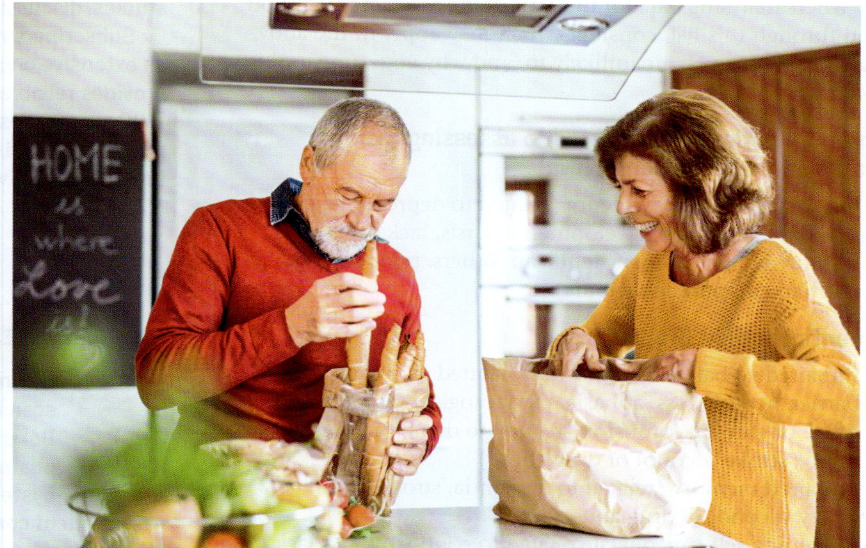

FIGURE 6-6 Older adulthood can be a rich and rewarding time to review life events. (Shutterstock.com/Halfpoint)

VALIDATING AND DOCUMENTING FINDINGS

Validate the mental status and psychosocial assessment data you have collected. This is necessary to verify that the data are reliable and accurate. Document the data following health care facility or agency policy.

CLINICAL TIP
When documenting your assessment findings, it is better to describe the patient's response than to label his or her behaviour.

Sample of subjective data

Mr X is concerned about forgetting students' names in his class over the past semester. Also misplaces objects more frequently than in the past. Concerned this will impair his abilities as a teacher. Memory loss and misplacing things increase as the day progresses. No history of stroke, meningitis or head injury. No family history of Alzheimer disease. Brother had bipolar disorder. Is able to perform normal activities of daily living but is finding it more difficult to concentrate on grading maths papers at night time. Becomes tired more quickly than in the past. Awakens two times a night but is able to go back to sleep within 30 minutes. Reports good appetite and normal bowel routine. Active in his community. Positive about current daily activities, including work, exercise and leisure. Expressed positive relationships with wife and children.

Sample of objective data

Mental status: Alert and oriented to person, place, day and time. Provided correct biographical information regarding: age (54 years), address and marital status (married). Holds a master's degree in education. Teaches Year 6 mathematics. Clean and well-groomed appearance. Good eye contact, with pleasant, cooperative disposition. Speech clear with moderate tone. Appears anxious over forgetting names and location of objects. Looking forward to retirement in about 8 years. Able to name familiar objects in examination room. Expresses clear, realistic, logical thought processes about the past and future. Recalls what he ate for breakfast and past dates of family members' birthdays. Repeated four unrelated words after 5 minutes, repeated one after 10 minutes, unable to repeat after a further 10 minutes. Explained what to do in an emergency situation in the classroom. Correctly drew the face of a clock. Scored 28 on the Mini–Mental State Examination (MMSE). Appears to have reached the psychosocial development level of 'generativity'. Expressed enjoyment and satisfaction in roles as husband, father, grandfather, teacher and church member.

Analysis of data

After collecting subjective and objective data pertaining to a general survey and vital signs, identify abnormal findings and the patient's strengths. Then cluster the data to reveal any significant patterns or abnormalities. These data may then be used to make clinical judgements about the patient.

DIAGNOSTIC REASONING: POSSIBLE CONCLUSIONS

Some possible conclusions related to the mental status examination and the assessment of the patient's psychosocial developmental level are discussed in the following text.

Below is a list of potential risks or problems you may identify when analysing data for this part of the assessment. As you read through this list, consider which may apply in the above example, and which are unlikely to, and why you came to this conclusion.

Potential patient risks related to assessing mental status and developmental level

- Risk of self-directed violence (related to depression, suicidal tendencies, developmental crisis, lack of support systems, loss of significant others, poor coping mechanisms and behaviours)

Potential patient problems

- Impaired verbal communication (related to language barrier, hearing loss, aphasia, psychological impairment)
- Acute or chronic confusion (related to dementia, head injury, stroke, alcohol or drug abuse)
- Impaired memory (related to dementia, stroke, head injury, alcohol or drug abuse)
- Grooming self-care deficit (related to confusion and lack of resources or support from carers)
- Disturbed thought processes (related to alcohol or drug abuse, psychotic disorder or organic brain dysfunction)
- Social isolation (related to inability to relate or communicate effectively with others)

Selected collaborative problems

After you group the data, it may become apparent that certain collaborative problems emerge. Remember that collaborative problems differ from nursing assessment in that they cannot be prevented by nursing interventions. However, these physiological complications of medical conditions can be detected and monitored by the nurse. In addition, the nurse can use doctor-and-nurse–prescribed interventions to minimise the complications of these problems. The nurse may also have to refer the patient in such situations for further treatment of the problem. Following is a list of collaborative problems that may be identified when obtaining a general impression:

- Stroke
- Increased intracranial pressure
- Seizures
- Meningitis
- Depression.

Medical problems

After you group the data, it may become apparent that the patient has signs and symptoms that require psychiatric or medical diagnosis and treatment. Refer to an appropriate specialist as necessary.

ONLINE RESOURCES

An extensive range of additional resources to enhance teaching and learning and to facilitate understanding may be found online at the text's accompanying website, located on thePoint at http://thepoint.lww.com. These include Watch and Learn videos, Concepts in Action animations, journal articles, case studies, discussion topics and quizzes.

Subscribers may also access Lippincott Procedures, an extensive online point-of-care procedure guide that provides reliable step-by-step instructions for more than 1700 procedures, including 450 evidence-based Australian procedures, and skills in a variety of speciality settings, together with a wealth of supporting information.

SIMULATED LEARNING

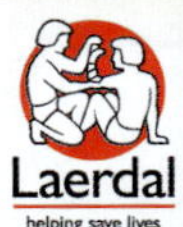

Having completed this chapter, explore the scenarios of Doris Bowman Parts 1 and 2. Doris is a 39-year-old female who is postoperative following a total abdominal hysterectomy. Incorporating the health assessment content in this chapter with your existing theoretical knowledge and clinical experience, progress through the simulation scenarios (this is best done in a small group). How would you manage Doris's care? When reflecting on your management of Doris, what do you think you did well and what do you think you can improve? Consider why you think this and also how you might manage a similar problem in the future.

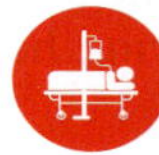

Throughout this chapter you have considered the case of Jenny Wilson, who has been experiencing sleeping difficulties, loss of appetite and a general feeling of anxiety. She has also had trouble concentrating. In the simulation scenario based on Jenny and available to your lecturer online, you will continue to assess Jenny in a simulated encounter. In this simulation you will be using the mental status assessment tools described in this chapter.

CASE STUDY

The case study demonstrates how to analyse mental and psychosocial assessment data for a specific patient. The critical thinking exercises included in the ancillary product on thePoint that complements this text also offer opportunities to analyse assessment data.

Jenny Wilson, a 61-year-old female, has come to the local family clinic where you work. She is accompanied by her husband Steve. When you ask her the reason for her visit she states, 'I am very nervous and not thinking straight.' She sits quietly, slumped over in her chair and often wrings her hands. Her face is expressionless, with minimal eye contact given. You notice that her hair appears unwashed and her clothes are ill fitting. Steve says he is worried about her because she doesn't leave the house much anymore.

Jenny reports sleep difficulties, loss of appetite and a general feeling of anxiety. When asked about her daily routine she tells you she is unable to concentrate and has a hard time completing actvities. She reports feeling confused, tired and depressed. She denies any plans to hurt herself.

Jenny Wilson is 170 cm centimetres tall and weighs 56 kg kilograms. Her vital signs are temperature 36.8 °C, pulse 82, respirations 18, and blood pressure 100/62 mmHg. She does not appear to be in any physical distress. Her gait is steady and strong.

Jenny appears to be alert and oriented to person, place, time and situation. However, you find you have to repeat questions because she is having difficulty concentrating. Her responses are brief and low in volume. She sometimes looks to her husband for reassurance. She is unable to recall recent events, including what she ate for dinner last night.

Jenny and Steve have been retired for 2 years. They have one daughter who is living overseas with her partner and their 6-month-old grandson.

The following concept map illustrates the diagnostic reasoning process.

Applying COLDSPA

COLDSPA can be used to explore the patient's symptoms of 'anxiety and confusion' as illustrated below.

Mnemonic	Question	Data provided	Missing data
Character	Describe the sign or symptom (feeling, appearance, sound, smell or taste, if applicable).	'Very nervous and not thinking straight.' Patient sits quietly and often wrings her hands. Dishevelled appearance, expressionless face and minimal eye contact.	
Onset	When did it begin?		When did these feelings first occur?
Location	Where is it? Does it radiate? Does it occur anywhere else?		Is there any place that you can feel calm or safe?
Duration	How long does it last? Does it recur?		Have these feelings been consistent since the onset?
Severity	How bad is it? How much does it bother you?	Difficulty sleeping, concentrating and completing chores. Unable to recall recent events from the day before.	
Pattern	What makes it better or worse?	Does not leave the house much anymore and has difficulty sleeping. Questions to her need to be repeated.	When do you feel most anxious? Is there anything that relieves or intensifies your feelings?
Associated factors/How it **A**ffects the patient	What other symptoms occur with it? How does it affect you?	Patient reports feeling confused, tired, depressed and generally anxious, with a loss of appetite.	

1) Identify abnormal findings and patient strengths

Subjective data

- 'I'm very nervous and not thinking straight'
- Reports sleep difficulties, loss of appetite and a general feeling of anxiety
- Tells you she is unable to concentrate and has a hard time completing household chores
- Reports feeling confused, tired and depressed
- Denies any plans to hurt herself
- Her husband informs you that she used to never leave the house without makeup and accessories, so he is worried about her

Objective data

- 61-year-old Caucasian female
- Appropriately dressed for the season and situation
- Looks pale and thin, appears stated age, hair dishevelled, not wearing jewellery or makeup
- Has very brief eye contact, often stares at the floor, face expressionless
- Wrings her hands often
- Appears alert and oriented to person, place, time and situation
- You have to repeat questions because she is having difficulty concentrating
- Speech is clear, but low in volume, and her responses are brief
- Sometimes looks at her husband for reassurance
- Unable to recall some recent events, including what she ate for dinner last night
- Unable to recall four objects 10 minutes after they were recited to her
- Able to answer remote memory questions
- 170 cm tall and weighs 56 kg
- Vital signs are tympanic temperature, 36.8°C; pulse, 82; respirations, 18; and blood pressure, 100/62 mmHg
- Does not appear to be in any physical distress
- Gait is steady and strong

2) Identify cue clusters

- Reports sleep difficulties, loss of appetite and a general feeling of anxiety
- Tells you she is unable to concentrate and has a hard time completing household chores
- You have to repeat questions because she is having difficulty concentrating
- Has very brief eye contact and often stares at the floor

- Reports sleep difficulties, loss of appetite and a general feeling of anxiety
- Reports feeling confused, tired and depressed
- Her husband informs you that she used to never leave the house without makeup and accessories, so he is worried about her
- Her hair is dishevelled and she is not wearing any jewellery or makeup
- Her face is expressionless
- She sits quietly, slumped over in her chair

- Reports loss of appetite
- Looks pale and thin
- 170 cm tall and weighs 56 kg

3) Draw inferences

Patient is nervous and experiencing anxiety related to an unknown cause.

Patient is possibly depressed. Refer to doctor for evaluation.

Patient may be undernourished.

4) List possible diagnoses

Anxiety

Imbalanced nutrition: less than body requirements

5) Check for defining characteristics

Major: Diminished productivity, insomnia, extraneous movement, scared, worried, apprehensive, confusion, impaired attention
Minor: Poor eye contact

Major: None
Minor: Aversion to eating

6) Confirm or rule out diagnoses

Confirm diagnosis because it meets the major and minor defining characteristics

Rule out at this time, but monitor patient's weight

7) Document conclusions

The following diagnosis is appropriate:
- Anxiety

Potential collaborative problems include the following:
- Risk of depression

References

Alzheimer's Association. (2019). Alzheimer's and dementia in Australia. Viewed October 2019 at https://www.alz.org/au/dementia-alzheimers-australia.asp#about.

American Psychiatric Association (APA). (2013). *Diagnostic and statistical manual of mental disorders* (5th ed.). Arlington, VA: American Psychiatric Publishing. (DSM-5).

David, L. (2014). Erikson's stages of development. Learning theories. Viewed October 2019 at https://www.learning-theories.com/eriksons-stages-of-development.html.

Erikson, E. H. (1950). *Childhood and society*. New York: Norton.

Erikson, E. H. (1963). *Childhood and society* (2nd ed.). New York: Norton.

Folstein, M. F., Folstein, S. E. & McHugh, P. R. (1975). Mini-mental state: A practical guide for grading the cognitive state of patients for the clinician. *Journal of Psychiatric Research, 12*(3), 189–198.

Folstein, M. F., Anthony, J., Parhad, I., Duffy, B. & Gruenberg, E. (1985). The meaning of cognitive impairment in the elderly. *Journal of the American Geriatrics Society, 33*, 228–235.

Kessler, R. C. & Mroczek, D. (1994). Final version of our Non-specific Psychological Distress Scale [memo dated 10/3/94]. Ann Arbort (MI): Survey Research Center of the Institute for Social Research. University of Michigan.

Kessler, R. C., Andrews, G., Colpe, L., et al. (2002). Short screening scales to monitor population prevalence and trends in non-specific psychological distress. *Psychological Medicine, 32*, 959–976.

Kessler, R. C., Barker, P. R., Colpe, L. J., Epstein, J. F., Gfroerer, J. C., Hiripi, E., et al. (2003). Screening for serious mental illness in the general population. *Archives of General Psychiatry, 60*(2), 184–189.

Rush, A. J., Trivedi, M. H., Ibrahim, H. M., Carmody, T. J., Arnow, B., Klein, D. N., et al. (2003). The 16-item Quick Inventory of Depressive Symptomatology (QIDS) Clinician Rating (QIDS-C) and Self-Report (QIDS-SR): A psychometric evaluation in patients with chronic major depression. *Biological Psychiatry, 54*, 573–583.

Stephan, B. C. M. (2014). Risk factors and screening methods for detecting dementia: A narrative review. *Journal of Alzheimer's Disease, 42*, S329–S338.

Teasdale, G. & Jennett, B. (1974). Assessment of coma and impaired consciousness: A practical scale (later called the 'Glasgow Coma Scale'). *Lancet, 2*(7872), 81–84.

Wing, J. K., Beevor, A. S., Curtis, R. H., Park, S. B. G., Hadden, S. & Burns, A. (1998). Health of the Nation Outcome Scales (HoNOS): Research and development. *British Journal of Psychiatry, 172*, 11–18.

Selected reading

Dementia Australia. (2017). Vascular dementia. Available at https://www.dementia.org.au/about-dementia/types-of-dementia/vascular-dementia.

Online resources

Alzheimer's Australia: www.fightdementia.org.au

Alzheimer's New Zealand: www.alzheimers.org.nz

Australian Mental Health Outcomes and Classification Network: www.amhocn.org

Dementia Australia: https://www.dementia.org.au/about-dementia/what-is-dementia/progression-of-dementia

National Health Priority Areas: www.aihw.gov.au/national-health-priority-areas

Te Pou o Te Whakaaro Nui: The National Centre of Mental Health Research, Information and Workforce Development, New Zealand: www.tepou.co.nz

World Health Organization: https://www.who.int/features/factfiles/mental_health/en/

CHAPTER 7

Assessing general status and vital signs

Assessing the status of an individual and completing their vital signs is best accomplished when the context of the person is known. In this chapter you will consider Mr Stephen Lucas and you will notice that the assessment begins with personal information.

CASE STUDY

Stephen Lucas is a 47-year-old male who has been admitted to the neurology ward after a transient ischaemic attack. He has a history of hypertension and atrial fibrillation that was diagnosed 2 years ago and has been controlled with enalapril and digoxin. Mr Lucas has six-monthly appointments with his general practitioner to ensure his scripts are filled. He is happily married to his wife of 25 years and has three children. Mr Lucas is a carpenter, is physically active and eats a healthy diet. Mrs Lucas recently lost her job and money has been 'a bit tight'; however, she starts a new job next week.

Structure and function

The general survey is the first part of the physical examination that begins the moment the nurse meets the patient. It requires nurses to use all of their observational skills while interviewing and interacting with patients. These observations will lead to clues about a patient's health status. The outcome of the general survey provides the nurse with an overall impression of the patient's wellbeing. The general survey includes observation of the patient's:

- Level of consciousness and orientation (Glasgow Coma Scale score; see Assessment tool 6-4)
- Skin condition and colour
- Vital signs (including pain and oxygen saturation)
- Speech
- Apparent age as compared with reported age
- Facial expression
- Behaviours, body movements and affect
- Dress and hygiene
- Posture and gait
- Physical development and body build
- Gender and sexual development.

The patient's vital signs are indicators of health. Usually when a vital sign is abnormal, something is wrong in at least one body system. Traditionally, vital signs have included the patient's temperature, pulse, respirations and blood pressure. Today, 'pain' is an essential part of vital signs assessment; however, there are risks associated with pain scores used in isolation (Solodiuk & Curley, 2017). The quality of the pain and its impact on daily life must also be assessed. Pain is inexpensive to assess and does not involve the use of fancy instruments, yet it can be an early predictor of impending disability that might have an impact on the patient's ability to function. For example, early assessment of a patient's chest pain may promote early treatment and prevention of complications and the high cost of cardiovascular damage and heart failure. Assessment of pain is discussed in Chapter 8. In addition, oxygen saturations are assessed as a vital sign in most clinical areas where hypoxaemia may occur, and level of consciousness is now commonly assessed in the clinical area.

CASE STUDY

Mrs Lucas tells you that she saw her husband fall to the ground and not wake up for 4 minutes. Mr Lucas recalls talking with his wife one minute and waking up in hospital the next. He says, 'I usually take my medication every day, but I stopped taking it five days ago as I just didn't get around to fulfilling the script and it didn't seem to help.' He also says: 'I've had a headache for 24 hours. I woke up with it yesterday morning. I have taken regular pain relief and last took some Panadol about 2 hours ago. I've got no problems with my vision but can feel my heart racing and have numbness in my fingers.' Mr Lucas points to the middle of his head as he describes his pain.

He looks flushed in the face; his temperature is 36.8 °C; and his heart rate is 155 beats/minute and irregular. He has a respiratory rate of 20 breaths/minute; his blood pressure is 195/105 mmHg; and his oxygen saturations are 99% on room air. On a scale of 0 to 10 (with 10 being the worst pain imaginable), Mr Lucas rates his headache as a 6 and he describes it as an ache that worries him. He is 190 cm tall, weighs 85 kg, is talking clearly, is dressed appropriately for the weather, looks his age, is clean and well groomed, and has a steady gait. He is alert and oriented.

He is currently awaiting a computed tomography scan and a carotid ultrasound. He now understands how important it is to take his medications.

CRITICAL THINKING

1. Identify cue clusters that relate to Mr Lucas's admission to hospital, and draw inferences on his general status, particularly in relation to his:
   - Onset of pain
   - Non-compliance with medications
   - Risk factors
   - Diagnosis.

OVERALL IMPRESSION OF THE PATIENT

The first time you meet a patient, you tend to remember certain obvious characteristics. Forming an overall impression consists of a systematic approach to the examination and recording these general characteristics and impressions of the patient. If possible, try to observe the patient and environment quickly before interacting with him or her. This gives you the opportunity to 'see' the patient before he or she assumes a social face or behaviour and allows you to glimpse any distress, sadness or pain before the patient (knowingly or unknowingly) masks it.

When you initially meet the patient, observe any significant abnormalities in the patient's skin colour, dress, hygiene, posture and gait, physical development, body build, apparent age and gender. Abnormalities may also be seen when assessing the patient's level of comfort, behaviour, body movements, affect, facial expression, speech and mental acuities. If your observations give you cause for concern, you will need to perform an in-depth assessment of the body area that appears to be affected. An unusual gait may prompt you to perform a detailed musculoskeletal assessment, or if a patient is showing behavioural or mental acuity changes, an in-depth mental status examination can be performed (as described in Chap. 6). Additional preparation involves creating a comfortable, non-threatening environment to relieve any anxiety the patient may have.

VITAL SIGNS

The nurse usually begins the 'hands-on' physical examination by taking vital signs. This is a common, non-invasive physical assessment procedure that most patients are accustomed to. Vital signs provide data that reflect the status of the cardiovascular, neurological, peripheral vascular and respiratory systems. When measuring the patient's vital signs it is important to explain to the patient what you are going to do, how long it is going to take and for the patient to remain as still as possible. This explanation can put the patient's mind at ease, decrease any anxiety he or she may have and help increase the accuracy of the data you are taking (as pulse, respirations and blood pressure are all influenced by anxiety and activity).

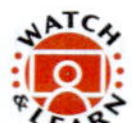

Measuring Oral Temperature, Radial Pulse, Apical Pulse, Respiratory Rate and Blood Pressure

Temperature

For the body to function on a cellular level, a core body temperature between 36.5°C and 37.7°C must be maintained. A core body temperature reading is accurate compared with taking a peripheral body temperature; however, it is more invasive. Core body temperatures are generally taken in critically ill patients and involve placing a temperature probe into the patient—for example, into their nasogastric tube, urinary catheter or pulmonary artery catheter. A peripheral body temperature, although less accurate, is more commonly used, allows for an approximate core temperature reading and simply is a good reflection of the core body temperature. A tympanic temperature (35.8°C to 38°C) is one of the most common sites to perform a temperature reading in the clinical setting, but temperature can be also be measured in the axilla (34.7°C to 37.3°C) or orally (35.5°C to 37.5°C). Although the rectal route is an accurate method for taking a temperature (as it is the closest to the core body temperature), it is not routinely performed. Several factors may cause normal variations in core body temperature. Strenuous exercise, stress, thyroid hormones and ovulation can raise the temperature, so too can the circadian rhythm, where the body temperature is lowest early in the morning (4 a.m. to 6 a.m.) and highest late in the evening (8 p.m. to midnight). Drinking a warm or cold drink or even smoking can also vary a patient's temperature. Hypothermia (lower than 35°C) may be seen in prolonged exposure to the cold, hypoglycaemia, hypothyroidism or starvation. Hyperthermia (higher than 38°C) may be seen in viral or bacterial infections, malignancies, trauma and various blood, endocrine and immune disorders.

OLDER ADULT CONSIDERATIONS

In the older adult, the temperature may range from 35°C to 36.4°C. Therefore, the older patient may not have an obviously elevated temperature with an infection or be considered hypothermic below 35.6°C.

PAEDIATRIC CONSIDERATIONS

A normal temperature range for a child is usually 37°C and up to 38°C. Unless you are using a tympanic thermometer specifically designed for children less than 3 years old, a digital or electronic thermometer under the arm is the safest way to take an infant's or toddler's temperature.

Pulse

When the heart contracts and forcefully pumps blood out of the ventricles into the aorta, a pulse can be felt. It is commonly called the *arterial pulse* or *peripheral pulse*. The body has many arterial pulse sites, some of which can be felt at the radial, brachial, temporal, carotid, apical, femoral and pedal sites (see Chap. 23 for more sites). The radial pulse gives a good overall picture of the patient's health status. Several characteristics should be assessed when measuring a pulse—the rate, rhythm, amplitude and contour, and elasticity. Amplitude can be quantified by the Pulse Amplitude Scale as follows:

0 Absent
1+ Weak
2+ Normal
3+ Increased
4+ Bounding.

If abnormalities are noted during assessment of the radial pulse, further assessment should be performed. For more information on assessing pulses and abnormal pulse findings, refer to Chapters 22 and 23.

PAEDIATRIC CONSIDERATIONS

The following ranges are considered normal pulse ranges for the paediatric patient:

- **3 months to 2 years: 80 to 150 beats/minute**
- **2 to 10 years: 70 to 110 beats/minute**
- **10 years and above: 55 to 90 beats/minute.**

Respirations

The respiratory rate and character are additional clues to the patient's overall health status. Respirations can be easily observed without alerting the patient by watching chest movement before removing the stethoscope after you have completed counting the apical beat. Notable characteristics of respirations are rate, rhythm and depth (see Chap. 20 for more information about respirations).

PAEDIATRIC CONSIDERATIONS

The following ranges are considered normal respiratory rate ranges for the paediatric patient:

- **6 months to 2 years: 20 to 30 breaths/minute**
- **3 to 10 years: 20 to 28 breaths/minute**
- **10 to 18 years: 12 to 20 breaths/minute.**

Blood pressure

Blood pressure reflects the pressure exerted on the walls of the arteries. This pressure varies with the cardiac cycle, reaching a high point with systole and a low point with diastole (Fig. 7-1). Therefore, blood pressure is a measurement of the pressure of the blood in the arteries when the ventricles are contracted (systolic blood pressure) and when the ventricles are relaxed (diastolic blood pressure). Blood pressure is expressed as the ratio of the systolic pressure over the diastolic pressure. A patient's blood pressure is affected by several factors:

- *Cardiac output*—Blood pressure increases with increased cardiac output and decreases with decreased cardiac output.
- *Distensibility of the arteries*—Blood pressure increases when more effort is required to push blood through stiffened arteries.
- *Blood volume*—Blood pressure increases with increased volume and decreases with decreased volume.
- *Blood velocity*—Blood pressure increases when blood flow is slowed because of resistance; it decreases when blood flow meets no resistance.
- *Blood viscosity (thickness)*—Blood pressure increases when the blood is thickened; it decreases with thinning of the blood.

A patient's blood pressure will normally vary throughout the day because of external influences. These include the time of day, caffeine or nicotine intake, exercise, emotions, pain and temperature (see Display 7-1). The size of cuff can also affect the accuracy of the blood pressure reading. The difference between systolic and diastolic pressure is termed the *pulse pressure.* The pulse pressure can be determined after the blood pressure is measured because it reflects the stroke volume—the volume of blood ejected with each heartbeat.

Blood pressure may also vary depending on the positions of the body and the arm. Blood pressure in a normal person who is standing is usually slightly higher to compensate for the effects of gravity. Blood pressure in a normal reclining person is slightly lower because of decreased resistance. A postural drop occurs if a patient's blood pressure drops by 20 mmHg from the sitting to standing position.

CLINICAL TIP

You should always avoid taking a blood pressure using a patient's arm if:

- **The patient has intravenous therapy because the pressure may cause pain or extravasation of the fluid, or**
- **The patient has had a mastectomy or suffers from lymphoedema, or**
- **The patient has an arteriovenous fistula or graft for haemodialysis.**

PAEDIATRIC CONSIDERATIONS

Systolic

The following ranges are considered normal systolic blood pressure ranges for the paediatric patient:

- **1 to 7 years = Age in years + 90**
- **8 to 18 years = (2 × age in years) + 90**

Diastolic

- **1 to 5 years = 56**
- **6 to 18 years = Age in years + 52**

See also Table 33-12 on blood pressure levels for girls and boys.

Pulse oximetry

Pulse oximetry is now considered to be a routine observation in the clinical setting. It can be used to monitor and detect the patient's oxygen saturation and is particularly important in detecting patient deterioration. Pulse oximetry should be measured when a patient requires oxygen therapy, has difficulty breathing, is cyanotic, is agitated or is at risk of oxygen desaturation. Infrared and red light are absorbed by haemoglobin and the reading depends on whether the haemoglobin

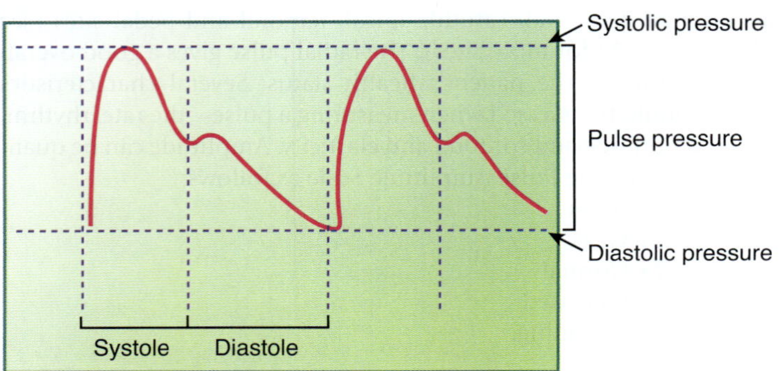

FIGURE 7-1 Blood pressure measurement identifies the amount of pressure in the arteries when the ventricles of the heart contract (systole) and when they relax (diastole).

DISPLAY 7-1 FACTORS CONTRIBUTING TO BLOOD PRESSURE

1. Cardiac output. The more blood the heart pumps, the greater the pressure in the blood vessels. For example, blood pressure increases during exercise.

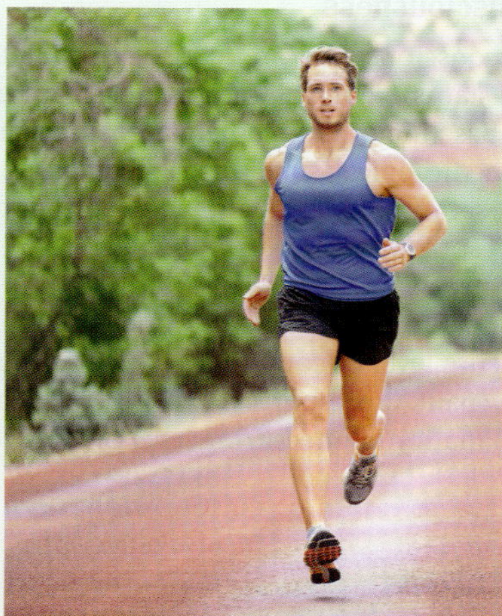

(Shutterstock.com/Maridav.)

2. Peripheral vascular resistance. An increase in resistance in the peripheral vascular system, as happens with people who have circulatory disorders, will increase blood pressure.

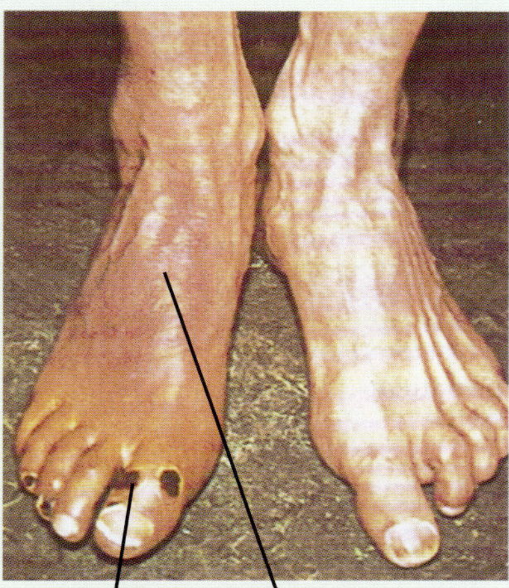

3. Circulating blood volume. An increase in volume will increase blood pressure. A sudden drop in blood pressure may indicate a sudden blood loss, as with internal bleeding.

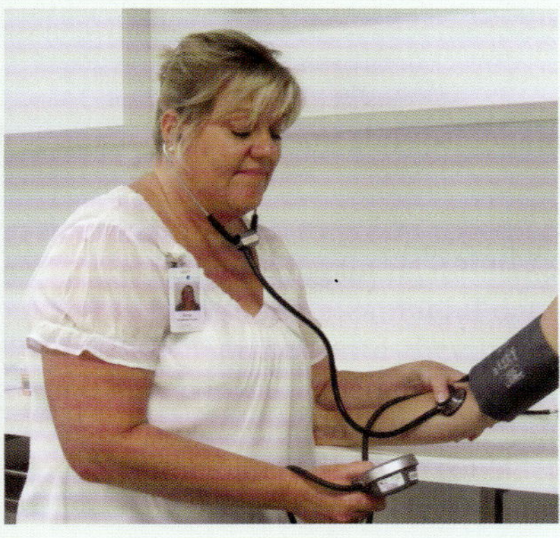

4. Viscosity. When the blood becomes thicker or more viscous (as with polycythaemia), the pressure in the blood vessels will increase.

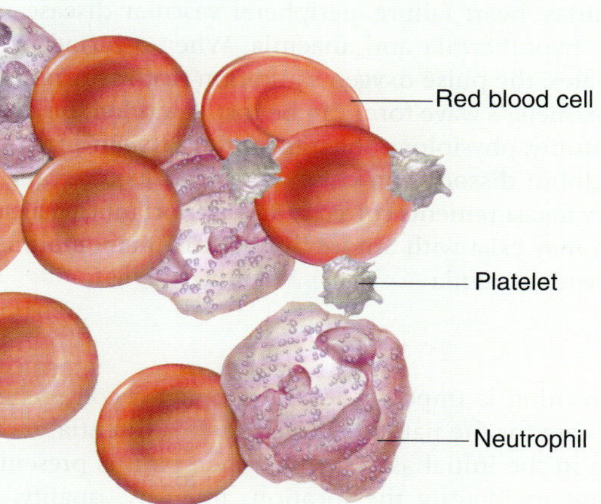

Densely packed red blood cells

5. Elasticity of vessel walls. An increase in stiffness of the vessel walls (e.g. atherosclerotic changes) will increase blood pressure.

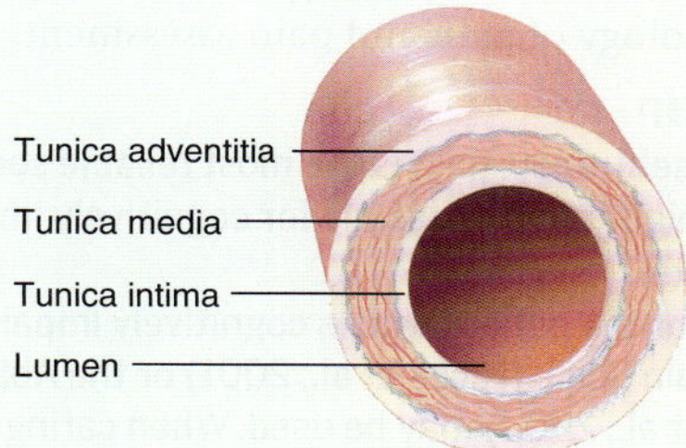

Normal coronary artery

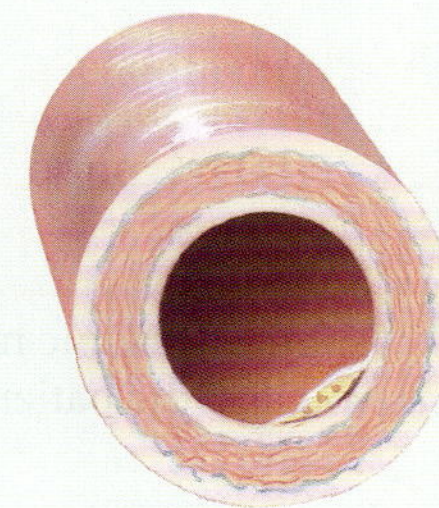

Fatty streak

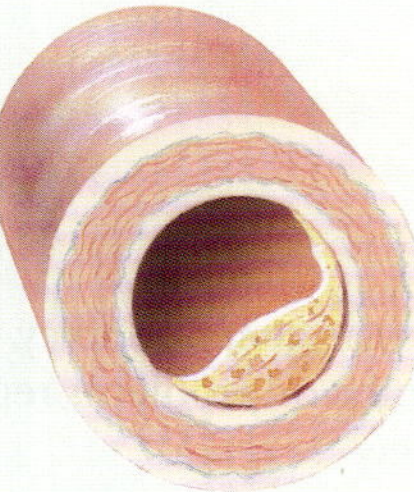

Fibrous plaque

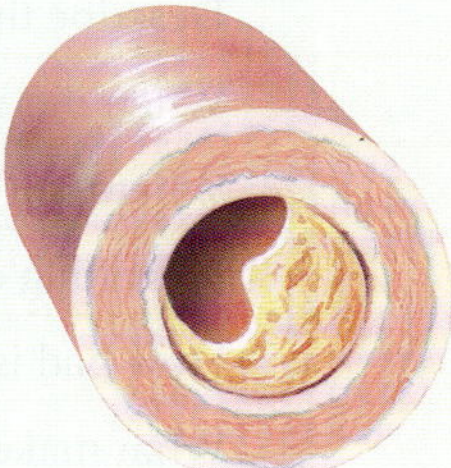

Complicated plaque

is saturated (oxygenated) or unsaturated (deoxygenated) with oxygen.

Pulse oximetry may be inaccurate because of several factors including, but not limited to, movement, bright light, nail polish, carbon monoxide poisoning, weak arterial pulse, arrhythmias, heart failure, peripheral vascular disease, hypotension, hypothermia and anaemia. When a blood pressure cuff inflates, the pulse oxygen saturation reading can decrease or the oximeter's wave form can be lost. Knowledge of respiratory anatomy, physiology, the transport of oxygen and the oxyhaemoglobin dissociation curve is needed to interpret pulse oximetry measurements correctly. It is important to realise that hypoxia may exist with a normal pulse oximetry reading in a patient with anaemia

Pain

Pain screening is important in developing a comprehensive plan of care for the patient. Therefore, it is essential to assess for pain in the initial assessment. When pain is present, it is important to identify the location, intensity, quality, duration and any alleviating or aggravating factors. Pain intensity measurement tools such as a 0 to 10 Likert scale (described in Chap. 8) may be used. Pain quality may be described as 'dull', 'sharp', 'radiating' or 'throbbing'. The mnemonic device 'COLDSPA' may help you to remember how to further assess pain if present (see below). Chapter 8 provides in-depth information on the aetiology of pain and pain assessment.

CLINICAL TIP

The ability to self-report pain is the most reliable source; however, doing so might not be possible for cognitively impaired or paediatric patients.

When caring for the patient who is cognitively impaired, the revised Faces Pain Scale (Hicks et al., 2001) or the Abbey Pain Scale (Abbey et al., 2004) may be used. When caring for the paediatric patient, the Faces Legs Activity Cry and Consolability (FLACC) scale (Merkel et al., 1997) is best used for neonates and infants. For children, the Faces Pain Scale and Wong–Baker Faces Pain Rating Scale (www.wongbakerfaces.org) can be used. In both instances, asking the patient's main carer how the patient normally responds to pain is a good way to begin the assessment.

Level of consciousness

The level of consciousness can be assessed to detect changes in neurological status. Neurological observations are generally performed as a baseline or in an emergency situation so that rapid changes in neurological status can be detected. They include measuring a set of vital signs and then assessing eye opening, best verbal response and best motor response. Pupil response to light can also be assessed. This assessment is known as the Glasgow Coma Scale (Teasdale & Jennett, 1974). Another tool used to measure level of consciousness is the mnemonic AVPU (alert, voice, pain, unresponsive). Refer to Chapter 29 for a detailed explanation of measuring level of consciousness.

CRITICAL THINKING

2. Using the COLDSPA mnemonic, complete the following table relevant to Mr Lucas's admission.

Data provided	Missing data
Character	
Onset	
Location	
Duration	
Severity	
Pattern	
Associated factors/How it Affects the patient	

COLDSPA

Symptom analysis mnemonic

During the general survey, the COLDSPA mnemonic may be particularly helpful in exploring unusual signs and symptoms or problems reported, as you and the patient ask and answer various questions during the health history interview.

Mnemonic	Question
Character	Describe the sign or symptom (feeling, appearance, sound, smell or taste, if applicable).
Onset	When did it begin?
Location	Where is it? Does it radiate? Does it occur anywhere else?
Duration	How long does it last? Does it recur?
Severity	How bad is it? How much does it bother you?
Pattern	What makes it better or worse?
Associated factors/How it Affects the patient	What other symptoms occur with it? How does it affect you?

Initial health history

QUESTION	RATIONALE
General survey questions	
What are your name, address and telephone number?	Answers to these questions provide verifiable and accurate identification data about the patient. They also provide baseline information about level of consciousness, memory, speech patterns, articulation or speech defects. For example, a patient who is unable to answer these questions has cognitive or neurological deficits.
How old are you?	Establishes baseline for comparing appearance and development to chronological age.
History of present health concern	
Do you have any present health concerns?	This allows the patient to voice his or her concerns and provides a focus for the examination.
Have you had any high fevers that occur often or persistently?	A pattern of elevated temperatures may indicate a chronic infection or blood disorder such as leukaemia.
Have you noticed any alteration to your heartbeat or feeling like your heart is either racing or skipping beats?	Alterations in heartbeat felt by a patient are called palpitations and can be caused by various circumstances including thyroid dysfunction, medication reaction or alteration in fluid volume.
Are you having any difficulty breathing or trouble catching your breath? If so, does this occur at rest or with mild, moderate or strenuous exercise?	Difficulty with breathing or dyspnoea can be a sign of chronic heart failure, pneumonia, asthma, chronic obstructive pulmonary disease or other chronic lung disease.
Do you have any pain? If yes, describe the pain using the COLDSPA mnemonic. **Character:** How does it feel (dull, sharp, aching, throbbing)? How does the area of pain look (shiny, bumpy, red, swollen, bruised)? **Onset:** When did it begin? **Location:** Where is it? Does it radiate? **Duration:** How long does it last? Does it recur? **Severity:** How bad is it? **Associated factors:** What makes it better? What makes it worse? What other symptoms occur with it?	Exploring the pain in depth helps the nurse to understand the cause and significance of the pain.
Personal history	
Do you know what your usual blood pressure is?	Knowing blood pressure indicates patient is involved in his or her own health care.
When and where did you last have your blood pressure checked?	Answer indicates if patient consults professionals for health care, if patient relies on possibly erroneous equipment in public places (e.g. chemists) or if patient has approved equipment at home that he or she is trained to use.

Continued on following page

Initial health history (continued)

QUESTION	RATIONALE
Personal history (continued)	
Are you aware if your heartbeat is unusually fast or slow?	Often a patient will know that his or her heartbeat frequently runs either high or low, especially if taking certain medications. In addition, well-trained athletes will often have a lower-than-average heartbeat because of their level of physical fitness. This is a normal variation in those individuals.
What medications do you take? Please list prescription and over-the-counter medications, vitamins and minerals and any herbal supplements taken routinely or on an as-needed basis.	Having a complete list of all medications, vitamins and herbal supplements is essential in assessing the general status of the patient. Many medications have side effects that can alter a patient's vital signs and may even affect general appearance. It is important to have the patient bring a list from home that contains all the information needed including names, dosages, route of administration and time given for all medications, vitamins and supplements.
What allergies do you have to medications, foods or the environment?	It is important to gather a patient's list of allergies in order to provide safe nursing care.
Family history	
Do you have any family history of heart disease, diabetes, thyroid disease, lung disease, high blood pressure or cancer? Are you aware of any other family history?	Frequently diseases such as heart disease, diabetes, thyroid disease, lung disease, hypertension or cancer can be hereditary; thus, it is important to ask about them when assessing the general status of your patient. Even if there is no personal history of these diseases, the patient's family history would put the patient at an increased risk of developing such diseases in the future.
Lifestyle and health practices	
What is your educational background?	This gives you a basis for communication and understanding your patient's level of comprehension.
Are you currently employed? If so, what is your occupation? If not, are you disabled or are you seeking employment?	An occupation can provide insight into the patient's condition and may lead to identification of significant health concerns.
How satisfied are you with your life?	Asking about life satisfaction can help illicit potential psychological problems such as anxiety or depression.
How often do you seek health care?	This question provides insight into the patient's health practices.
Do you use any tobacco products including cigarettes, chewing tobacco, snuff or dip?	Tobacco use causes vasoconstriction of blood vessels, which leads to hypertension and peripheral vascular disease. Tobacco use can also cause chronic lung disease and cancer.
Do you drink alcohol? If so, how much and how often? What type of alcohol do you drink? Do you use any illicit drugs? If so, which drugs and how often?	Excessive alcohol or illicit drug use may indicate poor lifestyle management and may suggest psychological illness. These behaviours can also lead to obesity or malnutrition depending on which substance is abused. For example, methamphetamines often cause anorexia and malnutrition, whereas alcoholism can lead to abdominal obesity.
Do you follow any special diet?	Patients with hypertension may follow a low-sodium (salt) diet. Those with obesity may follow a low-fat or low-cholesterol diet. Patients with diabetes may consume a specific number of kilojoules each day and not eat concentrated sweets or sugar. There are many different diets available to patients. Some are prescribed, while others are not. It is important to know what dietary restrictions patients have, as these diets directly affect the patient's general status.
Do you exercise regularly? What type of exercise do you do and how often?	Exercise status can directly affect the musculature and build of a patient.

Health assessment

COLLECTING OBJECTIVE DATA: PHYSICAL EXAMINATION

Preparing the patient

The general survey begins when the nurse first meets the patient. During this time the nurse observes the patient's posture, movements and overall appearance. To begin the interview for the physical examination, the patient should be in a comfortable sitting position in a chair, on the examination table or in a hospital bed. Prepare the patient for the physical examination by explaining its purpose. Then explain that vital signs will be taken.

Equipment

Common pieces of equipment used to perform assessments of vital signs are:

- Thermometer: tympanic or electronic (for oral, axilla or rectal use)
- Protective, disposable covers for type of thermometer used
- Sphygmomanometer or electronic blood pressure measuring equipment
- Stethoscope
- Watch with a second hand
- Pulse oximeter and appropriate probe
- Patient chart.

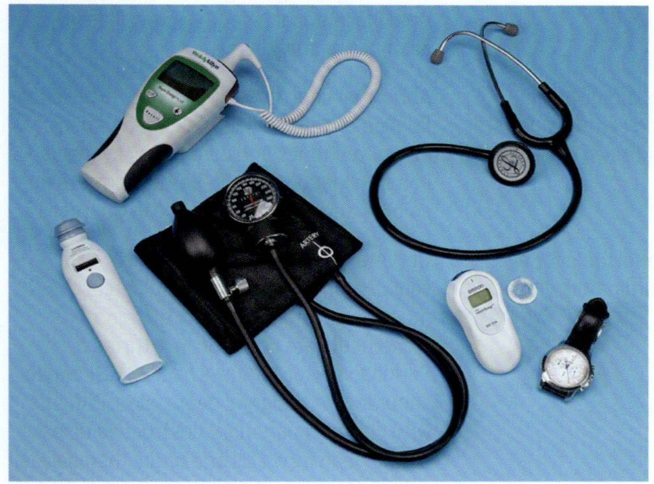

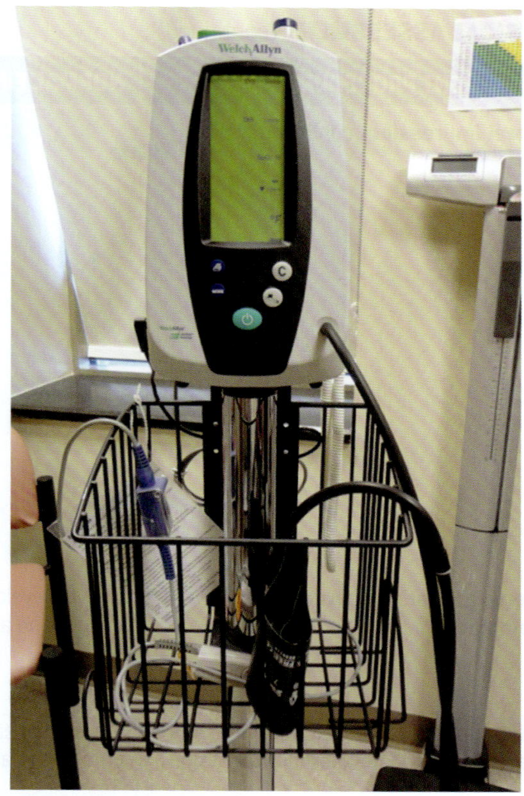

FIGURE 7-2 Mobile monitoring system.

Physical assessment

Identify the equipment needed to measure vital signs and the proper use of each piece of equipment. If available, use a mobile monitoring system (Fig. 7-2), which can be taken from room to room to perform multiple vital signs simultaneously. These devices often have an electronic sphygmomanometer (to measure non-invasive blood pressure) and an oxygen saturation monitor (that also monitors a pulse). You should take a manual pulse and blood pressure where possible.

You may assess mental status effectively using the Mental State Examination or Mini-Mental State Examination tools found in Assessment tool 6-1.

PHYSICAL ASSESSMENT

ASSESSMENT PROCEDURE	NORMAL FINDINGS	ABNORMAL FINDINGS
General impression		
Observe physical development, body build and fat distribution.	A wide variety of body types fall within a normal range: from small amounts of fat and muscle to larger amounts of fat and muscle. See Chapter 14 for more information. Body proportions are normal. Arm span (distance between finger tips with arms extended) is approximately equal. The distance from the head crown to the symphysis pubis is approximately equal to the distance from the symphysis pubis to the sole of the patient's foot.	A lack of subcutaneous fat with prominent bones is a sign of malnutrition. Abundant fatty tissue is seen in obesity. Decreased height and delayed puberty, with chubbiness, are seen in people with short stature and a hypopituitary disorder. Skeletal malformations with a decrease in height are seen in achondroplastic conditions. In gigantism, there is increased height and weight with delayed sexual development.

Continued on following page

PHYSICAL ASSESSMENT (continued)

ASSESSMENT PROCEDURE	NORMAL FINDINGS	ABNORMAL FINDINGS
General impression (continued)		
		Overgrowth of bones in the face, head, hands and feet with normal height is seen in hyperpituitarism (acromegaly). Extreme weight loss is seen in anorexia nervosa. Arm span is greater than height, and pubis to sole measurement exceeds pubis to crown measurement in Marfan syndrome. Excessive body fat that is evenly distributed is referred to as exogenous obesity. Central body weight gain with excessive cervical obesity (Buffalo hump) seen in Cushing syndrome is referred to as endogenous obesity. (See Abnormal findings 7-1, pages 105–106.)
Observe gender and sexual development.	Sexual development is appropriate for gender and age.	Abnormal findings include delayed puberty, male patient with female characteristics and female patient with male characteristics.
Compare patient's stated age with their apparent age and developmental stage.	Patient appears to be their stated chronological age.	Patient appears older than actual chronological age (e.g. as a result of hard life, manual labour, chronic illness, alcoholism, smoking).
Observe skin condition and colour.	Colour is even without obvious lesions: light to dark beige-pink in light-skinned patient; light tan to dark brown or olive in dark-skinned patients.	Abnormal findings include extreme pallor, flushed or yellow in light-skinned patient; loss of red tones and ashen grey cyanosis in dark-skinned patient. See abnormal skin colours and their significance in Chapter 15.
Observe posture and gait.	Posture is erect and comfortable for age. Gait is rhythmic and coordinated with arms swinging at side.	Curvatures of the spine (lordosis, scoliosis or kyphosis) may indicate a musculoskeletal disorder. Stiff, rigid movements are common in arthritis or Parkinson disease (see Chap. 28). Slumped shoulders may signify depression. Patients with chronic pulmonary obstructive disease tend to lean forwards and brace themselves with their arms. **OLDER ADULT CONSIDERATIONS** **In older adults, osteoporotic thinning and collapse of the vertebrae secondary to bone loss may result in kyphosis.** **In older men, gait may be wider based with arms held outwards. Older women tend to have a narrow base and may waddle to compensate for a decreased sense of balance. Steps shorten with decreased speed and arm swing. Mobility may be decreased, and gait may be rigid.**

PHYSICAL ASSESSMENT (continued)

ASSESSMENT PROCEDURE	NORMAL FINDINGS	ABNORMAL FINDINGS
Vital signs		
CLINICAL TIP **Prior to performing vital signs it is important that you wash your hands and explain what it is you are doing. On completion, return the patient to a comfortable position and document all findings.**		
TEMPERATURE		
The most commonly used thermometers are the tympanic thermometers. Electronic or digital thermometers are also used and allow a temperature to be taken by the oral or axillary route. Oral temperatures can be taken if a tympanic thermometer is not available. If an electronic or digital thermometer has a rectal probe, a rectal temperature can be taken but can be quite uncomfortable. In all instances hold the thermometer in place until it beeps or has a constant temperature reading on the display screen. Always ensure the correct disposable protective probe cover is placed on the thermometer. Never use a rectal thermometer for oral use.	 **OLDER ADULT CONSIDERATIONS** **Research has shown that, for older adults, normal body temperature values for all routes are consistently lower than values reported in younger populations (Lu et al., 2010).**	
For tympanic temperature, an electronic tympanic thermometer measures the temperature of the tympanic membrane quickly and safely. It is also a good device for measuring core body temperature because the tympanic membrane is supplied by a tributary of the artery (internal carotid) that supplies the hypothalamus (the body's thermoregulatory centre). Place the probe gently at the opening of the ear canal for 2 to 3 seconds until the temperature appears in the digital display (Fig. 7-3). **CLINICAL TIP** **To facilitate an accurate reading, tug on the patient's ear lobe to straighten the ear canal. Be aware that on some tympanic thermometers you may need to press a trigger button in order for a reading to be displayed.**	The tympanic membrane temperature is about 0.8°C higher than the normal oral temperature. 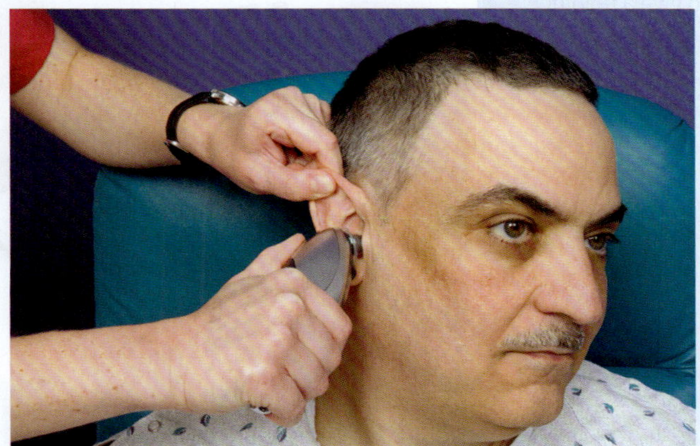 **FIGURE 7-3** Taking a tympanic temperature.	

Continued on following page

PHYSICAL ASSESSMENT (continued)

ASSESSMENT PROCEDURE	NORMAL FINDINGS	ABNORMAL FINDINGS
Vital signs (continued)		
To take axillary temperature, hold the digital thermometer or electronic thermometer under the axilla firmly by having the patient hold his or her arm down (Fig. 7-4). **CLINICAL TIP** **Although mercury-in-glass thermometers do exist in certain clinical settings, they are not commonly used because they are associated with safety risks such as exposure to broken glass or mercury. Care should be taken when using them. Ensure the thermometer is wiped with an alcohol swab, is dry, and the reading is less than 35°C prior to use.**	The axillary temperature is 0.5°C lower than the oral temperature. 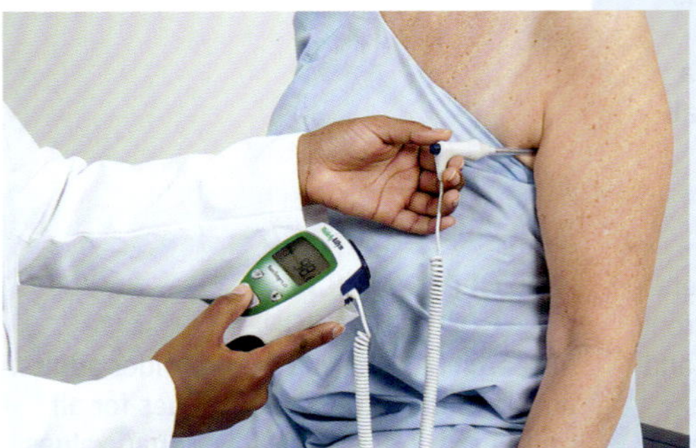 **FIGURE 7-4** Taking an axillary temperature.	
To take oral temperature, use an electronic thermometer with a disposable protective probe cover, or a digital thermometer (Fig. 7-5). Then place the thermometer under the patient's tongue to the right or left of the frenulum deep in the posterior sublingual pocket. Ask the patient to close his or her lips around the probe. Hold the probe until you hear a beep. Remove the probe and dispose of its cover by pressing the release button (Fig. 7-6). It can take up to 2 minutes for an electronic or digital thermometer to give a reading.	Oral temperature is 35.6°C to 37.7°C. 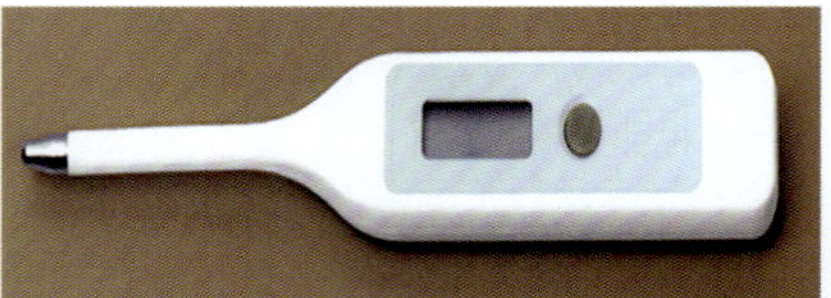 **FIGURE 7-5** Most digital thermometers do not have covers, so after using one for oral or axillary temperature, always clean it with an alcohol swab. 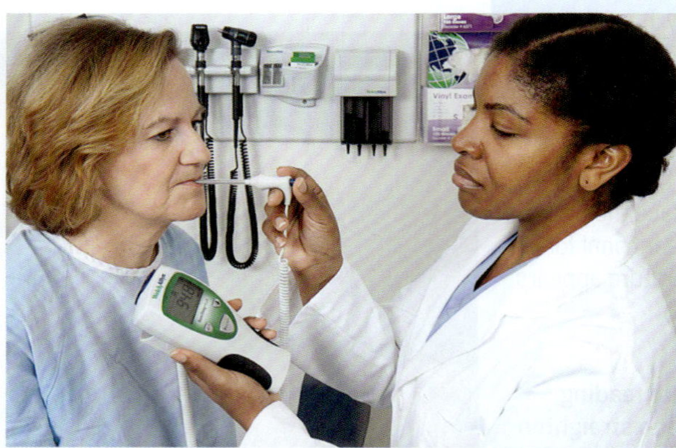 **FIGURE 7-6** Taking an oral temperature.	Oral temperature is below 35.6°C or over 37.7°C.

PHYSICAL ASSESSMENT (continued)

ASSESSMENT PROCEDURE	NORMAL FINDINGS	ABNORMAL FINDINGS
For rectal temperatures, if indicated, place disposable cover over temperature probe and lubricate. Wear gloves and insert thermometer 2.0 to 2.5 cm into rectum. Hold in place until temperature appears on display screen. **SAFETY TIP** **Use the rectal route only if other routes are not practical (e.g. patient cannot cooperate, is comatose, or cannot close mouth, or a tympanic thermometer is unavailable). Never force the thermometer into the rectum and never use a rectal thermometer for patients with severe coagulation disorders, recent rectal, anal, vaginal or prostate surgeries, diarrhoea, haemorrhoids, colitis or faecal impaction.**	The rectal temperature is between 0.4°C and 0.5°C higher than the normal oral temperature.	
PULSE		
Measure the radial pulse rate. Use the pads of your two middle fingers and lightly palpate the radial artery on the lateral aspect of the patient's wrist (Fig. 7-7). Count the number of beats you feel for 30 seconds if the pulse rhythm is regular. Multiply by two to get the rate. Count for a full minute if the rhythm is irregular or if taking a pulse for the first time. Then verify by taking an apical pulse as well.	A pulse rate ranging from 60 to 100 beats/minute is normal for adults. Tachycardia may be normal in patients who have just finished strenuous exercise. Bradycardia may be normal in well-conditioned athletes.	*Tachycardia* is a heart rate greater than 100 beats/minute. It may occur with fever, certain medications, stress and other abnormal states such as cardiac arrhythmias. *Bradycardia* is a heart rate less than 60 beats/minute. Sitting or standing for long periods may cause the blood to pool and decrease the pulse rate. Heart block or dropped beats can also manifest as bradycardia. Abnormal findings should be followed up with cardiac auscultation of the apical pulse (see Chap. 22 for more detail).

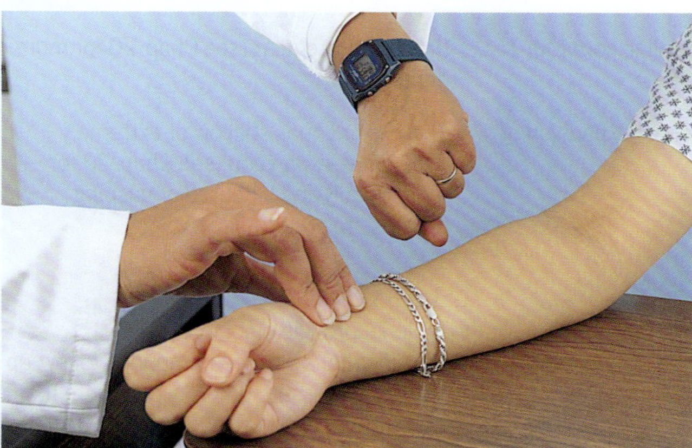

FIGURE 7-7 Timing the radial pulse rate. (© B. Proud.)

ASSESSMENT PROCEDURE	NORMAL FINDINGS	ABNORMAL FINDINGS
Evaluate pulse rhythm.	There are regular intervals between beats.	Irregular intervals between beats should be followed up with auscultation of the apical pulse (see Chap. 22). When describing irregular beats, indicate whether they are regular irregular or irregular irregular.

Continued on following page

PHYSICAL ASSESSMENT (continued)

ASSESSMENT PROCEDURE	NORMAL FINDINGS	ABNORMAL FINDINGS
Vital signs (continued)		
Assess amplitude and contour.	Normally pulsation is equally strong in both wrists. Upstroke is smooth and rapid with a more gradual downstroke.	A bounding or weak and thready pulse is not normal. Delayed upstroke is also abnormal. Follow up on abnormal amplitude and contour findings by palpating the carotid arteries, which provides the best assessment of amplitude and contour (see Chap. 23).
Palpate arterial elasticity.	Artery feels straight, resilient and springy. **OLDER ADULT CONSIDERATIONS** **The older patient's artery may feel harder and less straight.**	Artery feels rigid.
RESPIRATIONS		
Monitor the respiratory rate. Observe the patient's chest rise and fall with each breath. Count respirations for 30 seconds and multiply by 2 or count for 1 minute if performing respirations for the first time or if patient is dyspnoeic (refer to Chap. 20 for more information). **CLINICAL TIP** **If you place the patient's arm across the chest while palpating pulse, you can also count respirations. Do this by keeping your fingers on the patient's pulse even after you have finished taking the heart rate.**	Between 12 and 20 breaths/minute is normal. **OLDER ADULT CONSIDERATIONS** **In the older adult, the respiratory rate may range from 15 to 22 breaths/minute. The rate may increase with a shallower inspiratory phase because vital capacity and inspiratory reserve volume decrease with ageing.**	Fewer than 12 breaths/minute or more than 20 breaths/minute is abnormal.
Observe respiratory rhythm.	Rhythm is regular (if irregular, count for 1 full minute).	Rhythm is irregular (see Chap. 20 for more detail).
Observe respiratory depth.	There is equal bilateral chest expansion of 2.5 to 5 cm.	There is unequal, shallow or extremely deep chest expansion (see Chap. 20 for more detail) and laboured or gasping breaths are abnormal.
BLOOD PRESSURE		
Measure blood pressure (Fig. 7-8). Spotlight technique 7-1 and Display 7-2 provide guidelines.	Systolic pressure is <120 mmHg.	Table 7-1 provide blood pressure classifications and recommended follow-up criteria. A pressure difference of more than 10 mmHg between arms may indicate coarctation of the aorta or cardiac disease.

PHYSICAL ASSESSMENT (continued)

ASSESSMENT PROCEDURE	NORMAL FINDINGS	ABNORMAL FINDINGS
Measure on dominant arm first. Take blood pressure in both arms when recording it for the first time. Take subsequent readings in arm with highest measurement. **CLINICAL TIP** **Advise patient to avoid nicotine and caffeine for 30 minutes prior to measurement. Ask patient to empty bladder before evaluating and avoid talking to the patient while taking the reading. Each of these prevents elevating blood pressure prior to and during reading.**	Diastolic pressure is <80 mmHg; varies with individuals. A pressure difference of 10 mmHg between arms is normal.	 **OLDER ADULT CONSIDERATIONS** **More rigid, arteriosclerotic arteries account for higher systolic blood pressure in older adults. Systolic pressure over 140 mmHg, but diastolic pressure under 90 mmHg is called isolated systolic hypertension.**
If the patient takes antihypertensives or has a history of fainting or dizziness, assess for possible orthostatic hypotension. Measure blood pressure with the patient in a standing or sitting position after taking the pressure with the patient in a supine position. **CLINICAL TIP** **An ill patient may not be able to stand; sitting is usually adequate to detect if the patient truly has orthostatic hypotension.**	A drop of less than 20 mmHg from recorded sitting position is normal.	A drop of 20 mmHg or more from the recorded sitting blood pressure may indicate orthostatic (postural) hypotension. Orthostatic hypotension may be related to a decreased baroreceptor sensitivity, fluid volume deficit (e.g. dehydration) or certain medications (i.e. diuretics, antihypertensives). Symptoms of orthostatic hypotension include dizziness, light-headedness and falling. Further evaluation and referral to the patient's primary care provider are necessary.

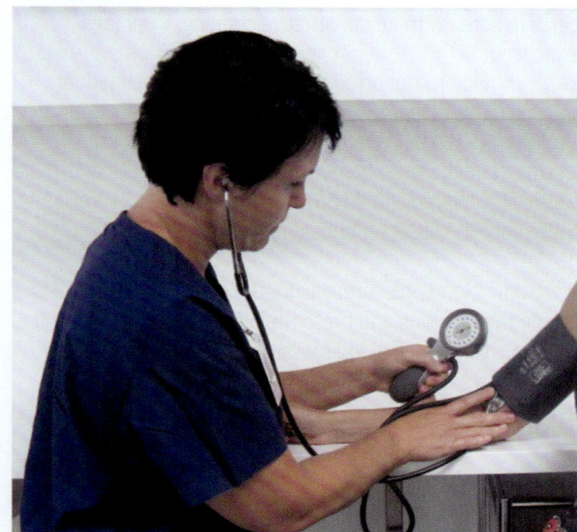

FIGURE 7-8 Measuring blood pressure.

SPOTLIGHT TECHNIQUE 7-1: MEASURING MANUAL BLOOD PRESSURE

Preparation

Before measuring the blood pressure, consider the following behavioural and environmental conditions that can affect the reading:

- Room temperature too hot or cold
- Recent exercise
- Alcohol intake
- Nicotine use
- Muscle tension
- Bladder distension
- Background noise
- Talking (either patient or nurse)
- Arm position.

Steps for measuring blood pressure

1. Assemble your equipment so that the sphygmomanometer, stethoscope, and your pen and recording sheet are within easy reach. Ask the patient what his or her normal blood pressure reading is for you to use as a baseline.
2. Assist the patient into a comfortable, quiet, restful position for 5 to 10 minutes. Patient may lie down or sit.
3. Remove the patient's clothing from the arm and palpate the pulsations of the brachial artery. (If the patient's sleeve can be pushed up to make room for the cuff, make sure that the clothing is not so constrictive that it would alter a correct pressure reading.)
4. Place the blood pressure cuff so that the midline of the bladder is over the arterial pulsation, and wrap the appropriately sized cuff smoothly and snugly around the upper arm, 2.5 cm above the antecubital area so that there is enough room to place the bell of the stethoscope. The bladder inside the cuff should encircle 80% of the arm circumference in adults and 100% of the arm circumference in children younger than age 13. A cuff that is too small may give a false or abnormally high blood pressure reading. Regular maintenance and calibration are required to ensure the accuracy of mercury and anaeroid sphygmomanometers and electric blood pressure monitoring devices.
5. Support the patient's arm slightly flexed at heart level with the palm up.
6. Palpate the radial artery with your fingers and, at the same time, inflate the cuff. Observe the pressure where the radial pulse disappears. This is known as a *palpable blood pressure* and gives you an idea of what the patient's systolic blood pressure might be. This step is useful to perform when initially checking a patient's blood pressure.
7. Put the earpieces of the stethoscope in your ears, then palpate the brachial pulse again and place the stethoscope lightly over this area. Position the gauge on the manometer at eye level.
8. Adjust the screw above the bulb to tighten the valve on the air pump, and make sure that the tubing is not kinked or obstructed.
9. Inflate the cuff by pumping the bulb to about 30 mmHg above the point at which the brachial pulse disappears. This will help you avoid missing an auscultatory gap.
10. Deflate the cuff slowly—about 2 mm per second—by turning the valve in the opposite direction while listening for the first of Korotkoff sounds.
11. Read the point, closest to an even number, on the mercury gauge at which you hear the first faint but clear sound. Record this number as the systolic blood pressure. This is phase I of Korotkoff sounds.
12. Next, note the point, closest to an even number, on the mercury gauge at which the sound becomes muffled (phase IV of Korotkoff sounds). Finally, note the point where the sound subsides completely (phase V of Korotkoff sounds). When both a change in sounds and a cessation of the sounds are heard, record the numbers at which you hear phase I, IV and V sounds. Otherwise, record the first and last sounds.
13. Deflate the cuff at least another 10 mmHg to make sure you hear no more sounds. Then deflate completely and remove.
14. Record readings to the nearest 2 mmHg.

Cuff selection guidelines

The 'ideal' cuff should have a bladder length that is 80% and a width that is at least 40% of the arm circumference (a length-to-width ratio of 2:1). A recent study comparing intra-arterial and auscultatory blood pressure concluded that the error is minimised with a cuff of 46% of the arm circumference. The recommended cuff sizes are:

- 12 × 22 cm for arm circumference of 22 to 26 cm, which is the 'small adult' size
- 16 × 30 cm for arm circumference of 27 to 34 cm, which is the 'adult' size
- 16 × 36 cm for arm circumference of 35 to 44 cm, which is the 'large adult' size
- 16 × 42 cm for arm circumference of 45 to 52 cm, which is the 'adult thigh' size.

Summary points for clinical blood pressure measurement

- The patient should be seated comfortably with their back supported and their upper arm bared without constrictive clothing. Their legs should not be crossed.
- The patient's arm should be supported at heart level, and the bladder of the cuff should encircle at least 80% of the arm circumference.
- The mercury column should be deflated at 2 to 3 mm per second, and the first and last audible sounds should be taken as systolic and diastolic pressure. The column should be read to the nearest 2 mmHg.
- Neither the patient nor the observer should talk during the measurement.

When taking an electronic blood pressure, ensure the correctly sized cuff is on the patient, turn on the machine and press the blood pressure button. It is safe practice to perform a manual blood pressure as well as an electronic blood pressure to see if there are any discrepancies.

(Based on information from Thomas G. Pickering, John E. Hall, Lawrence J. Appel, Bonita E. Falkner, John Graves, Martha N. Hill, Daniel W. Jones, Theodore Kurtz, Sheldon G. Sheps, & Edward J. Roccella. National Heart Foundation of Australia. (2016). *Guidelines for the diagnosis and management of hypertension in adults.* Available at https://www.heartfoundation.org.au/images/uploads/publications/PRO-167_Hypertension-guideline-2016_WEB.pdf.)

DISPLAY 7-2 IDENTIFYING KOROTKOFF SOUNDS

Phase I

It is characterised by the first appearance of faint, clear, repetitive, tapping sounds that gradually intensify for at least two consecutive beats. This coincides approximately with the resumption of a palpable pulse. The number on the pressure gauge at which you hear the first tapping sound is the systolic pressure.

Phase II

It is characterised as muffled or swishing; these sounds are softer and longer than phase I sounds. They also have the quality of an intermittent murmur. They may temporarily subside, especially in hypertensive people. The loss of the sound during the latter part of phase I and during phase II is called the auscultatory gap. The gap may cover a range of as much as 40 mmHg; failing to recognise this gap may cause serious errors of underestimating systolic pressure or overestimating diastolic pressure.

Phase III

It is characterised by a return of distinct, crisp and louder sounds as the blood flows relatively freely through an increasingly open artery.

Phase IV

It is characterised by sounds that are muffled, less distinct and softer (with a blowing quality).

Phase V

It is characterised by all sounds disappearing completely. The last sound heard before this period of continuous silence is the onset of phase V and is the pressure commonly considered to define the diastolic measurement. (Some clinicians still consider the last sounds of phase IV the first diastolic value.)

Note: The American Heart Association recommends that values in phase IV and phase V be recorded when both a change in the sounds and a cessation in the sounds occur.

These recommendations apply particularly to children under age 13, pregnant women and patients with high cardiac output or peripheral vasodilation. For example, such a blood pressure would be recorded as 120/80/64.

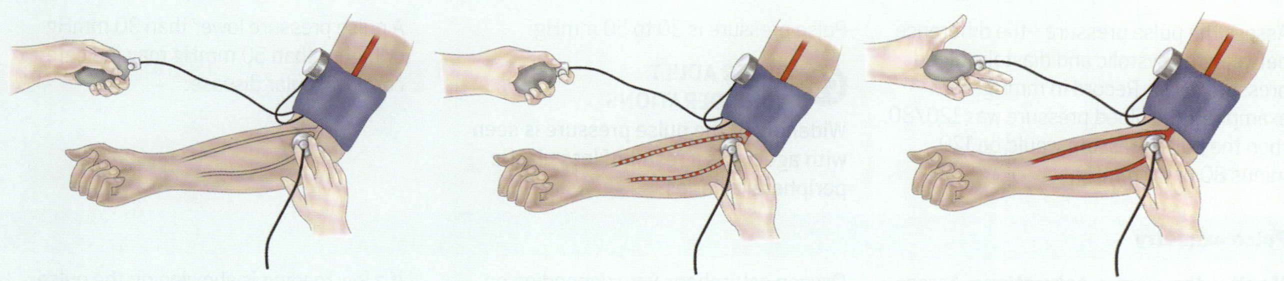

(Based on Muntner, P., Shimbo, D., Carey, R. M., Charleston, J. B., Gaillard, T., Misra, S., Myers, M. G., Ogedegbe, G., Schwartz, J. E., Townsend, R. R., Urbina, E. M., Viera, A. J., White, W. B. & Wright, J. T., Jr. (2019). Measurement of blood pressure in humans: A scientific statement from the American Heart Association. *Hypertension*, *73*(5), e35–e66.)

Table 7-1 Classification of clinic blood pressure levels in adults

Diagnostic category*	Systolic (mmHg)		Diastolic (mmHg)
Optimal	<120	and	<80
Normal	120–129	and/or	80–84
High-normal	130–139	and/or	85–89
Grade 1 (mild) hypertension	140–159	and/or	90–99
Grade 2 (moderate) hypertension	160–179	and/or	100–109
Grade 3 (severe) hypertension	≥180	and/or	≥110
Isolated systolic hypertension	>140	and	<90

*When a patient's systolic and diastolic blood pressure levels fall into different categories, the higher diagnostic category and recommended actions apply, 2016.

PHYSICAL ASSESSMENT (continued)

ASSESSMENT PROCEDURE	NORMAL FINDINGS	ABNORMAL FINDINGS
Vital signs (continued)		
CLINICAL TIP **To avoid patient discomfort and overinflation of the blood pressure cuff, perform a palpable blood pressure. This will give you an approximate systolic pressure. Place the blood pressure cuff on the patient and palpate the radial artery with your fingers. Inflate the cuff until you can no longer feel the radial artery. Note the pressure when the radial pulse disappears. When taking the patient's blood pressure over the brachial artery, inflate the cuff to 30 mmHg above this reading.**		
Assess the pulse pressure—the difference between the systolic and diastolic blood pressure levels. Record in mmHg. For example, if the blood pressure was 120/80, then the pulse pressure would be 120 minus 80 or 40 mmHg.	Pulse pressure is 30 to 50 mmHg. **OLDER ADULT CONSIDERATIONS** **Widening of the pulse pressure is seen with ageing as a result of less elastic peripheral arteries.**	A pulse pressure lower than 30 mmHg or higher than 50 mmHg may indicate cardiovascular disease.
Pulse oximetry		
Monitor the oxygen saturations. Assess the blood supply to the area where the probe is being attached (finger, toe, ear lobe or forehead). If the blood pressure is being taken, ensure that the probe is on the opposite arm; remove nail polish or constricting clothing. Turn on the machine and place the sensor probe on the patient's finger (or toe, ear lobe or forehead) (Fig. 7-9). Ask the patient to keep still, to reduce motion artefact. Wait until you are satisfied that you have an accurate reading. If continuous readings are necessary, check and rotate the probe at least every 2 hours to prevent pressure areas. Document the findings.	Oxygen saturations vary depending on the health and age of the patient. Ask the doctor to document what percentage the oxygen saturations should be for the individual patient.	If a low reading is showing on the pulse oximeter, recheck the position of the probe and the patient's perfusion. Where possible, encourage the patient to perform deep breathing and coughing exercises. If clinically needed, initiate appropriate action such as oxygen therapy.

PHYSICAL ASSESSMENT (continued)

ASSESSMENT PROCEDURE	NORMAL FINDINGS	ABNORMAL FINDINGS
CLINICAL TIP **Closely monitor the oximeter pulse rate with the palpable pulse rate to ensure accuracy.**	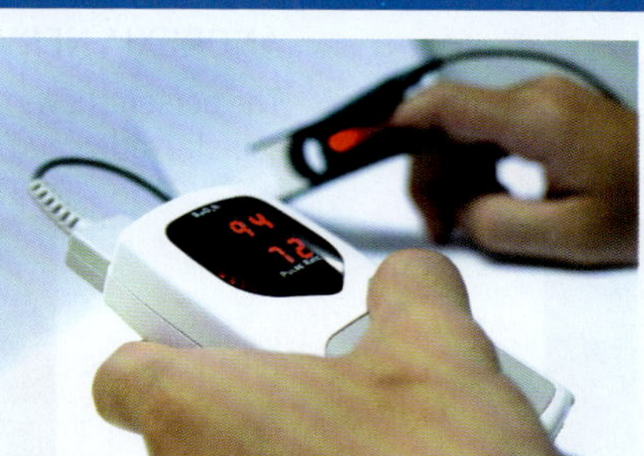 **FIGURE 7-9** Pulse oximeter. (Shutterstock.com/ toysf400)	
Pain		
Observe comfort level.	Patient assumes a relatively relaxed posture without excessive position shifting. Facial expression is alert and pleasant.	Facial expression indicates discomfort (grimacing, frowning). Patient may brace or holds body part that is painful. Breathing pattern indicates distress (shortness of breath, shallow, rapid breathing).
Ask the patient if he or she has any pain.	No subjective report of pain	Any subjective report of pain should be further explored using the mnemonic COLDSPA. **Refer to Chapter 8 for further assessment of pain.**

ABNORMAL FINDINGS 7-1 Deviations related to physical development, body build and fat distribution

DWARFISM

These images show the associated decreased height and skeletal malformations.

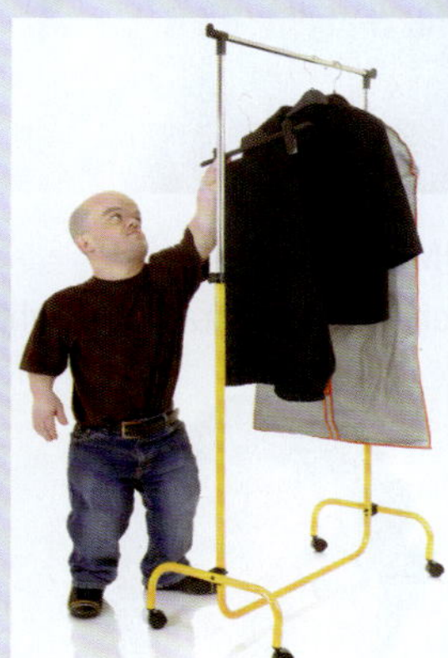

(Weber, J.R. & Kelley, J.H. [2017]. Health Assessment in Nursing, 6e, © Wolters Kluwer Health.)

ACROMEGALY

The affected person shows the characteristic overgrowth of bones in the face, head and hands.

A

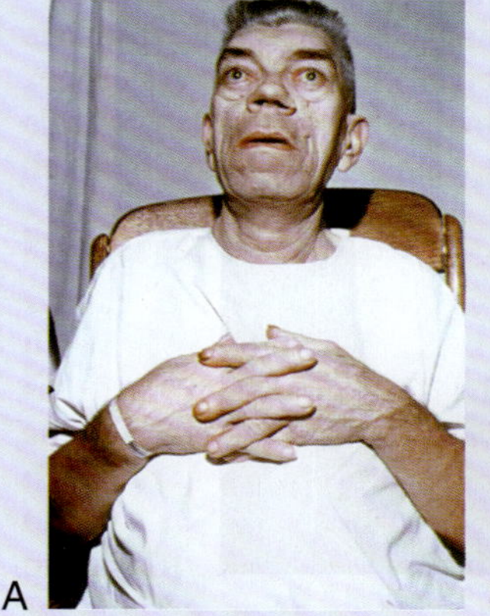

B

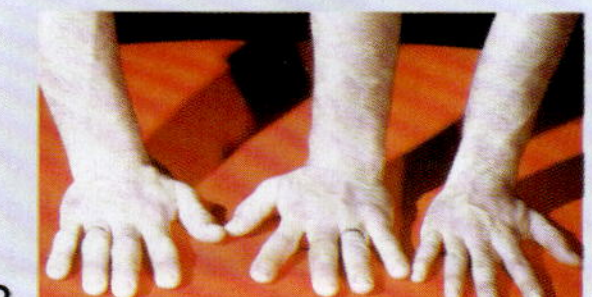

Continued on following page

ABNORMAL FINDINGS 7-1 Deviations related to physical development, body build and fat distribution (continued)

GIGANTISM

Note the disparity in height between the affected person and a person of the same age.

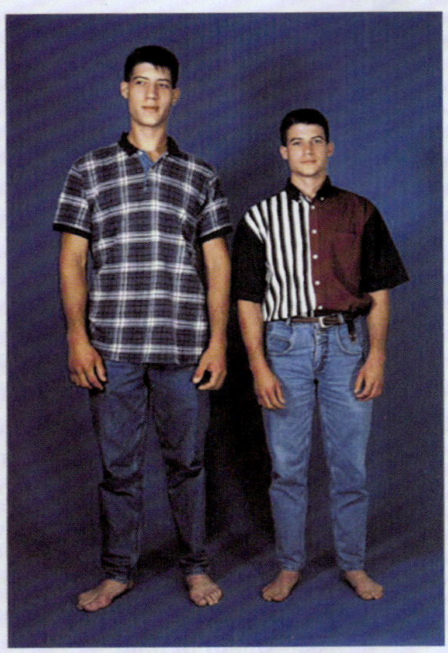

ANOREXIA NERVOSA

The person shows the emaciated appearance that follows self-starvation and accompanying extreme weight loss.

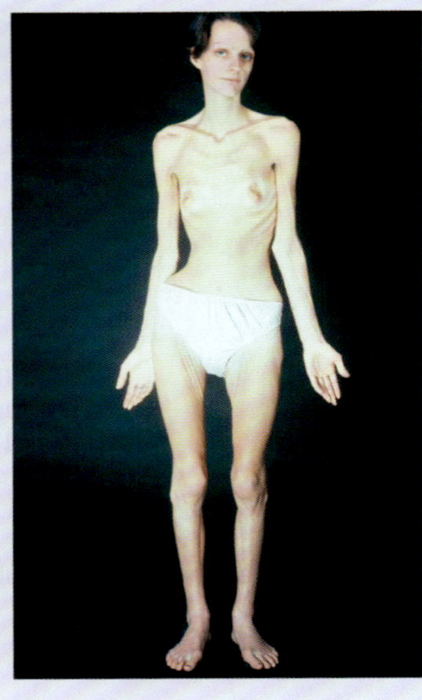

OBESITY

Obesity is defined as having an excessive amount of body fat. It increases the risk of diseases and health problems such as heart disease, diabetes and high blood pressure (Mayo Clinic, 2019).

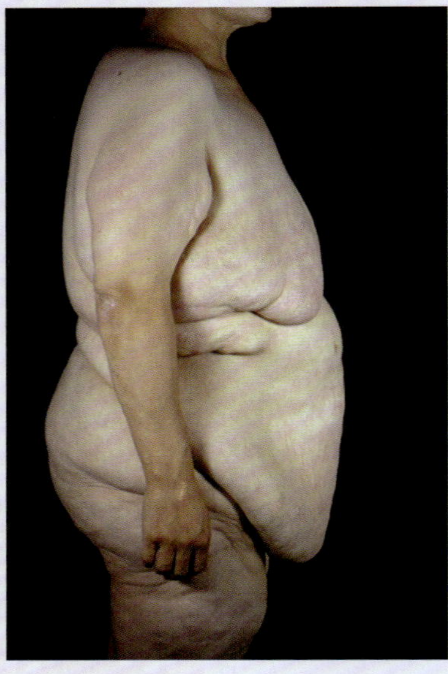

MARFAN SYNDROME

The elongated fingers are characteristic of this condition.

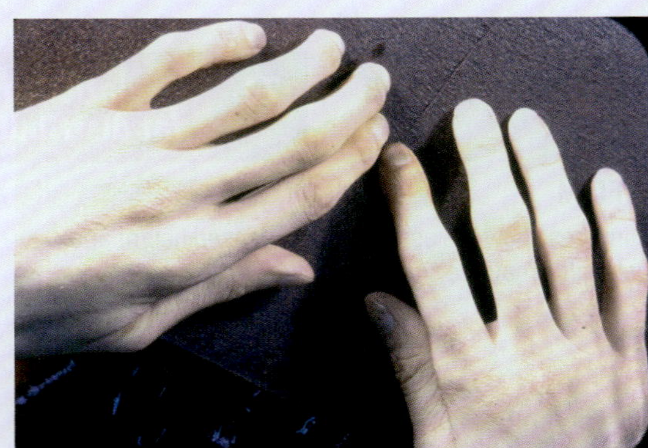

CUSHING SYNDROME

The affected patient reflects the centralised weight gain.

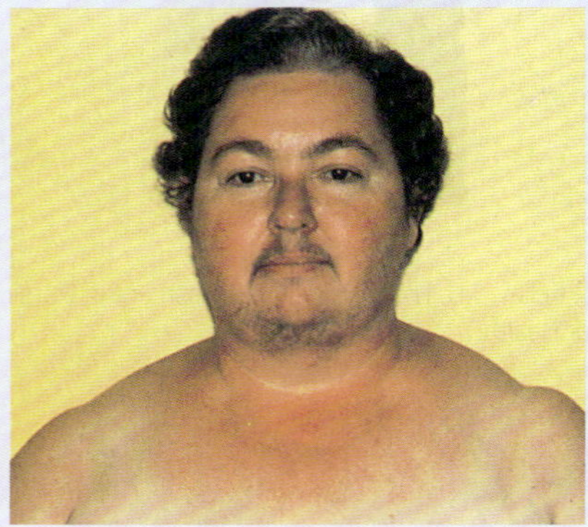

VALIDATING AND DOCUMENTING FINDINGS

Validate the assessment data you have collected. This is necessary to verify that the findings are reliable and accurate. Document the assessment findings according to hospital policy.

Clinical deterioration of patients in the acute care setting is an expectation of competent hospital care, resulting in a national approach for recognising and responding to clinical deterioration—*National safety and quality health service (NSQHS) Standard 9: Recognising and responding to clinical deterioration in acute health care*—developed by the Australian Commission on Safety and Quality in Health Care (ACSQHC), which prescribes the provision of appropriate and timely care to patients whose condition is deteriorating and to prevent further deterioration. This standard describes the systems for recognising and responding to clinical deterioration. It applies to all patients in acute health care services including adults, adolescents, children and babies, and to all types of patients including medical, surgical, maternity and mental health patients.

The Rapid Detection and Response Observation Chart based on a chart recommended by the ACSQHC (see Fig. 3-1 in Chap. 3) enables standardised documentation and reposting of vital signs. The patient's respiratory rate, oxygen saturation, oxygen flow rate and delivery method, heart rate, blood pressure, temperature, level of consciousness, and pain scores are documented with an appropriate frequency. Each observation has threshold limits and when an abnormality in the observation is detected, it triggers an escalation of care.

Below is a sample of both subjective and objective data of different patients. Use the samples to help complete Critical thinking exercise 3.

Sample of subjective data

The patient, Mr Stephens, reports hot flushes on occasion. He says he does not have any pain or pain concerns. He also describes his family life as 'happy' and his job as a teacher, 'fulfilling'. He just completed a master's degree in education and expresses interest in teaching English to high school students.

Sample of objective data

Ms Lilley has an erect posture and her gait is smooth. She is a neatly dressed female in light-weight clothes appropriate for the summer season. Clean nails, well groomed. Even distribution of fat and firm muscle. Patient is alert, friendly, cooperative and answers questions with good eye contact. Smiles and laughs appropriately. Speech is fluent, clear and moderately paced. Thoughts are free flowing. Able to recall recent events earlier in day (e.g. what she had for breakfast) without difficulty.

Oral temperature: 37°C; radial pulse: 84 per minute regular, bilateral, equally strong and resilient; respirations: 16 per minute regular, equal bilateral chest expansion; blood pressure: sitting position 120/78 mmHg right arm, 124/80 mmHg left arm; standing position 124/80 mmHg right arm, 126/82 mmHg left arm.

CRITICAL THINKING

3. From the information provided in the case study, and the samples of subjective and objective data, write down all of the subjective and objective data that are important for you to document about Mr Lucas.

Analysis of data

DIAGNOSTIC REASONING: POSSIBLE CONCLUSIONS

After collecting subjective and objective data pertaining to the general survey, mental status examination and vital signs, identify abnormal findings and patient strengths. Then cluster or organise the data to reveal any significant patterns or abnormalities. These findings may be used to make clinical judgements about the patient.

Potential patient risks

- Risk of activity intolerance (related to deconditioned status)
- Risk of self-harm (related to depression, suicidal tendencies, developmental crisis, lack of support systems, loss of significant others, poor coping mechanisms and behaviours)

Potential patient problems

- Impaired verbal communication (related to international language barrier, inability to clearly express self or understand others, hearing loss, aphasia, psychological impairment or organic brain disorder)
- Acute or chronic confusion or impaired memory (related to dementia, head injury, stroke, alcohol or drug abuse)
- Dressing and grooming self-care deficit (related to impaired upper-extremity mobility and lack of resources)
- Bathing and hygiene self-care deficit (related to inability to wash body parts or inability to obtain water)
- Disturbed thought processes (related to alcohol or drug abuse, psychotic disorder or organic brain dysfunction)
- Pain

CRITICAL THINKING

4. Following completion of Mr Lucas's general survey and vital signs:
   - List the possible actual or potential health problems requiring nursing interventions.
   - Check for defining characteristics.
   - Confirm or rule out diagnoses.

Selected collaborative problems

After grouping the data, certain collaborative problems may become apparent. These physiological conditions can be detected and monitored by the nurse or a doctor. In addition, the nurse can use doctor- and nurse-prescribed interventions to minimise the complications of these problems. The nurse may also have to refer the patient in such situations for further treatment of the problem. The following is a list of collaborative problems that may be identified when assessing vital signs:

- Hypertension
- Hypotension
- Arrhythmias
- Hyperthermia
- Hypothermia
- Tachycardia
- Bradycardia
- Tachypnoea
- Dyspnoea
- Hypoxia
- Hypoxaemia.

Medical problems

If, after grouping the data, it becomes apparent that the patient has signs and symptoms that may require medical diagnosis and treatment, referral to a doctor is necessary.

CRITICAL THINKING

5. Identify the potential collaborative problems and nursing diagnoses appropriate for Mr Lucas.

CASE STUDY

The case study demonstrates how to analyse vital signs data for a specific patient. The exercises included in the ancillary product on thePoint that complements this text offer further opportunities to enhance your skills.

Stephen Lucas is a 47-year-old male who has been admitted to the neurology ward after a transient ischaemic attack. He has a history of hypertension and atrial fibrillation that was diagnosed 2 years ago and has been controlled with enalapril and digoxin. He is happily married to his wife of 25 years and has three children. Mr Lucas is a carpenter, is physically active and eats a healthy diet. Mrs Lucas recently lost her job and money has been 'a bit tight'; however, she starts a new job next week.

Mrs Lucas tells you that she saw her husband fall to the ground and not wake up for 4 minutes. Mr Lucas recalls talking with his wife one minute and waking up in hospital the next. He says, 'I usually take my medications every day, but I stopped taking them 5 days ago as I had to pay the children's school fees and there was no money left to buy medicine.' He also says: 'I've had a headache.'

Applying COLDSPA

Applying COLDSPA for patient symptoms: 'Headache' for 24 hours. I've got no problems with my vision, but can feel my heart racing and have numbness in my fingers.' He looks flushed in the face; his temperature is 36.8 °C; and his heart rate is 155 beats/minute and irregular. He has a respiratory rate of 20 breaths/minute; his blood pressure is 195/105 mmHg; and his oxygen saturations are 99% on room air. On a scale of 0 to 10 (with 10 being the worst pain imaginable) Mr Lucas rates his headache as a 6 and he describes it as an ache that worries him. He is 190 cm tall, weighs 85 kg, is talking clearly, is dressed appropriately for the weather, looks his age, is clean and well groomed, and has a steady and strong gait. He is alert and oriented.

He is currently waiting for a computed tomography scan and a carotid ultrasound. He now understands how important it is to take his medications.

The following concept map illustrates the diagnostic reasoning process.

Mnemonic	Question	Data provided	Missing data
Character	Describe the sign or symptom (feeling, appearance, sound, smell or taste if applicable).	'I have a headache'	Describe the pain—sharp, dull, throbbing
Onset	When did it begin?	'I've had a headache for 24 hours'	I woke up with the headache.
Location	Where is it? Does it radiate? Does it occur anywhere else?		Where is the headache (ask patient to point to exact location)?
Duration	How long does it last? Does it recur?	The headache has been continuous for the past 24 hours	
Severity	How bad is it? or How much does it bother you?	6 out of 10, with 10 being the worst	
Pattern	What makes it better or worse?		What makes the headache better/ worse?
Associated factors/How it Affects the patient	What other symptoms occur with it? How does it affect you?	'I can feel my heart racing and have numbness in my fingers'	

1) Identify abnormal findings and patient strengths

Subjective data

- Diagnosed with hypertension and atrial fibrillation 2 years ago
- 'I have a headache'
- Rates pain 6/10
- Numbness in hands, heart racing
- Wife present when patient collapsed
- Wife lost her job and patient had no money to pay for his medications

Objective data

- Gait steady and strong
- Height 190 cm, weight 85 kg
- 47-year-old male
- Appropriately dressed, well-groomed and clean
- Alert and oriented
- Able to converse well and has clear speech
- Looks flushed in the face
- Vital signs: temperature 36.8°C, rapid AF/HR = 155 beats per minute, RR = 20 breaths per minute, BP = 195/105 mmHg, oxygen saturations = 99% on room air

2) Identify cue clusters

- Diagnosed with hypertension and AF
- Admitted with TIA
- Not able to pay for his medications
- Looks flushed, is hypertensive and in uncontrolled/rapid AF
- Unable to recall events of his unconscious collapse until he woke up in hospital

- Diagnosed with hypertension and AF
- For the past 24 hours has had a continuous headache, numbness in his fingers and his heart has been pounding
- Unable to recall events of his unconscious collapse until he woke up in hospital

3) Draw inferences

- Patient is not medicated and is aware of the importance of taking his medications
- Textbook picture of a TIA as diagnosed by doctor; monitor for collaborative problems

- Patient has risk factors for TIA; patient needs neurology referral
- Patient has onset of pain. Refer for investigation and diagnosis

4) List possible diagnosis

Ineffective health maintenance related to knowledge deficit in importance of taking medication

Acute pain-related headache, hypertension and not taking medications

5) Check for defining characteristics

Major: Increased blood pressure and pulse + AF

Minor: Heart pounding and numbness in fingers

Major: Has headache—verbal reports of pain 6/10 continuous

6) Confirm or rule out diagnoses

Confirm the diagnosis because it meets defining characteristics and is validated by the patient

Confirm the diagnosis because it meets the major defining characteristic

7) Document conclusions

Diagnoses that are appropriate for this patient include:

- Ineffective health maintenance related to knowledge deficit in importance of taking medication
- Acute pain-related headache, hypertension and not taking medications

Potential collaborative problems include the following:

- Hypertension
- Atrial fibrillation
- Transient ischaemic attack

ONLINE RESOURCES

An extensive range of additional resources to enhance teaching and learning and to facilitate understanding may be found online at the text's accompanying website, located on thePoint at http://thepoint.lww.com. These include Watch and Learn videos, Concepts in Action animations, journal articles, case studies, discussion topics and quizzes.

Subscribers may also access Lippincott Procedures, an extensive online point-of-care procedure guide that provides reliable step-by-step instructions for more than 1700 procedures, including 450 evidence-based Australian procedures, and skills in a variety of speciality settings, together with a wealth of supporting information.

SIMULATED LEARNING

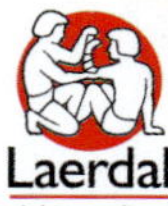

Having completed this chapter, explore the scenarios of Lloyd Bennett Parts 1 and 2. Lloyd is 76-year-old male who is postoperative following a hip arthroplasty; Lloyd required a blood transfusion. Incorporating the health assessment content in this chapter with your existing theoretical knowledge and clinical experience, progress through the simulation scenarios (this is best done in a small group). How would you manage Lloyd's care? When reflecting on your management of Lloyd, what do you think you did well and what do you think you can improve? Consider why you think this and also how you might manage a similar problem in the future.

References

Abbey, J., Piller, N., De Bellis, A., et al. (2004). The Abbey pain scale: A 1-minute numerical indicator for people with end-stage dementia. *International Journal of Palliative Nursing, 10*, 6–13.

Hicks, C. L., von Baeyer, C. L., Spafford, P., et al. (2001). The Faces Pain Scale—Revised: Toward a common metric in pediatric pain measurement. *Pain, 93*, 173–183. Faces Pain Scale. Viewed November 2019 at www.iasp-pain.org.

Lu, S., Leasure, A. & Dai, Y. (2010). A systematic review of body temperature variations in older people. *Journal of Clinical Nursing, 19*(1–2), 4–16.

Merkel, S. I., Voepel-Lewis, T., Shayevitz, J. R., et al. (1997). The FLACC: A behavioral scale for scoring postoperative pain in young children. *Pediatric Nursing, 23*, 293–297.

Muntner, P., Shimbo, D., Carey, R. M., et al. (2019). Measurement of blood pressure in humans: A scientific statement from the American Heart Association. *Hypertension, 73*(5), e35–e66. Available at https://www.ahajournals.org/doi/10.1161/HYP.0000000000000087.

National Heart Foundation of Australia. (2010 update). Guide to management of hypertension 2008 (Table 2, p. iii.). Sydney: Author. Available at www.heartfoundation.org.au.

National Heart Foundation of Australia. (2016). Guideline for the diagnosis and management of hypertension in adults. Available at https://www.heartfoundation.org.au/images/uploads/publications/PRO-167_Hypertension-guideline-2016_WEB.pdf.

Solodiuk, J. C. & Curley, M. A. Q. (2017). In defense of routine inpatient pain assessment. *The American Journal of Nursing, 117*(5), 11.

Teasdale, G. & Jennett, B. (1974). Assessment of coma and impaired consciousness: A practical scale (later called the 'Glasgow Coma Scale'). *The Lancet, 2*(7872), 81–84.

Selected readings

Diaz-Thomas, A. (2016). Hyperpituitarism. Available at https://emedicine.medscape.com/article/921568-overview.

Healthdirect. (2018a). Acromegaly. Available at https://www.healthdirect.gov.au/acromegaly.

Healthdirect. (2018b). Dwarfism. Available at https://www.healthdirect.gov.au/dwarfism.

Healthdirect. (2018c). High blood pressure (hypertension). Available at https://www.healthdirect.gov.au/high-blood-pressure-hypertension.

Healthdirect. (2018d). Hypothermia. Available at https://www.healthdirect.gov.au/hypothermia.

Healthdirect. (2018e). Low blood pressure (hypotension). Available at https://www.healthdirect.gov.au/low-blood-pressure-hypotension.

Healthdirect. (2018f). Obesity. Available at https://www.healthdirect.gov.au/obesity.

Healthdirect. (2018g). Tachycardia. Available at https://www.healthdirect.gov.au/tachycardia.

Healthdirect. (2019). Anorexia nervosa. Available at https://www.healthdirect.gov.au/anorexia-nervosa.

Mayo Clinic. (2019). Obesity. Available at www.mayoclinic.org/diseases-conditions/obesity/symptoms-causes/syc-20375742.

Online resources

Austin Health: www.austin.org.au/page?ID=568

Australian Commission on Safety and Quality in Health Care: www.safetyandquality.gov.au

Blood pressure measurement with manual blood pressure monitors: https://bihsoc.org/wp-content/uploads/2017/11/BP-Measurement-Poster-Manual-2017.pdf

Heart Foundation, guide to hypertension: www.heartfoundation.org.au

International Association for the Study of Pain (IASP): www.iasp-pain.org

Nursing Times, on patient deterioration and pain assessment: www.nursingtimes.net

Royal Children's Hospital, on fever: www.rch.org.au/kidsinfo/fact_sheets/Fever_in_children

CHAPTER 8

Assessing pain: The fifth vital sign

CASE STUDY

Alex Burra is a 58-year-old divorced man with two children; he works as an accountant. Two years ago, he had difficulty urinating. Tests revealed prostate cancer. Mr Burra underwent prostatectomy followed by cycles of chemotherapy a year ago. For the past 8 to 10 months, he has had continuous lower back pain and leg pain that is worse at night and while walking. He says, 'I sometimes feel that I will fall down while walking and at night I am awakened by stabbing, deep dull pain in my legs, so I don't sleep very well. Then during the day I feel tired and unable to proceed with my work.' Mr Burra also says that he is eating less and has lost about 6 kg in the past 3 months.

Conceptual foundations

DEFINITION

The International Association for the Study of Pain (IASP) defines pain as 'An unpleasant sensory and emotional experience associated with actual or potential tissue damage' (IASP, 2017). McCaffery and Pasero (1999) make an important addition to this definition by asserting that 'Pain is whatever the person says it is.' This is important to remember when assessing and treating pain.

Dunwoody et al. (2008) emphasise the importance and undertreatment of pain and recommended that pain be acknowledged as the fifth vital sign. This is because inadequate treatment of acute pain has been shown to result in physiological, psychological and emotional distress that can lead to chronic pain.

Pain is a combination of physiological phenomena but with psychosocial aspects that influence perception of the pain.

PATHOPHYSIOLOGY

The pathophysiological phenomena of pain are associated with the central and peripheral nervous systems. The source of pain stimulates peripheral nerve endings (nociceptors), which transmit the sensations to the central nervous system. Nociceptors are sensory receptors that detect signals from damaged tissue and chemicals released from the damaged tissue (Dafny, 1997–2019a). These pain receptors are located at the peripheral ends of both myelinated nerve endings of type A fibres or unmyelinated type C fibres. There are three types of nociceptors that respond to different stimuli: mechanosensitive nociceptors (of A-delta fibres), sensitive to intense mechanical stimulation (e.g. pliers pinching skin); temperature-sensitive (thermosensitive) nociceptors (of A-delta fibres), sensitive to intense heat and cold; and polymodal nociceptors (of C fibres), sensitive to noxious stimuli of mechanical, thermal or chemical nature (Patestas & Gartner, 2006). Some nociceptors may respond to more than one type of stimulus. Nociceptors are distributed in the body, skin, subcutaneous tissue, skeletal muscle, joints, peritoneal surfaces, pleural membranes, dura mater and blood vessel walls. Note that they are not located in the parenchyma of visceral organs. Physiological processes involved in pain perception include transduction, transmission, perception and modulation (Fig. 8-1).

Transduction of pain begins when a mechanical, thermal or chemical stimulus results in tissue injury or damage stimulating the nociceptors, which are the primary afferent nerves for receiving painful stimuli. Noxious stimuli initiate a painful stimulus that results in an inflammatory process leading to the release of cytokines and neuropeptides from circulating leucocytes, platelets, vascular endothelial cells, immune cells and cells from within the peripheral nervous system. This inflammatory process results in the activation of the primary afferent nociceptors (A-delta and C fibres). Furthermore, the nociceptors themselves release a substance P that enhances nociception, causing vasodilation, increased blood flow and oedema with further release of bradykinin, serotonin from platelets and histamine from mast cells. A-delta primary afferent fibres (small-diameter, lightly myelinated fibres) and C fibres (unmyelinated, primary afferent fibres) are classified as nociceptors because they are stimulated by noxious stimuli. A-delta primary afferent fibres transmit fast pain to the spinal cord within 0.1 second, which is felt as a pricking, sharp or electrical-quality sensation and usually is caused by

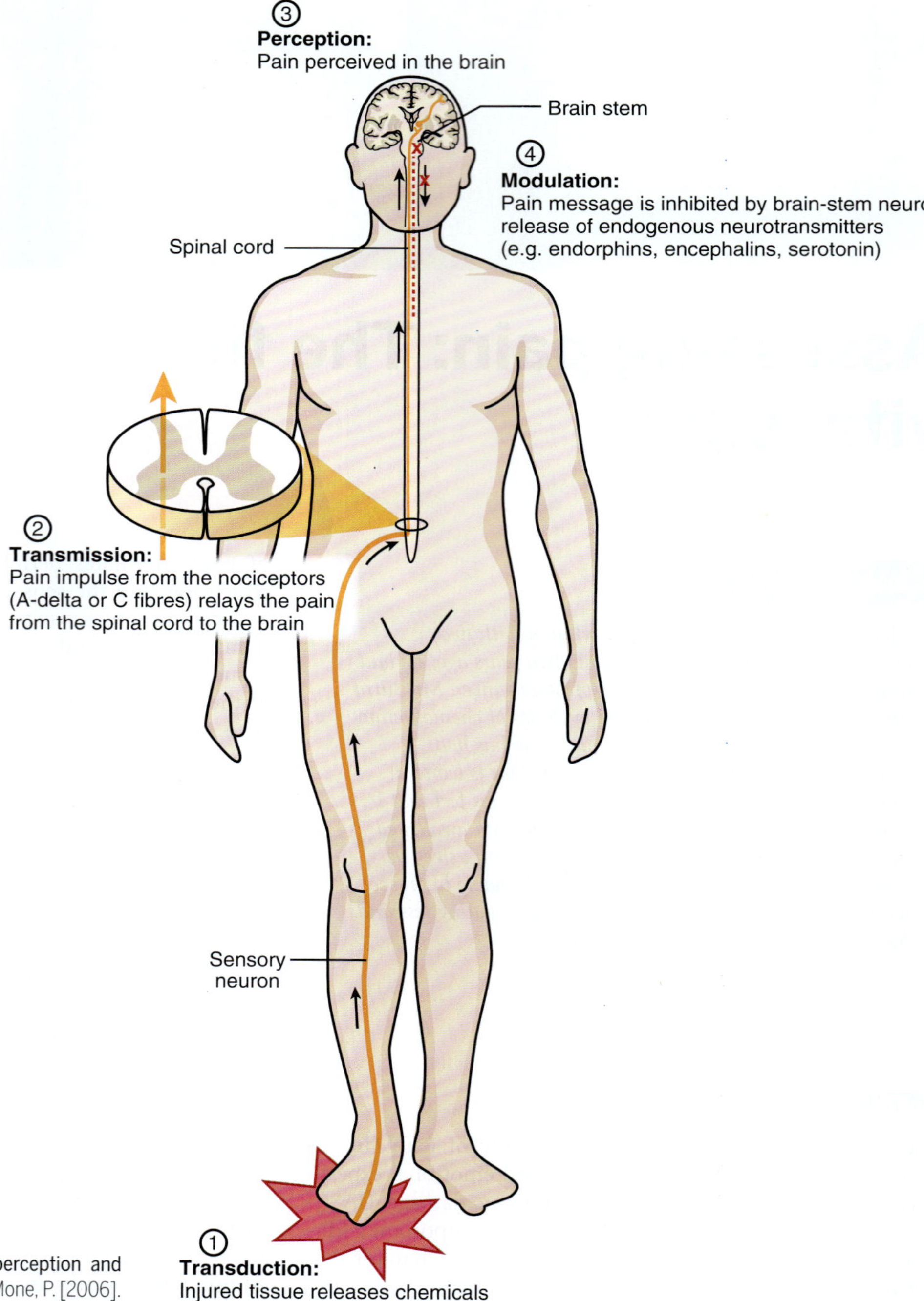

FIGURE 8-1 Transduction, transmission, perception and modulation of pain. (Taylor, C., Lillis, C. & LeMone, P. [2006]. *Fundamentals of nursing* [6th ed.]. Philadelphia: Lippincott Williams & Wilkins.)

mechanical or thermal stimuli. C fibres transmit slow pain within 1 second, which is felt as burning, throbbing or aching and is caused by mechanical, thermal or chemical stimuli, usually resulting in tissue damage. By the direct excitation of the primary afferent fibres, the stimulus leads to the activation of the fibre terminals.

The transmission process is initiated by this inflammatory process, resulting in the conduction of an impulse in the primary afferent neurons to the dorsal horn of the spinal cord. There, neurotransmitters are released and concentrated in the substantia gelatinosa (which is thought to host the gating mechanism described in the gate control theory) and bind to specific receptors. The output neurons from the dorsal horn cross the anterior white commissure and ascend the spinal cord in the anterolateral quadrant in ascending pathways (Fig. 8-2). There are several tracts within the anterolateral quadrant: spinothalamic, spinoreticular, spinomesencephalic, spinotectal and spinohypothalamic. The anterolateral tracts relay sensations of pain, temperature, non-discriminative (crude) touch, pressure and some proprioceptive sensation (Dafny, 1997–2019a). The pathways for the spinothalamic tract and its anterior and lateral portions are shown in Figure 8-2.

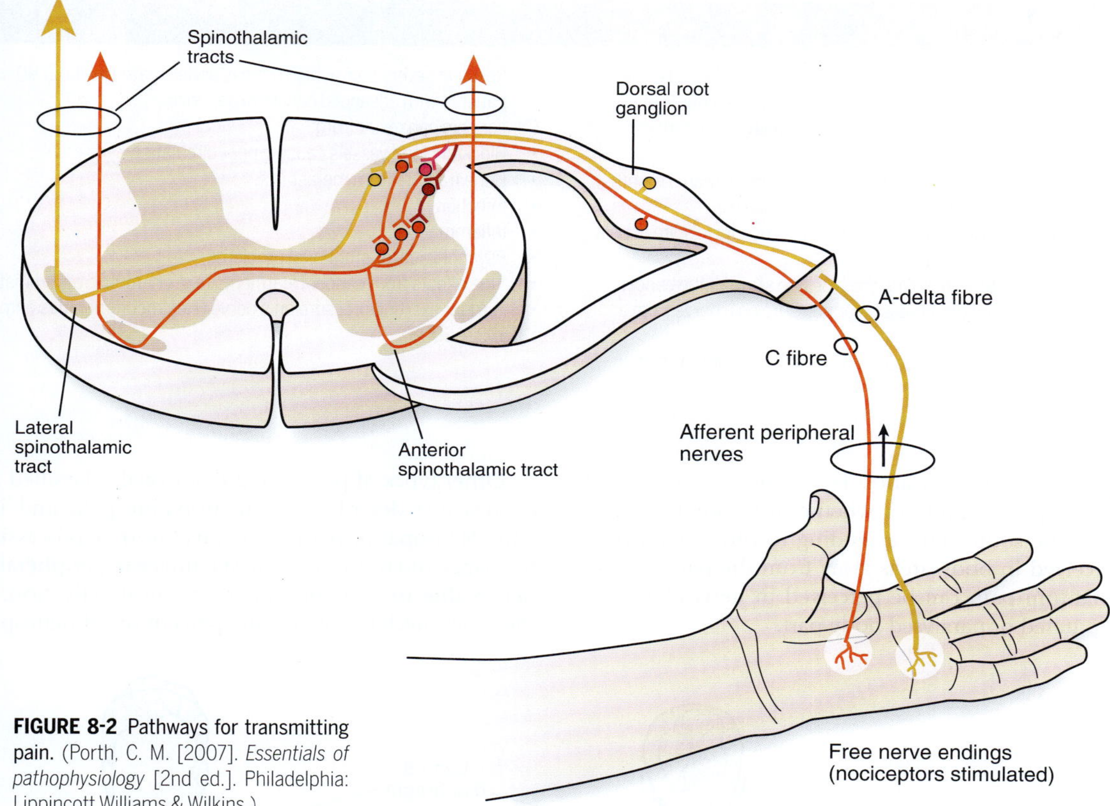

FIGURE 8-2 Pathways for transmitting pain. (Porth, C. M. [2007]. *Essentials of pathophysiology* [2nd ed.]. Philadelphia: Lippincott Williams & Wilkins.)

The emotional states of depression and anxiety directly affect the level of pain perceived and reported by patients. The hypothalamus and limbic system are responsible for the emotional aspect of pain perception, whereas the frontal cortex is responsible for the rational interpretation and response to pain.

Adjustment (modulation) of the pain experience occurs as messages relayed in the spinal cord change or inhibit the pain. The descending modulating pain pathways either increase (excite) or inhibit pain transmission. Endogenous neurotransmitters involved with modulating pain include endogenous opioids, such as endorphins and encephalin; serotonin; noradrenaline; gamma-aminobutyric acid; neurotensin; acetylcholine; and oxytocin (Dafny, 1997–2019b).

PHYSIOLOGICAL RESPONSES TO PAIN

Pain elicits a stress response in the human body that triggers the sympathetic nervous system, resulting in:

- Anxiety, fear, hopelessness, sleeplessness and thoughts of suicide
- A preoccupation with the pain, reports of pain, cries and moans, frowns and grimaces
- A decrease in cognitive function; mental confusion; and altered temperament and anxiety expressed as physical symptoms
- Dilated pupils
- Increased heart rate, peripheral, systemic and coronary vascular resistance, and increased blood pressure
- Increased respiratory rate and sputum retention, resulting in infection and atelectasis
- Decreased gastric and intestinal motility
- Decreased urinary output resulting in urinary retention, fluid overload and depression of all immune responses
- Increased antidiuretic hormone, adrenalin, noradrenaline, aldosterone and glucagon, and decreased insulin and testosterone
- Hyperglycaemia, glucose intolerance, insulin resistance and protein catabolism
- Muscle spasm resulting in impaired muscle function and immobility, perspiration.

CLASSIFICATION

Pain can be classified according to duration, location, aetiology and severity. Duration and aetiology are often classified together to differentiate between acute pain, chronic non-malignant pain and cancer pain.

- *Acute pain:* usually associated with a recent injury so that it comes on quickly but lasts a short time
- *Chronic non-malignant pain:* usually associated with a specific cause or injury and described as a constant pain that persists for more than 6 months
- *Cancer pain:* often due to the compression of peripheral nerves or meninges or from the damage to these structures following surgery, chemotherapy, radiation, or tumour growth and infiltration (see Display 8-1).

Classifications of pain by location include:

- **Cutaneous pain** (skin or subcutaneous tissue)
- **Visceral pain** (abdominal cavity, thorax, cranium)
- **Deep somatic pain** (ligaments, tendons, bones, blood vessels, nerves).

DISPLAY 8-1 CANCER PAIN

Cancer pain is a special category of pain because it may reflect all of the pain types at the same time or at different times during the course of the disease. Cancer pain may be caused by the cancer, its treatment or its metastases. Cancer pain can:

- Be acute (sudden and severe) or chronic (lasting more than 3 months)
- Include somatic pain, visceral pain and neuropathic pain
- Cause breakthrough pain (brief, severe pain that occurs in spite of pain medication) in many patients
- Depend on many factors, including the type and stage of the cancer
- Be triggered by blocked blood vessels or pressure on a nerve from a tumour
- Result from the side effects of treatments, such as surgery, radiation and chemotherapy
- Result in severe pain, which often is undertreated in about 90% of patients with advanced cancer experience.

Cancer pain can result from:

- Blocked blood vessels causing poor circulation
- Bone fracture from metastasis
- Infection
- Inflammation
- Psychological or emotional problems
- Side effects from cancer treatments (e.g. chemotherapy, radiation)
- Tumour exerting pressure on a nerve (Healthcommunities.com, 1998–2008).

Another aspect of pain location is whether it is perceived at the site of the pain stimuli, or whether it is radiating (perceived both at the source and extending to other tissues) or referred (perceived in body areas away from the pain source; Fig. 8-3). Phantom pain can be perceived in nerves left by a missing, amputated or paralysed body part.

Other types of pain that are not easily classified in the categories just described are neuropathic pain and intractable pain. Neuropathic pain causes an abnormal processing of pain messages and results from past damage to peripheral or central nerves due to sustained neurochemical activation. However, the exact mechanisms for the perception of neuropathic pain

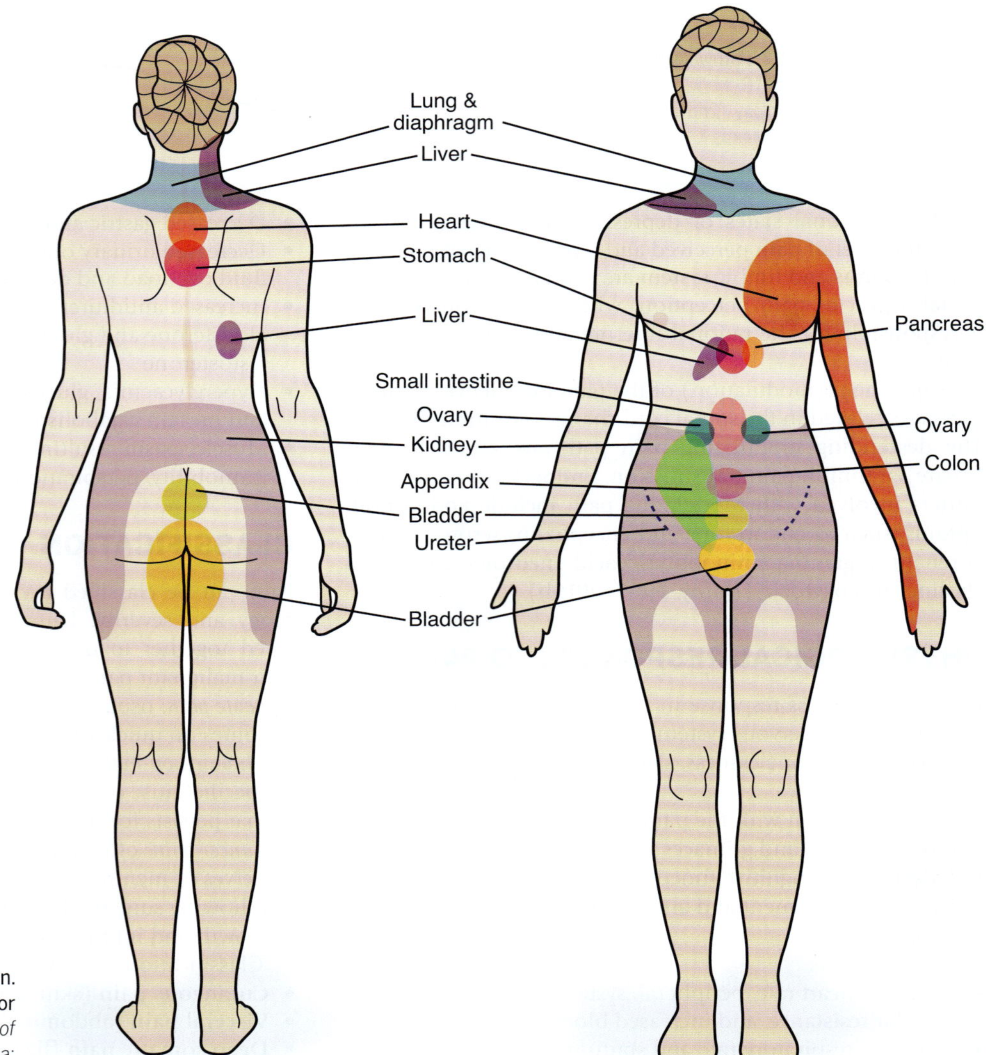

FIGURE 8-3 Areas of referred pain. **(Left)** Posterior view. **(Right)** Anterior view. (Porth, C. M. [2007]. *Essentials of pathophysiology* [2nd ed.]. Philadelphia: Lippincott Williams & Wilkins.)

are unclear. Intractable pain is defined by its high resistance to pain relief.

SEVEN DIMENSIONS OF PAIN

The experience of pain is quite complex. It is more than the physiological and neurochemical responses. Silkman (2008) describes the multidimensional complexity of pain in seven dimensions: physical, sensory, behavioural, socio-cultural, cognitive, affective and spiritual. The physical dimension refers to the physiological effects of pain; it includes the patient's perception of the pain and the body's reaction to the stimulus. The sensory dimension includes the quality of the pain and how severe the pain is perceived to be. This dimension also includes the patient's perception of the location, intensity and quality of the pain. The behavioural dimension refers to the verbal and non-verbal behaviours that the patient demonstrates in response to pain. The socio-cultural dimension describes the influences of the social context and cultural background of the patient on his or her pain experience. The cognitive dimension encompasses 'beliefs, attitudes, intentions, and motivations related to the pain and its management' (Silkman, 2008, p. 14). Of course, beliefs, attitudes, intentions and motivations are affected by all of the dimensions but can be associated with the management of the pain experience, which is dependent on cognition. The affective dimension concerns feelings, sentiments and emotions related to the pain experience. The pain can affect the emotions, and the emotions can affect the perception of pain. Finally, the spiritual dimension refers to the meaning and purpose that the person 'attributes to the pain, self, others, and the divine' (p. 15). For some suggested questions to assess each dimension, see Assessment tool 8-1.

PAIN ASSESSMENT

Before beginning to collect data from the patient, several additional elements of pain history must be considered. The developmental level or age of the person makes a difference in the assessment approach. Also, **culture** must be considered, as cultural beliefs about pain and its treatment vary widely. Cancer pain is often considered separately because it can be caused by many elements of the disease or treatment, or by other sources of pain not related to the disease (see Display 8-1). A thorough pain assessment includes questions about location, intensity, quality, pattern, precipitating factors and pain relief, as well as the effect of the pain on daily activities, what coping

ASSESSMENT TOOL 8-1 Pain dimensions: sample assessment questions

Here are examples of questions to ask your patient when assessing the seven dimensions of pain.

Dimension	Sample questions
Physical: effect of anatomical structure and physiological functioning on the experience of pain	What surgeries or other medical procedures have you had? What medical conditions do you have? What conditions brought you to the hospital or doctor's surgery in the past?
Sensory: qualitative and quantitative descriptions of pain	Where is the pain located? What does the pain feel like? How would you rate the pain on a scale of 0 to 10, with 10 being the worst pain imaginable? When did the pain begin? How long does the pain usually last?
Behavioural: verbal and non-verbal behaviours associated with pain	I notice that you are __________ (fill in the patient's behaviour, such as grimacing). Are you having pain?
Socio-cultural: effect of social and cultural backgrounds on the experience of pain	What is your country of origin? Do you have any special cultural or social practices that influence the decisions you make about health care? How do you manage your pain at home?
Cognitive: thoughts, beliefs, attitudes, intentions and motivations related to the experience of pain	How effective is the pain relief treatment you're currently getting? What's the highest level of education you've completed? What do you do for a living? What do you think is causing your pain? What do you think will relieve it?
Affective: feelings and emotions that result from pain	How does the pain affect your overall mood? Daily life and activities? Social activities and interactions? Personal relationships?
Spiritual: ultimate meaning and purpose attributed to pain, self, others and the divine	What's your religious affiliation? What religious or spiritual practices and preferences do you have? How do your religious or spiritual beliefs influence your health care decisions? How would you describe the support you receive from friends and loved ones?

(From Silkman, C. [2008]. Assessing the seven dimensions of pain. *American Nurse Today, 3*(2), 13–15.)

DISPLAY 8-2 COLDSPA

Example for pain

Use the COLDSPA mnemonic as a guideline to collect needed information for each symptom the patient shares. In addition, the following questions help elicit important information.

Mnemonic	Question	Patient response example
Character	Describe the sign or symptom (feeling, appearance, sound, smell or taste, if applicable).	'My right lower side hurts. It is a steady aching that is getting worse.'
Onset	When did it begin?	'Late last night.'
Location	Where is it? Does it radiate? Does it occur anywhere else?	'It started in the middle of my stomach and now it is worse on my right side. It does not hurt anywhere else.'
Duration	How long does it last? Does it recur?	'It has been ongoing since last night around 3 o'clock and is getting worse.'
Severity	How bad is it? How much does it bother you?	'It hurts to walk or even move. I would rate it 8 on a scale of 10 (with 10 being the worst).'
Pattern	What makes it better or worse?	'It hurts constantly and gets worse if I move.'
Associated factors/How it **A**ffects the patient	What other symptoms occur with it? How does it affect you?	'I feel nauseated and like I may vomit. I cannot do anything except stay still or it gets worse.'

strategies have been used and emotional responses to the pain. The COLDSPA mnemonic is one useful method for assessing pain (see Display 8-2).

Developmental level

The two extremes of development—paediatric (neonate to later childhood) and geriatric age groups—have characteristics that make pain assessment more difficult. The developmental stage therefore needs to be considered, particularly because pain has both sensory and emotional components, which will be determined by developmental level.

In Australia, the prevalence of chronic pain in children is reported to be between 25% and 35% (Pain Australia, 2013). Friedrichsdorf et al. (2016) report that chronic pain affects 20% to 35% of children. The prevalence of chronic pain in residents of Australian aged-care facilities is between 60% and 83% (Royal Australian College of General Practitioners, 2006). Fetuses, at least by 26 weeks gestation, are known to perceive pain and may feel pain as early as 20 weeks (Mahieu-Caputo et al., 2000). Extremely premature infants and full-term neonates feel pain.

Not knowing whether an infant, a neonate, a young child, an elderly or a person with cognitive impairment is feeling pain can lead to gross undertreatment of pain in these people. The results of undertreated pain are profound and may result in physical as well as psychological problems. In children, undertreated pain can lead to chronic pain conditions. These complications can be avoided if pain is assessed and treated properly.

Cognitively intact elders, parents of children and persons from certain cultures hold beliefs that may prevent a person's pain from being assessed and treated correctly. Some people believe that pain is a punishment for past sins or behaviours; some believe it is a natural part of the ageing process; and some believe that having pain indicates that a disease is getting worse or that death is near. These beliefs may lead to misleading answers to questions about pain. Some people fear the addictive effects of narcotics and opioids, and this concern may lead them to underreport pain. Learning how to assess pain and teaching patients and other carers about pain care are essential skills for nurses who provide high-quality care.

Pain in persons unable to provide a self-report

There are specific methods of assessing pain in infants and preverbal toddlers, people who are unconscious or have cognitive problems or intellectual disability, elders with dementia, and patients who are intubated.

For patients who unable to talk or those with cognitive impairment, Herr et al. (2011) recommend using the Hierarchy of Pain Assessment Techniques (McCaffery & Pasero, 1999). The hierarchy includes five items:

1. Try to get a self-report—if the patient is unable to provide one, go on to the other items
2. Search for potential causes of pain—these include pathological conditions, procedures such as surgery, wound care, positioning, skin invasion by needle or catheter, and other known inducers of pain
3. Observe patient behaviours—many measurement tools reflect pain-related behaviours of different patient types. See pain scales listed by Herr et al. (2011) and selected ones later in this chapter. *Note:* Patient behaviours may not accurately reflect pain intensity
4. Try surrogate reporting (family members, parents, carers) of pain and behaviour or activity changes—note that discrepancies may exist between self-reports of pain and surrogate reports. There may also be differences between surrogates and health care providers on judgements of pain and its intensity
5. Attempt an analgesic trial—a full protocol is recommended. After an analgesic is ordered, the nurse needs to observe for changes or differences in behaviour.

QUESTT principles for pain in children

Baker and Wong (1987) developed the mnemonic QUESTT for assessment of pain in children. The main points that underlie the mnemonic are that in clinical assessment of pain, regular and systematic assessment is essential; the healthcare provider should believe the patient's or family's report of the pain and should empower them by involving them in decision making. The mnemonic is as follows:

Question the child
Use pain rating scales

Evaluate behaviour and physiological changes
Secure parents' involvement
Take cause of pain into account
Take action and evaluate results.

Cultural expressions of pain

Pain is a universal human experience, but how people respond to it varies with the meaning they place on pain and the response to pain that is expected in their culture. Pain can have several meanings between cultures that lead to these different response patterns. Refer to the examples shown in Display 8-3, Cultural expressions of pain. Although these examples of differences in meaning and expression of pain show some of the cultural variations that are important for the nurse assessing for pain, the most important point is to avoid stereotyping. The nurse should keep in mind that although people from a particular cultural background tend to exhibit certain characteristics, many people of that culture will not. The nurse must assess what the person says about pain; what the person says about asking for pain medication; what the person says about the meaning pain has; how the person behaves when undergoing painful procedures; and how the person behaves when others are present or absent. In other words, treat each person as a unique individual, assess each patient, respect each patient's responses to pain, and treat all with dignity and consideration (see Chap. 10, Assessing culture).

A variety of issues can create barriers to pain assessment (see Display 8-4). For an excellent source for interventions to overcome cultural and communication barriers when caring for patients in pain, see 'What colour is your pain?' by Louise Kaegi (2004).

Health assessment

COLLECTING SUBJECTIVE DATA: THE NURSING HEALTH HISTORY

There are few objective findings on which the assessment of pain can rely. This is because pain is a subjective phenomenon and thus the main assessment depends on the patient's report. The patient's description of pain is quoted. The exact words used to describe the experience of pain are used to help in the diagnosis and management of pain. Display 8-5 lists common definitions of terms used by people to describe pain. The onset, duration, causes, alleviating and aggravating factors are also assessed. Then the quality, intensity and effects of pain on the physical, psychosocial and spiritual aspects are questioned. Past experience with pain, in addition to past and current therapies, is explored. Review Display 8-6 before assessing the patient's subjective experience of pain.

DISPLAY 8-3 CULTURAL EXPRESSIONS OF PAIN

Cultural group	Pain expression/beliefs
Asian	• Pain is natural • Use mind over body; positive thinking • Pain is honourable • Pain may be caused by past transgressions and helps to atone and achieve higher spirituality • Stigma against narcotic use may result in underreporting of pain
Hindu	• Pain must be endured as part of preparing for the next life in the cycle of reincarnation • Must remain conscious when nearing death to experience the events of dying and perhaps rebirth

Aboriginal and Torres Strait Islander peoples	• Pain experience is connected to the land, their 'kin' and the spirit world
	• For some, the origins of pain are connected to the wind and weather
	• For some, returning home to be with family may be more important than receiving treatment for pain
	• Some may suppress pain behaviours and demonstrate reluctance to discuss their pain experience
	• The numerical pain assessment tool may be inaccurate as some Aboriginal and Torres Strait Islander languages do not have a conceptual recognition of the numbers above five
	
	Asking about pain
	• Need to establish a 'trust relationship'
	• When asked about pain, the respondent may:
	  ◦ Turn away their head with eyes averted or downcast
	  ◦ Feign sleep
	  ◦ Choose not to discuss how their pain began, as it resulted from breaking cultural law
	  ◦ Choose not to respond, particularly if the answer is obvious. For example, asking someone with a bony fracture whether they have pain is a 'non-sense question' that is not worth responding to. In this situation, acknowledge the pain the person is experiencing and then perform a more detailed assessment
	  ◦ Be silent before answering, because for some Indigenous people it is polite to pause before a reply; accept the pause and wait.
	
	Behaviours
	Stereotyping and generalisation of pain behaviours are dangerous; this list encompasses commonly observed and reported behaviours. The person may:
	• Be reserved and non-obtrusive when experiencing pain (this is not an indication of high pain tolerance)
	• Be quieter than usual
	• Lie very still
	• Cry, shake their head and 'cluck' the tongue
	• Avert their gaze (Fenwick, 2006).

Continued on following page

DISPLAY 8-3 CULTURAL EXPRESSIONS OF PAIN (continued)

Cultural group	Pain expression/beliefs
Māori	Pain assessment of Māori needs to be based in the Māori model of health, *te whare tapa wha*. In this model, health is a multidimensional balance between spiritual, emotional, physical and family health. Commonly used descriptors of pain are acceptable: Magnusson and Fennell (2011) present this table:

Sensory	Emotional	Cognitive	Social
Boring	Angry	Suicidal	Dependent
Bruised	Crappy	Useless	Despair
Constant	Shattered	Unthinkable	Left out
Sprained	Stuffed	Unconscious	Restless
Sticking	Broken	Delirium	Quarrelsome

Many people, including those of Māori ethnicity, present aggressively when experiencing pain. Also, Māori have a tendency to take a subordinate stance when faced with health professionals whom they deem to be in a position of higher authority. This is manifest by not making eye contact and averting their eyes towards the floor or away from the health practitioner. Such behaviour can be regarded as hostile. Try sitting or standing alongside the patient rather than being confrontational by facing them directly.

Cultural group	Pain expression/beliefs
Pacific Islanders (Pasifika)	• Males are expected to have high pain tolerance and to not cry • Pacific peoples respect those with higher status, such as doctors, so they may answer questions with a simple yes or no. Alternatively, they may avoid answering the question because they don't want to waste the doctor's time. This can prevent a full understanding of the patient's pain, unless extra effort is made to inquire about the pain (Mauri Ora Associates, SAEJ Consultancy & Panapa Ehau, 2010) • Traditionally Pacific Islanders do not wear shoes and so become accustomed to the pain of walking on rocks, gravel, and rough, hard grass.

As a nurse it is important to recognise your own response to pain. How did you respond to pain in your family? What did you think about pain when you were a child? Did your parents respond the same way? What did they teach you about pain? Some people are raised to deny pain, seeing it as just a normal part of life. Others are raised to respond verbally and loudly to pain because it indicates an invasion of the body and is a sign that something bad has happened or will happen. Are you a stoic? Are you vocal and loud, moaning or crying, if pain is intense? Knowing your own response to pain lets you know a little about what you believe about pain. A perception that our responses and beliefs are 'normal' and those of others are not can lead to miscommunications between nurses and patients. To be a culturally competent nurse caring for patients in pain:

- Be aware of your own cultural and family values
- Be aware of your personal biases and assumptions about people with different values from yours
- Be aware and accept cultural differences between yourself and individual patients
- Be capable of understanding the dynamics of differences
- Be able to adapt to diversity (Weissman et al., 2004; Chap. 10, Assessing culture).

DISPLAY 8-4 BARRIERS TO PAIN ASSESSMENT

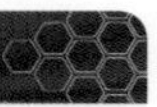

Barriers to correct pain assessment may be present and must be assessed as well. Cultural differences and physiological differences account for most of these. Consider cultural variation to exist in all patient populations and not just among persons from other countries. Also, gender differences are expressed differently in different cultures. Nurses' and other health care providers' beliefs about pain can also affect the assessment.

Barriers based on beliefs

- Acknowledging pain is not manly; it is a sign of weakness.
- Pain is a punishment (often thought to be from God) for past mistakes, sins or behaviours, and must be tolerated.
- Pain indicates that my illness is getting worse and that I am going to die soon. If I don't acknowledge it, it won't be so bad.
- Pain medications are addictive; cause awful side effects; and make me confused and sleepy or unconscious.
- All people have pain, especially as they age. This is just normal pain and I should not say anything about it.

Barriers based on physical conditions

- The disease, illness or injury for which the patient is being treated is not the source of the pain.
- Both the current disease and another disease are causing pain.
- The person expresses few, if any, pain-related behaviours once they have accommodated to prolonged chronic pain conditions.

Barriers based on health care providers' beliefs

- Patients who complain of pain frequently are just trying to get more pain medicine or are addicts wanting more narcotics.
- Patients who complain of pain but don't show physical and behavioural signs of pain don't need more pain medication, whether they are chronic-pain patients or acute-pain patients.
- Old people just have more pain.
- Confused or demented patients, or very young patients, neonates and fetuses don't feel pain.
- Patients who are sleeping don't have pain.
- Pain medication causes addiction.
- Pain medication cause respiratory depression and too many side effects.
- Giving as much pain medication as possible at night will make the patients sleep and not disturb the nurses.

DISPLAY 8-5 TERMS USED BY PEOPLE TO DESCRIBE PAIN

Quality

Sharp	Pain that is intense and knifelike in nature.
Dull	Pain that is not as intense or acute as sharp pain, possibly more annoying than painful. It is usually more diffuse than sharp pain.
Diffuse	Pain that covers a large area. Usually, the person is unable to point to a specific area without moving the hand over a large surface, such as the entire abdomen.
Shifting	Pain that moves from one area to another, such as from the lower abdomen to the area over the stomach.

Other terms used to describe the quality of pain include sore, stinging, pinching, cramping, gnawing, cutting, throbbing, shooting, vicelike pressure.

Severity

Severe or excruciating Moderate, slight or mild	These terms depend on the person's interpretation of pain. Behavioural and physiological signs help assess the severity of pain. On a scale of 1 to 10, slight pain could be described as being between about 1 and 3; moderate pain, between about 4 and 6; and severe pain, between about 8 and 10.

Periodicity

Continuous	Pain that does not stop
Intermittent	Pain that stops and starts again
Brief or transient	Pain that passes quickly

DISPLAY 8-6 TIPS FOR COLLECTING SUBJECTIVE DATA

- Maintain a quiet and calm environment that is comfortable for the patient being interviewed.
- Maintain the patient's privacy and ensure confidentiality.
- Ask the questions in an open-ended format.
- Listen carefully to the patient's verbal descriptions and quote the terms used.
- Watch for the patient's facial expressions and grimaces during the interview.
- DO NOT put words in the patient's mouth.
- Ask the patient about past experiences with pain.
- Believe the patient's expression of pain.

CASE STUDY

During the physical exam, Mr Burra entered the room limping. He then sat on the chair with his shoulders slumped. He changed his position every 2 to 3 minutes, looking anxious and uncomfortable, with frowns and grimaces as facial expressions. He rates his pain on the Visual Analogue Scale as 7/10. His vital signs are: heart rate 110 beats/minute, respiratory rate 22 breaths/minute and blood pressure135/85 mmHg.

CRITICAL THINKING

1. When talking about the 'quality' of pain, what do we mean?
2. What further questions would you ask Mr Burra to assess the quality of his pain?
3. What other pain symptoms does Mr Burra describe?
4. What inferences might you draw from Mr Burra's history and his description of his pain?

History of present health concern

Review the standards (Display 8-7) and tips for collecting subjective data (Display 8-6) before assessing the patient's subjective experience of pain.

QUESTION	RATIONALE
Are you experiencing pain now or have you in the past 24 hours?	To establish the presence or absence of perceived pain.
Where is the pain located?	The location of pain helps to identify the underlying cause.
Does it radiate or spread?	Radiating or spreading pain helps to identify the source. For example, chest pain radiating to the left arm is most probably of cardiac origin, whereas the pain that is pricking and spreading in the chest muscle area is probably musculoskeletal in origin.
Are there any other concurrent symptoms accompanying the pain?	Accompanying symptoms help to identify the possible source. For example, right lower quadrant pain associated with nausea, vomiting and the inability to stand up straight is possibly associated with appendicitis.

History of present health concern (continued)

QUESTION	RATIONALE
When did the pain start?	The onset of pain is an essential indicator for the severity of the situation and suggests a source.
What were you doing when the pain first started?	This question helps to identify the precipitating factors and what might have exacerbated the pain.
Is the pain continuous or intermittent?	Information elicited by this question helps to identify the nature of the pain.
If intermittent pain, how often do the episodes occur and for how long do they last?	Understanding the course of the pain provides a pattern that may help to determine the source.
Describe the pain in your own words.	Patients are quoted so that terms used to describe their pain may indicate the type and source. The most common terms used are: *throbbing*, *shooting*, *stabbing*, *sharp*, *cramping*, *gnawing*, *hot-burning*, *aching*, *heavy*, *tender*, *splitting*, *tiring*, *exhausting*, *sickening*, *fearful* and *punishing*.
What factors relieve your pain?	Relieving factors help to determine the source and the plan of care.
What factors increase your pain?	Identifying factors that increase pain helps to determine the source and ways of avoiding aggravating factors.
Are you on any therapy to manage your pain?	This question establishes any current treatment modalities and their effect on the pain. This helps in planning the future plan of care.
Is there anything you would like to add?	An open-ended question allows the patient to mention anything that has been missed or the issues that were not fully addressed by the questions listed.

Past health history

QUESTION	RATIONALE
Have you had any previous experience with pain?	Past experiences of pain may shed light on the history of the patient in addition to possible positive or negative expectations of pain therapies.
Does this pain have any special meaning to you?	Some cultures view pain as a punishment or view pain as the main symptom to be treated as opposed to treating the underlying disease.

Family history

QUESTION	RATIONALE
Does anyone in your family experience pain?	To assess possible family-related perceptions or any past experiences with persons in pain.
How does pain affect your family?	To assess how much the pain is interfering with the patient's family relations.

COLLECTING OBJECTIVE DATA: PHYSICAL EXAMINATION

Objective data are collected by using pain assessment tools. There are many assessment tools, some of which are specific to a type of pain. The main criteria in the choice of tool are its reliability and its validity. The tool must be clear and, therefore, easily understood by the patient; its use should require little effort from the patient or the nurse.

Preparing the patient

In preparation for the interview, patients are seated in a quiet, comfortable and calm environment with minimal interruption. Explain to the patient that the interview will entail

DISPLAY 8-7 JOINT COMMISSION STANDARDS FOR PAIN MANAGEMENT IN AUSTRALIA AND NEW ZEALAND

Measurement

1. Regular assessment of pain leads to improved acute pain management.
2. There is good correlation between the visual analogue and numerical rating scales.
3. Self-reporting of pain should be used whenever appropriate as pain is by definition a subjective experience.
4. The pain measurement tool chosen should be appropriate to the individual patient; developmental, cognitive, emotional, language and cultural factors should be considered.
5. Scoring should incorporate different components of pain including the functional capacity of the patient. In the postoperative patient this should include static (rest) and dynamic (e.g. pain on sitting, coughing) pain.
6. Uncontrolled or unexpected pain requires a reassessment of the diagnosis and consideration of alternative causes for the pain (e.g. new surgical or medical diagnosis, neuropathic pain).

Outcome measures in acute pain management

- Multiple outcome measures are required to adequately capture the complexity of the pain experience and how it may be modified by pain management interventions (Macintyre et al., 2010).

(MacIntyre, P., Schug, S., Scott, D., et al. [2010]. *Acute pain management: Scientific evidence*. Melbourne: Australia and New Zealand College of Anaesthetists and Faculty of Pain Medicine.)

OLDCARTS

OLDCARTS: Alternative mnemonic to COLDSPA

Another common mnemonic used to collect symptoms about pain is OLDCARTS.

Mnemonic	Question	Patient response example
Onset	When did it begin?	'Late last night.'
Location	Where is it? Does it radiate? Does it occur anywhere else?	'It started in the middle of my stomach and now it is worse on my right side. It does not hurt anywhere else.'
Duration	How long does it last? Does it recur?	'It has been ongoing since last night around 3 o'clock and is getting worse.'
Characteristic	Describe the sign or symptom (feeling, appearance, sound, smell or taste, if applicable).	'It is very sharp; it feels like a knife is sticking into me.' 'I feel sick and want to vomit.'
Aggravating factors	What makes it worse?	'Any movement hurts.'
Relieving factors	What makes it better?	'Keeping very still.'
Treatment	What treatment have you received for it? Did the treatment reduce the pain?	'I took 2 paracetamol tablets with codeine at 3 o'clock but they haven't helped much.'
Severity	How bad is it? How much does it bother you?	'I would rate it 8 on a scale of 10 (with 10 being the worst pain).'

Lifestyle and health practices

QUESTION	RATIONALE
What are your concerns about pain?	Identifying the patient's fears and worries helps in prioritising the plan of care and providing adequate psychological support.
How does your pain interfere with the following? • General activity • Mood or emotions • Concentration • Physical ability • Work • Relationships with other people • Sleep • Appetite • Enjoyment of life	These are the main lifestyle factors that pain interferes with. The more that pain interferes with the patient's ability to function in his or her daily activities, the more it will reflect on the patient's psychological status and thus the quality of life.

questions to clarify the picture of the pain experienced in order to develop the plan of care.

Pain assessment tools

Select one or more pain assessment tools appropriate for the patient. There are many pain assessment scales, such as:

- Visual Analogue Scale (VAS) (Fig. 8-4)
- Numeric Rating Scale (NRS) (Fig. 8-5)
- Numeric Pain Intensity Scale
- Verbal Descriptor Scale (Fig. 8-6)
- Simple Descriptive Pain Intensity Scale
- Graphic Rating Scale
- Verbal Rating Scale
- Faces Pain Scales (FPS, FPS—Revised [FPS-R]; see Chap. 33).

You can look at all of these and other scales at www.iasp-pain.org. Most of these scales have been shown to be reliable measures of patient pain. The three most popular scales are the NRS, the Verbal Descriptor Scale, and the FPS, although VASs are often mentioned as very simple.

Assessing pain in older adults, infants and children

The NRS has been shown to be best for older adults with no cognitive impairment, and the FPS-R for cognitively impaired adults (Flaherty, 2008).

It is hard to evaluate pain in neonates and infants. Behaviours that indicate pain are used to assess their pain. One tool for such assessment is the N-PASS (Neonatal Pain, Agitation and Sedation Scale [Hummel et al., 2008]). Another popular tool for assessing paediatric pain is the FLACC Scale (Face, Legs, Activity, Cry and Consolability); see Assessment tool 8-2.

Three pain assessment tools that serve well for the patient's initial assessment are the Initial Pain Assessment Tool (see Fig. 8-7; McCaffery & Pasero, 1999), the Brief Pain Inventory (Short Form; Cleeland & Ryan, 1994) and, specifically for paediatric pain assessment, the Initial Pain Assessment for Paediatric Use Only (Otto et al., 1996).

CRITICAL THINKING

5. Using the information that has been provided about Mr Burra and using your imagination complete a pain assessment.
6. How much relief do you think is he able to achieve at home?

Physical assessment

During examination of the patient, remember these key points:

- Choose an assessment tool that is reliable and valid to your culture.
- Explain to the patient the purpose of rating the intensity of pain.
- Ensure the patient's privacy and confidentiality.
- Respect the patient's behaviour towards pain and the terms used to express it.

Understand that different cultures express pain differently and maintain different pain thresholds and expectations.

VALIDATING AND DOCUMENTING FINDINGS

Validate the pain assessment data you have collected. This step is necessary to verify the reliability and accuracy of the data. Document the assessment data following the health care facility or agency policy.

FIGURE 8-4 Visual Analogue Scale (VAS). (*Source:* Riegel, B. [n.d.]. *Pain assessment*. Available at www.burnsurvivorsttw.org. Burn Survivors Throughout The World, Inc. is an international not-for-profit organisation offering a support team, advocacy, medical referrals, email and a chat room for burn survivors.)

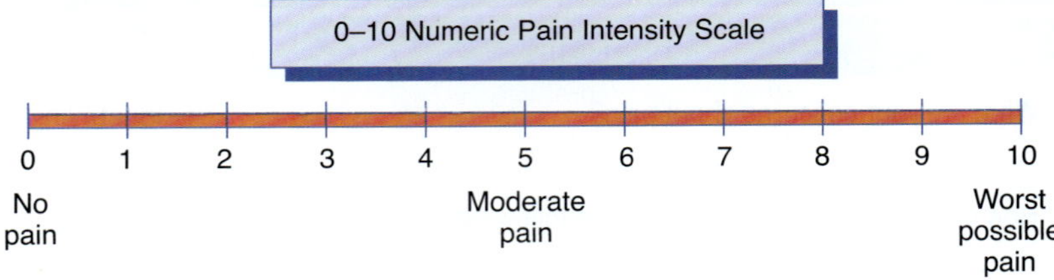

FIGURE 8-5 Numeric Rating Scale. (From Agency for Health Care Policy and Research [AHCPR], 1992.)

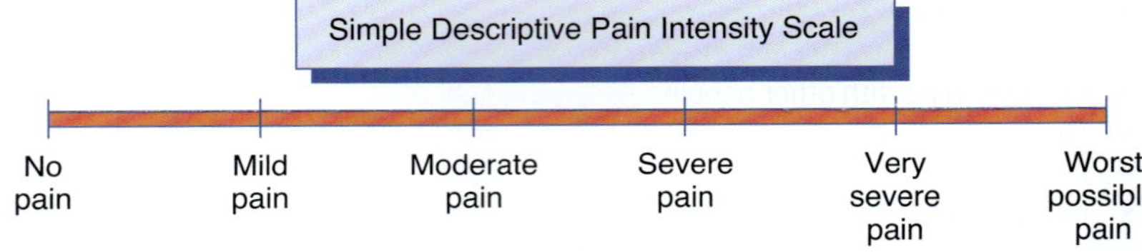

FIGURE 8-6 Verbal Descriptor Scale. (From Agency for Health Care Policy and Research [AHCPR], 1992.)

ASSESSMENT TOOL 8-2 rFLACC Behavioral Scale

		SCORE (circle most appropriate)
FACE	0=No particular expression or smile	**0**
	1=Occasional grimace/frown; withdrawn or disinterested; **appears sad or worried**	**1**
	2=Consistent grimace or frown; Frequent/constant quivering chin, clenched jaw; **Distressed-looking face; Expression of fright or panic**	**2**
	Individual behavior: ____________	
LEGS	0=Normal position or relaxed; Usual tone & motion to limbs	**0**
	1=Uneasy, restless, tense; **occasional tremors**	**1**
	2=Kicking, or legs drawn up; **marked increase in spasticity, constant tremors or jerking**	**2**
	Individual behavior: ____________	
ACTIVITY	0=Lying quietly, normal position, moves easily; Regular, rhythmic respirations	**0**
	1=Squirming, shifting back and forth, tense or guarded movements; **mildly agitated (eg. head back & forth, aggression); Shallow, splinting respirations, intermittent sighs.**	**1**
	2=Arched, rigid or jerking; **severe agitation; head banging; shivering (not rigors); Breath holding, gasping or sharp intake of breaths, severe splinting**	**2**
	Individual behavior: ____________	
CRY	0=No cry	**0**
	1=Moans or whimpers; **occasional complaint; occasional verbal outburst or grunt**	**1**
	2=Crying steadily, screams or sobs, frequent complaints; **repeated outbursts, constant grunting**	**2**
	Individual behavior: ____________	
CONSOLABILITY	0=Content and relaxed	**0**
	1=Reassured by occasional touching, hugging or being talked to. Distractable	**1**
	2=Difficult to console or comfort; **pushing away caregiver, resisting care or comfort measures**	**2**
	Individual behavior: ____________	
		Total:

- The revised FLACC can be used for all non-verbal children.
- The rFLACC contains the descriptors from the validated FLACC scale. The additional descriptors (in bold) are descriptors used in the validation of the tool in children with cognitive impairment (2002).
- To individualize the rFLACC, the clinician can review with parents or caregiver the descriptors within each category. Ask them if there are additional behaviors that are better indicators of pain in their child. Add these behaviors to the appropriate category of the tool. Indicate if the behavior is associated with a score of 0, 1 or 2.
- Each of the five categories (F) Face; (L) Legs; (A) Activity; (C) Cry; (C) Consolability is scored from 0-2, which results in a total score between zero and ten. The instructions for scoring the FLACC can be used to help score the rFLACC.
- **Patients who are awake**: Observe for at least 1-2 minutes. Observe legs and body uncovered. Reposition patient or observe activity, assess body for tenseness and tone. Initiate consoling interventions if needed
- **Patients who are asleep**: Observe for at least 2 minutes or longer. Observe body and legs uncovered. If possible reposition the patient. Touch the body and assess for tenseness and tone.

Whenever feasible, behavioral measurement of pain should be used in conjunction with self-report. When self-report is not possible, interpretation of pain behaviors and decision making regarding treatment of pain requires careful consideration of the context in which the behaviors are observed.

Assessment of rFLACC Behavioral Scores

0 = Relaxed and comfortable
1-3 = Mild discomfort
4-6 = Moderate pain
7-10 = Severe discomfort/pain

McCaffrey Initial Pain Assessment Tool

Date ____________

Patient's name ______________________ Age __________ Room ____________

Diagnosis ______________________ Doctor ______________________

Nurse ______________________

1. LOCATION: Patient or nurse marks drawing.

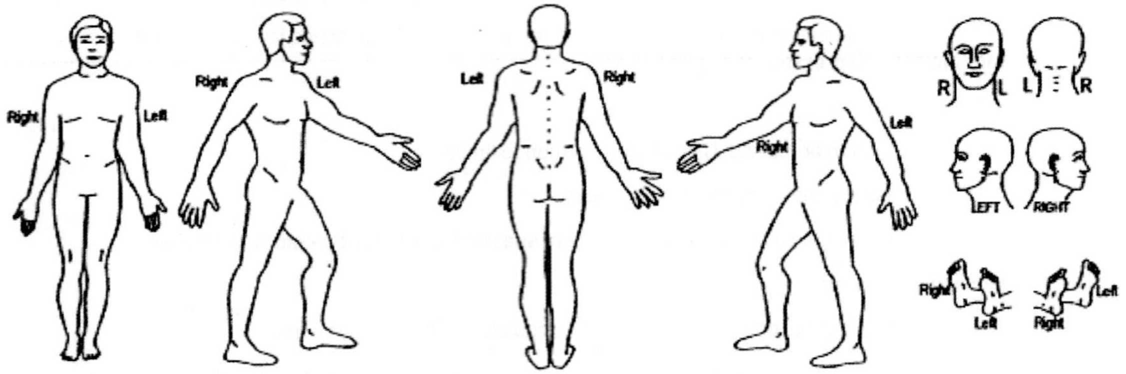

Right Left Right Left Left Right Left Right R L L R LEFT RIGHT Right Left Left Right

2. INTENSITY: Patient rates the pain. Scale used ______________________

   Present: ______________________

   Worst pain gets: ______________________

   Best pain gets: ______________________

   Acceptable level of pain: ______________________

3. QUALITY: (Use patient's own words, e.g. prick, ache, burn, throb, pull, sharp) ______________________

4. ONSET, DURATION, VARIATIONS, RHYTHMS: ______________________

5. MANNER OF EXPRESSING PAIN? ______________________

6. WHAT RELIEVES THE PAIN? ______________________

7. WHAT CAUSES OR INCREASES THE PAIN? ______________________

8. EFFECTS OF PAIN: (Note decreased function, decreased quality of life.)

   Accompanying symptoms (e.g. nausea) ______________________

   Sleep ______________________

   Appetite ______________________

   Physical activity ______________________

   Relationship with others (e.g. irritability) ______________________

   Emotions (e.g. anger, suicidal, crying) ______________________

   Concentration ______________________

   Other ______________________

9. OTHER COMMENTS: ______________________

10. PLAN: ______________________

May be duplicated for use in clinical practice. From McCaffrey, M. & Pasero, C. (1999). *Pain: Clinical manual* (2nd ed., p. 60).

FIGURE 8-7 McCaffrey Initial Pain Assessment Tool.

CRITICAL THINKING

7. We chose to use the Visual Analogue Scale to assess Mr Burra's pain. What other scales might be appropriate?
8. Do you think that pain assessment scales provide objective data?
9. If all your patients rate their pain the same, do you think that they have the same amount of pain?
10. Use the COLDSPA mnemonic to describe Mr Burra's pain. You will need to describe the location, intensity, quality, pattern, precipitating factors and pain relief, as well as the effect of the pain on daily activities, the coping strategies that have been used and emotional responses to the pain.

Sample of subjective data

Ms Berri is a 68-year-old female patient known previously as having osteoporosis. This visit, she presents with low back pain, burning in nature, radiating to her left lower leg and associated with tingling and numbness of the lower leg. The pain is continuous and is worse in the morning and after any movement. The pain is mostly relieved by pain medications and rest. 'Pain is making it hard for me at home. I'm not able to shower, dress and perform the daily household jobs. Also, I'm not able to concentrate on my work anymore. I can't sleep at night and don't seem to enjoy anything lately.' Using the Visual Analogue Scale, Ms Berri rates her pain to be 8/10.

Sample of objective data

Ms Berri comes in, leaning on her daughter, and has difficulty sitting down in the chair. Her posture is slumped and she moves in an agitated manner. She is frowning and grimacing most of the time. She is unable to concentrate and continue an idea. Her vital signs are: heart rate 108 beats/minute, respiratory rate 22 breaths/minute and blood pressure 135/80 mmHg.

Analysis of data

DIAGNOSTIC REASONING: POSSIBLE CONCLUSIONS

After collecting subjective and objective data pertaining to pain assessment, identify abnormal findings and patient strengths. Then cluster the data to reveal any significant patterns or abnormalities. These data may be used to make clinical judgements about the status of the patient's pain.

Listed below are some possible conclusions that could be drawn from an assessment of pain.

Potential patient risks

- Risk of activity intolerance (related to chronic pain and immobility)
- Risk of constipation (related to intake of non-steroidal anti-inflammatory agents or opiates or poor eating habits)
- Risk of spiritual distress (related to anxiety, pain, life change and chronic illness)
- Risk of powerlessness (related to chronic pain, health care environment and pain treatment–related regimen)

Potential patient problems

- Acute pain (related to injury agents: biological, chemical, physical or psychological)
- Chronic pain (related to chronic inflammatory process of rheumatoid arthritis)
- Ineffective breathing pattern (related to abdominal pain and anxiety)
- Fatigue (related to stress of handling chronic pain)
- Impaired physical mobility (related to chronic pain)
- Bathing and hygiene self-care deficit (related to severe pain)

Selected collaborative problems

After grouping the data, certain collaborative problems may become apparent. Remember that collaborative problems differ from nursing diagnoses in that they cannot be prevented by nursing intervention. However, these physiological complications of medical conditions can be detected and monitored by the nurse. In addition, the nurse can use doctor- and nurse-prescribed interventions to minimise the complications of these problems. The nurse may also have to refer the patient in such situations for further treatment of the problem. The following is a list of collaborative problems that may be identified when assessing pain:

- Angina
- Decreased cardiac output
- Endocarditis
- Peripheral vascular insufficiency
- Paralytic ileus or small bowel obstruction
- Sickling crisis
- Peripheral nerve compression
- Corneal ulceration
- Osteoarthritis
- Joint dislocation
- Pathological fractures
- Renal calculi.

Medical problems

If, after grouping the data, it becomes apparent that the patient has signs and symptoms that may require medical diagnosis and treatment, referral to a primary care provider is necessary.

PHYSICAL ASSESSMENT

ASSESSMENT PROCEDURE	NORMAL FINDINGS	ABNORMAL FINDINGS
General impression		
INSPECTION		
Observe posture.	Posture is upright when the patient appears to be comfortable, attentive and without excessive changes in position and posture.	Patient appears to be slumped with the shoulders not straight (indicates being disturbed or uncomfortable). Patient is inattentive and agitated. Patient might be guarding affected area and have breathing patterns reflecting distress.
INSPECTION		
Observe facial expression.	Patient smiles with appropriate facial expressions and maintains adequate eye contact.	Patient's facial expressions indicate distress and discomfort, including frowning, moans, cries and grimacing. Eye contact is not maintained, indicating discomfort. Nodding up and down or saying, 'yeah, yeah', may not indicate a patient's positive response to questions, but just listening or not wanting to be negative.
Inspect joints and muscles.	Joints appear normal (no oedema); muscles appear relaxed.	Oedema of a joint may indicate injury. Pain may result in muscle tension.
Observe skin for scars, lesions, rashes, changes or discolouration.	No inconsistency, wounds or bruising is noted.	Bruising, wounds or oedema may be the result of injuries or infections, which may cause pain.
Vital signs		
INSPECTION		
Measure heart rate.	Heart rate ranges from 60 to 100 beats/minute.	Increased heart rate may indicate discomfort or pain.
Measure respiratory rate.	Respiratory rate ranges from 12 to 20 breaths/minute.	Respiratory rate may be increased, and breathing may be irregular and shallow.
Measure blood pressure.	Blood pressure ranges from: Systolic: 100 to 130 mmHg Diastolic: 60 to 80 mmHg.	Increased blood pressure often occurs in severe pain.

Note: Refer to the chapter on physical assessment appropriate to the affected body area. Body system assessment will include techniques for assessing for pain, for example, palpating the abdomen for tenderness and performing range-of-motion tests on the joints.

CASE STUDY

The case study demonstrates how to analyse pain assessment data for a specific patient. The exercises included in the ancillary product on thePoint that complements this text offer further opportunities to enhance your skills.

Alex Burra is a 58-year-old divorced man with two children and works as an accountant. Two years ago, he had difficulty urinating. Tests revealed prostate cancer. Mr Burra underwent prostatectomy followed by cycles of chemotherapy a year ago. For the past 8 to 10 months, he has had continuous low back pain and leg pain that is worse at night and while walking. He says, 'I sometimes feel that I will fall down while walking and at night I am awakened by stabbing, deep dull pain in my legs, so I don't sleep very well. Then during the day I feel tired and unable to proceed with my work.' Mr Burra also says that he is eating less and has lost about 6 kg in the past 3 months.

During the physical examination, Mr Burra entered the room limping and sat on the chair with his shoulders slumped. He changed his position every 2 to 3 minutes, looking anxious and uncomfortable, with frowns and grimaces as facial expressions. He rates his pain on the Visual Analogue Scale as 7/10. His vital signs are: heart rate 110 beats/minute, respiratory rate 22 breaths/minute and blood pressure 135/85 mmHg.

The following concept map illustrates the diagnostic reasoning process.

Applying COLDSPA

Applying COLDSPA for patient symptoms: 'back and leg pain'.

Mnemonic	Question	Data provided	Missing data
Character	Describe the sign or symptom (feeling, appearance, sound, smell or taste, if applicable).	Low back and stabbing, deep, dull pain in legs	
Onset	When did it begin?	8 to 10 months ago	
Location	Where is it? Does it radiate? Does it occur anywhere else?	Lower back and legs	
Duration	How long does it last? Does it recur?	Continuous, gets worse at night and when walking	
Severity	How bad is it? How much does it bother you?	Patient rates pain on the Visual Analogue Scale to be 7/10. Limps when walking and changes position every 2 to 3 minutes to try to get comfortable. Grimaces and frowns. Sits with slumped shoulders.	
Pattern	What makes it better or worse?		What makes the leg and back pain worse or better?
Associated factors/How it Affects the patient	What other symptoms occur with it? How does it affect you?	Feels like he may fall when walking. Is tired and has trouble working during the day because he cannot sleep at night; the pain wakes him up. Decreased appetite and weight loss of 6 kg in the past 3 months.	

ONLINE RESOURCES

An extensive range of additional resources to enhance teaching and learning and to facilitate understanding may be found online at the text's accompanying website, located on thePoint at http://thepoint.lww.com. These include Watch and Learn videos, Concepts in Action animations, journal articles, case studies, discussion topics and quizzes.

Subscribers may also access Lippincott Procedures, an extensive online point-of-care procedure guide that provides reliable step-by-step instructions for more than 1700 procedures, including 450 evidence-based Australian procedures, and skills in a variety of speciality settings, together with a wealth of supporting information.

SIMULATED LEARNING

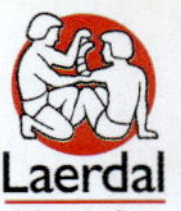

Having completed this chapter, explore the scenarios of Carl Shapiro Parts 1 and 2, Doris Bowman Parts 1 and 2, Marilyn Hughes Parts 1 and 2, Stan Checketts Parts 1 and 2 and Vernon Watkins Parts 1 and 2. Carl is a 54-year-old male presenting to the emergency department with a myocardial infarction. Doris is a 39-year-old female who is postoperative following a total abdominal hysterectomy. Marilyn is a 45-year-old lady who has broken her leg. Stan is a 64-year-old admitted with abdominal pain diagnosed as a bowel obstruction. Vernon is a 69-year-old man who is postoperative following a hemicolectomy and requires postoperative support. Incorporating the health assessment content in this chapter with your existing theoretical knowledge and clinical experience, progress through each simulation scenario (this is best done in a small group). How would you manage the care of each patient? When reflecting on your management of these virtual patients, what do you think you did well and what do you think you can improve? Consider why you think this and also how you might manage a similar problem in the future.

Throughout this chapter you have considered the case of Alex Burra, who has prostate cancer and low back pain. In the simulation scenario based on Alex and available to your lecturer online, you will continue to assess Alex and his pain in a simulated encounter. In this simulation you will be using the pain assessment tools described in this chapter.

1) Identify abnormal findings and patient strengths

Subjective data

- Diagnosed with prostate cancer; treated with surgery and chemotherapy 1 year ago
- Low back and leg pain while walking and at night
- Pain is stabbing, deep and dull
- 'Not able to sleep at night'
- 'I feel tired and unable to proceed with my work'
- Decreased appetite and weight loss
- Rates pain on the Visual Analogue Scale (VAS) to be 7/10 on average
- 'I am awakened by stabbing pain'

Objective data

- Entered the room limping
- Sat on the chair with his shoulders slumped
- Changes his position every 2 to 3 minutes
- Appears anxious and uncomfortable
- Frowns and grimaces
- Vital signs: HR = 110 beats/min, RR = 22 breaths/min, BP = 135/85 mmHg
- ROM tests of legs: Standing: lifts knees only 20° from straight position when asked to march in place. Lying: able to lift each leg with knee unbent 15° before pain starts; lying prone, able to lift each leg only 10° before pain.

2) Identify cue clusters

- Diagnosed with prostate cancer treated with surgery/chemotherapy 1 year ago
- Pain is stabbing, deep and dull; increasing for the past 8–10 months
- Pain on average 7/10 on the VAS
- Continuous low back pain and leg pain that exacerbates at night and while walking

- 'I sometimes feel that I will fall down while walking and at night I am awakened by stabbing deep dull pain in my legs'
- Limited ROM or legs w/pain
- Ability to lift knees in standing position for marching/walking decreased

- 'Not able to sleep at night'
- Pain exacerbates at night

- Increased respirations and pulse
- Frowns and grimaces as facial expressions
- Sat on the chair with his shoulders slumped
- Changes his position every 2 to 3 minutes
- 'I feel tired and unable to proceed with my work'
- Unable to sleep because of pain

3) Draw inferences

Patient has an onset of pain which is worrying him. Refer for medical investigation and diagnosis

Patient has difficulty in mobility affecting his work

Patient is awakened by his pain and his inability to sleep is affecting his performance during the day time

Patient is uncomfortable and shows facial expressions relating to being distressed and his posture is not straight; vital signs increased in line with discomfort or anxiety

4) List possible diagnoses

Chronic pain increasing related to unknown cause

Impaired physical mobility related to the pain

Sleep deprivation related to prolonged physical discomfort

Anxiety related to prolonged pain affecting daily activities

5) Check for defining characteristics

Major: 7/10 continuous and increasing deep stabbing and dull pain for the past 8–10 months

Major: Limited ROM limited ability to perform gross motor activities

Major: Daytime drowsiness, decreased ability to function, tiredness, anxious, inability to concentrate

Major: Restlessness, concern over effect of pain on lifestyle, anxious, increased respiration, increased pulse, sleep disturbance, increased blood pressure, awareness of physiological symptoms

6) Confirm or rule out diagnoses

Confirm the diagnosis because it meets the defining characteristics and is confirmed by the patient

Confirm the diagnosis because it meets the defining characteristics and is confirmed by the patient

Confirm the diagnosis because it meets the defining characteristics and is confirmed by the patient

Confirm the diagnosis because it meets the defining characteristics and is confirmed by the patient

7) Document conclusions

Diagnoses that are appropriate for this patient include:

- Chronic pain (increasing) related to unknown cause
- Impaired physical mobility related to the pain
- Sleep deprivation related to prolonged physical discomfort
- Anxiety related to prolonged pain affecting daily activities

Potential collaborative problems include the following:

Prostate cancer metastasis

References

Abbey, J., Piller, N., De Bellis, A., et al. (2004). The Abbey pain scale: A 1-minute numerical indicator for people with end-stage dementia. *International Journal of Palliative Nursing, 10*, 6–13.

Agency for Health Care Policy and Research (AHCPR). (1992). *Acute pain management: Operative or medical procedures and trauma.* Clinical practice guidelines no. 1 (AHCPR publication no. 92-0032). Rockville, MD: Agency for Healthcare Research and Quality.

Baker, D. & Wong, C. (1987). QUEST: A process of pain assessment in children. *Orthopaedic Nursing, 6*(1), 11–21.

Cleeland, C. S. & Ryan, K. M. (1994). Pain assessment: Global use of the Brief Pain Inventory. *Annals Academy of Medicine Singapore, 23*, 129–138.

Dafny, N. (1997–2019a). Pain principles. Section 2, Ch. 6. In J. H. Byrne (Ed.). *Neuroscience online* . Available at https://nba.uth.tmc.edu/neuroscience/s2/chapter06.html.

Dafny, N. (1997–2019b). Pain modulation and mechanisms. Section 2, Ch. 8. In J. H. Byrne (Ed.). *Neuroscience online*. Available at https://nba.uth.tmc.edu/neuroscience/s2/chapter08.html.

Dunwoody, C., Krenzischek, D., Pasero, C., et al. (2008). Assessment, physiological monitoring, and consequences of inadequately treated acute pain. *Pain Management Nursing, 9*(1), S11–S21.

Fenwick, C. (2006). Assessing pain across the cultural gap: Central Australian Indigenous peoples' pain assessment. *Contemporary Nurse, 22*(2), 218–227.

Fishman, B., Pasternak, S., Wallenstein, S. L., et al. (1987). The Memorial Pain Assessment Card. A valid instrument for the evaluation of cancer pain. *Cancer, 60*(5), 1151–1158.

Flaherty, E. (2008). Pain assessment for older adults. *The American Journal of Nursing, 108*(6), 45–47.

Friedrichsdorf, S. J., Giordano, J., Desai Dakoji, K., et al. (2016). Chronic pain in children and adolescents: Diagnosis and treatment of primary pain disorders in head, abdomen, muscles and joints. *Children (Basel), 3*(4). pii: 42.

Healthcommunities.com. (1998–2008). Cancer pain. Viewed November 2013 at www.healthcommunities.com/cancer-pain/cancer-pain-overview.shtml.

Herr, K., Coyne, P. J., McCaffery, M., et al. (2011). Pain assessment in the patient unable to self-report: Position statement with clinical practice recommendations. *Pain Management Nursing, 12*(4), 230–250.

Hummel, P., Puchalski, M., Creech, S. D., et al. (2008). Clinical reliability and validity of the N-PASS: Neonatal Pain, Agitation and Sedation Scale with prolonged pain. *Journal of Perinatology, 28*(1), 55–60.

International Association for the Study of Pain. (2017). IASP terminology. Available at https://www.iasp-pain.org/Education/Content.aspx?ItemNumber=1698.

Kaegi, L. (2004). What colour is your pain? Minority Nurse. Viewed November 2013 at www.minoritynurse.com/nurse-led-interventions/what-colour-your-pain.

Macintyre, P., Schug, S., Scott, D., et al. (2010). *Acute pain management: Scientific evidence.* Melbourne: Australia and New Zealand College of Anaesthetists (ANZCA) and Faculty of Pain Medicine.

Magnusson, J. E. & Fennell, J. A. (2011). Understanding the role of culture in pain: Māori practitioner perspectives relating to the experience of pain. *The New Zealand Medical Journal, 124*(1328), 41–51.

Mahieu-Caputo, D., Dommergues, M., Muller, F., et al. (2000). Fetal pain. *La Presse Médicale, 29*(12), 663–669. Available at http://opoids.com/endormorphins/foetpain.

Mauri Ora Associates, SAEJ Consultancy & Panapa Ehau. (2010). *Best health outcomes for Pacific Peoples: Practice implications.* Wellington: Medical Council of New Zealand. Available at www.mcnz.org.nz/assets/News-and-Publications/Statements/Best-health-outcomes-for-Pacific-Peoples.pdf.

McCaffery, M. & Pasero, C. (1999). *Pain: Clinical manual* (2nd ed.). St Louis: Mosby.

Otto, S., Duncan, S. & Baker, L. (1996). Initial pain assessment for pediatric use only. Distributed by the City of Hope Pain/Palliative Care Resource Center. Available at http://prc.coh.org/pain_assessment.asp.

Pain Australia. (2013). Prevalence and the human and social cost of pain. Pain Australia. Available at http://painaustralia.staging3.webforcefive.com.au/static/uploads/files/painaust-factsheet2-wfdahrmggvwp.pdf.

Patestas, M. & Gartner, L. P. (2006). Ascending sensory pathways. In M. A. Patestas & L. P. Gartner (Eds). *A textbook of neuroanatomy*. Hoboken, NJ: Blackwell Publishing. Available at www.blackwellpublishing.com/patestas/chapters/10.pdf.

Porth, C. M. (2007). *Essentials of pathophysiology* (2nd ed.). Philadelphia: Lippincott Williams & Wilkins.

Royal Australian College of General Practitioners. (2006). *Medical care of older persons in residential aged care facilities* (4th ed.). South Melbourne: Author.

Silkman, C. (2008). Assessing the seven dimensions of pain. *American Nurse Today, 3*(2), 12–15.

Voepel-Lewis, T., Zanotti, J., Dammeyer, J. A., et al. (2010). Reliability and validity of the Face, Legs, Activity, Cry, Consolability behavioral tool in assessing acute pain in critically ill patients. *American Journal of Critical Care, 19*(1), 55–61.

Weissman, D. E., Gordon, D. & Bidar-Sielaff, S. (2004). Cultural aspects of pain management. *Journal of Palliative Medicine, 7*(5), 715–717.

Selected reading

World Health Organization (WHO). (2019). Web statement on pain management guidance. Available at www.who.int/medicines/areas/quality_safety/guide_on_pain/en/

Online resources

Australian and New Zealand College of Anaesthetists (ANZCA): www.anzca.edu.au
Australian Pain Society: www.apsoc.org.au
International Association for the Study of Pain (IASP): www.iasp-pain.org
Memorial Sloan-Kettering Cancer Center: www.mskcc.org
Society for Paediatric Anaesthesia in New Zealand and Australia (SPANZA): www.spanza.org.au
Wong–Baker Faces Pain Rating Scale: www.wongbakerfaces.org

CHAPTER 9

Assessing victims of violence

Undertaking a health assessment for victims of violence requires a caring and compassionionate approach, recognising that the person has experienced some trauma—often at the hands of someone he or she has known and trusted. These assessments also require sound knowledge and skills in clinical assessment and accurate, comprehensive documentation of your findings. The following case study is expanded upon further throughout the chapter—keep the facts of this scenario in mind as you read the materials on assessing victims of violence.

CASE STUDY

Mrs Wallis, a 52-year-old woman, brought her 76-year-old mother to the emergency department. On examination her mother appeared thin, with poor hygiene; she had a black eye, and bruising at various stages of healing was evident on her chest, upper external thighs and forearms. Her affect was flat, but she appeared anxious.

Mrs Wallis's daughter claimed her mother was 'clumsy' and frequently fell over and 'bumped into things', which is how she sustained the injuries. A chest X-ray reveals healed rib fractures. She has a previous diagnosis of mild heart failure but has not taken any of the tablets prescribed to her for about 2 weeks.

CONCEPTUAL FOUNDATIONS

Family or domestic violence (FDV) refers to intentional acts of violence between people who are in a familial or an intimate relationship and includes domestic violence, child abuse and elder abuse. Although the term 'domestic violence' is most commonly used in Australia, the term 'family violence' is preferred by many Aboriginal and Torres Strait Islander communities (Mitchell, 2011a; 2011b).

Family or domestic violence extends across a range of behaviours, including social isolation, physical abuse, emotional abuse, financial abuse, threats, intimidation and sexual assault, damage to property and possessions, and injuring pets. Historically, family violence was viewed as a private matter, but, in reality, it is a crime, a breach of human rights and a public health problem with a significant impact on health care systems and welfare agencies.

The World Health Organization (WHO, 2008) estimates that the cost of violence is greater than 4% of the gross domestic products of many countries. A report titled 'The Cost of Violence against Women and Their Children in Australia,' published in 2016, estimated that the cost of this violence from 2015 to 2016 was $22 billion dollars. However, it was also noted that Torres Strait Islander women, pregnant women, women with disabilities and those experiencing homelessness were significantly underestimated in this estimate and that an additional $4 billion dollars should be added to the total to include these vulnerable groups. Family or domestic violence is also the major cause of homelessness for women experiencing or fleeing FDV in Australia (AIHW, 2018a), where it is estimated to cost victims, businesses and the health system billions of dollars annually (Campbell, 2011).

There is no universal definition of child abuse, and it varies according to who is defining the abuse. For example, health professionals tend to define child abuse in terms of clinical presentation, whereas legal definitions are more descriptive and inclusive of perpetrator behaviour. Every jurisdiction in Australia has legislation that defines child abuse and the process for mandatory reporting. There is no mandatory reporting of any form of abuse in New Zealand.

Elder abuse, sometimes referred to as elder mistreatment, includes physical abuse, neglect, self-neglect, psychological abuse, sexual abuse, institutional abuse and financial abuse. The abuse may be from the commission of abuse but is frequently from omission in cases of neglect when there is a failure of care providers to fulfil their obligations towards an older person.

THEORETICAL BACKGROUND

To discuss the theory of family violence, the concepts of violence and aggression need to be defined. A dictionary definition of *violence* is 'any unjust or unwarranted exertion of force or power' (*Macquarie Dictionary*). However, the WHO (2008) defines violence as 'the intentional use of physical force or power, threatened or actual, against oneself, another person, or against a group or community, that either results in or has a high likelihood of resulting in injury, death, psychological harm, maldevelopment or deprivation.' Violence tends to have a negative connotation when thought of as murder, torture or hate but has more of a positive connotation if associated with self-defence or acts of war. A key concept of the WHO definition is intent and, in addition to physical injury, includes psychological harm, maldevelopement and deprivation as potential outcomes of intentional violence (WHO, 2008). The Australian and New Zealand cultures condemn violence; however, some movies, music, television programs and literature glorify it. *Aggression* is defined by the *Macquarie Dictionary* as 'any offensive action or procedure'. Aggression also has both positive and negative connotations. The positive connotation is associated with the drive for success, as in aggressive men. The negative connotation is often associated with the notion of aggressive women, which may violate what is considered appropriate for gender norms.

This chapter briefly discusses five theories related to domestic violence: biological, psychoanalytical, social learning, cultural attitude and Walker's Cycle of Violence (1979, 1984) theories. The first four focus on the bases of violence, whereas Walker's cycle discusses the cyclic nature of violence.

Biological theory asserts that violence is an innate human characteristic, based on neurophysiological states. Historically, human instinct served to preserve the species, so that those men who were more violent survived.

Psychoanalytical theory states that violence results from the need to discharge hostility. In addition, frustration is the stimulus that leads to violence or aggression.

Social learning theory describes both aggression and violence as learned responses, which may be considered negative or positive, depending on the situation. These behaviours are learned not only from the family, but also from the community and society.

Some experts purport that cultural attitudes influence violence. For example, the acceptance of war as a justified means of resolving a conflict and corporal punishment as a method of discipline both developed from various cultural attitudes.

Walker's Cycle of Violence theory (1979, 1984) explains that abuse occurs in a predictable pattern. During the beginning of a relationship, couples are rarely apart and the relationship is very intense. The abuser displays possessiveness and jealousy and starts to separate the victim from supportive relationships. Criticism is the herald of phase 1, the tension-building phase. The abuser makes unrealistic demands. When the expectations are not satisfied, the criticism and ridicule escalate into shoving or slapping. The victims often blame themselves for failing to satisfy the unrealistic demands of the abuser. Phase 2, the acute battering stage, may be triggered by something minor but results in violence that can last up to 24 hours. The victim is rarely able to stop the abuse. Phase 3, the honeymoon phase, is described as a period of reconciliation. This phase begins after an incident of battery. The abuser is loving, promises never to abuse the victim again and is very attentive to the victim. Then the cycle begins again.

Culture, race and ethnicity must also be considered in the theory of family violence. One needs to conduct a cultural assessment (using assessment guidelines) before attempting to understand family violence. Health care providers are more likely to report child abuse in minority populations or in lower socio-economic levels (ANA, 1998). Studies show little difference in rates of abuse in racial groups when income levels are included (Hawkins, 1993). However, many cultures within Australia and New Zealand have different beliefs about what is acceptable violence, and this makes prevention, detection and assessment more complex and can possibly result in lower numbers of reported rates.

Types of family violence

Types of FDV include physical abuse, psychological abuse, financial abuse and sexual abuse as well as abandonment and neglect.

Physical abuse includes threats to harm as well as pushing, shoving, slapping, kicking, choking, punching and burning. It may also involve holding, tying or other methods of restraint. The victim may be left in a dangerous place without resources. The abuser may refuse to help the victim when sick, injured or in need. Physical abuse may also involve attacking the victim with household items (lamps, radios, curling irons, ashtrays, irons, etc.) or with common weapons (knives or guns). Indicators include bruising, abrasions, cigarette burns, bite marks, rope burns, lacerations and fractures.

Psychological abuse, also known as emotional abuse, may have greater and longer impact on the victim than physical abuse. Psychological abuse involves the use of constant insults or criticism, blaming the victim for things that are not the victim's fault, threats to hurt children or pets, emotional blackmail, isolation from supporters (family, friends or colleagues), deprivation, humiliation and intimidation. Stalking is another form of psychological abuse, which may involve physically stalking the victim or using social media to punish and humiliate the person (Woodlock, 2016). The abuse of technology has also been recognised as the new 'tool' in domestic violence, where abusive partners use their phones, tablets and computers to remotely control objects such as thermostats, lights and sound systems in the victims home (Woodlock, 2016). Legal definitions of psychological abuse differ from state to state, which results in an underestimated number of cases reported.

Financial abuse, also known as economic abuse, is the improper exploitation of another person's personal assets, properties or funds. Examples of this type of abuse include the cashing of another person's cheques without their authorisation or permission, forging signatures, and misusing or stealing money or possessions. Economic abuse may also occur if someone deceives another into signing a will or contract, coerces a person into signing a will or contract, or controls another person's money and demands a detailed accounting of the funds. Statistics of financial abuse are difficult to find particularly with respect to under-reporting by abused elders.

Sexual abuse involves forcing the victim to perform sexual acts against her or his will, pursuing sexual activity after the victim has said 'no', using violence during sex and using weapons vaginally, orally or anally (Holzer & Bromfield, 2010), and being forced to watch or otherwise engage in pornography.

CATEGORIES OF FAMILY VIOLENCE

Family or domestic violence

There is no national or global definition of FDV. Domestic violence has been defined in numerous ways depending on context and any legislative requirements across jurisdictions. Definitions of FDV are also subject to change as the range of behaviours considered to be abusive and the nature and type of relationships included evolve (ABS, 2013). Here domestic violence is defined as 'a continuum of behaviour ranging from verbal abuse, physical, and sexual assault, to rape and even homicide' (Shipway, 2004). Domestic violence is the most widespread form of violence in our society and includes all acts of violence, coercion and intimidation. The WHO estimates that 30% of women who have been in a relationship since the age of 15 years have experienced physical or sexual violence from an intimate partner (WHO, 2013). It is generally categorised as domestic or family violence or intimate partner violence, child abuse and elder abuse. There are no boundaries; millions of people are affected by domestic violence regardless of race, culture, age, gender or class; however, women and children are predominantly affected by FDV. The Australian Bureau of Statistics (ABS) recorded crime data revealed that in 2017 two out of five assaults were FDV related, with females experiencing the highest number of assaults, ranging from 67% in New South Wales to 81% in the Northern Territory (ABS, 2017). Women were nearly three times more likely to have experienced partner violence than men, with approximately 1 in 6 women (17% or 1.6 million) and 1 in 16 men (6.1% or 547,600) having experienced partner violence since the age of 15 years. The 2016–2017 Personal Safety Survey (PSS) revealed that women were eight times (5.1% or 48,020 women) more likely to experience sexual assault by a partner than men (0.6% or 53,000 men) (ABS, 2016).

More women than men seek medical assistance because of domestic violence; from 2009 to 2010, there were 2,847 hospital admissions across Australia due to an assault by a partner—of these hospital admissions 83% involved a female patient (AIHW, 2012). The *National plan to reduce violence against women and their children* estimates the economic cost of domestic violence in Australia is $13.6 billion dollars annually (Herbert, 2011), and this figure could rise to $15.6 billion by 2021, if extra steps are not taken (KPMG, 2009).

New Zealand has extremely high statistics of family violence. Nearly half of Māori woman admit to experiencing abuse in their relationship, compared with 24% of non-Māori (*Pākehā*) and 23% of Pasifika (Mayhew & Reilly, 2009). In 2014 the estimated cost of family violence in New Zealand was reported to be between $4.1 billion and $7 billion annually (Kahui & Snively, 2014). Kahui and Snively (2014) also suggest that if nothing is done to address this growing incidence of FDV the costs will escalate to $80 billion in the next 10 years. Annually, police spend $3.9 million on family violence–related homicide inquiries (Stringer, 2010). Over time, FDV escalates in both severity and frequency unless intervention occurs, and can even lead to death.

Most homicide incidents in Australia and New Zealand are domestic homicides, with the number increasing annually (Virueda & Payne, 2010). In Australia. 487 homicides occurred from 2012 to 2014, of which 200 were classified as domestic homicides, with 79% of the victims being female (Bryant & Bricknewll, 2017). In New Zealand, 686 people were killed in homicides from 2007 to 2016. One in five of these homicides were committed by a partner or a former partner, with 75% of the victims being female.

The impact of FDV on the mental health of both male and female victims of domestic violence has been well documented. However, there are also negative effects on the mental health of children when they have been exposed to domestic violence in the home, including depression, anxiety disorders and emotional and behavioural problems (Braaf, 2012). In addition, children raised in homes with FDV are more likely to use violence as adults (Lamberg, 2000).

In both Australia and New Zealand there are a number of agencies that provide specific support and assistance to women and children in domestic violence situations. Often these services will provide emergency and longer-term accommodation and support for those in need. Mitchell (2011a; 2011b) notes that defining the forms of violence by perpetrators against victims is complicated in Australia because of the different types of intimate and family relationships and living arrangements in the community. The National Action Plan to Reduce Violence against Women and Children in Australia can be accessed via the website of the Department of Social Services at www.dss.gov.au.

When examining the problem of FDV, it is common to focus on the woman as the victim. Men also suffer from victimisation, although this is commonly perceived as a rarity. However, the 2016 PSS indicates that in Australia, 1 in 16 men (547,600) experienced partner violence since the age of 15 years, with 1 in 17 experiencing physical abuse and 1 in 6 experiencing emotional abuse (ABS, 2016). Male victims report that if they inform the police about an incident the complaint may not be filed and that they are often ridiculed or not taken seriously. Male victims suffer effects of trauma similar to those experienced by female victims (Huckle, 1995); when men attempt to leave their abuser, they face many of the same problems as female victims. However, the effect of the violence tends to be different as men are far less likely than women to be fearful of the perpetrator. Unfortunately, men have fewer options for assistance because there are few, if any, facilities that offer shelter to male victims.

History of child abuse

As with other forms of FDV abuse there is no universal definition of child abuse. The WHO (2006) defines child abuse to include 'All forms of physical and/or emotional ill-treatment, sexual abuse, neglect or negligent treatment or commercial or other exploitation, resulting in actual or potential harm to the child's health, survival, development or dignity in the context of a relationship of responsibility, trust or power' (p. 9). In Australia, children are defined as those people under the age of 18 years (AIHW, 2018b).

Child abuse may be either by commission or by omission and is rarely an isolated incident. There are four broad categories of child abuse: neglect, emotional abuse, sexual abuse and physical abuse. There are significant economic and social costs related to cases of child abuse and neglect. According to the Australian Government's Australia's Welfare report (AIHW, 2017), more than $4 billion was spent nationally from 2015 to 2016 on child protection and out-of-home care services—an increase from the previous year of $240.2 million. This, along with the substantial negative impact of abuse and neglect on children, justifies the need for early intervention and prevention programs (Nair & Scott, 2013). The number of children receiving child protective services in Australia is rising annually. From 2016 to 2017, 168,352 children received child protection services—a 25% increase on figures from 2012 to 2013 (AIHW, 2018b).

In New Zealand there continues to be no mandatory reporting of child abuse, whereas in Ausralia there is mandatory reporting of child abuse in all jurisdictions, although there are some variations in policy and reporting processes, including who is mandated to report. Each state and territory has child protection legislation:

- *Children & Young People Act 2008* (ACT)
- *Children and Community Services Act 2004* (WA)
- *Children & Young Person (Care and Protection) Act 1998* (NSW)
- *Care & Protection of Children Act 2007* (NT)
- *Child Protection Act 1999* (Qld)
- *Children's Protection Act 1993* (SA)
- *Children, Young Persons and Their Families Act 1997* (Tas)
- *Children Youth and Families Act 2005* (Vic).

The Australian Institute of Health and Welfare's report 'Child Protection Australia: 2016–2017' (2018b) describes a rise in substantiated cases of child abuse from the previous year. During this time 379,459 notifications of suspected child abuse were received. The total number of substantiated cases was 67,968, which involved 49,315 children. The most common type of abuse reported was emotional abuse (30,745 or 48%), followed by neglect (18,149 or 24% 14,984), then physical abuse (11,043 or 16%) and, lastly, sexual abuse (7,863 or 12%). Female children were more likely to be sexually abused than males; children less than 1 year old were the most likely to be abused and neglected (16.4 per 1000) and children 15 to 17 years old, the least likely (4.6 per 1000) (AIHW, 2018b).

Elder abuse

The WHO (2008) defines elder abuse as 'a single or repeated act or lack of appropriate action, occurring within any relationship where there is an expectation of trust which causes harm or distress to an older person.' Forms of elder abuse include physical, social, spiritual, sexual, financial and psychological including behaviours of exploitation, abandonment, bullying and harassment or prejudicial attitudes that decrease quality of life and is demeaning to those over the age of 65 years. A number of risk factors for elder abuse stem from the older persons' relationships with others, the general community and society. These include, physical disability, poor mental health, cognitive impairment, lower socio-economic status, social isolation and dependence upon others. Elder abuse has been a largely hidden phenomenon until late in the 20th century. Unlike child abuse and domestic violence, elder abuse initially attracted little attention from government agencies, despite repeated exposure from welfare groups. The middle of the 1970s is generally recognised as the beginning point for the research and exposure of elder abuse (Sadler, 1994). The primary focus in these early days was the neglect and exploitation of vulnerable adults; however, attention shifted to the incidence of physical abuse during the 'rethinking' on domestic violence to a broader family violence model in the 1980s. Public awareness of elder abuse in Australia and New Zealand gained little traction until the 1990s, despite compelling efforts from social and welfare groups to place it on the political agenda.

Although individual Australian state and territory parliaments made some attempt to protect vulnerable adults through broadening domestic violence legislation to address family violence, the reporting of violent abuse on older family members remained voluntary and very much in the private domain. It was not until the public exposure of several elderly women in their 90s being subjected to sexual assault in a Victorian nursing home that the federal government took action and, through amendments to the *Aged Care Act 1997* (Cth), mandated the reporting of some elder abuse.

The *Aged Care Act 1997* (Cth) now requires all employees of Commonwealth-funded aged-care facilities to report suspected or witnessed sexual assault or use of excessive force on an older person resident in that facility. Whereas this protection is limited to a selected group of older people in Australia, mandatory reporting of elder abuse has not yet been enacted in New Zealand. In Australia, mandatory reporting does not apply to any form of financial or psychological abuse or neglect of older people, nor does it address the sexual assault and physical abuse of older people in the community or in private or state-run facilities. From 2017 to 2018, the Department of Health received 4,013 notifications under the compulsory reporting provisions of the *Aged Care Act 1997* (Cth). Of these, 3,773 were required to be reported under the Act—3,226 were for alleged or witnessed unreasonable use of force; 513 were for alleged or suspected sexual assault; and 34 were for both, representing approximately 1.6% of the 241,723 in residential care at the time (Australian Government Department of Health, 2018).

Although the true extent of elder abuse is unknown, based on international indications there is evidence to suggest that it is likely to be between 2% and 14% of the older population in Australia across all forms of abuse, with the prevalence of neglect higher (AIFS, 2016). Elder abuse is often difficult to assess because of the older person's isolation from the community, immobility and inability to report because of cognitive impairments. Elders are often unwilling to report their abuser because they do not trust law enforcement or they have a relationship with the abuser (i.e. son or daughter), which may create feelings of guilt, burden, dependence or fear of abandonment. They may be unsure whom to report the abuse to, doubt authorities' willingness to become involved or fear that without their carer they will end up in an institution. Many elders prefer to stay in their own home, even if it means suffering abuse at the hands of a carer.

Violence in the workplace

Unfortunately, the incidence of violence in workplaces is escalating, including in the health care industry (Hills et al., 2012). Whilst regular media reports indicate the rise of violence directly against health care staff the frequency and severity of these is likely to be underreported and understudied. One example of this increase is the number of code blacks called. For example, between 2016 and 2017 South Australian Government hospitals had 6,245 code blacks compared with 4,765 from 2015 to 2016. A direct consequence of occupational violence is that nurses, and all other health workers, may also find themselves victims of violence in their place of employment. Unfortunately, there have been several extreme cases of workplace violence in recent times: two nurses in separate incidents were held hostage at knife point by patients in 2017; a health nurse in a remote area of South Australia was abducted, raped and murdered in 2016; and a mental health nurse was stabbed to death in regional New South Wales in 2011 (Pich, 2017). Because of the nature of emergency departments (EDs), there are increased risks for staff, patients and visitors. Patients with mental illness and those who misuse alcohol or drugs increased waiting times for patients in pain, and individuals who have been involved in gang violence are often seen in the ED. Staffing is often inadequate; fatigue is common and tempers may not be controlled. Nurses may encounter the fears, frustration and harassment of patients.

Even with all the factors contributing to the potential for serious incidents, one of the greatest risks continues to be in caring for victims of FDV. Injured victims are often accompanied to the ED by the batterer. Because the batterer has already shown the ability to inflict injury, he or she should be considered dangerous. By accompanying the victim, the batterer is attempting to maintain control of the victim and prevent reports from being filed.

Because of the potential for violence, health care facilities should have a safety plan to control potential violence and to ensure safety of the staff, patients and visitors.

Nursing assessment of family violence

Although routine screening for a history of current or past abuse has been widely advocated to identify women affected by FDV (Barclay, 2007), it is not universal. Routine screening would ordinarily take the form of a series of questions asked of women presenting to health services such as antenatal clinics and EDs. Where routine screening is not adopted as a policy to identify those experiencing or at risk of FDV, it is worthwhile to initiate opportunistic screening where there is an index of suspicion (Laing, 2003). As already mentioned, there are four areas to assess to determine the presence of family violence: physical abuse, psychological abuse, financial abuse and sexual abuse.

With physical abuse, it is important to remember that abuse may start at any time during a relationship. The abuse may not be part of the presenting problem for which the patient is being seen but may be the cause or aetiology of the presenting problem. Consistent risk factors for women at risk have not been identified. Therefore, both abused and non-abused women require routine screening by health care providers.

Psychological abuse is difficult to assess because of the lack of a clearly defined diagnosis. The majority of children who suffer from psychological abuse often use effective coping mechanisms and will not exhibit any pathological behaviour.

Although you may not know the state of your patient's finances, you can look for possible indicators of financial abuse during your assessment. For example, the patient may be inadequately dressed, or he or she may have missing or broken dentures, hearing aids or glasses. The patient may be malnourished or dehydrated if he or she does not have access to adequate nutrition or hydration.

When sexual abuse is suspected, a complete physical examination is required. Disclosure of the incident may not occur for months or years after the sexual abuse event. Often sexual abuse such as fondling, oral sex or activity without penetration does not involve physical injury. If sexual abuse is suspected, a trained interviewer should conduct a forensic interview. Both the interview and physical examination are part of the actual health interventions that assist the patient to recover from the sexual abuse.

CASE STUDY

When interviewed alone, Mrs Wallis anxiously supported her daughter's story, adding that she didn't want to cause a fuss. When asked about her financial position, she confides that her daughter controls her funds because she [the daughter] has many bills from a failed business venture and is unemployed. When asked how her daughter coped with the pressure of being unemployed and in debt, the mother reveals that her daughter often goes down to the hotel for a drink with friends and to play the pokies.

CRITICAL THINKING

1. Does this case study raise any suspicions of possible abuse? If yes, in what form?
2. What specific information would you record to support a suspicion of elder abuse?

It is crucial that victims of domestic violence are provided with an adequate assessment of their health and welfare status. The following tables provide a useful structure to guide the assessment process and provide indicators of what are normal and abnormal findings.

ASSESSMENT PROCEDURE

ASSESSMENT PROCEDURE	NORMAL FINDINGS	ABNORMAL FINDINGS (INDICATORS OF VIOLENCE OR POTENTIAL VIOLENCE)
Family violence assessment		
Review the patient's past health history and physical examination records if available.	No indicators of abuse are present.	Records include documentation of past assaults; unexplained injuries; unexplained symptoms of pain, nausea and vomiting or choking feeling; repeated visits to emergency department or clinic for injuries; signs and symptoms of anxiety; use of sedatives or hypnotics; injuries during pregnancy; history of drug or alcohol abuse; history of depression or suicide attempts.

ASSESSMENT PROCEDURE (continued)

ASSESSMENT PROCEDURE	NORMAL FINDINGS	ABNORMAL FINDINGS (INDICATORS OF VIOLENCE OR POTENTIAL VIOLENCE)
Family violence assessment (continued)		
If partner/parent/carer is present at the visit, observe patient's interactions with partner.	Patient does not seem afraid of partner and answers questions independently. Partner appears supportive.	Partner criticises patient about appearance, feelings, or actions. Partner is not sensitive to patient's needs. Partner refuses to leave patient's presence. Partner attempts to speak for and answer questions for patient. Patient appears anxious and afraid of partner; is submissive or passive to negative comments from partner.
INTERVIEW		
Perform the rest of the examination without the partner, parent or carer present.		
Ask all patients: Has anyone in your home ever hurt you? Do you feel unsafe in your home? Are you afraid of anyone in your home? Has anyone made you do anything you didn't want to do? Has anyone ever touched you without you telling them it was OK for them to do so? Has anyone ever threatened you?	Patient answers 'no' to all questions.	'Yes' to any of the questions indicates abuse.
For intimate partner violence, begin the screening by telling the patient that it is important to routinely screen all patients for intimate partner violence because it affects so many women and men in our society. Ask the patient to fill out or help the patient fill out the Abuse Assessment Screen in Assessment tool 9-1.	Patient responds 'no' to all three questions. If the patient replies 'no' to screening questions and is not being abused, it is important for the patient to know that you are available if she ever experiences abuse in the future. Make statements that build trust such as 'If your situation ever changes, please call me to talk about it. I am happy to hear that you are not being abused. If that should ever change, this is a safe place to talk.' **CLINICAL TIP** **Sometimes no matter how carefully you prepare the patient and ask the questions, she or he may not disclose abuse.**	'Yes' to any of the questions strongly indicates initial disclosure of abuse. You should do the following: • Acknowledge the abuse and his or her courage. • Use supportive statements such as 'I'm sorry this is happening to you. This is not your fault. You are not responsible for this behaviour against you. You are not alone. You don't deserve to be treated this way. Help is available to you.' • Acknowledge his or her autonomy and right to self-determination. Reiterate confidentiality of disclosure.

Continued on following page

ASSESSMENT PROCEDURE (continued)

ASSESSMENT PROCEDURE	NORMAL FINDINGS	ABNORMAL FINDINGS (INDICATORS OF VIOLENCE OR POTENTIAL VIOLENCE)
INTERVIEW (continued)		
For child abuse, use the guidelines in Display 9-1. Question the child about safety including physical abuse, sexual abuse, emotional abuse and neglect. ***For elder mistreatment,*** start out by asking the elder to tell you about a typical day in their life. Be alert for indicators placing the elder at a high risk of abuse or neglect. Then ask: • Has anyone ever made you sign papers that you did not understand? • Are you alone often? • Has anyone refused to help you when you needed help? • Has anyone ever refused to give you or let you take your medications?	Patient shows no signs of abuse. Patient answers 'no' to all questions.	Patient indicates someone has hurt them (physically, sexually or emotionally). Child appears neglected. 'Yes' to any of the questions indicates abuse.
PHYSICAL EXAMINATION		
Perform a general survey. Observe general appearance and body build.	Patient appears to be his or her stated age and well developed.	Abused children may appear younger than stated age due to developmental delays or malnourishment. Older patients may appear thin and frail due to malnourishment.
Note dress and hygiene.	Patient is well groomed and dressed appropriately for season and occasion.	Poor hygiene and soiled clothing may indicate neglect. Long sleeves and pants in warm weather may be an attempt to cover bruising or other injuries. Victims of sexual abuse may dress provocatively.
Assess mental status.	Patient is coherent and relaxed. A child shows proper developmental level for age.	Patient is anxious, depressed, suicidal or withdrawn, or has difficulty concentrating. Patient has poor eye contact or soft passive speech. Patient is unable to recall recent or past events. Child does not meet developmental expectations.
Evaluate vital signs.	Vital signs are within normal limits.	Hypertension may be seen in victims of abuse.
Inspect skin.	Skin is clean, dry and free of lesions or bruises. **OLDER ADULT CONSIDERATIONS** **Skin fragility increases with age, bruising may occur with pressure and may mimic bruising associated with abuse. Be careful to distinguish between normal and abnormal findings.**	Patient has scars, bruises, burns, welts or swelling on face, breasts, arms, chest, abdomen or genitalia.

ASSESSMENT PROCEDURE (continued)

ASSESSMENT PROCEDURE	NORMAL FINDINGS	ABNORMAL FINDINGS (INDICATORS OF VIOLENCE OR POTENTIAL VIOLENCE)
PHYSICAL EXAMINATION (continued)		
	CULTURAL CONSIDERATIONS **Mongolian spots on the buttocks and backs of children occur in some populations and can be confused with signs of abuse. They are normal findings. Evidence of raised red areas—either circular (from cupping) or deep scratchlike areas (coining)—may be seen in some ethnic groups and are not considered abnormal. If they appear on a child, ask the person or the parent about these areas to clarify their source.**	
Inspect the head and neck.	Head and neck are free of injuries.	Patient has hair missing in clumps, subdural haematomas or rope marks or finger/hand strangulation marks on neck.
Inspect the eyes.	Eyes are free of injury.	Patient has bruising or swelling around eyes, unilateral ptosis of upper eyelids (due to repeated blows causing nerve damage to eyelids) or a subconjunctival haemorrhage.
Assess the ears.	Ears are clean and free of injuries.	Patient has external or internal ear injuries.
Assess the abdomen.	Abdomen is free of bruises and other injuries and is non-tender.	Patient has bruising in various stages of healing. Assessment reveals intra-abdominal injuries. A pregnant patient has received blows to abdomen.
Assess genitalia and rectal area.	Patient is free of injury.	Patient has irritation, tenderness, bruising, bleeding or swelling of genitals or rectal area. Discharge, redness or lacerations may indicate abuse in young children. Haemorrhoids are unusual in children and may be caused by sexual abuse. Extreme apprehension during examination may indicate physical or sexual abuse.
Assess the musculoskeletal system.	Patient shows full range of motion and has no evidence of injuries.	Dislocation of shoulder; old or new fractures of face, arms or ribs; and poor ROM of joints are indicators of abuse.
Assess the neurological system.	Patient demonstrates normal neurological function.	Abnormal findings include tremors, hyperactive reflexes and decreased sensations to areas of old injuries secondary to neurological damage.
Additional tools for victims of domestic violence		
If screening for family or domestic violence is positive, ask the patient if she (or he) has a safety plan and where she would like to go when she leaves your agency. Assess her (or him) for safety issues in her (or his) home using Assessment tool 9-2. Make a follow-up appointment and or referral as appropriate.	Patient has a plan.	If the patient says she (or he) prefers to return home, ask her if it is safe for her to do so, and have her complete the danger assessment tool in Assessment tool 9-3. Provide the patient with contact information for shelters and groups. Encourage her to call with any concerns.

ASSESSMENT TOOL 9-1 Abuse assessment screen

1. WITHIN THE LAST YEAR, have you been hit, slapped, kicked or otherwise physically hurt by someone? YES NO

   If YES, by whom? _________

   Total number of times _________

2. SINCE YOU'VE BEEN PREGNANT, have you been hit, slapped, kicked or otherwise physically hurt by someone? YES NO

   If YES, by whom? _________

   Total number of times _________

   MARK THE AREA OF INJURY ON THE BODY MAP. SCORE EACH INCIDENT ACCORDING TO THE FOLLOWING SCALE:

	SCORE
1 = Threats of abuse including use of a weapon	______
2 = Slapping, pushing: no injuries and/or lasting pain	______
3 = Punching, kicking, bruises, cuts and/or continuing pain	______
4 = Beating up, severe contusions, burns, broken bones	______
5 = Head injury, internal injury, permanent injury	______
6 = Use of weapon; wound from weapon	______

   If any of the descriptions for the higher number apply, use the higher number.

3. WITHIN THE LAST YEAR, has anyone forced you to have sexual activities? YES NO

   If YES, who? _________

   Total number of times _________

McFarlane & Parker, (1994). Abuse during pregnancy: Effects on Maternal Complications and Birth Weight in Adult and Teenage Women. Obsetetics & Gynecology.

DISPLAY 9-1 CONSIDERATIONS FOR INTERVIEWING CHILDREN

- It is important to establish a reassuring environment for the interview.
- Although you may be uncomfortable questioning the child about abuse, do not convey this in the interactions with the child.
- It is important that you receive any information the child may disclose to you with interest. Be calm and accepting without showing surprise or distaste.
- Do not coerce the child into answering questions by offering a reward to answer your questions.
- Establish the child's understanding or developmental stage by asking simple questions (Name, how to spell name, age, birth date, how many eyes do you have, etc.). Use the child's comprehensive abilities and any language limitations to structure your interview and questions. Use terms for body parts or acts that the child uses.
- Questions must be direct to extract information without being leading. Children will answer questions. The majority disclose to questions specific to direct inquiry about the person suspected of abuse or related to the type of abuse (Heger et al., 2000).
- Avoid questions that can be answered with a 'yes' or a 'no'. Give the child as many choices during the interview as possible. Use multiple-choice or open-ended questions.
- The less information you supply in your questions and the more information the child gives answering the questions increases the credibility of the information gathered during the interview.

ASSESSMENT TOOL 9-2 Assessing a safety plan

Ask the patient, do you:

- Have a packed bag ready? Keep it hidden but make it easy to grab quickly?
- Tell your neighbours about your abuse and ask them to call the police when they hear a disturbance?
- Have a code word to use with your kids, family and friends so they will know to call the police and get you help?
- Know where you are going to go, if you ever have to leave?
- Remove weapons from the home?
- Have the following gathered:
  - Cash
  - Medicare, pensioner cards/numbers for you and your children
  - Birth certificates for you and your children
  - Driver's licence
  - Rent and utility receipts
  - Bank account numbers
  - Insurance policies and numbers
  - Marriage licence
  - Jewellery
  - Important phone numbers
  - Copy of protection order

Ask children, do you:

- Know a safe place to go?
- Know who is safe to tell you are unsafe?
- Know how and when to call 000 in Australia or 111 in New Zealand? Know how to make a reverse-charges phone call?

Inform children that it is their job to keep themselves safe; they should not interject themselves into adult conflict.

If the patient is planning to leave:

- Remind the patient this is a dangerous time that requires awareness and planning.
- Review where the patient is planning to go, shelter options and the need to be around others to curtail violence.
- Review the patient's right to possessions and list of possessions to take.

ASSESSMENT TOOL 9-3 Danger assessment

Several risk factors have been associated with increased risk of homicides (murders) of women and men in violent relationships. We cannot predict what will happen in your case, but we would like you to be aware of the danger of homicide in situations of abuse and for you to see how many of the risk factors apply to your situation.

Using the calendar, please mark the approximate dates during the past year when you were abused by your partner or ex-partner. Write on that date how bad the incident was according to the following scale:

1. Slapping, pushing; no injuries and/or lasting pain
2. Punching, kicking; bruises, cuts and/or continuing pain
3. 'Beating up'; severe contusions, burns, broken bones
4. Threat to use weapon; head injury, internal injury, permanent injury, miscarriage or choking (use a © in the date to indicate choking/strangulation/cut off your breathing-example 4©)
5. Use of weapon; wounds from weapon

(If **any** of the descriptions for the higher number apply, use the higher number.)

Mark **Yes** or **No** for each of the following. ('He' refers to your husband, partner, ex-husband, ex-partner or whoever is currently physically hurting you.)

Yes	No		
____	____	1.	Has the physical violence increased in severity or frequency over the past year?
____	____	2.	Does he own a gun?
____	____	3.	Have you left him after living together during the past year? 3a. (If you have *never* lived with him, check here: ____)
____	____	4.	Is he unemployed?
____	____	5.	Has he ever used a weapon against you or threatened you with a lethal weapon? (If yes, was the weapon a gun? Check here: ____)
____	____	6.	Does he threaten to kill you?
____	____	7.	Has he avoided being arrested for domestic violence?
____	____	8.	Do you have a child that is not his?
____	____	9.	Has he ever forced you to have sex when you did not wish to do so?
____	____	10.	Does he ever try to choke/strangle you or cut off your breathing? 10a. (If yes, has he done it more than once, or did it make you pass out or black out or make you dizzy? Check here: ____)
____	____	11.	Does he use illegal drugs? By drugs, I mean 'uppers' or amphetamines, 'meth', speed, angel dust, cocaine, 'crack', street drugs or mixtures.
____	____	12.	Is he an alcoholic or problem drinker?

Continued on following page

ASSESSMENT TOOL 9-3 Danger assessment (countinued)

Yes	No		
____	____	13.	Does he control most or all of your daily activities? For instance, does he tell you who you can be friends with, when you can see your family, how much money you can use, or when you can take the car? (If he tries, but you do not let him, check here: ____)
____	____	14.	Is he violently and constantly jealous of you? (For instance, does he say: 'If I can't have you, no one can.')
____	____	15.	Have you ever been beaten by him while you were pregnant? (If you have never been pregnant by him, check here: ____)
____	____	16.	Has he ever threatened or tried to commit suicide?
____	____	17.	Does he threaten to harm your children?
____	____	18.	Do you believe he is capable of killing you?
____	____	19.	Does he follow or spy on you, leave threatening notes or messages, destroy your property or call you when you don't want him to?
____	____	20.	Have you ever threatened or tried to commit suicide?
			_____ Total 'Yes' answers

Thank you. Please talk to your nurse, advocate or counsellor about what the Danger Assessment means in your situation.

Campbell, J.C., (2004). Danger Assessment. Retrieved October 2019, from http://www.dangerassessment.org.

PREPARING FOR THE EXAMINATION

Before you can effectively begin to assess for the presence of FDV, you must first examine your feelings, beliefs and biases regarding violence. Violence is a prevalent family and community health problem that needs to be confronted by society today. No one under any circumstances should be physically, sexually or emotionally abused. As a nurse, it is imperative you become active in interrupting or ending cycles of violence. During your assessment, be aware of 'red flags' that may indicate the presence of FDV; these red flags are often hidden from others.

A second person

In emergency departments it is usual and recommended practice to include a second health professional in the interview. This helps to protect both the nurse conducting the interview and the patient. However, you should obtain consent from your patient, providing him or her with a clear explanation as to why this person is present.

INTERVIEW TECHNIQUES

Creating a safe and confidential environment is essential to obtain concise and valid subjective data from the patients who have experienced FDV. For any patient over the age of 3 years, ask any screening questions in a secure, private setting, with no one else present in the room. Do not screen if there are any safety concerns for the patient or for yourself.

Prior to screening, discuss any legal, mandatory reporting requirements or other limits to confidentiality. Screening may be done orally and in a written format or through computer-generated questions. Find a reliable interpreter if the patient does not speak a language you understand; however, avoid using a patient's relative or friend as the interpreter.

Remember to ask questions and allow the patient to answer completely. Do not interrupt the patient. Convey a concerned and non-judgemental attitude. Show appropriate empathy and allow the patient to have breaks when needed.

For additional communication strategies, please review the content of Chapter 2, Collecting subjective data.

CRITICAL THINKING

3. As the older woman does 'not want to cause a fuss', how would you raise the issue of mandatory reporting if it applied to Mrs Wallis's case?

VALIDATING AND DOCUMENTING FINDINGS

Validate any FDV data you have collected. This is necessary to verify that the data are reliable and accurate. Document your assessment data following the health care facility or agency policy.

Sample of subjective data

Patient reports injuries to head, neck and breasts. States, 'I am having difficulty talking.' Shares that she was beaten with a plastic cricket bat on her head; denies any loss of consciousness. Reports pain and soreness of her neck, and pain when speaking after being choked with a cord. Also reports multiple bites and bruising on both breasts. States, 'This has happened on a number of occasions for the past 3 years.' Denies any witnesses for any of the events.

Sample of objective data

Ears: right tympanic membrane scar noted at 3 o'clock position; Eyes: conjunctival haemorrhage bilaterally; Neck: circular pattern of bruising and abrasions noted around the neck.

Chest: respiration regular, 20 per minute; Breasts: right nipple, red, swollen with multiple abrasions noted around the areola; Abdomen: multiple bruises noted at various stages of healing.

CRITICAL THINKING

4. Using the case study on Mrs Wallis, write both a subjective and an objective account of her case.

Analysis of data

DIAGNOSTIC REASONING: POSSIBLE CONCLUSIONS

After collecting subjective and objective data pertaining to FDV, identify abnormal findings and patient strengths. Then cluster the data to reveal any significant patterns or abnormalities. These data may be used to make clinical judgements about the status of the patient.

After you have collected your assessment data, analyse the data using diagnostic reasoning skills. Use the case study on the following pages as a guide to analysing the assessment data for a specific patient.

Listed below are some possible conclusions that could be drawn from assessment of family or domestic violence (FDV). After collecting subjective and objective data pertaining to FDV, you will need to identify abnormal findings and cluster the data to reveal any significant patterns or abnormalities. These data will then be used to make clinical judgements (diagnoses, wellness, risk or actual) about the status of FDV in your patient's life. The following is a listing of selected patient problems you may identify when analysing data for assessment of FDV.

Potential patient risks

- Risk of impaired parent, infant or child family processes (related to the presence of domestic violence)
- Risk of violence (related to the presence of poor coping mechanisms and the misuse of alcohol and illegal drugs)
- Risk of sexually transmitted infections and human immunodeficiency virus (related to participation in forced sexual relationships)
- Risk of powerlessness (related to control of relationships, control of children and finances by abusive significant other)
- Risk of post-traumatic stress disorder (related to the inability to remove self from abusive intimate relationship).

Potential patient problems

- Dysfunctional grieving (related to loss of ideal relationship as evidenced by refusal to discuss feelings and prolonged denial)
- Impaired parenting (related to choosing to remain living in the presence of an abusive marriage or intimate relationship)
- Disturbed personal identity (related to inability to function effectively outside of a victimised abusive role)
- Rape-trauma syndrome (related to the forced violent penetration against the patient's will, secondary to the lack of a safety plan for the victim)
- Rape-trauma syndrome: silent reaction (related to inability to discuss occurrences of a victim of rape)
- Rape-trauma syndrome: compound reaction (related to inability to function effectively in everyday activities after being a victim of rape)
- Fear of losing an ineffective abusive intimate relationship (related to unrealistic expectations of self and others)
- Hopelessness (related to remaining in a prolonged abusive relationship and inability to seek counselling and healthy supportive relationships)
- Anxiety (related to inconsistency of behaviours and instability of abusive spouse or parent)
- Low self-esteem (related to lack of confidence related to presence of prolonged physical, sexual and emotional abuse).

Selected collaborative problems

After grouping the data, you may see various collaborative problems emerge. Remember that collaborative problems differ from nursing diagnoses in that they cannot be prevented by nursing interventions. However, these physiological complications of medical conditions can be detected and monitored by the nurse. In addition, the nurse can use doctor- and nurse-prescribed interventions to minimise the complications of these problems. The nurse may also have to refer the patient in such situations for further treatment of the problem. The following is a list of collaborative problems that may be identified when assessing a victim of family violence:

- Fractures
- Bruises
- Concussion
- Subdural haematoma
- Subconjunctival haemorrhage
- Intra-abdominal injury
- Depression
- Suicide
- Death.

Medical problems

Once the data are grouped, certain signs and symptoms may become evident and might require medical diagnoses and treatment. Refer to the primary health care provider as necessary.

ONLINE RESOURCES

An extensive range of additional resources to enhance teaching and learning and to facilitate understanding may be found online at the text's accompanying website, located on thePoint at http://thepoint.lww.com. These include Watch and Learn videos, Concepts in Action animations, journal articles, case studies, discussion topics and quizzes.

Subscribers may also access Lippincott Procedures, an extensive online point-of-care procedure guide that provides reliable step-by-step instructions for more than 1700 procedures, including 450 evidence-based Australian procedures, and skills in a variety of speciality settings, together with a wealth of supporting information.

CASE STUDY

The case study demonstrates how to analyse personal violence assessment data for a specific patient. The exercises included in the ancillary product on thePoint that complements this text offer further opportunities to enhance your skills.

Mrs Wallis, a 52-year-old woman, brought her 76-year-old mother to the emergency department. On examination her mother appeared thin, with poor hygiene; she had a black eye, and bruising at various stages of healing was evident on her chest, upper external thighs and forearms. Her affect was flat but she appeared anxious.

Mrs Wallis's daughter claimed that her mother was 'clumsy' and frequently fell over and bumped into 'things', which is how she sustained the injuries. A chest X-ray revealed healed rib fractures. She has a previous diagnosis of mild heart failure but has not had any of the tablets prescribed to her for about 2 weeks.

When interviewed alone, Mrs Wallis anxiously supported her daughter's story, adding that she didn't want to cause a fuss. When asked about her financial position, she confides that her daughter controls her funds because she [the daughter] has a lot of bills from a failed business venture and is unemployed. When asked how her daughter coped with the pressure of being unemployed and in debt, the mother reveals that her daughter often goes down to the hotel for a drink with friends and to play the pokies.

The following concept map illustrates the diagnostic reasoning process.

Applying COLDSPA

Applying COLDSPA for patient symptoms: 'chest pain'.

Mnemonic	Question	Data provided	Missing data
Character	Describe the sign or symptom (feeling, appearance, sound, smell or taste, if applicable).	'My chest hurts and I cannot breathe easily.'	
Onset	When did it begin?	'I had the same symptoms 6 months ago.' 'My daughter, when she is drunk, has been hitting and kicking me in the chest and stomach.' She indicates this has occurred 'several times' and shows fear for her own life.	
Location	Where is it? Does it radiate? Does it occur anywhere else?		Does your chest pain radiate? Do you have pain anywhere else?
Duration	How long does it last? Does it recur?		How long does this pain last? Does it recur?
Severity	How bad is it? How much does it bother you?		How bad is this chest pain? Does it limit your ability to move or go about your normal activites?
Pattern	What makes it better or worse?		Does this chest pain occur only when your daughter physically hurts you?
Associated factors/How it **A**ffects the patient	What other symptoms occur with it? How does it affect you?	The patient makes poor eye contact and looks at her daughter frequently while answering questions. The patient is frail and thin, with bruising and swelling over her right chest wall.	How has this abusive situation affected your activities of daily living?

1) Identify abnormal findings and patient strengths

Subjective data

- 'My chest hurts and I cannot breathe easily'
- Discloses that her daughter has been hitting her, and kicking her in the chest and stomach
- 'I know she is going to hurt me; I just don't know when'
- When questioned about old healed fracture, patient states, 'I did not come to the doctor when she hurt me because she threatened to take away all my money'

Objective data

- Frail, thin, 76-year-old female
- Family displays good hygiene and dress
- Her daughter assists her as she walks into the reception area
- When asked about her injuries, she has poor eye contact
- Daughter interrupts all conversations with health care workers
- Decreased breath sounds over right lung
- Large area of discolouration and swelling noted on the right chest wall
- Bruising on right side of the abdomen and right hip
- Full ROM, but movement elicits pain (per patient)
- X-rays reveal 2 fractured ribs

2) Identify cue clusters

- 'My chest hurts and I cannot breathe easily'
- Daughter assisted her as she walked into the reception area
- Discolouration and swelling noted on the right chest wall
- Bruising on right side of the abdomen and right hip
- X-rays reveal two fractured ribs
- Full ROM, but movement elicits pain (per patient)
- Discloses that her daughter has been hitting her, and kicked her in the chest and stomach several times

- 'She is going to hurt me and take my money; I just do not know when'
- When asked about her injuries, she has poor eye contact
- Daughter interrupts all conversations with health care workers

3) Draw inferences

Generalised pain, musculoskeletal pain
Shared daughter had hit her

Family displays conflict

4) List possible diagnosis

Acute pain related to repeated physical abuse

Interrupted family processes

5) Check for defining characteristics

Major: Verbal reports of pain, observed evidence (recent and old abusive injuries, limps when walking, visible bruising and abrasions)

Major: None

Minor: None

6) Confirm or rule out diagnoses

Confirm because it meets major characteristics

Rule out as this has been in existence for a period of time, as evidenced by repeated abusive, violent actions by daughter

7) Document conclusions

Diagnoses that are appropriate for this patient include:

- Acute pain related to physical abuse
- Impaired family relationship related to abusive daughter

Potential collaborative problems include the following:

- Fractures
- Haemorrhage
- Intra-thoracic injuries
- Intra-abdominal injuries
- Death

SIMULATED LEARNING

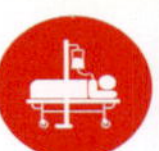

Throughout this chapter you have considered the case of Mrs Wallis, a victim of abuse. In the simulation scenario based on Mrs Wallis and available to your lecturer online, you will continue to assess Mrs Wallis in a simulated encounter. In this simulation you will be using the screening tools and assessment procedures described in this chapter.

References

Aged Care Act 1997 (Cth). Available at www.austlii.edu.au/au/legis/cth/consol_act/aca199757.

Australian Bureau of Statistics (ABS). (2013). Directory of family and domestic violence statistics. Cat 4533.0. Canberra: Author.

Australian Bureau of Statistics (ABS). (2016). Personal safety survey, Australia. Cat 4906.0. Canberra: Author.

Australian Bureau of Statistics (ABS). (2017). Recorded crimes, Victims Australia 2017. Cat 4510.0. Camberra: Author.

Australian Government Department of Health. (2018). 2017–18 Report on the operation of the *Aged Care Act 1997*. Canberra: Author. Available at www.health.gov.au.

Australian Institute of Family Studies. (2016). Elder Abuse: Understanding issues, frameworks and responses. Viewed April 2019 at https://aifs.gov.au/publications/elder-abuse.

Australian Institute of Health and Welfare. (2017). Australia's welfare 2017. Australia's welfare series no. 13. AUS 214. Canberra: Author.

Australian Institute of Health and Welfare. (2018a). Family, domestic and sexual violence in Australia 2018. Cat. no. FDV 2. Canberra: Author.

Australian Institute of Health and Welfare. (2018b). Child protection Australia 2016–17. Child welfare series no. 68. Cat. no. CWS 63. Canberra: Author.

Australian Institute of Health and Welfare (AIHW). (2012). Hospital separations due to injury and poisoning, Australia 2009–10. Injury research and statistics series no. 69. Cat. no. INJCAT 145. Canberra: Author.

American Nurses Association (ANA). (1998). *Culturally competent assessment for family violence*. Washington, DC: Author.

Barclay, L. (2007). Screening tool helps to identify mothers affected by intimate partner violence. Viewed December 2013 at www.medscape.com/viewarticle/568324.

Barclay, L. & Lie, D. (2007). New guidelines issued for evaluating physical abuse in children. *Medscape Medical News*. In Biller, H. (1995). The battered spouse made male. *Brown University Child Adolescent Behavior Letter*, March, 1–3.

Braaf, R. (2012). *Health impacts of domestic and family violence*. Australian Domestic & Family Violence Clearing House. Available at www.adfvc.unsw.edu.au.

Bryant, W. & Bricknewll, S. (2017). Homicide in Australia 2012-13 and 2013-14: National homicide monitoring program. Report. Canberra: Australian Institute of Criminology.

Campbell, R. (2011). The financial cost of domestic and family violence. Paper available online via the Australian Domestic & Family Violence Clearing House at www.adfvc.unsw.edu.au.

Hawkins, D. F. (1993). Inequality, culture, and interpersonal violence. *Health Affairs*, *12*(4), 80–95.

Heger, A. H., Emans, S. J. & Muram, D. (2000). *Evaluation of the sexually abused child: A medical textbook and photographic atlas*. New York: Oxford University Press.

Herbert, B. (2011). Domestic violence costs $13 billion a year. ABC News. Available at www/abc/net/au/news/2011-03-07/domestic-violence-costs-13bn-a-year/5728.

Hills, D. J., Joyce, C. M. & Humphreys, J. S. (2012). A national study of workplace aggression in Australian clinical medical practice. *The Medical Journal of Australia*, *197*(6), 336–340.

Holzer, P. & Bromfield, L. (2010). *Australian legal definitions: When is a child in need of protection?* Melbourne: National Child Protection Clearinghouse, Australian Institute of Family Studies.

Huckle, P. (1995). Male rape victims referred to a forensic psychiatric service. *Medicine, Science, and the Law*, *35*, 187–192.

Kahui, S. & Snively, S. (2014) Measuring the economic costs of child abuse and intimate partner violence to New Zealand. The Glenn Inquiry. MoreMedia Enterprises Wellington, New Zealand.

KPMG. 2009. The Cost of Violence against Women and their Children, Safety Taskforce, Department of Families, Housing, Community Services and Indigenous Affairs, Australian Government.

Laing, L. (2003). Routine screening for domestic violence in health services. Topic paper. Australian Domestic and Family Violence Clearinghouse. Available at https://www.researchgate.net/publication/237436573_Routine_Screening_for_Domestic_Violence_in_Health_Services/link/0f31753c6690db0781000000/download.

Lamberg, L. (2000). Domestic violence: What to ask, what to do. *JAMA*, *284*(5), 554.

Mayhew, P. & Reilly, J. L. (2009). Family violence: Statistics report. Families Commission research report no. 4/09. Wellington: Families Commission/Kōmihana ā Whānau. Viewed February 2020 at https://thehub.sia.govt.nz/assets/documents/family-violence-statistics-report.pdf.

Mitchell, L. (2011a). *Domestic violence in Australia: An overview of the issues*. Canberra: Department of Parliamentary Services.

Mitchell, L. (2011b). *Domestic violence in Australia: An overview of issues*. Canberra: Commonwealth Government Australia.

Nair, L. & Scott, D. (2013). *The economic costs of child abuse and neglect*. Melbourne: Australian Institute of Family Studies.

Pich, J. (2017). Violence against nurses is on the rise, but protections remain weak. The Conversation. Available at https://theconversation.com/violence-against-nurses-is-on-the-rise-but-protections-remain-weak-76019.

Sadler, P. (1994). What helps? Elder abuse interventions and research. *Australian Social Work*, *47*(4), 27–36.

Shipway, L. (2004). *Domestic violence: A handbook for health professionals*. London: Routledge.

Stringer, D. (2010). Police attend a family violence incident every seven minutes. Media release, New Zealand Police Association. Viewed December 2013 at www.policeassn.org.nz/newsroom/publications/featured-articles/police-attend-family-violence-incident-every-seven-minutes.

Virueda, M. & Payne, J. (2010). Homicide in Australia 2007–2008: National homicide monitoring program annual report. Canberra: Australian Institute of Criminology.

Woodlock, D. (2016). The abuse of technology in domestic violence and stalking. *Violence Against Women*, *23*(5), 584–602.

World Health Organization (WHO). (2006). *Preventing child maltreatment: A guide to taking action and generating evidence*. Geneva: Author. Available at www.who.int/violence_injury_prevention/publications/violence/child_maltreatment/en/.

World Health Organization (WHO). (2008). A global response to elder abuse and neglect. Viewed December 2013 at www.who.int/ageing/projects/elder_abuse/en.

World Health Organization (WHO). (2013). *Global and regional estimates of violence against women: Prevalence and health effects of intimate partner violence and non-partner sexual violence*. Geneva: Author. Viewed March 2019 at https://www.who.int/reproductivehealth/publications/violence/9789241564625/en/.

Selected readings

Australian Bureau of Statistics (ABS). (2018). Crime victimisation, Australia, 2017-2018. Cat no. 4530.0. Canberra: Author.

Forsyth, L. (2016). The cost of violence against women and children in Australia. Final Report. Australia: KPMG.

Nursing Research Consortium on Violence and Abuse. (2004). Abuse assessment screen. Handout.

Online resources

Advocare, for the rights of older people and people with disabilities: www.advocare.org.au

Australian Association of Maternal, Child and Family Health Nurses (AAMC & FHN): www.mcafhna.org.au

Australian Domestic & Family Violence Clearinghouse: www.adfvc.unsw.edu.au

Australian Government Department of Families, Housing, Community Services and Indigenous Affairs (FaHCSIA), Office for Women: www.fahcsia.gov.au/our-responsibilities/women/overview/office-for-women

Australian Government Department of Social Services. *National plan to reduce violence against women and their children*. Available at https://www.dss.gov.au/women/programs-services/reducing-violence/the-national-plan-to-reduce-violence-against-women-and-their-children-2010-2022

Australian Institute of Health and Welfare: www.aihw.gov.au

Australian National Sexual Assault and Domestic Family Violence Counselling Service 1800RESPECT: www.1800respect.org.au

Elder Abuse Action Australia: https://eaaa.org.au/

Family & Community Services, New Zealand: www.familyservices.govt.nz

Family Court of New Zealand, domestic violence and the law: www.justice.govt.nz

Journal of Elder Abuse & Neglect: www.tandfonline.com

Journal of Interpersonal Violence: www.sagepub.com

New Zealand Police/Nga Pirihimana O Aotearoa, family violence: www.police.govt.nz/advice/family-violence

CHAPTER 10

Assessing culture

Culture affects many aspects of life, including health and health practices. Culture affects many aspects of how people communicate the rituals and behaviours used to express spirituality, and the main events of life such as marriage, pregnancy, birth, death and other celebrations. Beyond culture, there are biological variations that affect disease susceptibility. Individuals may view themselves as 'normal' and view others who are not the same as 'other', or have 'cultural variations'. We all vary, with no one person or culture viewed as being the norm.

What do you believe causes illness? What do you believe is the correct way to treat minor or serious illnesses? Whom do you go to when you need to treat a minor illness, or to diagnose or treat a more serious illness? What barriers do you run into when you seek care? The answers to these questions vary based on the cultural context in which you grew up, or the influence of the contexts you have lived in later in life. Based on the idea that everyone has cultural variations, along with the large number of immigrants moving from one country to another, nurses must understand cultural variation as a basis for even minimally safe and effective care.

Why do nurses need to understand culture? Nurses interact with patients every day. A person who looks like you and comes from your community may actually hold very different beliefs about health and illness—beliefs about when and from whom to seek care, or about who makes the decision about health-related issues for the family. If someone who seems so similar to you could be so different, imagine the possible differences nurses might encounter when caring for people from obviously different cultural backgrounds.

CULTURAL CONTEXTS

Culture incorporates the following elements: family structure and function, spirituality and religion, and community. Together these form the major contexts for seeing a patient as an individual or a group, but inseparable from their background contexts of culture. The influence of culture, family, spirituality and community on the health status of the patient cannot be emphasised enough. The use of folk or traditional healers, spirituality, communication styles, familial roles, personal space, touch, nutrition, disease susceptibility, immigration, medication interactions and psychological factors needs to be considered when patients enter the health care setting (Brown et al., 2016). The nurse must perceive the patient within these contexts and be able to assess these when performing health assessments.

CONCEPTS AND RELATED TERMS

Nurses often ask, 'What is culture and why do we need to know something about it?' Other questions may include: How do culture and race differ? What about ethnicity? Minority? Do I have a culture? In order to answer these questions, we must first define some terms.

Culture may be defined as a shared system of values, beliefs and learned patterns of behaviour. Culture includes the knowledge, values, beliefs, art, morals, law, customs and habits of members of a society, including technology, education, social structures and political practices (Brown et al., 2016). The particular culture defines values (learned beliefs about what is held to be good or bad) and norms (learned behaviours that are perceived to be appropriate or inappropriate). So, culture is learned, shared and associated with adaptation to the environment, and it is universal. All people have a socially transmitted culture. Our own culture forms our worldview based on the values, beliefs and behaviours sanctioned by it. That worldview becomes, for us, reality and how we view the world locally and globally.

If an individual has limited interaction with other cultural groups, his or her cultural worldview is the limit of his or her experience. The perception that one's worldview is the only acceptable truth and that one's beliefs, values and sanctioned behaviours are superior to all others is called *ethnocentrism*. To avoid this, it is imperative for nurses to be aware of cultural differences in the health care requirements of all populations within Australia and New Zealand.

Many people are aware of other cultures and their different beliefs, values and accepted behaviours but do not recognise the great variation that can exist within any cultural group. Not recognising this variation tends to lead to stereotyping all members of a particular culture, expecting group members to hold the same beliefs and behave in the same way. There is a danger in stereotyping all members of one culture. The nurse who does not take the time to identify the individualities of

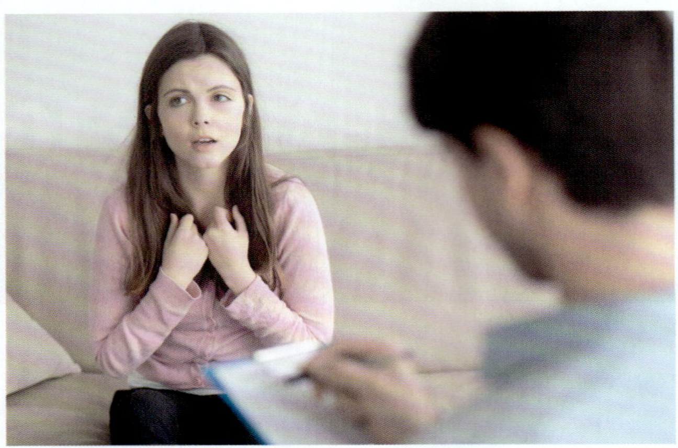

FIGURE 10-1 Nurses need to take the time to identify the individualities of their patients to avoid overlooking their specific health care needs. (Shutterstock.com/fizkes.)

his or her patients from one culture may overlook their specific health care needs and ultimately compromise the quality of nursing care provided (Stein-Parbury, 2017).

Ethnicity, or a person's ethnic identity, exists when the person identifies with a 'collective cultural group, largely based on the group's common heritage' (Wilson, 2014, p. 97). Put another way, ethnicity describes subgroups that have a common history, ancestry or other cultural identity and may relate to geographical origin such as Aboriginal and Torres Strait Islander peoples, Māori or Pasifika or country of origin for people who may be migrants or refugees but now living in another country.

Race is not a physical characteristic but a socially constructed concept that has meaning to a larger group. The concept of race 'originates from societal desire to separate people based on their looks and culture … [it is] a vague, unscientific term referring to a group of genetically related individuals who share certain physical characteristics' (Bigby, 2003, p. 2). These physical characteristics may include skin pigmentation, stature, hair texture and facial features and form the basis for the major race classifications used today: Caucasian, Negroid, Polynesian and Mongoloid (Wilson, 2014).

Minority refers to a group with smaller population numbers. These groups are often perceived, at times incorrectly, to have less power or influence within a society. Minority groups in Australia may include Aboriginal and Torres Strait Islander peoples, immigrants and refugees, with Māori, Pasifika and Asian people being the minority groups in New Zealand (Statistics New Zealand, 2012). The term 'minority' has a negative meaning in most uses, indicating a group that does not hold the 'majority' values or does not behave in 'appropriate' ways.

There are several reasons why nurses need to know and understand culture. For example, there is a history of disparity in the level of health care received by persons from certain racial groups and minorities, and there are also the problems of ethnocentrism and stereotyping mentioned earlier. Increasing diversity in Australian and New Zealand populations due to migration and humanitarian resettlement means that a significant proportion of our populations are born overseas, highlighting the importance of cultural awareness from a more global perspective. To provide high-quality health care, nurses need to be aware of culture in the context of the individual seeking care. This necessitates cultural competence.

STANDARDS OF PRACTICE

Although there are no universally accepted standards for cultural competence in practice, there is an expanding focus on this area of health professional practice, particularly with increased mobility and diversity in population groups, whether permanent or temporary, migrants or refugees. Professional codes of conduct, and education and practice guidelines across all the health professions should acknowledge the cultural and linguistically diverse populations we work with and with whom we share a duty to provide culturally appropriate care.

The Nursing Council of New Zealand/Te Kaunihera Tapuhi o Aotearoa (NCNZ) has established guidelines for cultural safety relating to nursing education and practice (NCNZ, 2011). In Australia, the Nursing and Midwifery Board of Australia has recently adopted the Code of Ethics for both nurses and midwives developed by the International Council of Nurses (ICN). The ICN articulates expectations for practice that acknowledges, 'inherent in nursing is a respect for human rights, including cultural rights, the right to life and choice, to dignity and to be treated with respect. Nursing care is respectful of and unrestricted by considerations of age, colour, creed, culture, disability or illness, gender, sexual orientation, nationality, politics, race or social status' (ICN, 2012, p. 1). The Centre for Cultural Competence Australia (CCCA) provides further discussion and specific education, training and other resources in relation to the provision of culturally appropriate care. They address the delivery of tangible outcomes, through practical acts of reconciliation, with the aim of improving the lives of Aboriginal and Torres Strait Islander peoples (CCCA, 2018).

Standards of practice for culturally competent nursing care have been developed by the Transcultural Nursing Society, based on the United Nations' and ICN's concepts of social justice and human rights also applicable at a health system level (Transcultural Nursing Society, 2011). The standards of practice are underpinned by 'the belief that every individual and group is entitled to fair and equal rights and participation in social, educational, economic, and, specifically in this context, health care opportunities. Through the application of the principles of social justice and the provision of culturally competent care, inequalities in health outcomes may be reduced' (Transcultural Nursing Society, 2018, p. 2). Douglas et al. (2014) highlight the challenges nurses face with the global migration of populations in relation to delivering care to patients with health care beliefs and practices that may differ. They have also put together the global guidelines for culturally competent care and how each can be applied in practice. Table 10-1 outlines the global guidelines for culturally competent care and how each can be applied in practice.

Various government and policy documents exist that serve as guiding frameworks and principles for the implementation of culturally appropriate care across health systems more broadly, these being equally relevant to individual health and allied professionals in various practice settings (National Health & Medical Research Council [NHMRC], 2006). The key message contained within these documents is that culturally appropriate care is a shared responsibility between everyone involved in health care delivery.

Table 10-1 Guidelines for the practice of culturally competent nursing care

Guideline	Description
Knowledge of cultures	Nurses shall gain an understanding of the perspectives, traditions, values, practices, and family systems of culturally diverse individuals, families, communities, and populations they care for, as well as knowledge of the complex variables that affect the achievement of health and well-being
Education and training in culturally competent care	Nurses shall be educationally prepared to provide culturally congruent healthcare. Knowledge and skills necessary for assuring that nursing care is culturally congruent shall be included in global healthcare agendas that mandate formal education and clinical training, as well as required ongoing, continuing education for all practicing nurses
Critical reflection	Nurses shall engage in critical reflection of their own values, beliefs, and cultural heritage in order to have an awareness of how these qualities and issues can impact culturally congruent nursing care
Cross-cultural communication	Nurses shall use culturally competent verbal and nonverbal communication skills to identify client's values, beliefs, practices, perceptions, and unique healthcare needs
Culturally competent practice	Nurses shall utilize cross-cultural knowledge and culturally sensitive skills in implementing culturally congruent nursing care
Cultural competence in healthcare systems and organizations	Healthcare organizations should provide the structure and resources necessary to evaluate and meet the cultural and language needs of their diverse clients
Patient advocacy and empowerment	Nurses shall recognize the effect of healthcare policies, delivery systems, and resources on their patient populations and shall empower and advocate for their patients as indicated. Nurses shall advocate for the inclusion of their patient's cultural beliefs and practices in all dimensions of their healthcare
Multicultural workforce	Nurses shall actively engage in the effort to ensure a multicultural workforce in healthcare settings. One measure to achieve a multicultural workforce is through strengthening of recruitment and retention effort in the hospital and academic setting
Cross-cultural leadership	Nurses shall have the ability to influence individuals, groups, and systems to achieve outcomes of culturally competent care for diverse populations. Nurses shall have the knowledge and skills to work with public and private organizations, professional associations, and communities to establish policies and guidelines for comprehensive implementation and evaluation of culturally competent care
Evidence-based practice and research	Nurses shall base their practice on interventions that have been systematically tested and shown to be the most effective for the culturally diverse populations that they serve. In areas where there is a lack of evidence of efficacy, nurse researchers shall investigate and test interventions that may be the most effective in reducing the disparities in health outcomes

Source: Douglas, M. K., Rosenkoetter, M., Pacquiao, D. F., Callister, L. C., Hattar-Pollara, M., Lauderdale, J., Milstead, J., Nardi, D. & Purnell, L. (2014). Guidelines for implementing culturally competent nursing care. *Journal of Transcultural Nursing*, 25(2), 110. Reprinted with permission from Sage Publications, Inc.

Regardless of culture, country of origin, manner of arrival or portrayal in popular media, the basic tenet of culturally appropriate care remains that any person is entitled to expect to receive care that is respectful of diversity, culturally appropriate and unbiased. For some specific population groups within Australia and New Zealand more particularly, the circumstances surrounding more recent migration or relocation, will be an important consideration. These population groups may have experienced associated trauma and distress and have subsequent increased risks of mental health concerns such as depression or post-traumatic stress disorder (Iqbal et al., 2012).

CULTURAL COMPETENCE

According to Stein-Parbury (2017, p. 106), 'cultural competence is a multidimensional concept currently used to describe the conditions necessary for appropriate delivery of healthcare that is culturally congruent.' To provide congruent health care, nurses need to be aware of the various cultures within Australia and New Zealand as well as the individual needs of members of each culture. Provision of care that is both person-centred and culturally competent must be tailored or adapted to meet the unique needs of each person's cultural beliefs and values. Person-centred care, being an integral part of cultural competence, is recognised in a number of components and allows the nurse to integrate cultural assessment into the health assessment of each person (Campinha-Bacote, 2011).

According to Campinha-Bacote (2007), there are five constructs in the cultural competence process: cultural awareness, cultural skill, cultural knowledge, cultural encounters and cultural desire. (For a model and description of Campinha-Bacote's 'The Process of Cultural Competence in the Delivery of Healthcare Services', go to her website at http://transculturalcare.net/the-process-of-cultural-competence-in-the-delivery-of-healthcare-services/.)

Cultural awareness

Cultural awareness is the 'deliberate, cognitive process in which the healthcare provider becomes appreciative and sensitive to

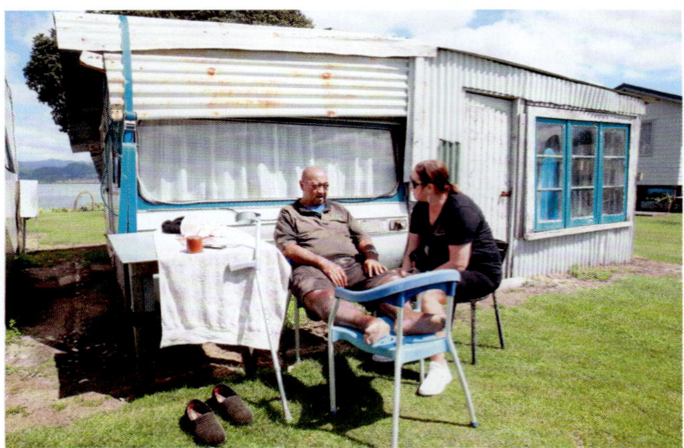

FIGURE 10-2 There are many variations among people, even between those from the same community. Thus, nurses should consider the needs of each individual when undertaking cultural assessment. (Stuff Limited.)

the values, beliefs, life ways, practices and problem-solving strategies of a patient's culture' (Campinha-Bacote, 2007). Put simply, cultural awareness is recognising there is a difference—a difference between cultures and among individuals within a culture (Fig. 10-2). But, first, cultural awareness involves 'self-examination and in-depth exploration of one's own cultural background' (Campinha-Bacote, 2007).

Nurses need to examine their own prejudices and biases towards other cultures and explore and reflect upon how their own cultural beliefs and background may affect their views of and interactions with patients from different cultures. By reflecting on their own beliefs and values surrounding culture, nurses can demonstrate cultural sensitivity. Cultural sensitivity is the capacity to understand and appreciate the legitimacy of differences and similarities that exist between cultures in a non-judgemental way, in addition to understanding how our own cultural beliefs and values impact on the care provided (Francis et al., 2013; Ramsden, 2002). Cultural awareness, cultural sensitivity and cultural safety can be considered as components of culturally competent practice and 'being' a culturally competent practitioner (Francis et al., 2013).

Cultural safety is a theoretical framework developed by Irihapeti Ramsden (a Māori nurse educator) as a process for understanding culture (Pairman et al., 2015). Cultural safety is 'an outcome of nursing and midwifery education that enables safe service to be defined by those that receive the service' (Ramsden, 2002, p. 117). The focus of safe service is on the experience the patient had, and this is what determines effective or culturally safe nursing care (Eckermann et al., 2009).

In the context of New Zealand, the Nursing Council of New Zealand (NCNZ, 2011) states that cultural safety extends beyond cultural awareness and sensitivity. It defines cultural safety as:

> the effective nursing practice of a person or family from another culture, and is determined by that person or family. Culture includes, but is not restricted to, age or generation; gender; sexual orientation; occupation and socioeconomic status; ethnic origin or migrant experience; religious or spiritual belief; and disability. The nurse delivering the nursing service will have undertaken a process of reflection on his or her own cultural identity and will recognise the impact that his or her personal culture has on his or her professional practice. Unsafe cultural practice comprises any action which diminishes, demeans or disempowers the cultural identity and well-being of an individual. (p. 7)

The key features of cultural safety include the transfer of power from nurse to patient and developing trust within a negotiated and equal partnership (Ramsden, 2002), adjusting the provision of care according to the needs of the patient and their family (Stein-Parbury, 2017) and recognising the presence of diversity within a culture along with the need for accurate assessment in the planning and implementation of nursing care (Farrell, 2017). As nurses become aware of cultural differences, they can be more sensitive to the needs of the person and their family and thus deliver nursing care in a culturally safe and appropriate manner.

The stages of cultural awareness are:

- **Unconscious incompetence:** not aware that one lacks cultural knowledge; not aware that cultural differences exist
- **Conscious incompetence:** aware that one lacks knowledge about another culture; aware that cultural differences exist but not knowing what they are or how to communicate effectively with people from different cultures
- **Conscious competence:** consciously learning about a person's culture and providing culturally relevant interventions; aware of differences; able to have effective transcultural interactions
- **Unconscious competence:** able to automatically provide culturally congruent care to people from a different culture; having much experience with a variety of cultural groups and having an intuitive grasp of how to communicate effectively in transcultural encounters.

Cultural skill

Cultural skill is 'the ability to collect relevant cultural data regarding the patient's health history and presenting problem as well as accurately performing a physical assessment' (Campinha-Bacote, 2007). Cultural skill involves learning how to complete cultural assessments and culturally based physical assessments and to interpret the data accurately.

Cultural knowledge

Cultural knowledge is 'the process of seeking and obtaining a sound educational foundation concerning the various worldviews of different cultures' (Campinha-Bacote, 2007). The person's worldview is the basis for his or her behaviours and interpretations of the world. For instance, the person's worldview will help to clarify his or her belief about what causes illness, what symptoms are defined as illness and what are considered appropriate interactions within cultural groups. These characteristics based on worldview, along with biological, psychological, social and environmental variations, constitute the content of cultural knowledge useful for the nurse assessing a person from a different culture.

Cultural encounters

A *cultural encounter* is 'the process that allows the healthcare provider to engage directly in face-to-face interactions with patients from culturally diverse backgrounds' (Campinha-Bacote, 2007). This process requires going beyond the study of a culture and limited interaction with three or four members of the culture. Repeated face-to-face encounters help to refine or modify the nurse's knowledge of the culture. The nurse must actively engage with people from different cultures with the intent to understand more about their culture.

Cultural desire

The motivation to engage in intercultural encounters and acquire cultural competence is known as *cultural desire*. Campinha-Bacote's revised model is based on the assumption that the starting point of cultural competence is cultural desire. In other words, to be a culturally competent health care provider, the nurse must sincerely desire to acquire the cultural knowledge and skill necessary for assessing the person effectively. The nurse must also seek repeated encounters with people of the culture so that awareness, knowledge and skill continually increase (Fig. 10-3). According to Pacquiao (2018, section 1.5), 'the goal of culturally competent care is the achievement of health equity, particularly for vulnerable populations who are most affected by the social determinants that lead to health inequity. In order to achieve health equity, culturally competent care must be grounded in the principles of social justice and human rights.'

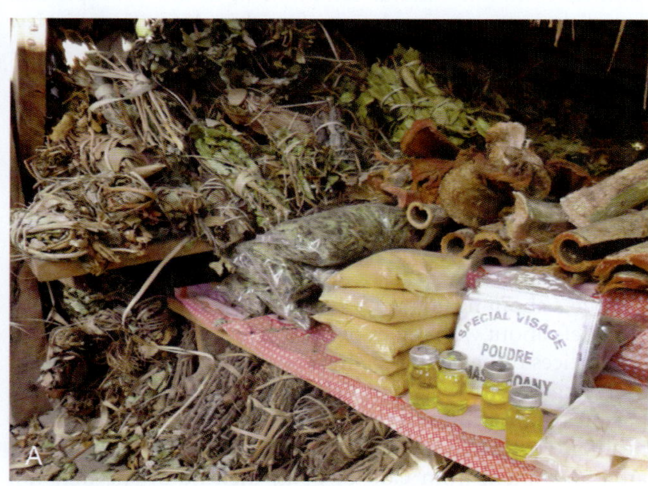

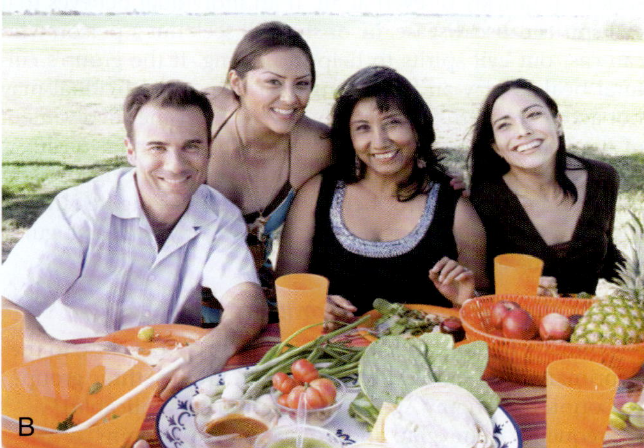

FIGURE 10-3 It is important to seek repeated encounters with people of various cultures so that awareness, knowledge and skill continually increase. Visiting a local herbal medicine market (A), or spending times with friends of another culture (B), are great ways to increase awareness, knowledge and skill.

CLINICAL TIP

Ask yourself about the level of your awareness, skill, knowledge and desire for cultural competence, and the patients you have encountered from cultures different from your own. The five constructs of cultural competence form the mnemonic ASKED (Awareness, Skill, Knowledge, Encounters, Desire). Use this mnemonic to examine your cultural competence. (The ASKED mnemonic can be found on Campinha-Bacote's website at http://transculturalcare.net/the-process-of-cultural-competence-in-the-delivery-of-healthcare-services/. Click on the 'Process of Cultural Competence Model'.)

CRITICAL THINKING

Use the following questions to help reflect on your level of growing cultural competence during practice:

1. How aware you are of your own biases and prejudices towards people different from yourself?
2. Can you complete a cultural assessment being sensitive to cultural differences and sensitivities?
3. How much do you know about different cultures and ethnic groups—about their beliefs, customs and biological variations?
4. What level of interest do you have in interacting with people from different cultures and ethnicities?
5. Are you really interested in becoming culturally competent? (Based on Campinha-Bacote, 2007.)

CULTURAL EMPATHY

According to Francis et al. (2013) health care professionals must be knowledgeable, clinically astute and able to provide empathic care. As health professionals we must also ensure we provide empathetic cultural care, but can we be empathetic to someone who has a different culture to our own? A group of researchers have developed an online resource with interactive activities as a way of addressing an empathetic approach to care of people from different cultures. The online resource is called The Virtual Empathy Museum (VEM) and holds numerous resources and simulations relating to empathy, including cultural competence and refugee health. Each evidence-based simulation presents authentic learning opportunities that explore the health care experiences of people from vulnerable and stigmatised groups. To access the resources, visit https://www.virtualempathymuseum.com.au/.

When entering the VEM, health professionals can walk in the shoes of someone from a different culture. The simulation scenario focuses on the empathic care of a person from a culturally and linguistically diverse background and includes 2D and 3D point-of-view films that present an unfolding scene in a hospital ward of a developing country where the environment, language and clinical practices are foreign and unfamiliar (VEM, 2018).

CULTURAL ASSESSMENT

Purposes and scope of assessment

The main purposes of assessing culture in a health care setting are:

- To learn about the person's beliefs and usual behaviours associated with health and illness, including beliefs

about disease causes, caregiving, expected treatments (Western medicine and folk practices), daily hygiene, food preferences and rituals, and religious beliefs relative to health care
- To compare the person's beliefs and practices with standard Western health care
- To compare the person's beliefs and practices with those of other people from a similar cultural background (to avoid stereotyping)
- To assess the person's health relative to the diseases prevalent in the specific cultural group.

Overview

When nurses encounter people from cultures different from their own, they become aware of certain aspects of a culture that are quite visible and obvious. There are, however, other aspects of a culture left hidden and discovered only following repeated or prolonged interactions between the person and nurse within the role of a therapeutic relationship. To illustrate this, the Iceberg Model of Culture (Hall, 1976) provides a visual explanation: just as only a small part of an iceberg protrudes above the water, so only a small part of each culture is visible and safe to those exploring the culture; the majority of the iceberg (or culture) is invisible below the water and can cause danger to those who are unaware of its existence. Aspects of culture that are visible, or so-called above the water, include food, music, dress and games, whereas those less visible or below the water include notions of modesty, leadership and family, concepts of time, rules of behaviour and the roles of men and women (Hall, 1976). When we are aware of what is 'below the water' we begin to understand the core values of a culture and the formative factors influencing and impacting on those values, which can be seen in the behaviours of people within that culture (Language and Culture Worldwide, 2015).

The purpose of a culturally inclusive health assessment is to identify the person's cultural background, including his or her ethnicity and religious beliefs, as well as customs and practices that influence the person's disease, illness and health state. Customs and practices that are important to identify during a cultural assessment include religious and dietary practices and health beliefs and practices.

The Centre for Culture, Ethnicity and Health (CEH) provides information on how to conduct a culturally inclusive health assessment, specifically relating to customs and practices. Identifying religious practices is important as the person may require access to religious leaders and a place to worship, and specific 'death and dying' customs and practices may need to be observed (CEH, 2011). Dietary practices may relate to food restrictions or point to cultural significance related to certain foods improving health (CEH, 2011). A person's health beliefs and practices need to be acknowledged and respected, together with applying a negotiated approach to implementing Western health care practices (CEH, 2011). For a more detailed explanation of how to conduct a culturally inclusive health assessment, visit the Centre for Culture, Ethnicity and Health website at www.ceh.org.au/resources/publications. The website also provides a broad range of specialist information and resources related to cultural diversity, health and wellbeing.

World populations are getting older, and it is important to consider the context of cultural diversity in aged care, particularly in the presence of conditions such as dementia. The Centre for Diversity in Aged Care website at www.culturaldiversity.com.au provides valuable resources and publications in relation to cultural and linguistic diversity in the specialist area of aged care.

Cultural assessment can involve incorporating elements of cultural assessment into any health assessment, or it can involve completing an individual cultural assessment in specific situations. To know what and when to include cultural components in health assessment, the nurse needs to know how to complete an entire cultural assessment. For this reason, many categories that may vary across cultures will be described. The nurse can then be aware of the possibilities for variation and select those that are most important for assessing each person. Many of these cultural variation categories are covered in transcultural nursing and cultural anthropology texts or can be found on the Internet. The more common cultural and biological variations encountered in the clinical setting will be described here.

Two main belief categories are included in a cultural assessment: those that affect the person's encounter with the health care system and provider, and those that affect the management of the disease, illness or health state. Of course, there is some overlap between these belief categories. Display 10-1 outlines common cultural variations in health concepts and promotion among populations found in Australia and New Zealand.

Cultural beliefs and values

- Dominant value orientation
- Beliefs about human nature
- Beliefs about relationship with nature
- Beliefs about purpose of life
- Beliefs about health, illness and healing
- Beliefs about what causes disease
- Beliefs about health
- Beliefs about who serves in the role of healer or what practices bring about healing

Assessing these beliefs will help the nurse to understand the person's approach to health care providers and to illness and healing. For instance, if an individual believes that diseases are punishment from God or gods, then he or she may not seek help quickly or even at all. If an individual believes that evil spirits cause disease, he or she will seek out a person who can cast out evil spirits to help in healing. If the group's cultural healers play an important role, then an individual may not accept Western-style health care without the involvement of the healer as well. If the individual believes that health is something that can be improved with exercise, eating the right foods and other 'healthy' behaviours, then seeking health care for early symptoms is usual. Refer to Display 10-2 as a guide for assessing a person's cultural beliefs.

Factors affecting approach to providers

- Ethnicity (assimilation or acculturation): How close to the primary culture does the person feel? To the ethnic group? Country of origin? Age at immigration (if applicable)? Frequency of travel to and from country of origin?
- Generational status: Age? Child, parent or grandparent? Family member or patient?
- Education level: Ability to understand spoken and written English? Ability to speak or write English? Acceptance of interpreter? Or interpreter of different age or gender?

DISPLAY 10-1 CULTURAL VARIATIONS IN HEALTH CONCEPTS AND PROMOTION

Cultural group	Concept of health	Health promotion
Aboriginal and Torres Strait Islander peoples[1]	Traditionally there is no word for health. Social and spiritual wellbeing relies holistically on relationships with and between people, the land and the creator.	Family and extended family are important. Illness is attributed to spiritual, grief, anger, or simply not known. Utilise home cures, bush medicine or traditional healers.
Māori[2]	Traditional health beliefs are holistic and health oriented. Spiritual wellbeing and contact with *whānau* (extended family) and the environment are important.	Not breaching the balance between *tapu* (sacred or restricted) and *noa* (common) aspects of life. Wellbeing is the balance between spiritual, social (including *whānau*), physical and emotional dimensions.
Samoan[3]	Holistic approach, including aspects of body, mind and spirit. Includes relationships with family, environment and spiritual world. Illness is seen as unavoidable and inevitable.	Concept of preventive health not well established in Samoa. May not believe that illness can be prevented.
African (refugees)[4]	Maintaining feelings of wellbeing, ability to fulfil role expectations, freedom from pain and excessive stress.	Proper diet, proper behaviour and exercise in fresh air are prescription for maintaining health; protect against excessive cold.
Greek[5]	Being healthy depends on having a positive mental attitude, and the spiritual belief that God will care for them. Avoid thinking about illness.	Use traditional remedies, such as herbal teas and aniseed. Presence of family is seen as vital to wellbeing. Illness is viewed as self-inflicted.
Chinese	Maintaining balance between *yin* (cool element) and *yang* (heat element) influences in the body and in the environment. Harmony is important to maintain body, mind and spirit.	One should eat a diet balanced with *yin* and *yang* foods and maintain harmony with friends and family.
Vietnamese[6]	Principles of harmony and balance within self. Overweight is a positive sign of good economic status and contentment.	Encompasses physical, spiritual, emotional and social factors. Consuming a lot of fresh vegetables, fruit, fish and meat. Keeping clean and warm.
Indian (Hindu)[7]	Maintaining balance between three *dosha*: *Vata* (wind), *Pitta* (bile) and *Kapha* (phlegm) (energy patterns that represent space, air, fire, water, earth). Based on Ayurveda medicine (holistic knowledge of life). A state of imbalance causes illnesses.	Rely on herbal remedies to prevent illness and cure illnesses. Nutrition is based on good hygiene and cooking using aromatic spices.
Lebanese (Muslim)[8]	Obligation to Islamic beliefs to maintain good health and prevent illness.	Caring for the body both physically and mentally, and for those who are dependent and vulnerable within the community.
Eastern Mediterranean and Central Africa (Iraq, Iran, Afghanistan, Somalia, Sudan, Ethiopia, Eritrea)[9]	Health is influenced by interaction of spiritual and religious factors that can enhance or reduce a person's power. Ill health may be seen as God's will.	Meeting obligations to Islamic beliefs are crucial to maintain balance. Cleanliness is important. Alcohol, as well as products containing alcohol, and illicit drugs are prohibited.

Sources: Dempsey et al. (2014): 1. Goold (2001); Reid (1982); 2. Durie (1998); 3. Lipson et al. (1996); 4. Papadopoulos, Lay, Lees & Gebrehiwot (2003); 5. Chan and Parker (2004); 6. Lipson et al. (1996); 7. Thakrar et al. (2008); 8. Brooke and Omeri (1999); 9. Camplin-Welch (2007).

DISPLAY 10-2 ASSESSING FOR CULTURAL BELIEFS

- What is the patient's country of origin? How long has the patient lived in this country? What is the patient's primary language and literacy level?
- What is the patient's ethnic background? Does he or she identify strongly with others from the same cultural background?
- What is the patient's religion, and how important is it to his or her daily life?
- Does the patient participate in cultural activities such as dressing in traditional clothing and observing traditional holidays and festivals?
- Are there any food preferences or restrictions?
- What are the patient's communication styles? Is eye contact avoided? How much physical distance is maintained? Is the patient open and verbal about symptoms?
- Who is the head of the family, and is he or she involved in decision making about the patient?
- What does the patient do to maintain his or her health?
- What does the patient think caused the current problem?
- Has the advice of traditional healers been sought?
- Have complementary and alternative therapies been used?
- What kind of treatment does the patient think will help? What are the most important results he or she hopes to get from this treatment?
- Are there cultural or religious rituals related to health, sickness or death that the patient observes?

From Farrell and Dempsey (2014). Farrell, M. & Dempsey, J. (2014). *Smeltzer & Bare's textbook of medical-surgical nursing* (3rd Australian and New Zealand ed.). Sydney: Lippincott Williams & Wilkins.

- Religion: Acceptance of care by provider of different gender, age or ethnic group? Level of modesty during care? Need for culturally specific healer to participate in care?
- Previous experience of care by the health care system? Positive or negative experience?
- Occupation and income level: Ability to pay or use insurance? Eligibility for medical subsidies? Embarrassment or fear due to inability to pay? Ability to follow prescribed care?
- Time dimensions: Focus on past, present or future? Orientation to time (importance of time versus immediate needs [arrives on time; arrives when convenient for self])?
- Space: Personal space distance? Comfortable with touch?
- Communication: Verbal, written language? Verbal and non-verbal language patterns? Eye contact? Who speaks to whom?

If the person seeking care is from a different cultural background from that of the nurse but is well acculturated to Western values, making assumptions that the person follows practices of their culture is stereotyping and may lead to conflict with the person. Family roles differ from culture to culture and may conflict with the beliefs of the health care systems in Australia and New Zealand regarding patient autonomy (Brown et al., 2016). In some cultures, it still may be the practice that older family members have more say in health care and treatment than the person themselves, even if that person is an adult (this might be especially true for females). Education level plays an important role in health care, but it is essential to assess language proficiency and the acceptance of an interpreter with specific characteristics. For example, some cultures do not allow a young person or a person of different gender to hear personal details. Religious rules and norms may affect who can assess, who can treat and what treatments are acceptable, among many other aspects of health care. Time, space and communication will be discussed in the following section.

Factors affecting disease, illness, health state

- Biomedical variations
- Nutrition/dietary habits
- Family roles and organisation, patterns
- Workforce issues
- High-risk behaviours
- Pregnancy and childbirth practices
- Death rituals
- Religious and spiritual beliefs and practices
- Health care practices
- Health care practitioners
- Environment

Biomedical variations are covered in the following section, as is a brief discussion of nutrition and dietary habits. Family content is addressed in Chapter 35, and religious and spiritual content in Chapter 13. Knowing what issues the culturally different person may have at work and what high-risk behaviours are common to the cultural group, as well as the environment from which the person comes, can give clues to the person's current health status. Assessing health care practices is discussed in the following section. As this is an assessment text, only the most common cultural and biological variations are covered here. More detailed content is available in transcultural nursing and cultural anthropology texts.

Communication and the culturally competent interview

When providing health care to people of cultures different from their own, nurses may be met with language barriers. Language barriers can make communication between the person and nurse difficult at times. Display 10-3 outlines how language barriers may be overcome during an assessment.

The first phase of assessment begins with meeting the person and involves observation and communication. These observations and communications between nurse and person

DISPLAY 10-3 OVERCOMING LANGUAGE BARRIERS

- Greet the patient using the last or complete name. Avoid being too casual or familiar. Point to yourself and say your name. Smile.
- Proceed in an unhurried manner. Pay attention to any effort by the patient or family to communicate.
- Speak in a low, moderate voice. Avoid talking loudly. Remember that there is a tendency to raise the volume and pitch of your voice when the listener appears not to understand. The listener may perceive that you are shouting or angry.
- Organise your thoughts. Repeat and summarise frequently. Use audio-visual aids when feasible.
- Use short, simple sentence structure and speak in the active voice.
- Use simple words such as 'pain' rather than 'discomfort'. Avoid medical jargon, idioms and slang. Avoid using contractions, such as *don't*, *can't*, *won't*.
- Use nouns repeatedly instead of pronouns. Example: Do not say: 'He has been taking his medicine, hasn't he?' Do say: 'Does Juan take his medicine?'
- Pantomime words (use gestures) and simple actions while verbalising them.
- Give instructions in the proper sequence. Example: Do not say: 'Before you rinse the bottle, wash it.' Do say: 'First, wash the bottle. Second, rinse the bottle.'
- Discuss one topic at a time and avoid giving too much information in a single conversation. Avoid using conjunctions. Example: Do not say: 'Are you cold and in pain?' Do say: (while pantomiming or gesturing): 'Are you cold?' 'Are you in pain?'
- Talk directly to the patient rather than to the person who accompanied him or her.
- Validate whether the person understands by having him or her repeat instructions, demonstrate the procedure or act out the meaning.
- Use any words you know in the person's language. This indicates that you are aware of and respect the patient's primary means of communicating.
- Try a third language. Many Indo-Chinese speak French. Europeans often know three or four languages, if you are familiar with the language.
- Be aware of culturally based gender and age differences and diverse socio-economic, educational and tribal or regional differences when choosing an interpreter.
- Obtain phrase books from a library or bookstore, make or purchase flash cards, contact hospitals for a list of interpreters, and use both formal and informal networking to locate a suitable interpreter. Although they are costly, some telecommunication companies provide translation services.

include many of the transcultural variations of time, space and communication, and biomedical variations. All communication is culturally based. Verbal communication can have many variations based on both language differences and usual tone of voice. For instance, a harsh tone of voice may be normal in some cultures and thought to be rude in others. Non-verbal communication has the most frequently misinterpreted variations. These variations include patterns of space, eye contact, body language, hand gestures, silence and touch. Time is also interpreted to be a form of communication when two people from different cultures perceive time differently.

Time

Time is perceived to be measurable (Western cultures) or fluid and flowing (Eastern cultures). Cultural groups tend to value time in the past, present or future. Those focused on past value practices that are unchanged from ancestors are often resistant to new ways. Those focused on the present put what is going on in the present above what will occur in the future. For instance, if a person has an appointment with you but is involved in a pleasurable activity at the time, then either the appointment will be missed or the person will arrive late. Family business, illness and funerals may be prioritised above appointments related to health care (Farrell, 2017). Those who are future oriented place value on deferring pleasure for a later gain. They value the care and treatment you offer in expectation of improvement (this reflects Western values). Time can also be viewed as a relative phenomenon. Aboriginal and Torres Strait Islander, and Māori cultures view time as 'cyclical continuity not lineal change: the past and future may be seen as integral parts to the present' (Farrell & Dempsey, 2014, p. 27).

Space

The area around a person is considered to be part of that person; more commonly referred to as personal space, it is the area into which others do not enter during personal interactions (Wilson, 2014). This concept of 'safe individual space' may be viewed quite differently by individuals and cultural groups; some people need more space to feel comfortable, others may react angrily if their space is threatened. As part of effective communication, it is important that respect for personal space expectations and preferences be considered in patient encounters. For example, people who live in rural areas, including Aboriginal Australians and Torres Strait Islander peoples, may prefer more personal space than those who live in urban areas (Farrell & Dempsey, 2014). Another variation is whether people face each other when talking or stand with their face slightly to the side or slightly away from each other. The quality of communication between individuals can be enhanced when there is an understanding of personal space and distancing characteristics (Purnell & Paulanka, 2013).

Eye contact and face positioning

Some cultures expect people who are talking to each other to maintain a fairly high level of eye contact. Those who look away and do not give 'good eye contact' are thought to be rude or inattentive. In Australia and New Zealand, direct eye contact while speaking is the dominant practice, but variations exist in other cultures (Wilson, 2014). For example, some people from Eastern countries tend to look down to show respect to the person talking. Some Pasifika and Māori may avert their eyes when speaking with a person who they view to be in a position of authority, as a way of showing respect and to demonstrate that they are listening closely to what the person is saying (Farrell & Dempsey, 2014). For further information, see the NCNZ's Code of Conduct and its guidelines on professional boundaries (both available at www.nursingcouncil.org.nz). Some African Americans look away when being spoken to but give a very high level of eye contact when speaking themselves. An Anglo American unfamiliar with this pattern may get the impression that the person does not care about what the carer is saying and is aggressive when talking. However, it is just a normal cultural variation in communication patterns. Other cultures that may regard direct eye contact as aggressive behaviour or impolite include Asians, Indochinese and Arabs (Wilson, 2014).

Body language and hand gestures

There are too many elements of body language and hand gestures to cover them all here; it is, however, important to consider how communication using hand gestures and facial expressions varies among cultures. Various cultures perceive the use of hands when communicating quite differently. For example, the flamboyant use of hand gesturing and raising the arms above the head or conversing with hands in pockets may be perceived negatively (Purnell & Paulanka, 2013). Similarly, the more open and welcoming Western gestures associated with greeting people or making introductions may be interpreted very differently by other cultures.

Silence

There are two types of silence. One is simply remaining silent for long periods; the other is used to space talking between two people carrying on a conversation. There are three patterns of the latter. In Eastern cultures there is a pause after each person speaks and before the next person speaks. The pause is thought to show respect and to allow for consideration of what has been said. In Western cultures speakers tend to interrupt this silence, leaving no pause between speakers; such cultures tend to be uncomfortable with silence. Yet in other cultures it is common for speakers to interrupt one another in conversation. This provides for overlap in speech. Within the culture, this indicates that the persons are deeply engaged in the conversation, but it can be perceived as rude by other cultures.

Touch

Touch is very culturally based. How much touch is comfortable and allowable, and by whom, is based on culture. Most modest and conservative cultures usually have religious rules about this. In many of these cultures, touch of females by males is restricted to male family members and may also be restricted among them. Even male health care providers, including doctors, may not be allowed to treat women from traditional Arab, Aboriginal and Torres Strait Islander and Māori backgrounds (Farrell & Dempsey, 2014). In some religions, there are prohibitions on touching people considered to be unclean. In some cultures, there are prohibitions about touching parts of the body, especially the head, or touching children because touch is a way to 'give the evil eye' to another. In the light of these cultural variations, the nurse should always ask permission before touching anyone.

Autonomy

Autonomy is assumed to be a right of all health care consumers, meaning that an individual has the right to know about the diagnosis and treatment plans and to make decisions for himself or herself. However, autonomy is not an accepted value in many societies. In paternalistic or patriarchal societies, the father or the family expects to be told of diagnoses and to make decisions about treatment. In many societies, women are not permitted to be decision makers. Do not assume that the person expects autonomy; clarify with the person and family. Patient autonomy is a legal issue in any health care setting, so the family and person will need to have a clear explanation of this. The information should be presented in such a way as to avoid a hostile response from 'the decision maker' in the family or the person being removed from the health care facility.

Diet and nutrition

What we eat, how we eat it and even when we eat are all culturally based. Dietary considerations in cultural assessment include the meaning of food to the individual, common foods consumed and rituals surrounding its consumption, the distribution of food throughout a 24-hour day, religious beliefs about certain foods, beliefs about food and health promotion, and nutritional deficiencies associated with the ethnic group. Asking people to drastically change their usual dietary habits can be difficult, even with knowledge of the interaction of diet and disease. What food means to the individual can also be very important. Food may be consumed to provide a sense of comfort or to bring the person closer to ethnic roots or family. Providing food may be perceived to reflect caring and love, just as withdrawing food may be considered akin to punishment.

The time at which the meal is served can seriously affect appetite. For those who usually eat lunch at 2 or 3 p.m., it is unappetising to see lunch served at 11 or 12 noon, and a 5 or 6 p.m. dinner is considered a late lunch rather than an evening meal. Religious beliefs affect what can and cannot be eaten, such as the prohibition of pork or pork products for some cultures. Asking about specific dietary requirements or preferences is part of cultural assessment.

Spirituality

Spirituality is closely associated with culture and includes religious practices, faith and a relationship with God or a higher being, and those things that bring meaning to life. See Chapter 13 for a detailed discussion of assessing spirituality.

Death rituals

As noted by Purnell and Paulanka (2013), death rituals include views of death, euthanasia and rituals for dying, burial and bereavement, and are unlikely to vary from the traditional cultural group's practices. Practices that affect health care include such customs as ritual washing of the body, the number of family members present at the death of a family member, religious practices required during or after dying, acceptance of life- or death-prolonging treatments, beliefs about withdrawing life support and beliefs about autopsy. Responses to death and grief vary. Some cultures expect loud wailing in grief with death, whereas others expect solemn, quiet grief. In addition, the expected duration of grief varies between cultures.

Pregnancy and childbearing

Accepted practices for family planning, pregnancy, birthing and parenting vary across cultures. As Purnell and Paulanka (2008, p. 30) noted, 'There are many culturally specific traditional, folk, and magicoreligious beliefs and taboos surrounding fertility control, pregnancy, childbearing, and postpartum practices.' These beliefs about conception, pregnancy and childbearing are passed from generation to generation.

Fertility control varies by culture and religion. Use of contraception, including sterilisation, is accepted by some, rejected by others and forcibly used in other cultures. Rituals to restrict sexuality are used in some cultures, including female genital mutilation (FGM) or ritual, female surgery involving the partial or complete removal of the external genitalia (World Health Organization [WHO], cited in Pairman et al., 2006). FGM is illegal in Australia and New Zealand. Previously suggested to be associated with certain religions, the practice is now condemned by many religious leaders (Pairman et al., 2015). Nonetheless, the practice continues in some countries; therefore, nurses and midwives must be alert to the possibility that women from certain regions of the world may have undergone this procedure and experience complications such as vesicovaginal fistula as a result.

Most societies have expectations and beliefs about acceptable maternal behaviours and lifestyle (Purnell & Paulanka, 2013). Pregnant women are expected to avoid potentially harmful elements in their environment such as very loud noises, smoking and drinking alcohol, consuming beverages high in caffeine and taking drugs, and be cautious about taking prescription and over-the-counter medications. Other cultures have pregnancy taboos, such as having the mother avoid reaching over her head to prevent the umbilical cord from going around the baby's neck, not buying baby clothes before the baby's birth and not permitting the father to see the mother or baby until the baby is cleaned.

Culture-based treatments

Culture-based treatments are often misinterpreted in Western health care settings, as they may produce marks on the skin that are interpreted as evidence of abuse (Fig. 10-4). Assuming abuse has occurred can have a negative impact on the nurse–patient relationship and may cause a culturally different person to reject Western-style health care in the future. Some of the more common Asian treatments are cupping, coining and moxibustion. Cupping, often used to treat back pain, involves placing heated glass jars on the skin. Cooling of the glass jars causes suction that leaves redness and bruising. Coining involves rubbing ointment into the skin with a spoon or coin. The rubbing leaves bruises or red marks but does not cause pain. Coining is used for 'wind illness' (a fear of being cold or of wind, which causes loss of yang), fever and stress-related illnesses such as headache. Moxibustion is the attachment of smouldering herbs to the end of acupuncture needles or placing the herbs on the skin; this causes scars that look like cigarette burns. Moxibustion is used to strengthen one's blood and the flow of energy, and generally to maintain good health.

Other treatments are related to different beliefs about what causes disease. In many cultures an imbalance between hot and cold is believed to cause disease, so treatment would be to take foods, drinks or medication of the opposite type (hot for a cold condition and cold for a hot condition). What is thought to be hot or cold bears no relation to temperature. Cancer, headache

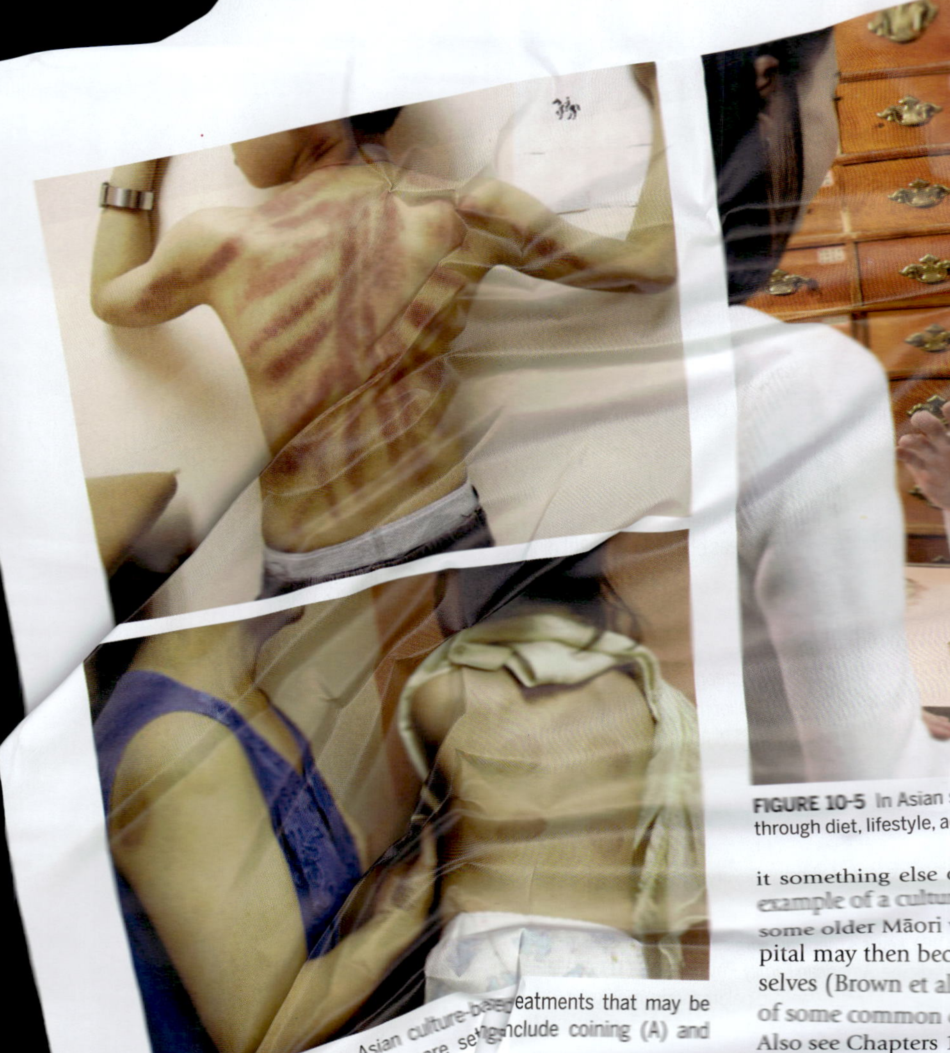

FIG... 4 Two common Asian culture-b... ...eatments that may be ...reted in Western health care se... include coining (A) and ...g (B).

and pneumonia are described ...d, whereas diabetes mellitus, hypertension and sore ... infection are hot. In Asian
societies, hot–cold is also ... with the body's energy of
yin–yang, which must ... alance for health. These are
balanced through die... ...upuncture and herbs.

Some standard ... ...ents are unacceptable in other
cultures. For exa... ...ing and psychiatric treatments
are resisted by ... ...y other cultures because mental
illness is con... ... There are also many Europeans
living in Au... ...ealand who do not openly discuss
mental h... ...e associated stigma still held about
people ... ...tal health problems (Wilson, 2014).

Cul... ...nes

C... ...nes are conditions that are specific to ... ccur as a combination of psychiatric or ... ysical symptoms. There is much debate ... syndromes are folk or traditional illnesses ... nges or local variations of Western mental ... or whether they are not syndromes at all but ... ways of explaining negative events in life.

...le might perceive the syndromes to be condi... ...fic symptoms, it is necessary to be familiar with ...ledging the person's belief that the symptoms ...order is important, even if Western medicine calls it something else or does not see it as a specific disease. An example of a culture-bound syndrome in Māori culture is that some older Māori who have had a family member die in hospital may then become fearful of hospitals and doctors themselves (Brown et al., 2016). See Display 10-4 for a description of some common culture-bound syndromes across the world. Also see Chapters 11 and 12 for more details.

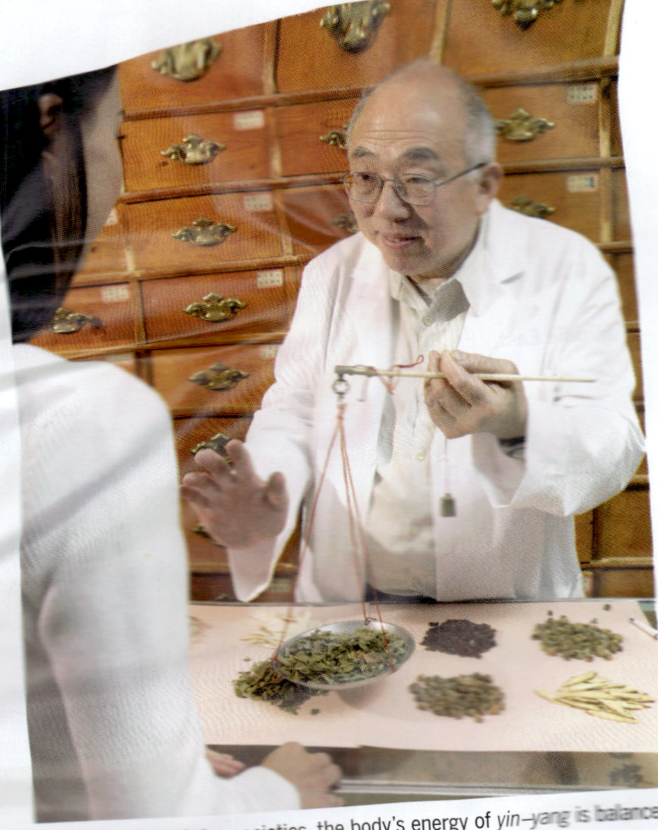

FIGURE 10-5 In Asian societies, the body's energy of *yin–yang* is balanced through diet, lifestyle, acupuncture and herbs.

Many culture-bound syndromes are based on different beliefs in what causes disease. Some of the culturally based beliefs about disease causation include yin–yang out of balance, hot–cold imbalance, and spirit possession (Fig. 10-5). Such beliefs in these as causes of disease may form the basis of culture-bound syndromes. The symptoms related to the conditions are often specific to a culture.

Health care practices

Purnell and Paulanka (2013) divide the assessment of health care practices into six categories: health-seeking beliefs and behaviours, responsibility for health care, folk and traditional practices, barriers to health care, cultural responses to health and illness, and blood transfusion and organ donation (see Display 10-5). The 14 items in Display 10-5 are easily understood as stated. However, pain and blood products will be discussed in detail in order to present a clearer explanation.

Pain

Pain assessment is considered the fifth vital sign in contemporary health care. Pain has psychological, social, spiritual and physical dimensions and is influenced and experienced differently across cultural groups (Narayan, 2010). Culture influences how individuals experience, express and respond to pain and will also guide their choice of treatment. Some believe that pain is punishment for wrongdoing; others believe it is atonement for wrongdoing. The response to pain is often based on cultural

DISPLAY 10-4 CULTURE-BOUND SYNDROMES

Common culture-bound syndromes by geographical area are listed below along with brief descriptions of each.

Australia

Sung	Some Aboriginal and Torres Strait Islander communities believe in and practise sorcery. This includes the belief that if a person is sung, he or she will fade away and die. Many Aboriginal and Torres Strait Islander peoples view hospitals as a place where you go to die and hospitals are therefore often feared. They also fear that if they die in hospital, their spirit will [illegible] trapped and unable to find its way home. A traditional healer needs to be called in such instances.

Middle East

Zar	Experience of spirit possession. Laugh, shout, weep, sing, hit head against wall. May be apathe[illegible] [illegible]wn, refuse food, unable to carry out daily tasks. May develop long-term relationship with possessing spirit (no[illegible] pathological in the culture).

Asian (South or East)

Amok (Malaysia)	Occurs among males (20 to 45 years old) after perceive[illegible] or insult. Aggressive outbursts, violent or homicida[illegible] aimed at people or objects, often with ideas of persecution. After [illegible] exhaustion, final return to previous state.
Koro (Malaysia, Southeast Asia)	Similar to conditions in China, Thailand and other areas. Fear that genita[illegible] into the body, possibly leading to death. Causes vary, including inappropriate sex, mass cases from belief that e[illegible] flu-vaccinated pork is a cause.
Latah (Malaysia)	Occurs after traumatic episode or surprise. Exaggerated startle response (usually in women). Screaming, cursing, dancing, hysterical laughter, may imitate people, hyper-suggestibility.
Shen kui (China) *Dhat* (India)	Similar conditions that result from the belief that semen (or 'vital essence') is [illegible]ing lost. Anxiety, panic, sexual complaints, fatigue, weakness, loss of appetite, guilt, sexual dysfunction [illegible] no physical findings.
Taijin kyofusho (Japan)	Dread of offending or hurting others by behaviour or physical condition such as [illegible]dour. Social phobia.
Wind illness (Asia)	Fear of wind, cold exposure causing loss of yang energy.

North America, Western Europe

Anorexia nervosa	Associated with intense fear of obesity. Severely restricted food and kilojoule intake.
Bulimia nervosa	Associated with intense fear of obesity. Binge eating and self-induced vomiting, laxative or diur[illegible]

Modified from these various sources: Brown et al. (2016). *Lewis's medical–surgical nursing: assessment and management of clinical pro*[illegible] Sydney: Elsevier. Juckett, G. (2005). Cross-cultural medicine. *American Family Physician, 72*(11). Available at http://www.aafp.org/afp/2005[illegible]7.html. O'Neill, D. (2002–2010). Culture specific diseases. Available at http://anthro.palomar.edu/medical/med_4.htm. Paniagua, F. & Yamada, A. (20[illegible] [illegible]ok *of multicultural mental health: Assessment and treatment of diverse populations* (2nd ed.). Burlington, MA: Academ[illegible] Press/Elsevier.

DISPLAY 10-5 HEALTH CARE PRACTICES

Health-seeking beliefs and behaviours

1. Identify predominant beliefs that influence health care practices.
2. Describe health promotion and prevention practices.

Responsibility for health care

3. Describe the focus of acute-care practice (curative or fatalistic).
4. Explore who assumes responsibility for health care in this culture.
5. Describe the role of health insurance in this culture.
6. Explore practices associated with the use of over-the-counter medications.

Folk and traditional practices

7. Explore combinations of magicoreligious beliefs, folk and traditional beliefs that influence health care behaviours.

Barriers to health care

8. Identify barriers to health care such as language, economics, accessibility and geography for this group.

Cultural responses to health and ill[illegible]

9. Explore cultural beliefs and responses to [illegible] interventions. Does pain have a special me[illegible]
10. Describe beliefs and views about mental illne[illegible]
11. Differentiate between the perceptions of ment[illegible] in this culture.
12. Describe cultural beliefs and practices related to c[illegible] rehabilitation.
13. Identify cultural perceptions of the sick role in this gr[illegible]

Blood transfusion and organ donation

14. Describe the acceptance of blood and blood products, org[illegible] and organ transplantation among this group.

Purnell, L. & Paulanka, B. (Eds). (2013). *Transcultural health care: A culturally competent approach* (4th ed.). Philadelphia: F.A. Davis. With kind permission of Dr. Larry Purnell, PhD, RN, FAAN.

values and may include culture-specific behaviours, some being stoic and others more expressive (Brady et al., 2016). Wilson (2014) reports that in some cultures the open expression of pain is encouraged, whereas other cultures frown upon open and free expression of emotions relating to the experience of pain. When the carer and person come from different cultures, interpreting the person's actual level of pain can be difficult. In addition, by explaining the therapeutic reasons for treating pain, a person from a stoic culture may be less reluctant to express or describe pain or consider other treatments.

Blood products

Use of blood products and blood transfusions is accepted by most religions except for Jehovah's Witnesses. Organ donation and autopsy are not accepted by certain cultural groups, including Christian Scientists, Orthodox Jews, Greeks and some Spanish-speaking groups (because of the belief that the person will suffer in the afterlife if organs are removed or autopsy is performed). The concepts of organ donation and transplants may be unfamiliar to some cultural groups; this highlights the importance of cultural awareness and sensitivity when considering how to introduce or discuss these issues in health care settings. In addition, some cultures may be suspicious of organ donation, believing that the donor will receive inadequate care so that organs can be harvested (Purnell & Paulanka, 2013).

Biological variations

Genetics and environment, and their interactions, cause humans to vary biologically. Gene variations cause obvious differences like eye colour and genetic diseases, such as trisomy 21. Genes are increasingly being identified as playing a role in most diseases, even if only to increase or decrease a person's susceptibility to infectious or chronic diseases. Environment has also been proven to cause disease, but modern Western thought on disease causation leans towards a mingling of genetics and environment. If, for example, a person has lungs that are genetically 'hardy', then exposure to smoking may not cause lung cancer or chronic lung disease. However, we know this is not necessarily true in all cases, as a significant percentage of the population develop lung cancer even when they have not been exposed to smoke (Australian Lung Foundation, 2018).

Physical variations (resulting from genetics or cultural behaviours) are included in the normal and abnormal findings in the physical assessment chapters throughout this book. Integrating the information helps the nurse to attend to the possible variations during all assessments rather than having to seek the information elsewhere if the person appears to be from a different culture.

One limitation of this approach needs to be acknowledged. Because characteristics vary along a continuum with many possible points of reference, it would be cumbersome to include every possible variation as the point from which a characteristic varies. Acknowledging that this is an imperfect approach, we have used the Australian and New Zealand population majority group as the point from which variation is assessed. As Australian and New Zealand population demographics change, the baseline point will have to change in future texts.

In his model of cultural competence, Purnell (Purnell & Paulanka, 2013) includes a category called biocultural ecology. This category refers to the person's physical, biological and physiological variations such as variations in drug metabolism, disease and health conditions. The term 'biocultural ecology' presents an interesting perspective. However, this text uses the term 'biological variation' to include human variation of a biological and physiological nature. Overfield (1995) divides the discussion of biological variation into sections, as follows:

I. Surface variations and anatomical differences
  A. Surface variation
    1. Colour
    2. Secretions
    3. Surface anatomy
  B. Anatomical variation
    1. Body proportions
    2. Bones
    3. Pelvic measurements and newborn size
    4. Pulmonary function
    5. Teeth
    6. Soft tissue
II. Developmental variation in childhood
  A. Body size and proportion differences
  B. Developmental maturity differences
  C. Environmental effects
  D. Surface features
  E. Common clinical measurements
  F. Disease differential
  G. Other variations
III. Developmental variation in adulthood
  A. Body size, shape and composition
  B. Surface manifestations
  C. Developmental changes
  D. Disease susceptibility
IV. Biochemical variation and differential disease susceptibility
V. Environmentally related variation
  A. Climate
  B. Altitude
  C. Diet
VI. Sexual variation

Additionally, there are culturally based syndromes of diseases that are perceived to exist in some cultures but not perceived to exist in other cultures or by the health care providers of other cultures.

Because an assessment text cannot discuss all the topics in biological variation, only a sampling is included in this text. The variations selected for inclusion are among those often seen or most likely to be misinterpreted.

Surface variation

Secretions as an example of a surface variation refer to the variation in apocrine and eccrine sweat secretions and the apocrine secretion of earwax. Sebaceous gland activity and secretion composition do not show significant variation.

Eccrine glands, distributed over the entire body, show no variation in number or distribution but do vary in activity based on environmental and individual adaptations (not by race). Persons born in the tropics have more functioning glands than those born in other areas and than those who move to the tropics later in life. Apocrine glands, opening into the hair follicles in the axilla, groin and pubic regions, around the anus, umbilicus and breast areola, and in the external auditory canal, vary with regard to the number of functioning glands. The amount of sweating and body odour may be directly related to the function of apocrine glands, although the odour is probably related to the decomposition of lipids in the secretions. Earwax, produced by the apocrine glands in the external ear, varies between dry and wet wax based on a genetic trait. Reasons for the many genetic variations are thought to also include climate and disease susceptibility.

Anatomical variation

Lower extremity venous valves vary between Native Africans and Caucasians. Native Africans have been noted to have fewer valves in the external iliac veins but many more valves lower in the leg than do Caucasians. The additional valves may account for the lower prevalence of varicose veins in this group (Overfield, 1995).

Developmental variation

Developmental differences appear to be related to both genetic and environmental influences. Infants and children from some racial groups tend to develop ahead of other groups in motor development. However, studies of the effect of socio-economic status indicate that lower-status children show earlier motor development than do higher-status children, irrespective of racial group (Overfield, 1995).

Biochemical variation and differential disease susceptibility

Drug metabolism differences, lactose intolerance and malaria-related conditions—such as sickle cell disease, thalassaemia, glucose-6-phosphate dehydrogenase (G-6-PD) deficiency and Duffy blood group—are considered biochemical variations. Overfield (1995), Campinha-Bacote (2007), and Purnell and Paulanka (2013) provide extensive reviews of ethnic–racial group differences in drug metabolism. As far as lactose intolerance is concerned, most of the world's population is lactose intolerant. The ability to digest lactose after childhood relates to a mutation that occurs mainly in those of North and Central European ancestry and in some Middle Eastern populations (Overfield, 1995). Malaria-related conditions occur more commonly in populations living in or near areas where mosquito-borne diseases are prevalent, such as the Mediterranean, Asia and Africa.

These brief examples show that health status and health assessment are greatly influenced by biological variations. Many of the chapters in this text include physical characteristics to be assessed that have normal variations or that vary in the way abnormalities are expressed. These variations are inserted into the physical assessment discussions. Also, many of the chapters include risk factor discussions addressing common illnesses associated with the content of the chapter.

Drug metabolism

There have been many studies on ethnic, racial and biological variations in drug metabolism. As Purnell and Paulanka (2013) noted, Chinese people are more sensitive to cardiovascular effects of some drugs and have increased absorption of antipsychotics, some narcotics and antihypertensives. Farrell and Dempsey (2014) suggest that care needs to be taken in prescribing medications, as there can be a genetic predisposition to different rates of metabolism, which can lead to people experiencing adverse reactions to a dose commonly considered normal. In addition, many conditions can alter drug metabolism; for instance, smoking accelerates it, malnutrition affects it, stress affects it and low-fat diets decrease absorption of some drugs. Cultural beliefs about taking medication also affect acceptance and compliance with dosage regimens.

Geographical and ethnic disease variation

In general, chronic diseases predominate in developed countries and infectious diseases predominate in developing countries. However, there is some genetic and ethnic variation in addition to the chronic versus infectious pattern. Often the studies in developing countries and on immigrants from these countries are limited. Patterns are known, however, and are often based on body size, lifestyle and genetics. For instance, vascular diseases tend to be higher in cultures and populations with larger body size and lifestyle habits such as smoking.

Osteoporosis is more prevalent in small-framed people such as Asians. Knowing that some groups will be more prone to a disease or condition can help the nurse to more carefully assess each person. However, increasing ethnic diversity in global populations more broadly means we must be cautious about making generalisations and further highlights the need to understand the cultural context and relationships between health, illness and culture (Willis & Elmer, 2011). Following are examples of geographical or ethnic disease variations for the physical systems.

Skin, hair and nails

Skin cancer is highly feared among skin diseases. Fair-skinned people and those with light eyes and freckles are at higher risk of developing skin cancer than those with naturally darker skin, although all people who are exposed to high levels of intense sunlight are at risk (Cancer Council Australia, 2019). Because ozone depletion is a factor in skin cancer risk, people living in Australia, New Zealand and southern Africa are among those at greater risk. Australia has one of the highest rates of skin cancer in the world, at nearly four times the rates in Canada, the U.S. and the U.K. (AIHW, 2019). Both Australia and New Zealand have increasing rates of melanoma compared with the rest of the world. Worldwide, 2 to 3 million cases of non-melanoma and 132,000 cases of melanoma skin cancer occur each year (WHO, 2018).

Although too much sun exposure can damage skin and eyes, too little can lead to a deficiency in vitamin D, which can weaken bones and affect overall health. Certain sections of the population are more likely to be at risk of vitamin D deficiency. These include naturally dark-skinned people (who need more ultraviolet [UV] exposure to produce adequate levels of vitamin D, as the pigment in their skin reduces UV penetration) and people who cover their skin for religious or cultural reasons. Others at risk include the elderly, people who are housebound or in institutional care, babies and infants of vitamin D–deficient mothers and those with osteoporosis (AIHW, 2019).

Head and neck

The most common causes of brain injury following trauma are those involving falls, vehicle accidents and assaults, with more males than females involved in accidents and assaults (Harrison, 2010). It is common knowledge that falls are the leading cause of injury-related hospitalisations. Less well known is that falls are now the most common cause of nearly half of all traumatic brain injuries (Beck et al., 2016; Rushworth, 2010). Cultural considerations are commonly related to dependence on poorly maintained cars and bicycles, lack of use of protective headgear, inadequate and unsafe housing, and unsafe practices involving alcohol, drugs and firearms.

Eyes

Visual impairment varies across age (greater after 50), gender (more in females) and geography (90% living in developing countries) (WHO, 2018). Among all who are visually impaired, the WHO estimates that 80% of all visual impairment can be avoided or cured (WHO, 2018).

The leading causes of visual impairment include uncorrected refractive errors and cataracts; other major causes include glaucoma, age-related macular degeneration, diabetic retinopathy, corneal opacity and trachoma (WHO, 2018). Certain groups within the Australian population are at greater risk of developing eye disease, including older people, people with a family history of eye disease, people with diabetes, and marginalised or disadvantaged people (AIHW, 2019).

Visual impairment due to infectious diseases has declined worldwide over the last 20 years; however, some Aboriginal and Torres Strait Islander communities continue to have a high prevalence of trachoma, an infectious disease linked to poor hygiene that may lead to blindness (Kirby Institute, 2017). Although active trachoma is preventable, screening rates for this disease have been reported to be as high as 11% in children between the ages of 1 and 14 living in some Aboriginal and Torres Strait Islander communities (Kirby Institute, 2017). Excessive exposure to UV radiation—an increased risk in Australia and New Zealand—can also lead to eye disease (AIHW, 2019).

Other eye diseases include corneal diseases and diseases in children, such as cataracts, prematurity retinopathy and vitamin A deficiency (AIHW, 2019).

Ear and hearing loss

Of the more than 4 million people across the world with hearing loss in both ears, 80% live in low- to middle-income countries (WHO, 2019). These numbers will increase as the global population ages; in Australia, hearing loss is one of the most common long-term conditions reported in those over 65 years old (AIHW, 2019).

The main cause of hearing loss in children is chronic middle ear infection. In Australia, chronic otitis media is far more common among Aboriginal and Torres Strait Islander children than among non-Aboriginal and Torres Strait Islander children (AIHW, 2019). At least 50% of all cases of hearing loss can be prevented through primary prevention (WHO, 2019). Other common causes of hearing loss at or before birth are genetic (through one or both parents) and include birth complications such as prematurity, reduced oxygen for the baby or the mother's infections (e.g. rubella, syphilis); use of drugs affecting the baby's hearing (more than 130 drugs including gentamicin); and severe jaundice, which can damage the baby's hearing. After birth, infectious diseases, ototoxic drugs, head or ear injury, wax or foreign body blockage, excessive noise and age can lead to hearing loss.

Mouth, nose and sinus

Oral diseases are prevalent in poorer populations in developed and developing countries. They include dental cavities, periodontal disease, tooth loss, oral mucosal and oropharyngeal lesions and cancers, human immunodeficiency virus (HIV) – related diseases, and trauma. Poor living conditions including diet, nutrition, hygiene, limited oral health care, and the use of alcohol, tobacco and tobacco-related products contribute to developing oral disease.

The incidence of oral cancer is variable across different countries and is attributed to environmental factors rather than genetics. Tobacco use and excessive alcohol intake are the main risk factors for oral cancer. Very high rates are reported in areas of South Asia where tobacco mixed with betel nut, lime, spices, perfumes and other substances is used for smoking and chewing and in some rituals (Kao et al., 2009). Chronic sinusitis is reported consistently as one of 10 most common long-term conditions in those over age 25 years (Australian Centre for Asthma Monitoring, 2011), affecting 12% of people in developed countries (Copeland et al., 2018).

Good oral health in childhood contributes to better teeth and gums in adulthood—less decay and the loss of fewer natural teeth. Although internationally Australia compares favourably on child dental decay, ranking 7th out of 27 Organisation for Economic Co-operation and Development (OECD) countries in 2002, the prevalence of tooth decay among young children continues to increase (Chrisopoulos & Harford, 2016).

Thorax and lungs

Australia and New Zealand have among the highest rates of hospitalisation for chronic obstructive pulmonary disease (COPD) in the world (OECD, 2017). Aboriginal and Torres Strait Islander Australians were hospitalised for respiratory diseases such as COPD at five times the rate of other Australians from 2006 to 2008 (Australian Centre for Asthma Monitoring, 2011). Lung cancer continues to be a leading cause of death in Australian men and women, and the leading cancer cause of death in New Zealand (AIHW, 2019; New Zealand Ministry of Health, 2019a). Lung cancer is directly related to smoking and to the quantity of cigarettes smoked. Direct smoke inhalation is responsible for 80% to 90% of all lung cancers, with a 35% risk for passive inhalation (Brown et al., 2016). COPD has a significant impact on the health of the Australian and New Zealand populations. In Australia, it is the fifth leading cause of death in men and women. In New Zealand, it is the third leading cause of death in men and the fourth for women. Aboriginal and Torres Strait Islander peoples are three times more likely to die from the disease than other Australians.

Within Australia, rates of tuberculosis (TB) have increased in some states, with high rates being reported in certain populations, even though there has been a decline in TB across the nation. Two major factors are suggested to have contributed to the resurgence of TB: the high rates of TB among people with HIV and the emergence of multidrug-resistant strains of Mycobacterium tuberculosis (Brown et al., 2016). TB remains a problem within Aboriginal and Torres Strait Islander communities, Māori and immigrants from endemic countries (WHO, 2016). Up to 85% of cases detected have occurred in migrants, with up to 20% of migrants being carriers of TB (inactive). As a result, all immigrants are routinely screened for TB prior to entering Australia (WHO, 2016).

Approximately 11% of Australians and 700,000 New Zealanders live with asthma (AIHW, 2018; Asthma Foundation New Zealand, 2019). Asthma rates are considered high by international standards in both countries, more so in New Zealand, where hospitalisation rates are much higher among Pacific peoples and Māori in New Zealand (Asthma Foundation New Zealand, 2019). Prevalence is higher among Aboriginal and Torres Strait Islander Australians and people living in the most disadvantaged localities.

According to the Australian Centre for Asthma Monitoring (2011), death rates are lower in Australia than in New Zealand and the U.K., but much higher than those in European countries.

Breasts and lymphatic system

The incidence of breast cancer has increased worldwide. The incidence rate for migrants and their offspring has been found to approach that of their adopted homeland rather than their country of origin, with environmental and lifestyle factors thought to contribute to the level of breast cancer risk (AIHW, 2019). In Australia in 2007, the main cause of death in females between the ages of 25 and 64 was breast cancer (12% of all deaths), declining to 6.5% in 2018 (AIHW, 2019). Men can also have breast cancer, but the incidence is so low that widespread studies for ethnic differences have not been undertaken.

Cultural beliefs about the causes of breast cancer, the meaning of breast cancer to the person and partner, the availability of or knowledge of services, fear due to the status of migration, and other barriers have been found to contribute to the lower use of screening services for breast cancer in some cultural groups (Khan et al., 2015).

Heart and neck vessels

Coronary heart disease remains the leading cause of death for people in Australia and New Zealand (AIHW, 2019; NZMOH, 2015); however, rates have been steadily declining in recent decades. Cardiovascular risk factors, combined with socio-economic conditions and ethnic differences, have been identified as contributing factors to the development of hypertension. Hypertension rates are higher in Aboriginal, Torres Strait Islander, Māori and Pasifika populations, with Aboriginals and Torres Strait Islander peoples experiencing not only a higher prevalence of associated risk factors, but also higher mortality from acute coronary events (AIHW, 2019).

Modifiable factors for increased risk of cardiovascular disease include tobacco smoking, physical inactivity, obesity, diet high in saturated fats and high alcohol consumption in addition to non-modifiable risk factors (age, sex, family history and ethnicity) (AIHW, 2019). There is also increasing awareness of the sociocultural, psychological and economic factors that contribute to these risk factors, including level of education, income and social supports, and broader living and working conditions (AIHW, 2019).

Peripheral vascular system

Peripheral vascular disease is set to become a major health care problem in Australia and New Zealand as the population ages (Brown et al., 2016). Most cases are asymptomatic, with a reported prevalence of 15% in Australia and other Western countries and as high as 30% in older populations (Conte & Vale, 2018).

Abdomen

Along with many developed and developing countries, Australia and New Zealand are experiencing an epidemic of obesity; obesity is now the most common nutritional problem within these populations. In Australia, approximately 63% of the adult population are considered overweight or obese (AIHW, 2019). The 2017–2018 New Zealand Health Survey found that 47.5% of Māori adults and 65% of Pasifika adults were obese (New Zealand Ministry of Health [NZMOH], 2019b).

Colorectal cancer is the third most commonly diagnosed cancer in Australia; representing 8.5% of all deaths from cancer in 2018 (AIHW, 2019). The incidence of gastric cancer is declining, although survival rates remain poor. New Zealand has one of the highest rates of bowel cancer in the world; colorectal cancer is the second most common form of cancer and cause of death (NZMOH, 2018). Western industrialised populations that consume low-fibre, highly refined carbohydrate diets experience a higher prevalence of diverticular disease (Brown et al., 2016).

Chronic kidney disease is far more common than we may realise in both Australia and New Zealand, with increasing numbers of the population affected but often unbeknown to them because 90% of normal kidney function can be lost before any symptoms are experienced (Kidney Health Australia, 2018). The incidence of end-stage renal disease (where kidney function has deteriorated to an extent that dialysis or transplant is required) is far higher in Aboriginal, Torres Strait Islander and Māori peoples than among the remainder of those populations (AIHW, 2019; NZMOH, 2015). The main causes of chronic kidney disease across both countries include diabetes, polycystic kidney disease, nephritis and hypertension (AIHW, 2019; NZMOH, 2015).

Female and male genitalia, anus, rectum and prostate

The risks associated with unprotected sexual activity include infections (such as Chlamydia, gonorrhoea, HIV and syphilis), unwanted pregnancy and some cancers (such as cervical and anal cancer). Unsafe sexual practices account for most disease burden associated with HIV and acquired immunodeficiency syndrome and cervical cancer, irrespective of geographic location or ethnicity (AIHW, 2018; Brawner et al., 2016). Important actions that can reduce these health risks include greater use of condoms and having fewer sexual partners. Over the past decade, rates of sexually transmitted infections have increased.

In 2018, Chlamydia continued to be the most notified sexually transmitted infection in Australia, with more than 95,000 new diagnoses reported in the National Notifiable Diseases Surveillance System; a large majority of these notifications came from the 15–29-year-old age group. An increase in rates of gonorrhoea and syphilis have been reported in parts of Australia since 2011 (AIHW, 2018). The most important feature of Chlamydia is that it is often a silent infection. In males, it can infect the prostate, urethra and testes, whereas females can develop infections of the cervix, uterus and pelvis, and complications may result in chronic pelvic pain, infertility and ectopic pregnancy (AIHW, 2018). Aboriginal and Torres Strait Islander women experience a disproportionate health burden in relation to reproductive outcomes, with higher rates of sexually transmitted infections, cervical cancer and pregnancy complications compared with other Australian women (AIHW, 2019).

Among males in 2018, prostate cancer was the most common type of newly diagnosed cancer (excluding basal cell carcinoma and squamous cell carcinoma). The increase in the incidence of prostate cancer in recent years correlates strongly with the increased use of prostate-specific antigen tests in screening for prostate cancer.

Musculoskeletal system

In both male and female, bone mineral density (BMD) peaks at around age 20 and then begins to decrease from ages 35 to 40 (Brown et al., 2016). BMD is higher in men and lowest in Asian people, with Europeans and Asians associated with a higher risk of osteoporosis and hip fractures (Brown et al., 2016; Leslie, 2012).

Nervous system

Cerebrovascular disease has neurological effects, but the cause is vascular. According to the Australian Institute of Health and Welfare (AIHW, 2019), being hospitalised for stroke was 1.7 times higher for Aboriginal and Torres Strait Islander peoples in 2018. The risk of dying from stroke was also 1.5 times higher among the Aboriginal and Torres Strait Islander population (AIHW, 2019).

CRITICAL THINKING

6. Identify a person either in your care or in your community who is from a different cultural background to you and conduct a cultural assessment, using the information you have gained from this chapter. What are this person's health beliefs and how do they differ from your own?
7. Upon completion of the cultural assessment, identify gaps in your own knowledge or areas of further interest for you to research. What could you do to address these gaps?
8. Gather various forms of print media and critically review how culture and cultural groups are portrayed in popular media. Are there any examples of misleading or incorrect information?

SUMMARY

Australia and New Zealand comprise a diverse demographic, including many minority groups and subgroups. Nurses working in such environments not only need to be aware of cultural diversity, but also must take steps to improve their knowledge of different cultures to ensure that they provide culturally competent care to those in need (Brown et al., 2016). To complete a culturally competent assessment, it is essential to interact with the person, showing respect for that individual, the family and their beliefs. Challenge yourself to learn about many of the cultural groups in your geographical area and interact with them to gain some understanding and appreciation for their worldviews. Use your knowledge when meeting and assessing each individual, but be alert for behaviours, descriptions or physical variations that need to be clarified as either normal for their culture or abnormal and needing further assessment.

ONLINE RESOURCES

An extensive range of additional resources to enhance teaching and learning and to facilitate understanding may be found online at the text's accompanying website, located on thePoint at http://thepoint.lww.com. These include Watch and Learn videos, Concepts in Action animations, journal articles, case studies, discussion topics and quizzes.

Subscribers may also access Lippincott Procedures, an extensive online point-of-care procedure guide that provides reliable step-by-step instructions for more than 1700 procedures, including 450 evidence-based Australian procedures, and skills in a variety of speciality settings, together with a wealth of supporting information.

References

Asthma Foundation New Zealand. (2019). Asthma in New Zealand. Available at https://www.asthmafoundation.org.nz/resources/asthma-in-new-zealand.

Australian Centre for Asthma Monitoring. (2011). Asthma in Australia. AIHW Asthma Series no. 4. Cat. no. ACM 22. Canberra: AIHW. Available at https://www.aihw.gov.au/getmedia/8d7e130c-876f-41e3-b581-6ba62399fb24/11774.pdf.

Australian Institute of Health & Welfare (AIHW). (2018). Australia's Health, 2018. Australia's health series no. 16. Cat. no. AUS 221. Canberra: AIHW.

Australian Institute of Health & Welfare (AIHW) (2019) Cancer in Australia 2019 Canberra: AIHW. Available at www.aihw.gov.au/reports/cancer/cancer-in-australia-2019/contents/summary.

Australian Lung Foundation. (2018). Lung cancer. Available at https://lungfoundation.com.au/wp-content/uploads/2018/09/Infographic-Lung-cancer-Oct2018.pdf.

Beck, B., Bray, J. E., Cameron, P. A., et al. (2016). Trends in severe traumatic brain injury in Victoria, 2006-2014. *The Medical Journal of Australia, 204*(11), 1.e1–1.e6.

Bigby, J. (Ed). (2003). *Cross-cultural medicine*. Philadelphia: American College of Physicians.

Brady, B., Veljanova, I. & Chipchase, L. (2016). Are multidisciplinary interventions multicultural? A topical review of the pain literature as it relates to culturally diverse patient groups. *Pain, 157*(2), 321–328.

Brawner, B. M., Alexander, K. A., Fannin, E. F., et al. (2016). The role of sexual health professionals in developing a shared concept of risky sexual behavior as it relates to HIV transmission. *Public Health Nursing, 33*, 139–150. doi:10.1111/phn.12216.

Brooke, D. & Omeri, A. (1999). Beliefs about childhood immunisation among Lebanese Muslim immigrants in Australia. *Journal of Transcultural Nursing, 10*, 229–236.

Brown, D., Edwards, H., Seaton, L., & Buckley, H. (2016). *Lewis's medical-surgical nursing: Assessment and management of clinical problems* (4th Revised ed.). Chatswood: Elsevier Australia.

Campinha-Bacote, J. (2007). *The process of cultural competence in the delivery of healthcare services* (5th ed.). Cincinnati, OH: Transcultural CARE Associates.

Campinha-Bacote, J. (2011). Delivering patient-centered care in the midst of a cultural conflict: The role of cultural competence. *Online Journal of Issues in Nursing, 16*(2), 5.

Camplin-Welch, V. (2007). Cross-cultural resource for health practitioners working with culturally and linguistically diverse clients (CALD). Viewed November 2013 at www.caldresources.org.nz/info/Cross_Cultural_Resource_Kit-Printable.pdf.

Cancer Council Australia. (2019). Risk and benefits of sun exposure. A joint statement from the Australasian College of Dermatologists, Australian and New Zealand Bone and Mineral Society, Osteoporosis Australia and Cancer Council Australia. Viewed April 2019 at https://www.cancer.org.au/policy-and-advocacy/position-statements/sun-smart/#jump_3.

Centre for Cultural Competence Australia (CCCA). (2018). Turning cultural awareness into change. Available at http://ccca.com.au.

Centre for Culture, Ethnicity and Health (CEH). (2017). Cultural considerations in inclusive health assessment. Available at https://www.ceh.org.au/wp-content/uploads/2017/07/CEH_TipSheet3_Mar2011_Web-002.pdf.

Chan, B. & Parker, G. (2004). Some recommendations to assess depression in Chinese people in Australasia. *The Australian and New Zealand Journal of Psychiatry, 38*(3), 141–147.

Chrisopoulos, S. & Harford, J. E. (2016). Oral Health and Dental Care in Australia: Key Facts and Figures 2015. Australian Institute of Health and Welfare and the University of Adelaide, Canberra, ACT, Australia.

Conte, S. M. & Vale, P. R. (2018). Peripheral Arterial Disease. *Heart, Lung and Circulation, 27*(4), 427–432. https://doi.org/10.1016/j.hlc.2017.10.014.

Copeland, E., Leonard, K., Carney, R., et al. (2018). Chronic rhinosinusitis: Potential role of microbial dysbiosis and recommendations for sampling sites. *Frontiers in Cellular and Infection Microbiology, 8*(57), doi:10.3389/fcimb.2018.00057.

Douglas, M., Rosenkoetter, M., Pacquiao, D., et al. (2014). Guidelines for Implementing Culturally Competent Nursing Care. *Journal of Transcultural Nursing, 25*(2), 109–121. doi:10.1177/1043659614520998.

Durie, M. H. (1998). *Whaiora*. Auckland: Oxford University Press.

Eckermann, A., Dowd, T. & Jeffs, L. (2009). Culture and ethnicity. In J. Crisp & C. Taylor (Eds). *Potter & Perry's fundamentals of nursing* (3rd ed., pp. 108–128). Sydney: Elsevier.

Farrell, M. (Ed). (2017). *Smeltzer & Bare's textbook of medical-surgical nursing* (4th Australian and New Zealand ed.). Sydney: Lippincott Williams & Wilkins/ Wolters Kluwer Health.

Farrell, M. & Dempsey, J. (2014). *Smeltzer & Bare's textbook of medical-surgical nursing* (3rd Australian and New Zealand ed.). Sydney: Lippincott Williams & Wilkins.

Francis, K., Chapman, Y., Hoare, K., et al. (2013). *Australia and New Zealand community as partner: Theory and practice in nursing* (2nd ed.). Sydney: Lippincott Williams & Wilkins.

Goold, S. (2001). Transcultural nursing: Can we meet the challenges of caring for the Australian Indigenous person? *Journal of Transcultural Nursing, 12*(2), 94–99.

Hall, E. T. (1976). *Beyond culture*. Garden City, NY: Anchor Press.

Harrison, H. G. (2010). *Injury of Aboriginal and Torres Strait Islander people due to transport, 2003–04 to 2007–08*. Canberra: Australian Institute of Health & Welfare. Available at www.aihw.gov.au/WorkArea/DownloadAsset.aspx?id=6442472783.

International Council of Nurses. (2012). The ICN code of ethics for nurses. Available at https://www.icn.ch/sites/default/files/inlinefiles/2012_ICN_Codeofethicsfornurses_%20eng.pdf.

Iqbal, N., Joyce, A., Russo, A., et al. (2012). Resettlement experiences of Afghan Hazara female adolescents: A case study from Melbourne, Australia. *International Journal of Population Research*, doi:10.1155/2012/868230. article ID 868230.

Juckett, G. (2005). Cross-cultural medicine. *American Family Physician, 72*(11), 2267–2274, Available at www.aafp.org/afp/20051201/2267.html.

Kao, S., Chu, Y., Chen, Y., et al. (2009). Detection and screening of oral cancer and pre-cancerous lesions. *Journal of the Chinese Medical Association, 72*(5), 227–233.

Khan, T. M., Leong, J. P., Ming, L. C., et al. (2015). Association of knowledge and cultural perceptions of Malaysian women with delay in diagnosis and treatment of breast cancer: A systematic review. *Asian Pacific Journal of Cancer Prevention, 16*(13), 5349–5357.

Kidney Health Australia. (2018). Kidney fast facts. Viewed April 2019 at https://kidney.org.au/cms_uploads/docs/kidney-fast-facts-fact-sheet.pdf.

Kirby Institute. (2017). *Australian trachoma surveillance report 2018*. Sydney: Kirby Institute. Available at https://kirby.unsw.edu.au/report/australian-trachoma-surveillance-report-2017.

Language and Culture Worldwide. (2015). The cultural iceberg. Available at https://www.languageandculture.com/cultural-iceberg.

Leslie, W. D. (2012). Ethnic Differences in Bone Mass—Clinical Implications. *The Journal of Clinical Endocrinology and Metabolism, 97*(12), 4329–4340. doi:10.1210/jc.2012-2863.

Lipson, J. G., Dibble, S. L. & Minarik, P. A. (Eds). (1996). *Culture and nursing care: A pocket guide*. San Francisco, CA: UCSF Nursing Press.

Narayan, M. C. (2010). Culture's effects on pain assessment and management. *American Journal of Nursing, 110*(4), 38–47.

National Health and Medical Research Council (NHMRC). (2006). Cultural competency in health: A guide for policy, partnerships and participation. Available at www.nhmrc.gov.au/guidelines/publications/hp19-hp26.

New Zealand Ministry of Health (NZMOH). (2015). *Tatau kahukura: Māori health chart book 2015* (3rd ed.). Wellington: Author. https://www.health.govt.nz/publication/tatau-kahukura-maori-health-chart-book-2015-3rd-edition.

New Zealand Ministry of Health (NZMOH). (2018). Bowel cancer. Viewed April 2019 at https://www.health.govt.nz/your-health/conditions-and-treatments/diseases-and-illnesses/bowel-cancer.

New Zealand Ministry of Health (NZMOH). (2019a). Lung cancer. Viewed April 2019 at https://www.health.govt.nz/your-health/conditions-and-treatments/diseases-and-illnesses/lung-cancer.

New Zealand Ministry of Health (NZMOH). (2019b). Obesity in New Zealand. Viewed April 2019 at https://www.health.govt.nz/publication/annual-update-key-results-2017-18-new-zealand-health-survey.

Nursing Council of New Zealand/Te Kaunihera Tapuhi o Aotearoa (NCNZ). (2011). Guidelines for cultural safety, the Treaty of Waitangi and Māori health in nursing education and practice. Available at www.nursingcouncil.org.nz/download/97/cultural-safety09.pdf.

O'Neill, D. (2002–2010). Culture-specific diseases. Available at http://anthro.palomar.edu/medical/med_4.htm.

Organisation for Economic Co-operation and Development. (2017). *Health at a glance 2017: OECD indicators*. Paris: OECD Publishing. Available at https://www.oecd-ilibrary.org/social-issues-migration-health/health-at-a-glance-2017_health_glance-2017-en.

Overfield, T. (1995). *Biological variation in health and illness: Race, age, and sex differences*. Menlo Park, CA: Addison-Wesley.

Pacquiao, D. (2018). Conceptual framework for culturally competent care. In M. Douglas, D. Pacquiao, & L. Purnell (Eds). *Global applications of culturally competent health care: Guidelines for practice*. Cham: Springer. Available from https://doi.org/10.1007/978-3-319-69332-3_1.

Pairman, S., Pincombe, J., Thorogood, C., et al. (2006). *Midwifery: Preparation for practice*. Sydney: Elsevier.

Pairman, S., Pincombe, J., Thorogood, C., et al. (2015). *Midwifery: Preparation for practice* (3rd ed.). Sydney: Elsevier.

Papadopoulos I., Lay M., Lees S., et al. (2003). The Impact of Migration on Health Beliefs and Behaviours: The case of Ethiopian refugees in the UK. *Contemporary Nurse, 15*(3), 210–221.

Purnell, L. & Paulanka, B. (Eds). (2008). *Transcultural health care: A culturally competent approach* (3rd ed.). Philadelphia: F.A. Davis.

Purnell, L. & Paulanka, B. (Eds). (2013). *Transcultural health care: A culturally competent approach* (4th ed.). Philadelphia: F.A. Davis.

Ramsden, I. M. (2002). Cultural safety and nursing education in Aotearoa and Te Waipounamu. Unpublished PhD thesis, Victoria University of Wellington.

Reid, J. (Ed). (1982). *Body, land and spirit: Health and healing in Aboriginal society*. St Lucia, Qld: University of Queensland Press.

Rushworth, N. (2010). Falls-related traumatic brain injury in older people: Under-recognised, under-diagnosed, highly fatal, highly preventable. *Aged Care Australia, 72*.

Statistics New Zealand. (2012). The 'browning' of New Zealand. Available at www.stats.govt.nz/browse_for_stats/population/mythbusters/browning-nz.aspx.

Stein-Parbury, J. (2017). *Patient and person: Interpersonal skills in nursing* (6th ed.). Sydney: Elsevier.

Thakrar, D., Das, R. & Sheikh, A. (2008). *Caring for Hindu patients*. London: Radcliffe Publishing.

Transcultural Nursing Society. (2011). Transcultural nursing standards of practice. Available at www.tcns.org/TCNStandardsofPractice.html.

Transcultural Nursing Society. (2018). Standards of Practice for Culturally Competent Nursing Care-Revised. Available at https://tcns.org/wp-content/uploads/2018/03/Standards_of_Practice_for_Culturally_Compt_Nsg_Care-Revised_.pdf.

Virtual Empathy Museum. (2018). Take a walk in my shoes. Available from https://www.virtualempathymuseum.com.au/.

Willis, K. & Elmer, S. (2011). Culture and health: Ethnic diversity in healing practices and health issues. In K. Willis & S. Elmer (Eds). *Society, culture and health: An introduction to sociology for nurses* (2nd ed., pp. 143–165). Melbourne: Oxford University Press.

Wilson, D. (2014). Cultural diversity. In J. Dempsey, S. Hillege, & R. Hill (Eds). *Fundamentals of nursing and midwifery: A person-centred approach to care* (2nd Australian and New Zealand ed.). Sydney: Lippincott Williams & Wilkins.

World Health Organization (WHO). (2016). Tuberculosis. Available at https://www.who.int/tb/areas-of-work/preventive-care/australia.pdf.

World Health Organization (WHO). (2018). Blindness and vision impairment. Available at https://www.who.int/news-room/fact-sheets/detail/blindness-and-visual-impairment.

World Health Organization (WHO). (2019). Deafness and hearing loss. Available at https://www.who.int/news-room/fact-sheets/detail/deafness-and-hearing-loss.

Selected readings

Australian Indigenous Health. (2018). Selected health conditions. Available at www.healthinfonet.ecu.edu.au/health-facts/overviews/selected-health-conditions.

Dempsey, J., Hillege, S. & Hill, R. (2014). *Fundamentals of nursing: A person-centred approach to care* (2nd ed.). Sydney: Lippincott Williams & Wilkins.

Kaiser Family Foundation. (2016). Key facts on health and health care by race and ethnicity. Available at https://www.kff.org/disparities-policy/report/key-facts-on-health-and-health-care-by-race-and-ethnicity/.

Online resources

Australian Indigenous Health*InfoNet*: www.healthinfonet.ecu.edu.au
Centre for Cultural Competence Australia: www.ccca.com.au
Centre for Culture, Ethnicity and Health: www.ceh.org.au
Centre for Diversity in Aged Care: www.culturaldiversity.com.au
Diversity Health Clearinghouse: http://203.32.142.106/clearinghouse
New Zealand Ministry of Health, Māori health: www.health.govt.nz/our-work/populations/maori-health
Transcultural CARE Associates (Dr Camphina-Bacote): www.transculturalcare.net
Transcultural Nursing & Health Care Consulting (Dr Akram Omeri): http://transculturalnursingandhcc.com.au
Transcultural Nursing Society: www.tcns.org

CHAPTER 11

Assessment in Aboriginal and Torres Strait Islander communities

This chapter presents information on how to approach a culturally competent nursing assessment when caring for Aboriginal and Torres Strait Islander peoples.

It discusses factors contributing to the high prevalence of ill health and premature deaths among this population, such as the social determinants resulting in the inequities in health that Aboriginal and Torres Strait Islander peoples have experienced historically since colonisation, and Australia's present-day commitment to 'Closing the Gap'.

The chapter offers practical guidance with some terminology and explanations to help nurses with factors involved in assessment, including communication, language, information sharing, informed consent and privacy.

The inclusion of Elsie's story is a way of raising key issues that may be faced by patients, their nurses and a wider health care team. Elsie's story and five other real but anonymous patient stories are provided as exercises to assist nurses in understanding and reflecting upon all of the above factors to enable them to conduct culturally competent assessments of people presenting from these communities.

Who are Aboriginal and Torres Strait Islander peoples?

ABORIGINALITY

The word 'Aborigine' comes from the Latin word *aborigine* meaning 'from the beginning'. As such, Dr Jenny Baker (Associate Professor in Aboriginal Health, University of Adelaide—retired) reminds us that 'Aborigine' should be a proud word because Aboriginal and Torres Strait Islander peoples have occupied the land now known as Australia for thousands of years since the Dreamtime, not merely for 230 years since colonisation.

In Australia, there is a three-part 'working definition' from the Department of Aboriginal Affairs' Report (1981) for the first national peoples of this continent, the Aboriginal and Torres Strait Islander peoples, which states:

> An Aboriginal or Torres Strait Islander is a person of Aboriginal or Torres Strait Islander descent [*part 1*] who identifies as an Aboriginal or Torres Strait Islander [*part 2*] and is accepted as such by the community in which he (she) lives [*part 3*]. (Cited in Gardiner-Garden, 2000, italics added).

This working definition has been accepted by Aboriginal and Torres Strait Islander organisations, government departments and agencies across Australia as the determinant of identity; however, the definition continues to be debated by Aboriginal and Torres Strait Islander peoples.

ETIQUETTE IN USING DESCRIPTORS

Aboriginal and Torres Strait Islander peoples have continued to use the adjective 'Aboriginal', despite its Latin origins, but insist that it be written with an uppercase first letter, as in the adjective 'English', and always be used with its following noun, as in 'Aboriginal person, people or community', and *not* simply 'Aboriginals' or 'Aborigines'. Similarly, an uppercase is used for the terms 'Torres Strait Islander' and 'Indigenous'. This etiquette is now required to be observed by all Australian governments, government institutions, public servants and documents.

Another etiquette observed by government and many non-government institutions, including hospitals, clinics and universities, and at meetings, conferences and other forums, is the *formal acknowledgement* of the traditional owners or custodians of the 'country', or land, on which the meeting is held. This ceremony is known as 'Welcome to Country'. There are multiple land areas across the continent of Australia that Aboriginal and Torres Strait Islander groups refer to as their 'country'.

As a first preference, the Welcome to Country ceremony is to be conducted by an Aboriginal and Torres Strait Islander person chosen by his or her community before the start of the meeting's proceedings. If this person is not available, then a non-Aboriginal and Torres Strait Islander person of the organisation responsible for the meeting will conduct a brief ceremony to acknowledge the traditional owners or custodians. This act continues to be an important aspect of reconciliation between non-Aboriginal and Torres Strait Islander Australians and Aboriginal and Torres Strait Islander peoples.

CRITICAL THINKING

1. Who are the traditional owners or custodians of the place where you are now?

CULTURAL NAMES

Many nations and communities across the world (and in Australia) retain their cultural identity. This is reflected by the terms they use to describe themselves, such as Māori, Inuit, Peruvian, Argentinean, Colombian, Fijian, Swiss, French, Dutch, Dane, Irish, English, Chinese and Vietnamese. Many nations and communities also have cultural subgroups who prefer to be referred to by their particular tribe, clan or language group name.

This practice is relevant also to Aboriginal and Torres Strait Islander peoples. According to their cultural identity and preference, a group or person may refer to themselves as 'Aboriginal', 'Aboriginal and Torres Strait Islander' or 'Indigenous'. For example, Dr Jenny Baker describes herself as a Nunga, an Aboriginal person, an Indigenous person and a Mirning person.

In the book *Survival in our own land* whose authors are Aboriginal and Torres Strait Islander peoples from South Australia (Mattingley & Hampton, 1998, p. xvi), we learn that 'Nunga' is the preferred collective term of many of the language groups. However, the Pitjantjatjara and Adnyamathanha peoples prefer to call themselves according to their particular cultural and language names, A<u>n</u>angu and Yura.

Therefore, it can be beneficial in health care settings if nurses know the preferred cultural names of their patients and their families. For example, an A<u>n</u>angu person would be offended if he or she is referred to as 'Nunga' or 'Koori'. Display 11-1 names some of the many diverse cultural and language groups across Australia.

For information about the traditional owners of the land where you live, work or attend meetings, see the map on the website of the Australian Institute of Aboriginal and Torres Strait Islander Studies at www.aiatsis.gov.au/asp/map.html (AIATSIS, 2019). Online reference sites such as the Telethon Institute's http://aboriginal.childhealthresearch.org.au/media/54859/part_1_chapter3.pdf (2013) and the Australian Museum's http://australianmuseum.net.au/Indigenous-Australia (2013) also outline the history, cultures and backgrounds of Aboriginal and Torres Strait Islander peoples.

DISPLAY 11-1 SOME ABORIGINAL AND TORRES STRAIT ISLANDER AUSTRALIAN LANGUAGE GROUPS

- Gunai and Kurnai peoples (Victoria)
- Kaurna and Ngarrindjeri (South Australia)
- Badjalang (New South Wales)
- Ngunnawal (Australian Capital Territory)
- Yolngu (Arnhem Land, Northern Territory)
- Wujal Wujal (Cape York Peninsula, Northern Queensland)
- Anmatjera people (Mount Leichhardt, Hann and Reynolds Ranges, Northern Territory)
- A<u>n</u>angu and Yarnangu (living on Ngaanyatjarra, Pitjantjatjara and Yankunytjatjara lands of the Western Desert language region)
- Ben Lomond people (Plangermaireener) (Tasmania)
- Tiwi people (Bathurst and Melville Islands)
- Kalaw Lagaw Ya, Kalau Kawau Ya, Kulkalgau Ya and Kawalgau Ya (dialects of the Torres Strait Islander peoples)

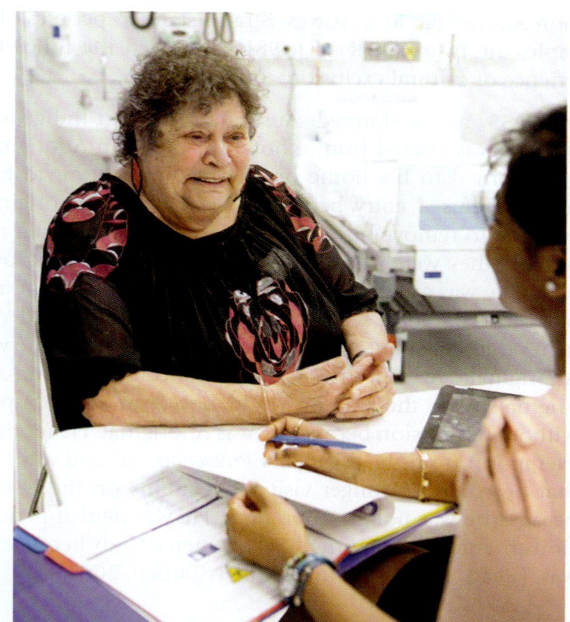

FIGURE 11-1 Consulting local Elders and community groups can provide a rich source of information on country, language, preferred terminology and cultural history. (Michael Mullan Photography, www.michaelmullan.com.au.)

You may also wish to consult the local Elders and community groups from the area where you work or live regarding their country, language, preferred terminology and cultural history (Fig. 11-1). They will appreciate your interest and the opportunity to meet and educate you.

History of Aboriginal and Torres Strait Islander peoples' health

The health issues faced by Aboriginal and Torres Strait Islander peoples across Australia today have their legacies in Australia's colonial history. As is so often the case, the 'victors' write the historical accounts of a nation from the point of view of their own cultural values and social and political perspectives. In recent times, challenges to the interpretations of Australia's colonial history have resulted in the so-called history wars (Evans & Thorpe, 2001; Reynolds, 1999). Although this discussion may seem a long way from relating to nursing assessment, it has still shaped the national consciousness and influenced how events need to be understood regarding the wellbeing and treatment of Aboriginal and Torres Strait Islander peoples today. For many, their 'Aboriginality' was debased after colonisation, forming part of the continuing struggle against a negative perception of their heritage.

IDENTITY UNRECOGNISED

In Australia, the history of identifying who was and was not an Aboriginal and Torres Strait Islander person was controlled by government authorities. This involved a punitive level of surveillance and control not experienced by the wider community of non-Aboriginal and Torres Strait Islander peoples. For example, the historian Read (1981) described the following experience of cultural exclusion:

> In 1935 a fair-skinned Australian of part-Indigenous descent was ejected from a hotel for being an Aboriginal. He returned to his home on the mission station to find himself refused entry because he was not an Aboriginal. He tried to remove his children but was told he could not because they were Aboriginal. He walked to the next town where he was arrested for being an Aboriginal vagrant and placed on the local reserve. During the Second World War he tried to enlist but was told he could not because he was Aboriginal. He went interstate and joined up as a non-Aboriginal. After the war he could not acquire a passport without permission because he was Aboriginal. He received exemption from the *Aborigines Protection Act*, and was told that he could no longer visit his relations on the reserve because he was not an Aboriginal. He was denied permission to enter the Returned Servicemen's Club because he was. (Read, 1981, cited in Gardiner-Garden, 2003)

EFFECTS OF THE AUSTRALIAN CONSTITUTION

The exclusion of people deemed to be of the 'Aboriginal race' was written into the 1901 Australian Constitution. Anderson (2001) highlighted this point when referring to a relevant clause in section 51 of the Constitution, which stated:

> The Parliament shall subject to this Constitution, have power to make laws for the peace, order, and good government of the Commonwealth with respect to: The people of any race, *other than the aboriginal race in any State*, for whom it is deemed necessary to make special laws. [italics added]

The italicised clause in this section was removed by national referendum in 1967, together with section 127, another exclusion clause, which stated:

> In reckoning the number of the Commonwealth, or of a State or other part of the Commonwealth, aboriginal natives shall not be counted.

Under these laws, Anderson (2001, p. 33) said, 'It would have been extremely difficult from a constitutional perspective to develop a nationally funded program in Aboriginal health.' This also meant that:

> For the first fifty years of federation, nearly all Commonwealth social welfare legislation excluded Aboriginal Australians, variously defined, from access [to it]. This included, for example: the *Invalid and Old Age Pensions Act 1908; Maternity Allowance Act 1912; Child Endowment Act 1941; Widows' Pension Act 1942; Unemployment and Sickness Benefits Act 1944*. Political marginalisation of Aboriginal Australians was realised when they were also excluded from the franchise in the *Commonwealth Franchise Act 1902* and the *Commonwealth Electoral Act 1918*.

These crucial aspects of constitutional history are raised here because nurses, other health professionals and students frequently ask why, in the first nearly two decades of the 21st century, there still needs to be special government policies and programs to address the disadvantage that Aboriginal and Torres Strait Islander peoples experience. Some examples are the formation of the Commonwealth Department of Health, Aboriginal and Torres Strait Islander Health (Department of Health, 2019), and funding for the delivery of primary health care through health services across Australia that are under the control of Aboriginal and Torres Strait Islander peoples.

Historical factors continue to influence current policy, but constitutional exclusion created a negative effect that contributed to the pervasive poverty, discrimination and disadvantage still evident in society today.

COLONISATION AND MODERNITY

Like Australia, the continents of South America, North America, Southeast Asia, the Indian subcontinent and many parts of Africa were colonised by Europeans. Colonisation has been a global phenomenon where particular nations have colonised and dominated other nations and their people across the world. This has divided populations of colonised countries into descendants of either the colonised or the colonisers and, of course, descendants who have 'mixed blood'.

Colonialism has precipitated enormous and calamitous changes for the Aboriginal and Torres Strait Islander peoples living in these regions. Prior to invasion, these people 'had their own knowledge and health systems', which healed illness, kept people well and enabled them to die with dignity (Kunitz, 1994). In 1989, the National Aboriginal Health Strategy Working Party stated:

> Prior to colonisation Aboriginal peoples had control over all aspects of their life. They were able to exercise self-determination in its purest form. They were able to determine their 'very being', the nature of which ensured their psychological fulfilment and incorporated the cultural, social and spiritual sense.

History contributes to our understanding of the causes of widespread ill health of people whose lands were colonised. However, from reports available, it would seem that their health up until 1788 was much better than that of the colonisers who began arriving by ship at that time. The impact of colonialism on the health and wellbeing of Aboriginal and Torres Strait Islander peoples has been only recently acknowledged, for example, the massacres on the frontier over land acquisition; the provision of small pox–infected blankets; the denial of access to fresh water; the replacement of traditional foods with flour, sugar and salt; and the removal of children from their mothers and families. Such atrocities and injustices were recognised by former Prime Minister Paul Keating in his significant 'Redfern Speech' delivered in 1992, which acknowledges the treatment of Aboriginal and Torres Strait Islander Australians from their perspective. To read his speech, go to http://antar.org.au/sites/default/files/paul_keating_speech_transcript.pdf.

A reliable, quality text that connects history and health is *Binang Goonj: Bridging cultures in Aboriginal health* (Eckermann et al., 2010). It is worthwhile visiting the website of the Australian Institute of Aboriginal and Torres Strait Islander Studies, of which the details are given at the end of this chapter.

SOCIAL DETERMINANTS OF HEALTH

It is important for everyone to have an understanding of what has contributed to the serious inequities in health and wellbeing that affects Aboriginal and Torres Strait Islander peoples. It is known that people's health and wellbeing are either supported or not, by the political, social and economic contexts in which the people live. These are known as the 'social determinants of health'. The World Health Organization (WHO, 2008) advises that:

> The social determinants of health are the conditions in which people are born, grow, live, work and age, including the health system. These circumstances are shaped by the distribution of money, power and resources at global, national and local levels, which are themselves influenced by policy choices. The social determinants of health are mostly responsible for health inequities—the unfair and avoidable differences in health status seen within and between countries.

The WHO, seeing health has a human right of all people, established the Commission on Social Determinants of Health in 2005 in response to increasing concerns about the persisting and widening inequities of health between countries, populations and groups. In 2008, the WHO Commission released its final report, *Closing the gap in a generation: Health equity through action on the social determinants of health.* In the opening paragraph of its Executive Summary, the Commission states:

> Social justice is a matter of life and death. It affects the way people live, their consequent chance of illness, and their risk of premature death. We watch in wonder as life expectancy and good health continue to increase in parts of the world and in alarm as they fail to improve in others. A girl born today can expect to live for more than 80 years if she is born in some countries—but less than 45 years if she is born in others. Within countries there are dramatic differences in health that are closely linked with degrees of social disadvantage. Differences of this magnitude, within and between countries, simply should never happen.

The findings and recommendations for 'Closing the Gap' in this report clearly relate to the social inequities experienced by Aboriginal and Torres Strait Islander Australians and their extreme poor health. To access this report online, go to www.who.int/social_determinants/en.

For a succinct overview of Aboriginal and Torres Strait Islander peoples' (ill) health since 1967, refer to the National Aboriginal Community Controlled Health Organisation (NACCHO)'s *Investing in healthy futures for generational change: NACCHO 10 Point Plan 2013–2030*, via www.naccho.org.au.

'Closing the Gap' in Australia

The national, state and territorial governments of Australia are jointly committed to meeting the challenge of the WHO Commission, which is to 'Close the Gap' by remedying the serious cultural, social, educational, economic and health inequities experienced by Aboriginal and Torres Strait Islander peoples.

A major starting point occurred when former Prime Minister Kevin Rudd, on behalf of the Australian Parliament, formally and publicly acknowledged and apologised to the Aboriginal and Torres Strait Islander peoples for what has happened to them since the first ships arrived.

Although some improvements have taken place since the apology, a lot still needs to be done according to the National Aboriginal Community Controlled Health Organisations (NACCHO). To access NACCHO's press release to the ABCon on 8 February 2018, go to www.nacco.org.au.

Federal apology

At 9.00 a.m. on Wednesday 13 February 2008, former Prime Minister Kevin Rudd made the much-belated 'Apology to Australia's Indigenous Peoples', the opening words of which are shown in Display 11-2. To read Prime Minister Rudd's entire apology online, go to www.aiatsis.gov.au/collections/exhibitions/apology/sorry.html.

Today, as a top priority and matter of urgency, all sectors of government have pledged to act to 'Close the Gaps' of inequity through, for example, policies, practices and funding programs to provide and support access to quality education and health care; employment and financial security; safe housing and land ownership; community safety; good nutrition; and all of the other essentials that people need to have a long, productive and healthy life.

DEFINITION OF ABORIGINAL AND TORRES STRAIT ISLANDER HEALTH

On its website, the Aboriginal Health & Medical Research Council of New South Wales (AH&MRC, 2011) defines 'Aboriginal health' as:

> … not just the physical well-being of an individual but refers to the social emotional and cultural well-being of the whole community in which each individual is able to achieve their full potential as a human being thereby bringing about the total well-being of their Community. It is a whole-of-life view and includes the cyclical concept of life-death-life.

ABORIGINAL AND TORRES STRAIT ISLANDER COMMUNITY-CONTROLLED HEALTH SERVICES

The AH&MRC (2011) states that 'Aboriginal community control' means:

> … the empowering of a community through the adoption of appropriate organisational structures which enable all Aboriginal people in the local Community the opportunity to be represented as members and to be involved in the decision-making process and, therefore, the right to participate and contribute to the goals, structure and operation of its health services.

With this background understanding of the history of colonisation and social determinants of ill health among Aboriginal and Torres Strait Islander peoples, nurses can be better able to offer them effective health assessment and care (Fig. 11-2).

Prevalence of ill health in Aboriginal and Torres Strait Islander communities

Many Aboriginal and Torres Strait Islander peoples live with multiple physical illnesses, which affect their psychological wellbeing. This problem is experienced not only by individuals but also by most of their family and wider community. The prevalence of physical as well as psychological illnesses inevitably diminish hopes of leading a healthy and full life in this

DISPLAY 11-2 FEDERAL APOLOGY TO ABORIGINAL AND TORRES STRAIT ISLANDER PEOPLES (EXTRACT)

At Parliament House, Canberra, in 2008, Prime Minister Kevin Rudd proposed a motion that was accepted by Parliament apologising for the mistreatment of Aboriginal and Torres Strait Islander peoples. His opening words to the nation were:

> I move—
>
> That today we honour the Indigenous peoples of this land, the oldest continuing cultures in human history.
>
> We reflect on their past mistreatment.
>
> We reflect in particular on the mistreatment of those who were Stolen Generations—this blemished chapter in our nation's history.
>
> The time has now come for the nation to turn a new page in Australia's history by righting the wrongs of the past and so moving forward with confidence to the future.
>
> We apologise for the laws and policies of successive Parliaments and governments that have inflicted profound grief, suffering and loss on these our fellow Australians.
>
> We apologise especially for the removal of Aboriginal and Torres Strait Islander children from their families, their communities and their country.
>
> For the pain, suffering and hurt of these Stolen Generations, their descendants and for their families left behind, we say sorry.
>
> To the mothers and the fathers, the brothers and the sisters, for the breaking up of families and communities, we say sorry.
>
> And for the indignity and degradation thus inflicted on a proud people and a proud culture, we say sorry.
>
> We the Parliament of Australia respectfully request that this apology be received in the spirit in which it is offered as part of the healing of the nation.
>
> For the future we take heart; resolving that this new page in the history of our great continent can now be written.
>
> We today take this first step by acknowledging the past and laying claim to a future that embraces all Australians.
>
> A future where this Parliament resolves that the injustices of the past must never, never happen again.
>
> A future where we harness the determination of all Australians, Indigenous and non-Indigenous, to close the gap that lies between us in life expectancy, educational achievement and economic opportunity.
>
> A future where we embrace the possibility of new solutions to enduring problems where old approaches have failed.
>
> A future based on mutual respect, mutual resolve and mutual responsibility.
>
> A future where all Australians, whatever their origins, are truly equal partners, with equal opportunities and with an equal stake in shaping the next chapter in the history of this great country, Australia.

population. Keeping strong is a daily challenge. In the words of an Aboriginal Elder, 'It's how it is for me and my family, so we just try and look after each other.'

There have been some important health gains such as reductions in the high levels of maternal, infant and child mortality and communicable diseases. However, the disproportionate prevalence of acute and chronic (physical and psychological) illness and premature deaths among Aboriginal and Torres Strait Islander peoples remains significant (Australian Institute of Health and Welfare [AIHW], 2011a; Emerson & Croucher, 2001; NACCHO 2013a, 2013b).

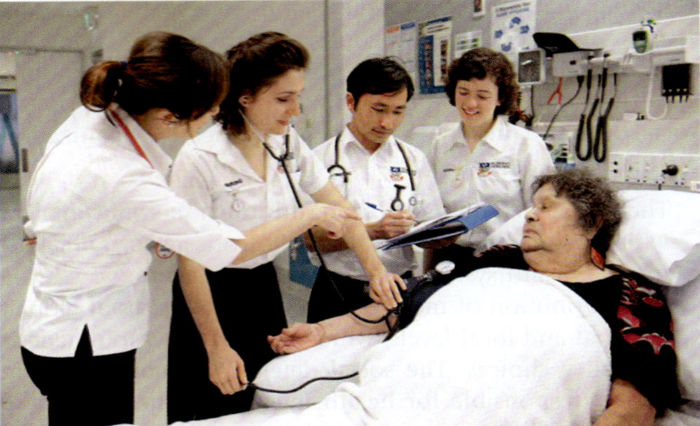

FIGURE 11-2 With improved cultural understanding, nurses are better able to offer effective health assessment and care to Indigenous patients. (Michael Mullan Photography, www.michaelmullan.com.au.)

In 2013, the gap in life expectancy between Aboriginal and Torres Strait Islander males and females and their non-Aboriginal and Torres Strait Islander counterparts continued (AIHW, 2011b, p. 6):

> For Australia, estimated non-Indigenous male life expectancy (78.7 years) is 11.5 years higher than for the male Indigenous population (67.2 years). For females, estimated non-Indigenous life expectancy (82.6 years) is 9.7 years higher than for Indigenous (72.9 years). The difference in Indigenous and non-Indigenous life expectancy is lower than the previous estimates have shown. This does not suggest any trend, rather that methodological changes have produced different estimates.

Chronic diseases play a major role in premature and preventable morbidity and mortality of Aboriginal and Torres Strait Islander Australians and Māori. In New Zealand, the National Advisory Committee on Health and Disability (2007, p. 10) reported that 'significant differences in life expectancy exist between Māori and non-Māori. Chronic conditions contribute to this disparity.'

In 2010, the AIHW (p. 18) reported the high prevalence of chronic diseases across the Aboriginal and Torres Strait Islander populations, stating that:

> For Indigenous Australians aged 35–54, chronic diseases are the cause of over 75% of the mortality gap, the main contributors being ischaemic heart disease, diseases of the liver (mainly in the form of alcoholic liver disease), diabetes mellitus and other forms of heart disease (mainly cardiomyopathy and heart failure).
>
> Chronic diseases are the cause of about 95% of the mortality gap for Indigenous Australians aged 55–74, mainly from ischaemic heart disease, diabetes, chronic lower respiratory diseases (mainly chronic obstructive pulmonary disease) and cancer of the respiratory and intrathoracic organs (mainly lung cancer).

It is necessary to consider that Aboriginal and Torres Strait Islander Australians and Māori who are affected by chronic disease are highly likely to also have co-existing chronic diseases from a relatively young age. Those comorbidities may involve physical and intellectual disabilities, injury and acute medical conditions, mental illness, and alcohol or drug problems (Kowanko et al., 2009).

Connolly (2011, pp. 18–19) reports that New Zealand Māori with chronic disease commonly experience multiple comorbidities:

> ... in view of the high degree of co-morbidity, even in a non-elderly population, single-disease management does not appear promising as a strategy to care for patients. In contrast, the burden is on primary care physicians and teams to provide the majority of care, not only for the target condition but for other conditions. Thus, management in the context of ongoing primary care and oriented more toward patients' overall health care needs appears to be a more promising strategy than care oriented to individual diseases.

There are multiple factors leading to the serious *gap* in mortality and morbidity rates between Aboriginal and Torres Strait Islander people and the general Australian population. Although individuals and communities have direct responsibility to address risks to their own health, such as tobacco smoking, many factors causing their extreme ill health are beyond community or individual control. Broadly, the factors contributing to the unacceptable levels of poor health are complex and multifactorial, encompassing a range of historical, socio-economic, environmental, cultural and access influences that remain today (Anderson et al., 2007; Stoneman & Taylor, 2007). This is described in the earlier section, 'Social determinants of health'.

CO-EXISTING HEALTH CONDITIONS: COMORBIDITY

Aboriginal and Torres Strait Islander peoples commonly suffer disproportionate levels of co-existing health conditions (comorbidities). It is not uncommon for younger patients to present with comorbidities that health care practitioners would otherwise expect to see in much older patients.

Nurses should be vigilant of the possibility of comorbidities when assessing all Aboriginal and Torres Strait Islander patients, whatever their current presentation or age. Timely identification and early treatment can improve health outcomes and minimise complications.

In 2005, the Australian Institute of Health and Welfare (pp. 1–2) reported that 'Cardiovascular disease (CVD), diabetes and chronic kidney disease (CKD) are serious illnesses that contribute significantly to deaths and levels of ill health' and that 'there are also complex causal relationships between these diseases, and each of them may be caused by, or be a complication of, one or both of the other.'

Cardiovascular disease, diabetes and CKD comorbidities are common, with people experiencing early onset, chronicity and death. For instance, the Australian Institute of Health and Welfare (2005, pp. 90–91) reported that:

> Compared with other Australians, Indigenous Australians, in particular those in remote communities have excessive chronic disease morbidity and mortality ... chronic kidney disease (CKD) is no exception to this. Indigenous Australians beginning kidney replacement therapy in 2001–03 were substantially younger than their non-Indigenous counterparts ... Overall there were more than eight times as many Indigenous treated end-stage kidney disease patients as would be expected based on the incidence rates in non-Indigenous Australians.

The impact of these and other comorbidities is great, resulting in poor quality of life, serious disability and premature death—irrespective of whether people live in urban, rural or remote communities.

Mental health problems and comorbidity

Many in this community face challenges to their psychological wellbeing (mental health) (AIHW, 2011a; de Crespigny & Valadian, 2010; de Crespigny et al., 2006). This can seriously complicate their physical conditions. In addition, poor psychological health can, in itself, be a major contributor to the development of CVD and other serious diseases (Hunter New England Health, 2008).

Dental health and comorbidity

Dental health problems are also pervasive and significant. During acute illness and hospitalisation, or in the context of general health care, poor oral health may be overlooked.

Dental problems can cause or complicate serious disease and must therefore be considered within all nursing assessments across the lifespan.

In 2004, the National Aboriginal Community Controlled Health Organisation (NACCHO) and National Rural Health Alliance Inc. (NRHA) stated in their joint media release (p. 6):

> Aboriginal and Torres Strait Islanders have poorer oral health than the rest of the community. Over 16 per cent are edentulous compared with the overall Australian figure of 10 per cent. Indigenous Australians have worse periodontal health, despite their lower average age, and Indigenous children are also much worse off in terms of dental disease and have a high level of untreated decayed teeth. Poor oral health often creates a situation where the overall health of a person is compromised. Too often poor oral health results in people adopting poor diet resulting in serious illness. Such illnesses include cardiovascular disease and diabetes.

Many of the Aboriginal and Torres Strait Islander community-controlled and government health services now provide dental services within their primary health care role, although there remain many urban, rural and remote communities without sufficient access to quality dental services.

Aboriginal and Torres Strait Islander peoples' experiences of health

Aboriginal and Torres Strait Islander peoples live collectively, with the common good of the group, clan, tribe and nation being their major focus and experience. Sharing stories and resources, having designated cultural and familial roles, and honouring the law of reciprocity are the 'glue' that keeps this system of life strong. This approach remains starkly different from how most Western cultures function, where the perspective of the individual is the major focus.

The cultural beliefs, views and traditions of Aboriginal and Torres Strait Islander, including what they understand about health, ill health and death, are thus important aspects that nurses need to acknowledge when caring for Aboriginal and Torres Strait Islander people. Nurses must also understand their patients' deep grief felt from the loss of so many 'brothers and sisters' who are ill or dying. This is a feeling of deep, mutual loss.

For the latest information on Aboriginal and Torres Strait Islander peoples, go to https://healthinfonet.ecu.edu.au/. For information about nursing and midwifery regarding babies, children, youth and adults in the Aboriginal and Torres Strait Islander population, go to www.catsinam.org.au.

ABORIGINAL AND TORRES STRAIT ISLANDER PEOPLES' STORIES

The story of Elsie is one of several included in this chapter to illustrate the various cultural and health care needs of an Aboriginal and Torres Strait Islander. Her story is true, although 'Elsie' is not her real name. First, consider how her cultural and health care needs were met. Then, as you proceed through the remainder of the chapter, reflect from time to time on Elsie's story and what else you might do if you were assessing her.

DOMAINS OF HEALTH AND WELLBEING

Among Aboriginal and Torres Strait Islander peoples, there are five key domains of health and wellbeing that co-exist within a never-ending cycle of life–death–life. These are:

1. Spiritual
2. Cultural
3. Social
4. Psychological
5. Physical.

Each of these domains needs to be functioning well for health to be maintained.

Although nurses may not be able to recognise or respond to all of these domains, they need to be aware and understand that they are fundamental to the experience of the patient and their family. It can be appropriate to suggest that patients be visited by a trusted Elder from their community or a Traditional Healer, someone who can assist them with their spiritual, cultural and social needs. This access may greatly enhance the patient's response to their health care experience, including their nursing assessment.

The following text discusses some issues regarding health and ill health within these five domains.

Spiritual

Spirituality is the foundation of the Aboriginal and Torres Strait Islander peoples' identity and that of their family and community. It binds and connects them with others, their land (country) and Dreaming. The contemporary life of these people continues to reflect the spiritual connections to all things (MacKean, 2005) and provides the strong spiritual bond that gives them resilience, a sense of purpose in life and space for healing. Spirituality is thus important in understanding their illness and capacity for recovery.

Cultural

Aboriginal and Torres Strait Islander peoples are the oldest-surviving cultures in the world; current estimates suggest they extend over 50,000 years. The people remain closely linked to land, sea and sky, and to one another. Within their cultural commonality there is diversity between particular nations,

CASE STUDY

Elsie's story

Elsie is a 49-year-old Aboriginal and Torres Strait Islander grandmother who lives with her extended family in an outer suburban community. She worked in the local newsagent until her poor health caused her to give up her job. She has many life stressors and deep grief from the loss of two sons, a sister, three brothers, her husband and other close family members through suicide, accidental death and serious illness—all of which were preventable or treatable. She has three remaining adult children and five grandchildren, with whom she is very close. As part of her 'Granny' role, she often cares for the children in her home, where they sleep with her at these times, as is common in Aboriginal and Torres Strait Islander society.

Elsie came to the local hospital yesterday with her sister 'Agnes' and adult niece 'Connie'. She had shortness of breath and a 'chesty' cough, unstable diabetes and ulcers on her lower legs. Elsie said she was feeling 'low'. She was admitted to the medical ward. She underwent nursing and medical assessments with a female nurse and female doctor, as was her stated cultural preference.

Her diagnoses were bronchitis, hypertension, diabetes, vascular disease (lower limb ulcers) and malnutrition. It was also considered that she may have long-standing depression due to grief. Agnes and Connie took it in turns to stay with Elsie throughout her admission, either sitting by her bed or sleeping at nearby residential quarters, depending on how Elsie was at the time.

Elsie was treated with respect. Agnes and Connie were present when the medical or nursing staff examined and talked with Elsie about her various problems, educated her about the various treatment choices, medicines and pathology tests required. The nurses agreed to arrange for an appropriate Traditional Healer to visit her whenever she needed one. Elsie, Agnes and Connie were involved in her discharge planning. She was discharged 6 days later to her home.

Her various medical conditions were treated and stabilised. Agnes and Connie were able to talk to the nursing and medical staff about how Elsie could be supported at home in terms of her nutrition, diabetes, other medical problems and safe medication use. The local home-visiting nurse had been introduced to Elsie and then arranged to visit her daily. The home-visiting nurse, general practitioner and pharmacist agreed to work together to monitor and support her with her nutrition, ulcer care, diabetes management and safe medication use. She decided not to see a psychiatrist or psychologist for 'depression', saying she would rather ask her Traditional Healer to continue helping her with her grief (depression).

tribes, and language and kinship (clan) groups. Wherever they live, they try at all times to maintain their Dreaming, kinship connections, knowledge, country, ceremonies, language and cultural responsibilities such as 'men's business' or 'women's business'. They continue to honour the cultural roles and responsibilities of 'Aunty', 'Uncle', 'Grandmother', 'Grandfather', 'Elder' and 'Traditional Healer'. These relationships are likely to be relevant to your patient even when they are *very* sick.

Social

Aboriginal and Torres Strait Islander family and kinship networks are fundamental to their social and emotional wellbeing. Social networks maintain the threads that bind families and groups together. These networks ensure the survival of individuals, families and community. Each patient will have their network made up of near and extended family. The presence of family is crucial to their feeling they will recover or experience a peaceful death.

Psychological

The psychological domain includes social as well as emotional wellbeing, which are interconnected with the other domains. There can be high levels of psychological distress in patients due to grief and trauma from the loss of many Elders, parents, children and other family members, and the impact of intergenerational poverty due to colonisation, racism and subsequent events.

Physical

Early pictures and photographs of Aboriginal and Torres Strait Islander peoples at the time the first ships arrived indicate they were physically healthy and robust. The colonisers considered them to be primitive and less than human. They were subsequently removed from their country and communities, and denied their traditional hunting, gathering and fishing lifestyles and strong community networks and culture. Subsequently, their physical health rapidly deteriorated. The introduction of foreign diseases, salt, sweet and fatty foods and psychoactive substances such as tobacco and alcohol have also caused high levels of sickness and death. The legacy is the appalling levels of ill health today (adapted from Department of Health and Ageing, 2007, pp. 1.10–1.12).

To read more about the important factors that continue to affect the health of Aboriginal and Torres Strait Islander peoples, go to the sections titled 'History of Aboriginal and Torres Strait Islander peoples', 'Social determinants of health' and 'Closing the Gap', National Aboriginal Community Controlled Health Organisation (NACCHO) and Congress of Aboriginal and Torres Strait Islander Nurses and Midwives (CATSINaM). An understanding of all of these background factors will help nurses to complete culturally competent nursing assessments.

Culturally competent nursing assessments

CULTURAL COMPETENCE

Living and working with Aboriginal and Torres Strait Islander peoples in multicultural Australia means that cultural competence is an essential and transferable component of nursing practice.

DISPLAY 11-3 RIGHTS OF PATIENTS IN A CULTURALLY COMPETENT NURSING ASSESSMENT

Culturally competent nursing assessment is based on the rights of all Aboriginal and Torres Strait Islander peoples to:

1. Receive health care that is culturally appropriate, respectful and non-judgemental
2. Have their 'health story' heard and responded to appropriately
3. Have their own and their family's cultural view of health (and illness) recognised and respected
4. Receive safe 'patient-centred' assessment and treatment for their illness, including comorbidities
5. Be educated and supported in being well informed, and able to give informed consent and make appropriate decisions regarding health care options
6. Receive relevant referral and complementary support from, for example, their Traditional Healer, Aboriginal and Torres Strait Islander community–controlled health service, general practitioner or other relevant service
7. Be referred to essential community services as required (e.g. step-down services, home nursing, physiotherapy and occupational therapy, safe medication support, housing and transport).

A hallmark of cultural competence is having respect for the patient and their family. This includes ensuring that no patient is stereotyped, stigmatised or labelled according to his or her culture, language, condition and other characteristics.

To be culturally competent we need to reflect on and understand our existing worldviews and how these influence our beliefs, perceptions and behaviours towards other people. Nurses who strive to be culturally competent are flexible in the ways they adapt their practice, including assessment, to the beliefs, practices and needs of the patient and their family. Display 11-3 lists the inherent rights of patients in a culturally competent nursing assessment.

Being culturally competent is a lifelong learning process for everyone. Ramsden (1992) developed a model titled 'Lifelong learning cycle of cultural competence', which shows that cultural competence is an evolving and cyclical process of awareness, ability, safety and knowledge. She based her work on the nature of and practices for cultural safety in New Zealand.

EMERGENCY PRESENTATION

In emergency situations, the immediate concern of the patient's family is for their loved one's life to be saved. Attending to cultural protocols and considerations are not the family's priority, so they need not be the nurse's at this time. However, the family will need to be well supported and informed as soon as the opportunity arises after the emergency.

Once the crisis is over, cultural issues are to be considered in the usual manner. This includes paying attention to the family's needs. In particular, at this time of stress and anxiety, it is essential to:

- Welcome the family members and orientate them to the service
- Offer them privacy and comfort
- Consult and inform them regarding any decisions that need to be made
- Ensure they are able give informed consent
- Offer access to a Traditional Healer, Elder or clergy as appropriate.

DISPLAY 11-4 SUGGESTED APPROACHES TO THE NURSING ASSESSMENT OF ABORIGINAL AND TORRES STRAIT ISLANDER PATIENTS AND THEIR FAMILY

1. Present yourself in a courteous, friendly and unhurried manner (even if time is limited). Address the patient and their family members by their formal name, such as Mr Jones or Mrs Smith. Continue in this way until they invite you to use their first name or 'nickname'. If their traditional name is difficult to pronounce, as many can be, ask them how they say it and try to repeat in front of them. Then write it down phonetically so you can practise it. They will appreciate this effort.
2. Acknowledge family members and offer them a seat or area near the patient.
3. Attempt to provide privacy for the patient and demonstrate respect for their confidentiality.
4. Sit or stand slightly side-on and at arm's length from the patient (or family member). This enables you to talk to each other without looking directly into one another's eyes. For some people, direct eye contact is forbidden because of gender, seniority or respect for your role or other reasons. You will soon detect if they are trying to look at you directly. This may happen once they feel more at ease, or because face-to-face eye contact is their usual practice.
5. Remain at arm's length until you see or feel it is acceptable to come closer. *Ask permission* to touch the patient before doing so, unless it is imperative clinically.
6. Always inform the patient when your proximity is necessary, such as taking observations and other aspects of assessment. Inform them that part of your role is to help and establish what their problems and needs are.
7. Do not speak loudly and use simple (not patronising) language and terminology. This can demonstrate your respect for the patient and assist you with determining (from their responses) what their language style is, as well as their level of understanding of your language. This will help you to establish whether they can hear you well, as well as build rapport and engage them. Depending on the patient's responses to the above interactions—verbal and non-verbal—you will be able to determine if an interpreter or cultural advisor is required.

NON-URGENT PRESENTATION

As with any patient in this situation, nurses will need to pay attention to the usual, essential components of their assessment, which, for the purposes of this chapter, are not discussed in detail. Rather, particular information and suggestions are given here that will help nurses undertake this process in culturally competent and clinically effective ways.

Engaging the patient

As with all patients, engaging the patient (and their family) is necessary. The aim is to build rapport, establish trust and reduce any fear about what is happening so that the assessment can be conducted (see Display 11-4).

There are some communication, language and other factors that are helpful to know about to manage an assessment. These are described in the following text.

CLINICAL TIP

During communication in assessments, consider the level of hearing your patient may have. It may also take patients some time to respond because they may be translating from your language to their first language and back again before they answer. Try to avoid the temptation to fill in silences with speech, and give patients enough time to think and respond comfortably.

Names

In some regions, patients need to consider the cultural implications of a particular question to ensure they can give the most appropriate response. For example, asking 'What is your name?' may require consideration for cultural reasons as to why you need their name. For instance, is their name needed for a form? Should they give their English or kinship name?

They may give the nurse a different first name from their usual one because of their cultural obligation to respect a recently deceased person from the same cultural or language group and whose first name was the same. For example, in Pitjantjatjara, the replacement name would sound like 'kumina'. If, for instance, you know the patient's name is usually 'Jacob Jones' and you hear him or his family refer to him as 'Kumina' Jones, you will know that this is the case and that you must do the same. It will be important to explain this to other members of the team and to document such in his case notes.

There will be other names used in this instance according to the person's particular cultural language group. Because this issue is important, it is useful to consult the local Elders, liaison officers or relevant team members where you work.

To make the assessment situation less worrying for patients and their family, you may ask what name they wish to be used at this time, and if it is likely to remain the same in the near future. The health care team will still need to know what names have already been recorded in their medical records if they have had previous attendances. These questions need to be explained to the patients because it is necessary for their treatment. Reassure them that you and the team will be able to use the replacement name during verbal interactions and formal meetings with others.

Spoken language

There are significant numbers of Aboriginal and Torres Strait Islander peoples whose first language is not English. They may speak in what is known as 'Aboriginal English', a valid variety of the English language (Australian Council of Teaching English as a Second Language [TESOL], 2006). This can be difficult to understand well, depending on inflection, choice of words and so on.

If a patient's accent, words and phrases are unfamiliar, nurses may find it difficult to understand what is being said. Learning a small number of key words of local Aboriginal English to prepare for this situation will be useful. However, you may still need to introduce an interpreter to assist.

Interpreters

Appropriate interpreters are becoming more available, and there are now interpreter services in various areas. Interpreters may be required for the assessment, informed consent, discussions regarding diagnosis and treatment options.

It is not advisable to rely on family members for a number of reasons, which include a poor understanding of words or terms used for particular parts of the body or body functions, medications or other medical terminology. Patient confidentiality and cultural and privacy issues can also be barriers to asking necessary questions.

For information about interpreter services for patients, consult the Aboriginal and Torres Strait Islander Hospital Liaison Service where you work, the local Aboriginal and Torres Strait Islander community-controlled health service or government services in your area.

Two useful websites are:

- Kimberley Interpreter Service: www.kimberleyinterpreting.org.au
- Ngaanyatjarra Pitjantjatjara Yankunytjatjara (NPY) Women's Council: www.npywc.org.au.

HEALTH LITERACY

This term describes people's shared understanding of health promotion, screening and early intervention, particular diseases and related information. Health literacy is relatively poor in the general population and much more so in the Aboriginal and Torres Strait Islander population. It is often necessary for nurses to discuss particular concepts of health and illness with their patients, yet these may not be sufficiently understood. The high school completion rate is significantly lower than in other Australian populations, leaving many with low literacy and numeracy levels. There are thus significant numbers of Indigenous adults and children who are unable to understand verbal information, reading materials and documentation such as consent forms that are commonly used in hospitals and other health services. This also relates to verbal and written instructions about prescribed and non-prescribed medication use (de Crespigny & Valadian, 2010; de Crespigny et al., 2011; Cusack et al., 2013).

Assessment can be an intervention

It is always useful to remember that assessment can also be an intervention. Through talking and sharing information and asking questions, opportunities can arise for you to offer important information and health education relevant to the patient's situation (see Display 11-5). It is also a time when family members can be educated and supported, too.

INFORMATION EXCHANGE

It is vital for nurses to take the time to explain to the patient and their family, as appropriate, what is happening and why. This interaction relies on effective information exchange.

DISPLAY 11-5 HANDY TIPS FOR EDUCATING ABORIGINAL AND TORRES STRAIT ISLANDER PATIENTS

Offer information verbally and in simple, large writing (because the patient may have poor hearing or eyesight, or literacy problems).

Use visual aids with real pictures or models of, for example:

- Anatomy—heart and circulation, skeleton, stomach, liver, kidneys and brain
- Types of medicines
- Commonly used equipment such as blood glucose test kits, the blood pressure machine, thermometers, stethoscopes, urinary catheters, the electrocardiogram machine, X-ray machines and IV equipment.

Communication tends to focus on one theme at a time; that is, it does not cover multiple issues in quick succession. There are often silences that indicate the person is thinking and not ignoring what has been said. It is helpful, when taking a health history, to use short verbal exchanges and, if possible, undertake the assessment in stages (depending on priorities for diagnosis and treatment), possibly over more than one session. Using slower-paced communication may seem contrary to the urgency of some clinical priorities; however, it may be a 'false economy' not to take this approach.

CLINICAL TIP

Short exchanges of information can be especially important when working with patients and families who are having greater difficulty with language and medical concept or are hearing or visually impaired.

Verbal conversation and communication styles

Nurses and other health professionals may face different styles of conversation, pronunciations and abbreviations used by Aboriginal and Torres Strait Islander peoples. Here are some examples that may be useful. In time, your own experience will help you increase your vocabulary and confidence.

Approach to questioning

English speakers commonly use and accept the direct question-and-answer style in health care contexts. For example:

- Why are you here?
- What's wrong?
- Have you got pain?
- Are you pregnant?

However, patients whose first language is not English, or who speak using Aboriginal English, generally structure their questions differently. Direct questions are seldom used, even when seeking important information. Indirect methods such as triggers or hints within a story are typically used when seeking or offering information. For example, you might hear an Aboriginal English speaker ask an indirect question of another by saying:

1. Not feeling good, *eh?* (Australia-wide)
2. Pain in the head, *inna?* (South Australia)
3. Expecting a baby, *unna?* (south-west Western Australia) (adapted from Department of Health and Ageing, 2007, pp. 1.22–1.28).

A style is used where a statement is made, followed by a question tag such as 'eh', 'inna' or 'unna'. Nurses can also use this style by asking "Not feeling good today, eh?" (or *inna* or *unna*, depending on the patient's language background).

'Agreeing' with questions

Aboriginal and Torres Strait Islander peoples generally strive to maintain easy relationships with others and try not to disappoint, offend or upset them. This is particularly the case if the other person is perceived to have authority, such as doctors and nurses. The patient and their family may answer 'yes' to a nurse's questions to avoid offending you—even if the answer should be 'no' For example, they might give a 'yes' response when asked such questions as 'Have you been taking your diabetes medication as prescribed by your doctor?' or 'Have you stopped smoking yet?' when in fact the real answer is 'no'.

A useful approach can be to distance your request from the individual personally by first making a third-person statement such as, 'Some people find it hard to manage their diabetes medicines' or 'Many people can find it is hard to stop smoking.' The patient may then start talking about someone else they know as a way of responding to you without feeling ashamed. You could then follow with another question related more to their experience by saying, 'Maybe you can tell me what has been happening for you lately' (Department of Health and Ageing, 2007, p. 1.29).

As with any such interaction, it is critical to appreciate there can be times when a patient's silence reflects feelings of shame or powerlessness. Being overly compliant by answering 'yes' too frequently may mean the patient feels afraid of offending you or of saying the wrong thing. The patient may actually not understand your questions, or perceive you to be 'superior' because of your role and knowledge and therefore expect you to know what is wrong and how to treat it without asking questions.

What may seem to be simple questions that can be answered quickly may in fact not be the case. It may take patients some time to comprehend what has been asked and devise their answer. This can be because they have been listening and thinking seriously about what you have asked, what it means and how best to respond. They may be translating from English to their first language and back to English before they can answer you.

There are also particular words that are important to understand in the assessment. These will differ according to the person's cultural or language group. For example, Table 11-1 lists Pitjantjatjara words that may be used in the north-west of South Australia.

Standard English words may be used differently by people who come from different family groups, communities and locations. For example, in Central Australia, people use the word 'cheeky' for someone who is rude, offensive or aggressive; it does not have the more light-hearted meaning in standard English. Similarly, the word 'deadly' is often used as a compliment, to indicate that someone or something is very good-looking, exciting or interesting.

Silence

Many English speakers tend to avoid or fill moments of silence by talking, perceiving silence to be a sign the conversation needs to be ended or that communication has broken down. However, silence is often accepted and sought during conversations between Aboriginal and Torres Strait Islander peoples. Try to avoid the temptation to fill silences and give patients enough time to think and respond comfortably (adapted from Department of Health and Ageing, 2007, pp. 1.28–1.30).

Table 11-1 Useful words in the Pitjantjatjara language

Yes: *oo-ah*	Ear: *pinna*
No: *weir*	Foot: *chinna*
Very sick or very hurt: *bega bulga*	Arm: *minna*
	Back: *jilderoo*
Teeth: *cudjudee*	Stomach: *tuny* (*tunee*)
Mouth: *da*	Eye: *coora*

Miscommunication

A nurse may inadvertently confuse, cause shame or offend a patient by using terms that they do not understand. This can occur by using terms Aboriginal and Torres Strait Islander peoples do not understand. An example is when a nurse walks up to the patient, saying 'I am going to take your obs', meaning to test for blood pressure, temperature and heart and breathing rates. However, the patient might not understand what 'obs' means and can misinterpret not only what 'obs' refer to, but also the nurse's body language as he or she approaches. The patient can become frightened by this situation, but feel they have to succumb to whatever is about to happen. They may become agitated and feel they need to resist by verbally or physically trying to push the nurse away.

The nurse must clearly and quietly approach the patient and explain and show them why these observations are needed and how they are performed. This can be effective when time has first been taken to build rapport.

Knowing there are common cultural norms (etiquette) shared by many helps nurses to work with these patients and family members. This includes paying attention to body language such as eye contact, and where various people sit and place themselves in relation to where you are. There are easy ways to gauge norms that do not rely on having an in-depth knowledge of every requirement. The advice given in Display 11-4 provides suggestions, many of which can apply to patients from any cultural or language background.

CLINICAL TIP

Remember to inform the patient and family of the reasons and processes of the assessment before asking questions and physically touching the patient.

Three-way talking

Aboriginal and Torres Strait Islander peoples may use what is known as 'three-way talking' when asking or offering information about themselves. That is, they may bring a third person with them, usually a family member whose cultural role is to be their spokesperson and advocate, who will be the person with whom you speak while the patient remains silent and observes and listens.

During assessment, three-way communication can be very valuable because interacting with an advocate allows for an exchange of information without embarrassment, even though the patient is present. The patient would previously have discussed with their family member what was to be talked about, any questions they wanted to have answered and how best to respond if the nurse or doctor raised particular issues.

This situation is one in which the patient has given implicit permission to the nurse, doctor and third person to discuss private matters that relate to their health. This is a confidential situation, just as it would be if the patient is present with only a nurse or other health professional.

Local terminology

The Royal Commission into Aboriginal Deaths in Custody from 1987 to 1991 found that a number of preventable deaths in police custody, hospitals and other settings were due to unrecognised alcohol intoxication, hypoglycaemia, head and other serious injuries, or life-threatening complications from alcohol withdrawal. These deaths were also due to poor familiarity among police and health care providers about local words and communication styles used by Aboriginal and Torres Strait Islander detainees, who were trying to tell others what was happening, such as acute pain or feeling very ill. For example, the terms 'dings' and 'horrors' are commonly used when talking about life-threatening complications of alcohol withdrawal, such as hallucinations, dehydration, electrolyte imbalance and severe tremors previously not recognised. Visit the Australian Human Rights Commission's website to view its report on Aboriginal and Torres Strait Islander peoples who died in custody from 1989 to 1996, at www.humanrights.gov.au.

Confidentiality

If a health care centre employs Aboriginal and Torres Strait Islander liaison officers or health care workers, do not assume that all patients can be referred to them simply because they are Aboriginal and Torres Strait Islander peoples. The patient and the worker need to be consulted separately to ensure there are no cultural rules or family issues preventing them from being brought together. The patient or their family and the staff member will guide you whether it is acceptable to be involved, and their decisions need to be respected. Therefore, it is always wise to check with the various parties before making the referral to the Aboriginal and Torres Strait Islander worker or liaison unit. Knowing the language group of the patient and where he or she comes from will be very useful to the liaison staff. The staff can then make inquiries as to who on their team would be most suited to assist the patient or offer guidance on what other options there may be.

Gender

In many Aboriginal and Torres Strait Islander communities, a person's gender can strongly influence the exchange (or not) of sensitive information—verbal, non-verbal and physical. Some issues, such as sexual health matters, are kept strictly separate along gender lines and commonly referred to as 'men's business' or 'women's business'. A man may be deeply offended if asked questions of a sensitive nature by a woman. A woman may similarly be offended by questioning from a male.

It is not always possible to accommodate gender matches between medical staff and patients. It is important to explain this practicality to the patient if it arises. Ensure the patient's privacy when asking personal questions and remain sensitive to his or her modesty while undertaking any discussions, observations or physical examinations. Be mindful of your own body language, and speak quietly, particularly if you are in a public space because a private area is not available. It is useful to explain your understanding of such situations and, where possible, offer an alternative such as when an appropriate male or female nurse can be arranged.

However, this does not mean that males and females cannot or should not have access to gender-based health information, for example, information about breast, cervical or prostate cancer screening, contraception, alcoholism, or pregnancy. It is important that such information is managed sensitively and appropriately, according to the wishes of the particular community and the individual. It is therefore vital to seek advice from Aboriginal and Torres Strait Islander male and female colleagues, local Elders and community advocates on how best to manage these topics in your workplace, and by whom.

Physical assessment

This often requires direct physical contact, for example, attending to wounds, taking vital signs, conducting examinations, taking samples of blood, urine, sputum or tissue, and assisting with X-rays, scans. Any of these actions can induce fear, particularly if the processes and reasons are not well understood by the patient and his or her family. This is an important time when great care needs to be taken to ensure the patient is informed and actually consents to these procedures.

Fear and anxiety

Be aware that patients may be very fearful of or superstitious about being in hospital. These feelings can be due to past experiences, particularly regarding family members who have died. One way in which patients may express their fear is by being hostile to you or other staff. It is important to understand the possible reasons for such behaviour and that patients' reactions might not be related to you personally. Being respectful and reassuring patients that you and the team are there to care for them may help to overcome their fear. Explaining to patients what will happen will also assist in reducing fear and encouraging them and their family to accept an assessment. Asking for an Elder or the liaison officer from their community may be necessary.

In addition to being ill and in need of nursing and medical attention, other issues can cause patient anxiety. For example, questions that carry historical and personal burdens can unintentionally affect them. Asking what seems a normal question such as 'How often do you see your family?' may cause distress for the patient who was removed from his or her family and has not been able to reconnect with them since (see the section 'Federal apology').

Harmlessly asking a person how many children he or she has is a common way of 'breaking the ice' and starting up a conversation with patients. However, although many people see this as a normal, friendly question, caution is necessary here. This is because many people in this community may have lost more than one of their children as newborns or babies, adolescents or adults. Their grief is deep.

CLINICAL TIP

Take care when asking patients any questions about their family members and children because it may unintentionally cause them anxiety.

Hope

Because of high levels of morbidity and mortality occurring in their communities, many seldom receive good news about their own health or that of family members. This contributes to a loss of hope for recovery and a long healthy life ahead. As one grandmother said, 'We expect bad news—it's our life' (personal conversation).

A diminished sense of hope for health and wellbeing is common among patients and their families, even when their illnesses can be treated and recovery is possible.

Nurses therefore need to recognise that, although their contact with patients can be a sensitive time, it does offer the chance to educate the patient and his or her families about managing their health problems and treatments, and reducing complications and unnecessary admissions to hospital. This meeting can also be an important time to arrange for a

Traditional Healer or Elder to be with them, to offer cultural and spiritual healing and support.

INFORMED CONSENT

The patient or family at some stage will be required to give informed consent for investigations, treatment and other reasons. At this time, care is needed by the nurse to ensure the patient and their family fully understand the issues at hand and are able to give informed consent. The parties will need to understand where the patient's particular details will be recorded, who has access and where they are stored. Patients will also need to know why, how and where their tissues and images will be taken and where these too are stored. They will be very concerned that their confidentiality is honoured and kept secure.

Clear and culturally appropriate organisational policy and guidelines are needed ahead of time so that clinicians, patients and families can attend to patient confidentiality appropriately. There may be language or literacy issues and poor understanding of the health problems associated with the patient's condition. A suitable cultural and language interpreter may be required and should be facilitated as a priority.

State or territorial health departments can supply information on consent guidelines.

Five patient stories

As you read through these fictitious patient stories below reflect on what has been discussed throughout the chapter. Consider how you could deliver culturally competent nursing assessment for these Aboriginal and Torres Strait Islander patients.

Try to identify the cultural influences, possible communication and other issues important to recognise and respond to on behalf of the patient and/or their family.

Display 11-6 provides a list of questions for you to consider at the end of each story.

DISPLAY 11-6 QUESTIONS TO CONSIDER WHEN REFLECTING ON ABORIGINAL AND TORRES STRAIT ISLANDER PATIENT STORIES

For each patient story, consider the following questions:

(a) What their family's priority would be according to whether the patient's condition was urgent?
(b) What would your priorities be, and why?
(c) What key cultural, communication and family issues existed that needed to be responded to and why?
(d) How could you help the patient to feel respected and more at ease with your nursing assessment?
(e) How would you enable yourself, the patient and family to engage in effective information exchange?
(f) How likely was it that the patient had spiritual, cultural and psychological (social and emotional) issues as well as physical illness or injury? How would you respond to these?
(g) How would you ensure that the patient or appropriate family members could provide informed consent?
(h) How would you enable the patient's family to be with them at this time?
(i) How would you know if it is appropriate to organise access to an appropriate interpreter, Elder or Traditional Healer for the patient?

CASE STUDY

Dave's story

Dave is a 32-year-old man who was brought to the local hospital by ambulance, having been injured in a car accident near his home. He lives and works in a small town south of Perth in Western Australia. He has a fractured leg, two broken ribs and several deep lacerations to his arm. His condition is stable, and he is receiving adequate pain relief. He will be going to theatre when the local doctor arrives in about 2 hours.

He is in your ward and you are responsible for his nursing assessment. You learn that:

- He is afraid of being in the hospital: 'It's a one-way-trip.'
- He wants his grandfather to come and stay with him but does not know how to contact him.
- He speaks English but has poor literacy and moderate hearing loss due to chronic otitis media in childhood.
- He has been told by his Aboriginal and Torres Strait Islander health worker back home that he is at risk of hypertension and diabetes. He has had bouts of depression ('deep sadness') since his younger brother and two uncles were killed in a car accident 3 years ago.
- He refuses your offer for him to meet Julie, the Aboriginal and Torres Strait Islander hospital liaison officer.
- He wants to see a traditional healer.

CRITICAL THINKING

2. How will you approach Dave's assessment? In your answer, consider the questions in Display 11-6.

CASE STUDY

Josie's story

Josie is a 19-year-old woman who has been brought to your emergency department by her two sisters and aunty. She has had a serious fall and is semiconscious because of a possible head injury. Some of the issues you encounter with Josie are:

- While trying to talk with Josie's relatives about what is happening, you find communication with them is difficult because of language barriers.
- You need to ask them questions about essential matters, such as is Josie
  - Pregnant?
  - Experiencing physical illnesses or mental health problems?
  - Taking any prescribed or other medicines such as antibiotics, diabetes medicine or painkillers?
  - Likely to have been consuming any alcohol or other drug on that day (e.g. tobacco or cannabis—marijuana)?
- You want to inform the family and assure them that treating Josie's acute and serious injury is the priority of the nursing and medical team.
- They will need to give informed consent for Josie's required medical treatment.

CRITICAL THINKING

3. How will you approach Josie's situation? In your answer, consider the questions in Display 11-6.

CASE STUDY

Mary's story

Mary is a 39-year-old Koori woman. She has recently been attending her local Aboriginal and Torres Strait Islander community–controlled health clinic for treatment of asthma, high blood pressure, diabetes and depression. She has also started treatment for serious dental caries and gum disease. She has just been admitted to your ward with acute bronchitis and a urinary tract infection. Her older sister Macy has been sitting with her since she arrived. She has been seen by the medical staff and begun treatment for her bronchitis and urinary tract infection. This involves IV antibiotic therapy.

You have introduced yourself and explain that you need to undertake her nursing assessment. However, you find that Mary:

- Makes no eye contact and turns her head away
- Looks very anxious.

Macy also seems anxious and whispers to you that she and Mary are both scared because family members have died in hospital.

CRITICAL THINKING

4. How will you approach Mary's assessment? In your answer, consider the questions in Display 11-6.

CASE STUDY

John's story

John is an 11-month-old Aṉangu boy who has been admitted to the children's hospital because of failure to thrive, dehydration and acute otitis media in his left ear. There is evidence of recent otitis media in his right ear. He is asleep now having had pain relief, breast milk and baby cereal. His 23-year-old mother and Granny are with him. They told the Aboriginal and Torres Strait Islander liaison officer that they need to stay with him at all times while he is in hospital. Both have also told her that they have been trying to keep John as healthy as possible. They are from a remote community in the north of South Australia, which has limited fresh water and food, and few educational or practical resources to support young mothers and fathers. However, the culture is strong and the grandmothers assist as much as they can. They have some family living in an outer suburb of Adelaide about 30 km from the hospital.

CRITICAL THINKING

5. How will you approach John's assessment? In your answer, consider the questions in Display 11-6.

CASE STUDY

Sandra's story

Sandra is a healthy 10-year-old Badjalang girl from a country town in New South Wales. She was brought to the local hospital after having been burnt this morning when a kettle of boiling water fell from the kitchen shelf as she reached for the cup. She probably has third-degree burns to her abdomen and feet. She was in a lot of pain when she first arrived by ambulance with her father and older sister, but has settled now having had initial pain relief, treatment for her burns and hydration. She is heavily sedated and will need extensive and prolonged treatment. Her father and sister speak their local language and Aboriginal English but do not read or write English well. There is an Aboriginal and Torres Strait Islander health worker in the health care team attached to the hospital. She says she knows the family.

CRITICAL THINKING

6. How will you approach Sandra's assessment? In your answer, consider the questions in Display 11-6.

Summary of key concepts

In conclusion, the key concepts that inform culturally respectful nursing care of Aboriginal and Torres Strait Islander peoples are as follows.

Who are Aboriginal and Torres Strait Islander peoples?

The working definition of Aboriginal and Torres Strait Islanders used in the Department of Aboriginal Affairs' report (1981) is that: 'An Aboriginal or Torres Strait Islander is a person of Aboriginal or Torres Strait Islander descent [*part 1*] who identifies as an Aboriginal or Torres Strait Islander [*part 2*] and is accepted as such by the community in which he (she) lives [*part 3*]' (cited in Gardiner-Garden, 2000).

Social determinants of health

The World Health Organization (WHO, 2008) has advised that:

> The social determinants of health are the conditions in which people are born, grow, live, work and age, including the health system. These circumstances are shaped by the distribution of money, power and resources at global, national and local levels, which are themselves influenced by policy choices. The social determinants of health are mostly responsible for health inequities—the unfair and avoidable differences in health status seen within and between countries.

'Closing the Gap' in Australia

The national, state and territorial governments of Australia are jointly committed to meeting the challenge of the WHO Commission report (2008) of 'Closing the Gap' by remedying the serious cultural, social, economic and health inequities experienced by Aboriginal and Torres Strait Islander peoples. A major corner stone for this occurred when former Prime Minister Kevin Rudd (2008), on behalf of the Australian Parliament, formally and publicly acknowledged and apologised to Aboriginal and Torres Strait Islander peoples for what has happened to them since the first ships arrived.

Definition of health

The Aboriginal Health and Medical Research Council of New South Wales (2011) defines Aboriginal and Torres Strait Islander health as:

> ... not just the physical well-being of an individual but refers to the social emotional and cultural well-being of the whole community in which each individual is able to achieve their full potential as a human being thereby bringing about the total well-being of their Community. It is a whole-of-life view and includes the cyclical concept of life-death-life.

Prevalence of ill health

Aboriginal and Torres Strait Islander peoples experience the worst health of all populations in Australia, often beginning from a very young age. It is highly likely that a patient will have more than one acute or chronic condition while also facing disadvantage and diminished social and emotional wellbeing. Many of their family members will likewise be affected.

Perception, beliefs and experience of health

Aboriginal and Torres Strait Islander peoples perceive and experience their health to be inseparable from their family and community. The five domains of health are:

- Spiritual
- Cultural
- Social
- Psychological
- Physical.

Culturally competent nursing assessment

Culturally competent nursing assessment is based on the rights of all Aboriginal and Torres Strait Islander people listed in Display 11-3.

ONLINE RESOURCES

An extensive range of additional resources to enhance teaching and learning and to facilitate understanding may be found online at the text's accompanying website, located on thePoint at http://thepoint.lww.com. These include Watch and Learn videos, Concepts in Action animations, journal articles, case studies, discussion topics and quizzes.

Subscribers may also access Lippincott Procedures, an extensive online point-of-care procedure guide that provides reliable step-by-step instructions for more than 1700 procedures, including 450 evidence-based Australian procedures, and skills in a variety of speciality settings, together with a wealth of supporting information.

References

Aboriginal Health & Medical Research Council of New South Wales (AH&MRC). (2011). Aboriginal health information. Viewed January 2019 at www.ahmrc.org.au/AboriginalHealthInformation.htm.

Anderson, I. (2001). The truth about Indigenous health policy. *Arena, 56*, 32–37.

Anderson, I., Baum, F. & Bentley, M. (Eds). (2007). *Beyond Bandaids: Exploring the underlying social determinants of Aboriginal health.* Darwin: Cooperative Research Centre for Aboriginal Health. Papers from the Social Determinants of Aboriginal Health Workshop, Adelaide, July 2004.

Australian Council of TESOL. (2006). Home page. Viewed January 2019 at www.tesol.org.au/Contact-Us.

Australian Human Rights Commission. (n.d.). Indigenous deaths in custody: Report summary. Viewed January 2019 at www.humanrights.gov.au/publications/indigenous-deaths-custody-report-summary.

Australian Institute of Aboriginal and Torres Strait Islander Studies (AIATSIS). (2019). Aboriginal Australia map. In D. Horton (Ed). *The encyclopaedia of Aboriginal Australia: Aboriginal and Torres Strait Islander history, society and culture.* Canberra: Aboriginal Studies Press. Available at www.aiatsis.gov.au/asp/map.html.

Australian Institute of Health and Welfare (AIHW). (2005). Chronic kidney disease in Australia 2005. Cat. no. PHE 68. Canberra: Author. Available at https://www.aihw.gov.au/reports/chronic-kidney-disease/chronic-kidney-disease-australia-2005/contents/table-of-contents.

Australian Institute of Health and Welfare (AHIW). (2010). Contribution of chronic disease to the gap in adult mortality between Aboriginal and Torres Strait Islander Peoples and other Australians. Cat. no. IHW 48. Canberra: Author.

Australian Institute of Health and Welfare (AIHW). (2011a). The health and welfare of Australia's Aboriginal and Torres Strait Islander people, an overview 2011. Cat. no. IHW 42. Canberra: Author. Available at https://www.aihw.gov.au/getmedia/677d394f-92e1-4ad5-92b4-c13951b88968/12222.pdf.aspx?inline=true

Australian Institute of Health and Welfare (AIHW). (2011b). Life expectancy and mortality of Aboriginal and Torres Strait Islander people. Cat. no. IHW 51. Canberra: Author.

Congress of Aboriginal and Torres Strait Islander Nurses and Midwives (CATSINaM). (2013). *Towards a shared understanding of terms and concepts: Strengthening nursing and midwifery care of Aboriginal and Torres Strait Islander peoples.* Canberra: Author.

Connolly, M. (2011). Alleviating the burden of chronic conditions in New Zealand (ABCC NZ Study). Auckland: Waitemata District Health Board. Viewed December 2013 at http://dhbrfhrc.govt.nz/media/documents_abcc/ABCC_Study_NZ_Literature_Review_2011.pdf.

Cusack, L., de Crespigny, C., & Wilson, C. (2013). Over-the-counter analgesic use by urban Aboriginal people in South Australia. *Health and Social Care in The Community, 21*(4), 373–380. https://doi.org/10.1111/hsc.12023.

de Crespigny, C. & Valadian, S. (2010). Caring for Indigenous people. In D. B. Cooper (Ed). *Introduction to mental health—Substance use* (Chapter 5). Abingdon, Oxon: Radcliffe Publishing.

de Crespigny, C., Kowanko, I., Murray, H., et al. (2006). A nursing partnership for better outcomes in Aboriginal alcohol, other drugs and mental health. Advances in Indigenous Health Care (special issue). *Contemporary Nurse Journal, 22*(2), 275–287.

de Crespigny, C., Wilson, C., Chong, A., et al. (2011). Over-the-counter (OTC) analgesic use by Aboriginal people in Adelaide. Report. Adelaide: School of Nursing, University of Adelaide.

Department of Aboriginal Affairs, Australian Government. (1981). *Report on a review of the administration of the working definition of Aboriginal and Torres Strait Islander.* Canberra: Constitutional Section, Department of Aboriginal Affairs.

Department of Health, Australian Government. (2019). Aboriginal and Torres Strait Islander health. Available at https://www.health.gov.au/health-topics/aboriginal-and-torres-strait-islander-health.

Department of Health and Ageing, Australian Government. (2007). *Alcohol treatment guidelines for Indigenous Australians*. Canberra: Commonwealth of Australia. Available at www.alcohol.gov.au.

Eckermann, A., Dowd, T., Chong, E., et al. (2010). *Binan goonj: Bridging cultures in Aboriginal health* (3rd ed.). Sydney: Churchill Livingstone/Elsevier.

Emerson, L. & Croucher, K. (2001). *Quality use of medicines in Aboriginal communities: Final report 2001*. Canberra: Pharmacy Guild of Australia.

Evans, R. & Thorpe, B. (2001). Indigenocide and the massacre of Aboriginal history. *Overland, 163*, 33–39.

Gardiner-Garden, J. (2003). Defining Aboriginality in Australia. Current Issues Brief No. 10 2002–03. Canberra: Parliament of Australia, Parliamentary Library. Available at https://www.aph.gov.au/binaries/library/pubs/cib/2002-03/03cib10.pdf.

Hunter New England Health. (2008). *HNE health cardiac services plan 2008–2012*. New Lambton, NSW: Hunter New England Health Planning Unit.

Keating, P. (1992). 'Redfern speech'. Viewed December 2013 at http://antar.org.au/sites/default/files/paul_keating_speech_transcript.pdf.

Kowanko, L., de Crespigny, C., Murray, H., et al. (2009). Improving coordination of care for Aboriginal people with mental health, alcohol and drug use problems: Progress report on an ongoing collaborative action research project. *Australian Journal of Primary Health, 15*, 1–7.

Kunitz, S. (1994). *Disease and social diversity: The European impact on the health of non-Europeans*. New York: Oxford University Press.

MacKean, T. (2005). Personal communication in Australian Government Department of Health and Ageing. In *Alcohol treatment guidelines for Indigenous Australians 2007*. Canberra: Commonwealth of Australia. Available December 2013 at www.alcohol.gov.au.

Mattingley, C., (Ed. & Researcher) & Hampton, K., (Co-Ed.). (1998). *Survival in our own land: 'Aboriginal' experiences in 'South Australia' since 1836 told by Nungas of South Australia (Aboriginal preferred citation)*. Netley, SA: Wakefield Press.

National Aboriginal Community Controlled Health Organisation (NACCHO). (2013a). *Investing in healthy futures for generational change: NACCHO 10 Point Plan 2013–2030*. Canberra: Author. Available at https://www.naccho.org.au/wp-content/uploads/2016/03/NACCHO-Healthy-Futures-10-point-plan-2013-2030.pdf.

National Aboriginal Community Controlled Health Organisation (NACCHO). (2013b). A brief overview of Aboriginal Health to 1967. Viewed November 2013 at www.naccho.org.au.

National Aboriginal Community Controlled Health Organisation (NACCHO) & National Rural Health Alliance Inc. (NRHA). (2004). Joint media release, 'Indigenous dental health is crying out for special treatment', NRHA eForum, 9 April 2004. Viewed December 2013 at http://ruralhealth.org.au/media-release/indigenous-dental-health-crying-out-special-treatment.

National Aboriginal Health Strategy Working Party. (1989). The national Aboriginal health strategy (NAHS). Canberra: National Aboriginal and Torres Strait Islander Health Council, Department of Health and Ageing.

National Advisory Committee on Health and Disability. (2007). *Meeting the needs of people with chronic conditions: Hapai te whanau mo ake ake tonu*. Wellington: Author.

Ramsden, I. M. (1992). Cultural safety in nursing education in Aotearoa. Presented at the Year of Indigenous Peoples Conference, Brisbane.

Read, P. (1981), cited in Gardiner-Garden J. [2000]. Defining Aboriginality in Australia. Current Issues Brief No. 10 2002-03. Canberra: Parliament of Australia, Parliamentary Library. Available at https://www.aph.gov.au/binaries/library/pubs/cib/2002-03/03cib10.pdf.

Reynolds, H. (1999). *Why weren't we told? A personal search for the truth about our history*. Ringwood, Vic.: Viking.

Rudd, K. (2008). Apology to Australia's Indigenous peoples. House of Representatives Official Hansard, 13 February 2008, pp. 167–173. Available via Hansard at http://parlinfo.aph.gov.au or alternatively at https://parlinfo.aph.gov.au/parlInfo/search/display/display.w3p;query=Id:%22chamber/hansardr/2008-02-13/0003%22.

Stoneman, J. & Taylor, S. (2007). Pharmacists' views on Indigenous health: Is there more that can be done? *Rural and Remote Health, 7*(743), 1–15.

World Health Organization, Commission on Social Determinants of Health (CSDH). (2008). *Closing the gap in a generation: Health equity through action on the social determinants of health*. Geneva. Available at https://apps.who.int/iris/bitstream/handle/10665/43943/9789241563703_eng.pdf;jsessionid=FCA973A23D5223E45E5005D6AE7423D0?sequence=1.

Online resources

Australian Indigenous Health*InfoNet*: www.healthinfonet.ecu.edu.au
Australian Institute of Aboriginal and Torres Strait Islander Studies (AIATSIS): www.aiatsis.gov.au
Australian Museum: http://australianmuseum.net.au/Indigenous-Australia
Centre for Cultural Competence Australia: www.ccca.com.au
Centre for Culture, Ethnicity and Health: www.ceh.org.au
Centre for Diversity in Aged Care: www.culturaldiversity.com.au
Congress of Aboriginal and Torres Strait Islander Nurses and Midwives (CATSIN): http://catsin.org.au
Government Department of Health: www.health.gov.au
National Aboriginal Community Controlled Health Organisation (NACCHO): www.naccho.org.au
National and State Policy Context for Primary Care Partnerships: www.health.vic.gov.au/pcps/downloads/nationalstatepolicy_infores.pdf
Telethon Institute for Child Health Research, Aboriginal health: http://aboriginal.childhealthresearch.org.au
Tiwi Land Council: www.tiwilandcouncil.com
Torres Strait Regional Authority: www.tsra.gov.au/the-tsra

CHAPTER 12

Assessment in Māori communities

The provision of appropriate health care services, including health assessment, to New Zealanders who identify as Māori requires an awareness of, and cultural sensitivity to, their background and issues that might affect them.

This chapter provides a brief overview of Māori history and the current status of Māori health relative to the population of New Zealand as a whole. It also presents the concepts underpinning the *Te Whare Tapa Whā* health model, Pae ora (healthy futures equity model) and the *Whānau Ora* approach to nursing care. The case studies illustrate relevant key issues that may be encountered by nurses, community health workers and their patients.

In 1987, *te reo Māori* (the Māori language) was recognised as one of the official languages of *Aotearoa* (land of the long white cloud, the Māori name for New Zealand). Its use helps to define New Zealand's sense of identity and culture. In this chapter, where a Māori word or term is used, its English meaning is given in parentheses in the first instance.

BACKGROUND

The Indigenous people of New Zealand are commonly known as Māori, although prior to colonisation in the 18th century by the *Pākehā* (non-Māori New Zealanders), there was no need for Māori to identify as a single entity; identification was by tribal and sub-tribal groups (Lai, 2010). Although some controversy still exists as to its usage, the term Māori is now generally accepted by most Indigenous New Zealanders (Lai, 2010), and the term is used throughout this chapter.

Legend has it that the original Māori people arrived in the Great Fleet from Polynesia (Howe, 2009a, 2009b). They first settled around the east coast of New Zealand. There remains debate about their early history and the date of their arrival; however, there is no debate about the fact they are the *Tangata Whenua* (the Indigenous people of the ancestral lands).

During the late 18th century, European traders and visitors began to reach New Zealand shores (Phillips, 2009). By the early 19th century, socio-economic conditions in Britain were such that many people, seeking a better life, made the decision to migrate to the New World, and so British settlers began to arrive in New Zealand (Phillips, 2010). By the middle of that century British immigration was actively being encouraged by the British government, marking the beginning of British cultural domination (Thomas & Nikora, 1992). As more British settlers arrived in New Zealand, land disputes arose between them and the local tribal groups, creating much unrest. In 1839, the British government dispatched a representative with instructions to acquire sovereignty over New Zealand (McLintock, 1966a). As a result, the Treaty of Waitangi was negotiated and signed with *rangatira* (chiefs) of Māori tribal groups in 1840. The treaty was an agreement intended to assure Māori of equal rights and consideration under the management of the Crown.

It was believed that the treaty would alleviate the unrest over land issues, but as more settlers demanded ownership of land, disputes became more aggressive (McLintock, 1966b). There were numerous accounts of land confiscations and brutal land seizures by the settlers, with Māori men, women and children being incarcerated and mistreated (Boast, 2009). Māori, a race of warriors, fought back and to this day remain in negotiations with the government over the return of confiscated and other tribal lands.

British colonisation throughout the 19th century and the first half of the 20th century altered the lives of Māori (Ellison-Loschmann & Pearce, 2006). The long-term negative effects on their health and wellbeing cannot be disputed; a sense of grief and loss is still felt by many Māori today because they perceive the cultural practices of the colonisers have become dominant and that tribal cultural practices have become marginalised (Simon, 2001). Māori have deep spiritual connections to the land, and its loss left them displaced, disconnected and impoverished, prone to psychological and emotional stresses, and increasingly vulnerable to illness and the diseases introduced by the immigrants from Britain and Europe (Durie, 1998). Many Māori died from introduced diseases: it is estimated that during this time the mortality rate from disease and warfare was as high as 30% of the Māori population (Durie, 1998). Dispossession of their lands subjected Māori to many years of disharmony at great expense to their health and wellbeing.

During the period of colonisation, government officials, missionaries and anthropologists were the decision makers in discussions about the best policies for Māori. The common recommendation was for assimilation of Māori into the dominant society of the *Pākehā*. To implement this policy, Māori were banned from speaking their native language in public places, including schools, and forced to speak the foreign language of English (National Library of New Zealand, 2010). Thus, Māori were deprived not only of their language, but also of the dimensions of culture and history inherent in language customs and worldview. As a consequence, Māori suffered the effects of lowered cultural, legal, economic and social status in their own country. Some Māori supported the changes brought about by assimilation but simply because they saw this as being 'the only way to survive the effects of colonisation' (personal communication). Today, many elderly Māori who were subjected to this regime feel a strong sense of grief about the loss of knowledge and stories of their forebears, which was their cultural and spiritual right, and they are now reclaiming their Māori culture.

Although Māori adapted to the *Pākehā* system, this rapid acculturation has had a major impact on their current health status (New Zealand Ministry of Health [NZMOH], 2019b, 2010a). Over time, Māori cultural beliefs and values have become weakened, although *whakapapa* (ancestral heritage, genealogical ties) remains a very strong cultural influence. For many Māori *whakapapa* is the living thread of existence that has fortified them against destruction.

Acknowledgement of Māori rights in New Zealand is a slow and evolving process. During the 1970s, New Zealand made a commitment to biculturalism that continues to grow steadily. Consequently, there have been significant changes in the relationship between Māori and *Pākehā*, as is evidenced today by the annual celebration of *te reo Māori* during Māori Language Week (New Zealand Ministry for Culture and Heritage, 2013), the existence of specialist media such as the Māori Television Service and a higher visibility of Māori in public life (Derby, 2012). However, past inequalities in the provision of education, health, employment and other social determinants have been identified as major indicators of the poor health outcomes for Māori today. For example, the New Zealand Health Survey reported that, in the years 2016 and 2017, many health conditions were more common for Māori adults than for other adults, including ischaemic heart disease, stroke, diabetes, medicated high blood pressure, chronic pain, gout and arthritis (NZMOH, 2017a). Health assessment in New Zealand, especially when concerned with Māori, demands consideration of and respect for Māori cultural history and an appreciation of worldview Māori concepts. Equally important is an understanding of the *Te Whare Tapa Whā* health model, together with the incorporation of *Whānau Ora* concepts of health care provision and the inclusion of Pae ora (equity concepts model 'healthy futures'), all of which are discussed in this chapter.

CURRENT STATE OF MĀORI HEALTH IN NEW ZEALAND

As a population group, Māori have on average the poorest health status of any ethnic group in New Zealand. Māori have poorer health outcomes across all age groups: they die younger and have higher rates of chronic disease than non-Māori. In addition, the Māori infant mortality rate is almost double that of the non-Māori rate, and Māori are negatively represented in mental health statistics and have higher rates of mortality and morbidity from injuries, accidents and suicide (NZMOH, 2015). The aspects of health status and outcomes outlined above result in a life course of higher disability rates for Māori across all ages. Statistics reveal that 14% of Māori children, 32% of young and working age Māori and 62% of Māori seniors live with one or more disabilities (NZMOH, 2019b).

Alongside these statistics sit three polarising aspects that have deep significance to the stability and health of Māori communities. Māori and Pasifika have disproportionately high levels of incarceration and over-representation, including women and young people at all levels of the criminal justice process (Stanley & Mihaere, 2019). Māori represent half of the prison population in New Zealand. Elements of institutional and structural discrimination and racism have been identified as significant impediments in both the justice and the health systems. These factors impact on health outcomes across all levels of Māori communities. Māori adults are twice as likely as non-Māori adults to have experienced any type of racial discrimination (NZMOH, 2015). In a cross-sectional analysis of the 2011 to 2012 adult New Zealand Health Survey,which focuses on experiences of racism, unmet health need and health care satisfaction, Harris et al. (2019) found that racism may act as a barrier to, and influence the quality of health care.

The third compelling social consequence that is affecting the health of Māori communities is the increasing use of 'P' (pure methamphetamine). The social impact and negative health effects related to the use of this drug affects all age groups of Māori society: grandparents, families, their unborn children and future generations (La Gasse et al., 2010). Longitudinal studies have not been undertaken to assess the impact of methamphetamine use on Māori communities; however, the 2015 to 2016 New Zealand health survey (NZMOH, 2016) indicates that the use of this drug is higher in the Māori population. The social and health challenges related to the use of methamphetamine have been the focus of a mental health and addictions inquiry (New Zealand Drug Foundation, 2018). The inquiry recommends that addiction and drug use should be treated as a health issue, decriminalising personal use and offering a broader range of health options. A strategy of 'health not handcuffs' is currently being implemented in New Zealand, with varying degrees of success.

The New Zealand government acknowledges the health inequalities and inequities that face Māori, and since the early 2000s there have been strategies in place to address health-related mortality and morbidity status. However, despite prioritised health service strategies and initiatives over the last 20 years, Māori health outcomes remain at 'unacceptable levels', according to Dr Ashley Bloomfield, Director-General of Health (Hauora, 2019; NZMOH, 2019b). Government directives and strategies related to Māori health incorporate Māori health and health and disability strategies and are centred on the principles set out in the Treaty of Waitangi: partnership, participation and protection (NZMOH, 2014b). The key guiding principles are:

- *Partnership*: Working together with *iwi* (larger Māori tribal groups), *hapū* (secondary tribal groups), *whānau* (extended family) and all Māori communities to develop strategies for Māori health gains and appropriate health and disability services
- *Participation*: Involving Māori at all levels of decision making, planning, development and delivery of health and disability services
- *Protection*: Working to ensure that Māori have at least the same level of health as non-Māori, and safeguarding Māori cultural concepts, values and practices. (NZMOH, 2014b)

The *New Zealand Public Health and Disability Act* (2000) established the strategic direction and goals for health and disability services in New Zealand. This measure included goals to improve health and disability outcomes for all New Zealanders and to reduce disparities 'by improving the health of Māori and other population groups' (NZMOH, 2000). In 2019, a review of the Health and Disability legislation (NZMOH, 2019b) was started, with the aim of moving the health system to a path of equity, responsiveness and sustainability. The review acknowledges past failures of the Health and Disability legislation to recognise and embed Māori worldviews in policy and outline a commitment to establishing strong and effective partnerships for the future.

In the context of Māori health statistics that have failed to demonstrate improvement over the last 20 years, Māori health leaders have invoked the Treaty of Waitangi and placed a claim to outline historical and contemporary issues related to the health system, specific health services and outcomes, including health equity, primary care, disability services and Māori health providers. The tribunal process outlines root cause analysis for issues that have an impact on the health and wellbeing of Māori across New Zealand (Hauora, 2019). This comprehensive review has provided opportunity for grievances around health services and outcomes of national significance to be highlighted for increased action.

Māori health model

The *Te Whare Tapa Whā* health model is often used to understand a range of health issues affecting Māori, from physical issues to psychological wellbeing (Durie, 1998). It describes the four equal and interactive dimensions of Māori wellbeing (see Fig. 12-1) using the symbol of the *Wharenui* (large meeting house). Each of the four cornerstones represents one of the four dimensions of Māori health: *Taha Tinana* (physical health), *Taha Wairua* (spiritual health), *Taha Whānau* (family health) and *Taha Hinengaro* (mental health). Each dimension must be strong and balanced: if one is absent or damaged, then the person or group may become unwell. *Te Whare Tapa Whā* provides a strong framework for health providers to consider the needs of patients and *whānau*. To appreciate the model and its relevance to health care delivered to Māori, it must be clear that comprehensive application to all dimensions requires extensive resources. To support the application of the concepts of the *Te Whare Tapa Whā* model, the Pae ora model for healthy futures was introduced in 2014 and is one the main features of *The guide to He Korowai Oranga: Māori Health strategy* (Fig. 12-2) (NZMOH, 2014a).

This model importantly has a stronger focus on the relevance of equity in health. It demonstrates that no improvements to health for Māori will occur unless the wider elements of environment are improved to allow individual and family health to flourish. Environment includes the wider determinates of employment, education, housing and more. Within the two perspectives of *Te Whare Tapa Whā* and Pae ora the *Whānau Ora* model of nursing care sits as a family-centred approach to health care delivery and is inclusive across Māori community environments.

Cohorts in need of focus

The age distribution of the Māori population, shown in Figure 12-3, presents a fascinating portrayal of Māori health in the past, present and future. It represents many stories of cultural loss, disease prevention capacity, possibilities for support for those with existing disease and, most importantly, the opportunity to enhance and change the lives of those under the age of 25 years.

The narrowing of the pyramid at the age of 30 to 50 for both males and females represents a devastating loss of life. This premature mortality has a major psychosocial impact on family life as extended families lose their parents and grandparents. The resultant loss of generational knowledge and support has led to reduced cultural transference and family support, as there are fewer elders to pass on cultural values, beliefs and *tikanga* (cultural correctness). This weakens the thread of culture and leaves young people in a state of grief, sadness and loss. Many Māori suffer deep depression with the loss of so many *whānau* members (personal observation). Ngata (2005) describes the individual's reliance on *whānau:* kinship ties maintain collective strength; each family member contributes to the health and wellbeing of the *whānau* group; and losses through sickness and death weaken the family network. It is not uncommon for families to experience multiple losses in quick succession, resulting in mental distress and financial hardship.

This section of the population pyramid suggests an area upon which health professionals should place a greater emphasis, as it is this group that could benefit from preventative health measures. Early assessment and management of health issues can, over time, have a positive impact on mortality rates for Māori. Prevention programs delivered at primary health and community levels have been shown to be effective in increasing awareness of risk factors for common diseases affecting Māori, such as cardiovascular and respiratory diseases, diabetes and cancers (NZMOH, 2019a). In their capacity as health service providers, nurses making health assessments are perfectly positioned to positively alter the future for this population group. Nurse-led community health programs focused on issues such as cardiovascular risk assessment, nicotine awareness, comprehensive diabetes education, nutrition, weight loss and exercise are well within the scope and capacity of nurses. Nurses must become more proactive, taking up the challenge to make a difference for the patients and families with whom they work.

The Māori population is a young one: 52% are under the age of 25 years, and young populations have children. This statistic should be considered in the light of the fundamental significance in *Te Ao Māori* (the Māori world) of the place of *whakapapa, whānau* (extended family) and *tamariki* (young children). Pihama (2011, p. 3) describes *Te Ao Māori* as a '*whakapapa*-based society that is grounded upon the cultural systems and structures of *whānau, hapū* and *iwi*', with each of these terms highlighting the significance and centrality of being pregnant and giving birth to the next generation. Within this societal context, Māori *tamariki* and *mokopuna* (grandchildren, children of nephews or nieces) are the centre of *Te Ao Māori*, and the blessing of children is highly regarded. The challenge this presents is that there are not enough support systems in place to adequately and appropriately care for these children, now and in the future. The urgent challenge for government and the New Zealand health sector is to develop and implement strategies that can comprehensively support the future of Māori, to enable them to lead healthy, happy and productive lives.

Health literacy is defined as the ability to obtain, process and understand basic health information in order to make

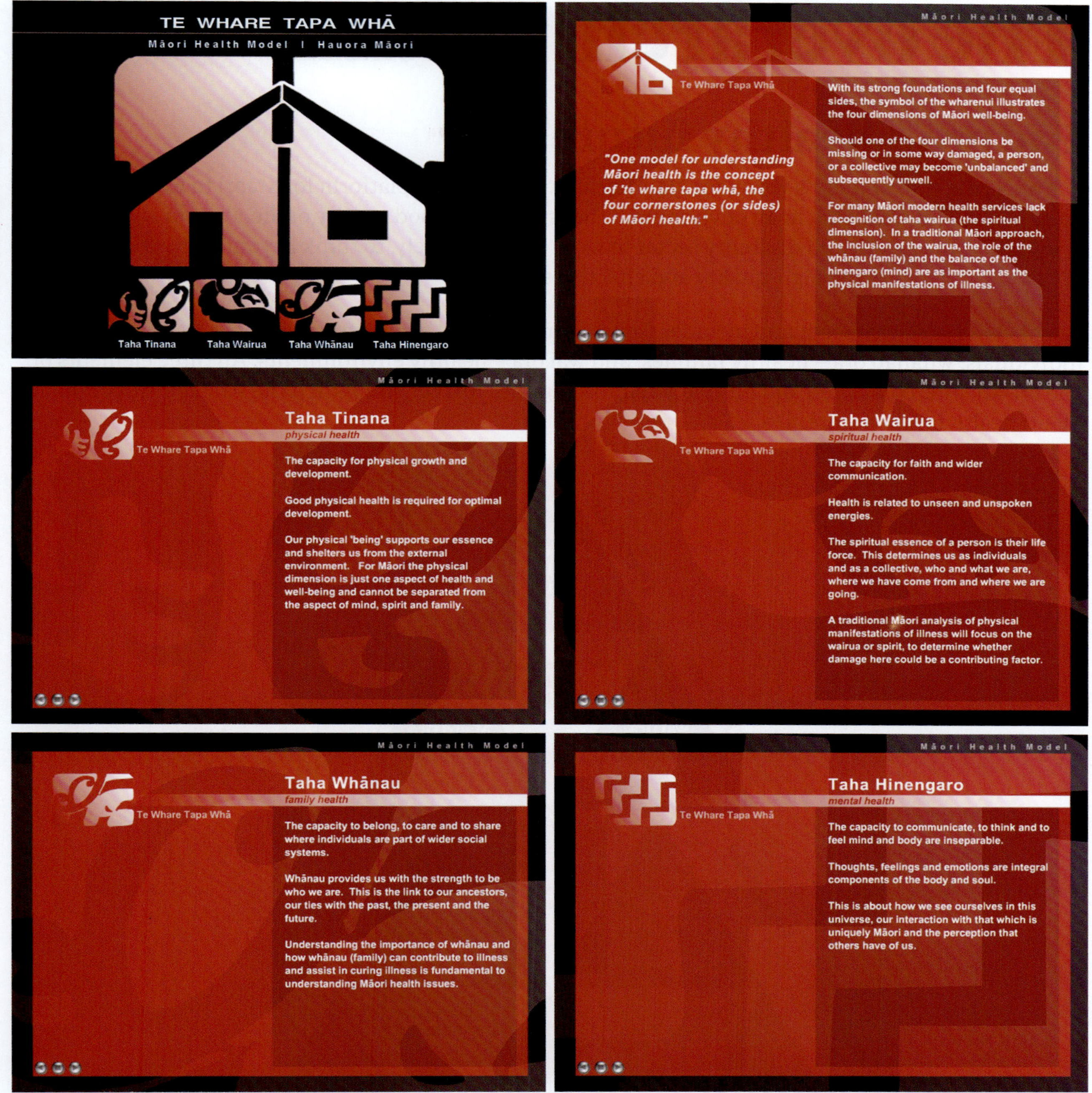

FIGURE 12-1 NZMOH. Māori health models – Te Whare Tapa Wha. www.health.govt.nz/our-work/populations/maori-health/maori-health-models. Reproduced with kind permission of New Zealand Ministry of Health. Updated 18 May 2017.

informed and appropriate health decisions (NZMOH, 2010a). Approximately 80% of Māori men and 73% of Māori women have health literacy levels, indicating they would not be adequately informed to make appropriate health decisions in typical situations.

These statistics highlight another area of focus for health practitioners, that is, to use multiple strategies to improve understanding of health messages because the level of individual and family health literacy can have a major impact on the successful management of patient health needs. A study by Lambert et al. (2014) suggested that health professionals had a limited understanding of health literacy and the consequences of low levels of literacy in indigenous peoples. The study concluded that reduced understanding and acknowledgement of barriers to literacy limited health professionals' ability to improve patients' health literacy skills to understand and support the management of their health conditions (Fig. 12-4). Misinterpretation or misunderstanding of health-related instructions or directions can lead to adverse events, including non-adherence to medication and treatment plans. Research suggests that poor health literacy levels in Māori are correlated with poor health outcomes via factors such as:

- Under-utilisation of preventative services such as screening programs

The overarching aim

Pae ora – healthy futures

Pae ora is the Government's vision for Māori health. It provides a platform for Māori to live with good health and wellbeing in an environment that supports a good quality of life. Pae ora encourages everyone in the health and disability sector to work collaboratively, to think beyond narrow definitions of health, and to provide high-quality and effective services.

Pae ora is a holistic concept and includes three interconnected elements: mauri ora – healthy individuals; whānau ora – healthy families; and wai ora – healthy environments. All three elements of pae ora are interconnected and mutually reinforcing, and further strengthen the strategic direction for Māori health for the future.

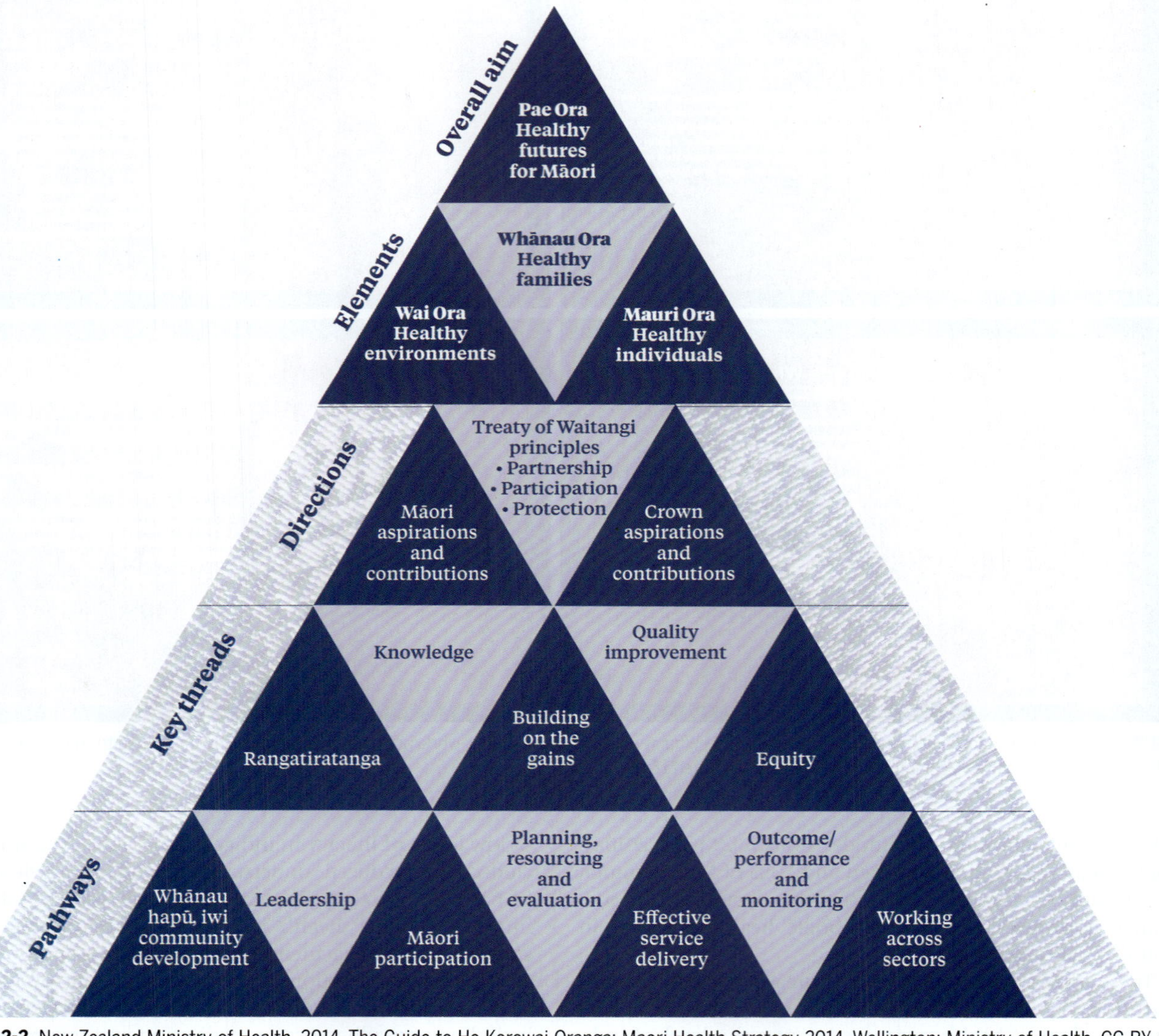

FIGURE 12-2 New Zealand Ministry of Health, 2014. The Guide to He Korowai Oranga: Maori Health Strategy 2014. Wellington: Ministry of Health. CC BY 4.0 International License.

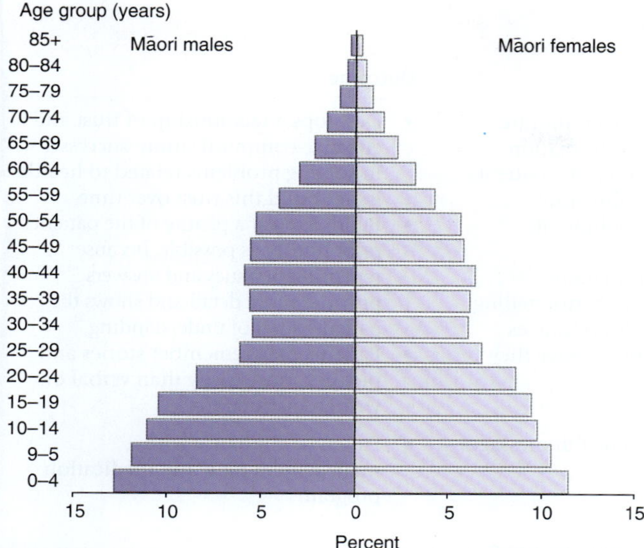

FIGURE 12-3 Age distribution of the Māori population, males and females, 2013. (Ministry of Health, 2015. *Tatau Kahukura: Maori Health Chart Book 2015* [3rd ed.]. Wellington: Ministry of Health and Statistics New Zealand. CC BY 4.0 International License.)

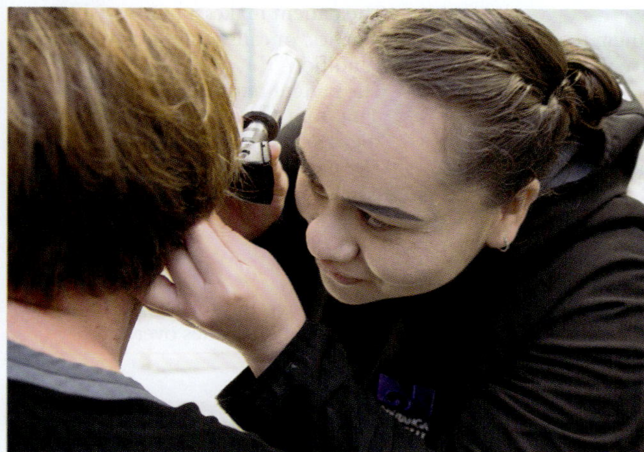

FIGURE 12-4 Nurses are able to help individuals and families improve their health literacy levels, which can have a major impact on their successful health management. (Stuff Limited.)

- Low comprehension levels regarding illnesses, treatment and medicines
- Lower ability to manage long-term or chronic conditions
- Higher probability of hospitalisations due to mismanagement of chronic conditions
- Higher use of emergency services
- Increased likelihood of workplace injury due to poor understanding of safety precautions. (NZMOH, 2010a)

In the short term, strategies to improve health literacy and understanding remain with health practitioners, who are in direct communication with patients and their communities. Assessment of a patient's health literacy level is as vital to the health assessment process as assessment of the patient's physical body systems. Recognising and accommodating everyone's literacy level when relaying complex health information will result in more positive outcomes. Table 12-1 outlines some successful strategies used by health practitioners today to improve understanding of health messages.

Whānau Ora service delivery

As a principal source of strength, support, security and identity play a central role in the wellbeing of Māori individually and collectively (NZMOH, 2009b). *Whānau Ora* has been defined as 'Māori families supported to achieve their maximum health and wellbeing' (Boulton & Gifford, 2014). The driving principle behind the Ministry of Health's *Whānau Ora* model is to improve Māori health by promoting healthy lifestyles and minimising disease by supporting and encouraging Māori to achieve maximum health and wellbeing. The *Whānau Ora* approach focuses on empowerment and self-determination of the *whānau*, with health providers facilitating the resources and support to realise change. This requires a shift in paradigm: instead of accepting related services, the approach is a more purposeful *whānau*-centred one, where people are empowered and assisted to make decisions and changes for themselves (NZMOH, 2010b).

Whānau Ora service delivery has been practised by Māori health providers since its inception some 20years ago. It is recognised that Māori and *iwi* health providers may be the most effective at delivering *Whānau Ora* services (NZMOH, 2019b). In 2010, the New Zealand government introduced plans to implement formal *whānau*-centred health initiatives and support the ongoing implementation of this type of service provision to encourage improvements in Māori health (NZMOH, 2010b). A recent review of the quality of New Zealand health care (Health, Quality & Safety Commision New Zealand, 2019) reveals deficits in achieving improvements in Māori health, and data reviewed show that focus drifts over time, suggesting widening patterns of inequity between Māori and non-Māori. This document refreshingly uses the 'life course' approach, which resounds with Māori health thinking, where experiences of life across the generations shape the health and wellbeing of the people. This quality review supports the work around *Whānau Ora* approaches and acknowledges that greater investment, leadership and partnership are required to realise the future health, education, cultural, social and economic aspirations of *whānau*.

Te Whare Tapa Whā, the guiding principles of Māori health, and Pae ora concepts of healthy futures, combine to transcend to a wider, more comprehensive service in the context of Māori health care provision and health service delivery. *Whānau* health should be viewed in the light of both approaches. The successful implementation of programs that encompass both approaches will deliver improvement for individuals, their *whānau* and their *iwi* in terms of their social, economic and cultural lives. Health care professionals should empower Māori to achieve wellbeing, encourage them to recognise and develop their strengths, and assist in building community development initiatives that offer sustainable long-term health outcomes for groups in their local community (Fig. 12-5).

The key principles of *Whānau Ora* service delivery are outlined in Display 12-1.

IMPORTANCE OF CULTURAL COMPETENCY AND SAFETY

Under the *Health Practitioners Competence Assurance Act* (2003), the Nursing Council of New Zealand (NCNZ) establishes and monitors standards and competencies that govern the

Table 12-1 Strategies to improve understanding of health messages

Goal	Strategy	Outcome
Assess the patient's level of literacy and previous health learning experiences	• Develop a relationship with the patient: inquire about their health history, family and situation • Use open-ended questions to ascertain the patient's understanding of the disease or health issue • Ask the same question again, but rephrase it differently • Use simple language; avoid medical jargon • Create scenarios or use simple analogy storytelling • Draw a picture, or use existing health resources • Ask the patient to repeat the health message they have been given	• Develops a relationship of trust and effective communication; successes in solving problems related to health issues build this trust over time • Builds as clear a picture of the patient's prior history as possible, because repetition of issues and answers provides more detail and shows the patient's level of understanding • Patients may remember stories and pictures more easily than verbal or written instructions
Improve the patient's understanding of health messages	• Take every opportunity to reinforce health messages or instructions • Reinforce concepts at each visit • Maintain consistency • Be confident and knowledgeable about the topic under discussion • Take the time to explain reinforce with online health videos • Use the internet to look up images to support the patient's understanding of health issues	• Patient compliance with management plan and medication program
Engage the patient in treatment and outcome plans	• Ask the patient to report back • Offer to call the patient or invite them to call • Set homework for the patient—give them something to watch out for by asking them to observe whether an intervention has helped or made the condition worse (e.g. monitoring weight, blood sugar) Encourage the use of health apps to assist health improvements. • Avoid being judgemental • Be fair and honest in communication and demonstrate a caring attitude	• The patient makes a return visit to practice, or calls with updates on condition • The patient returns to the clinic with data from homework (e.g. blood sugar recordings) • The patient feels relaxed and shares issues freely
Negotiate achievable health plans and treatment options	• Periodically review health plan and progress of issues	• Step-by-step improvements in health and social outcomes over time

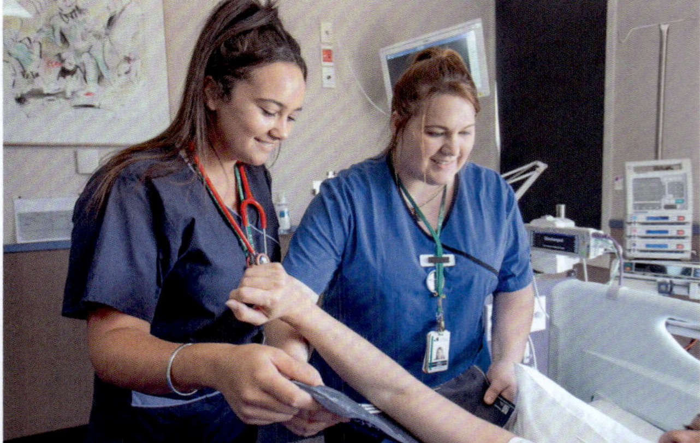

FIGURE 12-5 Health care professionals are in a position to empower Māori to achieve wellbeing and encourage them to recognise and develop their strengths. (Stuff Limited.)

practices of New Zealand nurses. The Medical Council of New Zealand has similar frameworks governing the competencies, conduct and standards of doctors. These comprehensive standards define the responsibilities of health care professionals in their provision of culturally safe practices.

DISPLAY 12-1 KEY PRINCIPLES OF *WHĀNAU ORA* SERVICE DELIVERY

- Focus on *whānau*
- Māori self-determination-supporting the individual and the community to achieve self-determination
- Development and growth of respectful relationships
- Recognition of the importance of *te Reo Māori*, *tikanga* and *Mātauranga Māori* (traditional knowledge of Māori cultural practices) to overall health and wellbeing
- Recognition of spiritual and cultural awareness as it applies to cultural competency in health environments
- Effective resourcing, and competent provision of services

Nurses must incorporate cultural safety when delivering nursing services to Māori by demonstrating that they:

- Acknowledge and respect the diversity of worldviews that may exist among Māori consumers of health services
- Understand the historical processes and social, economic and political power relationships that have contributed to the current status of Māori health

- Embody the principles of the Treaty of Waitangi, now an integral part of the *Public Health and Disability Act* (2000)
- Reflect the values inherent in *Kawa Whakaruruhau* (the philosophy of cultural safety within the context of nursing practice). (NCNZ, 2009)

The NCNZ (2009, p.7) defines cultural safety as:

> … the effective nursing practice of a person or family from another culture, [which] is determined by that person or family. Culture includes, but is not restricted to, age or generation; gender; sexual orientation; occupation and socio-economic status; ethnic origin or migrant experience; religious or spiritual belief; and disability.

The concepts of cultural competency and cultural safety are considered factors in the health care encounters over time; however, recent considerations of cultural competence demonstrate a narrow, potentially harmful disposition (Curtis et al., 2019). Concepts of cultural safety acknowledge the power imbalance between health practitioners and providers, cultural safety aligns to an awareness of difference, considering power deficits, utilising reflective practice and allowing the patient to engage, giving them a feeling of safety within the therapeutic encounter (Fig. 12-6). The wider considerations of cultural safety extend to and include accountability of the health care organisations, thereby ensuring a saturated offensive, aligning equity concepts across the health care boundaries.

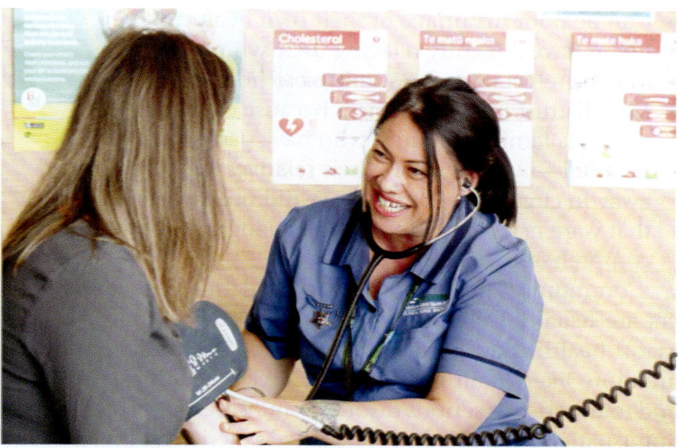

FIGURE 12-6 Nurses providing culturally competent care undertake a process of reflection on their own cultural identity and recognise the impact their own personal culture has on professional practice. (Stuff/Waikato Times.)

HEALTH SERVICE PROVIDERS

Māori and *iwi* health service providers

Under the *New Zealand Public Health and Disability Act* (2000), District Health Boards fund and support Māori health providers, which are owned and governed by Māori within their tribal boundaries. Māori Health providers have become a distinctive feature of the New Zealand health sector. Since the inception of this health delivery system in the mid-1990s, it has gained momentum and the number of Māori health service providers across New Zealand has grown to 280 (Hauora, 2019). Located in rural and urban areas, these providers deliver culturally appropriate and diverse services that offer health and social options to Māori families and individuals in such a way as to support concepts of empowerment. Māori cultural values, beliefs and practices are central to their operational activities, with a strong focus on *tikanga* and Māori models of wellbeing. Major factors in their success are that they:

- Are based within the communities they directly service
- Are predominantly Māori themselves
- Tend to have a better understanding of the needs of their communities than do other groups of providers.

Māori health providers act as navigators of the *Whānau Ora* health service delivery concepts. Their role is to assist *whānau* in identifying their strengths, needs and priorities, and to participate in developing solutions. They can also assist in making links to government agencies and specialist services, enabling faster access to solutions the *whānau* have identified. Broadly speaking, they offer three categories of service:

1. *Specialised practice units,* which focus on one or more areas of health service, such as breast screening or smoke cessation programs
2. *Comprehensive practice units,* which provide a mixture of personal and public health services, such as public health programs, mental health services or general practice
3. *Integrated provider units,* which offer a range of health and social services, such as housing or family support and education-linked programs. (NZMOH, 2009a)

Primary (mainstream) health service providers

Primary (or mainstream) health service providers are privately owned medical practices and are located throughout New Zealand. These practices deliver comprehensive care and remain a major contributor to Māori health services in community and urban areas. They play a vital role in ensuring that all New Zealanders including Māori have access to appropriate, timely and effective health care. The existence of Māori health providers does not reduce the onus on mainstream medical practices to provide comprehensive care to Māori, who have on average the poorest health status of any ethnic group in New Zealand and require enhanced access to quality primary care services. Mainstream community health care providers have strong relationships with the public hospital system, and in some community environments they have the resources to stabilise patients prior to referral to either district or base hospitals for further management and treatment.

EMERGENCY PRESENTATION IN THE HEALTHCARE SETTING

Emergency presentation in the primary health care environment

Assessment of emergency presentations in the primary health care environment can take place in a variety of settings and may require urgent referral to mainstream general practice or hospital. Emergency presentations for Māori in community settings are often difficult and can have poor outcomes. Some of the contributing factors to this are that Māori:

- May be reluctant to present to health services because of fear of ethnically biased treatment they may receive, often doing so only when their illness is well advanced

- Can be poor historians of their own health
- Often have difficulty relaying their symptoms
- May be reluctant to be admitted to hospital
- May distrust medical services because of memories of previous family members who have passed away in hospital—in many cases, their relatives may have passed away in circumstances that they did not understand or that were not relayed to them in a language they could comprehend.

Community health providers and medical practitioners are usually well aware of this reluctance to present. The Māori health chart book (NZMOH, 2015) reports that Māori are more likely than non-Māori to access health services later and to experience serious disorders and co-existing conditions. Some patients have had such negative experiences that they are less likely to access medical assistance when needed.

Research has highlighted the impact of racial discrimination on health outcomes. Harris et al. (2019) demonstrate the structuring of societal resources and health determinants. They examine the nature of racism outlining the societal, institutional and individual levels that provide multiple pathways where racism can have an impact on health, including access to health care and the quality of that health care received. There is evidence that Māori are sometimes not offered the same health care options as non-Māori. The Health, Quality & Safety Commission (2019) review identified disparities between Māori and non-Māori health, which reflect unequal distribution of socio-economic resource and unequal outcomes. A review by Sandiford et al. (2015) identified bias in coronary revascularisation rates for Māori and Pasifika. It should be recognised that in some cases Māori may choose not to take the treatment option, possibly because the fear of the unknown is too great. The thought of being separated from their support, along with fear related to past health experiences as an individual or to extended *whānau*, may influence their health choices and subsequently their health outcomes. The following case study demonstrates the worst outcome, but similar instances may be commonly seen in the community health environment.

CASE STUDY 1

Matu is a 60-year-old Māori man who is admitted to the district hospital with chest pain. His assessment discloses that he lives in an isolated coastal area where his family (three brothers and their families) have Māori land and are farmers. He has lived his whole life on the farm, within his close-knit community. He loves his lifestyle. He has never married and has no children but belongs to a large extended *whānau*. Following admission, his condition stabilised and he is commenced on best practice management for myocardial infarction. After 2 days the doctor explains, 'You are doing well, Matu, but I would like to send you to the city for further tests and possible heart surgery.' Matu refuses immediately and asks to go home. The doctor does not push him: he accepts Matu's decision. Matu is discharged, on medical management. Six months later, following a full-thickness myocardial infarct, he dies.

CRITICAL THINKING

1. Should the doctor have tried to convince Matu to have further treatment?
2. Should the doctor or nurse have asked Matu to explain his decision?
3. Should Matu have been given more information and time to consider his options?
4. What are the possible reasons and influences for Matu's decision?
5. What are the possible influences on or rationale for the doctor's decision?

Emergency presentation in the community outreach setting

The following list outlines the clinical review procedure for individuals presenting for assistance at outreach or community clinics; see also Table 12-2. The procedure can be used as a simple assessment for any patient. This basic assessment needs no equipment, but it can reveal a wealth of information to guide treatment and practice outcomes:

- Assess for life-threatening urgency, chest pain, sweating, pallor to mucous membranes, dyspnoea or tachypnoea, alteration in level of consciousness, alertness or lack of responsiveness to command.
- Listen carefully to the actual details of the presenting problem and issues surrounding the presentation; listen for information that may give clues to the extent of the presenting problem.
- Include and use family members who have presented with the patient to gather more information.
- Prioritise medical referral and include the patient and family members in communications with the patient.
- Be open to Māori or traditional explanations of health issues and treatments and seek their complementarity to mainstream or Western therapies.

CLINICAL TIP

Patients with complex chronic conditions with multiple comorbidities may deteriorate rapidly. Nurses should:

- **Be mindful of the risk of chronic conditions exacerbating to acute, life-threatening emergencies**
- **Ensure the patient is aware of the action plan in case of further deterioration.**

HEALTH ASSESSMENT IN THE COMMUNITY ENVIRONMENT

Health assessment in the community environment requires health professionals to take a wider view of the environment that presents. Community cases can challenge their established ethical, moral and clinical thinking. The ability to develop 'community eyes' and to use a wide range of skills to assist the patient or families in a meaningful way is a useful attribute.

Many problems that present will be 'the tip of the iceberg'; that is, they may not appear to be directly related to a health issue but may be indirectly affecting the overall wellbeing of the family or group. As the patients' and their families' advocate, the health professional should be constantly aware of the

Table 12-2 Emergency presentation in the community outreach setting

Basic examination	Clinical observation	Differential diagnosis
Assess life-threatening situation		
Undertake visual overall body scan	Observe for deviations from normal	General appearance, chest pain, sweating, rash, posture, skin colour and temperature
Complete respiratory system assessment	Assess respiratory rate and rhythm Check colour of nail beds and mucosa, lips, eyelids Anxiety level	Dyspnoea, tachypnoea Degree of cyanosis, other abnormality, clubbing Hyperventilation
Complete haemodynamic assessment	Observe skin colour, body temperature Feel pulse, volume, speed and rhythm Feel hands and feet—hot or cold or normal	Pallor, flushing, hot, cold Tachycardia—dehydration, shock Bradycardia—sick sinus syndrome Irregular—decompensated cardiac arrhythmia Cool—reduced circulation and cardiac output syndrome associated with shock or septicaemia Hot—overstimulated circulation, also associated with phase of septicaemia and shock
Complete neurological assessment	Check level of consciousness, alert, drowsy Assess ability to communicate, slurred speech, loss of muscle power in limbs, facial droop	Possible neurological event
History and presenting problem		
Listen carefully to the patient and relatives to get accurate picture Encourage and support *whānau*-centred connections Use community health worker to liaise with and support patient and *whānau* needs Assess social and cultural stressors	Listen for buzz words that may indicate more serious health deviation Assess degree to which these issues may be contributing to current illness	For example, haemoptysis, altered bowel habits or bleeding from bowel and night sweats Family disagreement or death in family Stress trigger to event; financial or living situation
Assess vital signs		
If equipment is available, check blood pressure, temperature, oxygen saturation and pulse Take electrocardiogram if rhythm disturbance is noted	Record and observe for further deviation; refer to medical team on their arrival	
Stabilise and refer on to medical services or local hospital via district ambulance		
Follow-up by community nursing staff via phone call or hospital visit is customary and ensures continuity of care and commencement of discharge planning		

rights of all of those involved and ensure they are receiving appropriate treatment.

Nurses should also be aware of their own values and beliefs, and ensure they are not imposing these on the individuals and *whānau* with whom they are working. It is important to be alert to the cultural sensitivities of individuals and the group, and to avoid causing offence—for example, by touching an individual's head without first obtaining their consent, or by moving a pillow from beneath a patient's feet and placing it beneath his or her head, because the head is viewed in *Te Ao Māori* as *tapu* (sacred or restricted) (Māuri Ora Associates, 2008). Causing such cultural offence may result in future access to the family being prohibited.

Complex community cases may take months or even years to achieve their objectives, and some never achieve all the goals identified by the *whānau*, who set the timelines. Prioritise issues of importance. Small improvements in social situations may have a major impact on the health of a family, and sometimes by improving one issue, many other issues disappear. For example, if a family group is living in poor, overcrowded housing, assistance in finding more appropriate accommodation will alleviate a multitude of other issues. Attention to small things can make a big difference: in some cases, they can be life-changing for the patient and their *whānau*.

Another factor that rural health service providers may need to consider is the influence of isolation. Working in community environments can be lonely for practitioners, and isolation can lead to burnout. It is important to build a team of like-minded care providers who share both a sense of commitment and philosophies of health care delivery. The team should be able to handle the level of care delivery that is identified in the community. In some cases, working in communities is a way of life, and the close, life-long connections formed between practitioners and the groups with whom they work can take health care to a new dimension.

Nursing in the primary care environment

A large proportion of health care is delivered in community environments in New Zealand, and this care is becoming more complex as patients age, live longer and undergo more complex medical procedures that are subject to early discharge from hospital environments. Urban to rural shifts of the population are also increasing health care needs in community environments, and consequently primary health care and secondary service responses are stretched. The health workforce across New Zealand faces challenges because of ageing and increasing number of retiring general practitioners (Royal New Zealand College of General Practitioners [RNZCGP], 2018), highlighting the urgent need to support solution-orientated workforce alternatives. Nurses play a central role in maintaining the stability of the workforce within these environments, especially in rural, isolated and marginalized populations.

Nursing has been undergoing a transformation, and this transformation has been about preparing nurses academically and clinically to advanced levels of practice to enable them to manage health interactions across the full spectrum of need, with improving access to health care, especially in community environments, the specific focus. Currently, the NCNZ Ministry of Health Chief Nurses Office the academic training facilities of nursing, and the New Zealand Nursing Organization have been working to implement nurse prescribing. Nurse prescribing has been gaining momentum for 20 years, and currently New Zealand nurses have pathways to three levels of nurse prescribers.

Nurse practitioners who are authorised prescribers are able to practise autonomously or in teams. They are authorised to diagnose, manage and treat patients, providing full episodes of care. Registered Nurse (RN) prescribers who are able to work in specialty areas or primary health care areas (e.g. diabetes nurse prescribers and long-term condition specialty nurses) must work with health care teams where they have access to medical or nurse practitioner supervision and have a limited pharmacopeia. The newest level of nurse prescribers is the RN prescriber in communities (NCNZ, 2019). This level of prescriber has been under a pilot program for some time and is now recognised as a viable model for supporting patient care in community environments. This prescribing nurse must be supported and work in primary health care teams and have a restricted pharmacopeia. These forms of advanced nurses will be able to support community populations gain access to health care in a timelier fashion.

Implications for Māori health in communities

It is acknowledged that Māori are most affected by limitations to access to health care, a situation that has been alluded to in this chapter. Issues of access to health care for Māori are complex and long-standing (Hauora, 2019). It has been proposed that primary care health services lack culturally sensitive approaches within their service delivery models. In the context of Māori health needs and attendance to general practice, there is imbalance and deficits around cultural safety and funding models, highlighting the financial outlay required to attend to the complexity of health issues and to provide continuing education and support sustainable health goals for Māori. Advanced nursing roles in New Zealand have a care delivery perspective that embraces models of care that holistically care for patients and families. It is these holistic *whānau*-centred models that incorporate equity that will create a brighter future for the health of Māori and their *whānau*.

CASE STUDY 2

A Māori health service provider receives a call from a concerned citizen, who asks to speak to a nurse. You take the call. The concerned citizen reports she has seen three Māori toddlers playing, unsupervised, on the side of a busy road. The caller gives you the address and description of the house where she believes they are living. This family is unknown to you.

CRITICAL THINKING

6. Using both the *Te Whare Tapa Whā* health model consideration of Pae ora and the *Whānau Ora* nursing concepts, how would you approach this case?
7. What would be your priorities to ensure the best outcomes for all?
8. Whose aid would you enlist to check that the children are safe and off the road, bearing in mind national guidelines on child protection and the need to build a relationship of trust with the family?
9. How would you protect the rights of this family?
10. Would you ask Māori wardens or a Māori support group to visit the house and check that the children are safe?

Points to consider when using the *Whānau Ora* nursing model

Refer to Figure 12-7.

- *Short-term options*: Provide options to alleviate the pressure of the presenting problem; arrange emergency food, shelter, medications and financial assistance
- *Relationships*: Develop trust, understanding, empowerment and collaboration with *whānau* or *family* supports and connections
- *Economic barriers*: Assess issues of existing medical expenses, limited financial resources and limited income, and review social benefit entitlements; assess the possible effect of *whakamā* (embarrassment, shame) as a cause of patient not presenting to the health service provider
- *Employment*: Explore possible employment opportunities, training and support to gain meaningful employment; review reduced opportunities related to the existing disease process, injury or mental health issues; explore options of social benefits
- *Housing, employment, cultural expressions and health needs*: Explore disadvantage related to transport, geographical isolation and telephone access to health service; develop long-term solutions with *whānau* or the individual over time.

CASE STUDY 2: EXTENSION

Case checklist

- Gather information
- Discuss and involve the community health worker
- Establish and develop relationship with the family

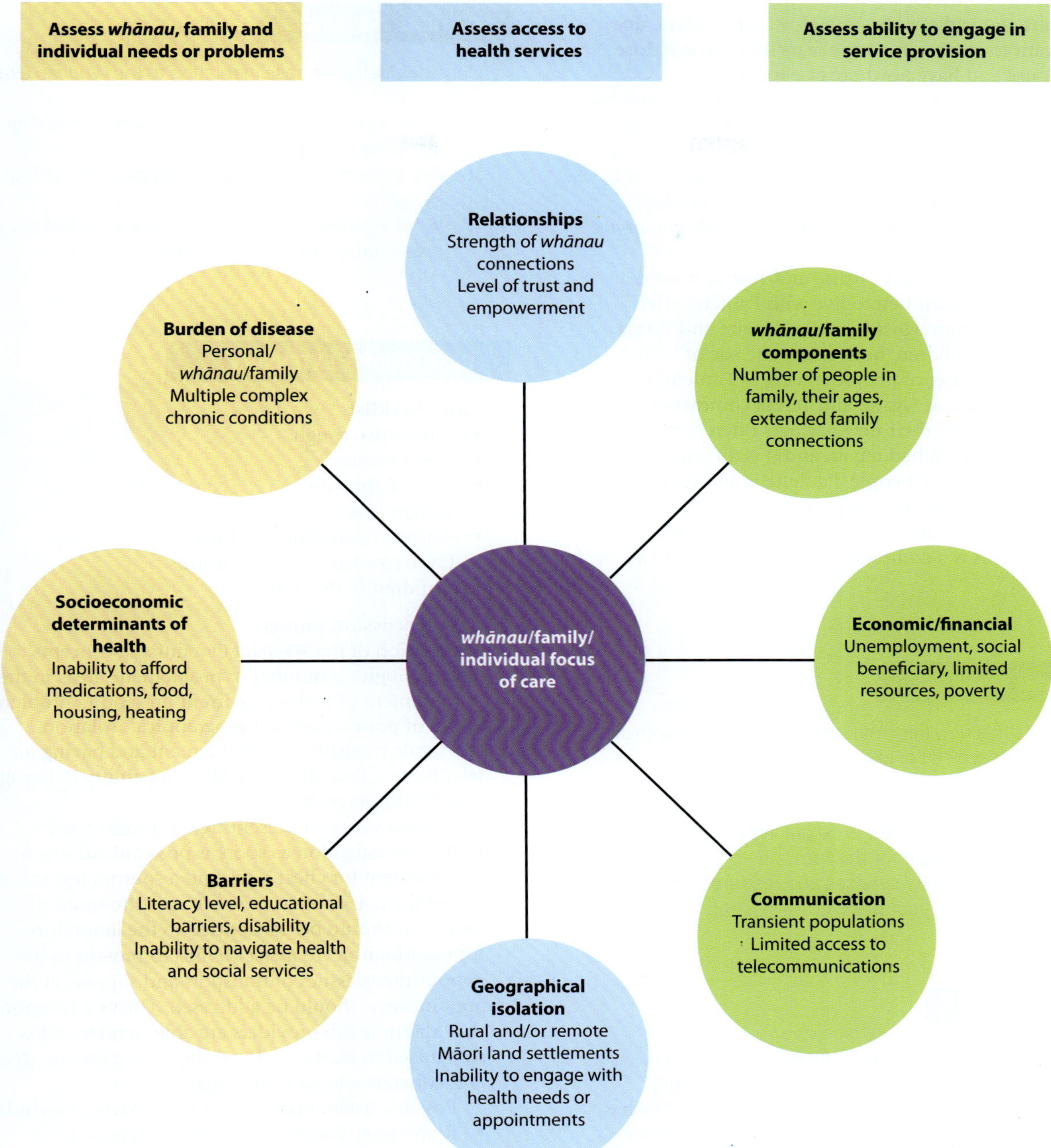

FIGURE 12-7 *Whānau Ora* or family nursing model for community environments.

- Assess family components, needs and issues
- Discuss the issues of most importance for stability
- Navigate the family towards options that will lead them to their goals

Additional case detail

Following up on the call from the concerned citizen, you have located the grandmother of the toddlers and met her. You now have the following case history.

Paulette is a 46-year-old Māori woman, a grandmother and mother. After separating from her husband 3 years ago, she found managing on her own very difficult. Deciding that she needed the support of *whānau*, she recently moved to the area because her brother and his family live there. She rents a three-bedroom house, the only one she can afford, but it is in a very dilapidated condition. It has no heating or curtains and leaks in the rain. However, Paulette does not want to complain, as she fears that she may lose the house and have nowhere else to go.

Paulette has three adult children living with her: two daughters and one son, Henare, who is now 21 years old. When Henare was 10, he lost his hearing. He has been deaf since then and has experienced subsequent learning difficulties. He has been under disability services for some years but lost contact with the service in the last 2 years.

Paulette's daughters, Ngaire and Teresa, moved back with their children to live with Paulette after experiencing marriage difficulties. Ngaire and Teresa each has two children, both under the age of 5. At times, the number of people staying in Paulette's house increases, as Ngaire and Teresa commence new relationships and their new partners often come to stay.

The house is in bad repair, and it is difficult to keep clean with so many people. Paulette is an extremely caring woman and very supportive of her family. She has just found a job in a local café and is happy to be working. This is a complex case and is identified as high-risk.

CRITICAL THINKING

11. Does this new information alter your initial approach to this case? If so, explain.
12. What are your main health concerns for this extended family?
13. What strategies need to be put in place to achieve a safe environment for this family?
14. What community services and resources would you incorporate in your plan?

CASE STUDY 3

You are running an outreach nurse-led clinic in a remote Māori settlement at the *marae* (meeting house). Melissa, age 28, presents to the clinic. She has a history of asthma. She tells you she ran out of her corticosteroid inhaler a week ago and is experiencing shortness of breath. With further questioning, she admits the shortness of breath has been worsening over the last 3 weeks and that she has also experienced increased cough (productive) and night sweats. She adds she feels anxious all the time. She reports reduced appetite and some weight loss. Further discussion discloses she moved to the city 6 months ago in search of a job, as there was no work available on the settlement. While in the city, she lived with *whānau*. However, she was unable to find work there, so just over a month ago she returned home and moved back into her mother's house on the settlement. This three-bedroom house is occupied by her mother, her two sisters and their six children. There is no telephone, and mobile reception is very poor.

CRITICAL THINKING

Consider Melissa's case in relation to the *Whānau Ora* program.

15. What would be your priorities around presenting symptomatology?
16. Are there any red flags with Melissa's presenting symptoms?
17. What are your responsibilities related to Melissa's presentation and health needs?

CASE STUDY 3: EXTENSION

Case checklist

- Productive cough
- Night sweats
- Loss of appetite
- Weight loss
- Asthma or shortness of breath
- Overcrowded living conditions
- Children in the house

Case discussion points

Application of the *Whānau Ora* nursing concepts to this case highlights a number of problematic areas in the management of Melissa's current presenting problem. Issues of poor access and geographical isolation, economic hardship, unemployment and having no telephone access all reduce Melissa's ability to engage with health services.

Melissa's current presenting symptoms need further investigation as soon as possible. An urgent appointment for chest X-ray and a sputum test should be obtained as soon as possible, and the sputum specimen should be transported to the laboratory for examination. To assist Melissa to present to this appointment, issues of transport and support at the appointment should be addressed. This is a component that Māori health providers are able to offer and is recognised to be successful at improving service access and adherence to treatment plans.

Possible differential diagnoses for Melissa include:

- Respiratory infection? Causative organism
- Exacerbation of asthma
- Pulmonary tuberculosis(TB)?

Tuberculosis is one of the most common notifiable infectious diseases in New Zealand. In 2011, 626 cases of TB were reported (Bissielo et al., 2012). Reasons for the persistence of TB as a public health problem are complex. They include immigration from countries where there is a high incidence of TB, social conditions favouring transmission of TB and the fact that identification and prophylaxis for all infected people is not practicable (NZMOH, 2017b) (Immunisation Advisory Centre, Auckland University). Worldwide, active pulmonary TB is highly contagious, and case management must follow strict guidelines for control, contact tracing, treatment and monitoring.

CASE STUDY 4

Veronica is a 48-year-old Māori woman who lives with her husband Hone and three children in public housing accommodation in a small rural town. Both Veronica and Hone have a long history of asthma. Their children, Lulu (age 3), Tane (7) and Joseph (10), also have asthma.

Veronica is employed as a care worker providing homecare services for people in the local community. Hone works at the local vegetable processing plant. They have a busy life and have close affiliations to their family *marae*. Veronica and Hone were born in this region, and their families are descendants of the local *Māori iwi*.

Veronica, Hone and their children are enrolled as patients of the local Māori health service provider and use the *koha* (donation) or free health clinics offered by this service. Children under 14 years can be seen without charge at community health services as well as receiving free prescriptions. Everyone in the family is affected by asthma. It is important the whole family observe their treatment regimens, which means they need to undergo regular assessment and medical prescriptions. The local general practitioner (GP) who attends the clinic has stipulated the family must present to get prescriptions and that there are no exceptions to this requirement.

Louise, the primary nurse in charge of the family's case, phones Veronica to discuss any potential problems with the GP's requirements. Veronica tells Louise one of her concerns is that she cannot take the children to the morning clinics as she is at work and they are at school. Another problem is that the children often lose their inhalers or have trouble identifying who owns which inhaler, so they can end up sharing inhalers. Veronica makes sure that the children take their medications regularly, as she knows first-hand the potential risks and consequences of uncontrolled asthma, but she highlights to Louise a problem with cost: purchasing inhalers for her entire family is an expense the family struggles to meet.

Louise arranges a home visit the following afternoon to make a plan to assist this *whānau* in achieving their health goals. The community health worker who will accompany her, Paula, has not yet met the family but knows of them through her connections.

Home visit

The issues for discussion are as follows:

- Assistance with access to the clinics
- Sharing of medications in the family
- Financial concerns related to the cost of the medications.

The children are all stable at present. It is summer and the weather is warm. Last winter the nursing team helped the family to find their current accommodation, because the house they had been living in was very damp and was exacerbating their asthma symptoms, as well as causing an increased number of cold and flu symptoms. Veronica reports that this house is much improved from their last home; it has a double-burning wood fire with a fan, which is in good working order, and this will be of great help throughout the winter. Through the family's connections to the *marae* and Māori land, they have good access to wood supply for the winter.

Veronica and Hone are both home with the children when Louise and Paula arrive. Discussion commences with introductions and greetings. Louise introduces Paula, who makes her *whakapapa* known to them. Veronica and Hone reply with information on their own origins and the group briefly acknowledge each other's family and connections. (It is important to make a connection with patients in some way. Within Māori culture, the sharing of background and identity is a critical element in establishing rapport and can effectively form the basis for therapeutic communication to develop. Māori individuals and families need to know that their health care professional is reliable and can be depended upon to deliver the services they promise.)

Improving access to the clinics

In considering the problem of access, Louise asks Veronica and Hone if they would consent to Paula collecting the children from school and taking them to clinic to get their prescriptions from the GP. Veronica and Hone could write a note to release them from school for half an hour. Louise and Paula would ensure that the children were returned to school in time. (Within community environments, health and education staff work closely together; collaboration between services operates to achieve positive results for children across the community.)

Sharing of medications within the family

This is not a perfect scenario, but it is easy to see how medication sharing happens with young children. Louise suggests that they request assistance from the community pharmacy to colour-code each child's prescription inhaler: pink for Lulu, blue for Tane and purple for Joseph. This will reduce cross-contamination of potential respiratory infections and assist with the evaluation of each child's medication usage, treatment compliance and degree of disease management.

Financial concerns

The New Zealand government has eased the financial burden related to prescription charges for children under 14, waiving the fee that existed previously for this age group. Financial concerns now rest on the cost of transport to attend appointments and the potential loss of wages from taking time off work to attend these visits with these children.

Disease management over time: Continuity of care

During subsequent consultations, Louise can ensure that Veronica, Hone and their children better manage their disease by:

- Referring them to the Māori asthma nurse for a family education session
- Incorporating evidenced-based best practice guidelines for asthma

- Reinforcing inhaler and spacer techniques
- Educating them regarding early recognition of asthma exacerbations or chest infection
- Preparing an action plan for an acute asthma event
- Educating them about healthy airways
- Promoting a smoke-free and pollutant-free environment
- Organising school-based education with teachers and students regarding asthma and its control in the school environment

Case discussion points and objectives

This case represents a *Whānau Ora* approach to nursing assessment in the community environment. These concepts are practised by problem-solving nurses who work directly with patients and their families in the community. Community situations are often far from perfect; however, simple common sense and education can improve outcomes. The important principle for nursing assessment and care in the Māori community is to ensure that respect and understanding of life problems are considered not from the health carer's personal perspective but from the perspective of the patient or family involved.

The following elements are integral to delivering effective health care in the community setting:

- Family or patient-centred care needs to be empowering; it requires the health professional to walk alongside patients and to offer options that may assist patients in managing difficult situations themselves.
- It is important to incorporate cultural connections into the care provided: using a community health worker who has long-standing connections in the region often quickly and effectively secures the formation of trusting relationships.
- The care factor—the formation of a trusting relationship with the patient or family—is vital. The health professional should demonstrate a caring and helpful attitude and reassure the patient and family about their ongoing support. Reflection of practice and critical analysis of return visits and contact often provide confirmation that a successful and meaningful relationship has been developed.

HOSPITAL ADMISSIONS FOR MĀORI

Being admitted to hospital is a traumatic event for many Māori. As to reasons for Māori reluctance to submit to hospital admission, Barton and Wilson (2012) cite visiting hours, suspicion and biomedical approaches. Restrictions to visiting hours in the hospital environment leave patients and family members feeling vulnerable, and often past experiences of family members passing in poorly explained or understood consequences contribute to higher levels of suspicion. In a retrospective cross-sectional assessment, Davis et al. (2006) examined the quality of care received by Māori while in hospital. Their findings suggest the hospital care Māori receive is marginally poorer than that received by New Zealand citizens of non-Māori or non-Pacific origin. Hospital systems throughout New Zealand have acknowledged that there are issues related to care provided to Māori in hospital environments. Wilson and Barton (2012), reviewing Māori experiences of hospitalisation, revealed Māori had shorter lengths of stay than non-Māori. Patients surveyed cited experiences that were not conducive to healing, and these patients requested to have early discharge.

Systems that include cultural and social needs are of high priority, including support while in hospital and inclusion of family in decision making and patient treatment plans. Furthermore, support and assistance with accommodation, transport and food are now considered and arranged for patients and their families. Māori who are hospitalised may be many kilometres from the support of their local extended *whānau*. Many families do not have the resources to support their relatives while they are in hospital, especially when the major health facilities are so far from home. Admission to hospital can impose heavy strains on families who are already stretched to their limit. Within community environments, staff working with these patients have close community relationships and extended knowledge of connections. It is this knowledge that can assist in hospital admission and the smooth transition between the primary and secondary services environment.

Display 12-2 outlines community health care priorities for Māori patients in hospital.

DISPLAY 12-2 COMMUNITY HEALTH CARE PRIORITIES FOR MĀORI PATIENTS WHO REQUIRE HOSPITALISED CARE

When providing community health care for Māori patients it is important to:

- Provide a culturally and clinically competent environment
- Give prompt attention to life-threatening situations
- Make prompt referral to mainstream medical services
- Ensure effective communication: engage, support and inform the patient and family of health plans
- Assist navigation of family supports—that is, transport, accommodation, travel assistance options and arrangements for care of children, elders and pets
- Assist with notification of extended *whānau* or other persons of cultural or religious importance
- Secure links with hospital staff regarding the case and issues related to the family situation
- Advise the Māori hospital liaison team of the patient's admission
- Make hospital visits or phone calls to support the patient and family, and provide progress updates
- Attend the hospital multidisciplinary meeting to assist with discharge planning
- Offer support at family planning meetings, if required
- Work with the patient and family to plan changes to the home environment and health needs at discharge
- Arrange the post-discharge home visit (within 3 days); review the treatment plan, follow up arrangements and requirements; and assist with medical practitioner or specialist follow-up appointments
- Assess the need for increased community support—issues related to medication adherence as well as understanding of the treatment plan and clinical stability
- Review the findings from home visit with the local medical practitioner assigned to the patient.

The community health team's responsibility for patients does not change if the patients are hospitalised; the time may present a short interlude where improvements or critical health issues need to be attended to, but the patient and family will continue to receive support and reassurance from the health team. This support includes cultural and clinical components. Families often request *karakia* (prayers) or *waiata* (songs) (Māuri Ora Associates, 2008) at the bedside, or an explanation of what is happening to them from a clinical point of view. This requires simple explanations; take the time to find out the treatment plan and relay it to the patient and *whānau*. In some cases, the family may have been informed of the treatment plan but are unable to comprehend the information given. Many times, it is not until patients are at home in their own environment that health messages and teachings are consolidated.

SUMMARY

In New Zealand, post-colonisation societal and governmental attitudes to Māori health have come a long way in a relatively short period. This is testimony to the many Māori leaders who have remained committed to the health and wellness of all Māori. Today, Māori have a higher standard of health than in previous post-colonisation generations, and they are actively involved in health policy and responsible for the provision of health services that endorse the recognition of *tikanga* Māori and Māori health perspectives.

This chapter has focused on health assessment in Māori communities. Health care delivery in community environments accounts for a major proportion of health interventions in New Zealand. The development of innovative community health services that also incorporate concepts of cultural beliefs and values is progressing, with the objectives of improving access to health services for Māori, stabilising and managing people with existing disease, preventing and slowing the progression of diseases that are causing high morbidity and mortality, and improving the health and lives of young Māori. The challenge for the government is to acknowledge and nurture these organisations and services to allow them to deliver care to their full potential.

Māori health providers are not taking over from mainstream providers; they work collaboratively or in partnership with mainstream providers, using available resources to address a recognised gap in service provision within their communities. Māori health providers are an example of one innovative model of health service delivery for Māori. The future will bring many new models of service delivery; some of these models will come from nursing arenas. Nurses have the capacity to improve community service delivery and, in the future, will provide local services to communities at a low cost, which will help improve access to health services for Māori. Nurses are well positioned to provide and deliver care that is culturally, spiritually and clinically competent. They can empower and coordinate individuals and *whānau* to address complex social issues that are impeding their ability to engage and grow. This is *Whānau Ora*, the model in action. New Zealand nurses must take up the challenge and make positive advances in reducing health inequity and inequalities wherever they are found.

ONLINE RESOURCES

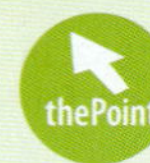

An extensive range of additional resources to enhance teaching and learning and to facilitate understanding may be found online at the text's accompanying website, located on thePoint at http://thepoint.lww.com. These include Watch and Learn videos, Concepts in Action animations, journal articles, case studies, discussion topics and quizzes.

Subscribers may also access Lippincott Procedures, an extensive online point-of-care procedure guide that provides reliable step-by-step instructions for more than 1,700 procedures, including 450 evidence-based Australian procedures, and skills in a variety of speciality settings, together with a wealth of supporting information.

References

Barton, P. & Wilson, D. (2012). Indigenous hospital experiences: A New Zealand case study. *Journal of Clinical Nursing, 21*, 2316–2326.

Bissielo, A., Lim, E. & Heffernan, H. (2012). *Tuberculosis in New Zealand: Annual report 2011*. Wellington: Institute of Environmental Science and Research, Wellington.

Boast, R. (2009). Story: Te tango whenuā—Māori land alienation. In *Te Ara: The encyclopedia of New Zealand* (online). Wellington: Ministry for Culture and Heritage.

Boulton, A. & Gifford, H. (2014). Whanau Ora; He Whakaaro Ā Whānau: Māori family views of family wellbeing. *The International Indigenous Policy Journal, 5*(1).

Curtis, E., Jones, R., Tipene-Leach, D., et al. (2019). Why cultural safety rather than cultural competency is required to achieve health equity; a literature review and recommended definition. *International Journal for Equity in Health, 18*, 174.

Davis, P., Lay-Yee, R., Dyall, L., et al. (2006). Quality of hospital care for Māori patients in New Zealand: Retrospective cross-sectional assessment. *The Lancet, 367*(9526), 1920–1925.

Derby, M. (2012). Māori–Pākehā relations—Māori renaissance. In *Te Ara: The encyclopedia of New Zealand* (online). Wellington: Ministry for Culture and Heritage.

Durie, M. (1998). *Whaiora: Māori health development* (2nd ed.). Auckland: Oxford University Press.

Ellison-Loschmann, L. & Pearce, N. (2006). Improving access to health care among New Zealand's Māori population. *American Journal of Public Health, 96*(4), 612–616.

Harris, R., Cormack, D. & Stanley, J. (2019). Experience of racism and associations of unmet need and healthcare satisfaction: The 2011/12 adult New Zealand health survey. *Australian and New Zealand Journal of Public Health, 43*, 1.

Hauora. (2019) Health services and outcomes inquiry. Available at https://waitangitribunal.govt.nz/inquiries/kaupapa-inquiries/health-services-and-outcomes-inquiry.

Health, Quality & Safety Commission New Zealand. (2019). A window on the quality of Aotearoa New Zealand health care 2019. Available at www.hqsc.govt.nz.

Howe, K. R. (2009a). Ideas of Māori origins: 1880s-1970s; Moriori origins; the Great Fleet. In *Te Ara: The encyclopedia of New Zealand* (online). Wellington: Ministry for Culture and Heritage.

Howe, K. R. (2009b). Ideas of Māori origins: 1920s-2000; new understanding. In *Te Ara: The encyclopedia of New Zealand* (online). Wellington: Ministry for Culture and Heritage.

La Gasse, L., Wouldes, T., Newman, E., et al. (2010). Prenatal methamphetamine exposure and neo natal neurobehavioural outcome in the USA and New Zealand. *Neurotoxicology and Teratology, 33*, 166–175.

Lai, J. C. (2010). *Māori culture in the modern world: Its creation, appropriation and trade. i-Call Research Centre working paper no. 2010/02*. Lucerne: University of Lucerne, Switzerland.

Lambert, M., Luke, J. Downey, B., et al. (2014). Health literacy: Health professionals' understandings and their perceptions of barriers that indigenous patients encounter. *Health Services Research, 14*, 614.

Māuri Ora Associates. (2008). *Best outcomes for Māori: Practice implications*. Wellington: Medical Council of New Zealand.

McLintock, A. H. (Ed). (1966a, updated 2009). Pre-colonial period. In *Te Ara: The encyclopedia of New Zealand* (online). Wellington: Ministry for Culture and Heritage.

McLintock, A. H. (1966b, updated 2009). Settlement from 1840 to 1852. In *Te Ara: The encyclopedia of New Zealand* (online). Wellington: Ministry for Culture and Heritage.

National Library of New Zealand. (2010). Māori Language Week, 2010. Available at www.natlib govt.nz/collections/online-exhibitions/maori-language-week-2010.

New Zealand Drug Foundation. (2018). 'Health not handcuffs campaign'. Available at https://www.drugfoundation.org.nz/about-us/.

New Zealand Ministry for Culture and Heritage. (2013). *Māori Language Week—Te Wiki o Te Reo Māori*. Wellington: Author.

New Zealand Ministry of Health (NZMOH). (2000). New Zealand Public Health and Disability Act (2000). Available at www.health.govt.nz/new-zealand-health-system/overview-health-system/statutory-framework.

New Zealand Ministry of Health (NZMOH). (2009a). *Ka Tika Ka Ora: Māori Health Provider Work Programme, 2009–2010*. Wellington: Author.

New Zealand Ministry of Health (NZMOH). (2009b). *Te Toi Hauora-Nui: Achieving excellence through innovative Māori health service delivery*. Wellington: Author.

New Zealand Ministry of Health (NZMOH). (2010a). *Kōrero Mārama health literacy and Māori: Results from the 2006 adult literacy and life skills survey*. Wellington: Author.

New Zealand Ministry of Health (NZMOH). (2010b). *Whānau Ora integrated service delivery: Report*. Wellington: Author.

New Zealand Ministry of Health (NZMOH). (2013). *The health of Māori adults and children. Brief*. Wellington: Author.

New Zealand Ministry of Health (NZMOH). (2014a). *The guide to He Korowai Oranga: Māori health strategy*. Wellington: Author.

New Zealand Ministry of Health (NZMOH). (2014b). *The Principles of the Treaty of Waitangi*. Available at https://www.health.govt.nz/our-work/populations/maori-health/he-korowai-oranga/strengthening-he-korowai-oranga/treaty-waitangi-principles.

New Zealand Ministry of Health (NZMOH). (2015). *Tatau KahukuraMāori health chart book* (3rd ed.). Wellington: Author.

New Zealand Ministry of Health (NZMOH). (2016). Amphetamine use 2015/16: New Zealand health survey. Available at www.health.govt.nz/publication/amphetamine-use-2015-16-new-zealand-health-survey.

New Zealand Ministry of Health (NZMOH). (2017a). New Zealand health survey. Available at https://www.health.govt.nz/nz-health-statistics/national-collections-and-surveys/surveys/new-zealand-health-survey.

New Zealand Ministry of Health (NZMOH). (2017b). Immunisation handbook (2nd ed.). Wellington: Author. Available at https://www.health.govt.nz/publication/immunisation-handbook-2017.

New Zealand Ministry of Health (NZMOH). (2019a). Improving the health of New Zealanders. Available at https://www.health.govt.nz/nz-health-statistics/national-collections-and-surveys/surveys/new-zealand-health-survey/improving-health-new-zealanders.

New Zealand Ministry of Health (NZMOH). (2019b). Health and disability system review interim review Hauora Manaaki ki Aotearoa whanui-Purango mo Tenei Wa. Wellington. Available at www.systemreview.health.govt.nz/interim-report.

Ngata, P. (2005) Death, dying and grief. In M. Schwass (Ed). *Last words: Approaches to death in New Zealand's cultures and faiths*. Wellington: Bridget Williams Books.

Nursing Council of New Zealand (NCNZ). (2009). *Guidelines for cultural safety, the Treaty of Waitangi and Māori health in nursing, education and practice*. Wellington: Nursing Council of New Zealand/Te Kaunihera Tapuhi o Aotearoa. Available at www.nursingcouncil.org.nz.

Nursing Council of New Zealand (NCNZ). (2019). Available at https://www.nursingcouncil.org.nz/Public/Nursing/Nurse_prescribing/NCNZ/nursing-section/Nurse_Prescribing.aspx.

Parliamentary Counsel Office New Zealand Legislation. (2003). Health Practitioners Competence Assurance Act (2003). Available at www.legislation.govt.nz.

Phillips, J. (2009). History of immigration: Early years. In *Te Ara: The encyclopedia of New Zealand* (online). Wellington: Ministry for Culture and Heritage.

Phillips, J. (2010). History of immigration: British immigration and the New Zealand Company. In *Te Ara: The encyclopedia of New Zealand* (online). Wellington: Ministry for Culture and Heritage.

Pihama, L. (2011). Overview of Māori teen pregnancy. Report prepared for the New Zealand Families Commission, Wellington. Auckland: Māori and Indigenous Analysis Ltd.

Royal New Zealand College of General Practitioners (RNZCGP). (2018). 2017 General practice workforce survey—Part 1. March, p. 3. Available at https://www.rnzcgp.org.nz/gpdocs/Workforce-Survey-2017-Report-1-final.pdf.

Sandiford, P., Bramley, D., El-Jack, S., et al. (2015). Ethnic differences in coronary artery revascularisation in New Zealand: Does the inverse care law still apply? *Heart, Lung & Circulation, 24*, 969–974.

Simon, V. (2001). *Characterising Māori nursing practice.* Unpublished Master's thesis, University of Waikato, Hamilton.

Stanley, E. & Mihaere, R. (2019). The problems and promise of international rights in the challenge to Māori imprisonment. *International Journal for Crime, Justice and Social Democracy, 8*(1), 1–17.

Thomas, D. R. & Nikora, L. W. (1992). From assimilation to biculturalism: Changing patterns in Māori-Pākehā relationships. In D. R. Thomans & A. Veno (Eds). *Community psychology and social change: Australian and New Zealand perspectives*. Palmerston North: Dunmore Press.

Wilson, D. & Barton, P. (2012). Indigenous hospital experiences: A New Zealand case study. *Journal of Clinical Nursing, 21*, 2316–2326.

Selected readings

State Services Commission. (2005a). *The story of the treaty*. Wellington: The Treaty of Waitangi Information Programme, State Services Commission.

State Services Commission. (2005b). *All about the treaty*. Wellington: The Treaty of Waitangi Information Programme, State Services Commission.

Online resources

National Council of Māori Nurses/Te Kaunihera o Nga Neehi Māori o Aotearoa: http://maorinursescouncil.nz

New Zealand Ministry of Health: www.health.govt.nz

New Zealand Ministry of Health, Māori Health: www.health.govt.nz/our-work/populations/maori-health

Te Puni Kōkiri: www.tpk.govt.nz/en

CHAPTER 13

Assessing spirituality and religious practices

CASE STUDY

Paula Li is a 39-year-old woman who lives with her three children and husband in a rural community. Paula attends church regularly and normally derives comfort from her faith. However, a recent cancer diagnosis is challenging her faith. You are talking with Paula after she has returned to the ward following radiotherapy for breast cancer.

Introduction to spiritual assessment

WHAT IS SPIRITUALITY?

Spirituality and religion are important factors in health and can influence health decisions and outcomes. Recent census data in Australia (Australian Bureau of Statistics [ABS], 2016) and New Zealand (Statistics New Zealand, 2013) show a small downward trend in reported religious affliation in both countries; however, religious affiliation remains at nearly 60% of Australians and 54% of New Zealanders. Whereas the number of Australians (8.2%) reporting non-Christian affiliations is increasing, the number of New Zealanders reporting non-Christian affiliations has slightly decreased (6.3%). Census reporting in Australia and New Zealand also indicate an increase in reporting of no religion (30% in Australia and 38.5% in New Zealand), and identify a rising cultural and linguisitic diversity, due to continuing non-European migrant and refugee growth. Greater cultural diversity has brought an increasing variety of religious and spiritual practices to the Australasian cultural milieu, which is evident in the rise in Muslim, Hindu, Buddhist and other religions and spiritual practices. There is also an increasing trend towards the use of non-religious spiritual practices in Australia (ABS, 2016; McCrindle, 2017; MacKinlay, 2010) and New Zealand (Nachowitz, 2007; Statistics New Zealand, 2013).

CLINICAL TIP

An awareness of the cultural, religious and spiritual diversity within a nurse's community will enable the nurse to provide care that focuses better on the patient's spiritual needs.

But what is religion? What is spirituality? People are often confused about religion and spirituality. The concepts overlap; however, although religion and spirituality share some common traits (i.e. seeking meaning and connection), there are some clear differences (Display 13-1). Dempsey et al. (2014) define *religion* as the rituals, practices and experiences shared within a group that involve a search for the sacred (God, Allah, etc.). For some faiths, this idea of religion encompasses the concept of spirituality and is a natural outflow of that idea. Others may view spirituality as a separate concept, possibly disconnected from any religious institution. In fact, the number of persons describing themselves as 'spiritual but not religious' has risen substantially over the past decade (Ammerman, 2013; McCrindle, 2017; Nielsen, 2009).

Spirituality encompasses a search for meaning, purpose and connectedness; it seeks to understand life's ultimate questions in relation to the sacred (Puchalski et al., 2014). It may include New Age philosophies and practices (e.g. Gaia philosophy or chakra balancing), or spiritual practices by Aboriginal and Torres Strait Islander Australians (Display 13-2) that connect people to the land (e.g. Australian Aboriginal 'Dreaming', the Torres Strait Islanders' Tagai stories or the Māori concept of *Mana* or spiritual essence).

Common to these spiritual philosophies and practices is the notion that spirituality pervades all aspects of life and is therefore an important element in maintaining health. Concepts of spiritual wellbeing (the status of spiritual health) and spiritual coping (the ability to withstand threats to spiritual wellbeing) increasingly characterise spirituality (Clark & Hunter, 2018). Thoughts about spirituality and religion may vary immensely from one patient to another, and changes in health often affect spiritual wellbeing. Indeed, significant changes in health can lead some patients to question the meaning and purpose of their lives (Mcharo, 2018). During a spiritual assessment, the nurse should keep an objective perspective with the goal of meeting patients at the point of their personal perceptions. Knowing how spiritual views can vary will help nurses to identify possible coping responses; otherwise, these resources might have gone unnoticed.

The literature also suggests that a person's focus on spirituality (religious or otherwise) increases when facing the process of dying (Stephenson & Berry, 2014). Many people find comfort from their spirituality; some will seek answers to

DISPLAY 13-1 FOUNDATIONAL KNOWLEDGE FOR SPIRITUAL ASSESSMENT

Religion
Definition: Rituals, practices and experiences involving a search for the sacred (God, Allah, etc.)* that are shared within a group.

Defining characteristics
- Formal
- Organised
- Group-oriented
- Ritualistic
- Objective, as in easily measurable (e.g. church attendance)

Spirituality
Definition: A search for meaning and purpose in life, which seeks to understand life's ultimate questions in relation to the sacred.

Defining characteristics
- Informal
- Non-organised
- Self-reflection
- Experience
- Subjective, as in difficult to consistently measure (e.g. daily spiritual experiences, spiritual wellbeing)

Spiritual assessment
Definition: Active and ongoing conversation that assesses the spiritual needs of the patient.

Defining characteristics
- Formal or informal
- Respectful
- Non-biased

Spiritual care
Definition: Addressing the spiritual needs of the patient as they unfold through spiritual assessment.

Defining characteristics
- Individualistic
- Patient oriented
- Collaborative

*Substitute God or Allah with universal spirit or higher power throughout this chapter as necessary to support the individual needs of the patient.

DISPLAY 13-2 INDIGENOUS SPIRITUALITY IN AUSTRALIA AND NEW ZEALAND

Aboriginal	Torres Strait Islander	Māori
Dreaming	***Tagai***	***Mana***
A system of knowledge, faith and practices derived from creation that pervades all aspects of Aboriginal life.	A connection to the Tagai stories that spiritually unifies people throughout the Torres Strait.	All living things are descended from the Gods, embodied within certain mountains, rivers and lakes.
Most beliefs centre on connection to either the earth, sea, people or culture.	Torres Strait Islanders are described in the stories as sea people who share a common way of life.	The *wairua* (soul) is in all things and spiritually ties Māori to the land.
Sets out the structures, rules and ceremonies of life.	The instructions of the Tagai provide order and structure in the world.	There is a spiritual essence (Mana) within humans, land, nature and even created objects and artefacts.

Source: Australian Museum, 2019; Korf, 2019; New Zealand in History, 2010.

questions of meaning, whereas others may experience distress around unresolved relationships with their family or their God (MacLeod et al., 2017). Questions around spirituality and death are very common in the palliative care context where the focus is on dignity, quality of remaining life, reducing suffering and the journey towards a peaceful death. It is important in these circumstances for the nurse to recognise the effect death and dying have on both the patient and the surviving family, especially in the case of a terminally ill child, and the need to maintain support to the emotional and spiritual needs of all involved (Nascimento et al., 2016).

WHY ASSESS SPIRITUALITY?

Public opinion and health care research give credence to the importance of the relationship between religion, spirituality and health. Many patients use spiritual resources during times of high stress (Dempsey et al., 2014). Religion and spirituality are associated with a person's greater wellbeing in the face of chronic disease management and adherence to medical regimens. Religion and spirituality can be powerful coping tools for a person facing acute and chronic health problems or end-of-life issues, and nurses should therefore be attentive to the spiritual practices and beliefs of their patients (Penman, 2018).

The positive effects of spirituality on health are well evidenced in the literature (Clark & Hunter, 2018; Moberg, 2011). Spiritual practices have the potential to encourage greater mental and physical health. Among certain populations, religion and spirituality have been related to lower levels of mortality, less heart disease, lower blood pressure, less depression, lower levels of stress, less alcohol and tobacco abuse, greater wellbeing and optimism, and positive health habits (Koenig et al., 2012; Kohn, 2010; Oman, 2018). Nurses generally have more opportunities to address spiritual concerns with patients because nurses are the primary points of contact for most patients in the hospital setting.

Nursing has a long history of incorporating spirituality into patient care. Florence Nightingale (1860 [1996]) wrote at length about a spiritual dimension that provided an inner strength. More recently, nursing theorists have used spirituality as a health determinant in the grand theories that guide nursing practice, and in a number of middle theories that focus on specific elements like spirituality that may be evident in the grand theories (Barnum, 2010). The Nursing and Midwifery Board of

Australia, Australian College of Midwives, Australian Nursing and Midwifery Federation (NMBA, 2017), and the Nursing Council of New Zealand (2012) have all recently adopted the International Council of Nurses Code of Ethics for Nurses (ICN, 2012). In adopting the International Code, these professional nursing bodies clearly recognise the importance of culturally sensitive nursing care that is respectful to the beliefs, religion and spirituality of patients. These references underlie a primary idea that nurses see their patients as holistic beings in body, mind and spirit.

Some religions encourage positive health behaviours and greater mental health, and provide a strong social support network. For example, the nurse may facilitate a referral of a patient newly diagnosed with Hodgkin lymphoma to an appropriate clergy member or hospital chaplain. Regardless of the form of spirituality incorporated into patient care, the nurse should be respectful, open and willing to discuss spiritual issues if he or she sees that doing so is appropriate (MacKinlay, 2010).

CLINICAL TIP
Plans for referral or intervention will develop out of the dialogue between the nurse and the patient.

Overview of spiritual assessment and nursing care

Spiritual assessment does not begin at the bedside. The nurse's knowledge of the cultural, religious and spiritual practices and temperament of the community and their own spirituality will lead to greater ease when discussing the patient's spirituality. To assist in assessing religion and spirituality, it would be useful to define the concepts as interconnected but separate ideas (see Fig. 13-1). With a growing proportion of the population identifying themselves as 'spiritual but not religious', the use of the correct instrument or framework will determine the accuracy of the assessment.

Many variations of spiritual practices exist. Spiritual practices may include prayer (Fig. 13-2), participation in church services (Fig. 13-3), meditation, yoga (Fig. 13-4), Tai Chi, dietary restrictions, pilgrimage, confessions, reflection, forgiveness and any other activity that provides meaning, purpose or

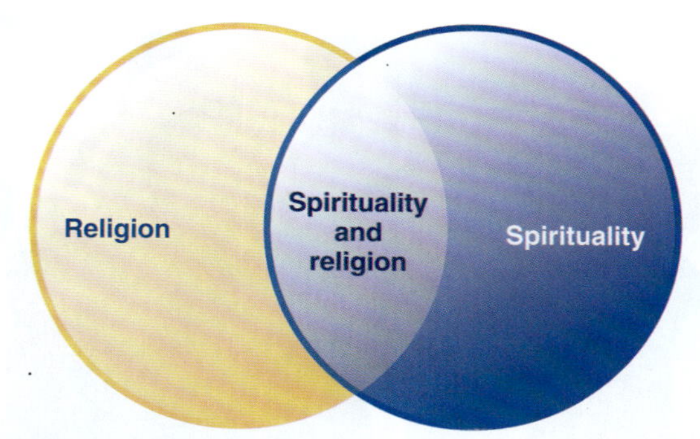

FIGURE 13-1 Interrelated yet separate concepts of religion and spirituality.

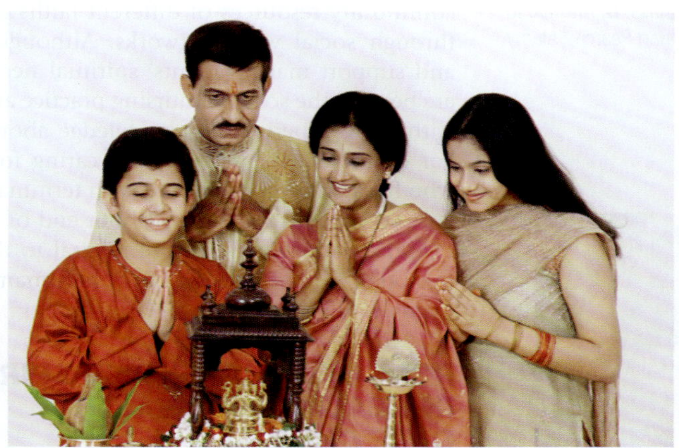

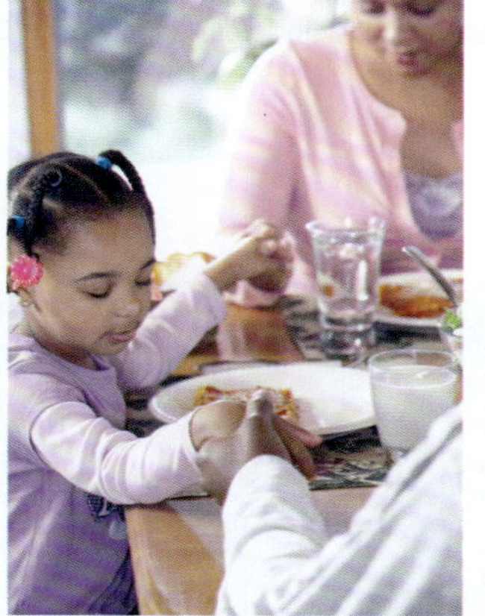

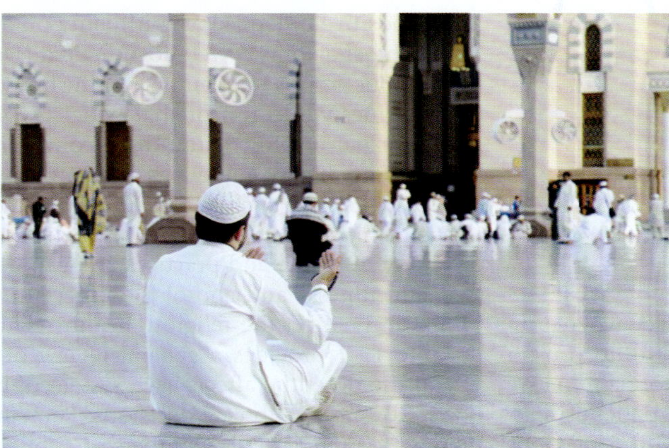

FIGURE 13-2 Prayer takes many forms.

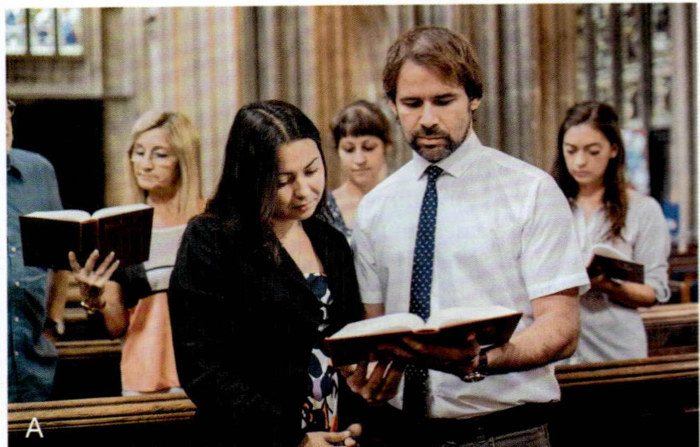

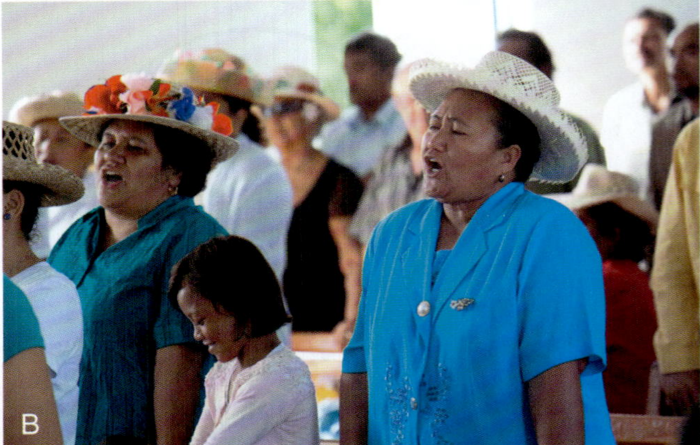

FIGURE 13-3 A, Many people find spiritual nourishment by participating in church services, such as singing in choirs and attending mass. **B,** Aitutaki in The Cook Islands. (**A,** Shutterstock.com/Rawpixel.com. **B,** Stuart Pearce / Alamy Stock Photo.)

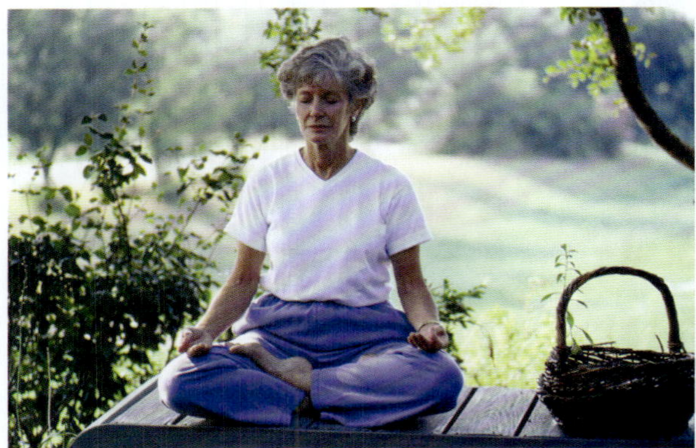

FIGURE 13-4 A woman meditates in a yoga position.

connection. If a patient identifies spiritual practices, where possible, they should be encouraged. It may be useful to consult the patient's family or spiritual advisor to explore alternative support avenues where accommodation of a patient's spiritual practices is not possible. Reconnecting with a previous spiritual practice may assist the patient in asserting a positive view of their situation. In addition, a working knowledge of the majority of faiths' ideals, beliefs and practices occurring in the nurse's community would provide a useful foundation for spiritual care.

The nurse should also consider specific cultural practices when assessing and providing spiritual care. Culturally sensitive care improves health care outcomes in Aboriginal and Torres Strait Islander communities (Laverty et al., 2017) and forms the centrepiece of the Australian government's National Aboriginal and Torres Strait Islander Health Plan 2013–2023 (Australian Government, 2013). Mason Durie's 1998 *Te Whare Tapa Whā* and Irahepeti Ramsden (2002) provide good examples of culturally sensitive health models that can guide the nurse in understanding the importance of spirituality to the health of Māori patients. When conducting any type of review of the denominations or faiths in a particular community, be aware that a patient's spiritual dimension is subjective and thus may vary greatly between people, even people of the same denomination, faith or cultural group. However, a general knowledge of the faiths may give context to some issues that certain religious groups face and provide time to develop appropriate interventions to meet those needs. A discussion with a hospital chaplain or clergy regarding the views of religious faiths in the nurse's community would also provide a greater understanding about the particular faith's view of health and give the nurse a resource for future referral or collaboration.

Collaboration and referral with chaplains or clergy are extremely important when dealing with religious issues in a health care setting. Many hospitals have staff chaplains, and community resources of different faiths are usually available through social work networks. Although nurses can assess and support many patients' spiritual needs, some situations are beyond the scope of nursing practice and require someone with more experience or knowledge about a particular faith. For example, a Christian nurse caring for a Muslim patient who has just been diagnosed with terminal cancer may not be able to speak to the patient about end-of-life issues, in which case the patient may require referral to the appropriate professional, whether that be his or her Imam or a Muslim nurse (Abdalla & Patel, 2010).

ROLE OF RELIGION AND SPIRITUALITY IN HEALTH AND HEALTH CARE CHOICES

The positive influence of spirituality on a person's health and health behaviours is well documented (Dempsey et al., 2014). Religious groups frequently view the body as a gift and encourage a lifestyle to mirror that belief. Avoidance of promiscuous sexual activity, shunning alcohol and tobacco use and following dietary guidelines each promote a healthy lifestyle. If patients have such beliefs, these behaviours can be encouraged and supported. Religious beliefs can express a wide variety of values and practices and can have rituals (i.e. birth, death, illness) and end-of-life aspects to them that may significantly affect the religion–health relationship of a person. Table 13-1 provides a general review of the major religions and the potential affects each system of belief might have on a follower's health care decisions. Remember, as with culture, never assume that all members of a religion adopt all aspects

Table 13-1 Major world religions and common health beliefs

	Overview	Illness	End of life	Nutrition
Buddhism Global: 6.9% AUS: 2.4%	Suffering is a part of human existence, but the inward death of the self and senses leads to a state beyond suffering and existence.	Prayer and meditation are used for cleansing and healing. Terminal illness may be seen as a unique opportunity to reflect on life's ultimate meaning and the meaning of one's relation with the world. Therefore, it is important that medication does not interfere with consciousness.	Life is the opportunity to cultivate understanding, compassion and joy for self and others. Death is associated with rebirth. Serene surroundings are important to the dignity of dying.	Many are strict vegetarians. Some holy days include fasting from dawn to dusk, but considerations are allowed for the frail and elderly for whom fasting could create problems.
Christianity Global: 31.2% AUS: 52%	Beliefs focus around the Old and New Testaments of the Bible and view Jesus Christ as the Saviour. Prayers may be directed to one or all of the Holy Trinity (God, Holy Spirit and Jesus Christ). Beliefs usually culturally developed, vary within denominations.	Most view illness as a natural process for the body and even as a testing of faith. Others may see illness as a curse brought on by living outside the laws of God and, therefore, retribution for personal evil.	There is belief in miracles, especially through prayer. Western medicine is usually held in high regard. Memorial services rather than funerals and cremation rather than burial are more common in Christian religions than in other sects.	No special or universal food beliefs are common to Christian religions, although there may be regional or cultural beliefs.
Hinduism Global: 15.1% AUS: 1.3%	Nirvana (oneness with God) is the primary purpose of the religion. Many have an altar in their home for worship.	Illness is the result of past and current life actions (karma). The right hand is seen as holy, and eating and intervention (IV) needs to be with the right hand to promote clean healing.	Death marks a passage because the soul has no beginning or end. At death the soul may be reborn as another person and one's karma is carried forwards. It is important for karma to leave this life with as little negativity as possible to insure a better life next birth. Holy water and basil leaves may be placed on the body; sacred threads may be tied around wrists or neck. The deceased arms should be straightened.	Many but not all are vegetarians. Many holy days include fasting.
Islam Global: 24.1% AUS: 2.2%	Mohammed is believed to be the greatest of all prophets. Worship occurs in a mosque. Prayer occurs five times a day: dawn to sunrise, noon, afternoon, sunset and evening. Prayers are done facing east towards the sacred place in Mecca and often occur on a prayer rug with ritual washing of hands, face and feet prior to prayer. Women are to be 'modest' and are not to view men, other than their husbands, naked.	Allah is in control of the beginning and end of life, and expressions of powerlessness are rare. To question or ask questions of health care providers is considered a sign of mistrust, so patients and family are less likely to ask questions.	All outcomes, whether death or healing, are seen as predetermined by Allah. It is important for dying patients to face east and to die facing east. Prayer is offered but need not be done by an Imam (religious leader).	Consumption of pork or alcohol is prohibited. Other meats must meet ritual requirements and many use Kosher meals (see Jewish nutrition in this table) because these meet the requirements of Islamic believers as well. During the holy days of Ramadan (29-day period), neither food nor drink is taken between sunrise and sunset, though frail or ill adults and young children are exempt.

Continued on following page

Table 13-1 Major world religions and common health beliefs (continued)

	Overview	Illness	End of life	Nutrition
Judaism Global: < 0.2% AUS: > 0.5%	Judaism includes religious beliefs and a philosophy for a code of ethics with four major groupings of Jewish beliefs: Reform, Reconstructionist, Conservative and Orthodox. Prayer shawls are common and are often passed between generations of family. The clergy are known as rabbi.	Restrictions related to work on holy days are removed to save a life. However, tests, signatures and assessments for medical needs that can be scheduled to avoid holy days are appreciated.	Psalms and the last prayer of confession (*vidui*) are held at the bedside. At death, arms are not crossed; any clothing or bandages with the patient's blood should be prepared for burial with the person. It is important that the whole person be buried together.	Orthodox or Kosher involves no mixing of meat with dairy; separate cooking and eating utensils are used for food preparation and consumption. Kosher laws include special slaughter and food handling. 'Keeping Kosher' is predominantly an Orthodox practice. When food has passed Kosher laws of preparation, a symbol (K) appears on the label. Many holy days include a fasting period.

Adapted with permission from Napier-Tibere, B. (2002). Diversity, healing and health care. Viewed May 2019 at bonsome.org—a website supported through grant funding from On Lok Senior Health, Inc., and Stanford University School of Medicine: Stanford Geriatric Education Center. Barrett, D., Kurlan, G. & Johnson, T. (2001). *World Christian encyclopedia: A comparative survey of churches and religions in the modern world* (2nd ed.). New York: Oxford. Hacket, C., & McClendon, D. (2017). Christians remain world's largest religious group, but they are declining in Europe. Viewed May 2019 at www.pewresearch.org. Pew Research Centre. (2019). Religious landscaspe study. Viewed May 2019 at pewforum.org/religion. Australian Bureau of Statistics (ABS). (2016). *2016 Census of population and housing.* Canberra: ABS.

of it. The patient's spiritual experiences or spiritual history are subjective and provide the best guide to conversations and decisions about referral or collaboration. Providing a quiet place or time of silence for the patient may encourage spiritual practices such as meditation, or the nurse may gather family members or clergy to participate in a prayer ritual.

Particular religious views may negatively affect health. Failure to seek timely medical care and withholding 'proper' medical care based on religious dogma remain prominent ethical dilemmas faced by health care providers. Christian Scientists frequently rely on prayer alone to heal illnesses, rarely seek mainstream medical care and have higher rates of mortality than the general population. A patient from the Jehovah's Witness faith may refuse a blood transfusion, blood product transfusion or certain immunisations because of their beliefs. Although Australian law provides general protections for the exercise of religious freedoms, the Family Court of Australia has the power to override parental decisions that are not in the best interests of the child (Babie et al., 2019). The Victorian Supreme Court provides a recent example of this power when in 2018 it made an order permitting health practitioners at a Victorian hospital to administer blood products to a 17-year-old Jehovah's Witness, despite objections from the patient and the patient's parents (Chosich, 2018). The decision cited a similar order made by the New South Wales Supreme Court in 2013 (Olding, 2013) that determined the 17-year-old was not legally of an age to make a decision to refuse life-saving treatment. Although this is a specific denominational example of a negative impact of religion on health, and adherence is not universal, there are also generalised manifestations of of the negative effects of religion. For example, a patient may experience depression or anxiety if they feel they do not meet the group's expectations, whereas certain spiritual practices, such as participation in complementary and alternative medical practices, may delay medical care (Barrett et al., 2001; Koenig, 2007).

If a nurse encounters a situation where religious or spiritual views have the potential to compromise adequate care, they should present the situation to a supervising staff member immediately. Refer complex cases to the ethics committee of the institution or organisation to ensure the implementation of appropriate measures. Refer to institutional or organisational handbooks for specific instructions regarding individual cases.

SELF-UNDERSTANDING OF SPIRITUALITY

Nurses who are more aware of their own spirituality are more likely to be comfortable discussing the potential spiritual needs of patients (Harrington, 2010; Koren & Papamiditriou, 2013; Ronaldson et al., 2012). Introspective reflection, through journal writing, meditation or discussions with interested persons, is a useful aid to understanding one's own beliefs and biases about the relationship between spirituality and health. Ask yourself:

1. What are my views on the interaction between spirituality and health?
2. How would I respond to someone in spiritual distress or to someone requesting an intervention relating to spirituality?
3. How can I provide spiritual care?

These reflections help to provide a deeper understanding of the nurse's spiritual dimension and build confidence for future discussions on spirituality. Although many nurses view spiritual assessment and care as an important part of nursing practice, training levels vary from institution to institution. However, nurses can train themselves to meet this vital need of the patient. The nurse who understands the content of a spiritual assessment can also use this knowledge to increase self-understanding.

APPROACH TO SPIRITUAL ASSESSMENT

A spiritual assessment is similar to the many other assessments nurses perform on a daily basis. Gaining relevant information about the patient's spirituality helps to identify potential problems and interventions that can improve patient care. Provided later in the chapter are examples of spiritual assessment tools and general, appropriate open-ended questions.

There is no absolute in the timing of a spiritual assessment. Some professionals recommend inclusion with the initial assessment, whereas others argue for a delayed assessment after the establishment of the nurse–patient relationship. Integrating both techniques may be the most useful approach because the spiritual assessment is not a static activity but rather an ongoing conversation between the nurse and the patient. An appropriate time to include general 'screening questions' on spirituality is during an initial assessment of a patient's relevant past medical history. General 'screening questions' can gauge the extent to which a patient integrates spirituality into his or her personal health care and resilience (e.g. 'from where do you draw strength and meaning in the good and bad times in your life' or 'Do you consider yourself to be a religious or spiritual person? If so, how is this related to your health or health care decisions?').

CLINICAL TIP

Briefly addressing a patient's spirituality will establish an open dialogue and provide a foundation for any possible intervention or care needed in the future.

The patient is the focus of the spiritual assessment. Therefore, the nurse does not have to be spiritual personally to take a spiritual assessment. Objectivity is a key component in a high-quality spiritual assessment. The questions posed in a spiritual assessment are inquiries for beliefs that could affect patient care. The nurse uses divulged information to support, encourage or lead patients in harmonising their personal relationships with spirituality and health. Some patients may not be connected to any religious group or have any interest in spirituality. These patients should be encouraged in whatever provides them strength in dealing with health care issues (connection with family, friends, nature, etc.). If a patient responds negatively to any aspect of the discussion on religion or spirituality, collaboration with the hospital clergy may assist the nurse in futher assessing the situation and understanding the needs of the patient.

CASE STUDY

You are talking to Paula after she has returned to the ward following radiotherapy for breast cancer. She appears upset and tells you she does not know how God can afflict her with cancer when she has a husband and a young family to take care of. You decide to collect some subjective data about Paula's spirituality.

CRITICAL THINKING

1. What questions would you ask Paula about her spirituality?
2. Considering Paula appears angry at God, would you ask questions about her relationship with God? Why or why not?

Spiritual assessment

SPIRITUAL ASSESSMENT TECHNIQUES

Spirituality is multidimensional. It is also unique to each individual. These variable characteristics of spirituality can present difficulties in an effective assessment. Many older spiritual assessment instruments originated from particular faith backgrounds and may have little cross-cultural relevance. Today the most useful spiritual assessment techniques should begin with general introductory questions and not be specific to any religious denomination so that nurses can tailor their spiritual care to the patient's specific spiritual needs.

Spiritual assessment may be formal or non-formal. It should seek to uncover the underlying factors that give coherence to a person's life without the imposition of a personal view or definition of spirituality (Rumbold, 2007). It is helpful to have a quick reference to guide assessment and begin a dialogue. Published acronyms related to the assessment of spirituality—for example, FICA in Assessment tool 13-1—can serve as excellent reminders when assessing a concept with many attributes. Techniques such as these are non-formal yet have somewhat systematic approaches. They are non-formal in that they ask open-ended questions and allow the patient to disclose pertinent information. They are systematic to the extent that the patient's responses guide future choices of questions, and they may cover numerous practices in which the patient may or may not be involved (prayer, organised religion, etc.).

Formal assessment tools, widely published in the nursing literature, are not freely available in the Australasian hospital setting. There are numerous nursing texts and articles that offer formal assessment tools (e.g. Barss, 2012; Dameron, 2005; Galek et al., 2005; Hodge, 2013; O'Brien, 2007; Royal College of Nursing, 2011), which could be consulted by any nurse wanting to increase his or her understanding and tools for spiritual assessment. Many of these describe paper-and-pencil self-response methods. Used in conjunction with other past medical history data, these measurements can uncover strengths or deficiencies that initially might have gone unnoticed. When, for example, a patient responds negatively to the statement, 'I find comfort in my religion or spirituality' during an initial history, the nurse could later incorporate this conversation and possibly reconnect the distressed patient with an effective source of spiritual support.

The remaining Assessment tools 13-2 and 13-3 and other tabled information provide guidelines for nurses to approach spiritual assessments. The positive and negative findings in no way cover all of the possible responses from a patient; use the information in these sections only as a guide.

ASSESSMENT TOOL 13-1 FICA spiritual assessment tool

F: Faith and beliefs
I: Importance and influence
C: Community
A: Address

Detailed questions relating to acronym:

F: What is your faith or belief?
Do you consider yourself spiritual or religious?
What things do you believe in that give meaning to your life?

I: Is it important in your life?
What influence does it have on how you take care of yourself?
How have your beliefs influenced your behaviour during this illness?
What role do your beliefs play in regaining your health?

C: Are you part of a spiritual or religious community?
Is this of a support to you?
Is there a person or group of people who you really love or who are really important to you?

A: How would you like me, your [nurse], to address these issues in your health care?

General recommendations when taking a spiritual history:

1. Consider spirituality as a potentially important component of every patient's physical wellbeing and mental health.
2. Address spirituality at each complete physical examination and continue addressing it at follow-up visits if appropriate. In patient care, spirituality is an ongoing issue.
3. Respect a patient's privacy regarding spiritual beliefs; do not impose your beliefs on others.
4. Make referrals to chaplains, spiritual directors or community resources as appropriate.
5. Be aware that your own spiritual beliefs will help you personally and will overflow in your encounters with those for whom you are to make the [nurse]–patient encounter a more humanistic one.

Adapted from Puchalski, C. (2001). Taking a spiritual history allows clinicians to understand patients more fully. In Solomon, M., Romer, A., Heller, K. & Weissman (Eds). *Innovations in end-of-life care: Practical strategies & international perspectives* (Vol. II). Larchmont, NY: Mary Ann Liebert.

ASSESSMENT TOOL 13-2 Daily spiritual experiences scale

The list that follows includes items you may or may not experience. Please consider if and how often you have these experiences; try to disregard whether you feel you should or should not have them. In addition, a number of items use the word 'God'. If this word is not a comfortable one, please substitute another idea that calls to mind the divine or holy for you.

Scoring:
1 = Many times a day 2 = Every day 3 = Most days 4 = Some days 5 = Once in a while 6 = Never or almost never

1.	I feel God's presence.	1	2	3	4	5	6
2.	I experience a connection to all of life.	1	2	3	4	5	6
3.	During worship or at other times when connecting with God, I feel joy which lifts me out of my daily concerns.	1	2	3	4	5	6
4.	I find strength in my religion or spirituality.	1	2	3	4	5	6
5.	I find comfort in my religion or spirituality.	1	2	3	4	5	6
6.	I feel deep inner peace and harmony.	1	2	3	4	5	6
7.	I ask for God's help in the midst of daily activities.	1	2	3	4	5	6
8.	I feel guided by God in the midst of daily activities.	1	2	3	4	5	6
9.	I feel God's love for me directly.	1	2	3	4	5	6
10.	I feel God's love for me through others.	1	2	3	4	5	6
11.	I am spiritually touched by the beauty of creation.	1	2	3	4	5	6
12.	I feel thankful for my blessings.	1	2	3	4	5	6
13.	I feel a selfless caring for others.	1	2	3	4	5	6
14.	I accept others even when they do things I think are wrong.	1	2	3	4	5	6
15.	I desire to be closer to or in union with Him.*	1	2	3	4	5	6
16.	In general, how close do you feel to God?*	1	2	3	4	5	6

*For questions 15 and 16, Scoring: 4 = not close at all, 3 = somewhat close, 2 = very close, 1 = as close as possible. Lower scores represent more daily spiritual experiences.

Adapted from Fetzer Institute. (1999). *Multidimensional measurement of religiousness/spirituality for use in health research.* Kalamazoo: John E. Fetzer Institute.

ASSESSMENT TOOL 13-3 Brief religious coping questionnaire (RCOPE)

Instructions for administration: Think about how you try to understand and deal with major problems in your life. To what extent is each involved in the way you cope?

Positive religious/spiritual coping subscale

1. I think about how my life is part of a larger spiritual force.
   1. A great deal
   2. Quite a bit
   3. Somewhat
   4. Not at all
2. I work together with God as partners to get through hard times.
   1. A great deal
   2. Quite a bit
   3. Somewhat
   4. Not at all
3. I look to God for strength, support and guidance in crisis.
   1. A great deal
   2. Quite a bit
   3. Somewhat
   4. Not at all

Negative religious/spiritual coping subscale

1. I feel that stressful situations are God's way of punishing me for my sins or lack of spirituality.
   1. A great deal
   2. Quite a bit
   3. Somewhat
   4. Not at all
2. I wonder if God has abandoned me.
   1. A great deal
   2. Quite a bit
   3. Somewhat
   4. Not at all
3. I try to make sense of the situation and decide what to do without relying on God.
   1. A great deal
   2. Quite a bit
   3. Somewhat
   4. Not at all

A more extensive form of the RCOPE exists and could be utilised for detailed analysis. Scale could be summed as a general screening tool, or individual items could be identified (e.g. abandonment) and incorporated into the clinical setting.

Adapted from Fetzer Institute. (1999). *Multidimensional measurement of religiousness/spirituality for use in health research.* Kalamazoo: John E. Fetzer Institute.

VALIDATING AND DOCUMENTING FINDINGS

A patient's spirituality often affects their health. There are numerous ways in which this occurs and that may go unnoticed without assessment. The nurse will collect subjective and objective data during assessment. Although spiritual wellbeing and distress are largely subjective findings derived from patient reporting, objective data can validate or call into question information presented to the nurse.

Sample of subjective data

A 39-year-old female recently admitted to the oncology ward for treatment of breast cancer. FICA spiritual assessment included in the initial exam. Patient reports a strong sense of hope and comfort from God; attends church regularly but is questioning her faith in relation to her cancer. She gladly accepts a visit from the hospital chaplain.

Sample of objective data

Patient has an affect that is consistent with spiritual distress. Avoids direct eye contact and cries while describing the difficulty she is having reconciling her spiritual beliefs with her cancer.

Analysis of data

DIAGNOSTIC REASONING: POSSIBLE CONCLUSIONS

After collecting subjective and objective data pertaining to spiritual assessment, identify the negative findings and the patient's strengths. Then cluster the data to reveal any significant patterns or distress. Use these data to make clinical judgements about the status of the patient's spiritual wellbeing and the patient's spiritual coping strategies. The following are some of the possible conclusions that the nurse may make after assessing the patient's spirituality.

Potential patient risks to spiritual wellbeing

- Risk of spiritual distress

Potential patient problems

- Spiritual distress related to questioning faith due to cancer

Selected collaborative problems

After grouping the data, certain collaborative problems may become apparent. Remember that collaborative problems are those that nursing intervention cannot prevent. However, the nurse can detect and monitor these physiological or other complications of medical or other conditions. In addition, the nurse can use doctor- and nurse-prescribed interventions to minimise the complications of these problems. The nurse may also have to refer the patient in such situations for further treatment of the problem. The following is a list of collaborative problems that the nurse may identify when assessing spirituality:

- Depression
- Alteration in body image
- Lymphoedema
- Pneumonitis.

Medical problems

If after grouping the data it becomes apparent that the patient has signs and symptoms that may require medical diagnosis and treatment, referral to a primary health care provider is necessary.

SPIRITUAL ASSESSMENT

ASSESSMENT PROCEDURE	POSITIVE FINDINGS	NEGATIVE FINDINGS
Listen to patient's story and seek clarification where needed. Support patient to develop trust. Ask patient: 'Do you consider yourself to be a religious or spiritual person? If so, how is this related to your health or health care decisions?'	Patient makes reference to involvement in religious groups or spiritual practices that have provided comfort and social support. Describes belief that prayer reduces stress and heals disease.	Reports lost connections to his or her religious group, while continuing to focus on the negative aspect of spirituality (e.g. suppressive religious rules). Comments and body language reveal a lack of hope with depressive symptomatology. Deficiencies in the social network are identified and appear to affect the patient's wellbeing and attitude towards recovery. Note: Not describing connections to a religious group does not indicate abnormal findings.
Observe non-verbal and verbal communication patterns in presence of others.	Eye contact is maintained (appropriate to cultural group) with non-verbal cues correlating with conversation.	Patient displays poor eye contact. The presence of others strongly influences information patient shares.
Begin to focus questions. Begin conversation with a general dialogue about global concepts such as hope, meaning, comfort, strength, peace, love and connection: • We have been discussing your support systems. • What are your sources of hope, strength, comfort and peace? • What do you hold onto during difficult times? • What sustains you and keeps you going? • For some people, their religious or spiritual beliefs act as a source of comfort and strength in dealing with life's ups and downs; is this true for you? Use FICA Spiritual Assessment tool, Assessment tool 13-1.	Reports spirituality giving a sense of peace that transcends illness or disease. Reports that meditation and exercise facilitate a sense of peace. Family frequently mentioned as source of strength and motivation. Patient places a strong emphasis on spirituality as a guiding force in life.	Describes no connection to others such as God, nature, family or peers. Shares pessimistic and fatalistic attitude towards recovery. Identifies limited coping resources with little desire to adapt new ones.
Continue to assess other dimensions of spirituality within groups. Ask about organisational (or formal) religious involvement. Reflect on previous conversations to direct questioning. Remember that not all persons who state they are religious or spiritual are involved with organised religious groups or ascribe to all the religious practices of that group. Note: If there is no connection to a religious group or faith tradition, skip or modify this section and the next. Ask the questions: • Do you consider yourself part of an organised religion? • How important is this to you? • What aspects of your religion are helpful and not so helpful to you? • Are you part of a religious or spiritual community? Does it help you? How?	Patient may report regular attendance at a local mosque, church or other religious meeting place and highlight importance of attendance as a recovery period in a very fast-paced life. States that involvement with others holding a similar worldview helps to give meaning and purpose to life.	Abnormal findings may include reporting involvement with 'new religious group' in the area but being unable to provide details regarding affiliation or purpose of religious group. Patient makes reference to extensive fasts and other activities that may be harmful to general health.

SPIRITUAL ASSESSMENT (continued)

ASSESSMENT PROCEDURE	POSITIVE FINDINGS	NEGATIVE FINDINGS
Ask transition question from organisational to personal beliefs. Ask patient to specify differences or similarities in own beliefs and the beliefs of the faith or denomination with which he or she is affiliated. Ask questions: • Do you have personal spiritual beliefs independent of organised religion? What are they? • Do you believe in God? What kind of relationship do you have with God? • What aspects of spirituality or spiritual practices do you find most helpful to you personally (e.g. prayer, meditation, reading scripture, attending religious services, listening to music, bushwalking, communing with nature)?	Describes personal beliefs that coincide with denominational beliefs. Denominational beliefs do not conflict with required medical care. Reports healthy and positive relationship with God. Desires to have time in the hospital to meditate and read scripture to gain focus and relieve stress.	Abnormal findings may include reporting very limited similarities between denomination and personal beliefs, past utilisation of prayer and listening to religious music, but currently has no avenue for the fostering of spirituality.
Directly address beliefs that may conflict or affect one's health care. Assist patients with expression of spiritual practices if appropriate. Attend to end-of-life issues if the condition dictates. Ask the questions: • Has being sick (or your current situation) affected your ability to do the things that usually help you spiritualy? (Or affected your relationship with God?) • As a nurse is there anything I can do to help you access the resources that usually help you? • Are you worried about any conflicts between your beliefs and your medical situation/care/decisions? • Would it be helpful for you to speak to a clinical chaplain/community spiritual leader? • Are there any specific practices or restrictions I should know about in providing your medical care? (e.g. dietary restrictions, use of blood products) • If the patient is dying: How do your beliefs affect the kind of nursing care you would like me to provide over the next few days/ weeks/months?	Patient views present diagnosis (e.g. cancer) as 'part of God's will for his or her life' or desires to continue nature walks and other spiritual practices to develop a closer relationship with God. Patient makes no reference to perceived abandonment or rejection that may lead to depression. Desires to have clergy from local church for visitation time. Patient asks the nurse to contact local clergy and provides telephone number.	Patient appears traumatised with diagnosis and views the illness as a fault of past lifestyle or a punishment. Refuses visits from local clergy and hospital chaplains. Declines conversation and just wants to be sent home to die.

SUMMARY

Spirituality is a multidimensional concept that can incorporate religion but more broadly includes those factors that bring meaning, purpose and connectedness. Understanding the cultural, religious and spiritual temperament of the community at large will assist the nurse in assessing a patient's spirituality and identifying meaningful strategies to provide culturally sensitive spiritual care. Spiritual assessment should be a normal part of any nursing assessment, achieved through non-formal and formal assessment tools. Regardless of the tool nurses use to open the discussion on spirituality, they need to be sensitive to the patient's needs and not impose their own beliefs.

CASE STUDY

The case study demonstrates how to analyse spiritual assessment data for a specific patient. The exercises included in the ancillary product on thePoint that complements this text offer further opportunities to enhance your skills.

Lindsay Baird is a 40-year-old woman who lives with her two children and husband outside of a rural community. Mrs Baird presents at the clinic today for a routine check of her hypertension. Upon reviewing the past medical and family history, it is noted that Mrs Baird is a Catholic and believes her spirituality to be a very important part of her medical care. Entering the room, Mrs Baird greets you gracefully and continues to respond to general health questions with ease. After proceeding through relevant medical history since the last visit, a 3-kg weight gain is noted with a correlating blood pressure notably higher than the last visit. Questioning the recent changes in her medical condition, Mrs Baird responds, 'I just haven't felt like doing any exercise lately.' Continuing to draw information out, you begin to ask questions related to stress levels, time restraints and motivation. Eventually Mrs Baird begins to tell the story of her family falling away from attending the church on a regular basis and the corresponding loss of support and motivation. She states, 'I used to gain such strength going to our church meetings. It was such an encouragement. We used to walk with one another and talk about what God is doing in our lives . . . now I just feel overwhelmed and busy all of the time . . . and I can't talk with anyone.'

The following concept map illustrates the diagnostic reasoning process.

Applying COLDSPA

Applying COLDSPA for patient symptoms: 'I just haven't felt like doing any exercise lately.'

Mnemonic	Question	Data provided	Missing data
Character	Describe the sign or symptom (feeling, appearance, sound, smell or taste if applicable).	Loss of motivation and social support network	
Onset	When did it begin?		When were you first separated from your church (or support group)?
Location	Where is it? Does it radiate? Does it occur anywhere else?	The patient reports negative physical and emotional consequences.	
Duration	How long does it last? Does it recur?		Have you been separated from your church (or support group) before? If so, how long and what was the outcome?
Severity	How bad is it? How much does it bother you?	Limited desire for exercise has resulted in weight gain.	
Pattern	What makes it better or worse?		Has anything made it better or worse?
Associated factors/How it Affects the patient	What other symptoms occur with it? How does it affect you?	The patient reports feeling overwhelmed and isolated.	

1) Identify abnormal findings and patient strengths

Subjective data

- Lack of adherence to the treatment regimen
- The information is not easily divulged
- Loss of previous strong ties to the religious group
- Patient describes lack of motivation to participate in health-promoting activities
- Heightened sense of stress due to the lost connections

Objective data

- Blood pressure elevation between visits
- Weight increased 3 kg from the previous visit
- Facial expressions changed to ones of concern as the conversation moved towards the patient's struggles

2) Identify cue clusters

- Loss of strong social ties
- Motivating force in health has been decimated

3) Draw inferences

Presented information implies displaced relationships are in need of addressing. Previous information of social ties to the religious organisation suggests intervention related to the patient's spiritual distress

4) List possible diagnoses

Spiritual distress related to the loss of connection to a spiritual and social support source

5) Check for defining characteristics

Major: Direct comments correlating the lack of treatment adherence to the loss of motivation and support.
Minor: Tone relays stress incurred from broken ties

6) Confirm or rule out diagnoses

Confirm the diagnosis. Encouraging the patient to reconnect to tried sources of social and spiritual support, or to seek new sources, may improve the patient's health condition through health promotion activities

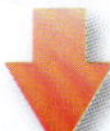

7) Document conclusions

Diagnoses that are appropriate for this patient include:

- Spiritual distress

ONLINE RESOURCES

An extensive range of additional resources to enhance teaching and learning and to facilitate understanding may be found online at the text's accompanying website, located on thePoint at http://thepoint.lww.com. These include Watch and Learn videos, Concepts in Action animations, journal articles, case studies, discussion topics and quizzes.

Subscribers may also access Lippincott Procedures, an extensive online point-of-care procedure guide that provides reliable step-by-step instructions for more than 1700 procedures, including 450 evidence-based Australian procedures, and skills in a variety of speciality settings, together with a wealth of supporting information.

SIMULATED LEARNING

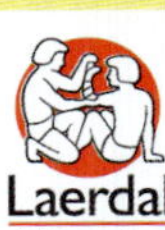

Having completed this chapter, explore the scenarios of Stan Checketts Parts 1 and 2. Stan is a 64-year-old admitted with abdominal pain diagnosed as a bowel obstruction. Incorporating the health assessment content in this chapter with your existing theoretical knowledge and clinical experience, progress through the simulation scenarios (this is best done in a small group). How would you manage Stan's care? When reflecting on your management of Stan, what do you think you did well and what do you think you can improve? Consider why you think this and also how you might manage a similar problem in the future.

References

Abdalla, M. & Patel, I. M. A. (2010). An Islamic perspective on ageing and spirituality. In *Ageing and spirituality across faiths and cultures* (pp. 112–123). London, UK: Jessica Kingsley.

Ammerman, N. T. (2013). Spiritual but not religious: Beyond binary choices in the study of religion. *Journal for the Scientific Study of Religion, 52*(2), 258–278.

Australian Bureau of Statistics (ABS). (2016). 2016 census of population and housing. Cat. no. 2024. Canberra: ABS. Retrieved 3 March 2018 via QuickStats via www.censusdata.abs.gov.au/census_services/getproduct/census/2016/quickstat/0.

Australian Government. (2013). National Aborginal and Torres Strait Islander Health Plan. Commonwealth of Australia. Available at www.health.gov.au/natsihp.

Australian Museum. (2019). Indigenous Australia: Spirituality. Available at http://australianmuseum.net.au/indigenous-Australians.

Babie, P., Neoh, J., Krumrey-Quine, J., et al. (2019). *Religion and Law in Australia* (2nd ed.). Netherlands: Wolters Kluwer.

Barnum, B. S. (2010). *Spirituality in nursing: The challenges of complexity* (3rd ed.). New York: Springer Publishing Company.

Barrett, D., Kurlan, G. & Johnson, T. (2001). *World Christian encyclopedia: A comparative survey of churches and religions in the modern world* (2nd ed.). New York: Oxford.

Barss, K. S. (2012). TRUST.: An affirming modelled for inclusive spiritual care. *Journal of Holistic Nursing, 30*(1), 24–34.

Chosich, C. (2018). Case Note: Consent to treatment and the best interests of the child. Viewed May 2019 at healhtlegal.com.au.

Clark, C. C. & Hunter, J. (2018). Spirituality, spiritual well-being, and spiritual coping in advanced heart failure. *Journal of Holistic Nursing*, 1–18.

Dameron, C. M. (2005). Spiritual assessment made easy: With acronyms. *Journal of Christian Nursing, 22*(1), 14–16.

Dempsey, J., Hillege, S. & Hill, R. (2014). *Fundamentals of nursing: A person-centred approach to care* (2nd ed.). Sydney: Lippincott Williams & Wilkins.

Durie, M. (1998). *Whaiora: Mãori health development* (2nd ed., p. 69). Auckland: Oxford University Press.

Fetzer Institute. (1999). *Multidimensional measurement of religiousness/spirituality for use in health research*. Kalamazoo: John E. Fetzer Institute.

Galek, K., Flannelly, K. J., Vane, A., et al. (2005). Assessing a patient's spiritual needs: A comprehensive instrument. *Holistic Nursing Practice, 19*(2), 62–69.

Harrington, A. C. (2010). Spiritual wellbeing for older people. In *Ageing and spirituality across faiths and cultures* (pp. 179–194). London, UK: Jessica Kingsley.

Hodge, D. R. (2013). Administering a two-stage spiritual assessment in healthcare settings: A necessary component of ethical and effective care. *Journal of Nursing Management*, Viewed December 2013 at www.ncbi.nlm.nih.gov/pubmed/23600740. in print.

International Council of Nurses (ICN). (2012). The ICN code of ethics for nurses. Available at www.icn.ch.

Koenig, H. (2007). When might religion or religious practices interfere with the health of a patient? In *Spirituality in patient care: Why, how, when & what* (2nd ed., pp. 108–122). Philadelphia: Templeton Foundation Press.

Koenig, H., King, D. & Carson, V. B. (2012). *Handbook of religion and health* (2nd ed.). New York: Oxford University Press.

Kohn, R. (2010). The ageing spirit. In *Ageing and spirituality across faiths and cultures* (pp. 57–67). London, UK: Jessica Kingsley.

Koren, E. M. & Papamiditriou, C. (2013). Spirituality of staff nurses: Application of modeling and role modeling theory. *Holistic Nursing Practice, 27*(1), 37–44.

Korf, J. (2019). Aboriginal spirituality and beliefs. Viewed April 2019 at creativespirits.info.

Laverty, M., McDermott, D. R. & Calma, T. (2017). Embedding cultural safety in Australia's main health care standards. *The Medical Journal of Australia, 207*(1), 15–17.

MacKinlay, E. B. (Ed). (2010). *Ageing and spirituality across faiths and cultures.* London: Jessica Kingsley.

MacLeod, R., Wilson, D. M., Crandall, J., et al. (2017). Death and anxiety among New Zealanders: The predictive roles of reigion, spirituality, and family connection. *Omega, 0*(0), 1–17.

McCrindle, M. (2017). Faith and belief in Australia: A national study on religion, spirituality and worldview trends. View May 2019 at https://mccrindle.com.au.

Mcharo, S. K. (2018). T.R.U.S.T. modelled for inclusive spiritual care: Critique of middle range theories. *Journal of Holistic Nursing, 36*(3), 282–290.

Moberg, D. O. (2011). *Expanding horizons of spirituality research*. Hartford, CT: Hartford Institute for Religion Research. Viewed December 2013 at http://hirr.hartsem.edu/sociology/spirituality-research.html.

Nachowitz, T. (2007). New Zealand as a multireligious society: Recent census figures and some relevant implications. *Aotearoa Ethnic Network Journal, 2*(2).

Napier-Tibere, B. (2002). Diversity, healing and health care. Viewed September 2004 at www.gasi-ves.org/pdf/1-total-cohort.pdf and viewed December 2013 at www.bonshome.org/diversity.htm.

Nascimento, L. S., Alvarenga, W. A., Caldiera, S., et al. (2016). Spiritual care: The nurses' expereincesin the pediatric intensive care unit. *Religions, 7*(27), doi:10.3390/rel7030027.

New Zealand in History (personal website of Robbie Whitmore). (2010). The Mãori: Religion and spirituality. Viewed December 2013 at http://history-nz.org/maori6.html.

Nielsen, P. (2009). Faith in Australia 2009. Available at www.smh.com.au/pdf/Nielsen%20Poll%20Faith%20Dec19.pdf.

Nightingale, F. (1860 [1996]). *Notes on nursing*. New York: Dover.

Northern Territory Government. Indigenous traditional religions. Office of Indigenous Policy. Viewed March 2019 at globaldialoguefoundation.org.l.

Nursing and Midwifery Board of Australia (NMBA). (2017). Change to ethical decision-making documents for nurses and midwives in Australia. Available at www.nursingmidwiferyboard.gov.au.

Nursing Council of New Zealand/Te Kaunihera Tapuhi o Aotearoa. (2012). Code of conduct for nurses. Available at http://nursingcouncil.org.nz/Nurses/Code-of-Conduct.

O'Brien, M. (2007). *Spirituality in nursing: Standing on holy ground* (3rd ed.). Boston: Jones & Bartlett.

Olding, R. (2013). Jehovah's Witness teen loses appeal over life saving transfusion. Sydney Morning Herald. Viewed December 2013 at www.smh.com.au/nsw/jehovahs-witness-teen-loses-appeal-over-lifesaving-transfusion-20130927-2uib6.html.

Oman, D. (2018). *Why religion and spirituality matter for public health: Evidence.* Switzerland: Springer International Publishing.

Penman, J. (2018). Finding paradise within: How spirituality protects care clients and carers from depression. *Journal of Holistic Nursing, 36*(3), 243–254.

Puchalski, C. (2001). Taking a spiritual history allows clinicians to understand patients more fully. In M. Solomon, A. Romer, K. Heller, et al. (Eds). *Innovations in end-of-life care: Practical strategies & international perspectives* (Vol. II). Larchmont, NY: Mary Ann Liebert.

Puchalski, C. M., Vitillo, R., Hull, S. K., et al. (2014). Improving the spiritual dimension of whole person care: Reaching national and international consensus. *Journal of Palliative Medicine, 17*(6), 642–656.

Ramsden, I. M. (2002). Cultural safety and nursing education in Aotearoa and Te Waipounamu. Unpublished dissertation, Victoria University Press.

Ronaldson, S., Hayes, L., Aggar, C., et al. (2012). Spirituality and spiritual caring: Nurses' perspectives and practice in palliative and acute care environments. *Journal of Clinical Nursing, 21*, 2126–2135.

Royal College of Nursing (RCN). (2011). *Spirituality in nursing care: A pocket guide.* London: Author.

Rumbold, B. D. (2007). A review of spiritual assessment in health care practice. *The Medical Journal of Australia, 186*(10, Suppl.), S60–S62.

Statistics New Zealand. (2013). Religious affiliation. In *2006 census data.* Viewed April 2019 at www.stats.govt.nz/Census/2013.archive.stats.govt.nzCensus/profile-and-summary-reports/quickstats-culture/identity/religion.aspx.

Stephenson, P. S. & Berry, D. M. (2014). Describing spirituality at the end of life. *Western Journal of Nursing Research, 39*(9), 1229–1247.

Selected readings

Abell, C. H., Garrett-Wright, D. & Abell, C. E. (2016). Nurses' perceptions of competence in providing spiritual care. *Journal of Holistic Nursing, 36*(1), 33–37.

Atkinson, C. (2015). Islamic values and nursing practice in Kuwait. *Journal of Holistic Nursing, 33*(3), 195–204.

Dobtratz, M. C. (2016). Building a middle-range theory of adaptive spirituality. *Nursing Science Quarterly, 29*(2), 146–153.

Hodge, D. R. & Wolosin, R. J. (2014). Hospitalised Asian patients and their spiritual needs: Developing a modelled of spiritual care. *Journal of Aging and Health, 26*(3), 380–400.

Lopez, V., Fischer, I., Larkin, D., et al. (2014). Spirituality, religiosity, and personal beliefs of Australian undergraduate nursing students. *Journal of Transcultural Nursing, 25*(4), 395–402.

Mamier, I., Taylor, E. J. & Winslow, B. W. (2018). Nurse spiritual care: Prevalence and correlates. *Western Journal of Nursing Research, 41*(4), 537–554.

Meaningful Ageing Australia. (2016). National Guidelines for Spiritual Care in Aged Care. Meaningful Ageing Australia, Parkville.

Musa, A. S. (2017). Spiritual care intervention and spiritual well-being. *Journal of Holistic Nursing, 35*(1), 53–61.

Online resources

Australians Together: australianstogether.org.au/indigenous-culture/aboriginal-spirituality

Center for Spirituality, Theology and Health, Duke University: https://spiritualityandhealth.duke.edu/

Creative Spirits: creativespirits.info

George Washington Institute for Spirituality and Health: www.gwish.org

Head to Health: Connecting with spirituality: https://headtohealth.gov.au/meaningful-life/connectedness/spirituality

Interfaith Health Program, Emory University: http://ihpnet.org

John Templeton Foundation: www.templeton.org

Larry Dossey (mind and body author): www.dosseydossey.com

Meaningful Ageing Australia: meaningfulageing.org.au

Pastoral and Spiritual Care of Older People: www.pascop.org.au

Spiritual Health Victoria: www.spiritualhealthvictoria.org.au

Spiritual Care, Health and Wellbeing: https://www.qld.gov.au/health/support/end-of-life/

University of Aberdeen Centre for Spirituality, Health and Divinity: www.abdn.ac.uk/sdhp/centre-for-spirituality-health-and-disability-182.php

University of Pennsylvania School of Medicine, Pastoral Care Faith Traditions and Health Care: www.uphs.upenn.edu/pastoral/pubs/traditions.html

CHAPTER **14**

Assessing nutrition

CASE STUDY

Mrs Visna Uddina, a 58-year-old lady of Indian descent, has a history of type 1 diabetes. When you weigh her during your weekly community home visit, you find she weighs 65 kg, which is 5 kg less than she weighed at your last visit. You try to weigh her at the same time of day each week—9.30 a.m. She usually has breakfast at 6.30 a.m. and takes 40 units of insulin at 7.30 a.m. Today she tells you she has been urinating 'a lot' and that she has felt lethargic and tired for the past 3 days, with nausea and 'just a little vomiting'. She also tells you that she has had headaches and blurred vision and that she feels dizzy sometimes. She says she has not been eating well but adds, 'I'm keeping my blood sugar up by drinking orange juice.'

NUTRITIONAL HEALTH: CURRENT PERSPECTIVES

Nutritional health is a vital contributor to a patient's overall physical and mental wellbeing, with both ends of the spectrum, under- and overnutrition, being risk factors for numerous health issues and increased mortality. Identifying factors that contribute to the risk of over- and undernutrition is a vital step in enabling management of the risk and promoting optimal health.

In Australia and New Zealand, optimal nutritional health is promoted through a number of national guidelines that are based on the most up-to-date scientific evidence available. Three of the most useful resources are the:

- Australian Government Department of Health and National Health and Medical Research Council's (NHMRC) *Australian dietary guidelines* and *Australian guide to healthy eating*, found at https://www.eatforhealth.gov.au/guidelines
- New Zealand Ministry of Health's (NZMOH) *Food and nutrition guidelines*, found at www.health.govt.nz
- NHMRC and NZMOH's *Nutrient reference values for Australia and New Zealand including recommended dietary intakes*, found at www.nhmrc.gov.au.

In 2013, the NHMRC released the revised *Australian dietary guidelines* and the *Australian guide to healthy eating*. The complementary promotional program is titled 'Eat for Health Program'. The guidelines are based on the best available evidence to provide information on the types and amounts of foods, food groups and dietary patterns that aim to promote health and wellbeing and reduce the risk of chronic disease and diet-related conditions. It is important to note the recommendations within these dietary guidelines apply to all healthy Australians, including those with common diet-related risk factors, but do not apply to the frail elderly or to individuals requiring specialised dietary advice for medical conditions. Subsets of recommendations are available for infants, children and pregnant women. Recently added are recommendations for Aboriginal and Torres Strait Islander peoples.

In New Zealand there are a series of guidelines relating to food and nutrition across the lifecycle and each includes a background paper outlining the applicable evidence and health education resources for use with the public. The population-specific food and nutrition guidelines relate to infants and toddlers, children and young people, pregnant and breastfeeding women, adults and older people.

A summary of the current available recommendations and guidelines is provided in Table 14-1.

Identification of nutritional risk

It is important to understand that poor nutritional health or malnutrition occurs at both extremes of a continuum (undernutrition and overnutrition) and that the tools to identify nutritional risk at each extreme will differ. It is also important to consider that, although both extremes of the continuum may be obvious to the trained observer, it is possible that what we observe may in fact be masking nutrient deficiency or toxicity. This chapter will deal only with the identification of quite straightforward under- and overnutrition. A full nutritional assessment by an Accredited Practising Dietitian (APD) would be recommended for more complex cases. Some general indications of nutritional status are provided in Assessment tool 14-1. Table 14-2 provides an outline of some symptoms of poor nutrition and their possible causes.

Malnutrition

Malnutrition has many forms including under- nutrition which is wasting, stunting or being underweight, having inadequate vitamins or minerals, overweight, obesity and diet-related non-communicable diseases.

Undernutrition

According to the World Health Organization (WHO), more than 460 million people are considered underweight. Of this number, approximately 224 million are children under age 5 (WHO, 2018b). Around 45% of deaths in children under 5

Table 14-1 Summary of current dietary recommendations and guidelines

Title	Author and date	Summary
Nutrient reference values (NRVs)	NHMRC and NZMOH, 2006	A set of evidence-based recommendations for intake of 33 nutrients for specific age and gender groups. In 2017, revisions of the NRV included updates to the fluoride recommendation for 0 to 8 years old and for sodium for adults. The recommendations are aimed at reducing the risk of inadequate intake in healthy individuals. Recommendations for preventing or avoiding chronic disease are also provided in a separate section. The NRVs form the basis for the development of healthy eating guides and dietary guidelines.
Australian dietary guidelines (ADGs)	NHMRC, 2013b	A set of five evidence-based guidelines providing up-to-date recommendations for health eating in children and adults, to reduce the burden of preventable diet-related chronic conditions. The guidelines are aimed at healthy, independent individuals, so caution should be exercised in using them with individuals who are not well.
Australian guide to healthy eating (AGHE)	NHMRC, 2017	The AGHE aims to encourage the consumption of a variety of foods from the five food groups and is consistent with the *Dietary guidelines for Australians*. There is a pictorial component of the AGHE to assist in nutrition education. The 'plate', as it is often referred to by nutrition professionals, highlights the five food groups, the types of foods and beverages contained in each group and the proportion of the daily diet that should be attributed to each food group. The AGHE is aimed at healthy individuals, to reduce the likelihood of diet-related conditions.
New Zealand Ministry of Health's *Food and nutrition guidelines*	NZMOH, 2013a	A series of five population-specific food and nutrition guidelines providing the evidence base for nutrition policy advice and supporting the implementation of strategies such as the New Zealand Health Strategy.

ASSESSMENT TOOL 14-1 General indicators of nutritional status

Good nutritional status	Poor nutritional status
Alert, energetic, good endurance, good posture	Withdrawn, apathetic, easily fatigued, stooped posture
Good attention span, psychological stability	Inattentive, irritable
Weight within range for height, age, body size	Overweight or underweight
Firm, well-developed muscles, healthy reflexes	Flaccid muscles, wasted appearance, paraesthesia, diminished reflexes
Skin glowing, elastic, good turgor, smooth	Skin dull, pasty, scaly, dry, bruised
Eyes bright, clear without fatigue circles	Eyes dull, conjunctiva pale, discolouration under eyes
Hair shiny, lustrous, minimal loss	Hair brittle, dull, falls out easily
Mucous membranes:	Mucous membranes:
pink-red, gums pink and firm, tongue pink and moderately smooth, no swelling	pale, gums are red, boggy and bleed easily, tongue bright dark red and swollen
Abdomen flat, firm	Abdomen flaccid or distended (ascites)
No skeletal changes	Skeletal malformations
	In children stunting, wasting, low weight for age

are associated with undernutrition from mostly under low to middle-income countries (WHO, 2018b). The causes of underweight nutritional status are low standards of living, number of family members exceeding four, parent's low education level, alcohol use, hunger, starvation, agricultural illiteracy, poor antenatal care, disease, poor sanitation and living facilities (Senthilkumar et al., 2018).

Undernutrition comes in four forms: wasting, known as low weight for height; stunting, which is low height for age; underweight, as measured by low weight for the patient's age; and deficiencies in vitamins or minerals (WHO, 2018b). Patients may present with a multitude of risk factors for undernutrition. These may include, but are not limited to, frequent hospitalisation, social isolation, poverty, disability preventing access to food and preparation of food, inability to self-feed, malabsorption (a disease state resulting in increased kilojoule requirements) and poor appetite. Another risk factor for wasting of the body is due to severe chronic illness known as cachexia (Fearon et al., 2011). Cancer cachexia is ongoing loss of skeletal muscle with or without fat loss (Fearon et al., 2011). Ultimately, the consequences are a frail individual who has lost significant weight because of an insufficient dietary intake and who is unable to function at his or her previous or optimal level. Numerous instruments have been developed to identify patients rapidly who may be at risk of undernutrition, and nursing professionals are in the ideal position to implement

Table 14-2 Evaluating nutritional disorders

Body system or region	Sign or symptom	Implications
General	• Weakness and fatigue • Weight loss	• Anaemia or electrolyte imbalance • Decreased kilojoule intake, increased kilojoule use or inadequate nutrient intake or absorption
Skin, hair and nails	• Dry, flaky skin • Dry skin with poor turgor • Rough, scaly skin with bumps • Bruising • Sore that won't heal • Thinning, dry hair • Spoon-shaped, brittle or ridged nails	• Vitamin A, vitamin B-complex or linoleic acid deficiency • Dehydration • Vitamin A deficiency • Vitamin C or K deficiency • Protein, vitamin C or zinc deficiency • Protein deficiency • Iron deficiency
Eyes	• Night blindness, corneal swelling, softening or dryness, Bitot spots (grey triangular patches on the conjunctiva) • Red conjunctiva	• Vitamin A deficiency • Riboflavin deficiency
Throat and mouth	• Cracks at the corner of mouth • Magenta tongue • Beefy, red tongue • Soft, spongy, bleeding gums • Swollen neck (goitre)	• Riboflavin or niacin deficiency • Riboflavin deficiency • Vitamin B12 deficiency • Vitamin C deficiency • Iodine deficiency
Cardiovascular	• Oedema • Tachycardia, hypotension	• Protein deficiency • Fluid volume deficit
Gastrointestinal	• Ascites	• Protein deficiency
Musculoskeletal	• Bone pain and bow leg • Muscle wasting	• Vitamin D or calcium deficiency • Protein, carbohydrate and fat deficiency
Neurological	• Altered mental status • Paraesthesia	• Dehydration and thiamine or vitamin B12 deficiency • Vitamin B12, pyridoxine or thiamine deficiency

Springhouse. (2007). *Nutrition made incredibly easy!* (2nd ed.). Philadelphia: Lippincott Williams & Wilkins.

Table 14-3 Recommended valid and reliable nutrition screening instruments for the identification of undernutrition in acute care and rehabilitation settings

Instrument	Scope
1. Malnutrition Screening Tool (MST) (Ferguson et al., 1999)	1. Incorporates recent weight loss and poor intake
2. Mininutritional assessment Short Form (MNA-SF) (Rubenstein et al., 2001)	2. Incorporates recent intake, weight loss, mobility, acute disease, psychological stress, neuropsychological issues, body mass index (BMI)
3. Malnutrition Universal Screening Tool (MUST) (Elia, 2003)	3. Incorporates BMI, weight loss and acute disease effect score
4. Nutrition Risk Screening (NRS-2002) (Kondrup et al., 2003)	4. Incorporates recent weight loss, poor intake, BMI, severity of disease, elderly

Queensland Government. (2017). Validated malnutrition screening and assessment tools: Comparison guide. Available at https://www.health.qld.gov.au/__data/assets/pdf_file/0021/152454/hphe_scrn_tools.pdf

these instruments and refer patients for dietary management. In areas with high rates of undernutrition in children under 5 years old, standard anthropometric measures are used to assess nutritional status (Ghosh-Jerath et al., 2017).

The Australian Government and the Department of Ageing (NHMRC, 2013b) published *Australian dietary guidelines: Eat for health,* which highlights suitable instruments for assessing, diagnosing and managing nutritional status. The New Zealand Ministry has created a set of guidelines for nutrition and physical activity titled *Eating and activity guidelines for New Zealand adults* (2015). An outline of the instruments recommended in the acute and rehabilitation settings is provided in Table 14-3 and a description of some of the measurements required to be undertaken as part of these instruments is provided in the physical assessment section. Note there are also recommendations for nutrition screening instruments in the community and residential care setting; however, discussion of these topics is beyond the scope of this chapter. If you are working in either of these settings, then your local APD should be able to provide some advice on the most appropriate nutrition screening instrument.

CRITICAL THINKING

1. Does Mrs Uddina require nutrition screening?

Overnutrition

Overweight and obesity are commonly defined by the calculation of *body mass index* (BMI), or the measurement of waist girth alone. BMI is an age-dependent calculator that compares the person's weight to his or her height and is calculated by dividing body weight (in kilograms) by the height (in metres squared) (WHO, 2018a). BMI is the same for both genders. Weight measurement is a method to check if someone is carrying excessive body fat around their girth (middle). The method of performing measurements required to calculate these indices are outlined in the physical assessment section, and the formulae for the calculations and recommended cut-offs are provided in Table 14-4. Note that these cut-offs are generally not appropriate for use in older adults because BMI is not reflective of natural loss of height and weight, which are used to measure BMI, because of age-related changes (Butler et al., 2017; Cohen et al., 2009).

A recent survey in Australia, reported over two-thirds (67%) of adults are overweight or obese, increasing from 63.4% during the period from 2014 to 2015 (Australian Bureau of Statistics, 2019). The proportion of adults categorised as obese, has also increased from 27.9% to 31.3% from 2014 (Australian Bureau of Statistics, 2019). More adult men (74.5%) than women (59.7%) are considered overweight or obese. In Australian children, one-quarter (24.9%) of those between ages 5 and 17 years were overweight or obese, with similar rates for both genders (Australian Bureau of Statistics, 2019). The prevalence of obesity in a recent New Zealand (NZ) survey found around 32% of adults were obese—an increase from 27% during the period from 2006 to 2007 (NZ Ministry of Health, 2017). Around one-third (30.5%) of Europeans, half (47%) of Māori and two-thirds (65%) of Pacific Islander adults are considered obese (NZ Ministry of Health, 2017). In NZ children, around one-eighth (12%)—an increase from 8% during the period from 2006 to 2007—are classified as obese. The rate of obesity for Māori children is 17% and 30% for Pacific children (NZ Ministry of Health, 2017).

Obesity is rapidly increasing in the world and is considered a risk factor for diabetes mellitus, hypertension, coronary artery disease and cancer (Hooper et al., 2018; Zitterman et al., 2014). Bariatric surgery is currently the most effective medical management for severe obesity in adults (Rahiri et al., 2018). In children, lifestyle interventions, goal setting, changes to eating habits, physical activities, self-monitoring, and stimulus control are required to effectively manage childhood obesity (Kim & Park, 2017).

A summary of evidence-based health promotion and disease prevention for obesity in Australia and New Zealand can be seen in Table 14-5.

CRITICAL THINKING

2. If nutrition screening is indicated for Mrs Uddina, which screening tool would be appropriate? Is there any additional information that you would need to gather?
3. On completing an appropriate nutrition screening tool, has Mrs Uddina been identified as being at nutritional risk?

Table 14-4 Calculation of indices necessary in nutrition screening

Body mass index (WHO, 2018a)	Body weight (kg)/[Height (m)]^2 Underweight: <18.5 kg/m^2 Desirable: 18.5–24.99 kg/m^2 (Older adults >22 kg/m^2) Overweight: 25–29.99 kg/m^2 Obese: >30 kg/m^2 Obese class 1: 30–34.99 kg/m^2 Obese class II: 35.00–39.99 kg/m^2 Obese class III: ≥40.00 units
Estimating stature from knee height (Chumlea et al., 1985)	White males 19–59 years old: Stature (cm) = (Knee height, cm × 1.88) + 71.85 White females 19–59 years old: Stature (cm) = (Knee height, cm × 1.86) – (Age, years × 0.05) + 70.25 White males ≥60 years old: Stature (cm) = (Knee height, cm × 2.06) + 59.01 White females ≥60 years old: Stature (cm) = (Knee height, cm × 1.91) – (Age, years × 0.17) + 75

Table 14-5 Evidence-based health promotion and disease prevention: Obesity

Obesity definition: Classification using body mass index (BMI)	Obesity is defined as *a condition of abnormal or excessive fat accumulation in adipose tissue to the extent that health may be impaired* (World Health Organization [WHO], 2018a). The most commonly used tool for obesity classification is the body mass index (BMI) (calculated as weight in kilograms divided by height in metres squared), where obesity is classified as a BMI ≥30 kg/m^2 (WHO, 2018a). These classifications for obesity are based primarily on the relationship between the marked increased in mortality observed when BMI is higher than 30 kg/m^2.
Causes of obesity	Causes of obesity are numerous and complex. One of the main causes is thought to be the chronic overconsumption of energy-dense food and drink, which leads to excess energy intake and consequent increases in adiposity. Increased sedentary behaviour also promotes adiposity by decreasing energy expenditure. In addition to diet and physical activity, it is recognised that additional physiological mechanisms are implicated in regulation of body weight such as changes in appetite regulation, energy intake and expenditure following weight loss (Sumithran et al., 2011; Rosenbaum et al., 2008). In addition, diet and physical activity behaviours may be directly and indirectly influenced by a wide range of environmental factors such as policies in health, the food industry, urban planning, transport, marketing and education, which also have an increasing role in the effects of obesity (WHO, 2018a).

Continued on following page

Table 14-5 Evidence-based health promotion and disease prevention: Obesity (continued)

Consequences of obesity	Obesity is a major risk factor for many chronic diseases, including type 2 diabetes, cardiovascular disease and some cancers. Sleep apnoea and reproductive problems are also associated with obesity. Weight loss and maintaining a healthy diet can help people decrease the likelihood of or prevent morbidity and mortality from obesity-related chronic disease. Obesity-related chronic diseases impose considerable burden on individuals, as well as families, communities and the broader economy, with evidence suggesting that obese individuals have medical costs approximately 30% greater than their healthy weight peers (Withrow & Alter, 2011).
Evidence-based obesity prevention in Australia and New Zealand	***Australian dietary guidelines: Eat for Health*** **(NHMRC 2013a) and New Zealand's *Food and nutrition guidelines* (NZMOH 2013a)** The NHMRC (2013a) states that much of the burden of disease due to poor nutrition in Australia and New Zealand is associated with an excess intake of energy-dense, nutrient-poor foods and an inadequate intake of nutrient-dense foods such as vegetables, fruit and wholegrain cereals. Both sets of guidelines are underpinned by scientific evidence of food, diet and health relationships and are intended for use among people with common diet-related risk factors such as obesity. The *Australian dietary guidelines* (NHMRC, 2013a) related only to weight management are included here: **Guideline 1** To achieve and maintain a healthy weight, it is important to be physically active and to consume nutritious food and drinks to meet one's energy needs. **Guideline 2** Enjoy a wide variety of nutritious foods from these five groups every day: • Vegetables and legumes and beans • Fruit • Grain (cereal) foods (wholegrain or high cereal-fibre varieties) • Lean meats and poultry, fish, eggs, tofu, nuts and seeds • Milk, yoghurt, cheese (reduced fat) Drink plenty of water. **Guideline 3** Limit intake of foods and drinks containing high saturated fat, added salt, added sugars and alcohol such as biscuits, cakes, pastries, pies, processed meats, commercial burgers, pizza, fried foods, potato chips, crisps and other savoury snacks; and sugar-sweetened soft drinks and cordials, fruit drinks, vitamin-waters, and energy and sports drinks.
Evidence-based approach to weight management in primary health care in Australia and New Zealand	Clinical practice guidelines for the management of overweight and obesity in adults, adolescents and children in Australia (NHMRC, 2013a) These guidelines have recently been developed to assist health professionals in assessment and management of people who are overweight or obese (NHMRC, 2013a). Routine assessment and monitoring of BMI is recommended for adults over 18 years old to identify obesity in primary care. Where obesity is indicated (BMI >30 kg/m^2), an individualised multidisciplinary approach to management is recommended that includes: management of comorbidities, advice and referral for lifestyle interventions (diet, exercise, behaviour) and, where appropriate, consideration of more intensive weight-loss interventions such as pharmacological and surgical interventions (NHMRC, 2013a). Routine assessment and monitoring of BMI is recommended for children between 2 and 18 years using the United States Centers for Disease Control and Prevention and WHO growth charts (WHO, 2006; Kuczmarski et al., 2002). It is recommended that children are referred for specialist assessment and input where a weight management program is indicated (NHMRC, 2013a). Clinical guidelines for weight management in New Zealand adults (NZMOH, 2009) provide similar evidence-based guidelines for the management of obesity in primary care.
Multidisciplinary teams	Where a multidisciplinary approach to obesity management is recommended (NHMRC, 2013a), other practitioners who might be involved include: • General practitioner • Dietitian • Exercise physiologist • Psychologist • Diabetes educator • Mental health nurse • Bariatric surgeon • Physiotherapist • Social worker • Occupational therapist

Table 14-5	Evidence-based health promotion and disease prevention: Obesity (continued)
Key practice points	The NHMRC's (2013a) key practice points for obesity assessment and treatment in adults are: 1. **Assessment** • Routinely calculate BMI and measure waist circumference. • Discuss with the patient their readiness to make lifestyle changes in behaviours such as diet and physical activity. • Emphasise that even small amounts of weight loss may improve health and wellbeing, and can be particularly beneficial for the management of comorbidities. 2. **Treatment** • Multi-component interventions are preferred because these address all three lifestyle areas related to obesity (nutrition, physical activity and psychological approaches to behavioural change). • Refer the patient appropriately to assist them in making lifestyle changes or for further intervention (e.g. referral to an Accredited Practising Dietitian to assist them to plan and implement dietary changes). • Support a self-management approach and provide ongoing monitoring.

Health assessment

COLLECTING SUBJECTIVE DATA: THE NURSING HEALTH HISTORY

The interview provides valuable information about the patient's nutritional status. Nutritional assessment begins with questions regarding the patient's dietary habits. Questions should solicit information about average daily intake of food and fluids, types and quantities consumed, where and when food is eaten, and any conditions or diseases that affect intake or absorption. Collection of this information can add to the evaluation of the patient's risk factors and point to health education needs. It is important to approach the patient in a respectful and non-judgemental manner because self-esteem and body-image issues arise in part from less-than-optimal nutritional choices.

History of present health concern	
QUESTION	**RATIONALE**
Height and weight	
What are your or your child's height and usual weight?	Answer provides a baseline for comparing patient's perception with actual and current measurements. Answer also indicates patient's knowledge of own health status.
Have you or your child lost or gained a considerable amount of weight recently? How much? Over what period of time?	Weight changes may point to changes in nutrition or hydration status or to an illness causing weight changes.
Diet	
Are you now or have you been on a diet recently? How did you decide which diet to follow? What kind of food does your child eat? Have your or your child changed their eating practices lately?	Whether or not the patient is following his or her own diet or a medically prescribed diet, the answer to the question helps to identify chronic dieters and patients with eating disorders.
How much fluid do you drink each day? How much fluid does your child/infant drink per day? How much of it is water? How many sugary, caffeinated or alcoholic beverages do you or your infant/child have each day?	Answers to these questions identify patients in terms of adequate, moderate or excessive consumption of various kinds of fluids; they also identify those at risk of dehydration.
Can you recall what you or your child ate in the last 24 hours? In the last 72 hours?	The patient's typical daily diet indicates his or her level of nourishment, likes and dislikes, and dietary habits. As such, it provides a basis for planning healthy menu choices. (See, for example, Assessment tool 14-2.)

Continued on following page

History of present health concern (continued)

QUESTION	RATIONALE
Any recent changes in appetite, taste or smell? Have you noticed changes to your infants/child's appetite? Any recent difficulties chewing or swallowing?	Changes to taste and smell and difficulty chewing or swallowing may reduce the patient's intake of food.
Have you or has your infant/child had any recent occurrences of vomiting, diarrhoea or constipation?	Each of these affects nutritional status.

Past health history

QUESTION	RATIONALE
Do you or your infant/child have any chronic illnesses?	Chronic illnesses, such as cancer or diabetes, may impact the patient's nutritional status.
Have you or your infant/child experienced any recent trauma, surgery or serious illness?	Each of these may increase the patient's nutritional needs but decrease the patient's ability to meet these needs.

Family history

QUESTION	RATIONALE
Are any members of your family obese or underweight?	Malnutrition often runs in families. In addition, families may have unhealthy eating patterns that contribute to obesity or underweight or vitamin and mineral deficiencies.
Do any family members have heart disease or diabetes?	Heart disease and diabetes run in families.

Lifestyle and health practices

QUESTION	RATIONALE
Does your religion or culture have diet restrictions or requirements?	Some cultures and religions dictate diet.
What current medications/vitamins/supplements are you or your infant/child taking?	Poor nutritional status can impair metabolism of some medications. Some medications may cause weight changes, nausea, vomiting, delayed or increased gastrointestinal motility, decrease the patient's absorption of nutrients. Adverse effects may occur when someone is taking cytotoxic or anti-Parkinson medications such as olfactory disturbances, diminished salivation or appetite. Anorexia is a common side effect of some medications. Some medications are not to be taken with milk or grapefruit juice (van Zyl, 2011).
Do you prepare your own meals? What kind of diet/formula is your infant taking? Is your child breast fed? What do you or your infant/child eat on a typical day? What fluids do you/infant/child consume and how much do you/infant/child drink?	A daily account of dietary and fluid intake provides insight into the patient's nutrition and hydration.
Do you have sufficient income for food?	Low income may compromise the patient's ability to purchase food or make healthy food choices (i.e. foods high in fat and low in nutrients are often inexpensive.)
Do you or child follow an exercise regimen?	Physical exercise is important to maintaining health.

ASSESSMENT TOOL 14-2 Speedy checklist for nutritional health

Some warning signs of poor nutritional health are noted in this checklist. Use it to find out if your patient is at nutritional risk. Read the statements below. Circle the number in the yes column for those that apply to the patient. For each yes answer, score the number in the box. Total the nutrition score.

	YES
Illness or condition that made patient change the kind and/or amount of food eaten	2
Eats fewer than two meals per day	3
Eats few fruits or vegetables, or milk products	2
Has three or more drinks of beer, liquor or wine almost every day	2
Tooth or mouth problems that make it hard to eat	2
Does not always have enough money to buy the food needed	4
Eats alone most of the time	1
Takes three or more different prescribed or over-the-counter drugs a day	1
Without wanting to, has lost or gained 4.5 kg in the last 6 months	2
Not physically able to shop, cook or feed self	2
TOTAL	

Total the nutritional score.

0–2	Good. Recheck the score in 6 months.
3–5	Moderate nutritional risk. See what can be done to improve eating habits and lifestyle. Recheck score in 3 months.
6 or more	High nutritional risk. Consult with doctor, dietitian or other qualified health or social service professional.

Note: Remember that warning signs suggest risk but do not represent diagnosis of any condition.

COLDSPA

Example for weight gain

Use the COLDSPA mnemonic as a guideline to collect needed information for each symptom the patient shares. In addition, the following questions help elicit important information.

Mnemonic	Question	Patient response example
Character	Describe the sign or symptom (feeling, appearance, sound, smell, or taste, if applicable).	Weight of 80 kg, height of 158 cm with a body mass index of 31
Onset	When did it begin?	'My weight has steadily increased over the past 5 years.'
Location	Where is it? Does it radiate? Does it occur anywhere else?	'Mostly in my abdomen and thighs.'
Duration	How long does it last? Does it recur?	N/A
Severity	How bad is it? How much does it bother you?	'I'm so tired of struggling with my weight. I look in the mirror and I can't believe it's me.'
Pattern	What makes it better or worse?	'I have tried almost every diet. Some work for a while and then I gain weight again.'
Associated factors/How it Affects the patient	What other symptoms occur with it? How does it affect you?	'I'm too tired to exercise. I don't even like to shop anymore because I hate trying on clothes. I look so fat.'

There are several infant and paediatric nutritional screening tools available: Paediatric Yorkhill Malnutrition Score (iPYMS), Subjective Global Nutritional Assessment (SGNA), Screening Tool Risk on Nutritional Status and Growth (STRONGkids) (Gerasimidis, 2017). Other tools used commonly in Australia are: Paediatric Nutrition Screening Tool (PNST), Paediatric Malnutrition Screening Tool, Electronic kids Dietary Index (E-Kindex), Nutrition screening tool for every pre-schooler / toddler (NutriSTEP, NutriSTEP toddler), Nutrition Screening for Childhood Cancer (SCAN) and Screening Tool for the Assessment of Malnutrition (STAMP) (Academy of Nutrition and Dietetics, 2018; Queensland Government, 2019). Also parents can be asked to fill out questionnaires on eating behaviour and habits including infant's diet type of milk, supplementary feeding, weaning diet, weight loss or gain or poor weight gain, gastrointestinal symptoms and daily activities (Gerasimidis, 2017).

Eating disorders such as anorexia nervosa and bulimia nervosa are undertreated in adolescents. SCOFF is a valid eating disorder screening tool (Hill et al., 2010). In the older population, where there is an emerging phenomenon of eating disorders in the elderly, especially in the residential care setting, the screening tools include the Geriatric Nutritional Risk Index (GNRI), Mini Nutritional Assessment-Short Form (MNA®-SF), Malnutrition Screening Tool (MST), Nutritional Risk Screening 2002 (NRS2002), Malnutrition Universally Screening Tool (MUST) Short Nutritional Assessment Questionnaire 65+ (SNAQ65+) and Australian Nutrition Screening Initiative (ANSI) (Ferguson et al., 1999; Vrdoljak, 2015; Winter et al., 2013). The first step in nutritional care for elderly is nutritional screening. For convenience and simplicity, the most common tool used to screen for malnutrition is the MNA-SF (Vrdoljak, 2015).

COLLECTING OBJECTIVE DATA: PHYSICAL EXAMINATION

Physical examination includes measuring weight and height and assessing hydration.

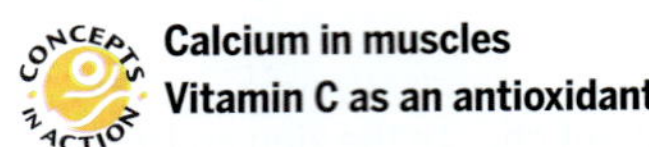

Calcium in muscles
Vitamin C as an antioxidant

In paediatric patients, nutritional physical assessment is collected using medical records, anthropometric measurements including patient's weight, length and head circumference. Nutrition-focused physical examination confirms muscle wasting, measurement of fat stores under skinfolds, subcutaneous fat loss, skin lesions and oedema. Other important information to collect includes chronic diseases, long-term tube feedings or total parenteral nutrition (Green Corkins, 2015).

Strategies to prevent and manage nutritional risk

Following the identification of nutritional risk or suboptimal nutritional status in a patient, there are a number of strategies that the nursing professional can implement with the potential of improving the patient's situation. The types and extent of strategies will depend on the setting in which the nursing professional works (e.g. hospital setting versus an outpatient setting), the patient's risk factors (risk factors for over- or undernutrition), and the resources available to the nursing professional and the patient themselves.

PHYSICAL ASSESSMENT

ASSESSMENT PROCEDURE	MEASUREMENT	ASSESSMENT PROCEDURE	MEASUREMENT
Measurements to complete nutrition screening instruments (Norton & Olds, 1996)			
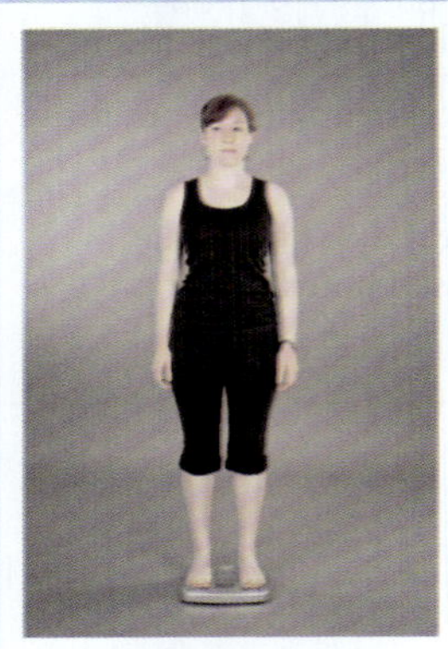 FIGURE 14-1 Measuring body weight.	**Body weight:** Measure using regularly calibrated electronic scales (bed, chair or stand on) with patient in light clothing and no shoes (Fig. 14-1). Record to the nearest 0.1 kg.	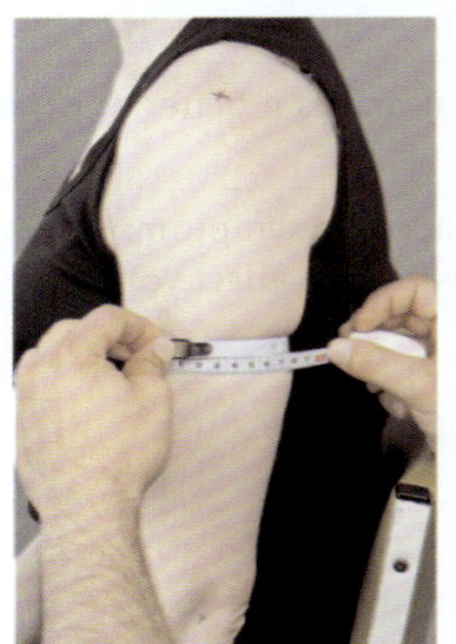 FIGURE 14-4 Measuring mid-arm circumference.	**Mid-arm circumference:** Using a steel tape measure, position the tape at the level of the mid-acromiale–radiale (Fig. 14-4). Record to the nearest 0.1 cm. The use of alternative tape measures (e.g. paper) is not recommended because they can be stretched and therefore give inaccurate readings.

PHYSICAL ASSESSMENT (continued)

ASSESSMENT PROCEDURE	MEASUREMENT	ASSESSMENT PROCEDURE	MEASUREMENT
Measurements to complete nutrition screening instruments (continued)			
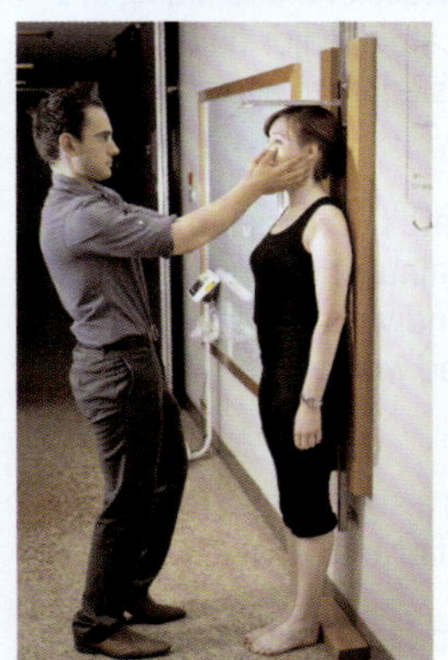 **FIGURE 14-2** Measuring standing height.	**Standing height:** Measure using a stadiometer or tape mounted to a wall when the patient is able to assume the appropriate position—feet together with heels, buttocks and upper part of the back touching the stadiometer or tape, with the patient looking directly ahead (Fig. 14-2). The measurement should be taken as the patient holds a deep breath. Record to the nearest 0.1 cm.	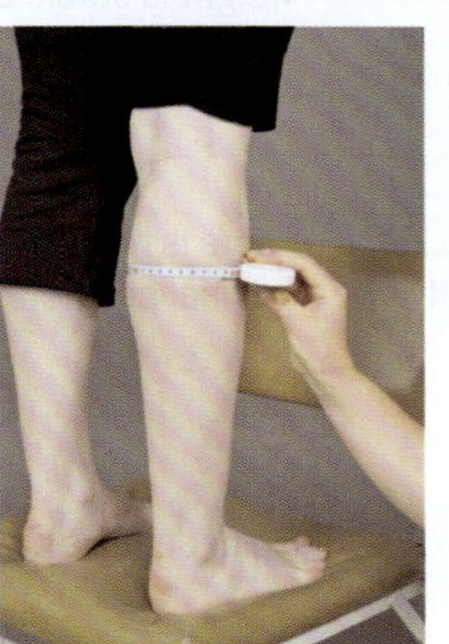 **FIGURE 14-5** Measuring calf circumference.	**Calf circumference:** Using a steel tape measure, position the tape at the maximum circumference of the calf (Fig. 14-5). Should be taken as the patient holds a deep breath. Record to the nearest 0.1 cm.
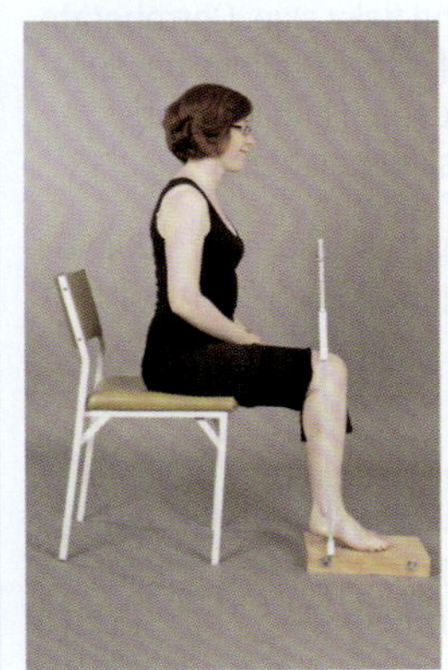 **FIGURE 14-3** Measuring knee height.	**Knee height:** An alternative measure to standing height, particularly useful for older adults or immobile patients who cannot assume the appropriate position for accurate measurement. Ideally measured on the left side unless affected by disease or disability, a calliper is positioned with one end under the heel and the sliding blade locked firmly in place approximately 5 cm behind the patella (Fig. 14-3). Record to the nearest 0.1 cm.	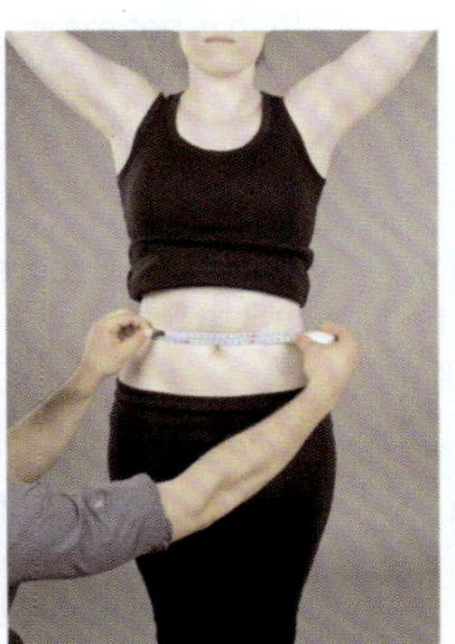 **FIGURE 14-6** Measuring waist circumference.	**Waist circumference:** Using a steel tape measure, assume a position directly in front of the patient and position the tape measure around the waist at the level of the narrowest point between the lowest rib and the iliac crest or alternatively at the mid-point if there is no obvious narrowing (Fig. 14-6). Take the measurement at the end of a normal expiration. Record to the nearest 0.1 cm.

PHYSICAL ASSESSMENT

ASSESSMENT PROCEDURE	NORMAL FINDINGS	ABNORMAL FINDINGS
Hydration		
INPATIENT SETTING: INTAKE AND OUTPUT		
Measure intake and output (I & O) in inpatient settings. Measure all fluids taken in by oral and parenteral routes, through irrigation tubes, such as medications in solution, and through tube feedings. Also measure all fluid output (urine, stool, drainage from tubes, perspiration). Calculate insensible loss at 800 to 1,000 mL daily, and add to total output.	Intake and output are closely balanced over 72 hours when insensible loss is included. **CLINICAL TIP** **Fluid is normally retained during acute stress, illness, trauma and surgery. Expect diuresis to occur in most patients in 48 to 72 hours.**	Imbalances in either direction suggest impaired organ function and fluid overload or inability to compensate for losses resulting in dehydration.

Continued on following page

PHYSICAL ASSESSMENT (continued)

ASSESSMENT PROCEDURE	NORMAL FINDINGS	ABNORMAL FINDINGS
ALL SETTINGS: FLUID-RELATED CHANGES		
Weigh patients at risk of hydration changes daily.	Weight is stable or changes less than 1 to 2 kg over 1 to 5 days.	Weight gains or losses of 2.5 to 4.5 kg in 1 week or less indicate a major fluid shift. A change of 1 kg is equal to a loss or gain of 1 L of fluid.
Check skin turgor. Pinch a small fold of skin, observing elasticity, and watch how quickly the skin returns to its original position.	There is no tenting and skin returns to original position.	Tenting can indicate fluid loss but is also present in malnutrition and loss of collagen in aged individuals. This finding must be correlated with other hydration findings.
Check for pitting oedema.	No oedema is present.	Pitting oedema is a sign of fluid retention, especially in cardiac and renal diseases.
Check muscle mass and strength	No wasting of muscles and normal full strength	Muscle wasting and reduced strength may be due to ongoing weight loss or cachexia.
Observe skin for moisture.	Skin is not excessively dry.	Abnormally dry and flaky skin. Corroborate such a finding with other findings because heredity and cholesterol and hormone levels determine skin moistness.
Assess venous filling. Lower the patient's arm or leg and observe how long it takes to fill. Then raise the arm or leg and watch how long it takes to empty.	Veins fill in 3 to 5 seconds. Veins empty in 3 to 5 seconds.	Filling or emptying that takes more than 6 to 10 seconds suggests fluid volume deficit.
Observe neck veins with patient in the supine position then with the head elevated above 45-degree angle.	Neck veins are softly visible in supine position. With head elevated above 45-degree angle, the neck veins flatten or are slightly visible but soft.	Flat veins in supine patient may indicate dehydration. Visible firm neck veins indicate distension possibly resulting from fluid retention and heart disease.
Inspect the tongue's condition and furrows.	Tongue is moist, plump with central sulcus and no additional furrows.	Tongue is dry with visible papillae and several longitudinal furrows, suggesting loss of normal third-space fluid and dehydration.
Gently palpate eyeball.	Eyeball is moderately firm to touch but not hard.	Eyeball is boggy and lacks normal tension, suggesting loss of normal third-space fluid and dehydration. **CLINICAL TIP** **A hard eyeball is more indicative of eye disease than of hydration abnormalities.**
Observe eye position and surrounding colouration.	Eyes are not sunken and no dark circles appear under them.	Sunken eyes, especially with deep dark circles, point to dehydration.

PHYSICAL ASSESSMENT (continued)

ASSESSMENT PROCEDURE	NORMAL FINDINGS	ABNORMAL FINDINGS
Hydration (continued)		
Auscultate lung sounds.	No crackles, friction rubs or harsh lung sounds are auscultated.	Loud or harsh breath sounds indicate decreased pleural fluid. Friction rubs may also be heard. Crackling indicates increased fluid, as in interstitial fluid sequestration (i.e. pulmonary oedema).
Take blood pressure with patient in standing, sitting and lying positions. Also palpate radial pulse.	There are no orthostatic changes; blood pressure and pulse rate remain within normal range for patient's activity level and status.	Blood pressure registers lower than usual or drops more than 20 mmHg from lying to standing position, thereby indicating fluid volume deficit, especially if the pulse rate is also elevated. Radial pulse rate +1 and thready denotes dehydration. Elevated pulse rate and blood pressure indicate overhydration.

For the overweight or obese patient, there are a number of strategies that could be implemented, depending on the extent of the patient's weight issue. In extreme cases, patients should be referred to an Accredited Practising Dietitian (APD) who has expertise in weight management. A referral to a medical professional with expertise and an interest in weight management should also be considered. Potential referrals should initially be discussed with the patient before making the referral, to ensure that the patient's consent is obtained. For overweight or obese patients, initial strategies that could be implemented include:

- Providing written resources on healthy eating, such as the *Australian guide to healthy eating* (NHMRC, 2017), with some verbal advice regarding a healthy diet
- Referring the patient to local community groups that promote physical activity (e.g. walking groups), particularly for patients who would benefit from peer support
- Referring the patient to ongoing dietary support and encouragement through regular review sessions with a community nutritionist or dietitian.

It is important to note that there are significant psychosocial issues for some patients with weight management issues that may affect their ability to be successful with weight loss. Some factors include inadequate support networks; mental health issues such as anxiety, depression and body image distortion; and past history of physical, sexual or verbal abuse. Referral to a psychologist or counselling service would be worthy of consideration in these cases.

For the undernourished patient, the strategies considered will depend on whether the nursing professional is in the acute setting, residential care or the community setting. Undernutrition is prevalent in each of these settings to varying extents, in particular among the elderly and in individuals with an illness, particularly chronic illness.

Acute setting

In the acute setting, most hospitals in Australia now have protected meal times as a method to improve food intake, provide feeding assistance and reduce interruptions (Porter et al., 2017). This is especially helpful for patient at risk of malnutrition, whereas hospitalised patients at risk of undernutrition should also have appropriate nutrition screening undertaken (see Table 14-3), which would then allow certain strategies to be implemented. The patient would then be referred to an APD for a full nutritional assessment, and the APD would then take responsibility for the nutritional management of the patient. However, there are a number of strategies that the nursing professional can implement prior to the APD becoming involved, particularly if there is an extended period before the dietitian is likely to be available for consultation, for example:

- *Ensuring the patient is receiving the correct diet.* Many hospitals have a high energy and protein diet for patients at risk of undernutrition, which the nursing professional could potentially order for the patient.
- *Ensuring appropriate assistance is available.* A crucial strategy for implementation by the nursing professional is to ensure that there is appropriate assistance available for the patient at meal times. Often, foods and drinks are served in packaging that may be difficult to open or hold, particularly prepackaged items, and rather than ask for assistance, the patient may leave the difficult item and hence have a reduced intake at meals. Simple strategies such as cutting foods, holding straws and ensuring items are within the patient's reach make a significant difference to the patient's ability to eat at meal times. The same applies to mid-meal snacks and drinks trolleys.
- *Providing encouragement and incentives during meal times.* The unwell patient will often have difficulties with consuming an adequate diet while in hospital; however, simple encouragement can often assist. Making sure that the patient is awake at meal times and encouraging them to try foods, particularly those that are higher in energy and protein, can improve overall intake. Encouraging intake between meals by reserving components of the meal (e.g. dessert) and offering them later can also assist, along with encouraging the patient to attempt any snack items or nutritional

supplements that have been ordered by the dietitian between meals. Often, large meals can be overwhelming and hence small amounts spread across the day result in a larger overall intake. Patients who undergo medical tests and procedures can miss many meal opportunities because they need to fast for the procedures or are away from the ward during a meal time. In these instances, meals should be retained for the patient and offered at an appropriate time after the procedure or period of fasting.

CASE STUDY

On assessment, you find Mrs Uddina has soft, sunken eyeballs and her tongue is dry and furrowed. Her blood pressure is 100/80 mmHg (usual is 150/70 mmHg); her pulse is 100 and respirations are 24. Her temperature is 37.5 °C. Her blood glucose level is 26 mmol/L (her usual is 14 to 16.5 mmol/L). Mrs Uddina refuses to check her blood glucose level herself. When asked why she did not call the nurse or doctor when she became ill, she stated, 'I didn't think it was that serious. I didn't have a high temperature.'

CRITICAL THINKING

4. What strategies could you implement as a nursing professional?

Residential care setting

In the residential care setting, many of the strategies listed above are applicable in maximising dietary intake; however, there are also additional strategies that may be possible:

- *Emphasising the social benefits of taking meals with others.* Social isolation is often a contributor to poorer nutritional health among individuals, particularly elderly individuals or those with a chronic illness. In the residential setting, individuals should be encouraged to spend meal times in the dining room with other residents and the social aspects of communal dining should be encouraged. This also enables easier monitoring of the residents' intake to facilitate timely intervention if indicated. Communal morning and afternoon tea could also be encouraged.
- *Providing high-energy or protein liquids or softer foods that are easy to swallow.* Many residential facilities routinely stock commercial nutritional supplements that can be used to maximise nutritional intake, particularly for residents who find it easier to drink, rather than eat. Although commercial supplements are useful, they are often expensive and if the resident is provided with them for a long period of time, they often experience 'flavour fatigue' leading to reduced consumption in the longer term. A good alternative to the commercial supplements, and something that should be trialled first, is the provision of nourishing fluids and snacks between meals. Nourishing fluids and snacks provide high energy and protein in a small volume. Some useful items are flavoured milk drinks and milkshakes, full-fat yoghurts and dairy desserts, scones with jam and cream, cheese and biscuits, and toast with spreads such as margarine, peanut butter and thickly spread honey or jam. An APD will be able to provide additional guidance on appropriate foods and drinks and methods of incorporating them into the patient's diet.
- *Varying mealtimes by including visitors.* Involving family members and friends who are external to the residential facility can often be useful in improving dietary intake. This could be in the form of family or friends joining the resident for the occasional meal; or, where possible, the resident could be taken out for a meal. Not only does this provide social interaction but it also increases variety in meals and exposure to different foods that may not be available in the facility. Encouraging family and friends to bring in the resident's favourite foods and drinks or particular items that cannot be provided by the facility can increase the resident's enjoyment in eating and improve intake.
- *Being aware of effects of the patient's cognitive level.* It is important for the nurse to be aware of psychosocial and cognitive issues in residential care patients that may limit the success of nutrition strategies. Some of these factors are delirium and apathy that may accompany the end of life, leading to food refusal and disinterest. Dementia is one of the most prevalent conditions in residential care; it affects the person's ability to meet required nutritional status as it impacts the person's ability to eat, drink and participate in meal activities. Some strategies used to support the person with dementia include food presentation on coloured plates, meal styles, training programs (e.g. Montessori or space retrieval), environmental adaptions (e.g. increased dining room lighting), music and animal-assisted therapy (Featherstonhaugh et al., 2019).
- *Referring at-risk patients to specialists for assessment.* Some residential facilities have an APD as part of their staff; however, this is not always the case. It is more common that residential facilities will have a consultation arrangement with an APD, who will visit the facility on an 'as needed' basis. It is important that residents who are identified as being nutritionally 'at risk' for both under and overnutrition are referred for expert nutritional assessment, particularly if the strategies outlined have been implemented with limited success.

Community setting

Undernutrition in a community-dwelling adult is usually suspected initially by community support providers or family and friends. Many of the strategies listed also apply to the community setting; however, the crucial difference lies within the individual's ability to access adequate nutritional assessment and support.

A community nurse can often be the initial health professional who identifies potential undernutrition and hence can implement some of the strategies discussed in this chapter, particularly those addressing social isolation and providing initial patient education on a high-energy and high-protein diet and small, frequent meals. The community nurse would also be instrumental in the regular monitoring of the individual. Potential difficulties may arise in ensuring that a full assessment and follow-up by an APD is done and also accessing commercial supplements that may be financially prohibitive.

Community-dwelling individuals identified as being undernourished or at risk of undernutrition should be referred to an

APD. Many community health services and hospitals have a dietetic service to which community health providers and general practitioners can refer. There are also a growing number of private practising dietitians who also work with patients with undernutrition. A list of private APDs can be accessed at www.daa.asn.au and access can be through self-referral or health-provider referral. Many private health insurance companies provide rebates for dietetic services and dietetic products; however, patients should check with their own insurance provider if they are eligibile for insurance. Access to commercial supplements can occur via a variety of methods for community-dwelling patients. Many government dietetic services, such as community health services and hospitals, can provide subsidised commercial supplements to patients whom they see on a regular basis, significantly reducing the financial costs associated with these products. Private practising dietitians may also be able to access subsidised products for some patients with particular benefits (e.g. Department of Veterans Affairs) or they may be subsidised through private health insurance.

MONITORING THE SUCCESS OF TREATMENT STRATEGIES

The outcomes of monitoring nutrition-intervention measurements can be described as: direct nutrition outcomes; clinical and health status outcomes; patient-centred outcomes; health care utilisation outcomes; and cost outcomes. The focus of this chapter is on direct nutrition outcomes and nutritional biochemistry that the nurse can be involved with while measuring or monitoring patients, such as those listed below.

- *Has an improvement in dietary intake been observed?* By simple observation, the nurse may be able to detect an increase or decrease in the amount or frequency of food and fluid consumed in the acute, rehabilitation or residential care setting. A more accurate method that will provide more comprehensive information to the dietitian about actual energy and protein intake (relevant particularly for undernutrition) or energy, fat, refined carbohydrate and fibre intake (relevant particularly for overnutrition) would be to complete a food chart. A food chart is designed to document all food and fluid consumed over 2 to 3 consecutive days. The dietitian can use this information, if sufficiently detailed, to estimate total energy, macro- and micronutrient intake, compare this with recommended amounts and make adjustments if necessary.

Other methods for monitoring improvement in dietary intake include measuring plate waste, 24-hour recall by the patient (inappropriate where poor cognition is a factor) and keeping a food diary.

- *Has there been an improvement in relevant nutrition anthropometry (measurement of size or shape of the human body)?* The simplest and most sensitive to change measure of nutrition anthropometry is body weight. Weight can be charted and any trend in either direction reported to the treating dietitian. Another measure increasing in popularity is the mid-arm circumference, which has been described in the physical assessment section.
- *Has there been an improvement in relevant nutritional biochemistry?* Reviewing certain laboratory tests can yield valuable information about the success of the dietary intervention. These tests can be useful for monitoring undernutrition, especially subtle changes before they are clinically evident. For example, a person can be obese yet undernourished because of poor food choices. In this situation, laboratory tests such as haemoglobin or protein levels may indicate anaemia or other nutritional disorders. When people are undernourished, the body's protein stores are affected. The proteins usually sacrificed early are those that the body considers to be less essential to survival: albumin, globulins, transport proteins, skeletal muscle proteins, blood proteins and immune globulins. These can be easily evaluated by blood tests.

CRITICAL THINKING

5. How would you monitor the impact of your interventions?

Communicating nutritional risk

Documentation is the key to communicating nutritional risk to other relevant health professionals. Nurses should document the findings of nutrition screening instruments administered and the action taken, if any. It is important to ensure high levels of awareness of nutrition risk and the likely consequences of inaction. Poor nutritional health can have an impact on the success of other medical or allied health interventions and ensuring successful interventions is therefore a team responsibility. Also integral to the team are the patients themselves and their families or support networks. The nurse professional can act as a vital liaison between team members and thereby optimise the nutritional outcomes for their patients.

CRITICAL THINKING

6. What plans would need to be considered to ensure Mrs Uddina's nutritional care is ongoing?

ONLINE RESOURCES

thePoint

An extensive range of additional resources to enhance teaching and learning and to facilitate understanding may be found online at the text's accompanying website, located on thePoint at http://thepoint.lww.com. These include Watch and Learn videos, Concepts in Action animations, journal articles, case studies, discussion topics and quizzes.

Subscribers may also access Lippincott Procedures, an extensive online point-of-care procedure guide that provides reliable step-by-step instructions for more than 1700 procedures, including 450 evidence-based Australian procedures, and skills in a variety of speciality settings, together with a wealth of supporting information.

CASE STUDY

The case study demonstrates how to analyse nutritional assessment data for a specific patient. The exercises included in the ancillary product on thePoint that complements this text offer further opportunities to enhance your skills.

Mrs Visna Uddina, a 58-year-old lady of Indian descent, has a history of type 1 diabetes. When you weigh her during your weekly community home visit, you find she weighs 65 kg, which is 5 kg less than she weighed at your last visit. You try to weigh her at the same time of day each week—9.30 a.m. She usually has breakfast at 6.30 a.m. and takes 40 units of insulin at 7.30 a.m. Today she tells you she has been urinating 'a lot' and that she has felt lethargic and tired for the past 3 days, with nausea and 'just a little vomiting'. She also tells you that she has had headaches and blurred vision and that she feels dizzy sometimes. She says she has not been eating well but adds, 'I'm keeping my blood sugar up by drinking orange juice.'

On assessment, you find Mrs Uddina has soft, sunken eyeballs and her tongue is dry and furrowed. Her blood pressure is 100/80 mmHg (usual is 150/70 mmHg); her pulse is 100, and respirations are 24. Her temperature is 37.5 °C. Her blood glucose level is 26 mmol/L (her usual is 14 to 16.5 mmol/L). Mrs Uddina refuses to check her blood glucose level herself. When asked why she did not call the nurse or doctor when she became ill, she stated, 'I didn't think it was that serious. I didn't have a high temperature.'

The following concept map illustrates the diagnostic reasoning process.

Applying COLDSPA

Applying COLDSPA for patient symptoms: 'urinating a lot and feels like she has a flu'.

Mnemonic	Question	Data provided	Missing data
Character	Describe the sign or symptom (feeling, appearance, sound, smell or taste, if applicable).	5-kg weight loss; frequent urination; flulike symptoms; nausea with some vomiting; soft, sunken eyeballs; dry, furrowed tongue; lower blood pressure than usual; high heart rate; increased respirations; low-grade fever; elevated blood glucose level, but not monitoring her glucose level (not eating much so reasons that she needs to keep 'blood sugar up by drinking orange juice').	
Onset	When did it begin?	Began sometime after last week's visit. Reports 3 days of lethargy and tiredness symptoms including nausea and vomiting, headaches, dizziness and blurred vision.	
Location	Where is it? Does it radiate? Does it occur anywhere else?		Do you have any pain? Where is the pain located? Does the pain move anywhere else?
Duration	How long does it last? Does it recur?		How often are you nauseated? How often do you urinate? How long the dizzy do spells last? Does the blurred vision come and go? How long do the headaches and pain last?
Severity	How bad is it? How much does it bother you?		How much do you urinate at a time? How much do you vomit at a time? On a scale of 0-10, 0 being no pain and 10 being worse pain ever, how would you rate your headaches? How thirsty do you feel?
Pattern	What makes it better or worse?		What are you eating and when? How do you feel before you drink orange juice? How much juice do you have and how often? How much insulin are you taking and when do you take it? Do you do anything for the headaches? Does it help? Do you do anything for the nausea and vomiting? Does it help?
Associated factors/How it Affects the patient	What other symptoms occur with it? How does it affect you?	Without a high fever, she didn't think her symptoms were very serious.	Are you hungry? Have you noticed any mood changes? Is your skin itchy or have you had skin infections, or wounds that do not heal? Have you noticed any weight loss? Do you suffer from leg cramps?

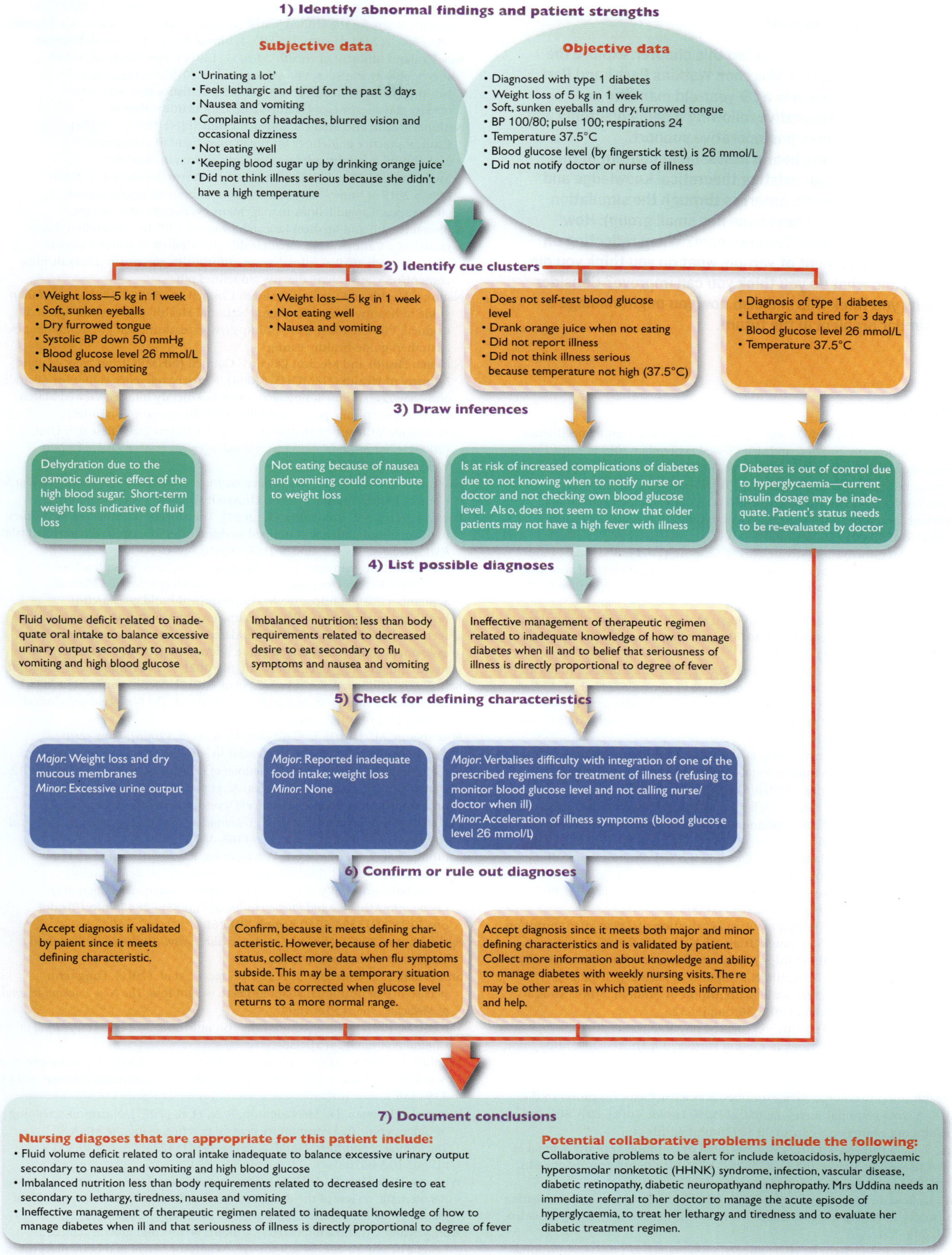

1) Identify abnormal findings and patient strengths

Subjective data

- 'Urinating a lot'
- Feels lethargic and tired for the past 3 days
- Nausea and vomiting
- Complaints of headaches, blurred vision and occasional dizziness
- Not eating well
- 'Keeping blood sugar up by drinking orange juice'
- Did not think illness serious because she didn't have a high temperature

Objective data

- Diagnosed with type 1 diabetes
- Weight loss of 5 kg in 1 week
- Soft, sunken eyeballs and dry, furrowed tongue
- BP 100/80; pulse 100; respirations 24
- Temperature 37.5°C
- Blood glucose level (by fingerstick test) is 26 mmol/L
- Did not notify doctor or nurse of illness

2) Identify cue clusters

- Weight loss—5 kg in 1 week
- Soft, sunken eyeballs
- Dry furrowed tongue
- Systolic BP down 50 mmHg
- Blood glucose level 26 mmol/L
- Nausea and vomiting

- Weight loss—5 kg in 1 week
- Not eating well
- Nausea and vomiting

- Does not self-test blood glucose level
- Drank orange juice when not eating
- Did not report illness
- Did not think illness serious because temperature not high (37.5°C)

- Diagnosis of type 1 diabetes
- Lethargic and tired for 3 days
- Blood glucose level 26 mmol/L
- Temperature 37.5°C

3) Draw inferences

Dehydration due to the osmotic diuretic effect of the high blood sugar. Short-term weight loss indicative of fluid loss

Not eating because of nausea and vomiting could contribute to weight loss

Is at risk of increased complications of diabetes due to not knowing when to notify nurse or doctor and not checking own blood glucose level. Also, does not seem to know that older patients may not have a high fever with illness

Diabetes is out of control due to hyperglycaemia—current insulin dosage may be inadequate. Patient's status needs to be re-evaluated by doctor

4) List possible diagnoses

Fluid volume deficit related to inadequate oral intake to balance excessive urinary output secondary to nausea, vomiting and high blood glucose

Imbalanced nutrition: less than body requirements related to decreased desire to eat secondary to flu symptoms and nausea and vomiting

Ineffective management of therapeutic regimen related to inadequate knowledge of how to manage diabetes when ill and to belief that seriousness of illness is directly proportional to degree of fever

5) Check for defining characteristics

Major: Weight loss and dry mucous membranes
Minor: Excessive urine output

Major: Reported inadequate food intake; weight loss
Minor: None

Major: Verbalises difficulty with integration of one of the prescribed regimens for treatment of illness (refusing to monitor blood glucose level and not calling nurse/doctor when ill)
Minor: Acceleration of illness symptoms (blood glucose level 26 mmol/L)

6) Confirm or rule out diagnoses

Accept diagnosis if validated by paient since it meets defining characteristic.

Confirm, because it meets defining characteristic. However, because of her diabetic status, collect more data when flu symptoms subside. This may be a temporary situation that can be corrected when glucose level returns to a more normal range.

Accept diagnosis since it meets both major and minor defining characteristics and is validated by patient. Collect more information about knowledge and ability to manage diabetes with weekly nursing visits. There may be other areas in which patient needs information and help.

7) Document conclusions

Nursing diagoses that are appropriate for this patient include:

- Fluid volume deficit related to oral intake inadequate to balance excessive urinary output secondary to nausea and vomiting and high blood glucose
- Imbalanced nutrition less than body requirements related to decreased desire to eat secondary to lethargy, tiredness, nausea and vomiting
- Ineffective management of therapeutic regimen related to inadequate knowledge of how to manage diabetes when ill and that seriousness of illness is directly proportional to degree of fever

Potential collaborative problems include the following:

Collaborative problems to be alert for include ketoacidosis, hyperglycaemic hyperosmolar nonketotic (HHNK) syndrome, infection, vascular disease, diabetic retinopathy, diabetic neuropathyand nephropathy. Mrs Uddina needs an immediate referral to her doctor to manage the acute episode of hyperglycaemia, to treat her lethargy and tiredness and to evaluate her diabetic treatment regimen.

SIMULATED LEARNING

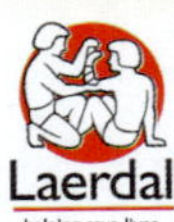

Having completed this chapter, explore the scenarios of Vernon Watkins Part 1 and Part 2. Vernon is a 69-year-old man who is postoperative following a hemicolectomy and requires postoperative support.

Incorporating the health assessment content in this chapter with your existing theoretical knowledge and clinical experience, progress through the simulation scenarios (this is best done in a small group). How would you manage Vernon's care? When reflecting on your management of Vernon, what do you think you did well and what do you think you can improve? Consider why you think this and also how you might manage a similar problem in the future.

References

Academy of Nutrition and Dietetics. (2018). Nutrition screening paediatrics: Tool components and descriptions. Viewed September 2019 at https://www.andeal.org/topic.cfm?menu=5767&cat=5922.

Australian Bureau of Statistics (ABS). (2019). National health survey: First results, 2017-18. ABS cat. no. 4364.0.55.001. Canberra: Australia. Viewed September 2019 at http://www.abs.gov.au/ausstats/abs@.nsf/mf/4364.0.55.001.

Butler, R., McClinchy, J., Morreale-Parker, C., et al. (2017). Body mass index (BMI) calculation in older people: The effect of using direct and surrogate measures of height in a community based setting. *Clinical Nutrition ESPEN, 22*, 112–115.

Chumlea, W. C., Roche, A. F. & Steinbaugh, M. L. (1985). Estimating stature from knee height for persons 60 to 90 years of age. *Journal of the American Geriatrics Society, 33*(2), 116–120.

Cohen, G., Jose, S. M. & Ahronheim, J. (2009). Body mass index: Pitfalls in elderly people. *Journal of the American Geriatrics Society, 57*(1), 170–172.

Elia, M. (2003). *Screening for malnutrition: A multidisciplinary responsibility. Development and use of the malnutrition universal screening tool ('MUST') for adults*. Redditch: BAPEN.

Fearon, K., Strasser, F., Anker, S. D., et al. (2011). Definition and classification of cancer cachexia: An international consensus. *The Lancet Oncology, 12*(5), 489–495. https://doi.org/10.1016/S1470-2045(10)70218-7.

Ferguson, M., Capra, S., Bauer, J. & Banks, M. (1999). Development of a valid and reliable malnutrition screening tool for adult acute hospital patients. *Nutrition, 15*, 458–464.

Featherstonhaugh, D., Haesler, E. & Bauer, M. (2019). Promoting mealtime function in people with dementia: A systematic review of studies undertaken in residential aged care. *International Journal of Nursing Studies, 96*, 99–118. https://doi.org/10.1016/j.ijnurstu.2019.04.005.

Gerasimidis, K. (2017). Development and evaluation of a new infant nutrition screening tool (iNEWS). Clinical Trials US National Library of Medicine. Viewed September 2019 at https://clinicaltrials.gov/ct2/show/NCT03323957.

Ghosh-Jerath, S., Singh, A., Jerath, N., Gupta, S. & Racine, E. F. (2017). Undernutrition and severe acute malnutrition in children. *British Medical Journal, 359*, https://doi.org/10.1136/bmj.j5632.

Green Corkins, K. (2015). Nutrition-focused physical examination in paediatric patients. *Nutrition in Clinical Practice, 30*(2), 203–209. https://doi.org/10.1177/0884533615572654.

Hooper, L., Anderson, A. S., Birch, J., et al. (2018). Public awareness and healthcare professional advice for obesity as a risk factor for cancer in the UK: A cross-sectional survey. *Journal of Public Health, 40*(4), 797–805. http://dx.doi.org.ezproxy.csu.edu.au/10.1093/pubmed/fdx145.

Kim, S.-H. & Park, M.-J. (2017). Management of childhood obesity. *Journal of Korean Medical Science, 60*(3), 233–241. http //dx.doi.org.ezproxy.csu.edu.au/10.5124/jkma.2017.60.3.233.

Hill, L., Reid, F., Morgan, J., et al. (2010). SCOFF, the development of an eating disorder screening questionnaire. *The International Journal of Eating Disorders, 43*, 344–351.

Kondrup, J., Rasmussen, H. H., Hamberg, O. & Stanga, Z. (2003). Nutritional Risk Screening (NRS 2002): A new method based on an analysis of controlled clinical trials. *Clinical Nutrition, 22*, 321–336.

Kuczmarski, R. J., Ogden, C. L., Guo, S. S., et al. (2002 update). 2000 CDC growth charts for the United States: Methods and development. *Vital Health Statistics, 11*(246). Hyattsville, MD: National Center for Health Statistics.

New Zealand Ministry of Health 2016/17. (2017). New Zealand Health survey obesity statistics. Viewed September 2019 at https://www.health.govt.nz/nz-health-statistics/health-statistics-and-data-sets/obesity-statistics?mega=Health%20statistics&title=Obesity.

National Health and Medical Research Council (NHMRC). (2013a). Clinical practice guidelines for the management of overweight and obesity in adults, adolescents and children in Australia. Melbourne: National Health and Medical Research Council. Viewed March 2019 at https://www.nhmrc.gov.au/about-us/publications/clinical-practice-guidelines-management-overweight-and-obesity.

National Health and Medical Research Council. (2013b). Australian dietary guidelines. Canberra: National Health and Medical Research Council. Viewed March 2019 at https://www.eatforhealth.gov.au/sites/default/files/content/n55_australian_dietary_guidelines.pdf .

National Health and Medical Research Council (NHMRC). (2017). Australian guide to healthy eating. Canberra: National Health and Medical Research Council. Viewed March 2019 at https://www.eatforhealth.gov.au/guidelines/australian-guide-healthy-eating.

National Health and Medical Research Council (NHMRC) and New Zealand Ministry of Health (NZMOH). (2006). Nutrient reference values for Australia and New Zealand including recommended dietary intakes. Viewed March 2019 at www.nhmrc.gov.au/guidelines/publications/n35-n36-n37.

New Zealand Ministry of Health (NZMOH), Clinical Trials Research Unit. (2009). *Clinical guidelines for weight management in New Zealand adults*. Wellington: Author.

Norton, K. & Olds, T. (1996). *Anthropometrica: A textbook of body measurement for sports and health courses*. Sydney: University of New South Wales Press.

Porter, J., Haines, T. P. & Truby, H. (2017). The efficacy of Protected Mealtimes in hospitalised patients: A stepped wedge cluster randomised controlled trial. *BMC Medicine, 15*, 25. doi:10.1186/s12916-017-0780-1.

Queensland Government. (2019). Paediatric Nutrition Screening Tool. Children's Health Queensland Hospital and Health Service. Viewed September 2019 at https://www.childrens.health.qld.gov.au/chq/health-professionals/paediatric-health-resources/nutrition-screening-tool/.

Queensland Government. (2017). Validated malnutrition screening and assessment tools: Comparison guide. Viewed March 2019 at https://www.health.qld.gov.au/__data/assets/pdf_file/0021/152454/hphe_scrn_tools.pdf.

Rahiri, J.-L., Gillon, A., Furukawa, S., et al. (2018). Media portrayal of Māori and bariatric surgery in Aotearoa/New Zealand. *The New Zealand Medical Journal, 131*(1479), 72–80.

Rosenbaum, M., Hirsch, J., Gallagher, D. A., et al. (2008). Long-term persistence of adaptive thermogenesis in subjects who have maintained a reduced body weight. *American Journal of Clinical Nutrition, 88*(4), 906–912.

Rubenstein, L. Z., Harker, J. O., Salva, A., et al. (2001). Screening for undernutrition in geriatric practice: Developing the short-form Mini-Nutritional Assessment (MNA-SF). *Journals of Gerontology Series A: Biological Sciences and Medical Sciences, 56*, M366–M372.

Senthilkumar, S. K., Chacko, T. V. & Suvetha, K. (2018). Nutritional status assessment of children aged 0–5 years and its determinants in a tribal community of Coimbatore district. *International Journal of Community Medicine and Public Health, 5*(7), 2836–2845. http://dx.doi.org/10.18203/2394-6040.ijcmph20182610.

Springhouse. (2007). *Nutrition made incredibly easy!* (2nd ed.). Philadelphia: Lippincott Williams & Wilkins.

Sumithran, P., Prendergast, L. A., Delbridge, E., et al. (2011). Long-term persistence of hormonal adaptations to weight loss. *The New England Journal of Medicine, 365*, 1597–1604.

van Zyl, M. (2011). The effects of drugs on nutrition. *South African Journal of Clinical Nutrition, 24*(3), S38–S41.

Vrdoljak, D. (2015). Malnutrition screening tools for elderly in general practice. *Acta Medica Croatica: Casopis Hravatske Akademije Medicinskih Znanosti, 69*(4), 339–345.

Winter, J., Flanagan, D., McNaughton, S. A., et al. (2013). Nutrition screening of older people in a community general practice, using the MNA-SF. *The Journal of Nutrition, Health & Aging, 17*(4), 322–325. doi:10.1007/s12603-013-0020-0.

Withrow, D. & Alter, D. A. (2011). The economic burden of obesity worldwide: A systematic review of the direct cost of obesity. *Obesity Reviews: An Official Journal of the International Association for the Study of Obesity, 12*(2), 131–141.

World Health Organization (WHO). (2006). WHO child growth standards: Length/height-for-age, weight-for-age, weight-for-height and body mass index-forage: Methods and development. Geneva. Viewed February 2019 at www.who.int/childgrowth/publications/technical_report_pub/en/index.html.

World Health Organization (WHO). (2018a). Body mass index (BMI) classification. Viewed September 2019 at https://apps.who.int/bmi/index.jsp?
World Health Organization (WHO). (2018b). Malnutrition fact sheet. Viewed September 2019 at https://www.who.int/news-room/fact-sheets/detail/malnutrition.
Zitterman, A., Becker, T., Gummert, J. F., et al. (2014). Body mass index, cardiac surgery and clinical outcome. A single-centre experience with 9125 patients. *Nutrition, Metabolism, and Cardiovascular Diseases, 24*(2), 168–175. https://doi.org/10.1016/j.numecd.2013.06.013.

Selected readings

Australian Department of Health. (2015). 2013 Australian dietary guidelines: Eat for health. Canberra: Australia. Viewed March 2019 at https://www.eatforhealth.gov.au/.
Australian Institute of Health and Welfare (AIHW). (2017). A picture of overweight and obesity in Australia 2017. Cat. no. PHE 216. Canberra: AIHW. Viewed March 2019 at https://www.aihw.gov.au/getmedia/172fba28-785e-4a08-ab37-2da3bbae40b8/aihw-phe-216.pdf.aspx?inline=true.
Health Direct. (2018). Body mass index (BMI) and waist circumference. Viewed October 2019 at https://www.healthdirect.gov.au/body-mass-index-bmi-and-waist-circumference.
Huse, O., Hettiarachchi, J., Gearon, E., et al. (2018). Obesity in Australia. *Obesity Research & Clinical Practice, 12*(1), 29–30. https://doi.org/10.1016/j.orcp.2017.10.002.
Marshall, S., Young, A. & Bauer, J. (2016). Nutritional screening in geriatric rehabilitation: Criterion (concurrent and predictive) validity of the Malnutrition Assessment—Short Form. *Journal of the Academy of Nutrition and Dietetics, 116*(5), 795–801.
Menigoz, K., Nathan, A., Heesch, K. C., et al. (2018). Ethnicity, length of residence and prospective trends in body mass index in a National sample of Australian adults 2006-2014. *Annals of Epidemiology, 28*(3), 160–168. https://doi.org/10.1016/j.annepidem.2018.01.006.
New Zealand Ministry of Health (NZMOH). (2015). *Eating and activity guidelines for New Zealand adults.* Wellington: New Zealand. Viewed March 2019 at https://www.health.govt.nz/publication/eating-and-activity-guidelines-new-zealand-adults.
New Zealand Ministry of Health (NZMOH). (2018). Obesity statistics. Viewed March 2019 at https://www.health.govt.nz/nz-health-statistics/health-statistics-and-data-sets/obesity-statistics.
Organisation for Economic Co-operation and Development (OECD). (2017). *Obesity update 2017.* Paris: OECD Publishing. Viewed March 2019 at https://www.oecd.org/els/health-systems/Obesity-Update-2017.pdf.
Zho, Q., Glasgow, N. J. & Wei, D. (2019). Health-related lifestyles and obesity among adults with and without disability in Australia: Implication for mental health care. *Disability and Health Journal, 12*(1), 106–113. https://doi.org/10.1016/j.dhjo.2018.08.007.

Online resources

Australian Department of Health and Ageing, Eat for Health program: www.eatforhealth.gov.au
Australian Institute of Health and Welfare, Overweight and obesity: https://www.aihw.gov.au/reports/overweight-obesity/overweight-and-obesity-an-interactive-insight/contents/what-is-overweight-and-obesity
Diabetes Australia: www.diabetesaustralia.com.au
Diabetes New Zealand: www.diabetes.org.nz
Dietitians Association of Australia: www.daa.asn.au
Dietitians New Zealand: www.dietitians.org.nz
Food Standards Australia New Zealand (FSANZ): www.foodstandards.gov.au
Glycaemic Index: www.glycemicindex.com
Heart Foundation Australia: www.heartfoundation.com.au
Heart Foundation of New Zealand: www.heartfoundation.org.nz
National Health and Medical Research Council, nutrition and diet: www.nhmrc.gov.au/about-us/publications/Australian-dietary-guidelines
Network of Alcohol & Other Drugs Agencies: www.nada.org.au
New Zealand Ministry of Health, food and nutrition guidelines: www.health.govt.nz/our-work/preventative-health-wellness/nutrition/food-and-nutrition-guidelines
New Zealand Nutrition Foundation: www.nutritionfoundation.org.nz
Australian Guide to Healthy Eating: https://www.eatforhealth.gov.au/guidelines/australian-guide-healthy-eating
Nutrition Australia: www.nutritionaustralia.org
Nutrient Reference Values for Australia and New Zealand: www.nrv.gov.au/resources
The New Weight Watchers: www.weightwatchers.com/au/

CHAPTER 15

Skin, hair and nails

CASE STUDY

Sara is a 22-year-old woman in her final year of an engineering degree. Sara is generally in good health, although she has a history of seasonal asthma exacerbated by exercise managed with salbutamol via a metered dose inhaler as required. Throughout her childhood Sara also experienced moderate eczema with focal points on her hands and wrists and in the area behind her knees. Sara tells you the eczema resolved before she started high school but even now she can get an occasional patch on her wrist that she treats with a topical steroid cream. Sara presents to the outpatient clinic of the university hospital with what she thinks might be an exacerbation of her eczema. She has a large patch of roughened skin on her scalp extending down on to her neck and on each elbow extending distally down each arm. For the last 6 months she has been applying the over-the-counter steroid cream regularly, but this has had no effect. The consultant dermatologist diagnoses Sara with plaque psoriasis.

Structure and function

The skin, hair and nails are external structures that serve a variety of specialised functions. The sebaceous and sweat glands originating within the skin also have many vital functions. Each structure's function is described separately.

SKIN

The skin is composed of three layers: the epidermis, dermis and subcutaneous tissue (Fig. 15-1A). The skin is thicker on the palms of the hands and soles of the feet and is continuous, with mucous membranes occurring at the orifices of the body. Subcutaneous tissue, which contains varying amounts of fat, connects the skin to underlying structures.

The skin is a physical barrier that protects the underlying tissues and structures from microorganisms, physical trauma, ultraviolet radiation and dehydration. It plays a vital role in temperature maintenance, fluid and electrolyte balance, absorption, excretion, sensation, immunity, and vitamin D synthesis. The skin also provides an individual identity to a person's appearance.

Epidermis

The epidermis (Fig. 15-1B), the outer layer of skin, is composed of four distinct layers: the stratum corneum, stratum lucidum, stratum granulosum and stratum germinativum. The outermost layer consists of dead, keratinised cells that render the skin waterproof. (Keratin is a scleroprotein that is insoluble in water. The epidermis, hair, nails, dental enamel are composed of keratin.) The epidermal layer is almost completely replaced every 3 to 4 weeks. The innermost layer of the epidermis (stratum germinativum) is the only layer that undergoes cell division and contains melanin (brown pigment) and keratin-forming cells. Skin colour depends on the amount of melanin and carotene (yellow pigment) contained in the skin and the volume of blood containing haemoglobin, the oxygen-binding pigment that circulates in the dermis. Albinism refers to a group of inherited disorders where there is a reduction or absence of melanin formation.

Dermis

The inner layer of skin is the dermis (Fig. 15-1). It is connected to the epidermis by means of papillae. These papillae form the base for the visible swirls or friction ridges that provide the unique pattern of fingerprints with which we are familiar. Ridges also appear on the palms of the hands, the toes and the soles of the feet. The dermis is a well-vascularised connective tissue layer containing collagen and elastic fibres, nerve endings and lymph vessels. It is also the origin of hair follicles, sebaceous glands and sweat glands.

Sebaceous glands

The sebaceous glands (Fig. 15-1A) develop from hair follicles and, therefore, are present over most of the body, excluding

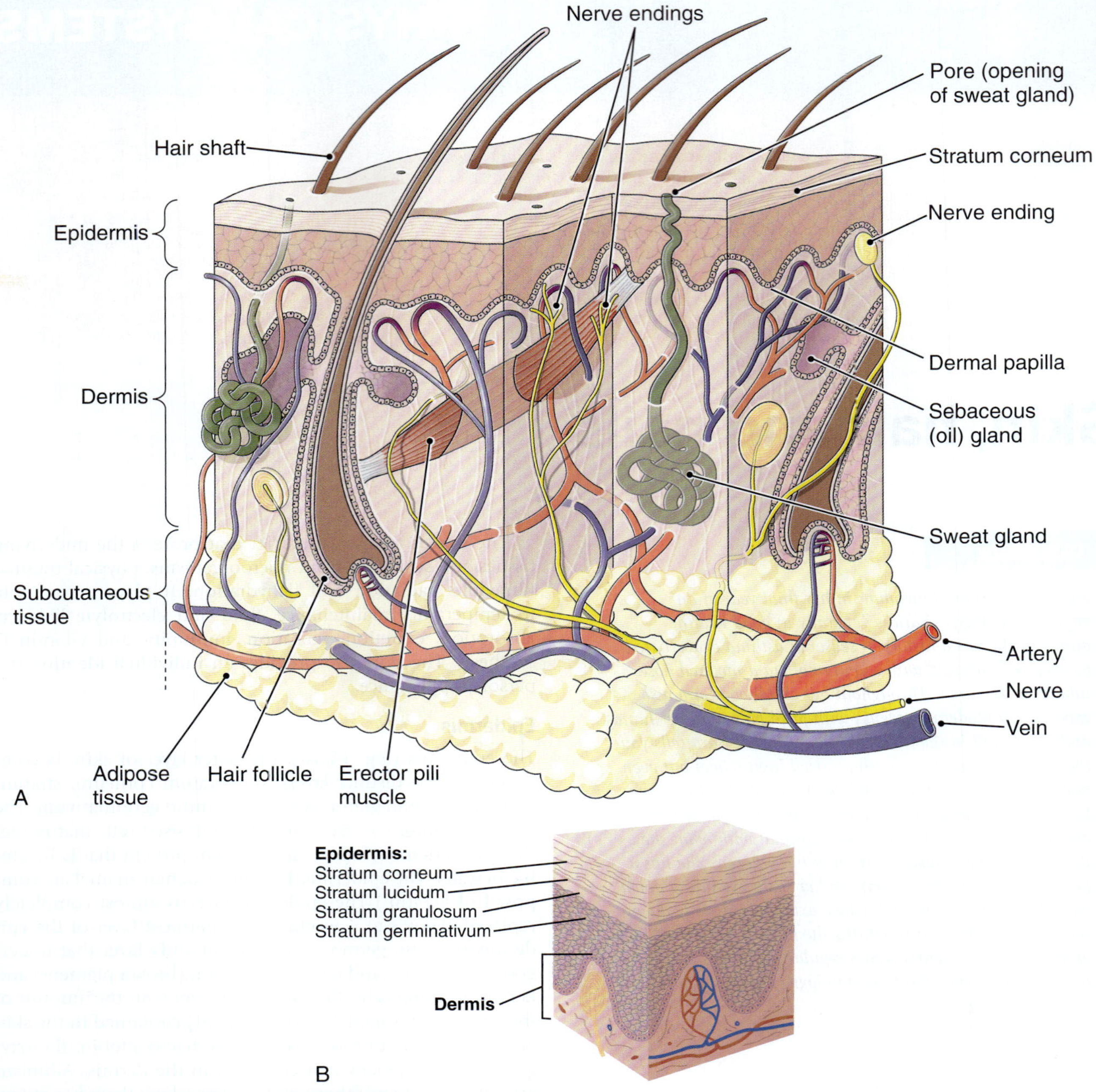

FIGURE 15-1 (A) The skin and hair follicles and related structures. **(B)** Layers of the epidermis. (Cohen, B. J. & Hull, K. L. (2015). *Memmler's structure and function of the human body* [11th ed.]. Philadelphia: Lippincott Williams & Wilkins.)

the soles and palms. They secrete an oily substance called sebum that lubricates hair and skin and reduces water loss through the skin. Sebum also has some fungicidal and bactericidal effects.

Sweat glands

Sweat glands (see Fig. 15-1A) are of two types: eccrine and apocrine. The eccrine glands are located over the entire skin surface and secrete an odourless, clear fluid, the evaporation of which is vital to the regulation of body temperature. The apocrine glands are concentrated in the axillae, perineum and areolae of the breast and are usually open through a hair follicle. They secrete a milky sweat. The interaction of sweat with skin bacteria produces a characteristic body odour. Apocrine glands are dormant until puberty, at which time they become active. In women, apocrine secretions are linked with the menstrual cycle.

Subcutaneous tissue

Merging with the dermis is the subcutaneous tissue, which is a loose connective tissue containing fat cells, blood vessels, nerves and the remaining portions of sweat glands and hair follicles (see Fig. 15-1A). The subcutaneous tissue assists with heat regulation and contains the vascular and lymphatic pathways for the supply of nutrients and removal of waste products from the skin.

HAIR

Hair consists of layers of keratinised cells and is found over much of the body except for the lips, nipples, soles of the feet, palms of the hands, labia minora and penis. Hair develops within a sheath of epidermal cells called the hair follicle. Hair growth occurs at the base of the follicle, where cells in the hair bulb are nourished by dermal blood vessels. The hair shaft is visible above the skin; the hair root is surrounded by the hair follicle (see Fig. 15-1). Attached to the follicle are the erector pili muscles, which contract in response to cold or fright, decreasing the skin's surface area and causing the hair to stand erect.

There are two general types of hair: vellus and terminal. Vellus hair is short, pale and fine and is present over much of the body. The terminal hair (particularly scalp and eyebrows) is longer and generally darker and coarser than the vellus hair. Puberty initiates the growth of additional terminal hair in both sexes on the axillae, perineum and legs. Hair colour varies and is determined by the type and amount of pigment production. The absence of pigment or the inclusion of air spaces within the layers of the hair shaft results in grey or white hair.

Hair serves useful functions. Scalp hair is a protective covering. Nasal hair and ear hair, as well as eyelashes and eyebrows, filter dust and other airborne debris.

NAILS

The nails, located on the distal phalanges of fingers and toes, are hard, transparent plates of keratinised epidermal cells that grow from a root underneath the skin fold called the cuticle (Fig. 15-2). The nail body extends over the entire nail bed and has a pink tinge as a result of the rich blood supply underneath. At the base of the nail is the lunula, a paler, crescent-shaped area. The nails protect the distal ends of the fingers and toes.

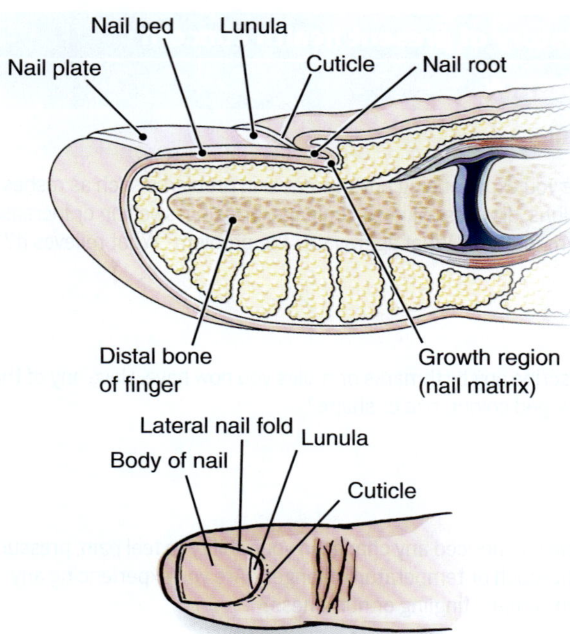

FIGURE 15-2 The nail and related structures.

Health assessment

COLLECTING SUBJECTIVE DATA: THE NURSING HEALTH HISTORY

Diseases and disorders of the skin, hair and nails can be local or may be caused by an underlying systemic problem. To perform a complete and accurate assessment, the nurse needs to collect data about current symptoms, the past medical history of the patient and his or her family, and their lifestyle and health practices. The information obtained provides clues to the patient's overall level of functioning in relation to their skin, hair and nails.

When interviewing patients for information regarding their skin, hair and nails, ask questions in a straightforward manner. Keep in mind that a non-judgemental and sensitive approach is needed if the patient has abnormalities that may be associated with poor hygiene or potentially unhealthy behaviours. Also, some skin disorders might be highly visible and potentially damaging to the person's body image and self-concept.

CASE STUDY

During the interview Sara tells you that she is desperately self-conscious about the lesions on her head and arms. She chooses clothing that hides the lesions, and avoids social occasions, particularly in summer. She is also currently avoiding intimate relationships.

CRITICAL THINKING

1. Considering Sara's perception of her physical appearance, what strategies would you use to make her comfortable in discussing her health issues with you?
2. What further questions might you ask Sara?

History of present health concern

QUESTION	RATIONALE
Skin	
Are you experiencing any current skin problems such as rashes, lesions, dryness, oiliness, drainage, bruising, swelling or increased pigmentation? What aggravates the problem? What relieves it?	Any of these symptoms may be related to a pathological skin condition. Bruises, welts or burns may indicate accidents or trauma or abuse. If these injuries cannot be explained or the patient's explanation seems unbelievable or vague, physical abuse should be suspected. Dry, itchy skin is a common concern in obese patients (Cowdell & Radley, 2014).
Describe any birthmarks or moles you now have. Have any of them changed colour, size or shape?	You need to know what is normal for the patient so that future variations can be detected. A change in the size or appearance of any skin mark, especially a mole, may indicate cancer. Asymmetry, irregular borders, colour variations, diameter greater than 0.5 cm and elevation are characteristics of cancerous lesions.
Have you noticed any change in your ability to feel pain, pressure, light touch or temperature changes? Are you experiencing any pain, itching, tingling or numbness?	Changes in sensation may indicate vascular or neurological problems such as peripheral neuropathy related to diabetes mellitus or arterial occlusive disease. Sensation problems may put the patient at risk of sustaining injuries including pressure injuries (see Promote health—Pressure injuries).
Do you have trouble controlling body odour? How much do you perspire?	Uncontrolled body odour or excessive or insufficient perspiration may indicate an abnormality with the sweat glands or an endocrine problem such as hypothyroidism or hyperthyroidism. Poor hygiene practices may account for body odour, and health education may be indicated. **OLDER ADULT CONSIDERATIONS** **Perspiration decreases with ageing because sweat gland activity decreases.** Any strong body odour may indicate an abnormality.
Do you have any body piercings, modifications, scarification or tattoos?	Piercing needles and modifications place patients at risk of infection (Breuner & Levine, 2017; Wong et al., 2012). Tattooing pigments can cause allergic reactions, keloids and scars. Patients should be informed regarding these risks.
Hair and nails	
Have you had any hair loss or change in the condition of your hair? Describe.	Patchy hair loss may accompany infections, stress, hairstyles that put stress on hair roots, and some types of chemotherapy. Generalised hair loss may be seen in various systemic illnesses such as hypothyroidism and in patients receiving certain types of chemotherapy or radiation therapy.  **OLDER ADULT CONSIDERATIONS** **A receding hairline or male pattern baldness may occur with ageing.**
Have you had any change in the condition or appearance of your nails? Describe.	Nail changes may be seen in systemic disorders such as malnutrition or with local irritation (e.g. nail biting). (See Promote health—Nail infections.) Bacterial infections cause green, black or brown nail discolouration. Yellow, thick, crumbling nails are seen in fungal infections. Yeast infections cause a white colour and separation of the nail plate from the nail bed.

Continued on page 236

COLDSPA

Example

Use the COLDSPA mnemonic as a guideline to collect needed information for each symptom the patient shares. In addition, the following questions help elicit important information.

Mnemonic	Question	Patient response example
Character	Describe the sign or symptom (feeling, appearance, sound, smell, or taste, if applicable).	Small 0.5 cm diameter raised brown spot
Onset	When did it begin?	3 months ago
Location	Where is it? Does it radiate? Does it occur anywhere else?	'On my right cheek next to my nose. I have had one like it on my lower back for a year.'
Duration	How long does it last? Does it recur?	'It never goes away.'
Severity	How bad is it? How much does it bother you?	'It scares me that it may be cancer.'
Pattern	What makes it better or worse?	'I cover the one on my face with a cosmetic. It bleeds if I scrub it.'
Associated factors/How it Affects the patient	What other symptoms occur with it? How does it affect you?	'It is ugly and embarrassing. It itches sometimes.'

PROMOTE HEALTH — PRESSURE INJURIES

OVERVIEW

A pressure injury is 'a localised injury to the skin and/or underlying tissue usually over a bony prominence, as a result of pressure, or pressure in combination with shear and/or friction' (Australian Wound Management Association, 2012, p. 15). Other terms used to describe a pressure injury include pressure ulcer, pressure sores, bed sores and decubitus ulcers. The contemporary term pressure injury is used to reflect the nature of preventable damage to the skin. (*Note:* The term 'pressure ulcer' is used for staging in Abnormal findings 15-1 as this reflects nomenclature used currently in North America.)

Although pressure injuries are commonly preventable, they continue to prove challenging for clinicians. An international point prevalence survey demonstrated a decrease in the overall prevalence of pressure injuries from 13.5% in 2006 to 9.3% in 2015 across all settings (VanGilder et al., 2017). In Australia, it is estimated that the incidence rate ranges from 6.4% to 11.7% in aged care facilities (Wilson et al., 2018). Pressure injuries cause considerable harm to patients, hindering recovery and frequently causing pain and the development of serious infections (Giroud et al., 2008). It is essential that nurses understand how to assess pressure injury risk correctly and implement interventions to prevent them. For an initial assessment of the potential to develop a pressure injury, see the Braden Scale (Assessment tool 15-1).

The Australian Wound Management Association (2012) has identified three conditions leading to pressure injury development: (1) pressure, (2) shear and (3) friction. The most significant contributing factor to pressure injury development is unrelieved pressure, but friction and shear may also contribute or worsen the condition.

NATIONAL SAFETY AND QUALITY HEALTH SERVICE STANDARDS

The National Safety and Quality Health Service (NSQHS) Standards set out minimum standards for quality and safety and provide quality assurance guidelines and improvement mechanisms to achieve them (Australian Commission on Safety and Quality in Health Care, 2012). The Standards aim to protect the public from harm by improving the quality of health service provision. The intention of 'Standard 8: Preventing and managing pressure injuries' is to provide a framework for an organisation-wide approach for screening and identification of modifiable risk factors and the implementation of preventative strategies.

Assess risk factors

Use an established risk assessment tool such as the Braden Scale (see Assessment tool 15-1), Norton Scale or Waterlow Score. Assess for the following risk factors:

- Perception: inability to perceive pressure
- Mobility: inability to move self, decreased activity level, unable to reposition
- Moisture: diaphoresis, incontinence, sweating from climate
- Nutrition: deficient (especially protein deficit) or excessive (obesity)
- Friction or shear against surfaces
- Tissue tolerance decreased: age, vascular incompetence, haemodynamic instability, impaired oxygenation, hypoglycaemia or hyperglycaemia related to diabetes mellitus, body weight, malnutrition, comorbidities
- Connection to equipment or therapeutic devices such as intravascular devices, catheters, orthotics or splints, monitoring cables

Teach risk reduction tips

- Inspect the skin at least daily and more often if at greater risk, using a risk assessment tool (such as the Braden Scale), and keep a flow chart to document.
- Bathe with mild soap or other agent; limit friction; use warm, not hot, water; set a bath schedule that is individualised.
- For dry skin: use moisturisers; avoid low humidity and cold air.
- Avoid vigorous massage.
- Use careful positioning, turning and transferring techniques to avoid shear and friction or prolonged pressure on any point.
- Refer nutritional supplementation needs to primary care provider or dietitian, especially if protein deficient.
- Refer incontinence condition to primary care provider.

Continued on following page

- Use incontinence skin cleansing methods as needed: frequency and methods of cleaning, avoiding dryness with protective barrier products.

For bed- or chair-bound patients:

- Reposition or teach to self-reposition every 15 minutes (chair) or 2 hours (bed).
- Use repositioning schedule.
- Use alternating pressure mattress or chair cushion.
- Use lifting devices if available to reduce shear.
- Use positioning with pillows or wedges to avoid bony prominence contact with surfaces and to maintain body alignment.
- For bed bound, avoid elevated head of bed except for brief periods.
- Provide structured teaching for patient, family and carers as necessary.
- Consider a referral to an occupational therapist.

PROMOTE HEALTH — NAIL INFECTIONS

OVERVIEW

Nails, both toe and fingernails, are susceptible to bacterial and fungal infections. Infections occur along the nail skin fold (paronychia), between the nail plate and the nail bed, or in the nail bed. Many other abnormal conditions cause nail changes; however, nail infections are often preventable. There are differences in how common conditions affect the nail. For instance, bacterial infections such as pseudomonas cause a green, brown or black discolouration with thickening and crumbling of the nail plate, and often separation of the plate from the bed. Yeast infections cause a white colour in the nail plate and may involve separation but without the debris or crumbling seen in the other conditions. When a nail is injured and a haematoma forms, blood accumulates under the plate and can allow infections to enter (see Abnormal findings 15-7).

Assess risk factors

- Nails in moist environment, especially walking in damp public locales (swimming pools, showers) or continuously wearing closed shoes; excessive perspiration
- Nail injury, trauma or irritation (tight footwear, exercise trauma, artificial nails, excessive hand washing, nail-biting)
- Repeated irritation (especially water, detergents)
- Immune system disorders such as diabetes mellitus, human immunodeficiency virus, or being on immunosuppressive medications
- Skin conditions such as psoriasis or lichen
- Some trades or professions (damp environments or shoe type required)
- Contagion from one digit to another or one person to another
- Possibly family predisposition.

Teach risk reduction tips

- Wear comfortable, well-fitted shoes.
- Avoid wearing closed shoes all the time.
- Wear socks that wick away moisture.
- Avoid going barefoot in damp public areas.
- Avoid too much perspiration or water.
- Avoid trauma to nails.
- Avoid unsanitary or unsafe nail care practices.
- If treatment has been started, do not stop until recovery is complete.

Past health history

QUESTION	RATIONALE
Describe any previous problems with skin, hair or nails, including any treatment or surgery and its effectiveness.	Current problems may be a recurrence of previous ones. Visible scars may be explained by previous problems.
Have you ever had any allergic skin reactions to food, medications, plants or other environmental substances?	Various types of allergens can precipitate a variety of skin eruptions.
Have you had a fever, nausea, vomiting, gastrointestinal or respiratory problems?	Some skin rashes or lesions may be related to viruses or bacteria.
For female patients: Are you pregnant? Are your menstrual periods regular? Are you perimenopausal or menopausal? Do you take hormone replacement therapy?	Some skin and hair conditions can result from hormonal imbalance (Herman et al., 2013).
Do you have a history of smoking and/or drinking alcohol?	A significant association between cigarette smoking, alcohol consumption and psoriatic males has been found (Rajagopalan et al., 2016).
What amount of daily sun exposure would you routinely have? Do you use sun screen routinely? Do you use tanning beds/solariums?	Inadequate sun exposure is associated with vitamin D deficiencies (Hoel et al., 2016). Frequent sun exposure is associated with an increased prevalence of skin cancers (Espinosa et al., 2015).
Do you have a history of anxiety, depression or any psychiatric problems?	Over one-third of dermatological disorders have significant psychiatric comorbidity (Dalgard et al., 2015; Jalenques et al., 2016). Depression often occurs in association with dermatological disease (Bahar et al., 2016; Chouliara et al., 2017; Greener, 2014).

Family history

QUESTION	RATIONALE
Has anyone in your family had a recent illness, rash or other skin problem or allergy? Describe.	Acne and atopic dermatitis tend to be familial. Viruses (e.g. chickenpox, measles) can be highly contagious. Some allergies may be identified from family history.
Has anyone in your family had skin cancer?	A genetic component is associated with skin cancer, especially malignant melanoma (see Promote health—Skin cancer).
Do you have a family history of keloids?	Keloid scars can provide functional challenges particularly over joints but are also aesthetically disfiguring which may be emotionally distressing (Trace et al., 2016).

Lifestyle and health practices

QUESTION	RATIONALE
How much sun exposure do you get? Do you sunbathe or use a sun bed (tanning booth)? If so, how much exposure do you get? What type of sunscreen protection do you use?	Sun exposure can cause premature ageing of skin and increase the risk of cancer. Hair can also be damaged by too much sun.

Continued on following page

PROMOTE HEALTH — SKIN CANCER

OVERVIEW

Skin cancer is one of the most common cancers. It occurs in three types: melanoma, basal cell carcinoma (BCC) and squamous cell carcinoma (SCC). BCC and SCC are non-melanomas. BCC is the most common skin cancer in Caucasians, and SCC is more common in darker-skinned people. Asians are less susceptible to skin cancers (Lee & Lim, 2003).

Malignant melanoma is the most serious skin cancer. Skin cancer is the most common form of cancer in New Zealand (Cancer Society of New Zealand, 2018). Although skin cancer is largely preventable, Australia and New Zealand have some of the highest rates of skin cancer in the world. According to SunSmart, an organisation jointly funded by Cancer Council Victoria and VicHealth, at least 66% of Australians will be diagnosed with skin cancer by the age of 70. More than 1,000 Australians are treated for skin cancer every day, and over 1,850 Australians die from skin cancer each year (SunSmart, 2018).

The major cause of skin cancer is exposure to ultraviolet (UV) radiation from the sun and other artificial sources such as solariums or sun beds. The use of sunbeds has been restricted globally to reduce the risk of skin cancer (WHO, 2017) and legislatively banned in all states of Australia (ARPANSA, n.d.). In Australia and New Zealand, sun exposure is the most common cause of skin cancer. Skin cancer can be effectively treated in most cases if treated early (Australian Institute of Health and Welfare [AIHW], 2017).

Assess risk factors

- Sun exposure, especially intermittent pattern with sunburn; risk increases if excessive sun exposure and sunburns began in childhood. Intermittent exposure to the sun or UV radiation is associated with the greatest risk for melanoma and for BCC, but overall amount of exposure is thought to be associated with SCC. SCC is most common on body sites with very heavy sun exposure, whereas BCC is most common on sites with moderate exposure (e.g. upper trunk or women's lower legs)
- Non-solar sources of UV radiation (tanning beds, solariums, sunlamps, high-UV geographical areas)
- Medical therapies such as psoralen plus UV-A phototherapy and ionising radiation
- Family or personal history and genetic susceptibility (especially for malignant melanoma)
- Moles, especially atypical lesions
- Pigmentation irregularities (albinism, burn scars)
- Fair skin that burns and freckles easily; lightly coloured hair; blue or grey eyes
- Age; risk increases with increasing age
- Actinic and cheilitis keratoses
- Male gender (for non-melanoma cancers), especially white men over 65 (AIHW, 2012)
- Chemical exposure (arsenic, tar, coal, paraffin, some oils for non-melanoma cancers)
- Human papillomavirus (non-melanoma cancers)
- Xeroderma pigmentosum (rare, inherited condition)
- Long-term skin inflammation or injury (non-melanoma)
- Alcohol intake (BCC); smoking (SCC)
- Inadequate niacin (vitamin B3) in diet
- Bowen disease (scaly or thickened patch) (SCC)
- Depressed immune system

Teach risk reduction tips

- Reduce sun exposure; seek shade.
- Always use sunscreen (SPF30 or higher) when sun exposure is anticipated and apply at least 20 minutes prior to sun exposure. Reapply second hourly.
- Wear long-sleeved shirts and wide-brimmed hats.
- Wear sunglasses that wrap around.
- Avoid sunburns.
- Understand the link between sun exposure and skin cancer and the accumulating effects of sun exposure on developing cancers.
- Examine the skin for suspected lesions. If there is anything unusual, seek professional advice as soon as possible (see Abnormal findings 15-5).
- Ensure that diet is adequate in vitamin B3.
- Talk with primary care provider about taking a vitamin D supplement (Cancer Council, 2019).

Lifestyle and health practices (continued)

QUESTION	RATIONALE
In your daily activities, are you regularly exposed to chemicals that may harm the skin (e.g. *paint, bleach, cleaning products, weed killers, insect repellents, petroleum*)? Do you use personal protective equipment when handling these products?	Any of these substances have the potential to irritate or damage the skin, hair or nails.
Do you spend long periods of time sitting or lying in one position?	Older patients, persons with disability and immobile patients who spend long periods of time in one position are at risk of pressure injuries.
Have you had any exposure to extreme temperatures?	Temperature extremes affect the blood supply to the skin and can damage the skin layers. Examples include frostbite and burns.
What is your daily routine for skin, hair and nail care? What products do you use (e.g. soaps, lotions, oils, cosmetics, self-tanning products, razor type, hair spray, shampoo, colouring, nail enamel)? How do you cut your nails?	Regular habits provide information on hygiene and lifestyle. The products used may also be a cause of an abnormality. Improper nail-cutting technique can lead to ingrown nails or infection. **OLDER ADULT CONSIDERATIONS** **Decreased flexibility and mobility may impair the ability of some elderly patients to maintain proper hygiene practices, such as nail cutting, bathing and hair care.**
What kinds of foods do you consume in a typical day? How much fluid do you drink each day? How much water do you drink each day?	A balanced diet is necessary for healthy skin, hair and nails. Adequate fluid intake is required to maintain skin elasticity.
Do skin problems limit any of your normal activities?	Certain activities such as hiking, camping and gardening may expose the patient to allergens. Moreover, exposure to the sun can aggravate conditions such as scleroderma. In addition, general home maintenance (e.g. cleaning, car washing) may expose the patient to certain cleaning products to which he or she is sensitive or allergic.
Describe any skin disorder that prevents you from enjoying your relationships.	Skin, hair or nail problems, especially if visible, may impair the patient's ability to interact comfortably with others because of embarrassment or rejection by others. Social stigma towards some dermatological disorders is widespread in Indian society (Chaturvedi et al., 2005).
How much stress do you have in your life? Describe.	Stress can cause or exacerbate skin abnormalities.
Do you perform a skin self-examination once a month?	If patients do not know how to inspect the skin, teach them how to recognise suspicious lesions early (see Self-assessment 15-1).

COLLECTING OBJECTIVE DATA: PHYSICAL EXAMINATION

The physical assessment of the skin, hair and nails provides the nurse with data that may reveal local or systemic problems or alterations in a patient's self-care activities. Local irritation, trauma or disease can alter the condition of the skin, hair or nails. Systemic problems related to impaired circulation, endocrine imbalances, allergic reactions or respiratory disorders may also be revealed by alterations to the skin, hair or nails. The appearance of the skin, hair and nails also provides the nurse with data related to health maintenance and self-care activities such as hygiene, exercise and nutrition.

A separate, comprehensive skin, hair and nail examination, preferably at the beginning of a comprehensive physical examination, ensures that you do not inadvertently omit part of the examination. While inspecting and palpating the skin, hair and nails, pay special attention to lesions and growths.

Preparing the patient

To prepare for the skin, hair and nail examination, ask the patient to remove all clothing and jewellery and put on an examination gown. In addition, ask the patient to remove nail enamel, artificial nails (if possible), wigs, toupees or hairpieces as appropriate.

Have the patient sit comfortably on the examination table or bed for the beginning of the examination. The patient may remain in a sitting position for most of the examination. However, to assess the skin on the buttocks and dorsal surfaces of the legs properly, the patient may lie on his or her side or abdomen.

Keep the room door closed or the bed curtain drawn to provide privacy. During the skin examination, expose only the body part being examined. Make sure that the room is a comfortable temperature. If available, sunlight is best for inspecting the skin. However, a bright light that can be focused on the patient works just as well. Explain what you are going to do and answer any questions the patient may have.

SELF-ASSESSMENT 15-1 HOW TO EXAMINE YOUR OWN SKIN

Coupled with a yearly skin examination by a doctor, self-examination of your skin once a month is the best way to detect early warning signs of the three main types of skin cancer: basal cell carcinoma, squamous cell carcinoma and melanoma. *Look for a new growth or any skin change.*

What you will need: a bright light, a full-length mirror, a hand mirror, two chairs or stools, a hair dryer, body maps, and a pencil.

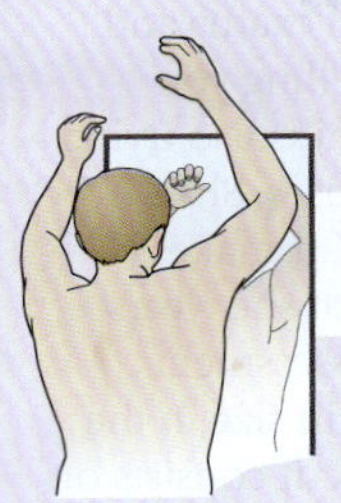

Focus on neck, chest, torso.
Women: check under breasts.

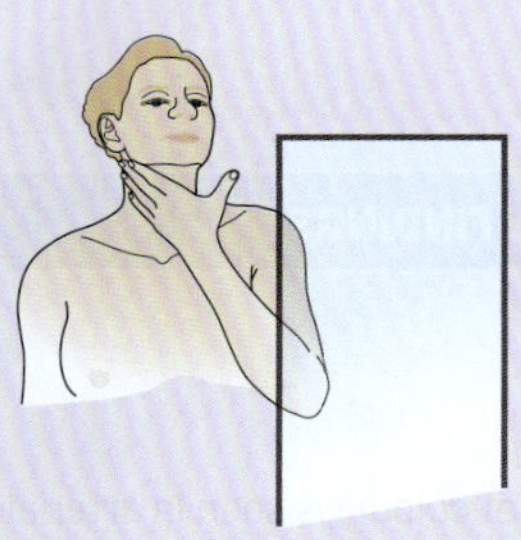

Examine head and face using one or both mirrors.
Use a blow dryer to inspect scalp.

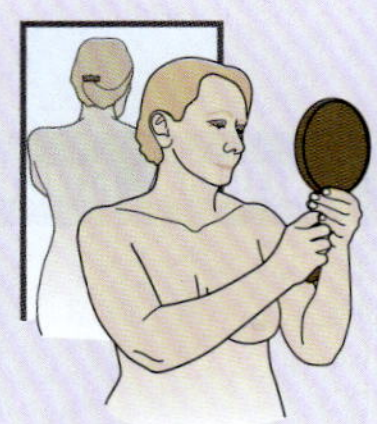

With back to the mirror, use hand mirror to inspect back of neck, shoulders, upper arms, back, buttocks, legs.

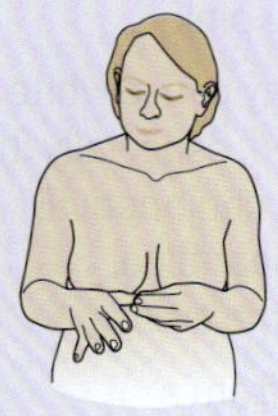

Check hands, including nails. In full-length mirror, examine elbows, arms and underarms.

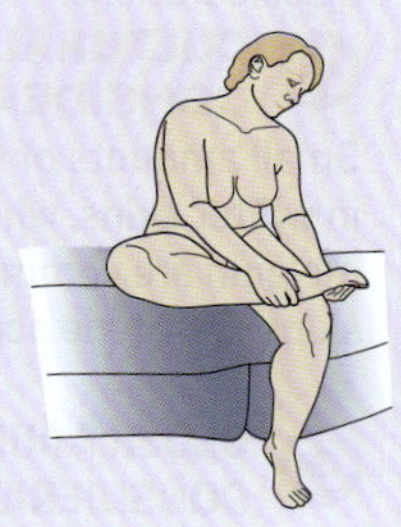

Sitting down, check legs and feet, including soles, heels and nails.
Use hand mirror to examine genitals.

Wear gloves when palpating any lesions because you may be exposed to exudate.

Patients from certain religious denominations (e.g. Jewish Orthodox, Islam) may require that the nurse be the same gender as the patient. Also, to respect the patient's modesty or desire for privacy, provide a long examination gown or robe.

Equipment

- Examination light
- Penlight
- Mirror for patient's self-examination of skin
- Magnifying glass
- Centimetre ruler
- Gloves (as required)
- Wood's light
- Examination gown or drape
- Braden Scale for Predicting Pressure Sore Risk
- Pressure Ulcer Scale for Healing (PUSH) tool to measure pressure ulcer healing

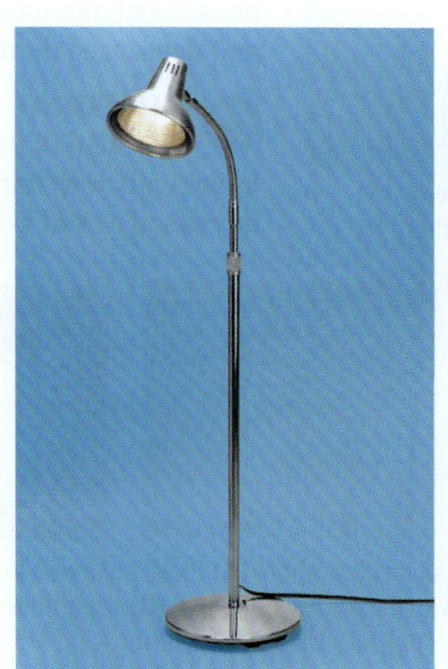

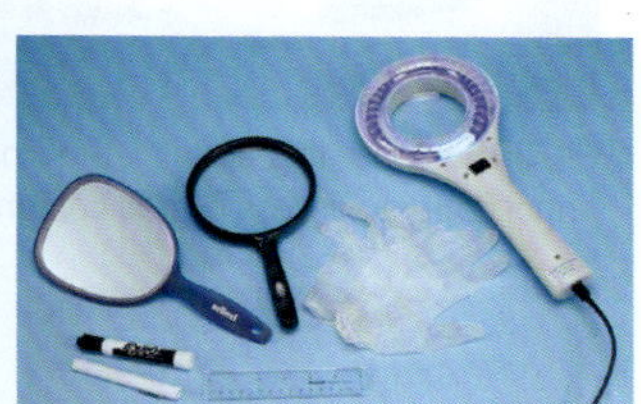

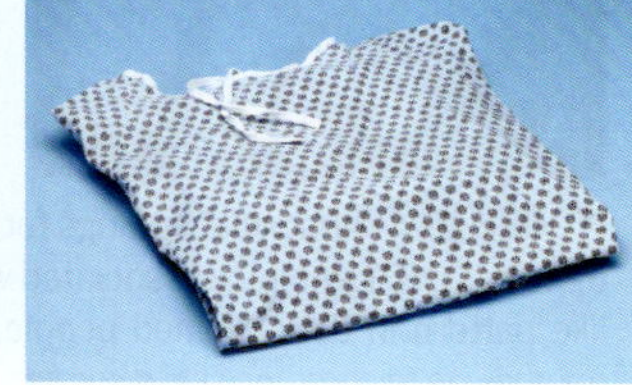

Physical assessment

When preparing to examine the skin, hair and nails, remember these key points:

- Inspect skin colour, temperature, moisture and texture.
- Check skin integrity.
- Be alert for skin lesions.
- Evaluate hair condition, including loss or unusual growth.
- Note nail bed condition and capillary refill.

CASE STUDY

Upon presentation Sara looks well nourished, wearing clean clothes. Her hair and nails are clean and well kept. She is quietly spoken and looks anxious. She tells you that she is under a lot of stress with her final exams and her skin problems. She starts crying while telling you about the amount of work she has to do while also trying to work part time to pay for her living expenses. She states that the psoriasis is 'getting her down'. It makes her feel self conscious and she modifies what she wears to try and cover up the areas. On physical assessment the scalp lesion is approximately 10 × 8 cm in size in the occipital region extending down to the neck. It consists of roughened, red, raised areas covered with silver coloured cells. Patchy alopecia is present around the plaques.

Both elbows have similar lesions of a similar size with satellite areas extending down to the wrists. Sara's vital signs are within normal physiological limits, and no other abnormalities are apparent at this time.

CRITICAL THINKING

3. Describe the morphology, configuration and distribution of lesions plaque psoriasis. Are Sara's findings (case study) consistent with a typical presentation of plaque psoriasis?
4. Outline the morphology of the following primary lesions: macule, papule, plaque, vesicle and pustule.

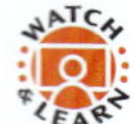

Physical assessment: Assessing the arms, hands and fingers

PHYSICAL ASSESSMENT

ASSESSMENT PROCEDURE	NORMAL FINDINGS	ABNORMAL FINDINGS
Skin		
INSPECTION		
Inspect general skin colouration (Fig. 15-3). Keep in mind that the amount of pigment in the skin accounts for the intensity of colour as well as hue. 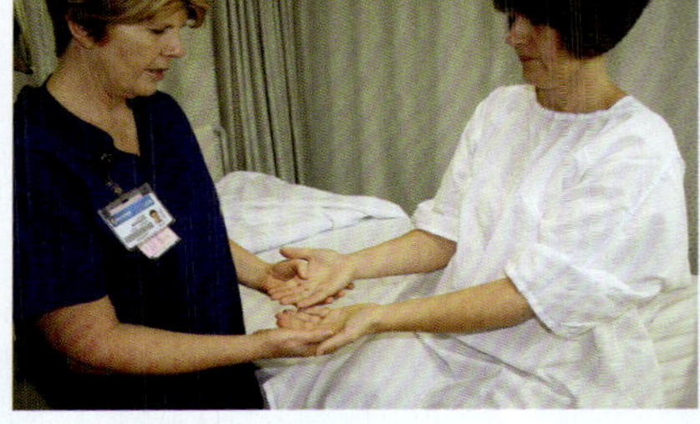 **FIGURE 15-3** Inspecting the palms is an opportunity to assess overall colouration.	Inspection reveals evenly coloured skin tones without unusual or prominent discolourations. **CULTURAL CONSIDERATIONS** **Small amounts of melanin are common in whiter skins, whereas large amounts of melanin are common in olive and darker skins. Carotene accounts for a yellow cast.** **OLDER ADULT CONSIDERATIONS** **The older patient's skin becomes pale because of decreased melanin production and decreased dermal vascularity.** **CULTURAL CONSIDERATIONS** **Individuals with fair complexions are at increased risk of skin cancer.**	**Pallor** (loss of colour) is seen in arterial insufficiency, decreased blood supply and anaemia. Pallid tones vary from pale to ashen without underlying pink. **Cyanosis** (Fig. 15-4A) may cause white skin to appear blue-tinged, especially in the perioral, nail bed and conjunctival areas. Dark skin may appear blue, dull and lifeless in the same areas. Central cyanosis results from a cardiopulmonary insufficiency whereas peripheral cyanosis may be a local problem resulting from vasoconstriction. **CLINICAL TIP** **To differentiate between central and peripheral cyanosis, look for central cyanosis in the oral mucosa.** **Jaundice** (Fig. 15-4B) in light- and dark-skinned people is characterised by yellow skin tones, from pale to pumpkin, particularly in the sclera, oral mucosa, palms and soles. **Acanthosis nigricans** (Fig. 15-4C) is roughening and darkening of skin in localised areas, especially the posterior neck.
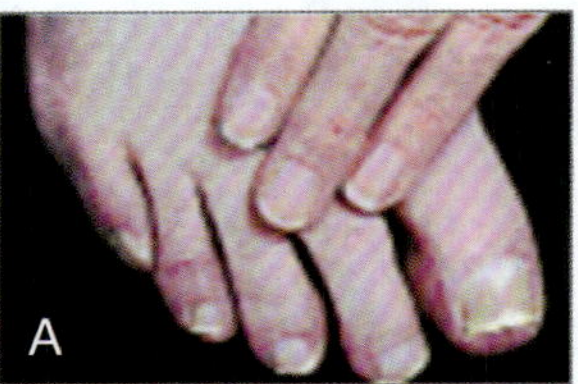 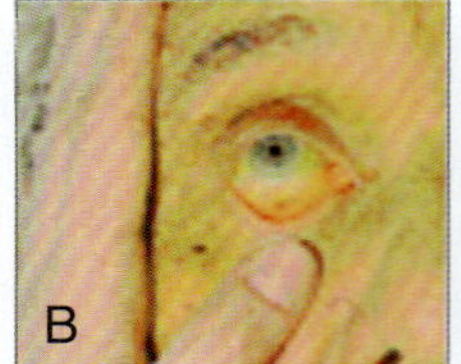 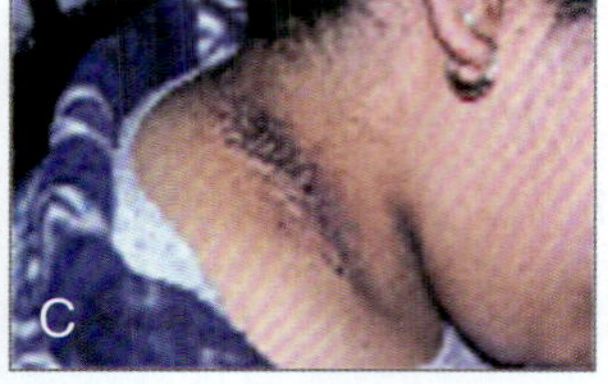 **FIGURE 15-4** Abnormal findings for skin colouration: **(A)** Bluish cyanotic skin associated with oxygen deficiency. **(B)** Jaundice associated with hepatic dysfunction. **(C)** Acanthosis nigricans, a linear streak-like pattern in dark-skinned people, suggests diabetes mellitus. (*Source:* Goodheart, H. P. [1999]. *A photoguide to common skin disorders: Diagnosis and management*. Baltimore: Williams & Wilkins.)		
While inspecting skin colouration, note any odours emanating from the skin.	Patient has slight or no odour of perspiration, depending on activity.	A strong odour of perspiration or foul odour may indicate disorder of sweat glands or infection. Poor hygiene practices may indicate a need for patient education or assistance with activities of daily living.

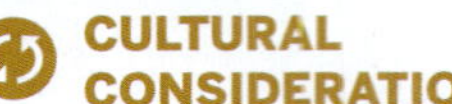

PHYSICAL ASSESSMENT (continued)

ASSESSMENT PROCEDURE	NORMAL FINDINGS	ABNORMAL FINDINGS
Inspect for colour variations. Inspect localised parts of the body, noting any colour variation. 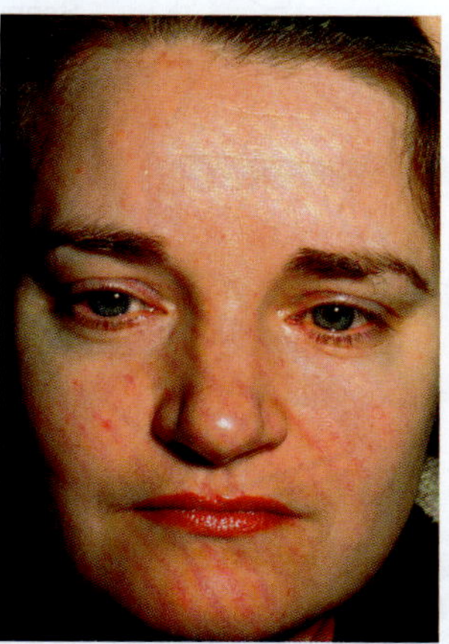 **FIGURE 15-5** Common variations: Butterfly rash of lupus erythematosus. (Science Photo Library/ Alamy Stock Photo.)	Keep in mind that some patients have suntanned areas, freckles or white patches known as vitiligo (Common variations 15-1). The variations are due to different amounts of melanin in certain areas. A generalised loss of pigmentation is seen in albinism. Dark-skinned patients have lighter-coloured palms, soles, nail beds and lips. Freckle-like or dark streaks of pigmentation are also common in the sclera and nail beds of dark-skinned patients. Congenital dermal melanocytosis or Mongolian Blue Spots are a type of birthmark seen in people of Asian, Indian and African descent. They are most commonly located on the back or buttocks and fade considerably with age. Care must be taken not to confuse these with bruising. **CULTURAL CONSIDERATIONS** **Light colour skinned patients may have darker pigment around the nipples, lips and genitalia.**	**Abnormal findings** include rashes, such as the reddish (in light-skinned people) or darkened (in dark-skinned people) butterfly rash across the bridge of the nose and cheeks (Fig. 15-5), characteristic of discoid lupus erythematosus. **Albinism** is a generalised loss of pigmentation. **Erythema** (skin redness and warmth) is seen in inflammation, allergic reactions or trauma. **Erythema in the dark-skinned patient may be difficult to see. However, the affected skin feels swollen and warmer than the surrounding skin.**
Check skin integrity, especially carefully in pressure point areas (see Fig. 15-6). Use the Braden Scale (see Assessment tool 15-1) to predict pressure injury risk. If any skin breakdown is noted, use the PUSH tool (see Assessment tool 15-2) to document the degree of skin breakdown. **CLINICAL TIP** **In the obese patient, carefully inspect skin on the limbs, in skin folds including under the breasts and in the groin area, where problems are frequent.**	Skin is intact, and there are no reddened areas.	Skin breakdown is initially noted as a reddened area on the skin that may progress to serious and painful pressure ulcers (see Abnormal findings 15-1 for stages of pressure ulcer development). Depending on the colour of the patient's skin, reddened areas may not be prominent, although the skin may feel warmer in the area of breakdown than elsewhere.

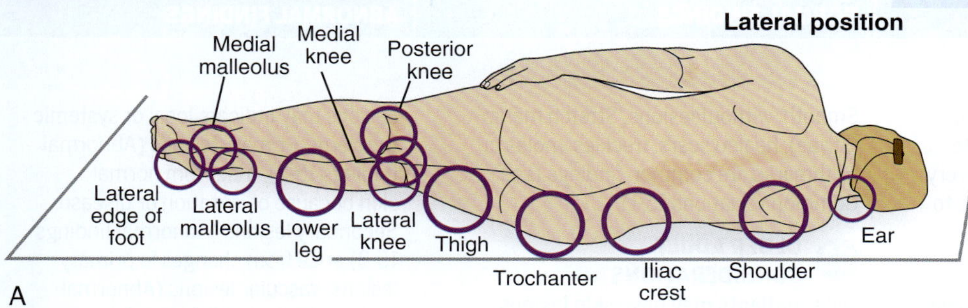

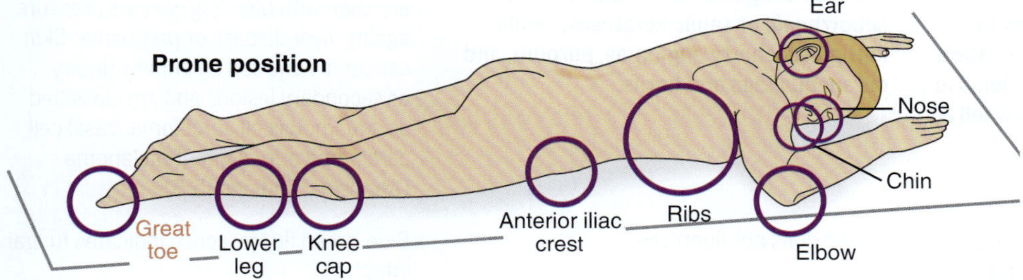

FIGURE 15-6 Common pressure ulcer sites.

Continued on following page

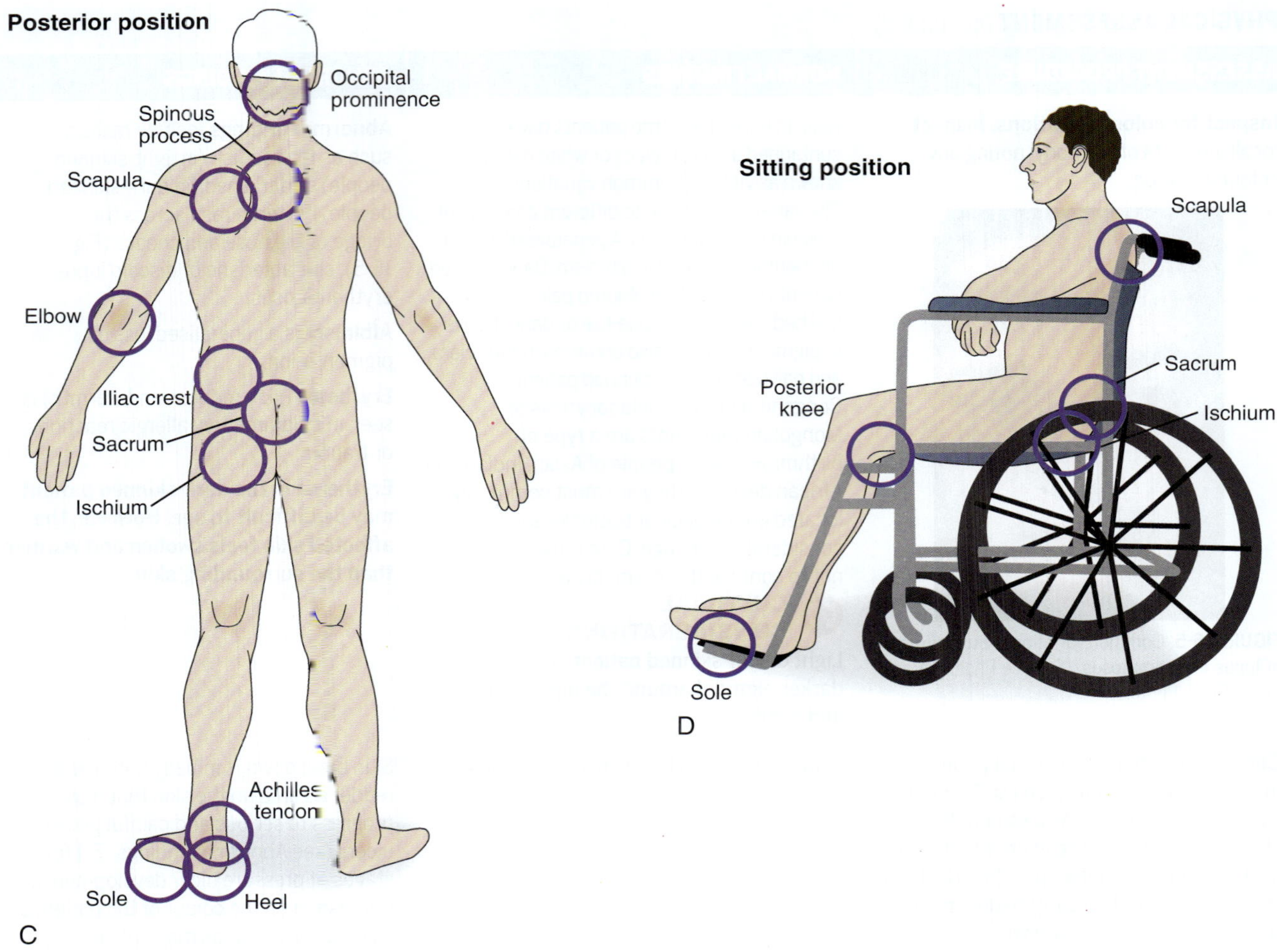

FIGURE 15-6 Common pressure ulcer sites. *(continued)*

PHYSICAL ASSESSMENT (continued)

ASSESSMENT PROCEDURE	NORMAL FINDINGS	ABNORMAL FINDINGS
Skin (continued)		
Inspect for lesions. Observe the skin surface to detect abnormalities. Note colour, shape and size of lesion. For very small lesions, use a magnifying glass to note these characteristics. **CLINICAL TIP** **When examining female or obese patients, lift the breasts (or ask the patient to lift them) and skin folds to inspect all areas for lesions. Perspiration and friction often cause skin problems in these areas in obese patients (Cowdell & Radley, 2014).**	Smooth, without lesions. Stretch marks (striae), healed scars, freckles, moles or birthmarks are common findings (see Common variations 15-1). **OLDER ADULT CONSIDERATIONS** **Older patients may have skin lesions because of ageing. Some examples are seborrhoeic or senile keratoses, senile lentigines, cherry angiomas, purpura, and cutaneous tags and horns.**	Lesions may indicate local or systemic problems. Primary lesions (Abnormal findings 15-2) arise from normal skin because of irritation or disease. Secondary lesions (Abnormal findings 15-3) arise from changes in primary lesions. Vascular lesions (Abnormal findings 15-4), reddish-bluish lesions, are seen with bleeding, venous pressure, ageing, liver disease or pregnancy. Skin cancer lesions can be either primary or secondary lesions and are classified as squamous cell carcinoma, basal cell carcinoma or malignant melanoma (Abnormal findings 15-5).
If you suspect a fungus, shine a Wood's light (an ultraviolet light filtered through a special glass) on the lesion.	Lesion does not fluoresce.	Blue-green fluorescence indicates fungal infection.

Continued on page 245

ASSESSMENT TOOL 15-1 Braden scale for predicting pressure sore risk

Patient's name ______________ Evaluator's name ______________ Date of assessment ____________

SENSORY PERCEPTION	**1. Completely limited**	**2. Very limited**	**3. Slightly limited**	**4. No Impairment**
Ability to respond meaningfully to pressure-related discomfort	Unresponsive (does not moan, flinch or grasp) to painful stimuli, due to diminished level of consciousness or sedation. OR Has limited ability to feel pain over most of body.	Responds only to painful stimuli. Cannot communicate discomfort except by moaning or restlessness. OR Has a sensory impairment that limits the ability to feel pain or discomfort over half of body.	Responds to verbal commands, but cannot always communicate discomfort or the need to be turned. OR Has some sensory impairment that limits ability to feel pain or discomfort in one or two extremities.	Responds to verbal commands. Has no sensory deficit that would limit ability to feel or voice pain or discomfort.
MOISTURE	**1. Constantly moist**	**2. Very moist**	**3. Occasionally moist**	**4. Rarely moist**
Degree to which skin is exposed to moisture	Skin is kept moist almost constantly by perspiration, urine, etc. Dampness is detected every time patient is moved or turned.	Skin is often, but not always, moist. Linen must be changed at least once per shift.	Skin is occasionally moist, requiring an extra linen change approximately once per day.	Skin is usually dry. Linen requires changing only at routine intervals.
ACTIVITY	**1. Bedfast**	**2. Chairfast**	**3. Walks occasionally**	**4. Walks frequently**
Degree of physical activity	Confined to bed.	Ability to walk severely limited or non-existent. Cannot bear own weight and/or must be assisted into chair or wheelchair.	Walks occasionally during day, but for very short distances, with or without assistance. Spends majority of each shift in bed or chair.	Walks outside room at least twice per day and inside room at least once every 2 hours during waking hours.
MOBILITY	**1. Completely immobile**	**2. Very limited**	**3. Slightly limited**	**4. No limitation**
Ability to change and control body position	Does not make even slight changes in body or extremity position without assistance.	Makes occasional slight changes in body or extremity position but unable to make frequent or significant changes independently.	Makes frequent, though slight, changes in body or extremity position independently.	Makes major and frequent changes in position without assistance.
NUTRITION	**1. Very poor**	**2. Probably inadequate**	**3. Adequate**	**4. Excellent**
Usual food intake pattern	Never eats a complete meal. Rarely eats more than half of any food offered. Eats 2 servings or less of protein (meat or dairy products) per day.	Rarely eats a complete meal and generally eats only about half of any food offered. Protein intake includes only 3 servings of meat	Eats over half of most meals. Eats a total of 4 servings of protein (meat, dairy products) per day. Occasionally will refuse a meal,	Eats most of every meal. Never refuses a meal. Usually eats a total of 4 or more servings of meat and dairy products. Occasionally eats

Continued on following page

ASSESSMENT TOOL 15-1 Braden scale for predicting pressure sore risk (continued)

NUTRITION	1. Very poor	2. Probably inadequate	3. Adequate	4. Excellent			
	Takes fluids poorly. Does not take a liquid dietary supplement. OR Is NPO and/or maintained on clear liquids or IVs for more than 5 days.	or dairy products per day. Occasionally will take a dietary supplement. OR Receives less than optimum amount of liquid diet or tube feeding.	but will usually take a supplement when offered. OR Is on a tube feeding or TPN regimen that probably meets most nutritional needs.	between meals. Does not require supplementation.			
FRICTION AND SHEAR	**1. Problem**	**2. Potential problem**	**3. No apparent problem**				
	Requires moderate to maximum assistance in moving. Complete lifting without sliding against sheets is impossible. Frequently slides down in bed or chair, requiring frequent repositioning with maximum assistance. Spasticity, contractures or agitation leads to almost constant friction.	Moves feebly or requires minimum assistance. During a move, skin probably slides to some extent against sheets, chair, restraints or other devices. Maintains relatively good position in chair or bed most of the time but occasionally slides down.	Moves in bed and in chair independently and has sufficient muscle strength to lift up completely during move. Maintains good position in bed or chair.				
				TOTAL SCORE			

ASSESSMENT TOOL 15-2 PUSH tool to measure pressure ulcer healing

PUSH Tool 3.0

Patient name ______________________ Patient ID# ______________

Ulcer location ______________________ Date ______________

Directions: Observe and measure the pressure ulcer. Categorise the ulcer with respect to surface area, exudate and type of wound tissue. Record a subscore for each of these ulcer characteristics. Add the subscores to obtain the total score. A comparison of total scores measured over time provides an indication of the improvement or deterioration in pressure ulcer healing.

LENGTH × WIDTH (in cm²)	0 0	1 <0.3	2 0.3–0.6	3 0.7–1.0	4 1.1–2.0	5 2.1–3.0	Subscore
		6 3.1–4.0	7 4.1–8.0	8 8.1–12.0	9 12.1–24.0	10 >24.0	
EXUDATE AMOUNT	0 None	1 Light	2 Moderate	3 Heavy			Subscore
TISSUE TYPE	0 Closed	1 Epithelial tissue	2 Granulation tissue	3 Slough	4 Necrotic tissue		Subscore
							TOTAL SCORE

ASSESSMENT TOOL 15-2 PUSH tool to measure pressure ulcer healing (continued)

Length × width: Measure the greatest length (head to toe) and the greatest width (side to side) using a centimetre ruler. Multiply these two measurements (length × width) to obtain an estimate of surface area in square centimetres (cm^2). Caveat: Do not guess! Always use a centimetre ruler and always use the same method each time the ulcer is measured.

Exudate amount: Estimate the amount of exudate (drainage) present after removal of the dressing and before applying any topical agent to the ulcer. Estimate the exudate (drainage) as none, light, moderate or heavy.

Tissue type: This refers to the types of tissue that are present in the wound (ulcer) bed. Score as a '4' if there is any necrotic tissue present. Score as a '3' if there is any amount of slough present and necrotic tissue is absent. Score as a '2' if the wound is clean and contains granulation tissue. A superficial wound that is re-epithelialising is scored as a '1'. When the wound is closed, score as a '0'.

4—Necrotic tissue (eschar): Black, brown or tan tissue that adheres firmly to the wound bed or ulcer edges and may be either firmer or softer than surrounding skin.

3—Slough: Yellow or white tissue that adheres to the ulcer bed in strings or thick clumps, or is mucinous.

2—Granulation tissue: Pink or beefy-red tissue with a shiny, moist, granular appearance.

1—Epithelial tissue: For superficial ulcers, new pink or shiny tissue (skin) that grows in from the edges or as islands on the ulcer surface.

0—Closed/resurfaced: the wound is completely covered with epithelium (new skin).

Source: National Pressure Ulcer Advisory Panel. Available at www.npuap.org.

PHYSICAL ASSESSMENT (continued)

ASSESSMENT PROCEDURE	NORMAL FINDINGS	ABNORMAL FINDINGS
Skin (continued)		
If you observe a lesion, note its location, distribution and configuration. Measure the lesion with a centimetre ruler.	Normal lesions may be moles, freckles, birthmarks, and the like. They may be scattered over the skin in no particular pattern.	In abnormal findings, distribution may be diffuse (scattered all over), localised to one area or in sun-exposed areas. Configuration (see Abnormal findings 15-6) may be discrete (separate and distinct), grouped (clustered), confluent (merged), linear (in a line), annular and arciform (circular or arcing), or zosteriform (linear along a nerve route).
PALPATION		
Palpate skin to assess texture. Use the palmar surface of your three middle fingers to palpate skin texture.	Skin is smooth and even.	Rough, flaky, dry skin is seen in hypothyroidism. Obese patients often report dry, itchy skin.
Palpate to assess thickness. If lesions are noted when assessing skin thickness, put gloves on and palpate the lesion between the thumb and finger. Observe for exudate or other characteristics.	Skin is normally thin but calluses (rough, thick sections of epidermis) are common on areas of the body that are exposed to constant pressure.	Very thin skin may be seen in patients with arterial insufficiency or in those on steroid therapy.
Palpate to assess moisture. Check under skin folds and in unexposed areas.	Skin surfaces vary from moist to dry depending on the area assessed. Recent activity or a warm environment may cause increased moisture.	Increased moisture or diaphoresis (profuse sweating) may occur in conditions such as fever or hyperthyroidism or with hyperhidrosis. Decreased moisture occurs with dehydration or hypothyroidism.
CLINICAL TIP Some nurses believe that using the dorsal surfaces of the hands to assess moisture leads to a more accurate result.	**OLDER ADULT CONSIDERATIONS** The older patient's skin may feel dryer than a younger patient's skin because sebum production decreases with age.	Clammy skin is typical in shock or hypotension.

Continued on following page

PHYSICAL ASSESSMENT (continued)

ASSESSMENT PROCEDURE	NORMAL FINDINGS	ABNORMAL FINDINGS
Skin (continued)		
Palpate to assess temperature. Use the dorsal surfaces of your hands to palpate the skin (Fig. 15-7). **CLINICAL TIP** **You may also want to palpate with the palmar surfaces of your hands because these surfaces of the hands and fingers may be more sensitive to temperature.**	Skin is normally a warm temperature.	Cold skin may accompany shock or hypotension. Cool skin may accompany arterial disease. Very warm skin may indicate a febrile state or hyperthyroidism.
Palpate to assess mobility and turgor. Ask the patient to lie down. Using two fingers, gently pinch the skin on the sternum or under the clavicle (Fig. 15-8). *Mobility* refers to how easily the skin can be pinched. *Turgor* refers to the skin's elasticity and how quickly the skin returns to its original shape after being pinched.	Skin pinches easily and immediately returns to its original position. **OLDER ADULT CONSIDERATIONS** **The older patient's skin loses its turgor because of a decrease in elasticity and collagen fibres. Sagging or wrinkled skin appears in the facial, breast and scrotal areas.**	Decreased mobility is seen with oedema. Decreased turgor (a slow return of the skin to its normal state taking longer than 30 seconds) is seen in dehydration.
Palpate to detect oedema. Use your thumbs to press down on the skin of the feet or ankles to check for oedema (swelling related to accumulation of fluid in the tissue).	Skin rebounds and does not remain indented when pressure is released.	Indentations on the skin may vary from slight to great and may be in one area or all over the body. See Chapter 23 on the peripheral vascular system for a full discussion of oedema.
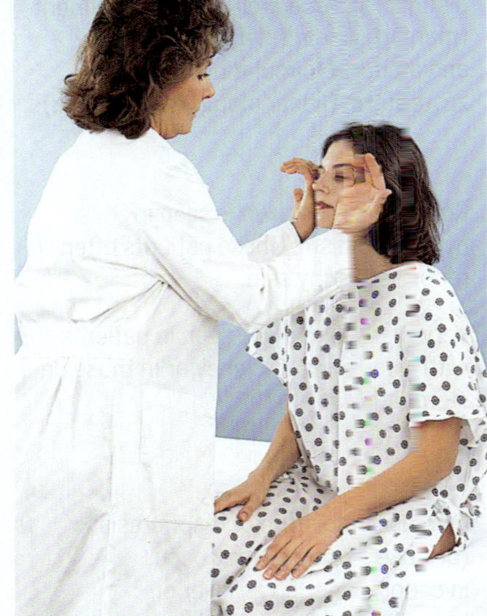 **FIGURE 15-7** Assessing temperature and moisture. (© B. Proud.)	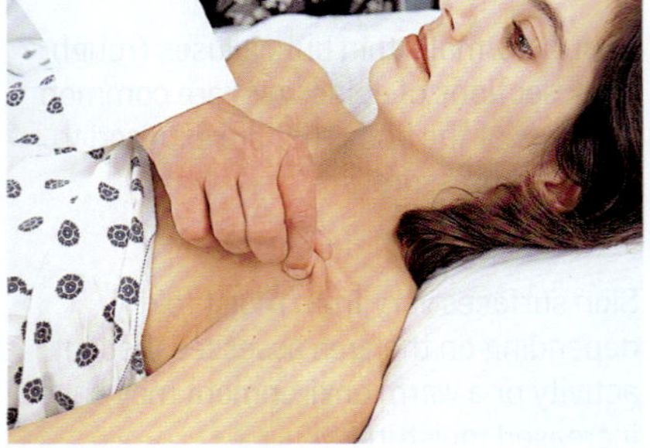 **FIGURE 15-8** Palpating to assess skin turgor and mobility. (© B. Proud.)	
Scalp and hair		
INSPECTION AND PALPATION		
Have the patient remove any hair clips, hair pins or wigs. Then inspect the scalp and hair for general colour and condition.	Natural hair colour, as opposed to chemically coloured hair, varies among patients from pale blond to black to grey or white. The colour is determined by the amount of melanin present.	 **OLDER ADULT CONSIDERATIONS** **Nutritional deficiencies may cause patchy grey hair in some patients.**

PHYSICAL ASSESSMENT (continued)

ASSESSMENT PROCEDURE	NORMAL FINDINGS	ABNORMAL FINDINGS
Scalp and hair (continued)		
At 2-cm intervals, separate the hair from the scalp and inspect and palpate the hair and scalp for cleanliness, dryness or oiliness, parasites and lesions (Fig. 15-9). Wear gloves if lesions are suspected or if hygiene is poor. 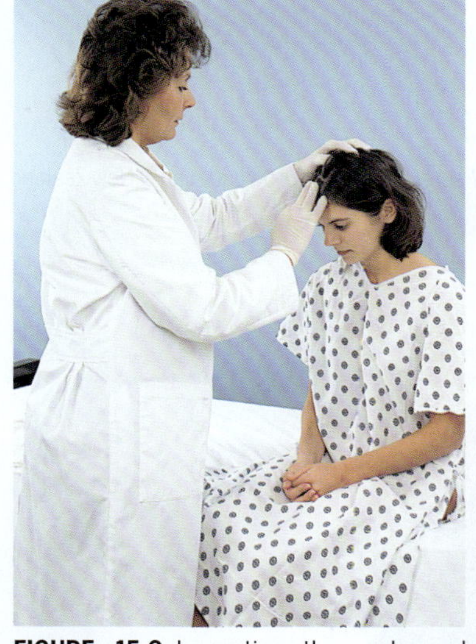 **FIGURE 15-9** Inspecting the scalp and hair. (© B. Proud.)	Scalp is clean and dry. Sparse dandruff may be visible. Hair is smooth and firm, somewhat elastic. However, as people age, hair feels coarser and drier. 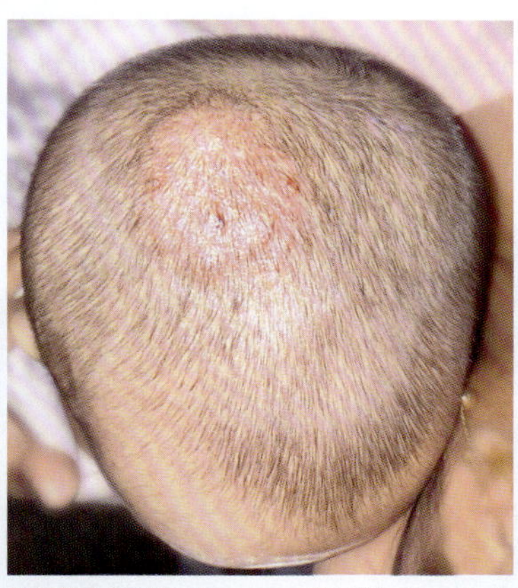 **FIGURE 15-10** Tinea capitis (Shutterstock.com/Zay Nyi Nyi).	Excessive scaliness may indicate dermatitis. Raised lesions may indicate infections or tumour growth. Dull, dry hair may be seen with hypothyroidism and malnutrition. Poor hygiene may indicate a need for patient education or assistance with activities of daily living. Pustules with hair loss in patches are seen in tinea capitis, a contagious fungal disease (ringworm, Fig. 15-10). Infections of the hair follicle (folliculitis) appear as pustules surrounded by erythema (Fig. 15-11).

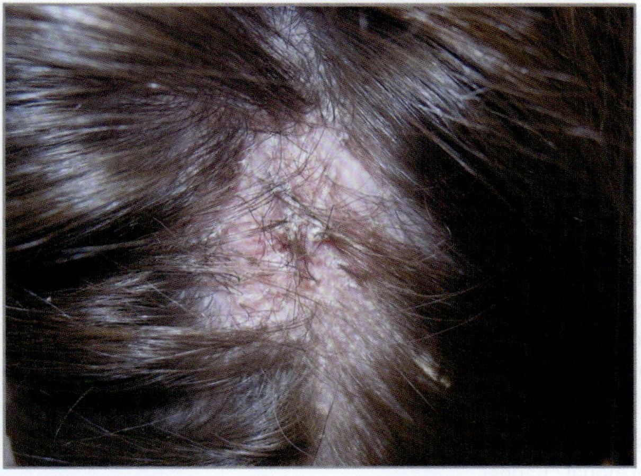

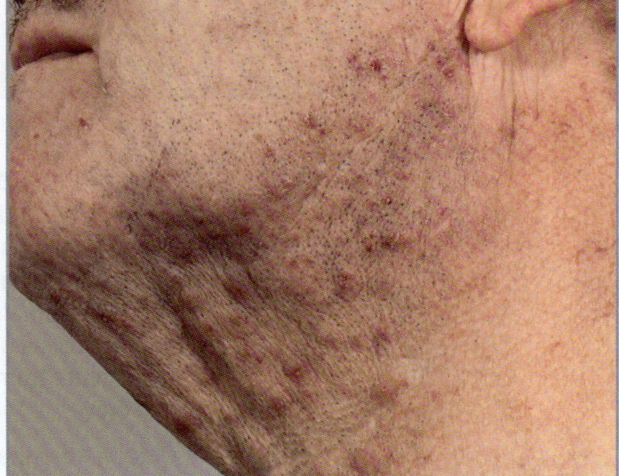

FIGURE 15-11 **(A)** Folliculitis of the scalp. **(B)** Folliculitis of the beard area. (**A,** Stedman, Stedman's Medical Dictionary, 28e, © 2005, Wolters Kluwer Health; **B,** Dermnet.nz/© Prof. Raimo Suhonen.)

ASSESSMENT PROCEDURE	NORMAL FINDINGS	ABNORMAL FINDINGS
Inspect amount and distribution of scalp, body, axillae and pubic hair. Look for unusual growth elsewhere on the body.	Varying amounts of terminal hair cover the scalp, axillary, body and pubic areas according to normal gender distribution. Fine vellus hair covers the entire body except for the soles, palms, lips and nipples. Normal male pattern balding is symmetrical (Fig. 15-12).	Excessive generalised hair loss may occur with infection, nutritional deficiencies, hormonal disorders, thyroid or liver disease, drug toxicity, hepatic or renal failure. It may also result from chemotherapy or radiation therapy. Patchy hair loss (Fig. 15-13) may result from infections of the scalp, discoid or systemic lupus erythematosus, and some types of chemotherapy.

Continued on following page

PHYSICAL ASSESSMENT (continued)

ASSESSMENT PROCEDURE	NORMAL FINDINGS	ABNORMAL FINDINGS
Scalp and hair (continued)		

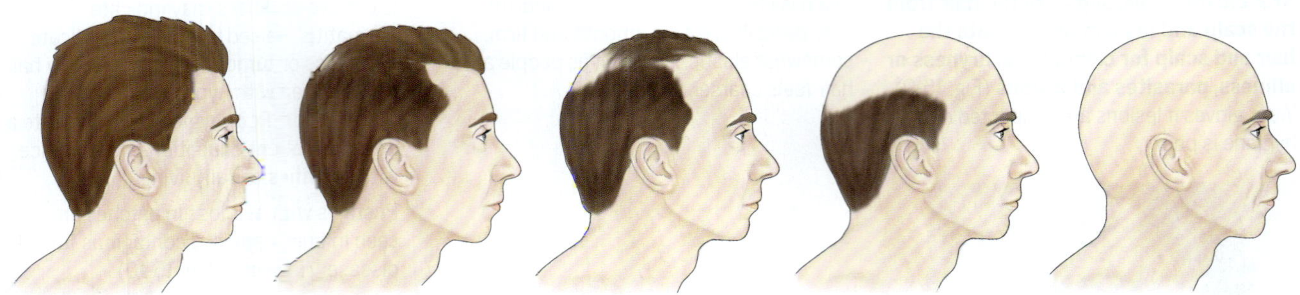

FIGURE 15-12 Male pattern balding. (From Farrell, M. & Dempsey, J. [2014]. *Smeltzer & Bare's textbook of medical-surgical nursing* [3rd Australian & New Zealand ed.]. Sydney: Lippincott Williams & Wilkins.)

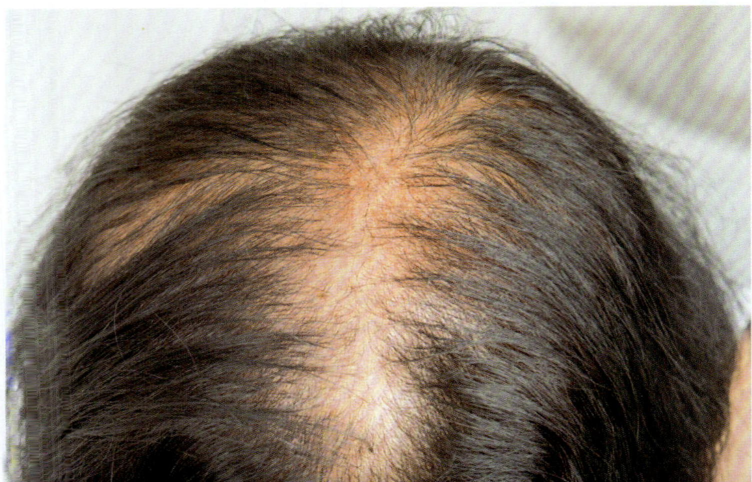

FIGURE 15-13 Patchy hair loss. (Shutterstock.com/srisakorn wonglakorn.)

ASSESSMENT PROCEDURE	NORMAL FINDINGS	ABNORMAL FINDINGS
	 **OLDER ADULT CONSIDERATIONS** **Older patients have thinner hair because of a decrease in hair follicles. Pubic, axillary and body hair also decrease with ageing. Alopecia is seen, especially in men. Hair loss occurs from the periphery of the scalp and moves to the centre.** Older women may have terminal hair growth on the chin owing to hormonal changes.	Hirsutism (facial hair on females) is a characteristic of Cushing disease and results from an imbalance of adrenal hormones, or it may be a side effect of steroids.
Nails		
INSPECTION		
Inspect nail grooming and cleanliness.	Nails are clean and manicured.	Dirty, broken or jagged fingernails may be seen with poor hygiene practices. They may also result from the patient's hobby or occupation.

PHYSICAL ASSESSMENT (continued)

ASSESSMENT PROCEDURE	NORMAL FINDINGS	ABNORMAL FINDINGS
Nails (continued)		
Inspect nail colour and markings.	Pink tones should be seen. Some longitudinal ridging is normal. **CULTURAL CONSIDERATIONS** **Dark-skinned patients may have freckles or pigmented streaks in their nails.**	Pale or cyanotic nails may indicate hypoxia or anaemia. Splinter haemorrhages may be caused by trauma. Beau lines occur after acute illness and eventually grow out. Yellow discolouration may be seen in fungal infections or psoriasis. Nail pitting is also common in psoriasis (Abnormal findings 15-7).
Inspect shape of nails.	There is normally a 160-degree angle between the nail base and the skin.	Early clubbing (180-degree angle with spongy sensation) and late clubbing (greater than 180-degree angle) can occur from chronic hypoxaemia. Spoon nails (concave) may be present with iron deficiency anaemia (Abnormal findings 15-7).
PALPATION		
Palpate nail to assess texture.	Nails are hard and basically immobile. **CULTURAL CONSIDERATIONS** **Dark-skinned patients may have thicker nails.** **OLDER ADULT CONSIDERATIONS** **Older patients' nails may appear thickened, yellow and brittle because of decreased circulation in the extremities.**	Thickened nails (especially toenails) may be caused by decreased circulation.
Palpate to assess texture and consistency, noting whether nail plate is attached to nail bed.	Nails are smooth and firm; nail plate should be firmly attached to nail bed.	Paronychia (inflammation) indicates local infection. Detachment of nail plate from nail bed (onycholysis) is seen in infections or trauma.
Test capillary refill in nail beds by pressing the nail tip briefly and watching for colour change (Fig. 15-14).	Pink tone returns immediately to blanched nail beds when pressure is released.	There is slow (greater than 2 seconds) capillary nail bed refill (return of pink tone) with respiratory or cardiovascular diseases that cause hypoxia.

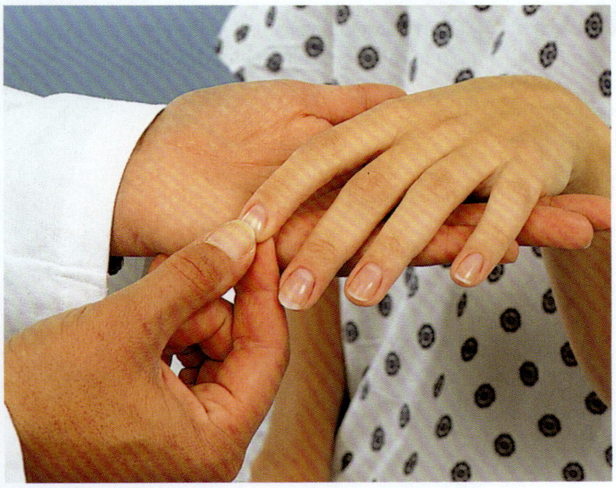

FIGURE 15-14 Testing capillary refill. (© B. Proud.)

COMMON VARIATIONS 15-1 COMMON SKIN VARIATIONS

Many skin assessment findings are considered normal variations in that they are not health- or life-threatening. For example, freckles and birthmarks are common variations in fair-skinned patients. Scars and vitiligo are not exactly normal findings because scars suggest a healed injury or surgical intervention and vitiligo may be related to dysfunction of the immune system. However, they are common and usually insignificant. Other common findings appear below.

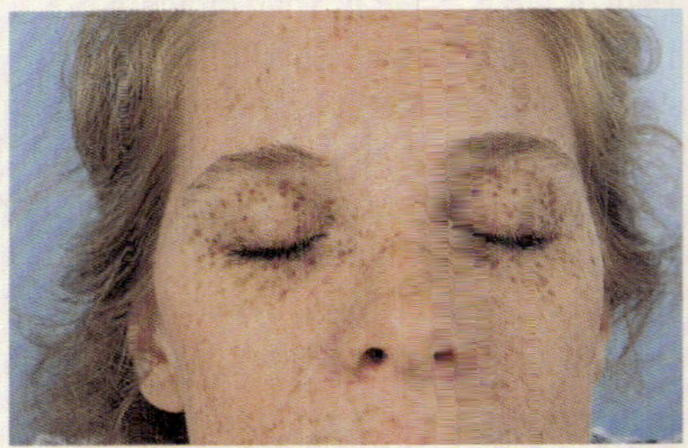

Freckles—flat, small macules of pigment that appear following sun exposure. (© B. Proud.)

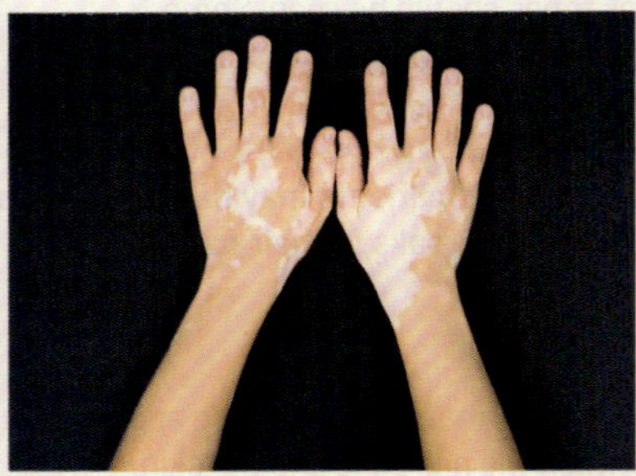

Vitiligo of the hands. (Shutterstock.com/Jelena Bekvelac.)

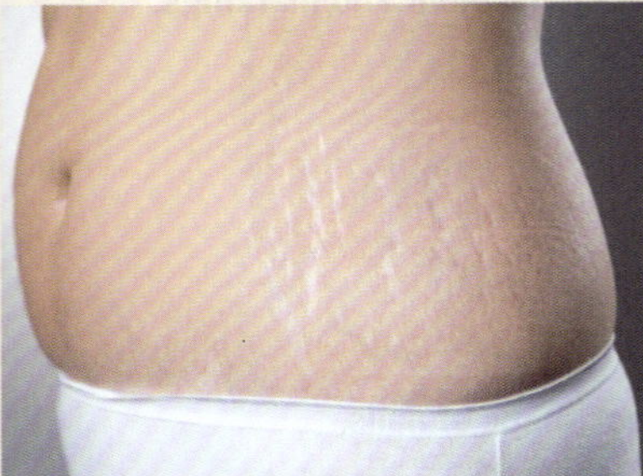

Striae (sometimes called stretch marks). (Shutterstock.com/staras.)

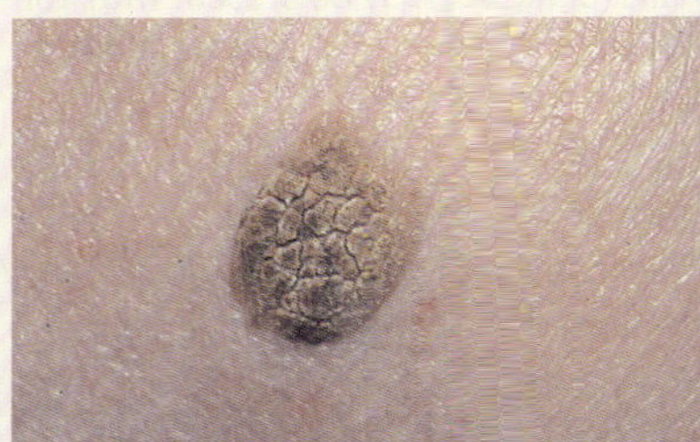

Seborrheic keratosis, a warty or crusty pigmented lesion. (With permission from Goodheart, H. P. [1999]. *A photoguide to common skin disorders: Diagnosis and management*. Baltimore: Williams & Wilkins.)

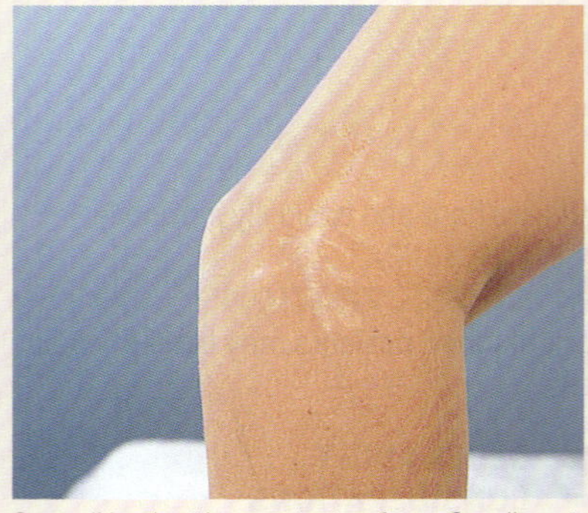

Scar. (Used with permission from Goodheart, H., & Gonzalez, M. E. (2016). Goodheart's photoguide to common pediatric and adult skin disorders (4th ed.). Philadelphia, PA: Wolters Kluwer.)

Mole (also called nevus), a flat or raised tan or brownish marking up to 6 mm wide.

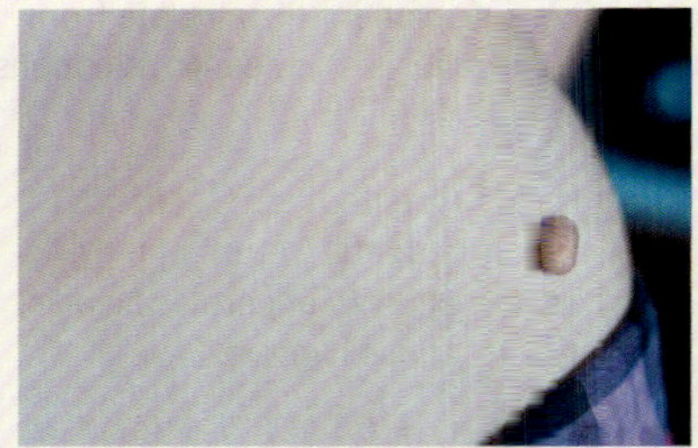

Cutaneous tags, raised yellow papules with a depressed centre. (Shutterstock.com/Manee_Meena.)

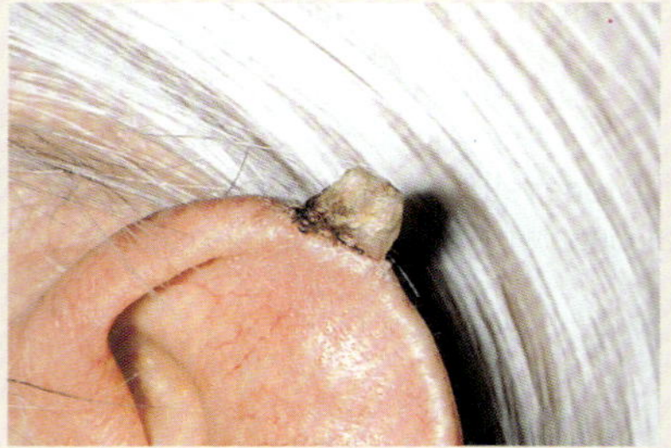

Cutaneous horn. (Used with permission from Goodheart, H., & Gonzalez, M. E. (2016). Goodheart's photoguide to common pediatric and adult skin disorders (4th ed.). Philadelphia, PA: Wolters Kluwer.)

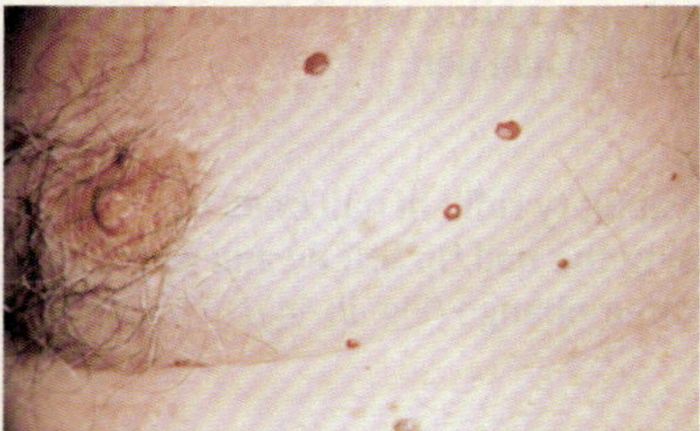

Cherry angiomas, small raised spots (1 to 5 mm wide) typically seen with ageing.

ABNORMAL FINDINGS 15-1 **Identification of pressure ulcer stage**

PRESSURE INJURY AND STAGES

A pressure injury is localized damage to the skin and underlying soft tissue usually over a bony prominence or related to a medical or other device. The injury can present as intact skin or an open ulcer and may be painful. The injury occurs as a result of intense pressure, prolonged pressure or pressure in combination with shear. The tolerance of soft tissue for pressure and shear may also be affected by microclimate, nutrition, perfusion, co-morbidities and condition of the soft tissue.

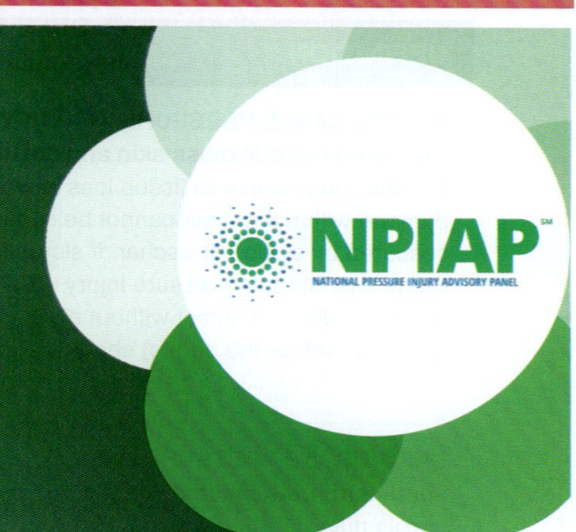

DEFINITION	SCHEMATIC DRAWING	EXAMPLE
STAGE 1 PRESSURE INJURY **Non-blanchable erythema of intact skin** Intact skin with a localized area of non-blanchable erythema, which may appear differently in darkly pigmented skin. Presence of blanchable erythema or changes in sensation, temperature, or firmness may precede visual changes. Color changes do not include purple or maroon discoloration; these may indicate deep tissue pressure injury.	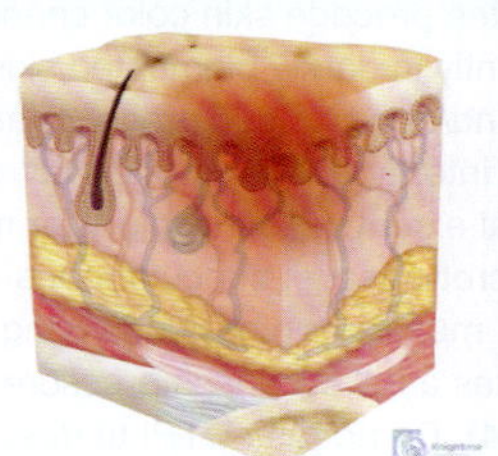	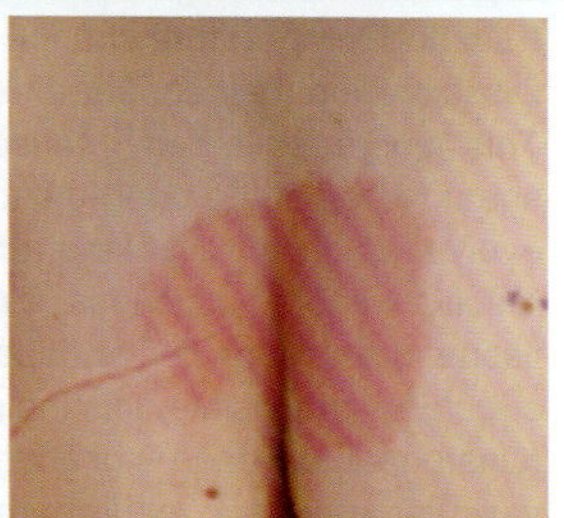
STAGE 2 PRESSURE INJURY **Partial-thickness skin loss with exposed dermis** Partial-thickness loss of skin with exposed dermis. The wound bed is viable, pink or red, moist, and may also present as an intact or ruptured serum-filled blister. Adipose (fat) is not visible and deeper tissues are not visible. Granulation tissue, slough and eschar are not present. These injuries commonly result from adverse microclimate and shear in the skin over the pelvis and shear in the heel. This stage should not be used to describe moisture associated skin damage (MASD) including incontinence associated dermatitis (IAD), intertriginous dermatitis (ITD), medical adhesive related skin injury (MARSI), or traumatic wounds (skin tears, burns, abrasions).	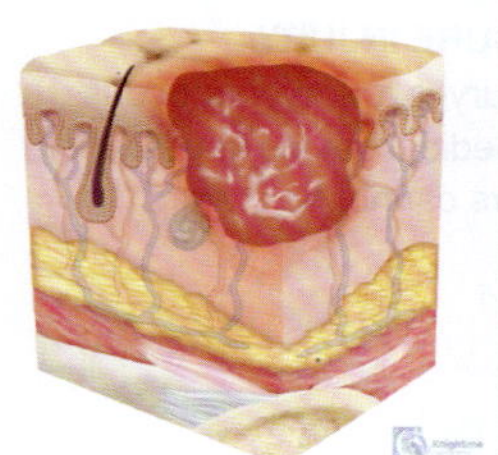	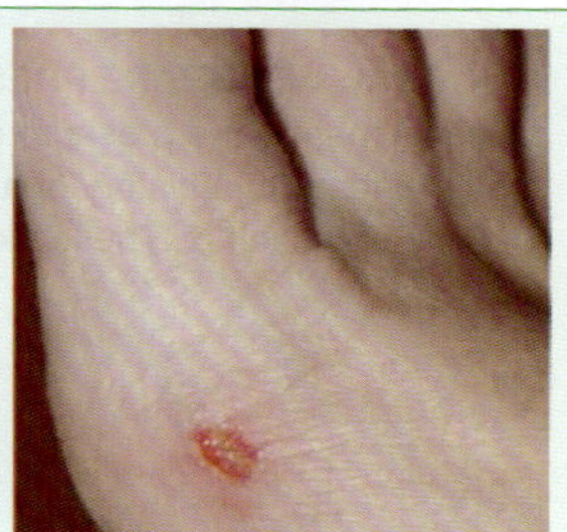
STAGE 3 PRESSURE INJURY **Full-thickness skin loss** Full-thickness loss of skin, in which adipose (fat) is visible in the ulcer and granulation tissue and epibole (rolled wound edges) are often present. Slough and/or eschar may be visible. The depth of tissue damage varies by anatomical location; areas of significant adiposity can develop deep wounds. Undermining and tunneling may occur. Fascia, muscle, tendon, ligament, cartilage or bone are not exposed. If slough or eschar obscures the extent of tissue loss this is an Unstageable Pressure Injury.	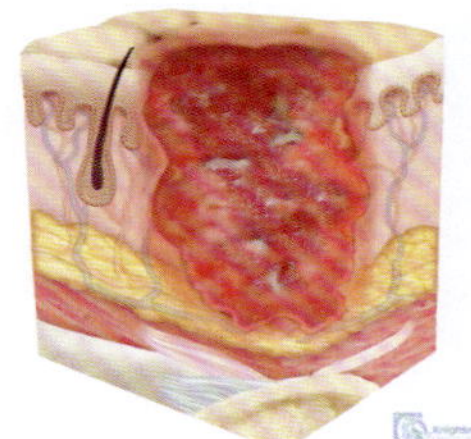	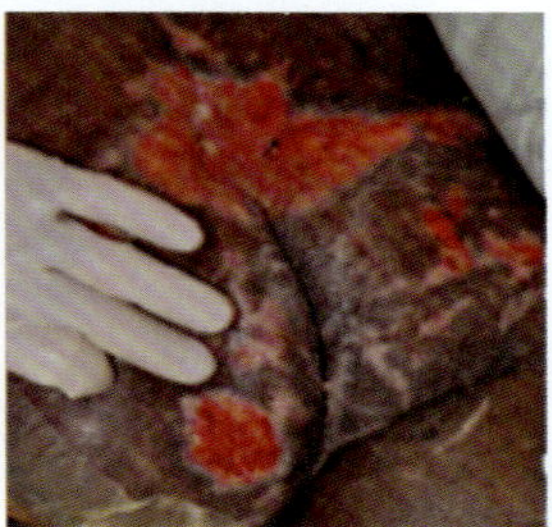
STAGE 4 PRESSURE INJURY **Full-thickness loss of skin and tissue** Full-thickness skin and tissue loss with exposed or directly palpable fascia, muscle, tendon, ligament, cartilage or bone in the ulcer. Slough and/or eschar may be visible. Epibole (rolled edges), undermining and/or tunneling often occur. Depth varies by anatomical location. If slough or eschar obscures the extent of tissue loss this is an Unstageable Pressure Injury.	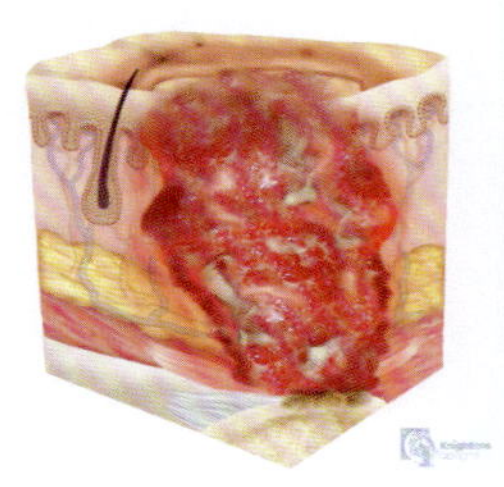	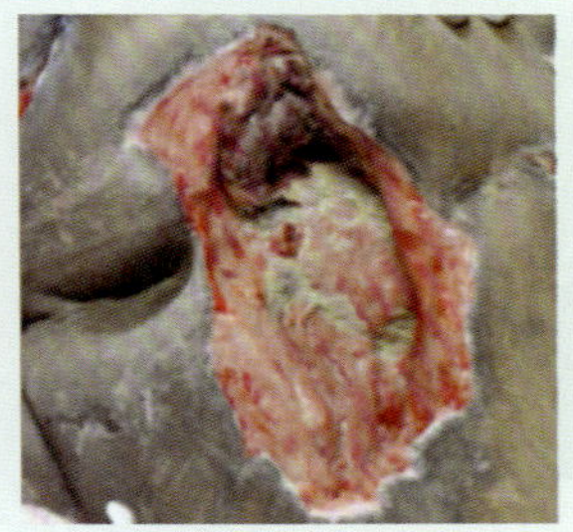

Continued on following page

ABNORMAL FINDINGS 15-1 Identification of pressure ulcer stage (continued)

DEFINITION	SCHEMATIC DRAWING	EXAMPLE
UNSTAGEABLE PRESSURE INJURY **Obscured full-thickness skin and tissue loss** Full-thickness skin and tissue loss in which the extent of tissue damage within the ulcer cannot be confirmed because it is obscured by slough or eschar. If slough or eschar is removed, a Stage 3 or Stage 4 pressure injury will be revealed. Stable eschar (i.e. dry, adherent, intact without erythema or fluctuance) on an ischemic limb or the heel(s) should not be softened or removed.	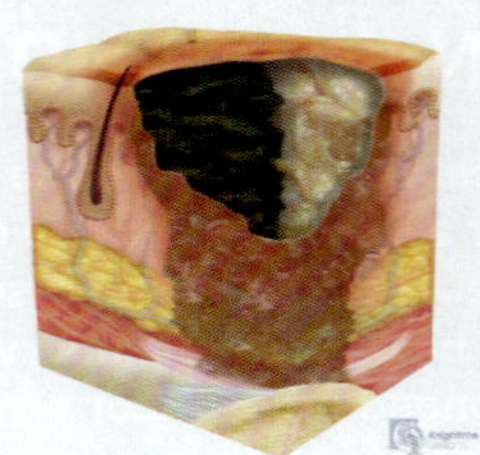	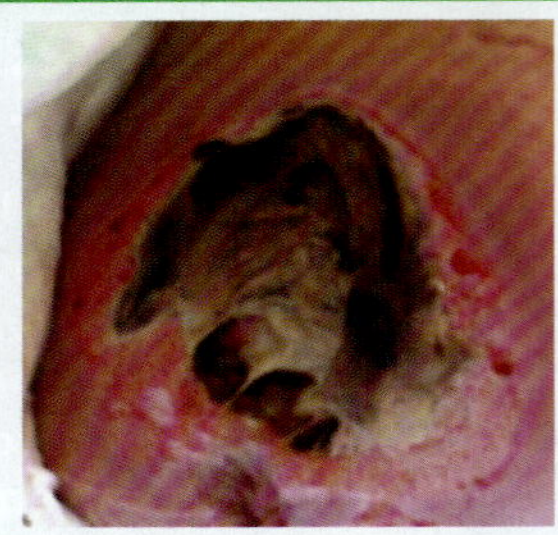
DEEP TISSUE PRESSURE INJURY **Persistent non-blanchable deep red, maroon or purple discoloration** Intact or non-intact skin with localized area of persistent non-blanchable deep red, maroon, purple discoloration or epidermal separation revealing a dark wound bed or blood filled blister. Pain and temperature change often precede skin color changes. Discoloration may appear differently in darkly pigmented skin. This injury results from intense and/or prolonged pressure and shear forces at the bone-muscle interface. The wound may evolve rapidly to reveal the actual extent of tissue injury, or may resolve without tissue loss. If necrotic tissue, subcutaneous tissue, granulation tissue, fascia, muscle or other underlying structures are visible, this indicates a full thickness pressure injury (Unstageable, Stage 3 or Stage 4). Do not use DTPI to describe vascular, traumatic, neuropathic, or dermatologic conditions.	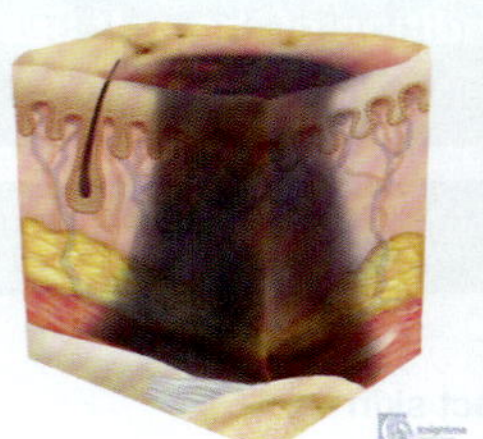	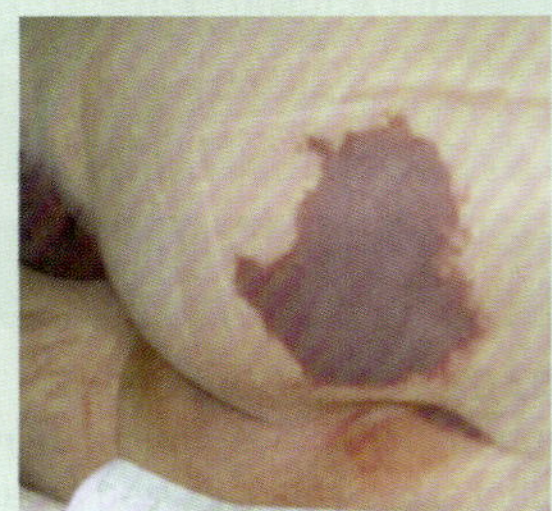
MUCOSAL MEMBRANE PRESSURE INJURY Mucosal membrane pressure injury is found on mucous membranes with a history of a medical device in use at the location of the injury. These ulcers cannot be staged .	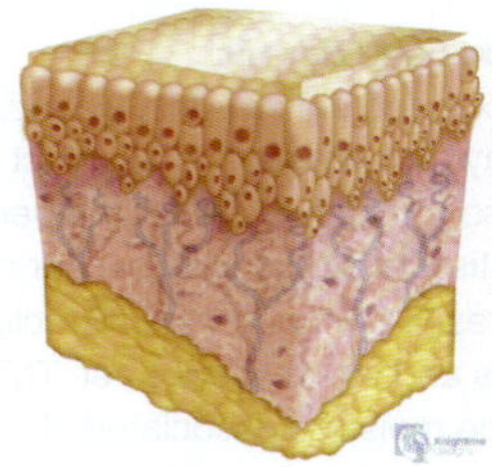	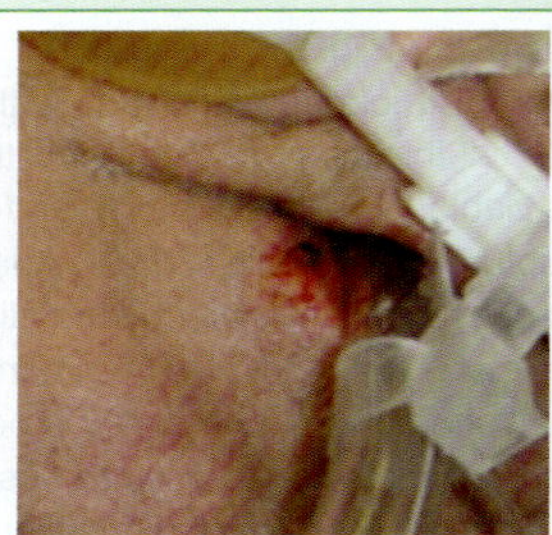

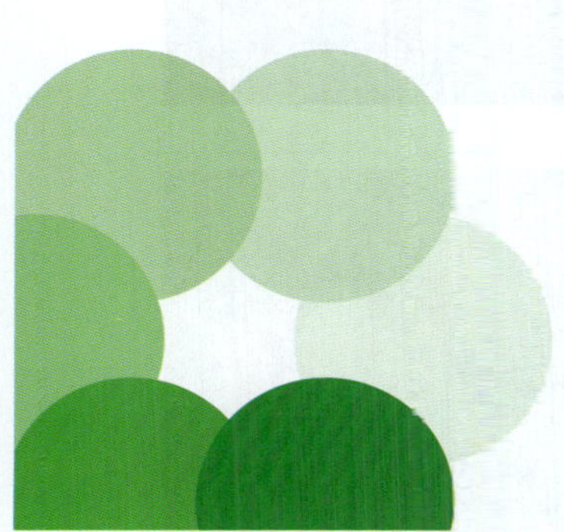

ABNORMAL FINDINGS 15-2 Primary skin lesions

Primary skin lesions are original lesions arising from previously normal skin. Secondary lesions can originate from primary lesions.

TYPE AND DESCRIPTION	EXAMPLES	ILLUSTRATION	PHOTOGRAPH OF EXAMPLE
Macule, patch • Flat, non-palpable skin colour change (skin colour may be brown, white, tan, purple, red) • Macule: <1 cm, circumscribed border • Patch: >1 cm, may have irregular border	• Freckles • Flat moles • Petechiae • Rubella • Vitiligo • Port wine stains • Ecchymosis	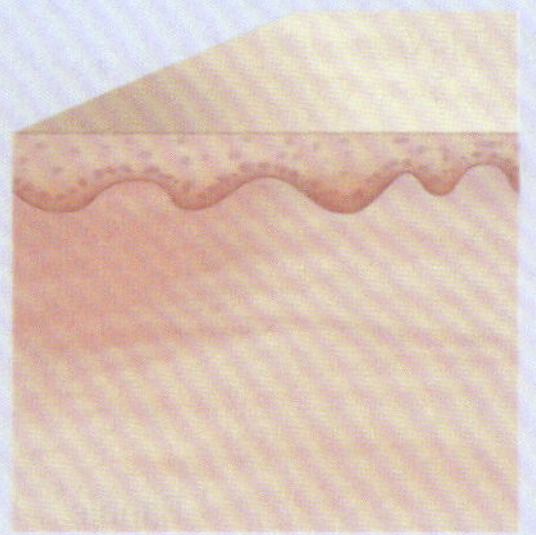 Macule	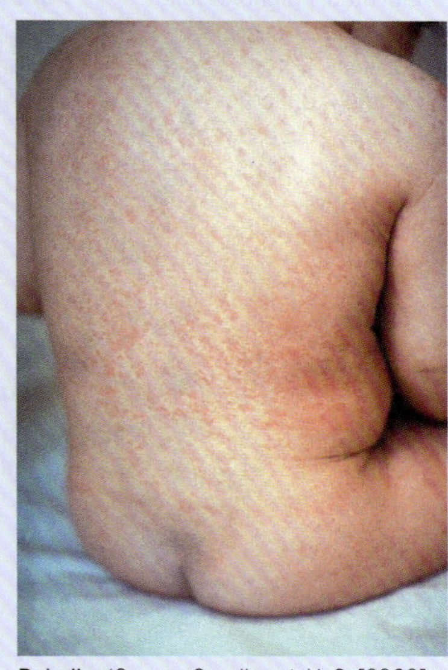 **Rubella.** (*Source:* Goodheart, H. G. [2009]. *Goodheart's photoguide to common skin disorders:* Diagnosis and management [3rd ed.]. Philadelphia: Lippincott Williams & Wilkins.)
		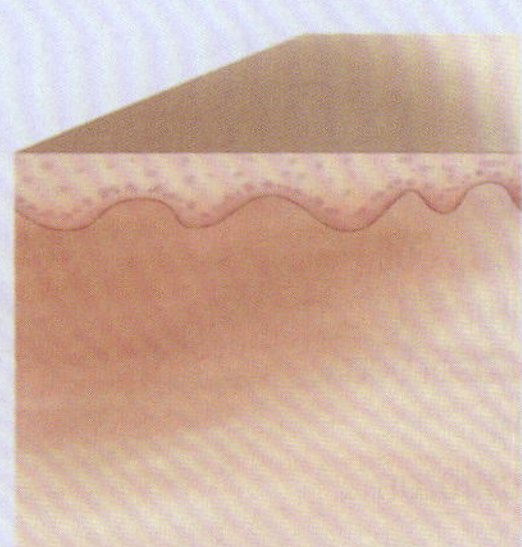 Patch	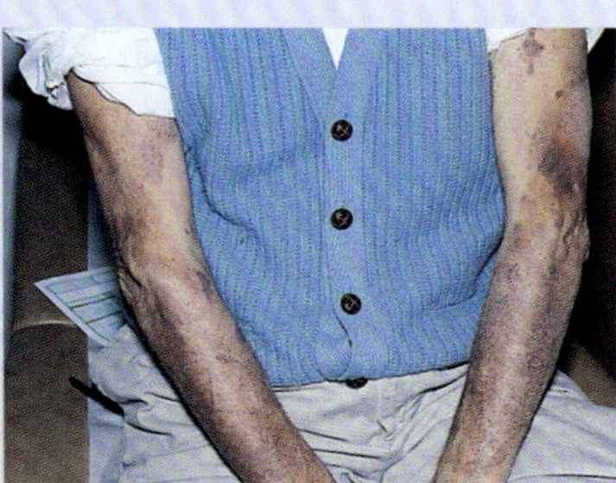 **Ecchymoses** (from prolonged topical corticosteroid use).

Continued on following page

ABNORMAL FINDINGS 15-2 Primary skin lesions (continued)

TYPE AND DESCRIPTION	EXAMPLES	ILLUSTRATION	PHOTOGRAPH OF EXAMPLE
Papule, plaque • Elevated, palpable, solid mass; circumscribed border • Papule: <0.5 cm • Plaque: >0.5 cm (may be coalesced papules with flat top)	***Papules:*** • Elevated naevi • Warts • Lichen planus	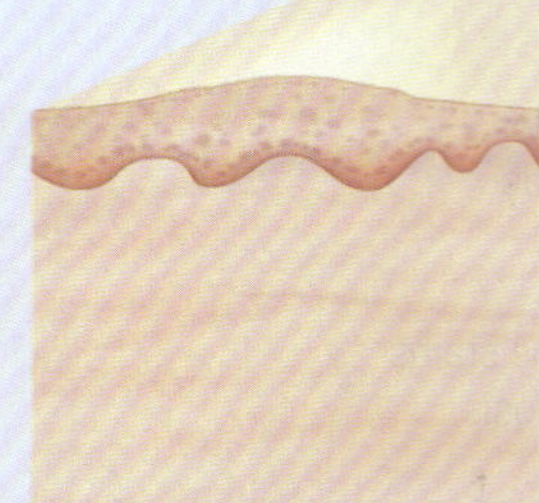 Papule	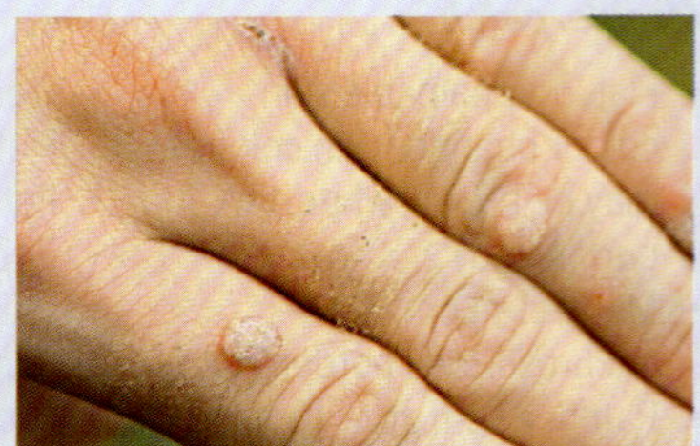 **Warts, circumscribed elevations caused by a virus.** (Shutterstock.com/Marcel Jancovic.)
	Plaques: • Psoriasis • Actinic keratosis	Plaque	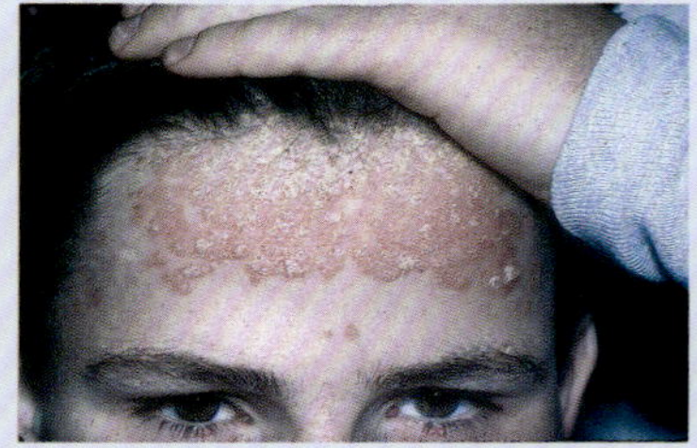 **Psoriasis vulgaris.** (*Source:* Goodheart, H. G. [2009]. *Goodheart's photoguide to common skin disorders: Diagnosis and management* [3rd ed.]. Philadelphia: Lippincott Williams & Wilkins.)
Nodule, tumour • Elevated, solid, palpable mass • Extends deeper into dermis than a papule • Nodule: 0.5–2 cm; circumscribed • Tumour: >1–2 cm; does not always have sharp borders	***Nodules:*** • Lipoma • Squamous cell carcinoma • Poorly absorbed injection • Dermatofibroma	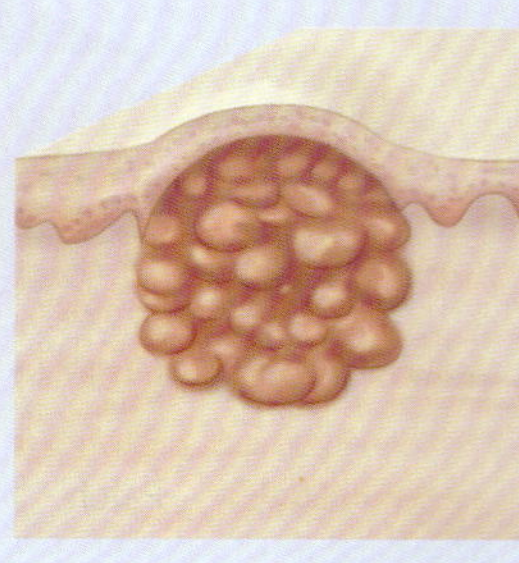 Nodule	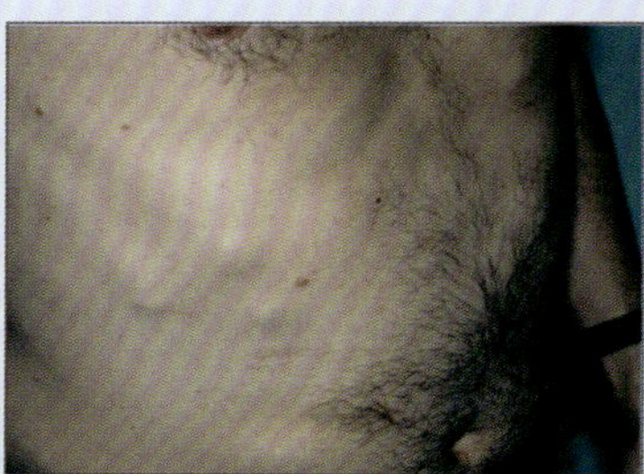 **Lipomas. Multiple rubbery flesh-coloured nodules are palpable on this patient.** (*Source:* Goodheart, H. G. [2005]. *Goodheart's photoguide to common skin disorders.* Philadelphia: Lippincott Williams & Wilkins.)

ABNORMAL FINDINGS 15-2 Primary skin lesions (continued)

TYPE AND DESCRIPTION	EXAMPLES	ILLUSTRATION	PHOTOGRAPH OF EXAMPLE
	Tumours: • Larger lipoma • Carcinoma	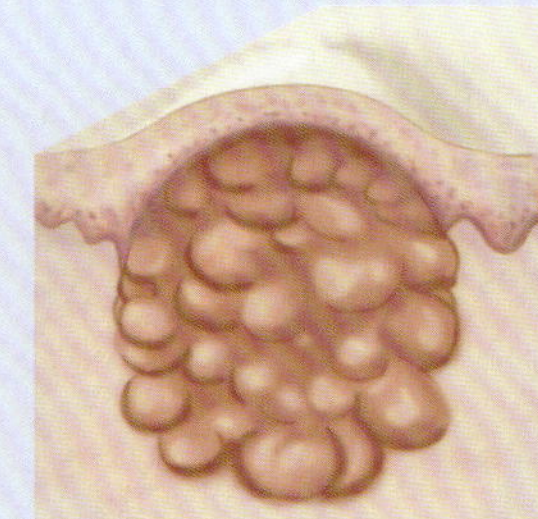 Tumour	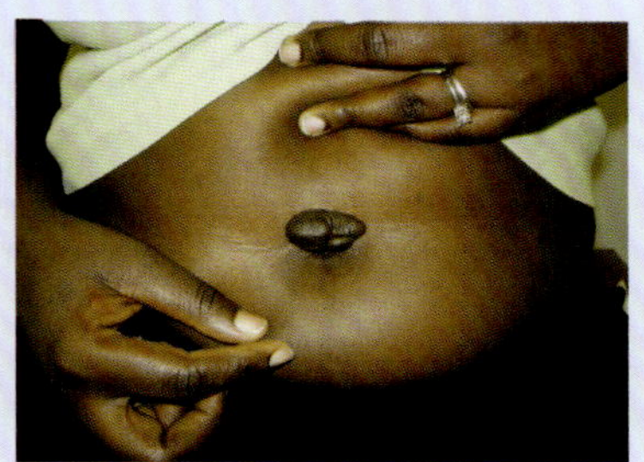 **Keloid.** (*Source:* Goodheart, H. G. [2009]. *Goodheart's photoguide to common skin disorders: Diagnosis and management* [3rd ed.]. Philadelphia: Lippincott Williams & Wilkins.)
Vesicle, bulla • Circumscribed elevated, palpable mass containing serous fluid • Vesicle: <0.5 cm • Bulla: >0.5 cm	***Vesicles:*** • Herpes simplex/ zoster • Varicella (chickenpox) • Poison ivy • Second-degree burn	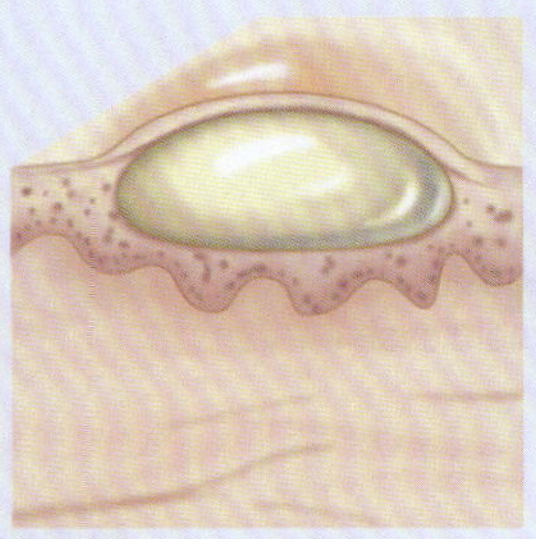 Vesicle	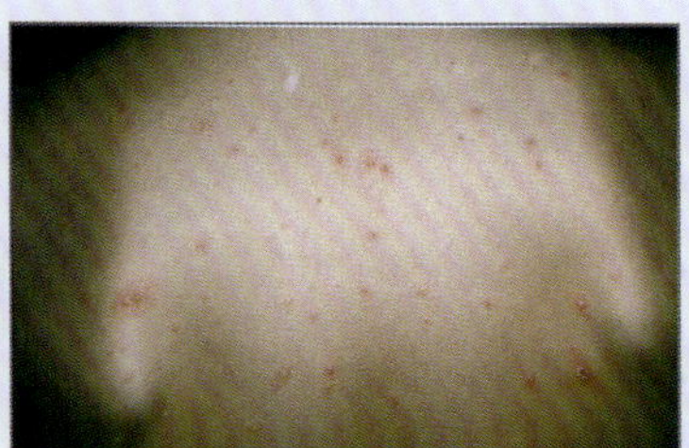 **Varicella. Vesicles and crusts.** (*Source:* Goodheart, H. G. [2005]. *Goodheart's photoguide to common skin disorders.* Philadelphia: Lippincott Williams & Wilkins.)
	Bulla: • Pemphigus, contact dermatitis, large burn blisters, poison ivy, bullous impetigo	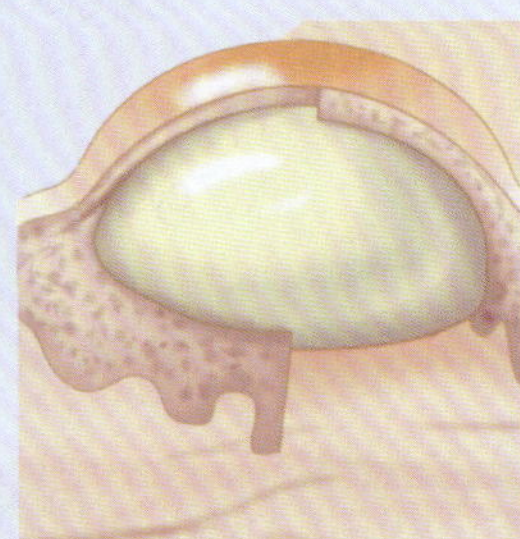 Bulla	
Wheal • Elevated mass with transient borders • Often irregular • Size and colour vary • Caused by movement of serous fluid into the dermis • Does not contain free fluid in a cavity (e.g. vesicle)	• Urticaria (hives) • Insect bites	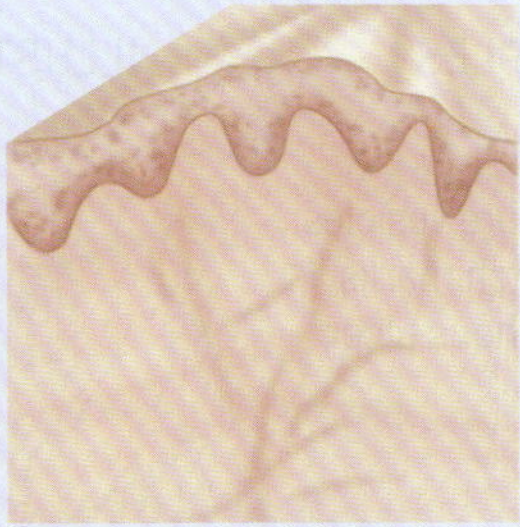 Wheal	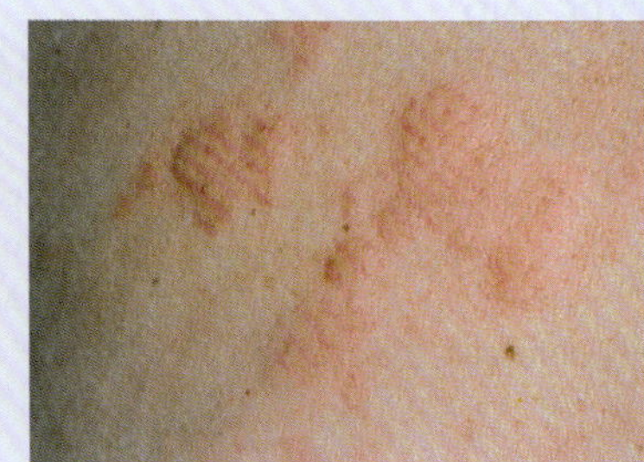 **Urticaria.** (*Source:* Hall, B. J. & Hall, J. C. [2010]. *Sauer's manual of skin diseases* [10th ed.]. Philadelphia: Lippincott Williams & Wilkins.)

Continued on following page

ABNORMAL FINDINGS 15-2 Primary skin lesions (continued)

TYPE AND DESCRIPTION	EXAMPLES	ILLUSTRATION	PHOTOGRAPH OF EXAMPLE
Pustule • Pus-filled vesicle or bulla	• Acne • Impetigo • Furuncles • Carbuncles	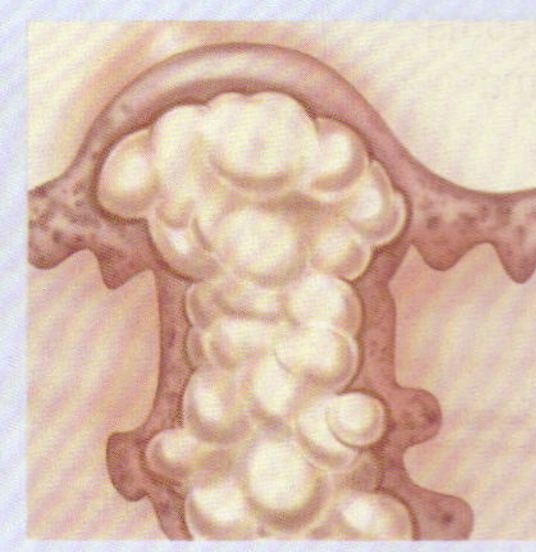 Pustule	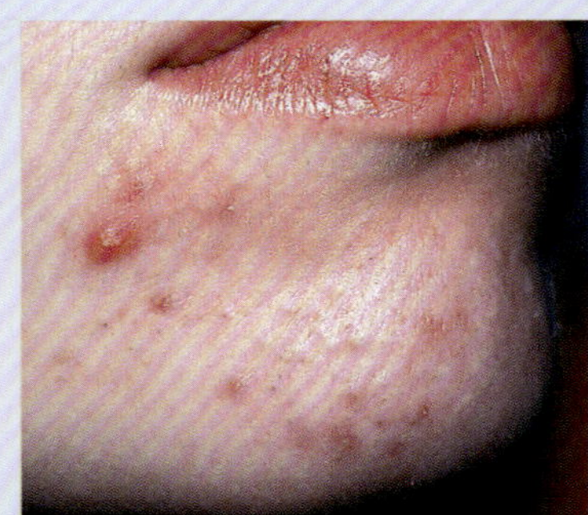 Inflammatory acne lesions. Papules, pustules and closed comedones are all present on this patient. (*Source:* Goodheart, H.G. [2009] *Goodheart's photoguide to common skin disorders.* Philadelphia: Lippincott Williams & Wilkins.)
Cyst • Encapsulated fluid-filled or semisolid mass • Located in the subcutaneous tissue or dermis	• Sebaceous cyst • Epidermoid cyst	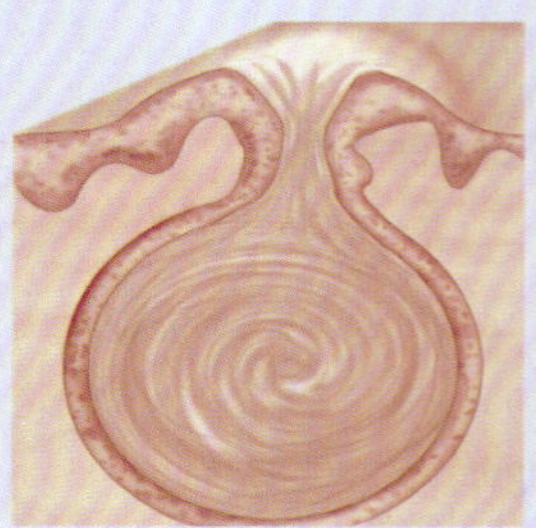 Cyst	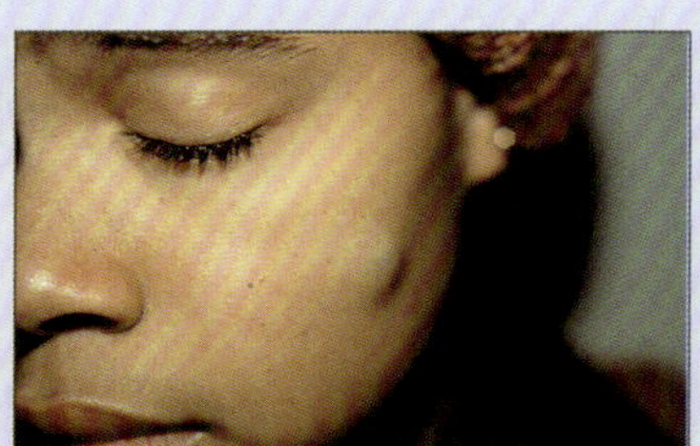 Epidermoid cysts are nodular.

ABNORMAL FINDINGS 15-3 Secondary skin lesions

Secondary skin lesions result from changes in primary lesions.

TYPE AND DESCRIPTION	EXAMPLES	ILLUSTRATION	PHOTOGRAPH OF EXAMPLE
Erosion • Loss of superficial epidermis • Does not extend to the dermis • Depressed, moist area	• Rupture vesicles • Scratch marks • Aphthous ulcer	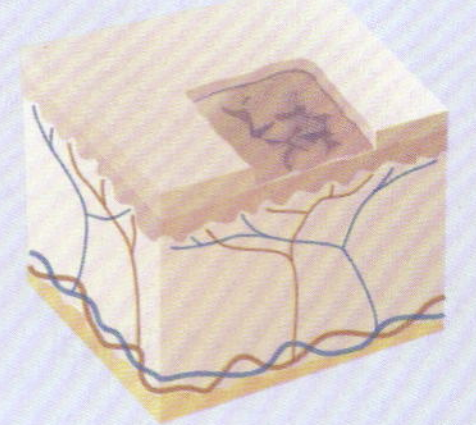 Erosion	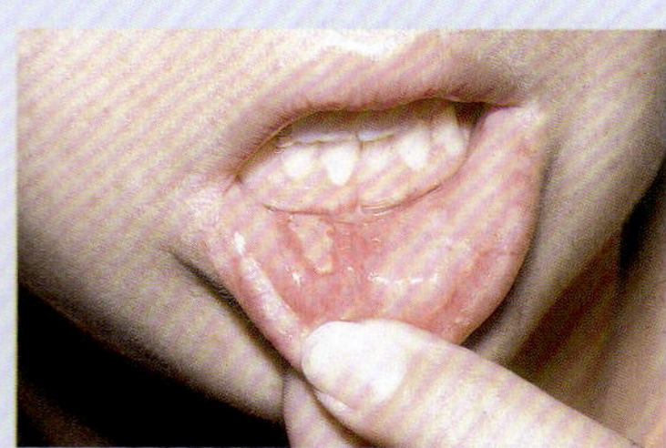 Aphthous ulcer. (*Source:* Goodheart, H. G. [2009]. *Goodheart's photoguide to common skin disorders: Diagnosis and management* [3rd ed.]. Philadelphia: Lippincott Williams & Wilkins.)

ABNORMAL FINDINGS 15-3 Secondary skin lesions (continued)

TYPE AND DESCRIPTION	EXAMPLES	ILLUSTRATION	PHOTOGRAPH OF EXAMPLE
Ulcer • Skin loss extending past epidermis • Necrotic tissue loss • Bleeding and scarring possible	• Stasis ulcer of venous insufficiency • Pressure ulcer	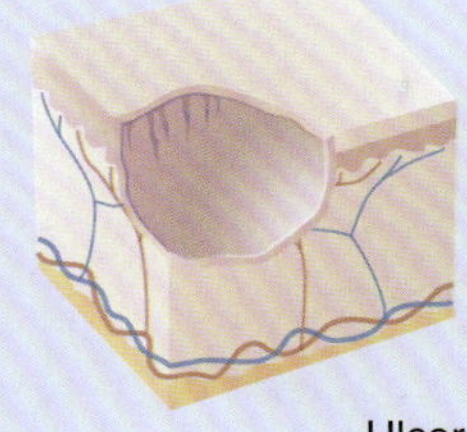 Ulcer	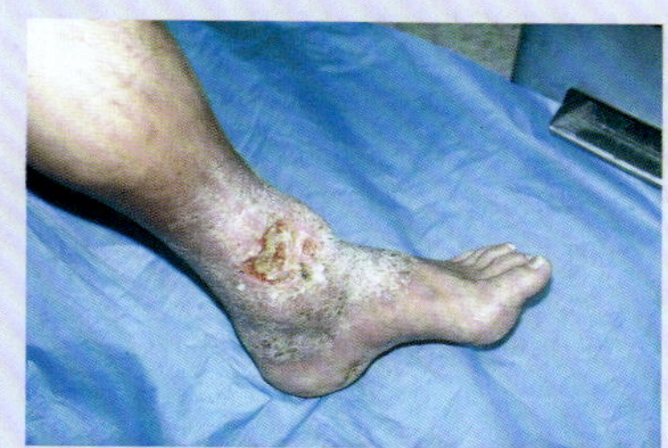 Stasis dermatitis with venous stasis ulcer. (*Source:* Goodheart, H. G. [2009]. *Goodheart's photoguide to common skin disorders: Diagnosis and management* [3rd ed.]. Philadelphia: Lippincott Williams & Wilkins.)
Scar (cicatrix) • Skin mark left after healing of wound or lesion • Represents replacement by connective tissue of the injured tissue • Young scars: red or purple • Mature scars: white or glistening	• Healed wound • Healed surgical incision	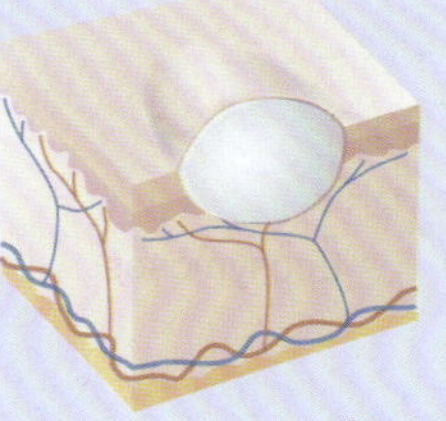 Scar	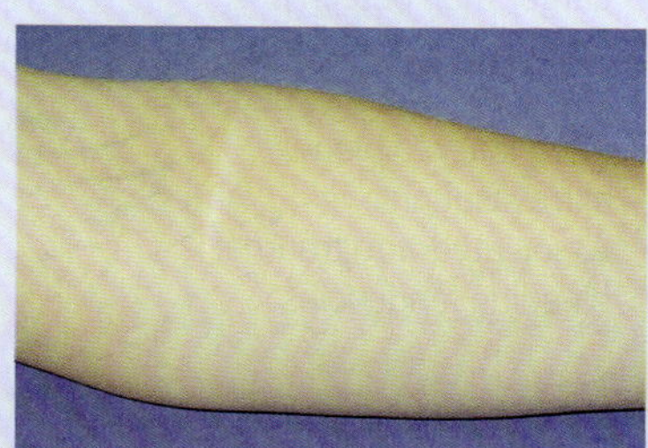 Mature healed wound.
Fissure • Linear crack in the skin • May extend to the dermis	• Chapped lips or hands • Athlete's foot	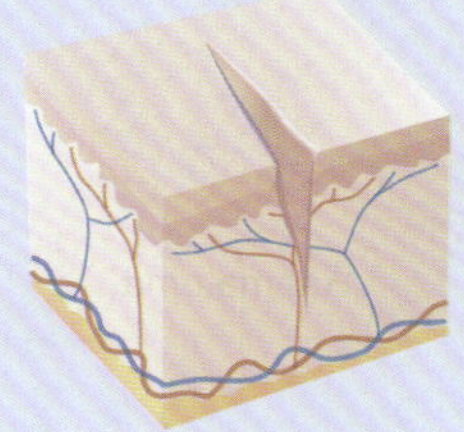 Fissure	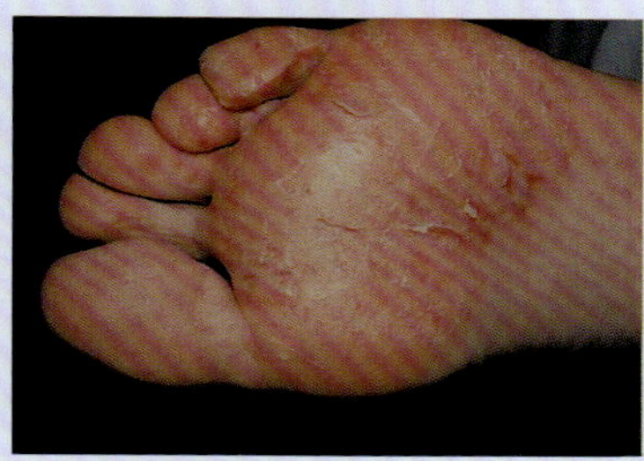 Athlete's foot.

ABNORMAL FINDINGS 15-4 Vascular skin lesions

Vascular skin lesions are associated with bleeding, ageing, circulatory conditions, diabetes, pregnancy and hepatic disease among other problems.

TYPE AND DESCRIPTION	ILLUSTRATION	PHOTOGRAPH OF EXAMPLE
Petechia (pl. petechiae) • Round red or purple macule • Small: 1–2 mm • Secondary to blood extravasation • Associated with bleeding tendencies or emboli to skin	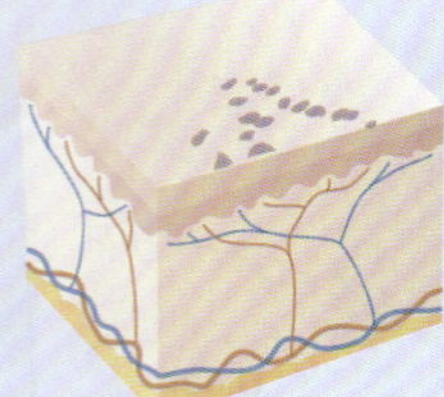 Petechiae (Shutterstock.com/TisforThan.)	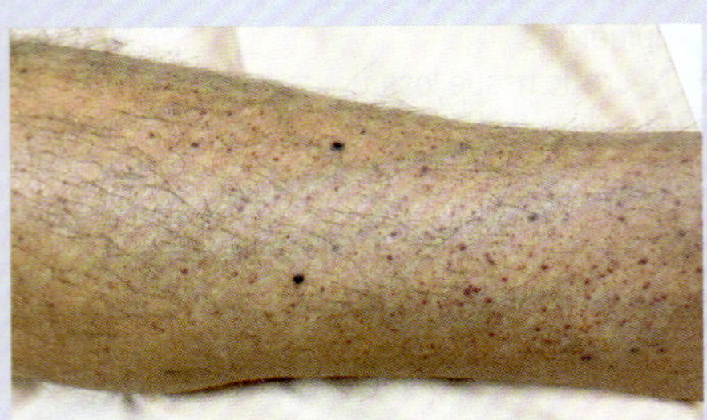 **Petechiae.** (Dermik Laboratories.)
Ecchymosis (pl. ecchymoses) • Round or irregular macular lesion • Larger than petechia • Colour varies and changes: black, yellow and green hues • Secondary to blood extravasation • Associated with trauma, bleeding tendencies	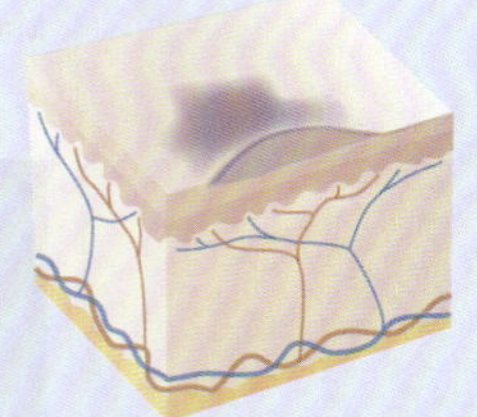 Ecchymoses	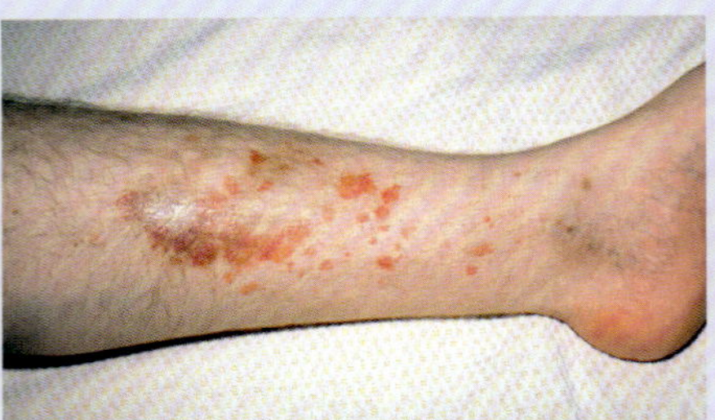 **Purpura.** (Alamy Stock Photo/Mediscan.)
Haematoma • A localised collection of blood creating an elevated ecchymosis • Associated with trauma	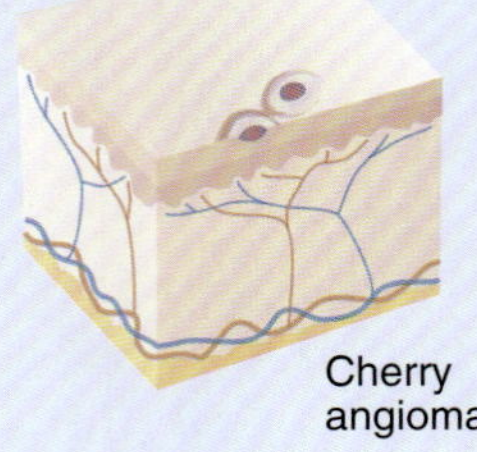 Haematoma	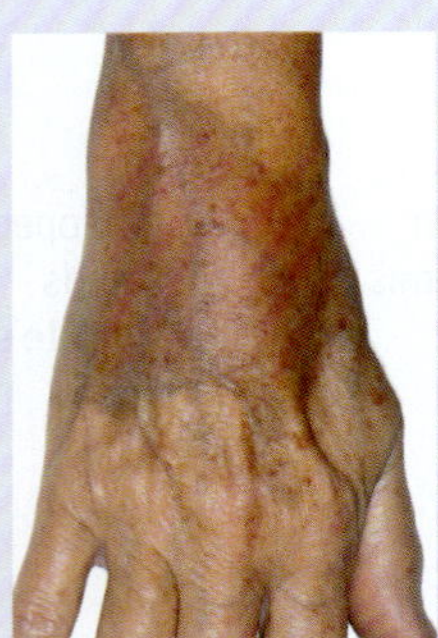 **Alamy.** (Alamy Stock Photo/Science Photo Library.)
Cherry angioma • Papular and round • Red or purple • Noted on trunk, extremities • May blanch with pressure • Normal age-related skin alteration • Usually not clinically significant	Cherry angioma	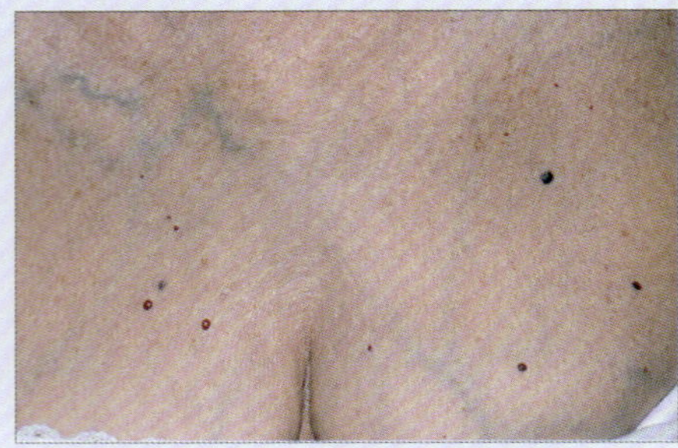

ABNORMAL FINDINGS 15-4 Vascular skin lesions (continued)

TYPE AND DESCRIPTION	ILLUSTRATION	PHOTOGRAPH OF EXAMPLE
Spider angioma • Red, arteriole lesion • Central body with radiating branches • Noted on face, neck, arms, trunk • Rare below waist • May blanch with pressure • Associated with liver disease, pregnancy and vitamin B deficiency	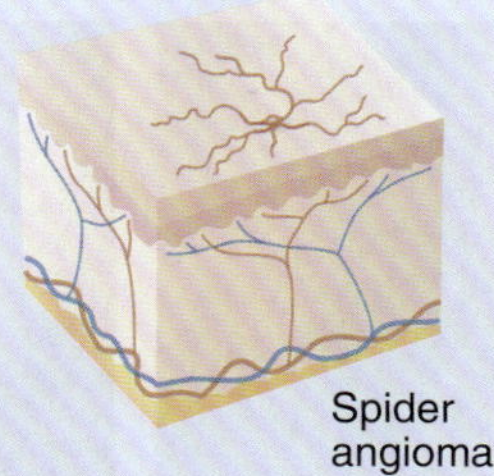	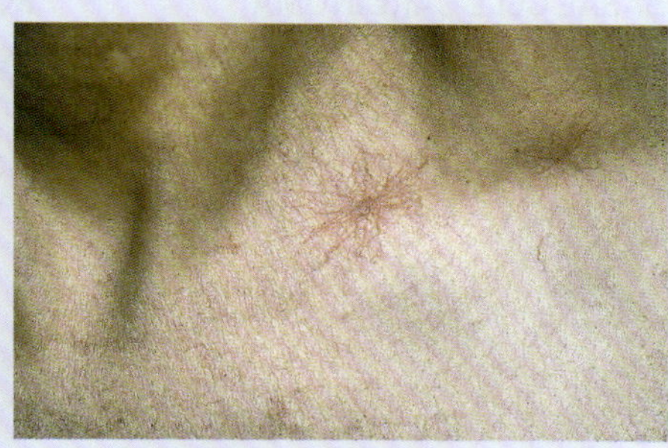 **Spider angioma.** (*Source:* Goodheart, H. G. [2009]. *Goodheart's photoguide to common skin disorders: Diagnosis and management* [3rd ed.]. Philadelphia: Lippincott Williams & Wilkins.)
Telangiectasis (venous star) • Shape varies: spiderlike or linear • Colour bluish or red • Does not blanch when pressure is applied • Noted on legs, anterior chest • Secondary to superficial dilation of venous vessels and capillaries • Associated with increased venous pressure states (varicosities)	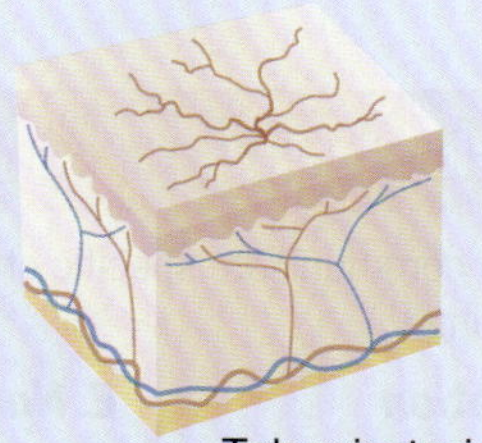	**Spider telangiectasias.** (*Source:* Goodheart, H. G. [2009]. *Goodheart's photoguide to common skin disorders*. Philadelphia: Lippincott Williams & Wilkins.)

ABNORMAL FINDINGS 15-5 Skin cancer

With the exception of malignant melanoma, most skin cancers are readily managed. Malignant melanoma can be fatal if not identified and treated early, which is one reason why an annual professional health assessment and regular skin self-assessment can be life-saving procedures.

Malignant melanoma is usually evaluated according to the mnemonic ABCDE: A for asymmetrical; B for borders that are irregular (uneven or notched); C for colour variations; D for diameter exceeding 3 to 6 mm; and E for elevated, not flat. Danger signs of malignant melanoma include any of the above factors. However, smaller areas may indicate early stage melanomas. Other warning signs include itching, tenderness or pain, and a change in size or bleeding of a mole. New pigmentations are also warning signs (Cancer Council Australia, 2019).

Asymmetry

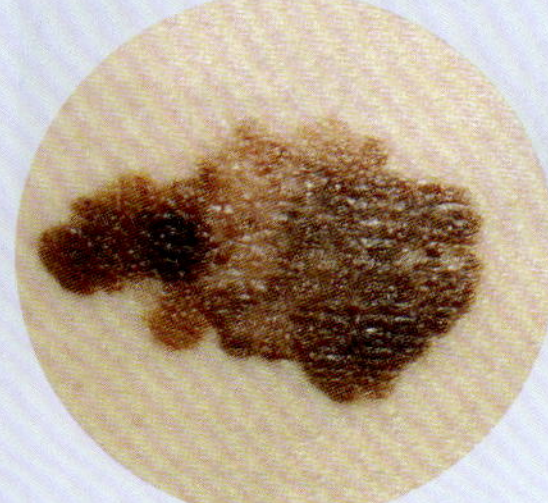

(PHIL-CDC/NCI www.cancer.gov.)

Borders

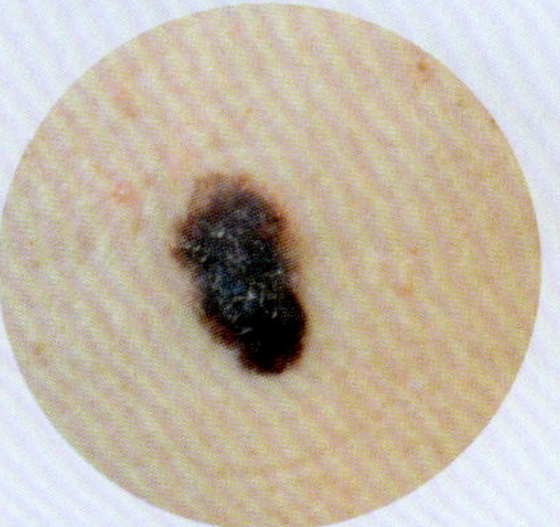

(Shutterstock.com/Nasekomoe.)

Colour

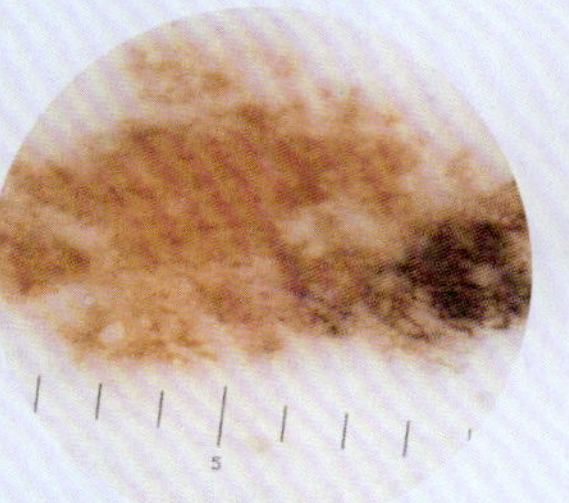

(Shutterstock.com/Nasekomoe.)

Diameter, Elevated

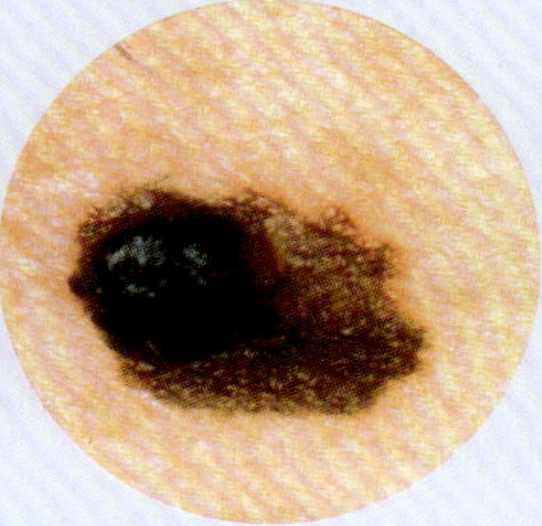

(Wikimedia Commons/NCI www.cancer.org.)

Continued on following page

ABNORMAL FINDINGS 15-5 Skin cancer (continued)

The most commonly detected skin cancers include basal cell carcinoma, squamous cell carcinoma and melanoma (all illustrated below).

BASAL CELL CARCINOMA

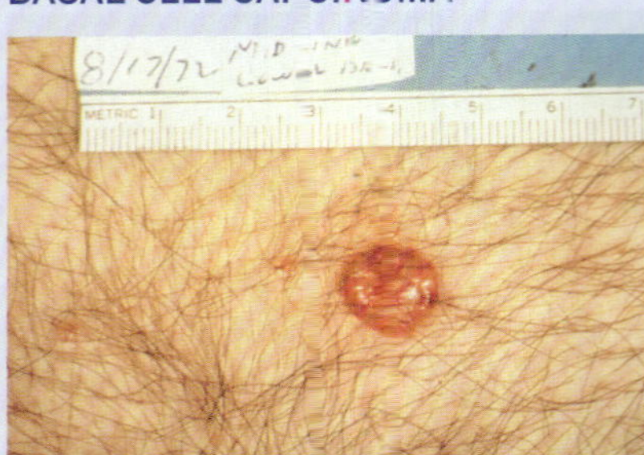

(Wikimedia Commons/NCI www.cancer.org.)

SQUAMOUS CELL CARCINOMA

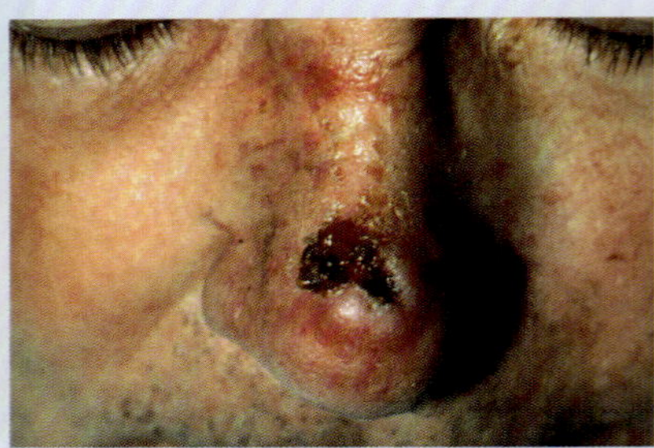

(PHIL-CDC/NCI www.cancer.gov.)

MELANOMA

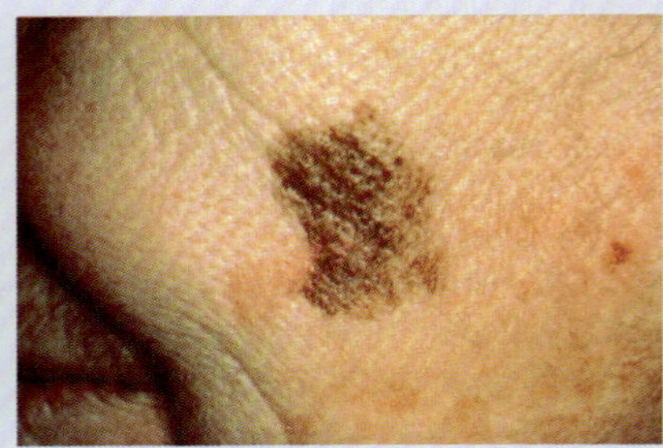

(Wikimedia Commons/NCI www.cancer.org.)

ABNORMAL FINDINGS 15-6 Configurations of skin lesions

Describing lesions by shape distribution or configuration is one way to communicate specific characteristics that can help to identify causes and treatments. Some common configurations include the following.

A. Linear configuration

Straight line, as in a scratch or streak. An example is dermatographism.

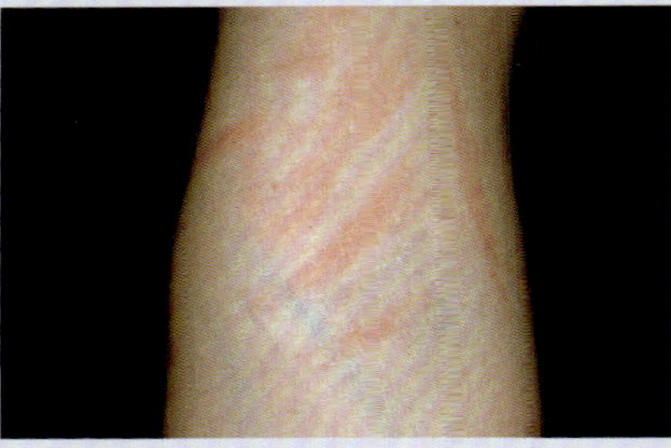

C. Clustered configuration

Lesions grouped together. An example is herpes simplex.

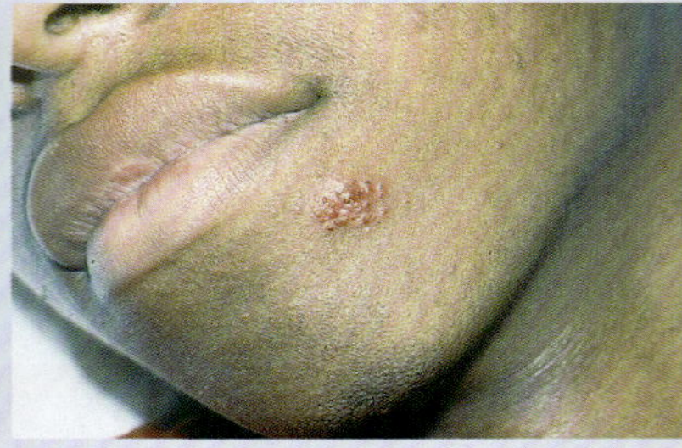

E. Nummular configuration

Coin-shaped lesions. An example is nummular eczema.

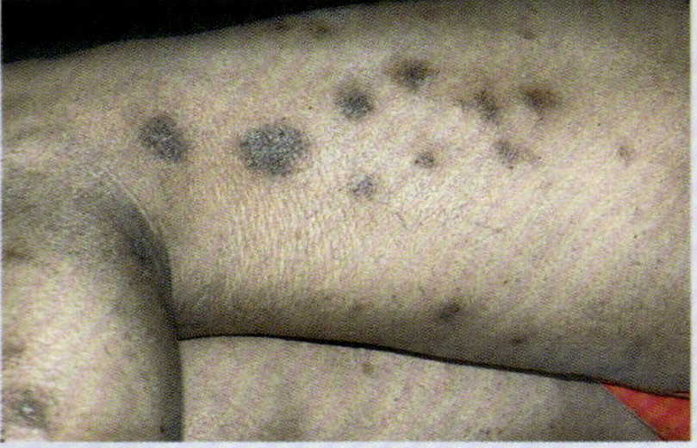

B. Annular configuration

Circular lesions. An example is tinea corporis.

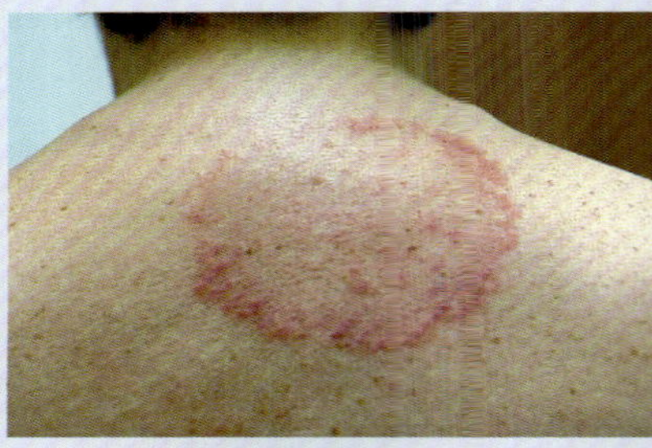

D. Discrete configuration

Individual and distinct lesions. An example is multiple nevi.

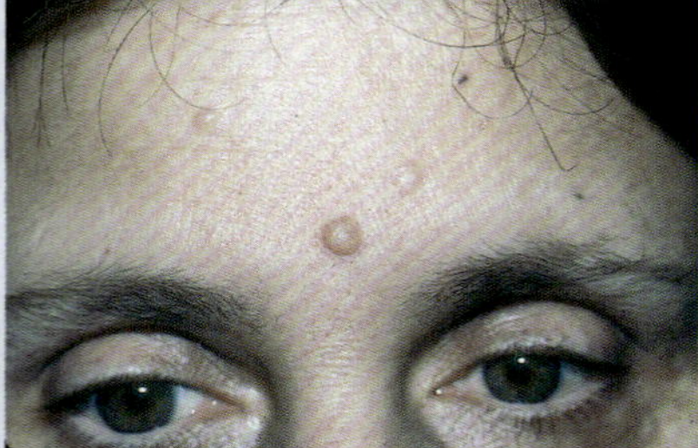

F. Confluent configuration

Smaller lesions run together to form a larger lesion. An example is tinea versicolor.

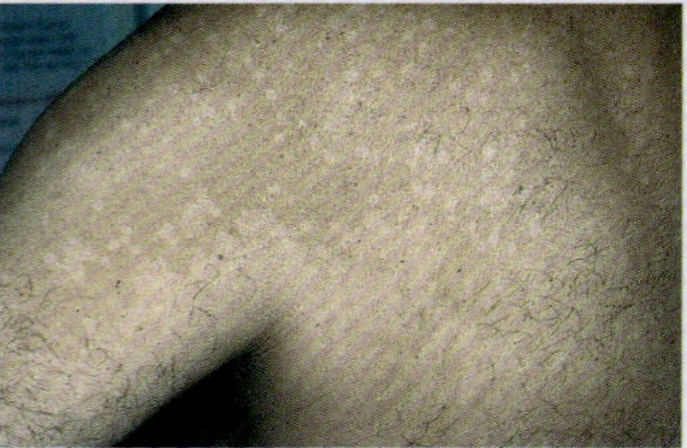

Photos used with permission from Goodheart, H. (2009). *Goodheart's photoguide to common skin disorders: Diagnosis and management* (3rd ed.). Philadelphia: Lippincott Williams & Wilkins.

ABNORMAL FINDINGS 15-7 Common nail disorders

Many patients have nails with lines, ridges, spots and uncommon shapes that suggest an underlying disorder. Some examples follow.

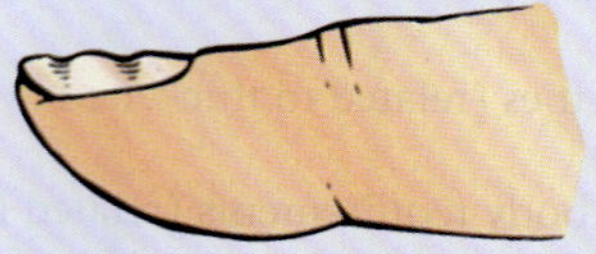

A. Beau's lines (acute illness)

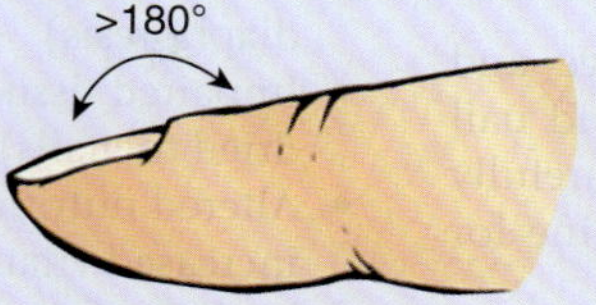

D. Late clubbing (oxygen deficiency)

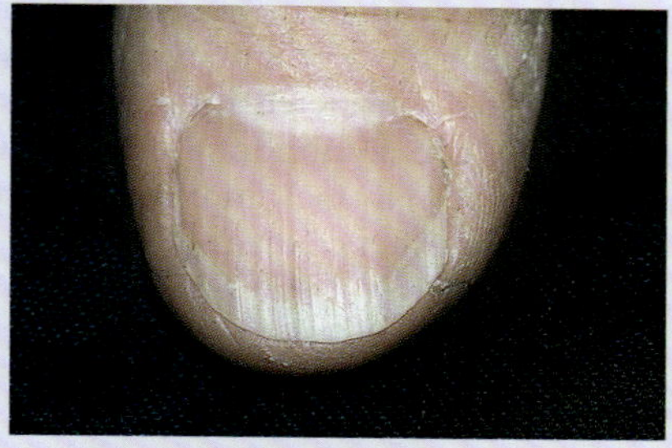

G. Longitudinal ridging. Parallel ridges running lengthwise. May be seen in the elderly and some young people with no known aetiology.

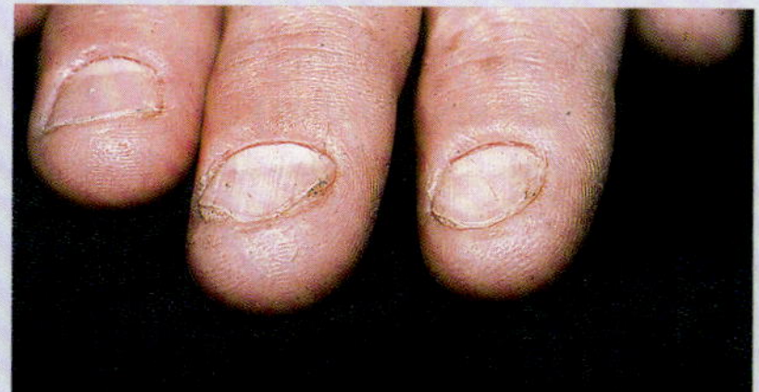

B. Koilonychia. Spoon-shaped nails that may be seen with trauma to cuticles or nail folds, or in iron deficiency anaemia, endocrine or cardiac disease.

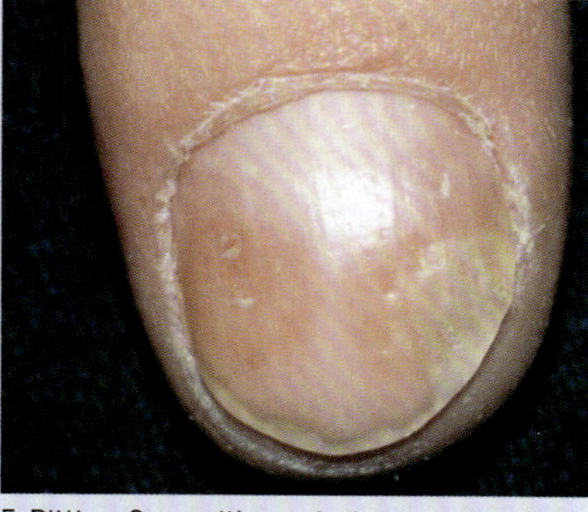

E. Pitting. Seen with psoriasis.

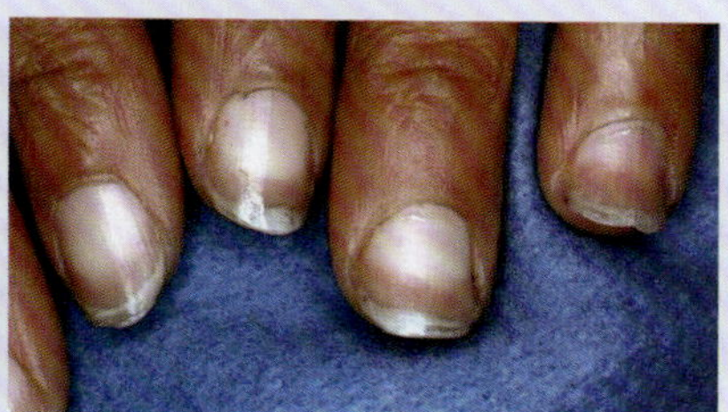

H. Half-and-half nails. Nails that are half white on the upper proximal half and pink on the distal half. May be seen in chronic renal disease.

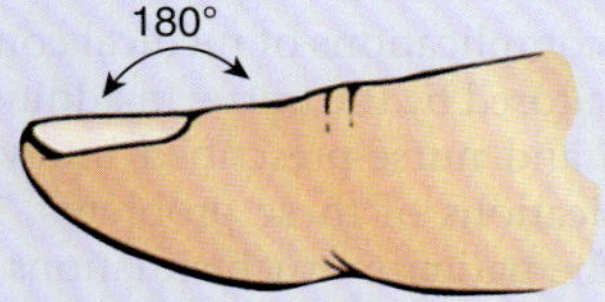

C. Early clubbing (oxygen deficiency)

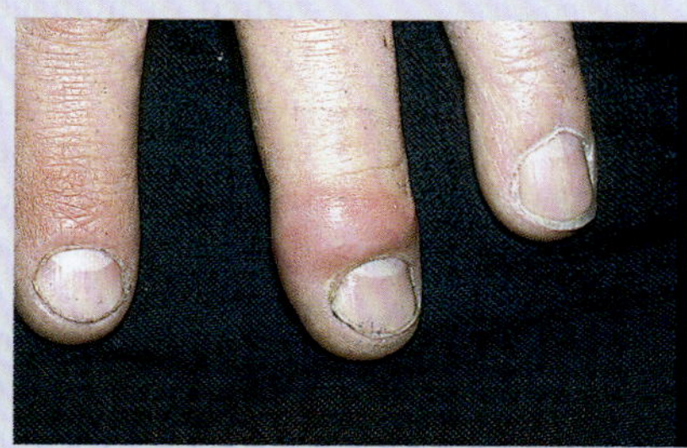

F. Paronychia. Local infection.

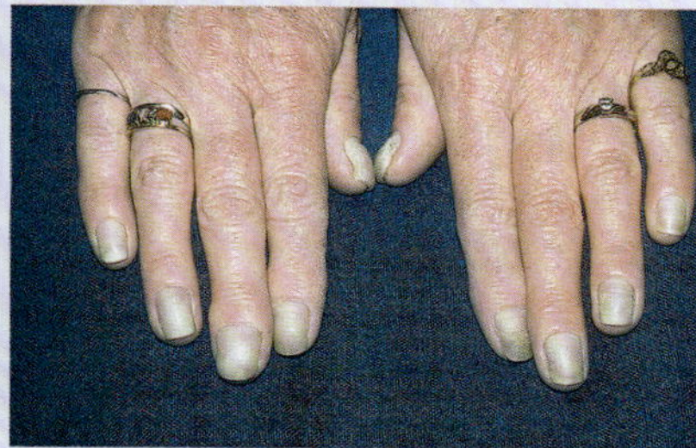

I. Yellow nail syndrome. Yellow nails grow slow and are curved. May be seen in AIDS and respiratory syndromes.

Half-and-half nails used with permission from Hall, B. J. & Hall, J. C. (2010). *Sauer's manual of skin diseases* (10th ed.). Philadelphia: Lippincott Williams & Wilkins. All other photographs used with permission from Goodheart, H. (2009). *Goodheart's photoguide to common skin disorders: Diagnosis and management* (3rd ed.). Philadelphia: Lippincott Williams & Wilkins.

VALIDATING AND DOCUMENTING FINDINGS

Validate your normal and abnormal findings with the patient, other health care workers or your clinical preceptors.

The following is a summary of areas of coverage and findings that are considered normal in a skin, hair and nail assessment. Of course, abnormal findings would be carefully documented, too. Normal findings can act as a baseline for findings that may later change.

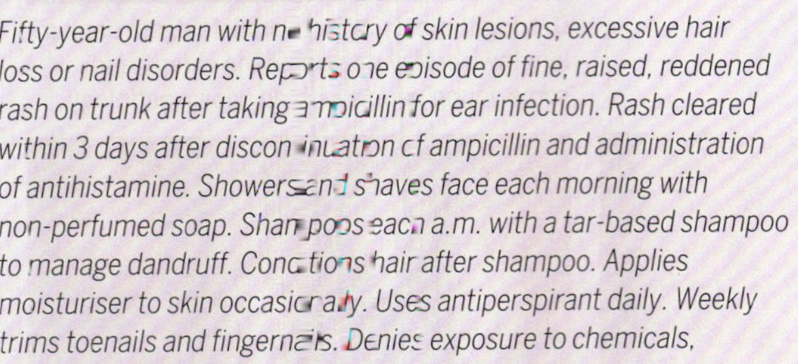

Sample of subjective data

Fifty-year-old man with no history of skin lesions, excessive hair loss or nail disorders. Reports one episode of fine, raised, reddened rash on trunk after taking ampicillin for ear infection. Rash cleared within 3 days after discontinuation of ampicillin and administration of antihistamine. Showers and shaves face each morning with non-perfumed soap. Shampoos each a.m. with a tar-based shampoo to manage dandruff. Conditions hair after shampoo. Applies moisturiser to skin occasionally. Uses antiperspirant daily. Weekly trims toenails and fingernails. Denies exposure to chemicals, abrasives or excessive sunlight.

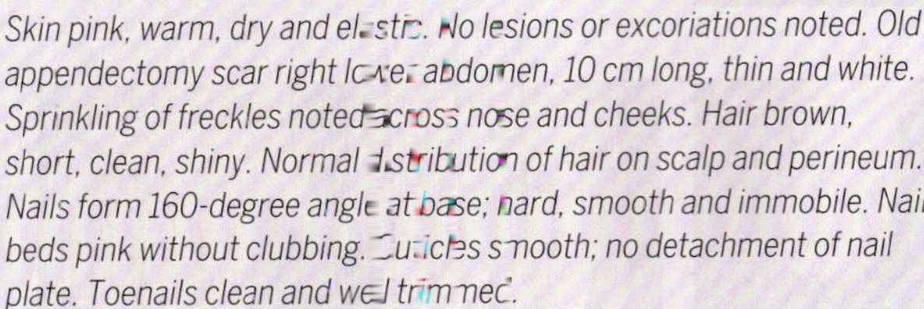

Sample of objective data

Skin pink, warm, dry and elastic. No lesions or excoriations noted. Old appendectomy scar right lower abdomen, 10 cm long, thin and white. Sprinkling of freckles noted across nose and cheeks. Hair brown, short, clean, shiny. Normal distribution of hair on scalp and perineum. Nails form 160-degree angle at base; hard, smooth and immobile. Nail beds pink without clubbing. Cuticles smooth; no detachment of nail plate. Toenails clean and well trimmed.

After you have collected your assessment data, you will need to analyse the data using diagnostic reasoning skills. Refer to the discussion of the diagnostic reasoning process in Chapter 5.

Analysis of data

DIAGNOSTIC REASONING: POSSIBLE CONCLUSIONS

After collecting subjective and objective data pertaining to the skin, hair and nails, identify abnormal findings and patient strengths. Then cluster the data to reveal any significant patterns or abnormalities. Listed below are some possible conclusions that the nurse may make after assessing a patient's skin, hair and nails.

Potential patient risks

- Impaired skin integrity (related to prolonged sun exposure)
- Imbalanced body temperature (related to severe diaphoresis)
- Impaired tissue integrity of toes (related to thickened, dried toenails)
- Altered nutrition: less than body requirements (related to increased vitamin and protein requirements necessary for healing of a wound)
- Infection (related to scratching of rash, multiple body piercings, skin tattooing)

Potential patient problems

- Ineffective health maintenance (related to lack of hygienic care of the skin, hair and nails; immobility; poor nutrition, incontinence)
- Disturbed body image (related to scarring, rash, or other skin condition that alters skin appearance)
- Disturbed sleep pattern (related to persistent itching of the skin)
- Deficient fluid volume (related to excessive diaphoresis secondary to excessive exercise and high environmental temperatures)

Selected collaborative problems

After grouping the data, certain collaborative problems may become apparent. Remember that collaborative problems differ from nursing diagnoses in that they cannot be prevented or managed with independent nursing interventions. However, these physiological complications of medical conditions can be detected and monitored by the nurse. In addition, the nurse can use physician- and nurse-prescribed interventions to minimise the complications of these problems. The nurse may also have to refer the patient in such situations for further treatment of the problem. The following is a list of collaborative problems that may be identified when assessing the skin, hair and nails:

- Allergic reaction
- Skin rash
- Insect or animal bite
- Septicaemia
- Hypovolaemic shock
- Skin infection
- Skin lesion
- Ischaemic skin injuries
- Graft rejection
- Haemorrhage
- Burns.

Medical problems

After grouping the data, it may become apparent that the patient has signs and symptoms that require medical diagnosis and treatment. Referral to a primary care provider is necessary.

CASE STUDY

The case study demonstrates how to analyse skin, hair and nail assessment data for a specific patient. The exercises included in the ancillary product on the Point that complements this text offer further opportunities to enhance your skills.

Sara McFadden, a 22-year-old student is in generally good health. She presents with recent onset of large lesions on her scalp and elbow regions which she has been trying to treat with over the counter steroid creams. The provisional diagnosis from the dermatologist is plaque psoriasis. A skin biopsy has been taken for confirmation. There appears to be a significant impact on Sara's self image and well being as a consequence of her skin disorder. She describes how she avoids social occasions and dresses carefully to cover the lesions. During the interview Sara reveals that she avoids exposing her skin to sunlight and is very careful with the products she applies to her skin, favouring simple unperfumed sorbolene. She also applies sunscreen daily. Sara is very tearful and describes feeling 'ugly'. She is worried that she won't be successful in securing a position after graduation as she is lacking in confidence. Your physical examination reveals a pale, anxious-appearing young woman. You note a lesion on the occipital region of the scalp extending down to the neck. The lesion is raised, irregular, red in colour, with a silvery surface. There are patchy regions of alopecia in and around the lesions. Satellite patches of a smaller size extend down the neck. Similar lesions are located over each elbow with patches extending down to the wrist. Her vital signs are within normal physiological limits.

The following concept map illustrates the diagnostic reasoning process.

Applying COLDSPA

Applying COLDSPA for patient symptoms: 'I have a red rash on my face.'

Mnemonic	Question	Data provided	Missing data
Character	Describe the sign or symptom (feeling, appearance, sound, smell or taste, if applicable).	Red, scaly, plaques	
Onset	When did it begin?		When did this lesion first appear?
Location	Where is it? Does it radiate? Does it occur anywhere else?	Located over the occipital region, posterior neck, elbows and forearms	
Duration	How long does it last? Does it recur?		Have you ever had this type of lesion or other rashes before?
Severity	How bad is it? How much does it bother you?	Significant impact on self-esteem and wellbeing. Socially isolating self.	
Pattern	What makes it better or worse?		Has anything made it better or worse?
Associated factors/How it **A**ffects the patient	What other symptoms occur with it? How does it affect you?	Patient 'feels ugly.' Patchy alopecia.	

1) Identify abnormal findings and patient strengths

Subjective data

- Generally in good health
- Treating lesions with over the counter steroid cremes
- Avoids social occasions and dresses to cover lesions
- Avoids exposing skin to sunlight
- Applies unperfumed sorbolene to her skin + sunscreen daily
- Worried won't secure employment post-graduation

Objective data

- Skin lesions appear to have significant impact on Sarah's self image
- Tearful and describes herself as 'ugly'
- Pale and anxious
- Scalp lesion on occiput extending down to neck (raised, irregular, red with silvery surface)
- Patchy alopecia
- Satellite patches of alopecia extending down to neck
- Lesions on bilateral elbows extending to wrists
- Vitals within normal range

2) Identify cue clusters

- Diagnosis of 'plaque psoriasis'
- Scalp lesion on occiput extending down to neck (raised, irregular, red with silvery surface)
- Patchy alopecia
- Satellite patches of alopecia extending down to neck
- Lesions on bilateral elbows extending to wrists

- Skin lesions appear to have significant impact on Sarah's self image
- Tearful and describes herself as 'ugly'
- Anxious
- Scalp lesion on occiput extending down to neck (raised, irregular, red with silvery surface)
- Patchy alopecia
- Satellite patches of alopecia extending down to neck
- Lesions on bilateral elbows extending to wrists

- Sought outpatient clinic assessment and management

- Pale and anxious
- Worried won't secure employment post-graduation

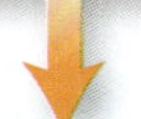

3) Draw inferences

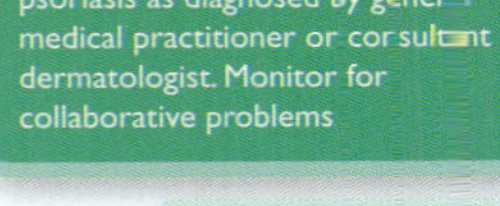

Textbook picture for plaque psoriasis as diagnosed by general medical practitioner or consultant dermatologist. Monitor for collaborative problems

Changes in physical appearance are affectingself-perception.

Possibly seeking information about managing her illness

Perceives current position depends on attractive appearance

4) List possible patient problems

Disturbed body imager elated to changes in physical appearance

Ineffective individual coping related to changes in physical appearance and newly diagnosed disease

Health-seeking behaviour

Anxiety related to possible loss of work position secondary to perceived unattractiveness

5) Check for defining characteristics

Major: Verbal negative response to actual change in structure
Minor: Negative feelings about body

Major: None
Minor: None

Major: None
Minor: None

Major: Sought out dermatology outpatient clinic
Minor: None

Major: Physical appearance (unspecified anxiety) and self-deprecation (about physical appearance)
Minor: None

6) Confirm or rule out patient problems

Accept diagnosis because it meets defining characteristics and is validated by patient

Rule out diagnosis because it has none of the defining characteristics; however, more data should be collected regarding her support systems and coping behaviours

Confirm diagnosis because it meets major defining characteristics and is validated by patient

This is ambiguous. The patient sought out the dermatology outpatient clinic for more information, but after she was already diagnosed, rather than for health promotion before the fact. Collect more data before accepting this diagnosis

Accept diagnosis because it meets defining characteristics, but collect more data to confirm this diagnosis. Fear may be more appropriate, but data needed for that as well

7) Document conclusions

The following problems are appropriate for this patient:

- Body image disturbance related to changes in physical appearance
- Anxiety related to fear of not securing employment post-graduation and feeling 'ugly'

Potential collaborative problems include the following:

- Skin infection/scarring
- Ischaemic ulcers

ONLINE RESOURCES

An extensive range of additional resources to enhance teaching and learning and to facilitate understanding may be found online at the text's accompanying website, located on thePoint at http://thepoint.lww.com. These include Watch and Learn videos, Concepts in Action animations, journal articles, case studies, discussion topics and quizzes.

Subscribers may also access Lippincott Procedures, an extensive online point-of-care procedure guide that provides reliable step-by-step instructions for more than 1700 procedures, including 450 evidence-based Australian procedures, and skills in a variety of speciality settings, together with a wealth of supporting information.

References

American Cancer Society. (2012). Cancer facts & figures. Available at www.cancer.org/acs/groups/content/@epidemiologysurveilance/documents/document/acspc-036845.pdf.

Australian Institute of Health and Welfare (AIHW). (2012). Cancer incidence projections, Australia 2011 to 2020. Canberra, Australia: Author.

Australian Institute of Health and Welfare (AIHW). (2017). Cancer in Australia, Cancer series no. 101. Cat.no. CAN 100. Canberra: Author.

Australian Radiation Protection and Nuclear Safety Agency (ARPANSA). (n.d.). https://www.arpansa.gov.au/understanding-radiation/radiation-sources/more-radiation-sources/solaria.

Australian Wound Management Association. (2012). *Pan Pacific clinical practice guidelines for the prevention and management of pressure injuries*. Osborne Park, WA: Cambridge Publishing.

Bahar, R., et al. (2016). The prevalence of anxiety and depression in patients with or without hyperhidrosis. *Journal of the American Academy of Dermatology, 75*(6), 1126–1133.

Bishop, A., Witts, S. & Martin, T. (2018). The role of nutrition in successful wound healing. *Journal of Community Nursing, 32*(4), 44–50.

Braden, B. (2012). The Braden Scale for Predicting Pressure Sore Risk: Reflections after 25 years. *Advances in Skin and Wound Care, 25*(2), 61.

Braden, B. & Bergstrom, B. (1988). Braden Scale for Predicting Pressure Sore Risk. Available at https://bradenscale.com/.

Breuner, C. C. & Levine, D. A. (2017). Adolescent and young adult tattooing, piercing and scarification. *Pediatrics, 140*(4), e20171962.

Cancer Council. (2019). Vitamin D. Available from https://www.cancer.org.au/preventing-cancer/sun-protection/vitamin-d/.

Cancer Council Australia. (2019). Melanoma. Viewed October 2019 at https://www.cancer.org.au/about-cancer/types-of-cancer/skin-cancer/melanoma.html.

Chaturvedi, S. K., Singh, G. & Gupta, N. (2005). Stigma experience in skin disorders: An Indian perspective. *Dermatologic Clinics, 23*(4), 635–642.

Cowdell, F. & Radley, K. (2014). What do we know about skin-hygiene care for patients with bariatric needs? Implications for nursing practice. *Journal of Advanced Nursing, 70*(3), 543–552.

Dalgard, F. J., et al. (2015). The psychological burden of skin diseases: A cross-sectional multicentre study among dermatological out-patients in 13 European countries. *The Journal of Investigative Dermatology, 135*(4), 984–991.

Espinosa, P., Pfeiffer, R. M., Garcia-Casado, Z., et al. (2015). Risk factors for keratinocyte skin cancer in patients diagnosed with melanoma, a large retrospective study. *European Journal of Cancer, 53*, 116–124.

Farrell, M. & Dempsey, J. (Eds). (2016). *Smeltzer & Bare's textbook of medical-surgical nursing* (3rd Australian & New Zealand ed.). Sydney: Lippincott Williams & Wilkins.

Garcia, A. D. (2012). Home care. Ch. 10. In B. Pieper, with the National Pressure Ulcer Advisory Panel (NPUAP) (Eds). *Pressure ulcers: Prevalence, incidence and implications for the future*. Washington, DC: NPUAP.

Giroud, K., Harrison, M. B. & VanDenKerkof, E. (2008). The symptom of pain with pressure ulcers: A review of the literature. *Ostomy/Wound Management, 54*(5), 30–42.

Goodheart, H. P. (1999). *A photoguide to common skin disorders: Diagnosis and management*. Baltimore: Williams & Wilkins.

Goodheart, H. G. (2005). *Goodheart's photo guide of common skin disorders*. Philadelphia: Lippincott Williams & Wilkins.

Goodheart, H. P. (2009). *Goodheart's photoguide to common skin disorders: Diagnosis and management* (3rd ed.). Philadelphia: Lippincott Williams & Wilkins.

Hall, B. J. & Hall, J. C. (2010). *Sauer's manual of skin diseases* (10th ed.). Philadelphia: Lippincott Williams & Wilkins.

Herman, J., Rost-Roskowska, M. & Skotnicka-Graca, U. (2013). Skin care during the menopause period: Non-invasive procedures of beauty studies. *Postepy Dermatologii i Alergologii, 30*(6), 388–395.

Hoel, D., Berwick, M., de Gruijl, F., et al. (2016). The risks and benefits of sun exposure 2016. *Dermato-Endocrinology, 8*(1), e1248325.

Jalenques, I., et al. (2016). High prevalence of psychiatric disorders in patients with skin-restricted lupus: A case-control study. *The British Journal of Dermatology, 174*(5), 1051–1060.

Lee, C. S. & Lim, H. W. (2003). Cutaneous disease in Asians. *Dermatology Clinics, 21*(4), 669–677.

National Pressure Ulcer Advisory Panel. (2019). NPUAP-EPUAP guidelines for pressure ulcer prevention and treatment. Available at www.npuap.org.

National Pressure Ulcer Advisory Panel, European Pressure Ulcer Advisory Panel & Pan Pacific Pressure Injury Alliance. (2014). Prevention and treatment of pressure ulcers: Quick reference guide. Emily Haesler (Ed.). Cambridge Media: Osborne Park, Western Australia.

SunSmart. (2018). Skin cancer. Available at www.sunsmart.com.au/skin_cancer.

Trace, A. P., Enos, C. W., Mantel, A., et al. (2016). Keloids and hypertrophic scars: A spectrum of clinical challenges. *American Journal of Clinical Dermatology, 17*(3), 201–223.

VanGilder, C., Lachenbruch, C., Algrim-Boyle, C., et al. (2017). The international pressure ulcer prevalence survey: 2006-2015. *Journal of Wound, Ostomy, and Continence Nursing, 44*(1), 20–28.

Wilson, L., Kapp, S. & Santamaria, N. (2018). The direct cost of pressure injuries in an Australian residential aged care setting. *International Wound Journal, 16*(1), 64–70.

Wong, S. S.-Y., Wong, S. C.-Y. & Yuen, K.-Y. (2012). Infections associated with body modification. *Journal of the Formosan Medical Association, 111*, 667–681.

WHO. (2017). Artificial tanning devices: Public health interventions to manage sunbeds. Viewed October 2019 at https://www.who.int/uv/publications/artificial-tanning-devices/en/.

Selected readings

Aquino, M. & Rosner, G. (2019). Systemic contact dermatitis. *Clinical Reviews in Allergy & Immunology, 56*(1), 9–18.

Baranoski, S. & Ayello, E. A. (2016). *Wound care essentials: Practice principles* (4th ed.). Springhouse, PA: Wolters Kluwer.

Bates-Jensen, B. M., McCreath, H. E., Nakagami, G., et al. (2017). Subepidermal moisture detection of heel pressure injury: The pressure ulcer detection study outcomes. *International Wound Journal, 15*(2), 297–309.

Beitz, J. M. (2014). Providing quality skin and wound care for the bariatric patient: An overview of clinical challenges. *Ostomy/Wound Management, 60*(1), 12–21.

Cai, E. D., Swetter, S. M. & Savin, K. Y. (2018). Association of multiple primary melanomas with malignancy risk: A population-based analysis of the Surveillance, Epidemiology, and End Results Program database from 1973-2014. *Journal of the American Academy of Dermatology*, doi:10.1016/j.jaad.2018.09.027.

Cancer Council Australia. (2018). About skin cancer. Available at www.cancer.org.au/cancersmartlifestyle/SunSmart/Aboutskincancer.htm.

Cancer Society of New Zealand. (2018). Cancer types. Available at https://cancernz.org.nz/.

Chouliara, Z., Stephen, K. & Buchanan, P. (2017). The importance of psychosocial assessment in dermatology: Opening Pandora's box. *Dermatological Nursing, 16*(4), 30–34.

Citty, S., Cowan, L., Wingfield, Z., et al. (2019). Optimizing nutrition care for pressure injuries in hospitalised patients. *Advances in Wound Care, 8*(7), 309–322.

Connor, C. J. (2017). Management of the psychological comorbidities of dermatological conditions: Practitioners' guidelines. *Clinical, Cosmetic and Investigational Dermatology, 10*, 117–132.

Connor, C. J., Liu, V. & Fiedorowicz, J. G. (2015). Exploring the physiological link between psoriasis and mood disorders. *Dermatology Research and Practice*, 1–11.

Dusingize, J. C., et al. (2017). Cigarette smoking and the risks of basal cell carcinoma and squamous cell carcinoma. *The Journal of Investigative Dermatology, 137*(8), 1700–1708.

Farley, C. L., Hoover, C. & Rademeyer, C.-A. (2019). Women and tattoos: Fashion, meaning and implications for health. *Journal of Midwifery and Women's Health, 64*(2), 154–169.

Gordon, L. G. & Rowell, D. (2014). Health system costs of skin cancer and cost-effectiveness of skin cancer prevention and screening: A systematic review. *European Journal of Cancer Prevention, 24*(2), 141–149.

Greener, M. (2014). Beneath the surface: Dermatology and psychiatry. *Progress in Neurology and Psychiatry, 18*(1), 16–18.

Hay, R. (2018). Therapy of skin, hair and nail fungal infections. *Journal of Fungi, 4*(99), 1–13.

Hay, R. J. & Ashbee, H. R. (2016). *Fungal infections. Rooks textbook of dermatology* (9th ed.). New Jersey.: J Wiley & Sons.

Jackson, D., et al. (2017). Pain associated with pressure injury: A qualitative study of community-based, home-dwelling individuals. *Journal of Advanced Nursing, 73*(12), 3061–3069.

Khalesi, M., et al. (2015). Basal cell carcinoma on sun-protected vs. sun-exposed body sites: A comparison of phenotypic and environmental factors. *Photodermatology, Photoimmunology & Photomedicine, 31*(4), 202–211.

Kottner, J. & Surber, C. (2016). Skin care in nursing: A critical discussion of nursing practice and research. *International Journal of Nursing Studies, 61*, 20–28.

Kourtis, A. P., Hatfield, K., Baggs, J., et al. (2019). Vital signs: Epidemiology and recent trends in methicillin-resistant and in methicillin-susceptible *Staphylococcus aureus* bloodstream infections—United States. *MMWR. Morbidity and Mortality Weekly Report, 68*, 214–219. http://dx.doi.org/10.15585/mmwr.mm6809e1.

Longhurst, P. (2019). Stigmatisation and societal pressure in patients with skin conditions. *Journal of Aesthetic Nursing, 8*(5), 212–216.

Mingoia, J., Hutchinson, A., Gleaves, D. H., et al. (2017). Use of social networking sites and associations with skin tone dissatisfaction, sun exposure and sun protection in a sample of Australian adolescents. *Psychology & Health, 32*(12), 1502–1517.

Moore, S. P., et al. (2015). Cancer incidence in Indigenous people in Australia, New Zealand, Canada, and the USA: A comparative population based study. *The Lancet Oncology, 16*(15), 1483–1492.

Newall, N., Lewin, G. F., Bulsara, M. K., et al. (2017). The development and testing of a skin tear risk assessment tool. *International Wound Journal, 14*, 97–103.

Nicol, N. H. (2016). *Dermatology nursing essentials* (3rd ed.). Philadelphia: Lippincott Williams & Wilkins.

Padula, W. V. & Black, J. M. (2019). The standardised pressure injury prevention protocol for improving nursing compliance with best practice guidelines. *Journal of Clinical Nursing, 28*(3/4), 367–371.

Pompili, M., Innamorati, M., Forte, A., et al. (2017). Psychiatric comorbidity and suicidal ideation in psoriasis, melanoma and allergic disorders. *International Journal of Psychiatry in Clinical Practice, 21*(3), 209–214.

Rajagopalan, P., et al. (2016). How does chronic cigarette smoke exposure affect human skin? A global proteomics study in primary human keratinocytes. *Omics: A Journal of Integrative Biology, 20*(11), 615–626.

Rosen, R. & Stewart, T. (2017). Results of a 10-year follow up study of botulinum toxin A therapy for primary axillary hyperhidrosis in Australia. *Internal Medicine Journal, 48*, 343–347.

Seger, E. W., Wechter, T., Strowd, L., et al. (2019). Relative efficacy of systemic treatments for atopic dermatitis. *Journal of the American Academy of Dermatology, 80*(2), 411–416.

Skin Cancer Foundation. (2018). Skin cancer facts. Available at www.skincancer.org/skin-cancer-information/skin-cancer-facts#melanoma.

Van Onselen, J. (2019). Frequently asked questions on skin cancer and melanoma. *Independent Nurse, 7*, 17–20.

Online resources

Australian Alopecia Areata Foundation Inc. www.aaaf.org.au
Australasian Lymphology Association: www.lymphoedema.org.au
Australasian Podiatry Council: www.apodc.com.au
Australasian Wound and Tissue Repair Society (AWTRS): www.awtrs.org
Australian Association of Stomal Therapy Nurses: www.stomaltherapy.com
Australian Institute of Health and Welfare: www.aihw.gov.au
Cancer Council Australia: www.cancer.org.au
Cancer Society of New Zealand: www.cancernz.org.nz
Centers for Disease Control and Prevention: www.cdc.gov/cancer/skin
Eczema Association of Australasia: www.eczema.org.au
National Cancer Institute: www.cancer.gov
National Pressure Ulcer Advisory Panel: www.npuap.org
National Psoriasis Association https://www.psoriasis.org
New Zealand Dermatological Society (DermNet NZ): www.dermnetnz.org
New Zealand Wound Care Society: www.nzwcs.org.nz
SunSmart: www.sunsmart.com.au
Vascular Birthmarks Foundation https://birthmark.org/
Wounds Australia: www.awma.com.au

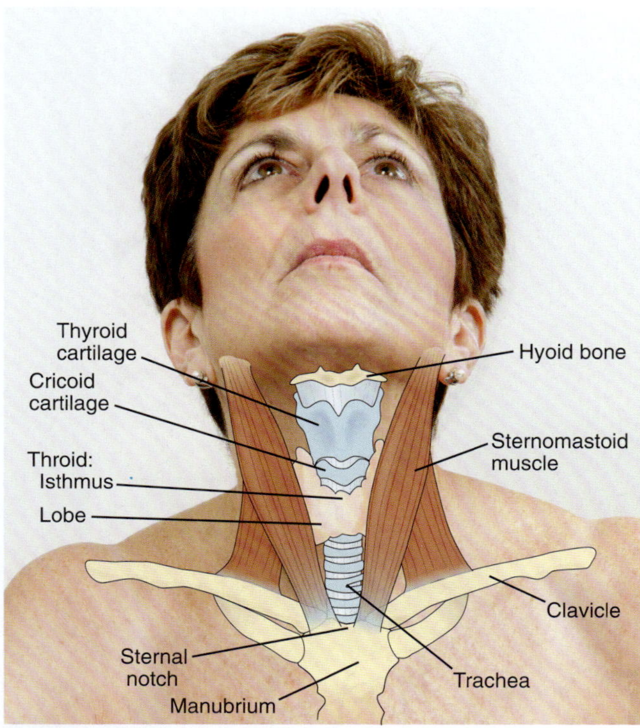

FIGURE 16-2 Structures of the neck.

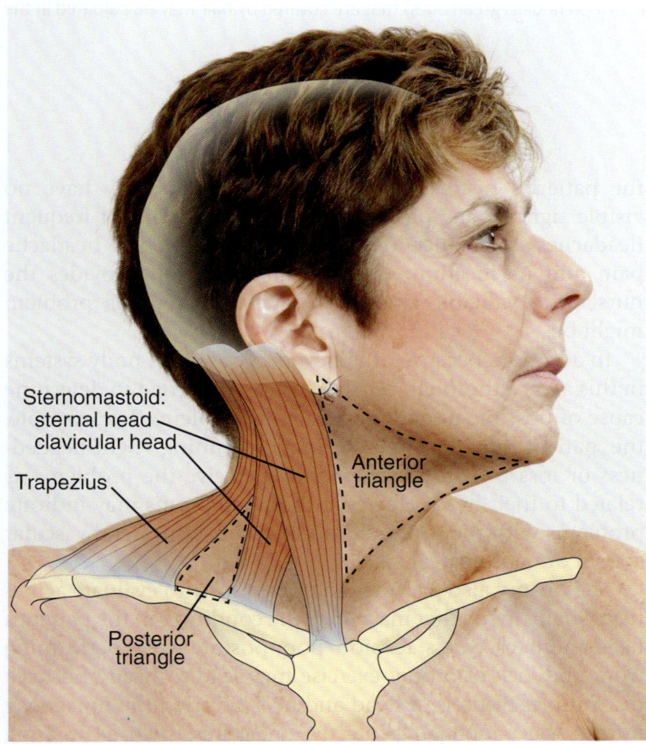

FIGURE 16-3 Neck muscles and landmarks.

LYMPH NODES OF THE HEAD AND NECK

Several lymph nodes are located in the head and neck (Fig. 16-5). Lymph nodes filter lymph, a clear substance composed mostly of excess tissue fluid, after the lymphatic vessels collect

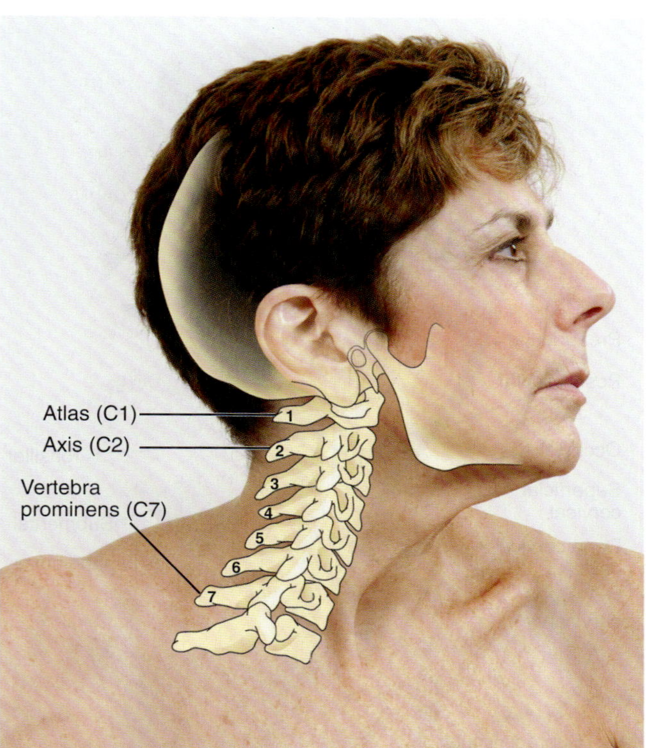

FIGURE 16-4 Cervical vertebrae.

it but before it returns to the vascular system. This filtering action removes bacteria and tumour cells from lymph. In addition, lymphocytes and antibodies are produced in the lymph nodes as a defence against invasion by foreign substances. They usually appear in clusters that vary in size from 2 to 100 individual nodes. The size and shape of lymph nodes vary, but most are less than 1 cm long and are buried deep in the connective tissue, which makes them non-palpable in normal situations.

If the nodes become overwhelmed by microorganisms, as happens with an infection such as mononucleosis, they swell

CRITICAL THINKING

There is a small widening in the internal carotid artery called the carotid sinus. It is located just above the point where the artery branches from the common carotid artery. The carotid sinus contains baroreceptors, which monitor blood pressure and provide an important negative feedback mechanism informing the neural regulation of blood pressure. When carotid pressure increases, the central nervous system responds by decreasing sympathetic impulses and increasing parasympathetic impulses.

1. What effect would decreasing sympathetic impulses have on heart rate and vascular tone? How would this impact blood pressure?
2. Can baroreceptors of the carotid sinus differentiate between rising blood pressure and pressure changes resulting from palpation during neck examination?
3. When palpating lymph nodes deep in connective tissue, why would it be important to avoid massaging the carotid sinus?

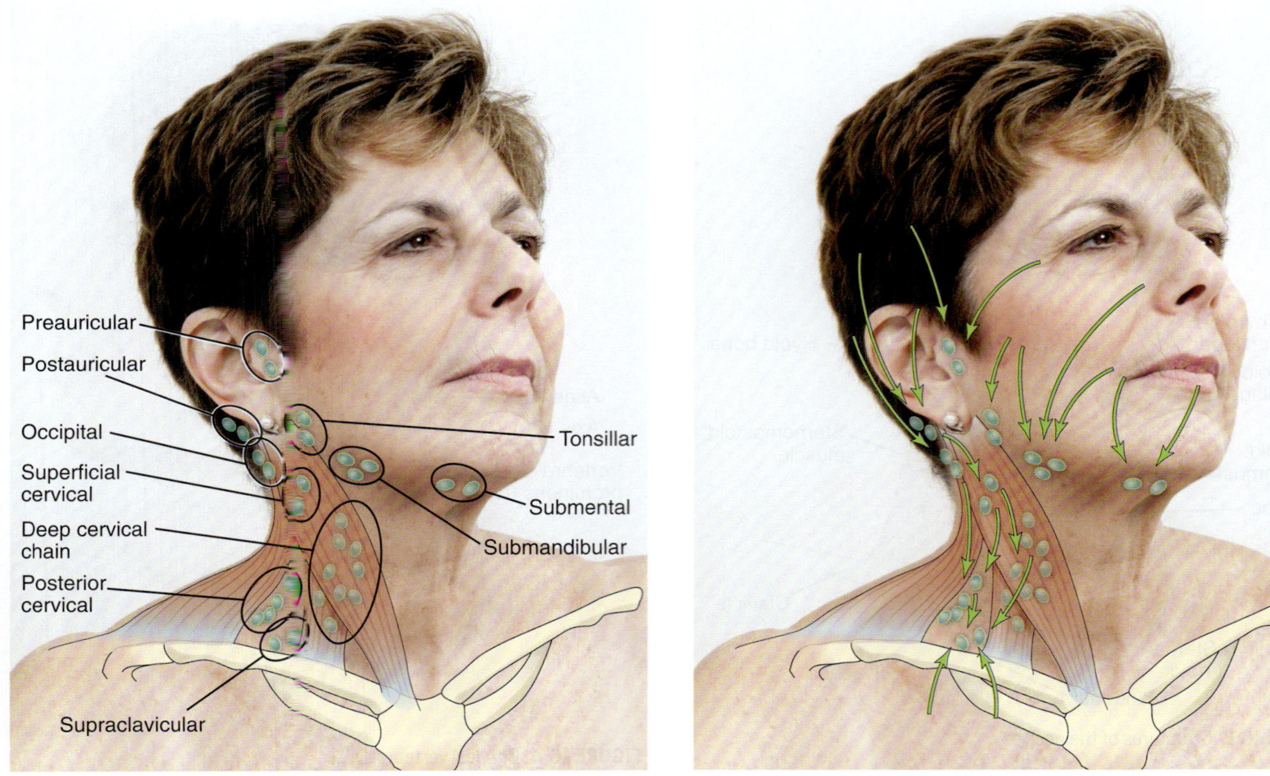

FIGURE 16-5 Lymph nodes in the neck **(left)**. Direction of lymph flow **(right)**. *Note:* Lymph nodes (green dots) that are covered by hair may be palpated in the scalp under the hair.

and become painful, but if cancer metastasises to the lymph nodes, they may enlarge but not be painful. Normally lymph nodes are not palpable, or they may feel like very small beads.

Sources vary in their reference to the names of lymph nodes. The most common head and neck lymph nodes are referred to as follows:

- Preauricular
- Postauricular
- Tonsillar
- Occipital
- Submandibular
- Submental
- Superficial cervical
- Posterior cervical
- Deep cervical
- Supraclavicular.

When an enlarged lymph node is detected during assessment, the nurse needs to know from which part of the head or neck the lymph node receives drainage to assess if an abnormality (e.g. infection, disease) is in that area.

Health assessment

COLLECTING SUBJECTIVE DATA: THE NURSING HEALTH HISTORY

Abnormalities that cannot be directly observed in the physical appearance of the head and neck are often detected in the patient's history. For example, a patient may have no visible signs of any problems but may complain of frequent headaches. A detailed description of the type of headache pain and its location, intensity and duration provides the nurse with valuable clues to what the underlying problem might be.

In addition, because of the overlap of several body systems in this area, a thorough nursing history is needed to detect the cause of possible underlying systemic problems. For example, the patient experiencing dizziness, spinning, light-headedness or loss of consciousness may perceive the problems as related to their head. However, these symptoms may indicate problems with the heart and neck vessels, peripheral vascular system or neurological system.

The history also provides an opportunity to evaluate activities of daily living that may affect the condition of the patient's head and neck. Stress, tension, poor posture while performing work and lack of proper exercise may lead to head and neck discomfort. To prevent head and neck injuries, the nurse may inform the patient of protective measures, such as wearing helmets, seatbelts and hard hats, during the history portion of the assessment.

Finally, when discussing the patient's head, neck and facial structures, recognise that the appearance of these structures often has a great influence on the patient's self-image.

The following table material contains a selection of questions you may ask and areas you may cover with an average patient.

CASE STUDY

You are concerned Vesna may be experiencing anxiety about going home, have a fever or perhaps be experiencing pain.

CRITICAL THINKING

4. Considering Vesna's recent surgery, what questions would help explore potential problems related to the operation?
5. What specific questions would you ask Vesna about her symptoms?
6. Would you ask questions about her lifestyle and history? Why or why not?

History of present health concern

QUESTION	RATIONALE
Pain	
Do you experience neck pain?	Neck pain may accompany muscular problems or cervical spinal cord problems. Stress and tension may increase neck pain. Sudden head and neck pain seen with elevated temperature and neck stiffness may be a sign of meningeal inflammation. **OLDER ADULT CONSIDERATIONS** **Older patients who have arthritis or osteoporosis may experience neck pain and a decreased range of motion.**
Do you experience headaches? Describe.	A precise description of the symptoms can help to determine possible causes of the discomfort. Temporomandibular joint syndrome is a major cause of chronic headaches. See Table 16-1 for a discussion of typical findings for migraine, tension, cluster and tumour-related headaches.
Do you have any facial pain? Describe.	Trigeminal neuralgia (tic douloureux) is manifested by sharp, shooting, piercing facial pains that last from seconds to minutes. Pain occurs over the divisions of the fifth trigeminal cranial nerve (the ophthalmic, maxillary and mandibular areas).
Do you have any difficulty moving your head or neck?	Diseases and disorders involving head and neck muscles may limit mobility and affect daily functioning.
Other symptoms	
Have you noticed any lumps or lesions on your head or neck that do not heal or disappear? Describe their appearance and location.	Lumps and lesions that do not heal or disappear may indicate cancer.
Have you experienced any dizziness, light-headedness, spinning sensation or loss of consciousness? Describe.	Problems with the neck vessels (such as carotid artery occlusion), neurological system (such as inner ear disease) or cardiovascular system (heart block) may cause these symptoms. These symptoms imply a risk of injury.
Have you noticed a change in the texture of your skin, hair or nails? Have you noticed changes in your energy level, sleep habits or emotional stability? Have you experienced any palpitations, blurred vision or changes in bowel habits?	Alterations in thyroid function are manifested in several ways. An increase in thyroid hormone production (hyperthyroidism) can result in insomnia, thinning hair, palpitations and weight loss. A decrease in thyroid hormone production (hypothyroidism) can result in insomnia and will have the opposite effects of thickening skin and nails, decreased energy levels and constipation.

Continued on page 273

Table 16-1 Kinds and characteristics of headaches

Sinus	Cluster	Tension	Migraine	Tumour related
Character				
Deep, constant, throbbing pain; pressure-like pain in one specific area of face or head (e.g. behind the eyes); face tender to the touch	May be accompanied by tearing, eyelid drooping, reddened eye or runny nose	Symptoms of anxiety, tension and depression may be present	Accompanied by nausea, vomiting and sensitivity to noise or light	Neurological and mental symptoms and nausea and vomiting may develop
Onset and precipitating factors				
Occurs with or after a cold or acute sinusitis or acute febrile illness with purulent discharge from the nose	• Sudden onset • May be precipitated by ingesting alcohol	• No prodromal stage • May occur with stress, anxiety or depression	• May have prodromal stage (visual disturbances, vertigo, tinnitus, numbness or tingling of fingers or toes) • Precipitated by emotional disturbances, anxiety or ingestion of alcohol, cheese, chocolate or other foods and substances to which patient is sensitive	• No prodromal stage • May be aggravated by coughing, sneezing or sudden movements of the head
Location				
May occur in one area of the face or along eyebrow ridge and below the cheek bone	Localised in the eye and orbit and radiating to the facial and temporal regions	Usually located in the frontal, temporal or occipital region	Located around eyes, temples, cheeks or forehead; may affect only one side of the face and include facial weakness; in rare cases extending to include limb weakness on the affected side	Varies with location of tumour
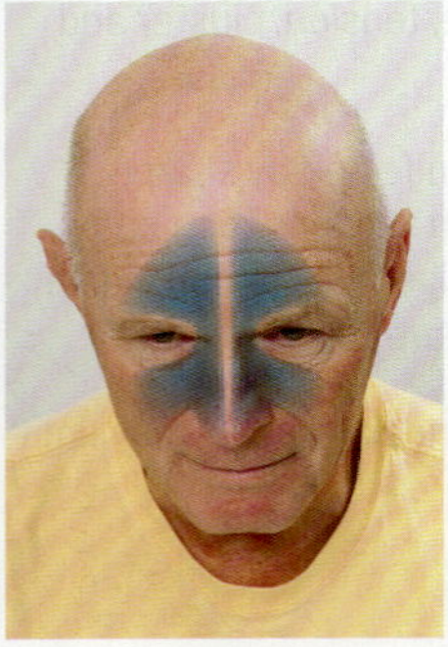 Sinus headache	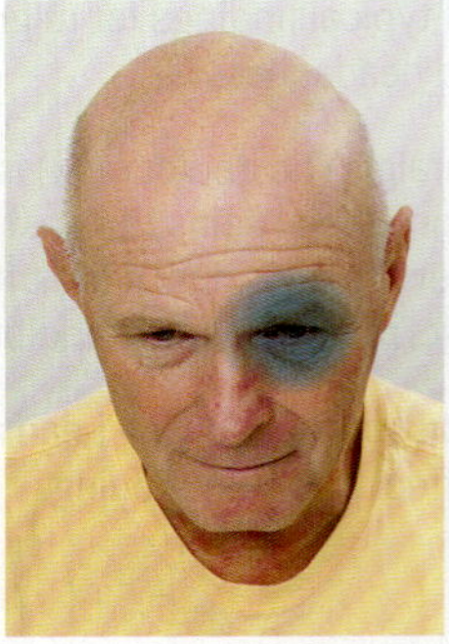 Cluster	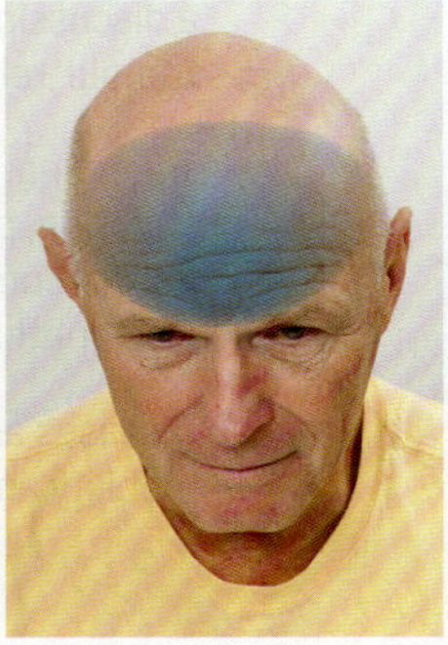 Tension	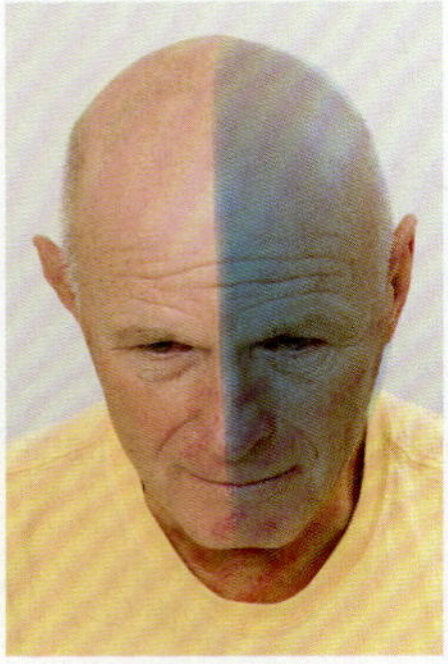 Migraine	
Duration				
Lasts until associated condition is resolved	Typically occurs in the late evening or night	Lasts days, months or years	Lasts up to 3 days	Commonly occurs in the morning and lasts for several hours
Severity				
Moderately severe; not generally debilitating	Intense and stabbing	Dull, aching, tight, diffuse	Throbbing, severe, recurring	Aching, steady, variable in intensity

Table 16-1 Kinds and characteristics of headaches (continued)

Sinus	Cluster	Tension	Migraine	Tumour related
Pattern				
Pain worse with sudden movements of the head, bending forwards, lying down, in the morning (due to mucus collecting and draining all night) or with sudden temperature changes (going from warm to cold environment)	Movement or walking back and forth may relieve the discomfort	Symptomatic relief may be obtained by local heat, massage, analgesics, antidepressants and muscle relaxants	Rest may bring relief	Headache usually subsides later in the day
Associated factors				
Symptoms of sinusitis, such as nasal drainage and congestion, fever and halitosis (foul-smelling breath)	Cluster headaches occur more in young males	Tension headaches affect women more often than men	Migraines occur more often in women	

COLDSPA

Example

Use the COLDSPA mnemonic as a guideline to collect needed information for each symptom the patient shares. In addition, the following questions help elicit important information.

Mnemonic	Question	Patient response example
Character	Describe the sign or symptom (feeling, appearance, sound, smell or taste, if applicable).	'I have trouble turning my head to the right.'
Onset	When did it begin?	'Two days ago, when I woke up in the morning, and it is getting worse.'
Location	Where is it? Does it radiate? Does it occur anywhere else?	'In the back of my neck and it radiates to my right shoulder with movement.'
Duration	How long does it last? Does it recur?	'It is OK if I just sit still, but it hurts more if I turn.'
Severity	How bad is it? How much does it bother you?	'It is difficult to drive because I can't see over my shoulder to change lanes.'
Pattern	What makes it better or worse?	'Ibuprofen and a heating pad or warm shower help a little.'
Associated factors/How it Affects the patient	What other symptoms occur with it? How does it affect you?	'I can't do my work on the computer without being irritated with it.'

Past health history

QUESTION	RATIONALE
Describe any previous head or neck problems (trauma, injury, falls) you have had. How were they treated (surgery, medication, physical therapy)? What were the results?	Previous head and neck trauma may cause chronic pain and limitation of movement. This may affect functioning.
Have you ever undergone radiation therapy for a problem in your neck region?	Radiation therapy has been linked to the development of thyroid cancer. Radiation to the neck area may also cause oesophageal strictures leading to difficulty with swallowing.

Family history

QUESTION	RATIONALE
Is there a history of head or neck cancer in your family?	Genetic predisposition is a risk factor for head and neck cancers.
Is there a history of migraine headaches in your family?	Migraine headaches commonly have a familial association.

Continued on following page

Lifestyle and health practices

QUESTION	RATIONALE
Do you smoke or chew tobacco? If yes, how much?	Tobacco use increases the risk of head and neck cancer.
Do you wear a helmet when riding a horse, bicycle, motorcycle or other open sports vehicle (e.g. four-wheeler, go-cart)? Do you wear a hard hat for hazardous occupations?	Failure to use safety precautions increases the risk of head and neck injury (see Promote health—Traumatic brain injury for more information).
What is your typical posture when relaxing, during sleep and when working?	Poor posture or body alignment can lead to or exacerbate head and neck discomfort.
In what kinds of recreational activity do you participate? Describe the activity.	Contact or aggressive sports may increase the risk of a head or neck injury.
Have any problems with your head or neck interfered with your relationships with others or the role you occupy at home or at work?	Head and neck pain may interfere with relationships or prevent patients from completing their usual activities of daily living.

PROMOTE HEALTH **TRAUMATIC BRAIN INJURY**

OVERVIEW

Research undertaken in 2008 by the Australian Institute of Health and Welfare (AIHW) estimated the direct costs of hospital care for patients experiencing traumatic brain injury (TBI) at $184 million. Over 26,000 episodes of inpatient care totalling nearly 206,000 days were reported in the period from 2004 to 2005 (Helps et al., 2008). In Australia, between 2002 and 2012, 164,126 children were hospitalised because of a TBI, with the most common reasons being falls (45.2%) and road trauma (16%) (Bierbaum et al., 2019). The cost of hospitalisation in children with TBI was nearly half a billion dollars over a 10-year period, with an increase for children between ages 11 and 16 years (Bierbaum et al., 2019). Across all age groups the rates of hospitalisation for males were two and a half times those of females (AIHW, 2018). Feign et al. (2013) reviewed the incidence of TBI in New Zealand and reported the total incidence of TBI was 790 cases per 100,000 per person per year. Children between ages 0 and 14 years and adolescents between ages 15 and 24 years constituted 70% of all cases. TBI affected males more than females (risk ratio 1.77, 95% confidence interval 1.58–1.97). Most TBI were due to falls (38%), mechanical forces (21%), transport accidents (20%) and assaults (17%), with Feign et al. also stating people of Māori heritage were more at risk than non-Māori people (p. 53). In Australia, falls resulting in head injuries increased 7% per year from 2002–2003 to 2014–2015, with approximately 26,693 people admitted to hospital in the period from 2014 to 2015 (AIHW & Pointer, 2018). The rates of TBI were 706 for males and 731 for females in 100,000 per population in 2014/15 (AIHW & Pointer, 2018). Rates of falls in the community were 1,814 in 100,000 compared with 10,090 in 100,000 per population (AIHW & Pointer, 2018). A more recent review of hospitalisations due to road accidents found 6,840 people were admitted with sustained head injuries from 2014 to 2015 (AIHW, 2018). Overall, 1% to 2% of TBI cases resulted in death (Australian Bureau of Statistics, 2018; Jagnoor & Cameron, 2014). Each year, however, many Australians survive TBI to be discharged from hospital with disabilities. Approximately 430,000 Australians with disabilities attributed to acquired brain injuries were reported in 2003 (AIHW, 2007). In one Australian state, it has been estimated that 11,000 have acquired brain injuries, of which 4,000 have serious disabilities (Queensland Health, 2017).

RISK FACTORS

- Transportation accidents
- Violence or assault
- Mechanical forces, e.g., falls (especially in the elderly and children)
- Male gender
- Failure to use protective equipment (helmets, seatbelts)
- Participation in contact or other sports, such as soccer, football, boxing, ice hockey, baseball, skiing, skateboarding or snowboarding, horse riding or motorcycling.

TEACH RISK REDUCTION TIPS

- Use safe driving techniques.
- Never drive while under the influence of alcohol, drugs or medications that cause drowsiness.
- Wear protective gear such as helmets and seatbelts.
- Avoid violent or potentially violent environments when possible.
- Work with community agencies to modify violent environments; develop anger management programs and drug-free programs.
- Modify one's residence to prevent falls, especially for the elderly and children.
- Acquire and learn safe use of adaptive equipment for safe mobility inside and outside the home.
- Avoid dangerous contact sports likely to cause brain injury; wear protective equipment when engaging in such activities.
- Make sure children's playgrounds are shock absorbent (hardwood mulch or sand).

COLLECTING OBJECTIVE DATA: PHYSICAL EXAMINATION

Examining the head allows the nurse to evaluate the overlying protective structures (cranium and facial bones) before evaluating the underlying special senses (vision, hearing, smell and taste) and the functioning of the neurological system. This examination can detect head and facial shape abnormalities, asymmetry, structural changes or tenderness. Assessment of both the head and the neck assists the nurse in detecting enlarged or tender lymph nodes. Thyroid enlargement, nodules, masses or tenderness may be detected by palpating the thyroid gland. Palpation may also detect abnormalities of the neck and facial muscles.

Preparing the patient

Prepare the patient for the head and neck examination by instructing him or her to remove any wig, hat, hair ornaments, pins, rubber bands, jewellery and head or neck scarves.

CULTURAL CONSIDERATIONS

Take care to consider cultural norms for touch when assessing the head. For example, in New Zealand the head is considered sacred (*tapu*) by Māori, and in Asian cultures touching the head is seen as offensive, with patting a child's head deemed inappropriate. For reasons such as these, some cultural groups may prohibit the touching of the head, or touching of the feet before touching the head (Purnell, 2013).

Ask the patient to sit in an upright position, with his or her back straight and shoulders held back. Explain the importance of remaining still during most of the inspection and palpation of the head and neck. However, explain that they will be requested to move and bend the neck for examination of muscles and for palpation of the thyroid gland. Be aware that some patients may be anxious as you palpate the neck for lymph nodes, especially if they have a history of cancer that caused lymph node enlargement. Remember also to be careful when palpating to avoid stimulating the carotid sinus (see earlier Critical Thinking question). Tell the patient what you are doing and share your assessment findings.

Another important thing to keep in mind as you examine the head and neck is that normal facial structures and features tend to vary widely among individuals and cultures.

Equipment

- Gloves
- Small cup of water
- Stethoscope

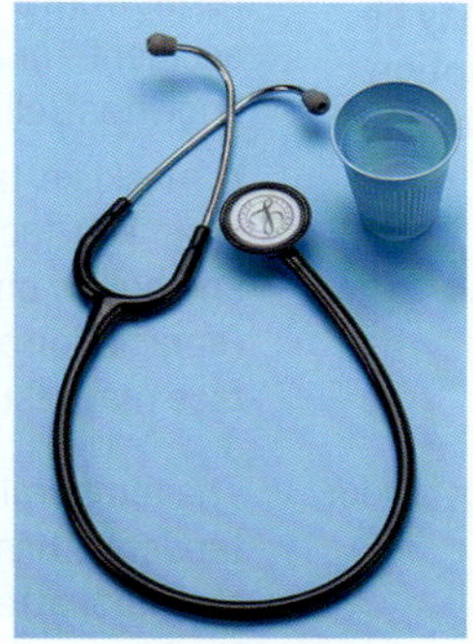

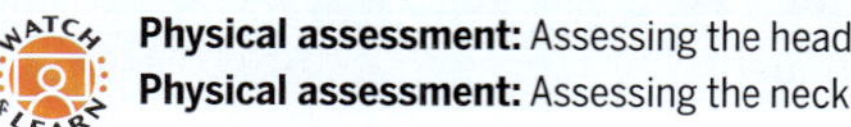

Physical assessment: Assessing the head
Physical assessment: Assessing the neck

CASE STUDY

You are concerned Vesna may be experiencing anxiety about going home, have a fever or perhaps be experiencing pain. However, Vesna is afebrile and states she is comfortable, with no anxiety about heading home today. She expresses concern that she has been fidgety and perspiring for some months, even before the operation. Although she had planned to see her local doctor about her restlessness, she has been too busy with work and study. Vesna states she has lost some weight recently despite being hungry all the time and eating more than usual and that her neck has been a little 'puffy'. As you have already noted on inspection, there was some diffuse swelling of the anterior neck consistent with Vesna's perception of puffiness.

CRITICAL THINKING

Most health assessments are based around common sense.

7. Prior to reading the physical assessment section, reread the 'Structure and function' section. What do you think would be the important things to assess or examine specific to a patient's head and neck?
8. Considering this and the data presented thus far, how would you assess Vesna's presenting complaint?

PHYSICAL ASSESSMENT

ASSESSMENT PROCEDURE	NORMAL FINDINGS	ABNORMAL FINDINGS
Head and face		
INSPECTION AND PALPATION		
Inspect the head. Inspect for size, shape and configuration.	Head size and shape vary, especially in accord with ethnicity. Usually the head is symmetrical, round, erect and in midline. No lesions are visible.	The skull and facial bones are larger and thicker in acromegaly, which occurs when there is an increased production of growth hormone. Acorn-shaped, enlarged skull bones are seen in Paget disease of the bone.
Inspect hair and the scalp.	Scalp can be normal, oily, dry or mixed. No lesions, bruising, swelling or discolouration should be visible. Hair should be soft and smooth to the touch. Colour and thickness vary between individuals.	Scalp that has swelling or oedema, bruising, scaling, redness, itching or dry. Certain medications and conditions can interfere with hair growth (alopecia or loss or thinning), hair colour, hair loss, hair texture.

Continued on following page

ASSESSMENT PROCEDURE	NORMAL FINDINGS	ABNORMAL FINDINGS
Head and face (continued)		
Inspect for involuntary movement.	Head should be held still and upright.	Tremors associated with neurological disorders may cause a horizontal jerking movement. An involuntary nodding movement may be seen in patients with aortic insufficiency. Head tilted to one side may indicate unilateral vision or hearing deficiency or shortening of the sternomastoid muscle.
Palpate the head. Palpate for consistency. **CLINICAL TIP** **Wear gloves to protect yourself from possible drainage.**	The head is normally hard and smooth without lesions.	Lesions or lumps on the head may indicate recent trauma or cancer.
Inspect the face. Inspect for symmetry, features, movement, expression and skin condition. **CLINICAL TIP** **The nasolabial folds and palpebral fissures are ideal places to check facial features for symmetry.**	The face is symmetrical with a round, oval, elongated or square appearance. No abnormal movements noted. **OLDER ADULT CONSIDERATIONS** **In older patients, facial wrinkles are prominent because subcutaneous fat decreases with age. In addition, the lower face may shrink, and the mouth may be drawn inwards as a result of resorption of mandibular bone, also an age-related process.**	Asymmetry in front of the earlobes occurs with parotid gland enlargement from an abscess or tumour. Unusual or asymmetrical orofacial movements may be from an organic disease or neurological problem, which should be referred for medical follow-up. Drooping of one side of the face may result from a stroke—or cerebrovascular accident—or a neurological condition known as Bell palsy (Fig. 16-6). A 'masklike' face marks Parkinson disease; a 'sunken' face with depressed eyes and hollow cheeks is typical of cachexia (emaciation or wasting); and a pale, swollen face may result from nephrotic syndrome.
Palpate the temporal artery, which is located between the top of the ear and the eye (Fig. 16-7).	The temporal artery is elastic and not tender. **OLDER ADULT CONSIDERATIONS** **The strength of the pulsation of the temporal artery may be decreased in the older patient.**	The temporal artery is hard, thick and tender with inflammation, as seen with temporal arteritis (inflammation of the temporal arteries that may lead to blindness).
Palpate the temporomandibular joint. To assess the temporomandibular joint (TMJ), place your index finger over the front of each ear as you ask the patient to open her mouth (Fig. 16-8).	Normally there is no swelling, tenderness or crepitation with movement. Mouth opens and closes fully (3 to 6 cm between upper and lower teeth). Lower jaw moves laterally 1 to 2 cm in each direction.	Limited range of motion, swelling, tenderness or crepitation may indicate TMJ syndrome. **CLINICAL TIP** **When assessing TMJ syndrome, be sure to explore the patient's history of headaches, if any.**

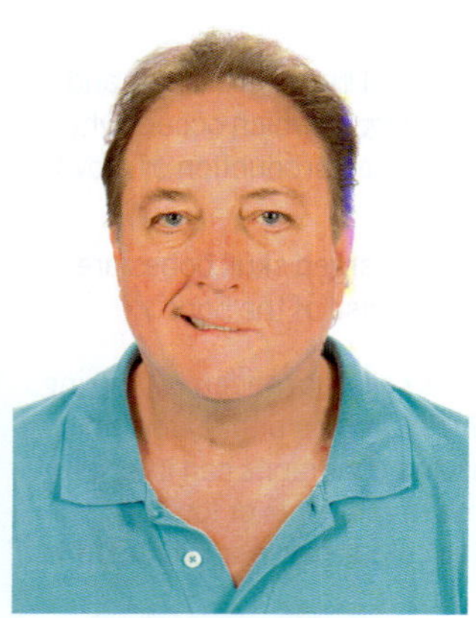

FIGURE 16-6 One-sided facial paralysis characterises Bell palsy. (Shutterstock.com/Steven Frame.)

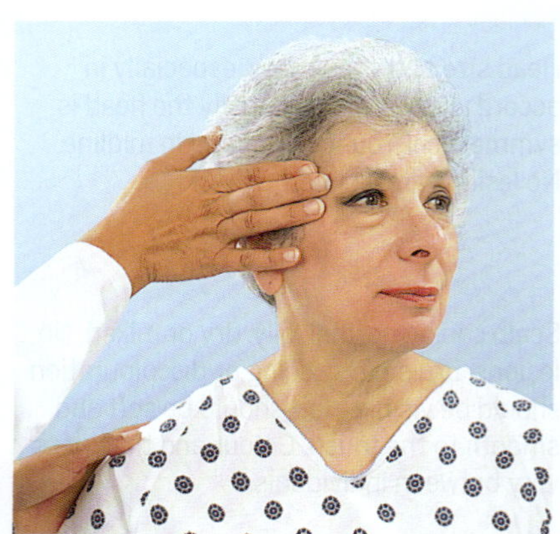

FIGURE 16-7 Palpating the temporal artery. (© B. Proud.)

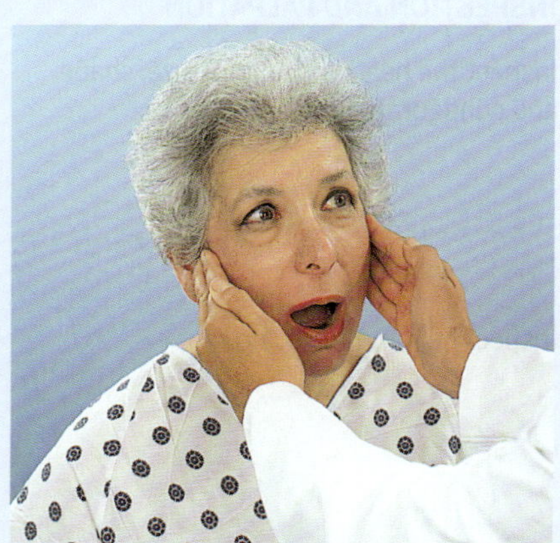

FIGURE 16-8 Palpating the temporomandibular joint. (© B. Proud.)

PHYSICAL ASSESSMENT (continued)

ASSESSMENT PROCEDURE	NORMAL FINDINGS	ABNORMAL FINDINGS
The neck		
INSPECTION		
Inspect the neck. Observe the patient's slightly extended neck for position, symmetry and lumps or masses. Shine a light from the side of the neck across to highlight any swelling.	Neck is symmetrical with head centred and without bulging masses.	Swelling, enlarged masses or nodules may indicate an enlarged thyroid gland (Fig. 16-9), inflammation of lymph nodes or a tumour.
Inspect movement of the neck structures. Ask the patient to swallow a small sip of water. Observe the movement of the thyroid cartilage, thyroid gland (Fig. 16-10).	The thyroid cartilage, cricoid cartilage and thyroid gland move upwards symmetrically as the patient swallows.	Asymmetrical movement or generalised enlargement of the thyroid gland is considered abnormal.
Inspect the cervical vertebrae. Ask the patient to flex the neck (chin to chest, ear to shoulder, twist left to right and right to left, and backward and forward).	C7 (vertebrae prominens) is usually visible and palpable. 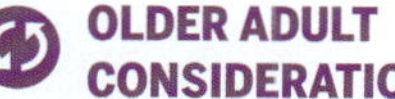 **OLDER ADULT CONSIDERATIONS** **In older patients, cervical curvature may increase because of kyphosis of the spine. Moreover, fat may accumulate around the cervical vertebrae (especially in women). This is sometimes called a 'Dowager hump' this may also be seen in people on long term corticosteroids.**	Prominence or swellings other than the C7 vertebrae may be abnormal.
Inspect range of motion. Ask the patient to turn the head to the right and to the left (chin to shoulder). touch each ear to the shoulder, touch chin to chest and lift the chin to the ceiling.	Normally neck movement should be smooth and controlled with 45- degree flexion, 55-degree extension, 40-degree lateral abduction and 70-degree rotation. **OLDER ADULT CONSIDERATIONS** **Older patients usually have somewhat decreased flexion, extension, lateral bending and rotation of the neck.** This is usually due to arthritis.	Muscle spasms, inflammation or cervical arthritis may cause stiffness, rigidity and limited mobility of the neck, which may affect daily functioning.

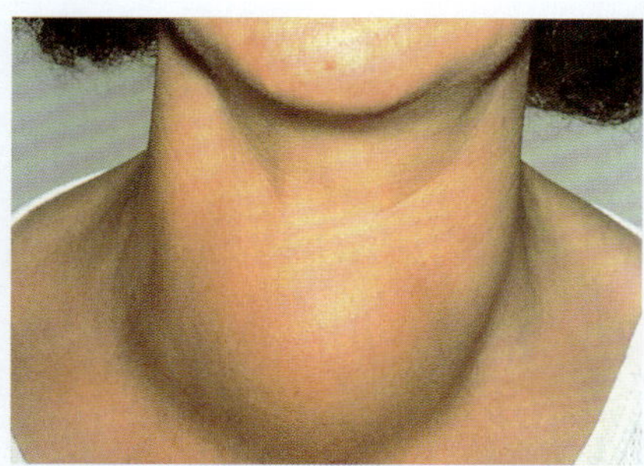

FIGURE 16-9 Diffuse enlargement of the thyroid gland.

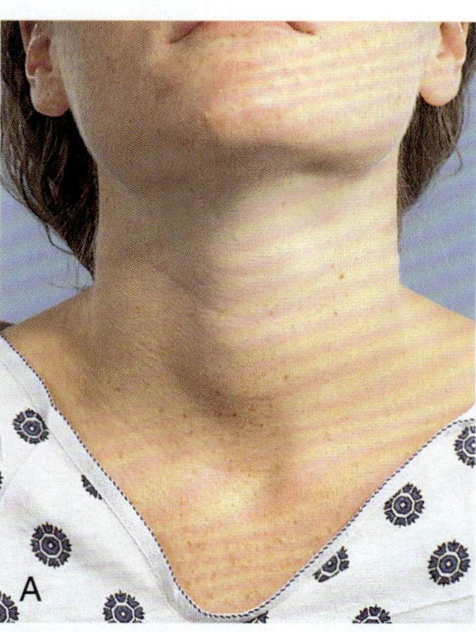

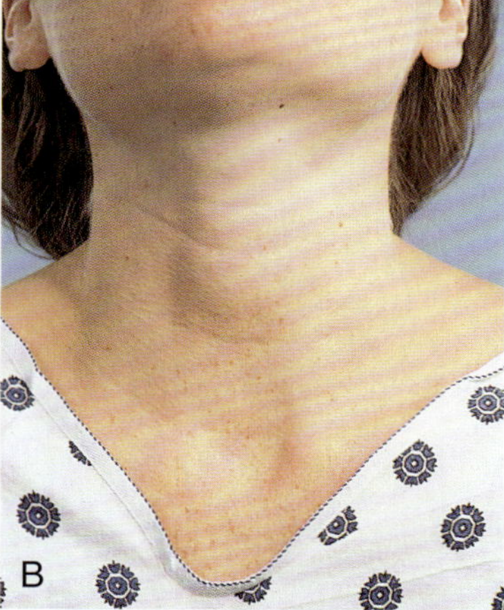

FIGURE 16-10 Inspecting the neck. **(A)** Slightly extended neck discloses internal structures. **(B)** Neck structures move (rise and fall). (© B. Proud.)

Continued on following page

PHYSICAL ASSESSMENT (continued)

ASSESSMENT PROCEDURE	NORMAL FINDINGS	ABNORMAL FINDINGS
The neck (continued)		
PALPATION		
Palpate the trachea. Place your finger in the sternal notch. Feel each side of the notch and palpate the tracheal rings (Fig. 16-11). The first upper ring above the smooth tracheal rings is the cricoid cartilage.	Trachea is midline.	The trachea may be pulled to one side in cases of a tumour, thyroid gland enlargement, aortic aneurysm, pneumothorax, atelectasis or fibrosis.
Palpate the thyroid gland. Locate key landmarks with your index finger and thumb: *Hyoid bone* (arch-shaped bone that does not articulate directly with any other bone; located high in anterior neck). *Thyroid cartilage* (under the hyoid bone; the area that widens at the top of the trachea), also known as the 'Adam's apple'. *Cricoid cartilage* (smaller upper tracheal ring under the thyroid cartilage).	Landmarks are positioned midline.	Landmarks deviate from midline or are obscured because of masses or abnormal growths.
To palpate the thyroid, use a posterior approach. Stand behind the patient and ask her or him to lower the chin to the chest and turn the neck slightly to the right. This will relax the patient's neck muscles. Then place your thumbs on the nape of the patient's neck with your other fingers on either side of the trachea below the cricoid cartilage. Use your left fingers to push the trachea to the right. Then use your right fingers to feel deeply in front of the sternomastoid muscle (Fig. 16-12).	Unless the patient is extremely thin with a long neck, the thyroid gland is usually not palpable. However, the isthmus may be palpated in midline. If the thyroid can be palpated, the lobes are smooth, firm and non-tender. The right lobe is often 25% larger than the left lobe.  **OLDER ADULT CONSIDERATIONS** **If palpable, the older patient's thyroid may feel more nodular or irregular because of fibrotic changes that occur with ageing; the thyroid may also be felt lower in the neck because of age-related structural changes.**	In cases of diffuse enlargement, such as hyperthyroidism, Graves' disease or an endemic goitre, the thyroid gland may be palpated. An enlarged, tender gland may result from thyroiditis. Multiple nodules of the thyroid may be seen in metabolic processes. However, rapid enlargement of a single nodule suggests a malignancy and must be evaluated further.

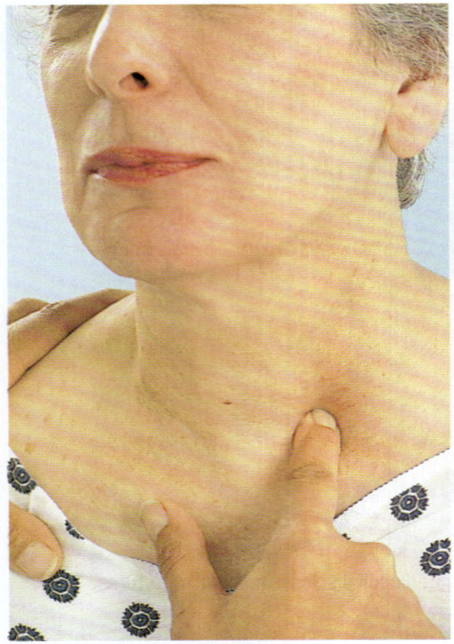

FIGURE 16-11 Palpating the trachea. (© B. Proud.)

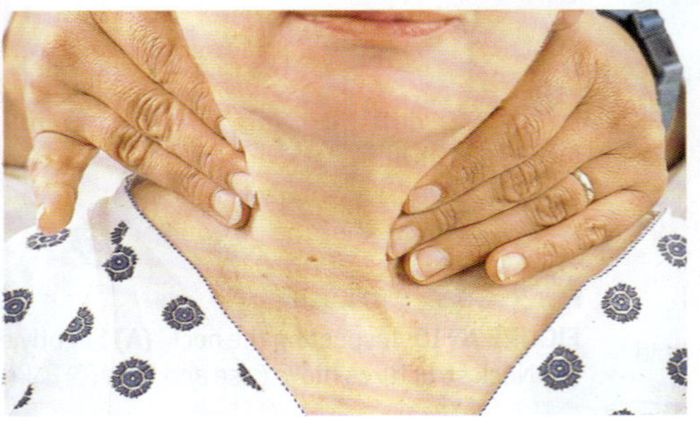

FIGURE 16-12 Palpating the thyroid. (© B. Proud.)

PHYSICAL ASSESSMENT (continued)

ASSESSMENT PROCEDURE	NORMAL FINDINGS	ABNORMAL FINDINGS
Ask the patient to swallow as you palpate the right side of the gland. Reverse the technique to palpate the left lobe of the thyroid.	Glandular thyroid tissue may be felt rising underneath your fingers. Lobes should feel smooth, rubbery and free of nodules.	Coarse tissue or irregular consistency may indicate an inflammatory process. Nodules should be described in terms of location, size and consistency (see Spotlight technique 16-1).
AUSCULTATION		
Auscultate the thyroid only if you find an enlarged thyroid gland during inspection or palpation. Place the bell of the stethoscope over the lateral lobes of the thyroid gland (Fig. 16-13). Ask the patient to hold his or her breath (to obscure any tracheal breath sounds while you auscultate).	No bruits are auscultated.	A soft, blowing, swishing sound auscultated over the thyroid lobes is often heard in hyperthyroidism because of an increase in blood flow through the thyroid arteries.
Lymph nodes of the head and neck		
Spotlight technique 16.1 describes general technique for palpating the lymph nodes.		
Palpate the preauricular nodes (in front of the ear), postauricular nodes (behind the ears), occipital nodes (at the posterior base of the skull).	There is no swelling or enlargement and no tenderness.	Enlarged nodes are abnormal.
Palpate the tonsillar nodes at the angle of the mandible on the anterior edge of the sternomastoid muscle (Fig. 16-14).	No swelling, no tenderness, no hardness is present.	Swelling, tenderness, hardness, immobility are abnormal.
Palpate the submandibular nodes located on the medial border of the mandible (Fig. 16-15).	No enlargement or tenderness is present.	Enlargement and tenderness are abnormal.

CLINICAL TIP
Do not confuse the submandibular nodes with the lobulated submandibular gland.

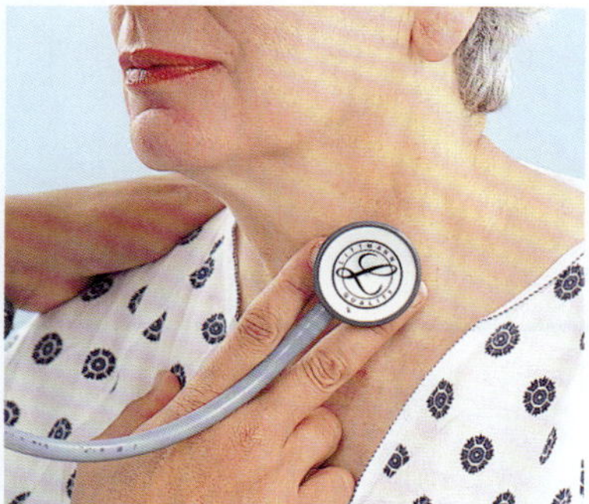

FIGURE 16-13 Auscultating for bruits over the thyroid gland. (© B. Proud.)

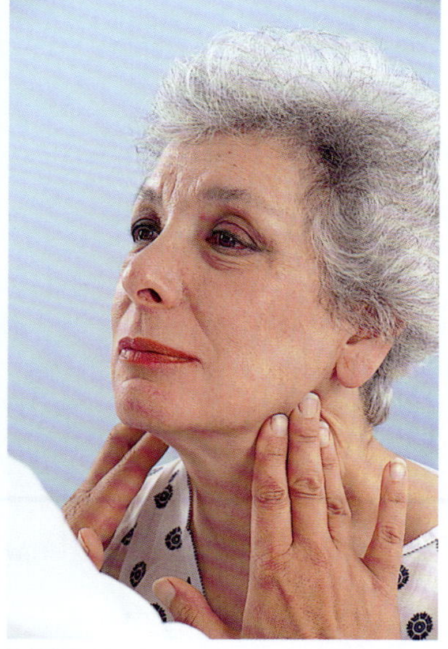

FIGURE 16-14 Palpating the tonsillar nodes. (© B. Proud.)

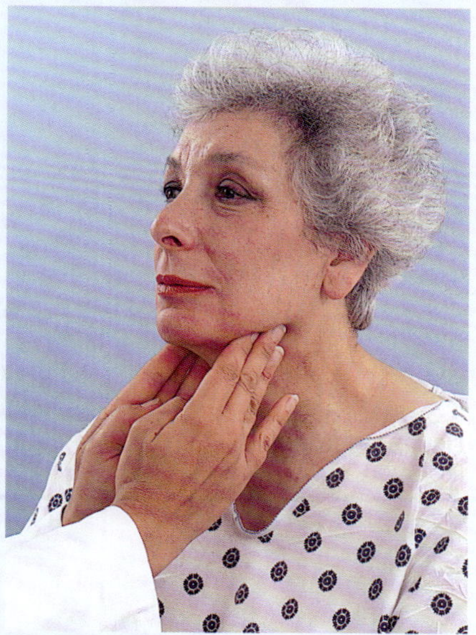

FIGURE 16-15 palpating the submandibular nodes. (© B. Proud.)

Continued on following page

PHYSICAL ASSESSMENT (continued)

ASSESSMENT PROCEDURE	NORMAL FINDINGS	ABNORMAL FINDINGS
The neck (continued)		
Palpate the submental nodes, which are a few centimetres behind the tip of the mandible **CLINICAL TIP** **It is easier to palpate these nodes using one hand.**	No enlargement or tenderness is present.	Enlargement and tenderness are abnormal.
Palpate the superficial cervical nodes in the area superficial to the sternomastoid muscle.	No enlargement or tenderness is present.	Enlargement and tenderness are abnormal.
Palpate the posterior cervical nodes in the area posterior to the sternomastoid and anterior to the trapezius in the posterior triangle.	No enlargement or tenderness is present.	Enlargement and tenderness are abnormal.
Palpate the deep cervical chain nodes deeply within and around the sternomastoid muscle.	No enlargement or tenderness is present.	Enlargement and tenderness are abnormal.
Palpate the supraclavicular nodes by hooking your fingers over the clavicles and feeling deeply between the clavicles and the sternomastoid muscles (Fig. 16-16). 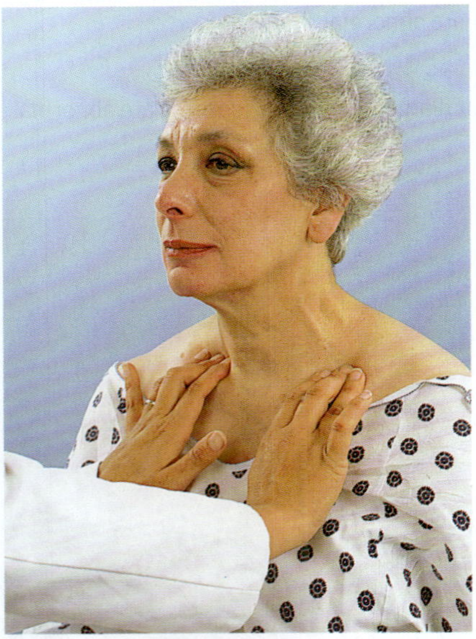 **FIGURE 16-16** Palpating the supraclavicular nodes. (© B. Proud.)	No enlargement or tenderness is present.	An enlarged, hard, non-tender node, particularly on the left side, may indicate a metastasis from a malignancy in the abdomen or thorax.

SPOTLIGHT TECHNIQUE 16-1 PALPATING LYMPH NODES

General guidelines for palpation

Have the patient remain seated upright. Then palpate the lymph nodes with your fingerpads in a slow walking, gentle, circular motion. Ask the patient to bend the head slightly towards the side being palpated to relax the muscles in that area. Compare lymph nodes that occur bilaterally. As you palpate each group of nodes, assess their size and shape, delimitation (whether they are discrete or confluent), mobility, consistency and tenderness. Choose a palpation sequence. This chapter presents a sequence that proceeds in a superior to inferior order (from 1 to 10).

CLINICAL TIP

Which sequence you choose is not important. What is important is that you establish a sequence that does not vary from assessment to assessment. This helps to guard against skipping a group of nodes.

Characteristics of. the lymph nodes

While palpating the lymph nodes, note the following:

- Size and shape
- Delimitation
- Mobility
- Consistency
- Tenderness and location.

Size and shape

Normally lymph nodes, which are round and smaller than 1 cm, are not palpable. In older patients especially, the lymph nodes become fibrotic, fatty and smaller because of a loss of lymphoid elements related to ageing. (This may decrease the older person's resistance to infection.)

When lymph node enlargement exceeds 1 cm, the patient is said to have lymphadenopathy, which may be caused by acute or chronic infection, an autoimmune disorder or metastatic disease. If one or two lymphatic groups enlarge, the patient is said to have *regional lymphadenopathy.* Enlargement of three or more groups is *generalised lymphadenopathy.* Generalised lymphadenopathy that persists for more than 3 months may be a sign of human immunodeficiency virus infection.

Delimitation

Normally lymph node delimitation (the lymph node's position or boundary) is discrete. In chronic infection, however, the lymph nodes become confluent (they merge). In acute infection, they remain discrete.

Mobility

Typical lymph nodes are mobile both from side to side and up and down. In metastatic disease, the lymph nodes enlarge and become fixed in place.

Consistency

Somewhat more fibrotic and fattier in older patients, the normal lymph node is soft, whereas the abnormal node is hard and firm. Hard, firm, unilateral nodes are seen with metastatic cancers.

Tenderness and location

Tender, enlarged nodes suggest acute infections; normally lymph nodes are not sore or tender. Document the location of the lymph node being assessed.

CASE STUDY

On the nursing admission assessment, Vesna's height is 175 cm and her weight is 47 kg. She states, 'This is about 7 kg lower than my normal weight.' When you consult the standard weight charts, you discover that she is underweight for her height and frame. Vesna's vital signs are blood pressure 140/85 mmHg; pulse 100; respirations 18; temperature 37.2°C. She does not know what her usual blood pressure is. Her thyroid gland appears slightly enlarged when palpated, and a bruit is detected upon auscultation. She denies any throat pain or difficulty swallowing. The remaining aspects of Vesna's physical examination findings appear to be within normal limits.

CRITICAL THINKING

9. You are concerned about Vesna's diffuse neck swelling. Her thyroid gland appears slightly enlarged when palpated. What other physical assessment technique could you use to assess the thyroid gland?
10. How can you explain the reported increase in appetite and unexplained weight loss? What could they be attributed to?

VALIDATING AND DOCUMENTING FINDINGS

Validate the head and neck assessment data that you have collected. This is necessary to verify that the data are reliable and accurate. Document the assessment data following health care facility or agency policy.

The following subjective and objective data are included as examples you can follow in practising data collection and documentation.

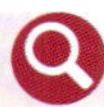

Sample of subjective data

No history of head or neck problems, trauma or surgery. No head or facial pain. Has not experienced episodes of light-headedness or dizziness. Does not chew or smoke tobacco. Is studying to be a physiotherapist and works in a coffee shop part time. Does yoga three times a week to relieve stress. Rides a bike to work and wears a bike helmet. Has no complaints about current condition of head and neck.

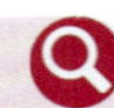

Sample of objective data

Head symmetrically round, hard and smooth without lesions or bumps. Face oval, smooth and symmetrical. Temporal artery elastic and non-tender. Temporomandibular joint palpated with full range of motion without tenderness. Neck symmetrical with centred head position and no bulging masses. C7 is visible and palpable with neck flexed. Has smooth, controlled, full range of motion of neck. Thyroid gland non-visible but palpable when swallowing. Trachea in midline. Lymph nodes non-palpable except for a few deep cervical less than 1 cm bilaterally.

After you have collected your assessment data, you will need to analyse the data using diagnostic reasoning skills. Refer to the discussion of the diagnostic reasoning process in Chapter 5.

Analysis of data

DIAGNOSTIC REASONING: POSSIBLE CONCLUSIONS

After collecting subjective and objective data pertaining to the head and neck assessment, you will need to identify abnormal findings and cluster the data to reveal any significant patterns or abnormalities. These data will then be used to make clinical judgements about the status of the patient's head and neck. Clinical judgements are developed through the application of diagnostic reasoning skills (see Chap. 5). Listed below are some of the possible conclusions that the nurse may make after assessing a patient's head and neck.

Potential patient risks

- Risk of injury to head and neck (related to poor posture and to not wearing protective devices, e.g. head gear during contact sports, seatbelts, eye goggles).

Potential patient problems

- Ineffective health maintenance (related to lack of knowledge of the importance of wearing protective gear during contact sports; to wearing seatbelts while driving or riding as a passenger; and to lack of knowledge of the effects and dangers associated with smoking and using smokeless tobacco)
- Ineffective cerebral tissue perfusion (related to impaired circulation to the brain)
- Imbalanced nutrition: less than body requirements (related to increased metabolism secondary to hyperthyroidism)
- Imbalanced nutrition (related to decreased metabolism secondary to hypothyroidism)
- Activity intolerance (related to fatigue and weakness, secondary to slowed metabolic rate, secondary to hypothyroidism)
- Constipation (related to hyperthyroidism or hypothyroidism)
- Disturbed body image (related to injury)
- Impaired swallowing (related to mechanical obstruction of the head and neck, secondary to tissue swelling, tracheostomy or abnormal growth; or to lack of gag reflex, paralysis of facial muscles or decreased cognition)

Selected collaborative problems

After grouping the data, certain collaborative problems may become apparent. Remember that collaborative problems cannot be prevented by nursing interventions alone. However, these physiological complications of medical conditions can be detected and monitored by the nurse. In addition, the nurse can use doctor- and nurse-prescribed interventions to minimise the complications of these problems. The nurse may also have to refer the patient in such situations to other members of the multidisciplinary team for further treatment of the problem. The following is a list of collaborative problems that may be identified when assessing the head and neck of a patient.

- Hypocalcaemia
- Hypercalcaemia
- Corneal abrasion (related to inability to close eyelids, secondary to exophthalmos)
- Thyroid crisis
- Thyroid dysfunction
- Cerebral vascular accident
- Seizures
- Cranial nerve impairment (5th trigeminal, 7th facial, 11th spinal accessory)
- Increased intracranial pressure.

Medical problems

If after grouping the data it becomes apparent that the patient has signs and symptoms that may require medical diagnosis and treatment, referral to a primary care provider is necessary.

ONLINE RESOURCES

An extensive range of additional resources to enhance teaching and learning and to facilitate understanding may be found online at the text's accompanying website, located on thePoint at http://thepoint.lww.com. These include Watch and Learn videos, Concepts in Action animations, journal articles, case studies, discussion topics and quizzes.

Subscribers may also access Lippincott Procedures, an extensive online point-of-care procedure guide that provides reliable step-by-step instructions for more than 1700 procedures, including 450 evidence-based Australian procedures, and skills in a variety of speciality settings, together with a wealth of supporting information.

CASE STUDY

The case study demonstrates how to analyse head and neck assessment data for a specific patient. The exercises included in the ancillary product on thePoint that complements this text offer further opportunities to enhance your skills.

Vesna Duric is an underweight 23-year-old woman with a 6-year history of endometriosis; she is 1 day postoperative following a laparoscopy and diathermy of endometrial cysts. You are helping Vesna prepare for discharge when you notice mild anterior neck swelling; you also notice beads of perspiration on Vesna's forehead even though the room is cool, and that she is fidgeting. You are concerned Vesna may be experiencing anxiety about going home, have a fever or perhaps be experiencing pain. However, Vesna is afebrile and states she is comfortable, with no anxiety about heading home today. She expresses concern that she has been fidgety and perspiring for some months, even before the operation. Although she had planned to see her local doctor about her restlessness, she has been too busy with work and study. Vesna states she has lost some weight recently despite being hungry all the time and eating more than usual and that her neck has been a little 'puffy'. As you have already noted on inspection, there was some diffuse swelling of the anterior neck consistent with Vesna's perception of puffiness.

On the nursing admission assessment, Vesna's height is 175 cm and her weight is 47 kg. She states, 'This is about 7 kg lower than my normal weight.' When you consult the standard weight charts, you discover that she is underweight for her height and frame. Vesna's vital signs are blood pressure 140/85 mmHg; pulse 100; respirations 18; temperature 37.2 °C. She does not know what her usual blood pressure is. Her thyroid gland appears slightly enlarged when palpated, and a bruit is detected upon auscultation. She denies any throat pain or difficulty swallowing. The remaining aspects of Vesna's physical examination findings appear to be within normal limits.

The following concept map illustrates the diagnostic reasoning process.

Applying COLDSPA

Applying COLDSPA for patient symptoms: 'hungry all the time, diffuse swelling in neck'.

Mnemonic	Question	Data provided	Missing data
Character	Describe the sign or symptom (feeling, appearance, sound, smell or taste, if applicable).	'I am hungry all the time.' Patient appears thin, fidgety and is perspiring on her forehead in a cool room.	
Onset	When did it begin?		When did you first start feeling hungry all the time? When did you first start losing weight?
Location	Where is it? Does it radiate? Does it occur anywhere else?		Have you noticed the swelling in your neck? When did this begin?
Duration	How long does it last? Does it recur?		What times of the day are you more or less hungry?
Severity	How bad is it? How much does it bother you?	'I have lost weight.'	How much weight have you lost?
Pattern	What makes it better or worse?		Is there anything that relieves your hunger?
Associated factors/How it Affects the patient	What other symptoms occur with it? How does it affect you?	'I have been planning to see my local doctor for a while but had to cancel because of the surgery.'	What other symptoms have you noticed with the weight loss? Any excessive thirst or urinating?

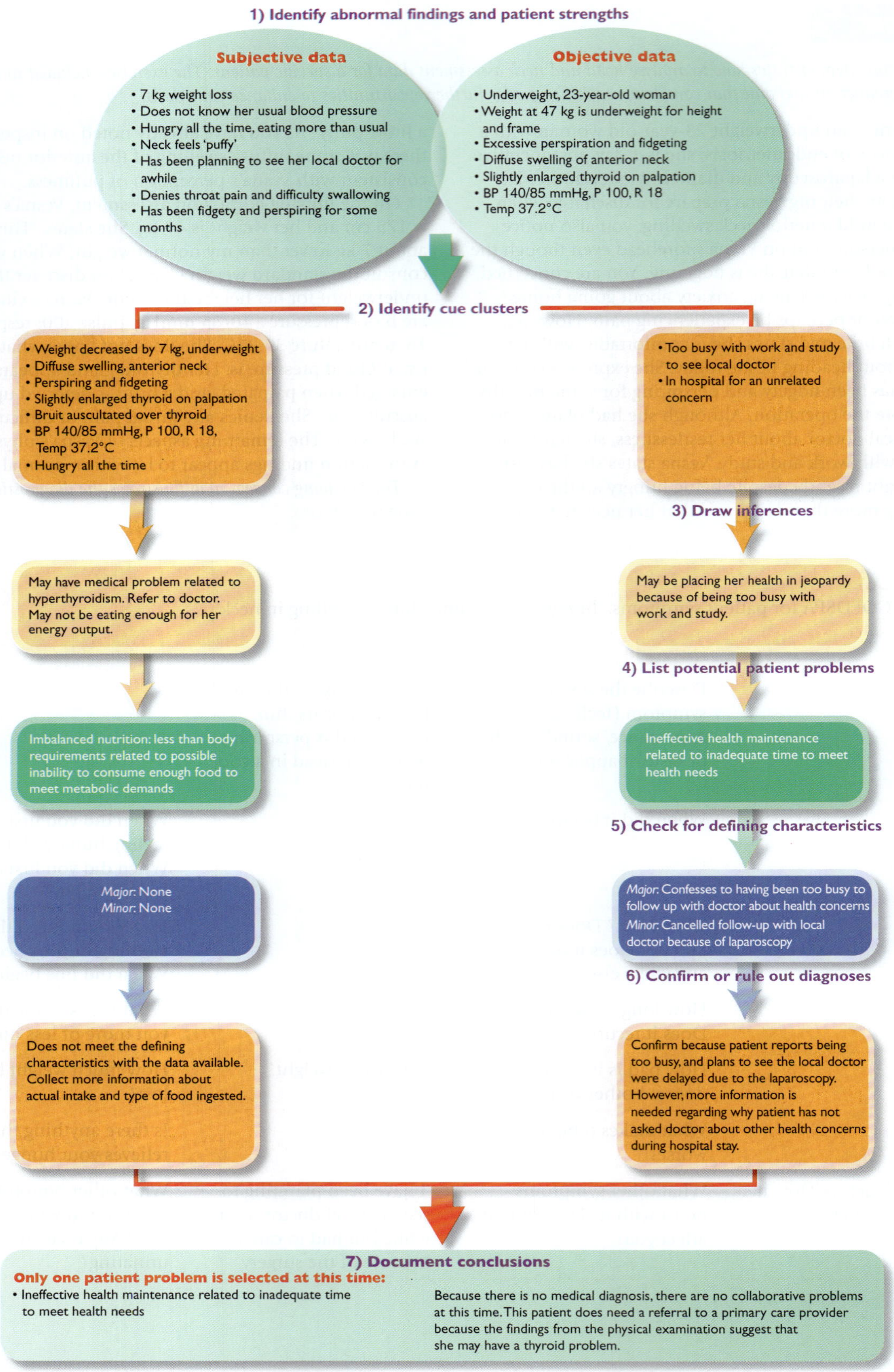

1) Identify abnormal findings and patient strengths

Subjective data

- 7 kg weight loss
- Does not know her usual blood pressure
- Hungry all the time, eating more than usual
- Neck feels 'puffy'
- Has been planning to see her local doctor for awhile
- Denies throat pain and difficulty swallowing
- Has been fidgety and perspiring for some months

Objective data

- Underweight, 23-year-old woman
- Weight at 47 kg is underweight for height and frame
- Excessive perspiration and fidgeting
- Diffuse swelling of anterior neck
- Slightly enlarged thyroid on palpation
- BP 140/85 mmHg, P 100, R 18
- Temp 37.2°C

2) Identify cue clusters

- Weight decreased by 7 kg, underweight
- Diffuse swelling, anterior neck
- Perspiring and fidgeting
- Slightly enlarged thyroid on palpation
- Bruit auscultated over thyroid
- BP 140/85 mmHg, P 100, R 18, Temp 37.2°C
- Hungry all the time

- Too busy with work and study to see local doctor
- In hospital for an unrelated concern

3) Draw inferences

May have medical problem related to hyperthyroidism. Refer to doctor. May not be eating enough for her energy output.

May be placing her health in jeopardy because of being too busy with work and study.

4) List potential patient problems

Imbalanced nutrition: less than body requirements related to possible inability to consume enough food to meet metabolic demands

Ineffective health maintenance related to inadequate time to meet health needs

5) Check for defining characteristics

Major: None
Minor: None

Major: Confesses to having been too busy to follow up with doctor about health concerns
Minor: Cancelled follow-up with local doctor because of laparoscopy

6) Confirm or rule out diagnoses

Does not meet the defining characteristics with the data available. Collect more information about actual intake and type of food ingested.

Confirm because patient reports being too busy, and plans to see the local doctor were delayed due to the laparoscopy. However, more information is needed regarding why patient has not asked doctor about other health concerns during hospital stay.

7) Document conclusions

Only one patient problem is selected at this time:

- Ineffective health maintenance related to inadequate time to meet health needs

Because there is no medical diagnosis, there are no collaborative problems at this time. This patient does need a referral to a primary care provider because the findings from the physical examination suggest that she may have a thyroid problem.

References

Australian Bureau of Statistics. (2018). 3303.0–Causes of death, Australia, 2017. Canberra.

Australian Institute of Health and Welfare (AIHW). (2018). Hospitalised injury due to land transport crashes. Cat. no. INJCAT 195. Injury research and statistics series no. 115. Canberra: AIHW.

Australian Institute of Health and Welfare (AIHW) & Pointer, S. (2018). Trends in hospitalisation injury due to falls in older people, 2002-03 to 2014-15 Cat no. INJCAT 191. Injury research and statistics series no. 111. Canberra: Author.

Australian Institute of Health and Welfare (AIHW). (2007). Disability in Australia: Acquired brain injury. Bulletin 55, December 2007. Adelaide: Author.

Bierbaum, M., Lystad, R. P., Curtis, K., et al. (2019). Incidence and severity of head injury hospitalisations in Australian children over a 10 year period. *Health Promotion Journal of Australia, 30*(2), 189–198.

Feign, V. L., Theadom, A., Barker-Collo, S., et al. (2013). Incidence of traumatic brain injury in New Zealand. *The Lancet, 12*(1), 53–64. doi:10.1016/S1474-4422(12)7026404.

Helps, Y., Henley, G. & Harrison, J. E. (2008). Hospital separations due to traumatic brain injury. Australia 2004–05. Injury research and statistics series number 45 (Cat. no. INJCAT 116).

Jagnoor, J. & Cameron, I. D. (2014). Traumatic brain injury support for injured people and their careers. *Australian Family Physician, 43*(11), 758–763.

Purnell, L. D. (2013). *Transcultural health care: A culturally competent approach* (4th ed.). Philadelphia: FA Davis.

Queensland Health. (2017). Acquired Brain Injury Outreach Service. Available at https://www.health.qld.gov.au/abios/asp/what_is_abi.

Selected readings

Farrell, M. & Dempsey, J. (2014). *Smeltzer & Bare's textbook of medical-surgical nursing* (3rd Australian and New Zealand ed.). Sydney: Lippincott Williams & Wilkins.

Sparkes, L., Bassett, J. & Jacob, E. (2014). *Checklists for clinical nursing skills* (1st Australian and New Zealand ed.). Sydney: Lippincott Williams & Wilkins.

Online resources

Acquired Brain Injury Outreach Service Queensland: www.health.qld.gov.au/abios/

Australian and New Zealand Head & Neck Cancer Society: https://anzhncs.org

Australian Thyroid Foundation: https://www.thyroidfoundation.org.au

Brain Foundation: https://brainfoundation.org.au

Brain Injury Australia: https://www.braininjuryaustralia.org.au

Brain Injury Centre: http://www.braininjurycentre.com.au/

Brain Injury Rehabilitation Network New South Wales Agency for Clinical Innovation: https://www.aci.health.nsw.gov.au/networks/brain-injury-rehabilitation

Brain Injury New Zealand: https://www.brain-injury.nz/

Brain Injury South Australia: http://braininjurysa.org.au/

Headache Australia: http://headacheaustralia.org.au

Headway Brain Injury Auckland: https://www.headway.org.nz/

Headwest Western Australia: www.headwest.asn.au/

National Disability Insurance Scheme: www.ndis.gov.au/

Thyroid Australia: www.thyroidfoundation.org.au/

CHAPTER 17

Eyes

CASE STUDY

Mr Sami Nowra is a 41-year-old Aboriginal and Torres Strait Islander Australian who presents with a history of blurred vision in his right eye. His health history includes type 2 diabetes mellitus (not well controlled with diet or exercise) and mild hypertension (well controlled with medication). Mr Nowra is a director for a national Aboriginal and Torres Strait Islander film company and his work involves him spending a considerable amount of time using computers and digital equipment. Because his work involves a lot of screen and fine-print reading, his wife advised him to go to the health clinic for assessment.

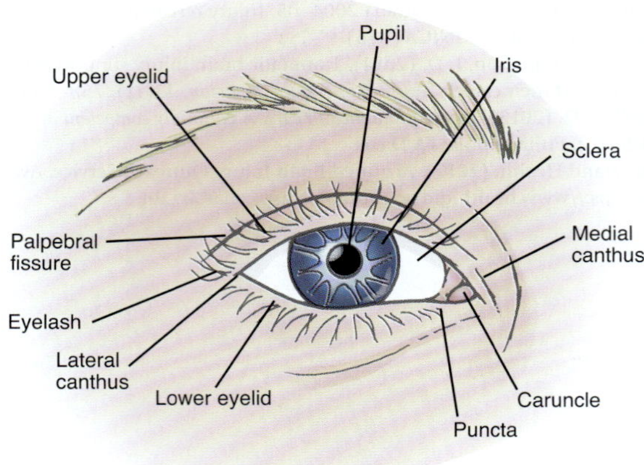

FIGURE 17-1 External structures of the eye.

Structure and function

The eye transmits visual stimuli to the brain for interpretation and, in doing so, functions as the organ of vision. The eyeball is located in the eye orbit, a round, bony hollow formed by several different bones of the skull. In the orbit, the eye is surrounded by a cushion of fat. The bony orbit and fat cushion protect the eyeball.

To perform a thorough assessment of the eye, you need a good understanding of the external structures of the eye, the internal structures of the eye, the visual fields and pathways, and the visual reflexes.

EXTERNAL STRUCTURES OF THE EYE

The eyelids (upper and lower) are two moveable structures composed of skin and two types of muscle: striated and smooth. Their purpose is to protect the eye from foreign bodies and limit the amount of light entering the eye. In addition, they serve to distribute tears that lubricate the surface of the eye (Fig. 17-1). The upper eyelid is larger, more mobile and contains *tarsal plates* made up of connective tissue. These plates contain the *meibomian glands,* which secrete an oily substance that lubricates the eyelid.

The eyelids join at two points: the lateral (outer) canthus and the medial (inner) canthus. The medial canthus contains the puncta, two small openings that allow drainage of tears into the lacrimal system, and the caruncle, a small, fleshy mass that contains sebaceous glands. The white space between open eyelids is called the palpebral fissure. When closed, the eyelids should touch. When open, the upper lid position should be between the upper margin of the iris and the upper margin of the pupil. The lower lid should rest on the lower border of the iris. No sclera should be seen above or below the limbus (the point where the sclera meets the cornea).

Eyelashes are projections of stiff hair curving outwards along the margins of the eyelids; they filter dust and dirt from air entering the eye.

The conjunctiva is a thin, transparent, continuous membrane that is divided into two portions: a *palpebral* portion and a *bulbar* portion. The palpebral conjunctiva lines the inside of the eyelids, and the bulbar conjunctiva covers most of the anterior eye, merging with the cornea at the limbus. The point at which the palpebral and bulbar conjunctivae meet creates a folded recess that allows movement of the eyeball. This transparent membrane allows for inspection of underlying tissue and serves to protect the eye from foreign bodies.

The lacrimal apparatus consists of glands and ducts that serve to lubricate the eye (Fig. 17-2). The *lacrimal gland,* located in the upper outer corner of the orbital cavity just above the eye, produces tears. As the lid blinks, tears wash across the eye, then drain into the *puncta,* which are visible on the upper and lower lids at the inner canthus. Tears empty into the *lacrimal canals* and are channelled into the *nasolacrimal sac* through the *nasolacrimal duct.* They drain into the nasal meatus.

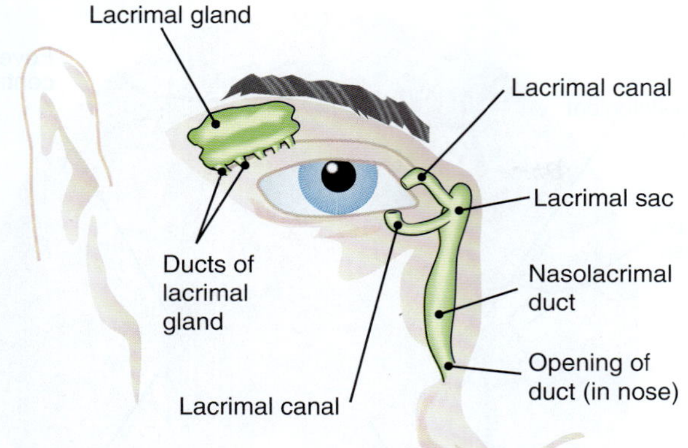

FIGURE 17-2 The lacrimal apparatus consists of tear (lacrimal) glands and ducts.

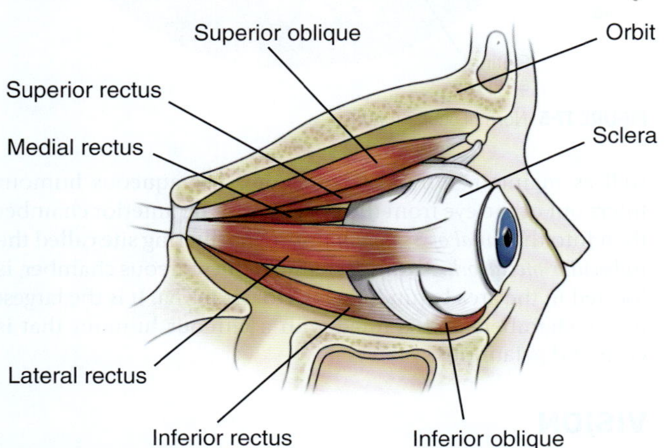

FIGURE 17-3 Extraocular muscles control the direction of eye movement. (Cohen, B. J. & Taylor, J. [2009]. Memmler's structure and function of the human body [9th ed.]. Philadelphia: Lippincott Williams & Wilkins.)

The extraocular muscles are the six muscles attached to the outer surface of each eyeball (Fig. 17-3). These muscles control six different directions of eye movement. Four rectus muscles are responsible for straight movement and two oblique muscles are responsible for diagonal movement. Each muscle coordinates with a muscle in the opposite eye. This allows for parallel movement of the eyes and thus the binocular vision characteristic of humans. Innervation for these muscles is supplied by three cranial nerves: the oculomotor (III), trochlear (IV) and abducens (VI).

INTERNAL STRUCTURES OF THE EYE

The eyeball is composed of three separate coats or layers (Fig. 17-4). The external layer consists of the sclera and cornea. The sclera is a dense, protective, white covering that physically supports the internal structures of the eye. It is continuous anteriorly with the transparent cornea (the 'window of the eye'). The cornea permits the entrance of light, which passes through the lens to the retina. It is well supplied with nerve endings, making it responsive to pain and touch.

CLINICAL TIP

Because of this sensory property, contact with a wisp of cottonwool stimulates a blink in both eyes known as the corneal reflex. This reflex is supported by the trigeminal nerve, which carries the afferent sensation into the brain, and the facial nerve, which carries the efferent message that stimulates the blink.

The middle layer contains both an anterior portion, which includes the iris and the ciliary body, and a posterior layer, which includes the *choroid*. The *ciliary body* consists of muscle tissue that controls the thickness of the lens, which must be adapted to focus on objects near and far away.

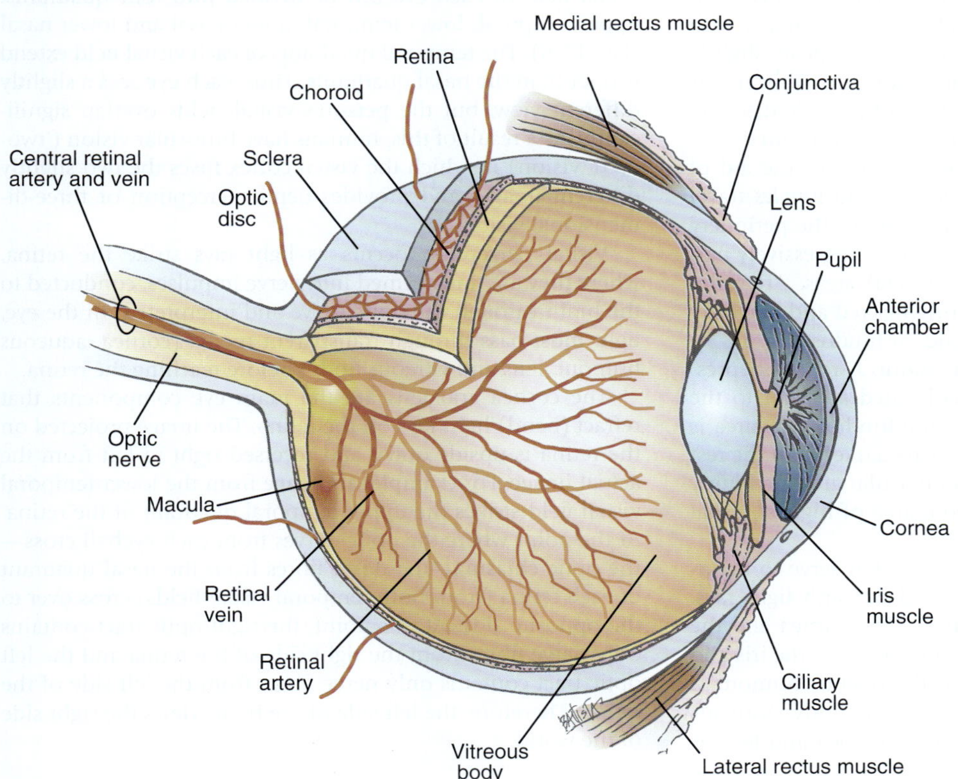

FIGURE 17-4 Anatomy of the eye.

The iris is a circular disc of muscle containing pigments that determine eye colour. The central aperture of the iris is called the pupil. Muscles in the iris adjust to control the pupil's size, which in turn controls the amount of light entering the eye. The muscle fibres of the iris also decrease the size of the pupil to accommodate for near vision and dilate the pupil when far vision is needed.

The lens is a biconvex, transparent, avascular, encapsulated structure located immediately posterior to the iris. Suspensory ligaments attached to the ciliary body support the position of the lens. The lens functions to refract (bend) light rays onto the retina. Adjustments must be made in refraction depending on the distance of the object being viewed. The refractive ability of the lens can be changed by a change in shape of the lens (which is controlled by the ciliary body). The lens bulges to focus on close objects and flattens to focus on far objects.

The chorioid layer contains the vascularity necessary to provide nourishment to the inner aspect of the eye and prevents light from reflecting internally. Anteriorly, it is continuous with the ciliary body and the iris.

The innermost layer, the retina, extends only to the ciliary body anteriorly. It receives visual stimuli and sends them to the brain. The retina consists of numerous layers of nerve cells, including the cells commonly called rods and cones. These specialised nerve cells are often referred to as 'photoreceptors' because they are responsive to light. The rods are highly sensitive to light, regulate black and white vision and function in dim light. The cones function in bright light and are sensitive to colour.

The optic disc is a cream-coloured, circular area located on the retina towards the medial or nasal side of the eye. It is where the optic nerve enters the eyeball. The optic disc can be seen with the use of an ophthalmoscope (an instrument used to magnify and examine the interior of the eye, including the lens, retina and optic nerve; this is an advanced skill so it is not directly addressed in this text, although it is covered in summary) and is normally round or oval in shape, with distinct margins. A smaller circular area that appears slightly depressed is referred to as the physiological cup. This area is approximately one-third the size of the entire optic disc and appears somewhat lighter or whiter than the disc borders.

The retinal vessels can be readily viewed with the aid of an ophthalmoscope. Four sets of *arterioles* and *venules* travel through the optic disc, bifurcate and extend to the periphery of the fundus. Vessels are dark red and grow progressively narrower as they extend out to the peripheral areas. Arterioles carry oxygenated blood and appear brighter red and narrower than the veins. The general background, or fundus (Fig. 17-5), varies in colour, depending on skin colour. A retinal depression known as the fovea centralis is located adjacent to the optic disc in the temporal section of the fundus. This area is surrounded by the macula, which appears darker than the rest of the fundus. The fovea centralis and macular area are highly concentrated with cones and form the area of highest visual resolution and colour vision.

The eyeball contains several chambers that serve to maintain structure, protect against injury and transmit light rays. The anterior chamber is located between the cornea and the iris, and the posterior chamber is the area between the iris and the lens. These chambers are filled with aqueous humour, a clear liquid substance produced by the ciliary body. Aqueous humour helps to cleanse and nourish the cornea and lens as well as maintain intraocular pressure. The aqueous humour filters out of the eye from the posterior to the anterior chamber then into the *canal of Schlemm* through a filtering site called the *trabecular meshwork*. Another chamber, the vitreous chamber, is located in the area behind the lens to the retina. It is the largest of the chambers and is filled with a vitreous humour that is clear and gelatinous.

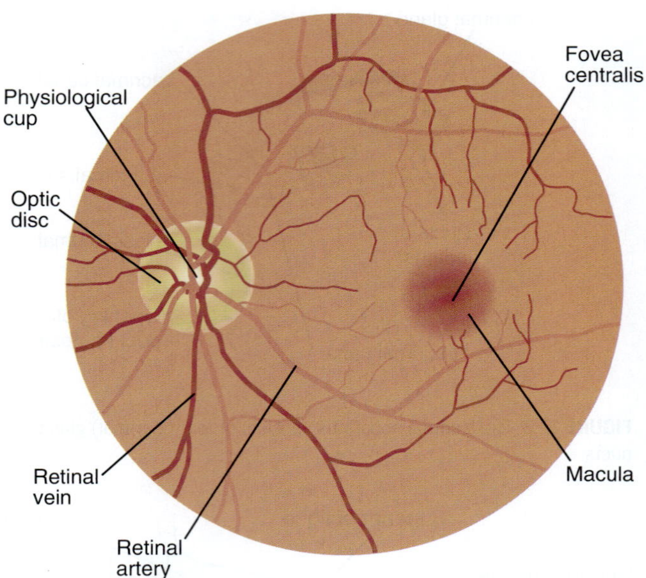

FIGURE 17-5 Normal ocular fundus.

VISION

Visual fields and visual pathways

A **visual field** refers to what a person sees with one eye. The visual field of each eye can be divided into four quadrants: upper temporal, lower temporal, upper nasal and lower nasal (Fig. 17-6). The temporal quadrants of each visual field extend further than the nasal quadrants. Thus, each eye sees a slightly different view, but the person's visual fields overlap significantly. As a result of this, humans have binocular vision ('two-eyed' vision) in which the visual cortex fuses the two slightly different images and provides depth perception or three-dimensional vision.

Visual perception occurs as light rays strike the retina, where they are transformed into nerve impulses, conducted to the brain through the optic nerve and interpreted. In the eye, light must pass through transparent media (cornea, aqueous humour, lens and vitreous body) before reaching the retina.

The cornea and lens are the main eye components that refract (bend) light rays on the retina. The image projected on the retina is upside down and reversed right to left from the actual image. For example, an image from the lower temporal visual field strikes the upper temporal quadrant of the retina. At the point where the optic nerves from each eyeball cross—the optic chiasma—the nerve fibres from the nasal quadrant of each retina (from both temporal visual fields) cross over to the opposite side. At this point, the right optic tract contains only nerve fibres from the right side of the retina and the left optic tract contains only nerve fibres from the left side of the retina. Therefore, the left side of the brain views the right side of the world.

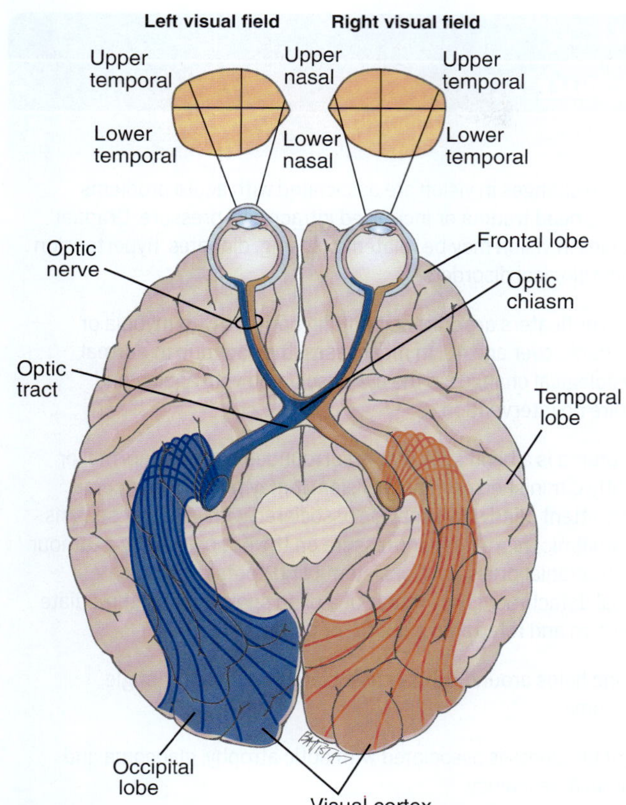

FIGURE 17-6 Visual fields and visual pathways. Each eye has a slightly different view of the same field. However, the views overlap significantly, which accounts for binocular vision.

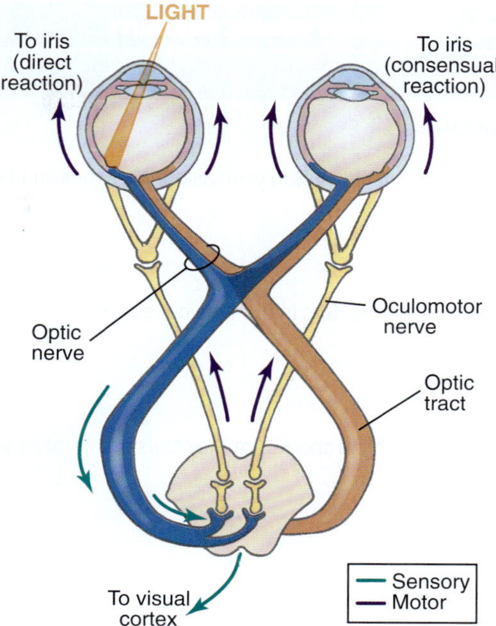

FIGURE 17-7 The pupils admit light that travels over the visual pathways. If a light focuses on only one eye, the pupil responds to ensure that the light needed for vision can enter but not so much that eye damage would result. The other pupil responds in the same manner. This phenomenon of direct pupillary response and consensual pupillary response is a reflex governed by the oculomotor nerve.

Visual reflexes

The pupillary light reflex causes pupils immediately to constrict when exposed to bright light. This can be seen as a *direct reflex*, in which constriction occurs in the eye exposed to the light, or as an *indirect or consensual reflex*, in which exposure to light in one eye results in constriction of the pupil in the opposite eye (Fig. 17-7). These protective reflexes, mediated by the oculomotor nerve, prevent damage to the delicate photoreceptors by excessive light.

Accommodation is a functional reflex allowing the eyes to focus on near objects. This is accomplished through movement of the ciliary muscles, which causes an increase in the curvature of the lens. This change in shape of the lens is not visible. However, convergence of the eyes and constriction of the pupils occur simultaneously and can be seen.

Health assessment

COLLECTING SUBJECTIVE DATA: THE NURSING HEALTH HISTORY

Beginning when the nurse first meets the patient, assessment of vision provides important information about the patient's ability to interact with the environment. Changes in vision are often gradual and go unrecognised by patients until a severe problem develops. Therefore, asking patients specific questions about their vision may help with early detection of disorders. With recent advances in medicine and surgery, early detection and intervention are increasingly important.

First, gather data from the patient about his or her current level of eye health. Also discuss any past problems and family history related to the eye. Collecting data concerning environmental influences on vision, as well as how any problems are influencing or affecting the patient's usual activities of daily living, is also important. Answers to these types of questions help to evaluate a patient's risk of vision loss and, in turn, present ways that the patient may modify or reduce the risk of eye problems.

CASE STUDY

You are talking with Mr Nowra about his concerns of blurred vision in his right eye. You recognise that this is the time to collect some subjective data.

CRITICAL THINKING

1. What specific questions would you ask Mr Nowra about his vision problem?
2. What questions would you ask to determine lifestyle alterations as a result of this problem?
3. What questions would help elicit a history for this problem?

Note: When considering specific questions to ask patients, be aware of common issues that may be attributed to the patient's background. For example, New Zealand Māori experience many of the same comorbidities as Aboriginal and Torres Strait Islander groups, such as hypertension, diabetes mellitus and eye infections like trachoma.

History of present health concern

QUESTION	RATIONALE
Visual problems	
Describe any recent changes in your vision. Were they sudden or gradual?	Sudden changes in vision are associated with acute problems such as head trauma or increased intracranial pressure. Gradual changes in vision may be related to ageing, diabetes, hypertension or neurological disorders.
Do you see spots or floaters in front of your eyes?	Spots or floaters are common among patients with myopia or in patients over age 40. In most cases, they are due to normal physiological changes in the eye associated with ageing and require no intervention.
Do you experience blind spots? Are they constant or intermittent?	A scotoma is a blind spot that is surrounded by either normal or slightly diminished peripheral vision. It may be from glaucoma. Intermittent blind spots may be associated with vascular spasms (ophthalmic migraines) or pressure on the optic nerve by a tumour or intracranial pressure. Consistent blind spots may indicate retinal detachment. Any report of a blind spot requires immediate attention and referral to a doctor or optometrist.
Do you see halos or rings around lights?	Seeing halos around lights is associated with narrow-angle glaucoma.
Do you have trouble seeing at night?	Night blindness is associated with optic atrophy, glaucoma and vitamin A deficiency.
Do you experience double vision?	Double vision (diplopia) may indicate increased intracranial pressure due to injury or a tumour.
Other symptoms	
Do you have any eye pain or itching? Describe.	Burning or itching pain is usually associated with allergies or superficial irritation. Throbbing, stabbing or deep, aching pain suggests a foreign body in the eye or changes within the eye. Most common eye disorders are not associated with actual pain; therefore, any reported eye pain should be referred immediately.
Do you have any redness or swelling in your eyes?	Redness or swelling of the eye is usually related to an inflammatory response caused by allergy, foreign body or bacterial or viral infection.
Do you experience excessive watering or tearing of the eye? One eye or both eyes?	Excessive tearing (epiphora) is caused by exposure to irritants or obstruction of the lacrimal apparatus. Unilateral epiphora is often associated with foreign body or obstruction. Bilateral epiphora is often associated with exposure to irritants, such as makeup or facial cleansers, or it may be a systemic response.
Have you had any eye discharge? Describe.	Discharge other than tears from one or both eyes suggests a bacterial or viral infection.

Past health history

QUESTION	RATIONALE
Have you ever had problems with your eyes or vision?	A history of eye problems or changes in vision provides clues to the current health of the eye.
Have you ever had eye surgery?	Surgery may alter the appearance of the eye and the results of future examinations.
Describe any past treatments you have received for eye problems (medication, surgery, laser treatments, corrective lenses). Were these successful? Were you satisfied?	Patient may not be satisfied with past treatments for vision problems.

COLDSPA

Example for eye pain

Use the COLDSPA mnemonic as a guideline to collect needed information for each symptom the patient shares. In addition, the following questions help elicit important information. Refer to Chapter 8 for further details of how to conduct a comprehensive pain assessment.

Mnemonic	Question	Patient response example
Character	Describe the sign or symptom (feeling, appearance, sound, smell or taste, if applicable).	'My right eye really hurts.'
Onset	When did it begin?	'A couple of hours ago, when I accidentally poked my key in my eye.'
Location	Where is it? Does it radiate? Does it occur anywhere else?	'Only my right eye.'
Duration	How long does it last? Does it recur?	'It hurts constantly.'
Severity	How bad is it? or How much does it bother you?	'It makes it difficult to drive and is quite painful.'
Pattern	What makes it better or worse?	'It hurts when I blink and feels better if I keep my eye shut.'
Associated factors/How it **A**ffects the patient	What other symptoms occur with it? How does it affect you?	'My right eye is watery and my vision is blurry.'

Family history

QUESTION	RATIONALE
Is there a history of eye problems or vision loss in your family?	Many eye disorders have familial tendencies. Examples include glaucoma, refraction errors and allergies.

Lifestyle and health practices

QUESTION	RATIONALE
Are you exposed to conditions or substances in the workplace or home that may harm your eyes or vision (e.g. chemicals, fumes, smoke, dust or flying sparks)? Do you wear safety glasses during exposure to harmful substances?	Injuries or diseases may be related to exposure in the workplace or home. These problems can be minimised or avoided altogether with hazard identification and implementation of safety measures.
Do you wear sunglasses during exposure to the sun?	Exposure to ultraviolet radiation puts the patient at risk of the development of cataracts (opacities of the lenses of the eyes; see Promote health—Cataracts, glaucoma and age-related macular degeneration). Consistent use of sunglasses during exposure minimises the patient's risk.
What types of medications do you take?	Some medications, such as corticosteroids, lovastatin, pyridostigmine bromide, quinidine, risperidone and rifampicin, have ocular side effects.
Has your vision loss affected your ability to care for yourself? To work?	Vision problems may interfere with the patient's ability to perform usual activities of daily living. The patient may be unable to read medication labels or fill insulin syringes. If the vision problem is severe, the patient's ability to perform hygiene practices or prepare food may be affected. Vision problems may affect a patient's ability to work if the job is one that depends on sight, such as pilot or bus driver.

Continued on following page

Lifestyle and health practices (continued)

QUESTION	RATIONALE
When was your last eye examination?	A thorough eye examination is recommended for healthy patients every 2 years. Patients with eye disorders or vision problems should be examined more frequently according to their optometrist's recommendations.
Do you have a prescription for corrective lenses (glasses or contacts)? Do you wear them regularly? If you wear contacts, how long do you wear them? How do you clean them?	The amount of time the patient wears the corrective lenses provides information on the severity of the visual problem. Patients who do not wear the prescribed corrective lenses are susceptible to eye strain. Improper cleaning or prolonged wearing of contact lenses can lead to infection and corneal damage.

PROMOTE HEALTH **CATARACTS, GLAUCOMA AND AGE-RELATED MACULAR DEGENERATION**

OVERVIEW

Cataracts are the leading cause of blindness worldwide, followed by glaucoma. Part of the ViSiON 2020 Global initiative of the World Health Organization (WHO) is devoted to reducing cataract, glaucoma and macular degeneration, which cause approximately 285 million people worldwide to be visually impaired (WHO, 2013).

A cataract is an opacity or clouding of the eye's lens. The opacity can develop in various parts of the lens. Glaucoma is a group of diseases that may begin with no symptoms but lead to vision loss through optic nerve damage. Glaucoma involves loss of retinal ganglion cells, causing optic neuropathy. Increased intraocular pressure is often but not always associated with glaucoma. Age-related macular degeneration is a group of diseases characterised by breakdown of the centre portion of the retina known as the macula.

Risk factors—cataracts

- Increasing age, especially over age 50
- Prolonged exposure to ultraviolet B (UV-B) light, especially in latitudes closer to the equator
- Diabetes mellitus
- Cigarette smoking
- Alcohol use
- Diet low in antioxidants, especially vitamins E and B
- High blood pressure
- Eye injury or surgery
- Steroid use
- Female gender

Risk factors—glaucoma

- Increased intraocular pressure (IOP)
- Age, usually over age 40
- Family history (genetics or similar environment)
- Race or ethnicity: Caucasian of northern European ancestry (pseudoexfoliative glaucoma); Asian (angle closure glaucoma); African (increased IOP, develops at an earlier age)
- Atherosclerosis
- Near or far sightedness (each predisposes to different type of glaucoma)

Risk factors—age-related macular degeneration

- Age (25% of those ages 65 to 74 and 33% of those over age 74)
- Cigarette smoking
- Female gender and early menopause
- High blood pressure or cardiovascular disease
- Diet high in mono- or polyunsaturated fats, or linoleic vegetable fats, especially those found in snack foods
- Prolonged sun exposure

Teach risk reduction tips

As many of the same causes result in these three eye diseases, preventive strategies overlap.

- Wear sunglasses and a hat in the sun (even on cloudy days; squinting does not eliminate ultraviolet light entering the eye).
- Wear protective eye equipment when appropriate.
- Quit smoking.
- Limit alcohol intake.
- Eat a diet high in antioxidant vitamins. Lutein and zeaxanthin are important nutrients for the macular and can be found in dark green leafy vegetables.
- Take a vitamin supplement of vitamin C (400 IU), vitamin E (15 IU), vitamin A (25,000 IU), zinc (80 mg) and copper (2 mg) if supported by your doctor.
- Avoid high fat intake, even monounsaturated fats.
- Eat fish (for macular degeneration in particular).
- Have eyes examined regularly (every 4 years for ages 40 to 65; every 1 to 2 years for those over age 65); new therapies have been developed to slow glaucoma if detected early.
- Seek medical care for the following symptoms:
  - Painless blurring of vision
  - Light sensitivity
  - Poor night vision
  - Double vision in one eye
  - Need for brighter light to read
  - Fading or yellowing of colours.

Centre for Eye Research Australia, 2014a, 2014b, 2014c.

COLLECTING OBJECTIVE DATA: PHYSICAL EXAMINATION

The purpose of the eye and vision examination is to identify any changes in vision or signs of eye disorders in an effort to initiate early treatment or corrective procedures. Collected objective data should include assessment of eye function through specific vision tests, inspection of the external eye and inspection of the internal eye using an ophthalmoscope.

For the most part, inspection and palpation of the external eye are straightforward and simple to perform. The vision tests and use of the ophthalmoscope require a great deal of skill, and thus practice, for the examiner to be capable and confident during the examination. It is a good idea for the beginning examiner to practise on friends, family or colleagues to gain experience and to become comfortable performing the examinations. However, use of an ophthalmoscope is an advanced clinical skill and will be addressed as an overview in this text, not as a detailed clinical skill.

Preparing the patient

Explain each vision test thoroughly to guarantee accurate results. For the eye examination, position the patient so that he or she is seated comfortably. An experienced examiner will move very close to the patient's face during examination of the internal eye with the ophthalmoscope to view the retina and internal structures. You will need to explain to the patient that this may be slightly uncomfortable, and explain in detail what you are doing and answer any questions the patient may have.

Equipment

- Snellen or E chart
- Hand-held Snellen card or near vision screener
- Penlight
- Opaque cards
- Disposable gloves (wear as needed to prevent spreading infection or coming into contact with exudate)
- Ophthalmoscope (outlined in Equipment spotlight 17-1; however, as this instrument is used for advanced eye assessment, an overview only is provided in this chapter).

Physical assessment

Before performing eye examination, review and recognise structures and functions of the eyes. While performing the examination, remember these key points:

- Perform vision tests competently and record the results
- Recognise and distinguish normal variations from abnormal findings (be aware that some variations will be readily apparent with the initial observation or inspection component of your physical assessment, for example, hyphaema, where red blood cells collect in the lower half of the anterior chamber following blunt trauma (Fig. 17-8).

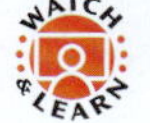

Physical assessment: Assessing the eyes

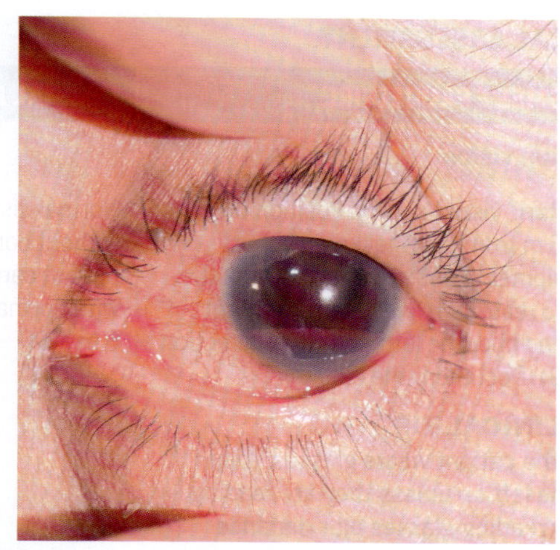

FIGURE 17-8 Hyphaemia. (Shutterstock.com/ARZTSAMUI.)

CASE STUDY

Over the last 2 months Mr Nowra reports experiencing increasing difficultly undertaking work because of vision problems. He states, 'It's getting harder to see the detail on the screen when reviewing and editing the film, especially when it's dark or the film is a night scene. After working for a couple of hours I get a headache over my right eye.' On examination he had a visual acuity of 6/9 in the right eye and 6/6 in the left eye. The lens in the right eye shows a small white opacity, and the left eye appears normal.

CRITICAL THINKING

4. Physical assessment for visual problems needs to be quite focused. How would you undertake a physical assessment for Mr Nowra's eyes?

EQUIPMENT SPOTLIGHT 17-1 OPHTHALMOSCOPE: TOOLS FOR ADVANCED CLINICIANS

Inspection of the internal eye structures is an advanced clinical skill. Although not used by the novice practitioner, the ophthalmoscope is a hand-held instrument that allows the examiner to view the fundus of the eye by the projection of light through a prism that bends the light 90 degrees. There are several lenses arranged on a wheel that affect the focus on objects in the eye. The examiner can rotate the lenses with his or her index finger. Each lens is labelled with a negative or positive number, a unit of strength called a diopter. Red numbers indicate a negative diopter and are used for myopic (nearsighted) patients. Black numbers indicate a positive diopter and are used for hyperopic (farsighted) patients. The zero lens is used if neither the examiner nor the patient has refractive errors.

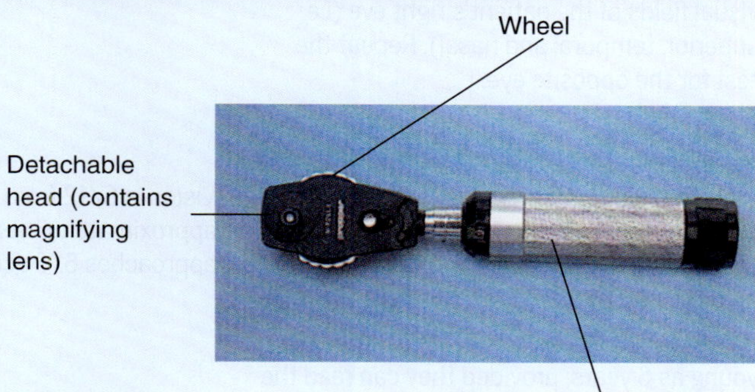

PHYSICAL ASSESSMENT

ASSESSMENT PROCEDURE	NORMAL FINDINGS	ABNORMAL FINDINGS
Evaluating vision		
Test distant visual acuity. Position the patient 6 m from the Snellen or E chart (see Equipment spotlight 17-2) and ask the patient to read each line until the patient cannot decipher the letters or their direction (Fig. 17-9). Document the results. **CLINICAL TIP** **If the patient wears glasses, they should be left on unless they are reading glasses (reading glasses blur distance vision).** During this vision test, note any patient behaviours (i.e. leaning forward, head tilting or squinting) that could be unconscious attempts to see better.	Normal distant visual acuity is 6/6 with or without corrective lenses. This means the patient can distinguish what the person with normal vision can distinguish from 6 m away.	*Myopia* (impaired far vision) is present when the second number in the test result is larger than the first (6/12). The higher the second number, the poorer the vision. A patient is considered legally blind when vision in the better eye with corrective lenses is 6/60 or less. Any patient with vision worse than 6/9 should be referred for further evaluation.
Test near visual acuity. Use this test for middle-aged patients and others who complain of difficulty reading. Give the patient a hand-held vision chart (e.g. Jaeger reading card, Snellen card or comparable chart) to hold 35 cm from the eyes. Have the patient cover one eye with an opaque card before reading from top (largest print) to bottom (smallest print). Repeat test for other eye. **CLINICAL TIP** **The patient who wears glasses should keep them on for this test.**	Normal near visual acuity is 35/35 (with or without corrective lenses). This means the patient can read what the normal eye can read from a distance of 35 cm.	*Presbyopia* (impaired near vision) is indicated when the patient moves the chart away from the eyes to focus on the print. It is caused by decreased accommodation. 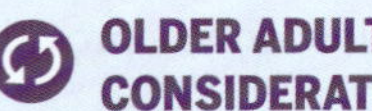 **OLDER ADULT CONSIDERATIONS** **Presbyopia is a common condition in patients over age 45.**
Test visual fields for gross peripheral vision. To perform the confrontation test, position yourself approximately 60 cm away from the patient at eye level. Have the patient cover his or her left eye while you cover your right eye. Look directly at each other with your uncovered eyes. Next fully extend your left arm at midline and slowly move one finger (or a pencil) upwards from below until the patient sees your finger (or pencil) (Fig. 17-10). Test the remaining three visual fields of the patient's right eye (i.e. superior, temporal and nasal). Repeat the test for the opposite eye.	With normal peripheral vision, the patient should see the examiner's finger at the same time the examiner sees it. Normal visual field degrees are approximately as follows: Inferior: 70 degrees Superior: 50 degrees Temporal: 90 degrees Nasal: 60 degrees	A delayed or absent perception of the examiner's finger indicates reduced peripheral vision (Abnormal findings 17-1). The patient should be referred for further evaluation.
PAEDIATRIC EXAMINATION		
Place the older infant, preschool, school-age or adolescent patient on the examination table. The younger infant or toddler can be held by the carer. Use the adult Snellen chart for children as young as 6 years, provided they can read the alphabet. The E chart is used for a patient over age 3 years or any child who cannot read the alphabet.	Vision is 6/12 from ages 2 to approximately 6 years, whereby it approaches 6/6 acuity.	The child should be referred to an opthamologist when results are: 6/12 or greater in a child age 3 years; 6/9 or greater in a child 6 years or older; vary by two or more lines between eyes.

EQUIPMENT SPOTLIGHT 17-2 VISION CHARTS

Snellen chart

Used to test distant visual acuity, the Snellen chart consists of lines of different letters stacked one on top of the other. The letters are large at the top and decrease in size from top to bottom. The chart is placed on a wall or door at eye level in a well-lighted area. The patient stands 6 m from the chart and covers one eye with an opaque card (which prevents the patient from peeking through the fingers). Then the patient reads each line of letters until he or she can no longer distinguish them.

E chart

If the patient cannot read or has a disability that prevents verbal communication, the E chart is used. The E chart is configured just like the Snellen chart but the characters on it are only Es, which face in all directions. The patient is asked to indicate by pointing which way the open side of the E faces. If the patient wears glasses, they should be left on, unless they are reading glasses (reading glasses blur distance vision).

Test results

Acuity results are recorded somewhat like blood pressure readings—in a manner that resembles a fraction (but in no way is interpreted as a fraction). A common example of an acuity test score is 6/6. The top, or first, number is always 6, indicating the distance from the patient to the chart. The bottom, or second, number refers to the last full line the patient could read. Usually the last line on the chart is the 6/6 line. The examiner needs to document whether the patient wore glasses during the test. If any letters on a line are missed, encourage the patient to continue reading until he or she cannot distinguish any letters, but record the number of letters missed by using a minus sign. If the patient missed two letters on the 6/9 line, the recorded score would be 6/9 –2.

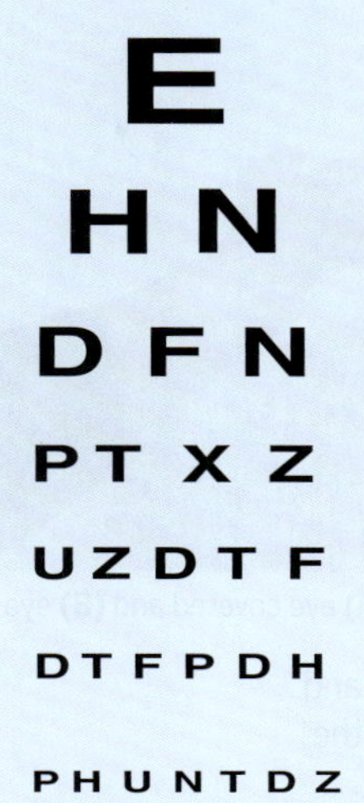

Snellen chart.

E chart.

PHYSICAL ASSESSMENT (continued)

ASSESSMENT PROCEDURE	NORMAL FINDINGS	ABNORMAL FINDINGS
Testing extraocular muscle function		
Perform corneal light reflex test. This test assesses parallel alignment of the eyes. Hold a penlight approximately 30 cm from the patient's face. Shine the light towards the bridge of the nose while the patient stares straight ahead. Note the light reflected on the corneas.	The reflection of light on the corneas should be in the exact same spot on each eye, which indicates parallel alignment.	Asymmetrical position of the light reflex indicates deviated alignment of the eyes. This may be due to muscle weakness or paralysis (see Abnormal findings 17-2).

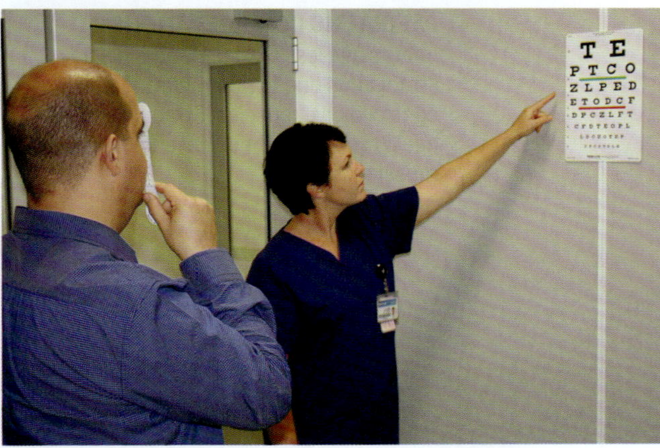

FIGURE 17-9 Testing distant visual acuity.

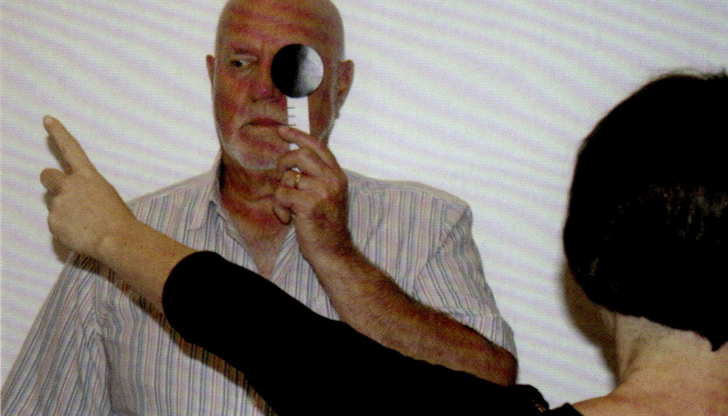

FIGURE 17-10 Performing confrontation test to assess visual fields.

ASSESSMENT PROCEDURE	NORMAL FINDINGS	ABNORMAL FINDINGS
Perform cover test. The cover test detects deviation in alignment or strength and slight deviations in eye movement by interrupting the fusion reflex that normally keeps the eyes parallel.	The uncovered eye should remain fixed straight ahead. The covered eye should remain fixed straight ahead after being uncovered.	The uncovered eye will move to establish focus when the opposite eye is covered. When the covered eye is uncovered, movement to re-establish focus occurs. Either of these findings indicates a deviation in alignment of the eyes and muscle weakness (see Abnormal findings 17-2).

Continued on following page

PHYSICAL ASSESSMENT (continued)

ASSESSMENT PROCEDURE	NORMAL FINDINGS	ABNORMAL FINDINGS

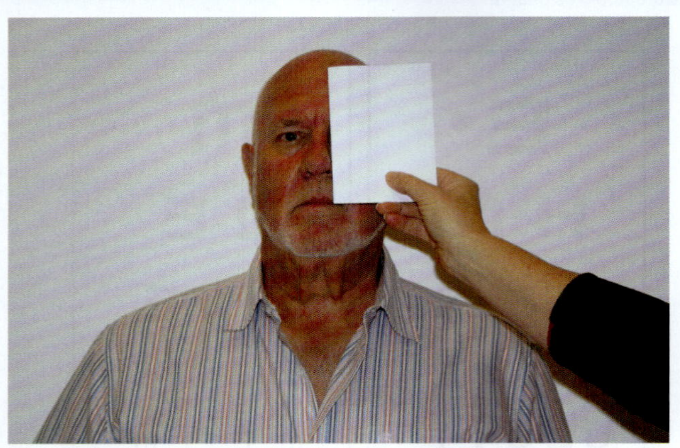

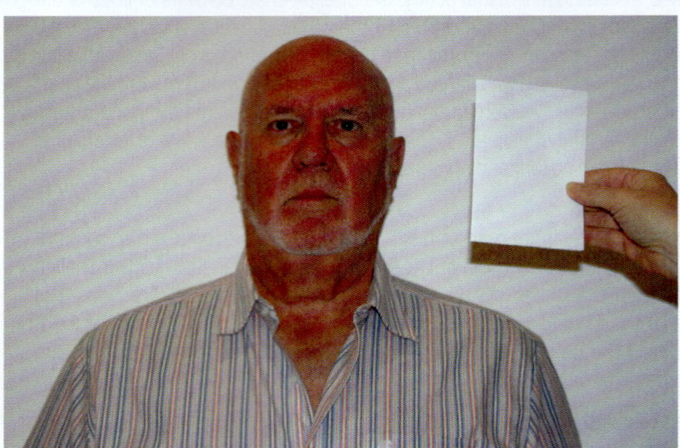

FIGURE 17-11 Performing cover test with **(A)** eye covered and **(B)** eye uncovered.

ASSESSMENT PROCEDURE	NORMAL FINDINGS	ABNORMAL FINDINGS
Ask the patient to stare straight ahead and focus on a distant object. Cover one of the patient's eyes with an opaque card (Fig. 17-11). As you cover the eye, observe the uncovered eye for movement. Now remove the opaque card and observe the previously covered eye for any movement. Repeat test on the opposite eye.		*Phoria* is a term used to describe misalignment that occurs only when fusion reflex is blocked. *Strabismus* is constant malalignment of the eyes. *Tropia* is a specific type of misalignment: *esotropia* is an inward turn of the eye, and *exotropia* is an outward turn of the eye.
Perform the positions test. This test assesses eye muscle strength and cranial nerve function. Instruct the patient to focus on an object you are holding (approximately 30 cm from the patient's face). Move the object through the six cardinal positions of gaze in a clockwise direction and observe the patient's eye movements (Fig. 17-12).	Eye movement should be smooth and symmetrical throughout all six directions.	Failure of eyes to follow movement symmetrically in any or all directions indicates a weakness in one or more extraocular muscles or dysfunction of the cranial nerve that innervates the particular muscle (see Abnormal findings 17-2). *Nystagmus,* an oscillating (shaking) movement of the eye may be associated with an inner ear disorder, multiple sclerosis, brain lesions or narcotics use. **PAEDIATRIC CONSIDERATIONS** Infants age less than 6 months display strabismus due to poor neuromuscular control of eye muscles. Strabismus after age 6 months is abnormal and indicates muscle weakness.

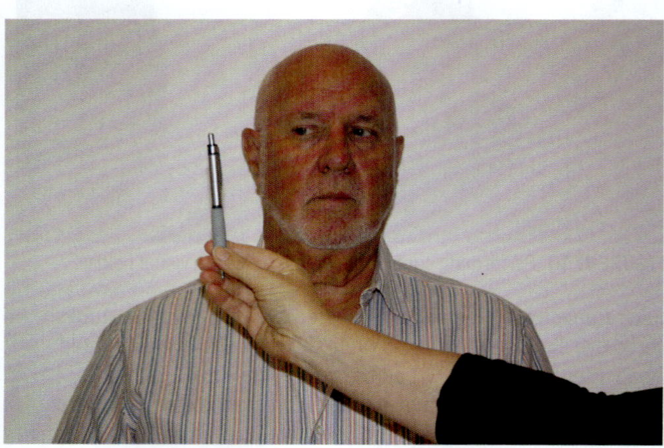

FIGURE 17-12 Performing positions test.

PHYSICAL ASSESSMENT (continued)

ASSESSMENT PROCEDURE	NORMAL FINDINGS	ABNORMAL FINDINGS
External eye structures		
INSPECTION AND PALPATION		
Inspect the eyelids and eyelashes.		
Note width and position of palpebral fissures.	The upper lid margin should be between the upper margin of the iris and the upper margin of the pupil. The lower lid margin rests on the lower border of the iris. No white sclera is seen above or below the iris. Palpebral fissures may be horizontal.	Drooping of the upper lid, called ptosis, may be attributed to oculomotor nerve damage, myasthenia gravis, weakened muscle or tissue or a congenital disorder (see Abnormal findings 17-3). Retracted lid margins, which allow for viewing of the sclera when the eyes are open, suggest hyperthyroidism.
Assess ability of eyelids to close.	The upper and lower lids close easily and meet completely when closed.	Failure of lids to close completely puts patient at risk of corneal damage.
Note the position of the eyelids in comparison with the eyeballs. Also note any unusual: • Turnings • Colour • Swelling • Lesions • Discharge.	The lower eyelid is upright with no inward or outward turning. Eyelashes are evenly distributed and curve outwards along the lid margins. Xanthelasma, raised yellow plaques located most often near the inner canthus, are a normal variation associated with increasing age and high lipid levels.	An inverted lower lid is a condition called an *entropion*, which may cause pain and injure the cornea as the eyelash brushes against the conjunctiva and cornea. *Ectropion*, an everted lower eyelid, results in exposure and drying of the conjunctiva. Both conditions (see Abnormal findings 17-3) interfere with normal tear drainage. **OLDER ADULT CONSIDERATIONS** **Though usually abnormal, entropion and ectropion are common in older patients.**
Observe for redness, swelling, discharge or lesions.	Skin on both eyelids is without redness, swelling or lesions.	Redness and crusting along the lid margins suggest seborrhoea or blepharitis, an infection caused by *Staphylococcus aureus*. Hordeolum (stye), a hair follicle infection, causes local redness, swelling and pain. A chalazion, an infection of the meibomian gland (located in the eyelid), may produce extreme swelling of the lid, moderate redness, but minimal pain (see Abnormal findings 17-3).
Observe the position and alignment of the eyeball in the eye socket.	Eyeballs are symmetrically aligned in sockets without protruding or sinking.	Protrusion of the eyeballs accompanied by retracted eyelid margins is termed *exophthalmos* (see Abnormal findings 17-3) and is characteristic of Graves disease (a type of hyperthyroidism). A sunken appearance of the eyes may be seen with severe dehydration or chronic wasting illnesses.

Continued on following page

PHYSICAL ASSESSMENT (continued)

ASSESSMENT PROCEDURE	NORMAL FINDINGS	ABNORMAL FINDINGS
Inspect the bulbar conjunctiva and sclera. Have the patient keep his or her head straight while looking from side to side then up towards the ceiling (Fig. 17-13). Observe clarity, colour and texture.	Bulbar conjunctiva is clear, moist and smooth. Underlying structures are clearly visible. Sclera is white.	Generalised redness of the conjunctiva suggests *conjunctivitis* (pink eye). Areas of dryness are associated with allergies or trauma.
CULTURAL CONSIDERATIONS **Darker-skinned patients may have sclera with yellow or pigmented freckles.**	**OLDER ADULT CONSIDERATIONS** **Yellowish nodules on the bulbar conjunctiva are called pinguecula. These harmless nodules are common in older patients and appear first on the medial side of the iris and then on the lateral side.**	*Episcleritis* is a local, non-infectious inflammation of the sclera. The condition is usually characterised by either a nodular appearance or by redness with dilated vessels (see Abnormal findings 17-3).
Inspect the palpebral conjunctiva. **CLINICAL TIP** **This procedure is stressful and uncomfortable for the patient. It is usually only done if the patient complains of pain or 'something in the eye.'**		
Put on gloves for this assessment procedure. First inspect the palpebral conjunctiva of the lower eyelid by placing your thumbs bilaterally at the level of the lower bony orbital rim and gently pulling down to expose the palpebral conjunctiva (Fig. 17-14). Avoid pressuring the eye. Ask the patient to look up as you observe the exposed areas.	The lower and upper palpebral conjunctivae are clear and free of swelling or lesions.	Cyanosis of the lower lid suggests a heart or lung disorder.

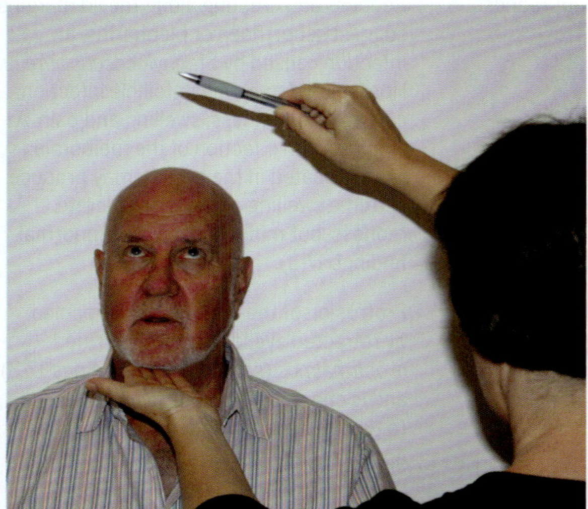

FIGURE 17-13 Inspecting the bulbar conjunctiva.

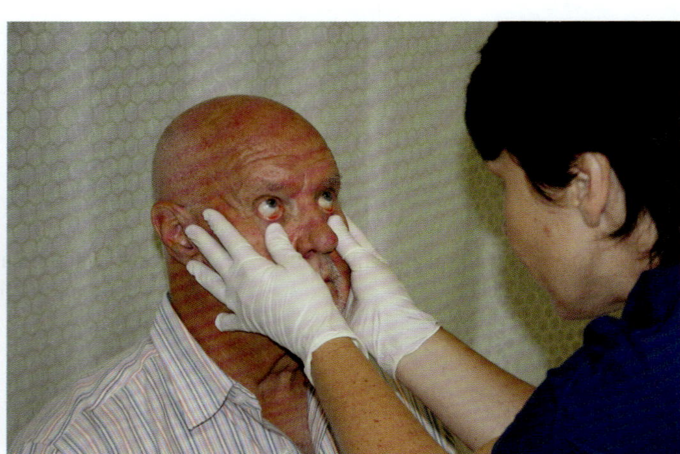

FIGURE 17-14 Inspecting palpebral conjunctiva: lower eyelid.

ASSESSMENT PROCEDURE	NORMAL FINDINGS	ABNORMAL FINDINGS
External eye structures (continued)		

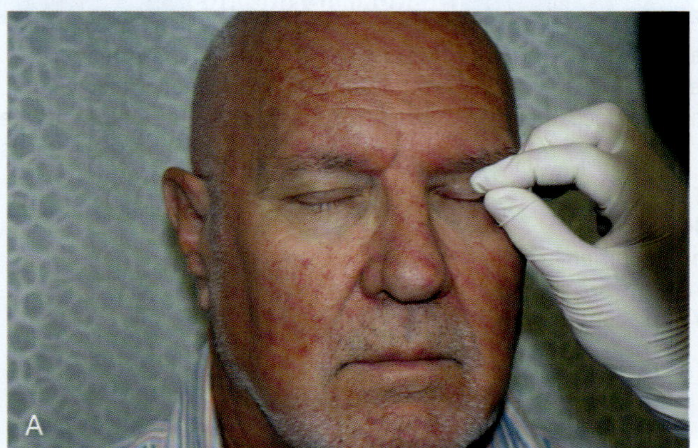

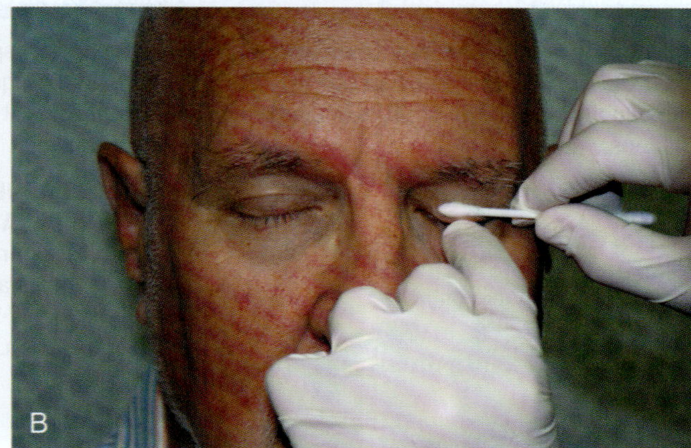

FIGURE 17-15 Everting the upper eyelid.

ASSESSMENT PROCEDURE	NORMAL FINDINGS	ABNORMAL FINDINGS
Evert the upper eyelid. Ask the patient to look down with their eyes slightly open. Gently grasp the patient's upper eyelashes and pull the lid downwards (Fig. 17-15A). Place a cotton bud approximately 1 cm above the eyelid margin and push down with the applicator while still holding the eyelashes (Fig. 17-15B). Hold the eyelashes against the upper ridge of the bony orbit just below the eyebrow, to maintain the everted position of the eyelid. Examine the palpebral conjunctiva for swelling, foreign bodies or trauma. Return the eyelid to normal by moving the lashes forward and asking the patient to look up and blink. The eyelid should return to normal.	Palpebral conjunctiva is free of swelling, foreign bodies or trauma.	A foreign body or lesion may cause irritation, burning, pain swelling of the upper eyelid.
Inspect the lacrimal apparatus. Assess the areas over the lacrimal glands (lateral aspect of upper eyelid) and the puncta (medial aspect of lower eyelid).	No swelling or redness should appear over areas of the lacrimal gland. The puncta is visible without swelling or redness and is turned slightly towards the eye.	Swelling of the lacrimal gland may be visible in the lateral aspect of the upper eyelid. This may be caused by blockage, infection or an inflammatory condition. Redness or swelling around the puncta may indicate an infectious or inflammatory condition. Excessive tearing may indicate a nasolacrimal sac obstruction.
Palpate the lacrimal apparatus. Put on disposable gloves to palpate the nasolacrimal duct to assess for blockage. Use one finger and palpate just inside the lower orbital rim (Fig. 17-16).	No drainage should be noted from the puncta when palpating the nasolacrimal duct.	Expressed drainage from the puncta on palpation occurs with duct blockage. **PAEDIATRIC CONSIDERATIONS** Lacrimal ducts should be patent by age 3 months. If a child is unable to produce tears at age 3 months, this is an abnormal finding.

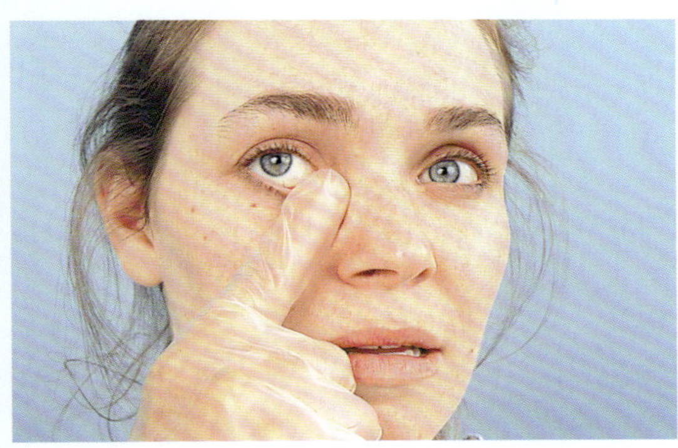

FIGURE 17-16 Palpating the lacrimal apparatus.
(© B. Proud.)

Continued on following page

PHYSICAL ASSESSMENT (continued)

ASSESSMENT PROCEDURE	NORMAL FINDINGS	ABNORMAL FINDINGS
Inspect the cornea and lens. Shine a light from the side of the eye for an oblique view. Look through the pupil to inspect the lens. 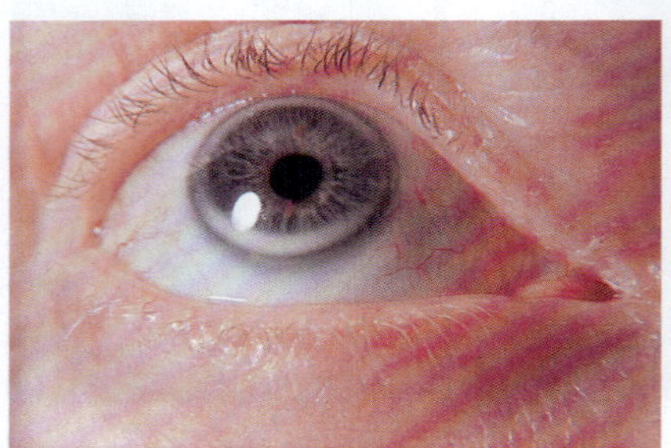 **FIGURE 17-17** Arcus senilis.	The cornea is transparent with no opacities. The oblique view shows a smooth and overall moist surface; the lens is free of opacities.  **OLDER ADULT CONSIDERATIONS** **Arcus senilis, a normal condition in older patients, appears as a white arc around the limbus (Fig. 17-17). The condition has no effect on vision.**	Areas of roughness or dryness on the cornea are often associated with injury or allergic responses. Opacities of the lens are seen with cataracts (see Abnormal findings 17-4).
Inspect the iris and pupil. Inspect shape and colour of iris and size and shape of pupil. Measure pupils against a gauge (Fig. 17-18) if they appear larger or smaller than normal or if they appear to be two different sizes. 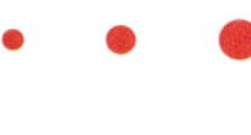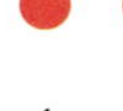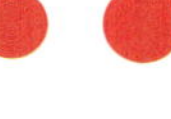 **FIGURE 17-18** Pupillary gauge measures pupils (dilation or constriction) in millimetres (mm).	The iris is typically round, flat and evenly coloured. The pupil, round with a regular border, is centred in the iris. Pupils are normally equal in size (3 to 5 mm). An inequality in pupil size of less than 0.5 mm occurs in 20% of patients. This condition, called *anisocoria,* is normal.	Typical abnormal findings include irregularly shaped irises, miosis, mydriasis and anisocoria. (For a description of these abnormalities and their implications, see Abnormal findings 17-5.) If the difference in pupil size changes throughout pupillary response tests, the inequality of size is abnormal.
Test pupillary reaction to light. Test for direct response by darkening the room and asking the patient to focus on a distant object. To test direct pupil reaction, shine a light obliquely into one eye and observe the pupillary reaction. Shining the light obliquely into the pupil and asking the patient to focus on an object in the distance ensures that pupillary constriction is a reaction to light and not a near reaction.	The normal direct pupillary response is constriction. **CLINICAL TIP** **Use a pupillary gauge to measure the constricted pupil. Then document the finding in a format similar to (but not) a fraction. The top (or first) number indicates the pupil's eye at rest, and the bottom (or second) number indicates the constricted size; for example, OS (left eye, *oculus sinister*) 3/2; OD (right eye, *oculus dexter*) 3/1.**	Monocular blindness can be detected when light directed to the blind eye results in no response in either pupil. When light is directed into the unaffected eye, both pupils constrict.
Assess consensual response at the same time as direct response by shining a light obliquely into one eye and observing the pupillary reaction in the opposite eye. **CLINICAL TIP** **When testing for consensual response, place your hand or another barrier to light (e.g. index card) between the patient's eyes to avoid an inaccurate finding.**	The normal consensual pupillary response is constriction.	Pupils do not react at all to direct and consensual pupillary testing.

PHYSICAL ASSESSMENT (continued)

ASSESSMENT PROCEDURE	NORMAL FINDINGS	ABNORMAL FINDINGS
External eye structures (continued)		
Test accommodation of pupils. Accommodation occurs when the patient moves his or her focus of vision from a distant point to a near object, causing the pupils to constrict. Hold your finger or a pencil about 30 to 38 cm from the patient. Ask the patient to focus on your finger or pencil and to remain focused on it as you move it closer in towards the eyes (Fig. 17-19).	The normal pupillary response is constriction of the pupils and convergence of the eyes when focusing on a near object (accommodation and convergence). 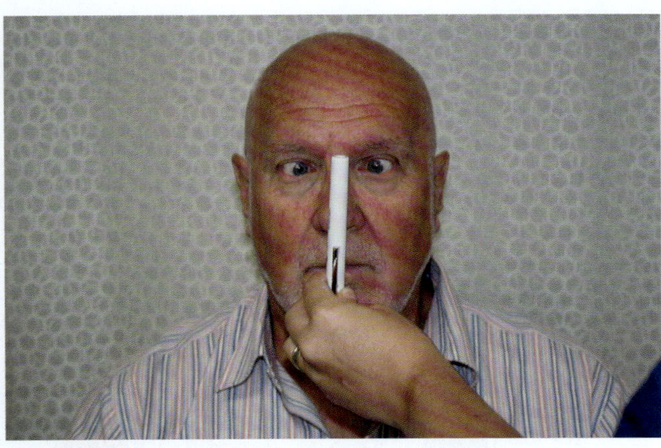 **FIGURE 17-19** Testing accommodation of pupils.	Pupils do not constrict; eyes do not converge.

CRITICAL THINKING

5. What aspects of eye assessment are vital for Mr Nowra's vision problem?
6. You identify concerns with Mr Nowra's assessment data. What approach will you take to assist Mr Nowra in accessing further assessment or management for his vision problem?

Sample of subjective data

Patient denies recent changes in vision. Denies excessive tearing, redness, swelling or pain in eyes. Denies spots, floaters or blind spots. States no problem with seeing at night. No previous eye surgeries. No family history of eye problems. Denies exposure to conditions or substances that harm the eyes. Mostly wears sunglasses when exposed to sunlight. Does not wear corrective lenses. Last eye examination was 1 year ago.

VALIDATING AND DOCUMENTING FINDINGS

Validate the eye assessment data that you have collected. This is necessary to verify that the data are reliable and accurate. Note that in documenting you may see vision separated into the right and left eye and referred to in the Latin terms of *oculus dexter* or OD (right eye) and *oculus sinister* or OS (left eye).

The following subjective and objective data samples do not relate specifically to Mr Nowra and are included as examples you can follow in practising data collection and documentation for Mr Nowra and other patients.

Sample of objective data

Acuity tested by Snellen chart: OD (right eye) 6/6, OS (left eye) 6/6. Visual fields full by confrontation. Corneal light reflex shows equal position of reflection. Eyes remain fixed throughout cover test. Extraocular movements smooth and symmetrical with no nystagmus. Eyelids in normal position with no abnormal widening or ptosis. No redness, discharge or crusting noted on lid margins. Conjunctiva and sclera appear moist and smooth. Sclera white with no lesions or redness. No swelling or redness over lacrimal gland; puncta is visible without swelling or redness; no drainage noted when nasolacrimal duct is palpated. Cornea is transparent, smooth and moist with no opacities; lens is free of opacities. Irises are round, flat and evenly coloured. Pupils are equal in size and reactive to light and accommodation. Pupils converge evenly.

ABNORMAL FINDINGS 17-1 Visual field defects

When a patient reports losing full or partial vision in one or both eyes, the nurse can usually anticipate a lesion as the cause. Some abnormal findings associated with visual field defects are illustrated here. The darker areas signify vision loss.

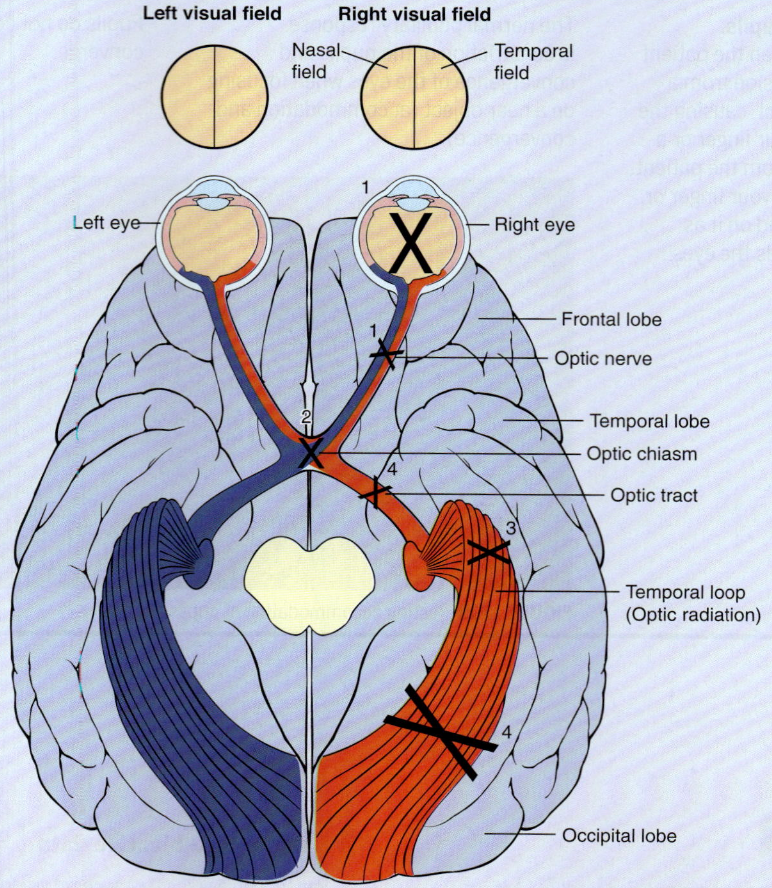

FINDING	POSSIBLE SOURCE	EXAMPLE *Left eye*	 *Right eye*
1. Unilateral blindness (e.g. blind right eye)	Lesion in (right) eye or (right) optic nerve		
2. Bitemporal hemianopia (loss of vision in both temporal fields)	Lesion of optic chiasm		
3. Left superior quadrant anopia or similar loss of vision (homonymous) in quadrant of each field	Partial lesion of temporal loop (optic radiation)		
4. Right visual field loss—right homonymous hemianopia or similar loss of vision in half of each field	Lesion in right optic tract or lesion in temporal loop (optic radiation)		

ABNORMAL FINDINGS 17-2 Extraocular muscle dysfunction

Abnormalities found during an assessment of extraocular muscle function are described below.

CORNEAL LIGHT REFLEX TEST ABNORMALITIES

Pseudostrabismus

Normal in young children, the pupils will appear at the inner canthus (because of the epicanthic fold).

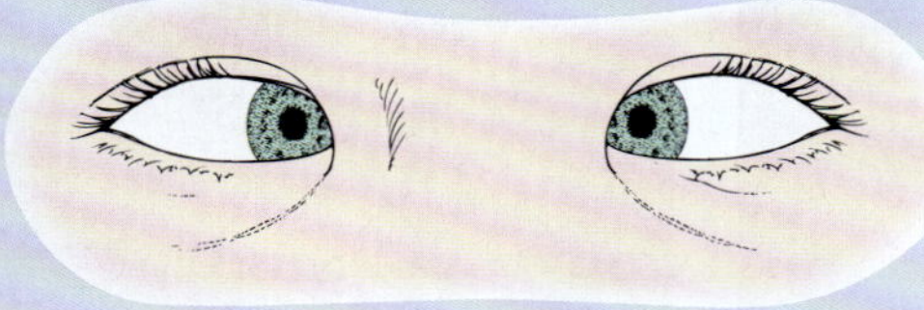

Strabismus (or tropia)

A constant malalignment of the eye axis, strabismus is defined according to the direction towards which the eye drifts and may cause amblyopia.

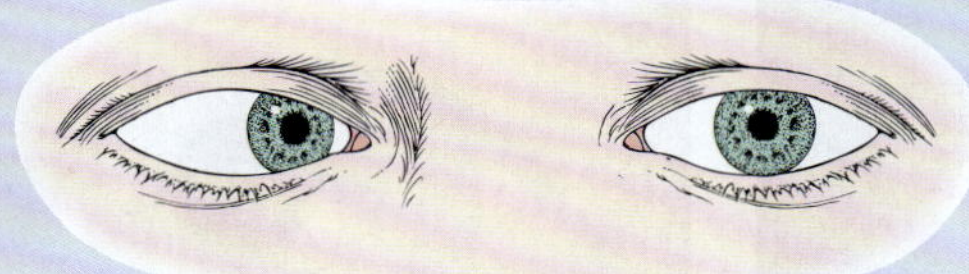

Esotropia (eye turns inwards).

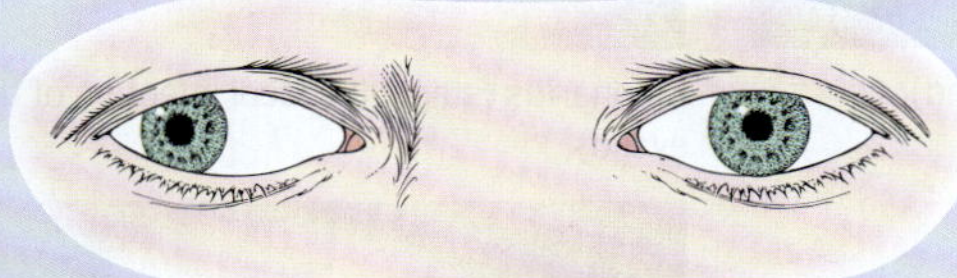

Exotropia (eye turns outwards).

COVER TEST ABNORMALITIES

Phoria (mild weakness)

Noticeable only with the cover test, phoria is less likely to cause amblyopia than strabismus. Esophoria is an inward drift and exophoria an outward drift of the eye.

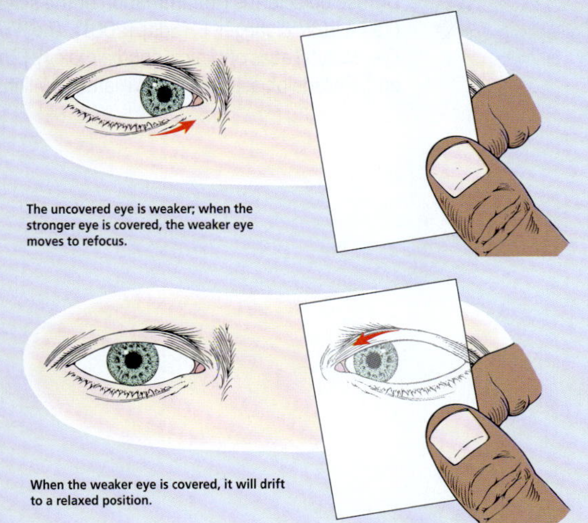

The uncovered eye is weaker; when the stronger eye is covered, the weaker eye moves to refocus.

When the weaker eye is covered, it will drift to a relaxed position.

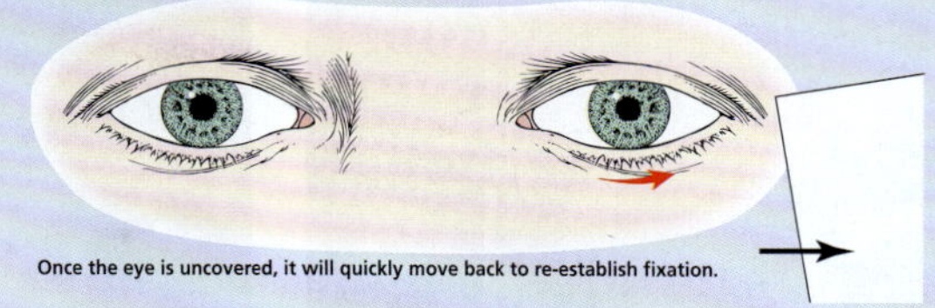

Once the eye is uncovered, it will quickly move back to re-establish fixation.

POSITIONS TEST ABNORMALITIES

Paralytic strabismus

Noticeable with the positions test, paralytic strabismus is usually the result of weakness or paralysis of one or more extraocular muscles. The nerve affected will be on the same side as the eye affected (for instance, a right eye paralysis is related to a right-side cranial nerve). The position in which the maximum deviation appears indicates the nerve involved.

Sixth nerve paralysis: The eye cannot look to the outer side.

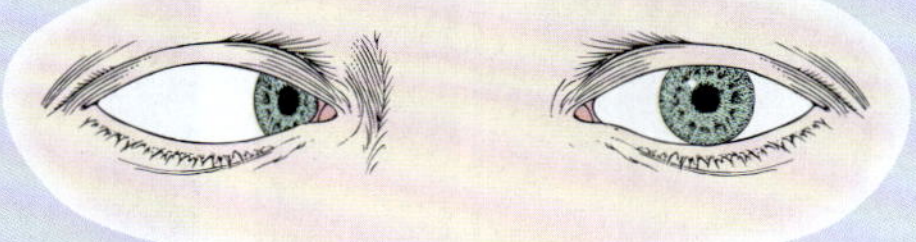

In left sixth nerve paralysis, the patient tries to look to the left. The right eye moves left, but the left eye cannot move left.

Fourth nerve paralysis: The eye cannot look down when turned inwards.

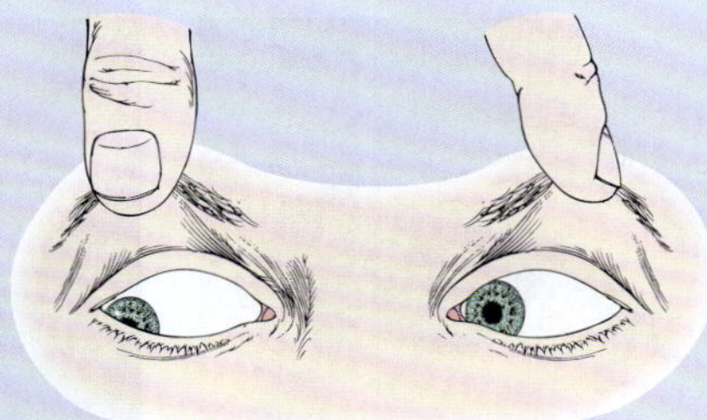

A patient with left fourth nerve paralysis looks down and to the right.

Third nerve paralysis: Upward, downward and inward movements are lost. Ptosis and pupillary dilation may also occur.

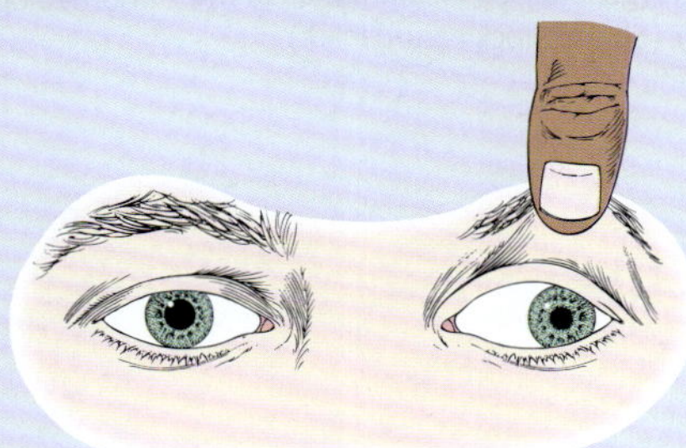

A patient with left third nerve paralysis looks straight ahead.

ABNORMAL FINDINGS 17-3 Abnormalities of the external eye

Some easily recognised abnormalities that affect the external eye are illustrated below.

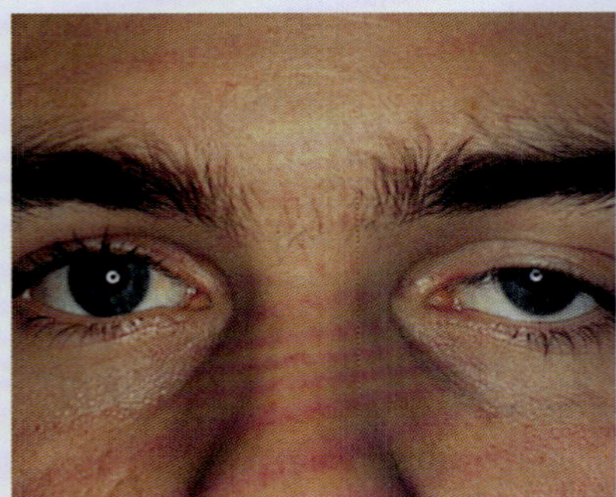

Ptosis (drooping eye).

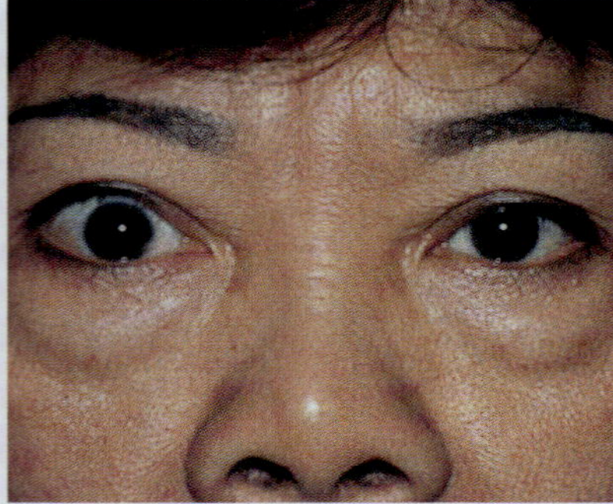

Exophthalmos (protruding eyeballs and retracted eyelids).

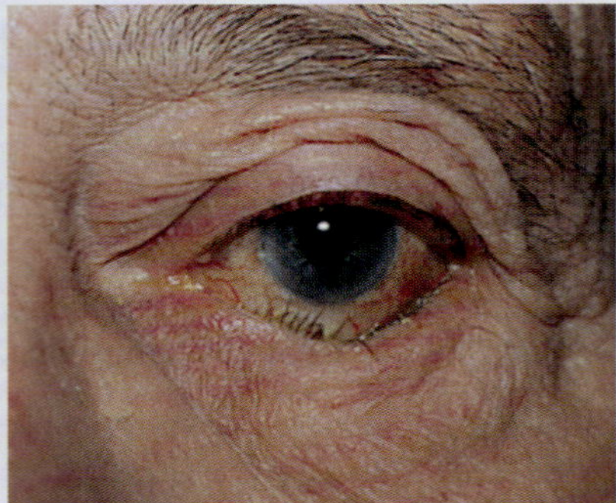

Entropion (inwardly turned lower eyelid).

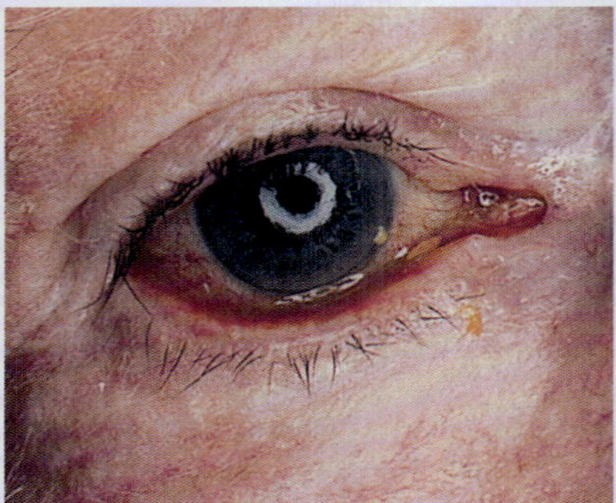

Ectropion (outwardly turned lower lid).

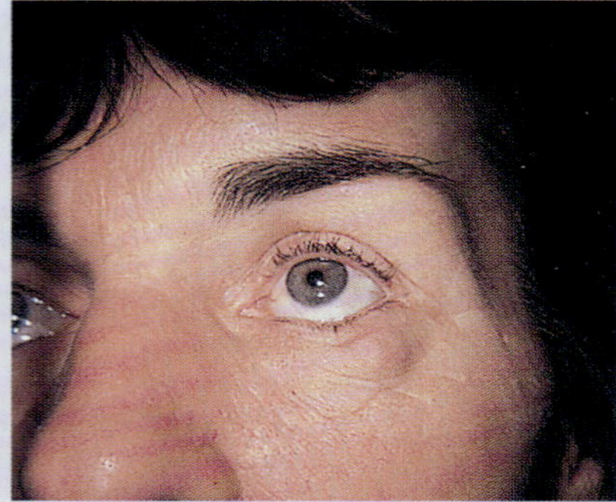

Chalazion (infected meibomian gland).

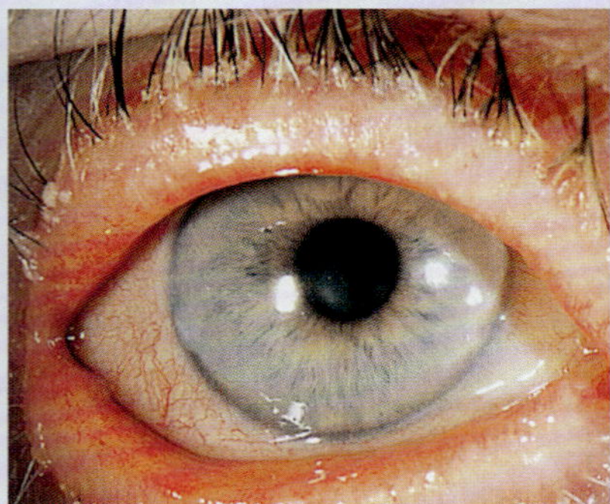

Blepharitis (staphylococcal infection of the eyelid).

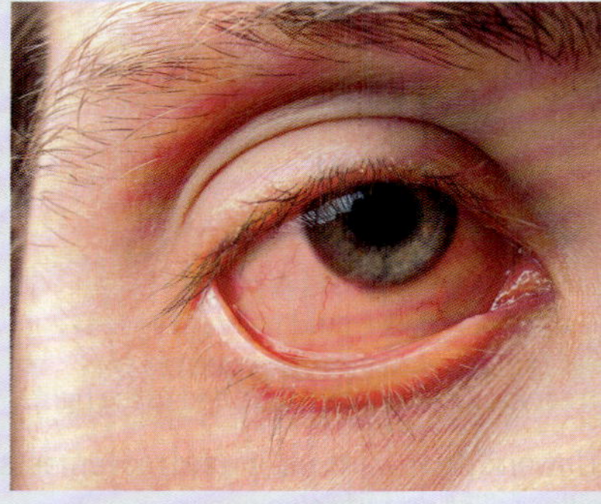

Conjunctivitis (generalised inflammation of the conjunctiva). (Shutterstock.com/daniiD.)

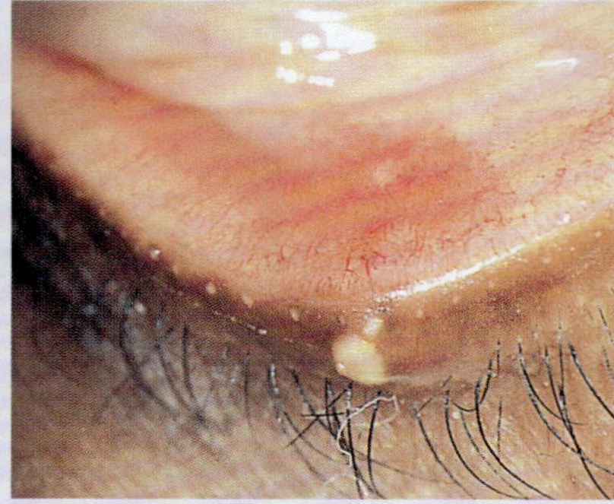

Hordeolum (stye).

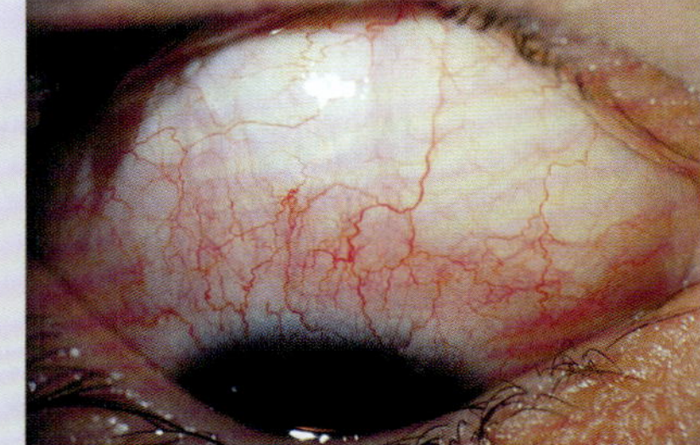

Diffuse episcleritis (inflammation of the sclera). (Tasman, W. & Jaeger, E. [Eds]. [2001]. *The Wills Eye Hospital atlas of clinical ophthalmology* [2nd ed.]. Philadelphia: Lippincott Williams & Wilkins.)

ABNORMAL FINDINGS 17-4 Abnormalities of the cornea and lens

Representative abnormalities of the cornea are illustrated below as a corneal scar and a pterygium. Lens abnormalities are represented by a nuclear cataract and a peripheral cataract. Usually, cataracts are most easily seen by the naked eye.

CORNEAL ABNORMALITIES

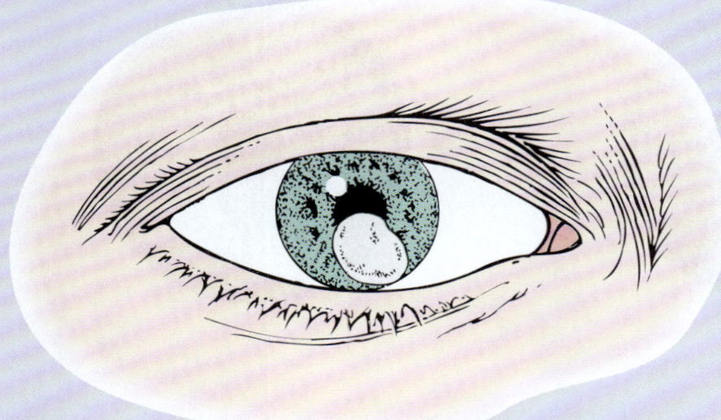

A corneal scar, which appears greyish, usually is due to an old injury or inflammation.

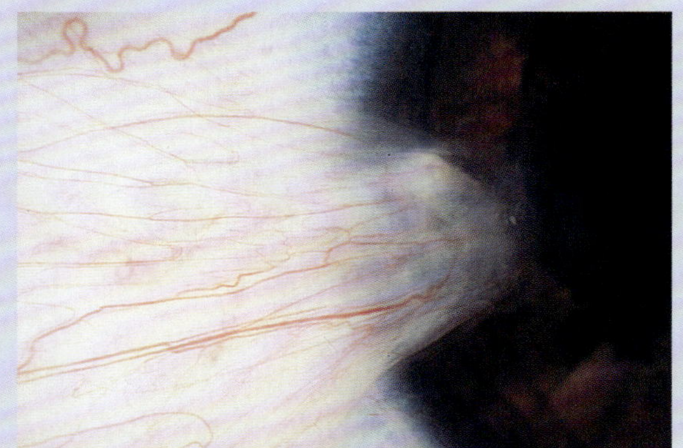

Early pterygium, a thickening of the bulbar conjunctiva that extends across the nasal side. (Tasman, W. & Jaeger, E. [Eds]. [2001]. *The Wills Eye Hospital atlas of clinical ophthalmology* [2nd ed.]. Philadelphia: Lippincott Williams & Wilkins.)

LENS ABNORMALITIES

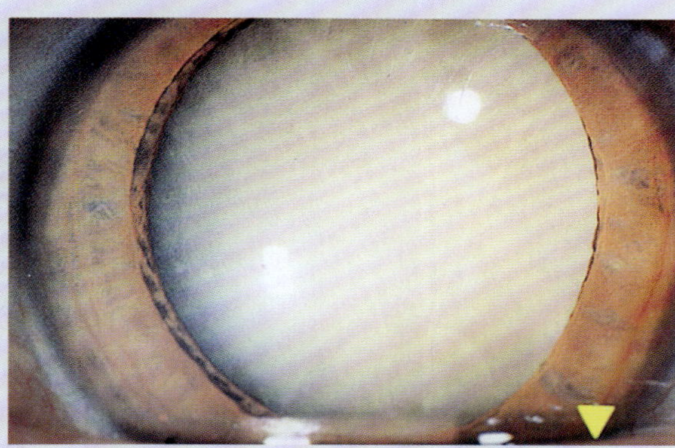

Nuclear cataracts appear grey when seen with a penlight; they appear as a black spot against the red reflex when seen through an ophthalmoscope.

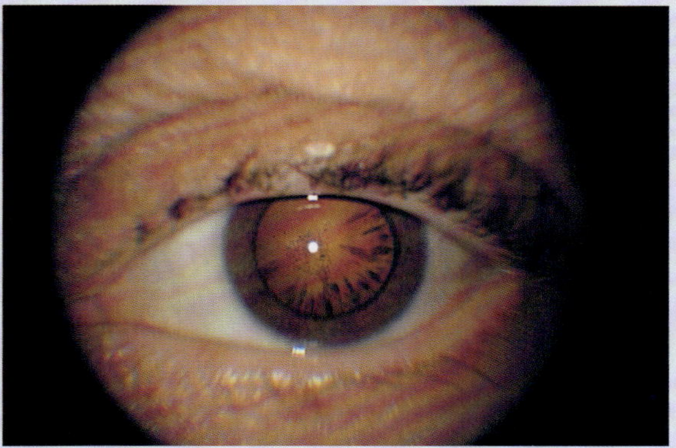

Peripheral cataracts look like grey spokes that point inwards when seen with a penlight; they look like black spokes that point inwards against the red reflex when seen through an ophthalmoscope. (Tasman, W. & Jaeger, E. [Eds]. [2001]. *The Wills Eye Hospital atlas of clinical ophthalmology* [2nd ed.]. Philadelphia: Lippincott Williams & Wilkins.)

ABNORMAL FINDINGS 17-5 Abnormalities of the iris and pupils

IRREGULARLY SHAPED IRIS

An irregularly shaped iris causes a shallow anterior chamber, which may increase the risk for narrow-angle (closed-angle) glaucoma.

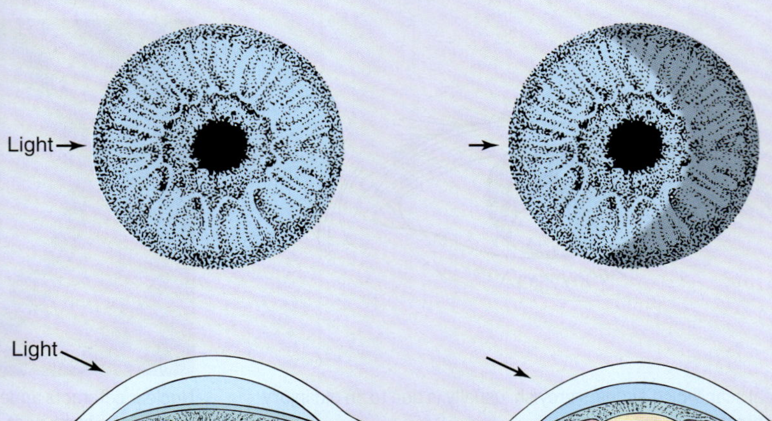

MIOSIS

Also known as pinpoint pupils, miosis is characterised by constricted and fixed pupils—possibly a result of narcotic drugs or brain damage.

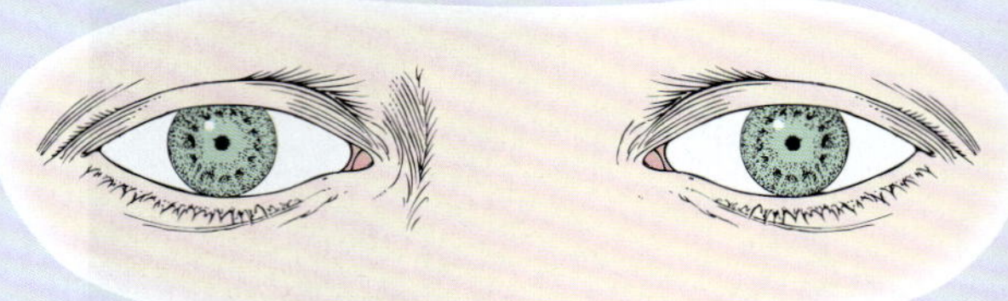

ANISOCORIA

Anisocoria is pupils of unequal size. In some cases, the condition is normal; in other cases, it is abnormal. For example, if anisocoria is greater in bright light compared with dim light, the cause may be trauma, tonic pupil (caused by impaired parasympathetic nerve supply to iris) and oculomotor nerve paralysis. If anisocoria is greater in dim light compared with bright light, the cause may be Horner syndrome (caused by paralysis of the cervical sympathetic nerves and characterised by ptosis, sunken eyeball, flushing of the affected side of the face and narrowing of the palpebral fissure).

MYDRIASIS

Dilated and fixed pupils, typically resulting from central nervous system injury, circulatory collapse or deep anaesthesia.

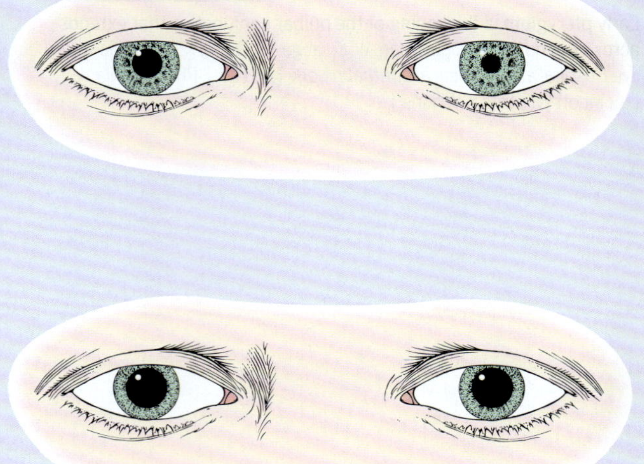

Analysis of data

DIAGNOSTIC REASONING: POSSIBLE CONCLUSIONS

After collecting subjective and objective data pertaining to the eyes, identify abnormal findings and patient strengths. Then cluster the data to reveal any significant patterns or abnormalities. These data may be used to make clinical judgements about the status of the patient's eyes.

Potential patient risks

- Risk of injury (related to impaired vision secondary to the ageing process)
- Risk of eye injury (related to decreased tear production secondary to the ageing process)
- Risk of loss of independence for self-care (related to vision loss)

Potential patient problems

- Ineffective health management
- Alteration in activities of daily living (related to poor vision)
- Acute pain (related to injury from eye trauma, abrasion or exposure to chemical irritant)
- Social isolation (related to inability to interact effectively with others secondary to vision loss)

Selected collaborative problems

After grouping the data, it may become apparent that certain collaborative problems emerge. Remember that collaborative problems cannot be prevented by nursing interventions. However, these physiological complications of medical conditions can be detected and monitored by the nurse. In addition, the nurse can use doctor- and nurse-initiated interventions to minimise the complications of these problems. The nurse may also have to refer the patient in such situations for further treatment of the problem. The following is a list of collaborative problems that may be identified when assessing the eye:

- Foreign body in eye
- Acute red eye
- Corneal ulceration or abrasion.

Medical problems

After grouping the data, it may become apparent that the patient has signs and symptoms that require medical diagnosis and treatment. Referral to a primary care provider is necessary. Some examples of complaints or symptoms that require immediate referral for urgent diagnosis and treatment include:

- Sudden vision loss
- Acute unilateral vision loss with severe pain, nausea or vomiting
- Patient complaint of seeing halos or rings of light
- Pain, photophobia, unilateral red eye
- Penetrating eye injury
- Hyphaema (blood collecting in the anterior chamber).

ONLINE RESOURCES

thePoint

An extensive range of additional resources to enhance teaching and learning and to facilitate understanding may be found online at the text's accompanying website, located on thePoint at http://thepoint.lww.com. These include Watch and Learn videos, Concepts in Action animations, journal articles, case studies, discussion topics and quizzes.

Subscribers may also access Lippincott Procedures, an extensive online point-of-care procedure guide that provides reliable step-by-step instructions for more than 1700 procedures, including 450 evidence-based Australian procedures, and skills in a variety of speciality settings, together with a wealth of supporting information.

CASE STUDY

The case study demonstrates how to analyse eye assessment data for a specific patient. The exercises included in the ancillary product on thePoint that complements this text offer further opportunities to enhance your skills.

Mr Sami Nowra is a 41-year-old Aboriginal and Torres Strait Islander Australian who presents with a history of blurred vision in his right eye. His health history includes type 2 diabetes mellitus (not well controlled with diet or exercise) and mild hypertension (well controlled with medication). Mr Nowra is a director for a national Aboriginal and Torres Strait Islander film company and his work involves him spending a considerable amount of time using computers and digital equipment. Because his work involves a lot of screen and fine-print reading, his wife advised him to go to the health clinic for assessment.

You are talking with Mr Nowra about his concerns of blurred vision in his right eye. You recognise that this is the time to collect some subjective data. Over the last 2 months he reports experiencing increasing difficulty to undertake his work because of vision problems. He states, 'It's getting harder to see the detail on the screen when reviewing and editing the film, especially when it's dark or the film is a night scene. After working for a couple of hours I get a headache over my right eye.' On examination he has a visual acuity of 6/9 in the right eye and 6/6 in the left eye. The lens in the right eye shows a small white opacity, and the left eye appears normal.

The following concept map illustrates the diagnostic reasoning process.

Applying COLDSPA

Applying COLDSPA for patient symptoms: 'vision changes'.

Mnemonic	Question	Data provided	Missing data
Character	Describe the sign or symptom (feeling, appearance, sound, smell or taste, if applicable).	Blurred vision in the right eye. 'It's getting harder to see the detail on the screen when reviewing and editing the film, especially when it's dark or the film is a night scene. After working for a couple of hours I get a headache over my right eye.'	
Onset	When did it begin?	Over the last 2 months he reports experiencing increasingly difficulty to undertake his work.	
Location	Where is it? Does it radiate? Does it occur anywhere else?	Right eye. The lens in the right eye shows a small white opacity, and the left eye appears normal.	
Duration	How long does it last? Does it recur?	Over the last 2 months he reports experiencing increasing difficulty to undertake his work.	Do you have this visual disturbance all the time?
Severity	How bad is it? Or How much does it bother you?	On examination he has a visual acuity of 6/9 in the right eye and 6/6 in the left eye.	Can you describe how severe this problem is for you? Is it always the same or does the severity of the vision problem change (e.g. worse at night)?
Pattern	What makes it better or worse?		Does anything improve or make a difference to your vision?
Associated factors/How it Affects the patient	What other symptoms occur with it? How does it affect you?	He is a director for a national Aboriginal and Torres Strait Islander film company and work involves him spending a considerable amount of time using computers and digital equipment.	Does this change in your vision impact on your life outside of work?

1) Identify abnormal findings and patient strengths

Subjective data

- Blurred vision in right eye
- 'It's getting harder to see the detail on the screen when reviewing and editing the film, especially when it's dark or the film is a night scene'
- Over the last two months he reports increasing difficulty to work
- 'After working for a couple of hours I get a headache over my right eye'

Objective data

- 41-year-old Aboriginal and Torres Strait Islander Australian male
- Married
- Health history: type 2 diabetes mellitus (not well controlled with diet and exercise), mild hypertension (well controlled with medication)
- Work involves considerable computer work
- Visual activity OS 6/9, OD 6/6
- Right eye shows small white-coloured opacity over the lens area
- Left eye appears normal

2) Identify cue clusters

- Worried about vision changes
- Vision changes affecting work/ability to complete work
- 41-year-old male, Aboriginal and Torres Strait Islander Australian

- Vision affecting work
- Reports headache after 2+ hours of working
- Visual activity OS 6/9, OD 6/6
- Visible opacity over right (lens) eye
- Health history of diabetes mellitus type 2 and hypertension
- Aboriginal and Torres Strait Islander Australian

3) Draw inferences

Ability to work and possible permanent loss of vision can affect ability to continue in employment and supporting self and family

Risk factors and presenting symptoms indicate need for referral for management of cataract

4) List potential patient problems

Self-care/self-concept disruption and fear of visual impairment

Requiring further care, needing referral to ophthalmologist. Manage symptoms of visual impairment

5) Check for defining characteristics

Inability to perfom work duties; inability to perform some self-care

Attends follow-up referrals; implements management strategies to reduce impact of vision impairment (if available)

6) Confirm or rule out diagnoses

Confirm: deterioration in performance of work duties/self-care due to visual disturbance

N/A

7) Document conclusions

Diagnoses that are appropriate for this patient include:

- Fear related to unknown progression of visual impairment
- Risk of injury related to lack of awareness of potential dangers due to changes in vision
- Disturbed self-concept related to potential altered role performance secondary to visual loss

Potential collaborative problems include the following:

- Blindness
- Increased intraocular pressure

Medical diagnosis is yet to be made. Patient should be referred to an ophthalmologist for further examination

References

Centre for Eye Research Australia. (2014a). Glaucoma. Viewed January 2019 at www.cera.org.au/community/your-eye-health/glaucoma/.

Centre for Eye Research Australia. (2014b). Cataract. Viewed January 2019 at www.cera.org.au/community/your-eye-health/cataract/.

Centre for Eye Research Australia. (2014c). Age-related macular degeneration. Viewed January 2019 at www.cera.org.au/community/your-eye-health/age-related-macular-degeneration-amd/.

Tasman, W. & Jaeger, E. (Eds). (2001). *The Wills eye hospital atlas of clinical ophthalmology* (2nd ed.). Philadelphia: Lippincott Williams & Wilkins.

World Health Organization (WHO). (2013) Universal eye health- A global action plan 2014-2019. Viewed February, 2019 at https://www.who.int/blindness/AP2014_19_English.pdf?ua=1.

Selected readings

Closing the Gap in Eye Health and Vision Care by 2020. Vision 2020: The Right to Sight Australia. View January 2019 at http://www.vision2020australia.org.au/uploads/resource/294/Closing-the-Gap-in-Eye-Health-and-Vision-Care-by-2020_FINAL.pdf.

Harvey, N. (2018). Sensory perception. In A. Berman (Ed). *Kozier and Erb's fundamentals of nursing : concepts, process and practice* (4th Australian ed.). Melbourne, Vic: Pearson Australia.

Keel, S., Xie, J., Foreman, J., et al. (2019). Prevalence of glaucoma in the Australian National Eye Health Survey. *The British Journal of Ophthalmology, 103*(2), 191–195.

Kilduff, C. & Lois, C. (2016). Red eyes and red-flags: Improving ophthalmic assessment and referral in primary care. *BMJ Open Quality, 5*, doi:10.1136/bmjquality.u211608.w4680. u211608.w4680.

Marieb, E. & Hoehn, K. (2018). *Human anatomy & physiology* (Global ed.). Harlow, England: Pearson Education Limited.

Morgan, C. & Upadhyaya, R. (2015). Sensory function. In S. Meiner (Ed). *Gerentologic nursing* (5th ed.). Maryland Heights, MO: Elsevier.

Mwangi, N. & Mutie, D. (2018). Emergency management: penetrating eye injuries and intraocular foreign bodies. *Community Eye Health, 31*(103), 70–71.

Prior, J. & Fisher, M. (2017). Sensory alterations. In J. Crisp, C. Douglas, G. Rebeiro, et al. (Eds). *Potter & Perry's fundamentals of nursing 5e* (Australia and New Zealand ed.). Chatswood, NSW: Elsevier Australia a division of Reed International Books Australia Pty Ltd.

Shaw, M. & Lee, A. (2017). *Ophthalmic Nursing* (5th ed.). Boca Raton, FL: CRC Press.

U.S. National Institutes of Health (NIH). (2016). Eye movement disorders. MedlinePlus, Viewed January 2019 at www.nlm.nih.gov/medlineplus/eyemovementdisorders.html.

Online resources

Association of Blind Citizens of New Zealand (ABC NZ): www.abcnz.org.nz
Australian Blindness Forum: www.australianblindnessforum.org.au
Blind Citizens Australia (BCA): www.bca.org.au
Centre for Eye Research Australia: https://www.cera.org.au/research/glaucoma-research/
Department of Health and Ageing: Eye Health http://www.health.gov.au/internet/main/publishing.nsf/Content/eye-healthDiabetes Australia: www.diabetesaustralia.com.au
Diabetes New Zealand: www.diabetes.org.nz
Glaucoma Australia: https://www.glaucoma.org.au/
Indigenous Eye Health: https://mspgh.unimelb.edu.au/centres-institutes/centre-for-health-equity/research-group/ieh
Vision 20/20 Australia: www.vision2020australia.org.au
Vision Australia: www.visionaustralia.org.au
Vision eye institute: Children's Eye Health https://visioneyeinstitute.com.au/services/childrens-eye-health/
World Health Organization: Blindness and Vision impairment www.who.int/topics/blindness/en

CHAPTER 18

Ears

CASE STUDY

Mrs Josephine Carmino is 67 years old and lives alone in a two-bedroom apartment. She lives on a fixed income from her pension.

You are talking with Mrs Carmino while she is waiting for her daughter to collect her following a colonoscopy earlier today. You notice that she does not always answer your questions, only answering you after you raise your voice and repeat the question. You also notice that Mrs Carmino talks very softly when she instigates the conversation.

Structure and function

The ear is the sense organ of hearing and equilibrium. It consists of three distinct parts: the external ear, the middle ear and the inner ear. The tympanic membrane separates the external ear from the middle ear. Both the external ear and the tympanic membrane can be assessed by direct inspection and by using an otoscope (using this instrument is an advanced skill, so it is not directly addressed in this text, although it is covered in summary). However, the middle and inner ear cannot be directly inspected. Instead, these parts of the ear are assessed by testing hearing acuity and the conduction of sound.

Before learning assessment techniques, it is important to understand the anatomy and physiology of the ear.

STRUCTURES OF THE EAR

External ear

The external ear is composed of the auricle or pinna and the external auditory canal (Fig. 18-1). The external auditory canal in a child is initially short and straight; with age and consequent growth, it becomes S-shaped in the adult. The outer part of the canal curves up and back and the inner part of the canal curves down and forwards. Modified sweat glands in the external ear canal secrete cerumen, a waxlike substance that keeps the tympanic membrane soft. Cerumen has bacteriostatic properties and its sticky consistency serves as a defence against foreign bodies. The tympanic membrane, or eardrum, has a translucent, pearly grey appearance and serves as a partition stretched across the inner end of the auditory canal, separating it from the middle ear. The membrane itself is concave and located at the end of the auditory canal in a tilted position such that the top of the membrane is closer to the auditory meatus than the bottom. The distinct landmarks (Fig. 18-2A) of the tympanic membrane include:

- Handle and short process of the malleus—the nearest auditory ossicle that can be seen through the translucent membrane
- Umbo—the base of the malleus, but also serves as a centre point landmark
- Cone of light—the reflection of the otoscope light seen as a cone due to the concave nature of the membrane
- Pars flaccida—the top portion of the membrane, which appears to be less taut than the bottom portion
- Pars tensa—the bottom of the membrane, which appears to be taut.

Middle ear

The middle ear, or tympanic cavity, is a small, air-filled chamber in the temporal bone. It is separated from the external ear by the eardrum and from the inner ear by a bony partition containing two openings, the round and oval windows. The middle ear contains three auditory ossicles: the malleus, the incus and the stapes (see Fig. 18-1). These tiny bones are responsible for transmitting sound waves from the eardrum to the inner ear through the oval window. Air pressure is equalised on both sides of the tympanic membrane by means of the eustachian tube, which connects the middle ear to the nasopharynx (see Fig. 18-1).

Inner ear

The inner ear, or labyrinth, is fluid-filled and is made up of the bony labyrinth and an inner membranous labyrinth. The bony labyrinth has three parts: the cochlea, the vestibule and the semicircular canals (see Fig. 18-1). The inner cochlear duct contains the spiral organ of Corti, which is the sensory organ for hearing. Sensory receptors, located in the vestibule and in the membranous semicircular canals, sense position and head movements to help maintain both static and dynamic equilibrium. Nerve fibres from these areas form the vestibular nerve, which connects with the cochlear nerve to form the eighth cranial nerve (acoustic or vestibulocochlear nerve).

HEARING

Sound vibrations travelling through air are collected by and funnelled through the external ear and cause the eardrum to vibrate. Sound waves are then transmitted through auditory

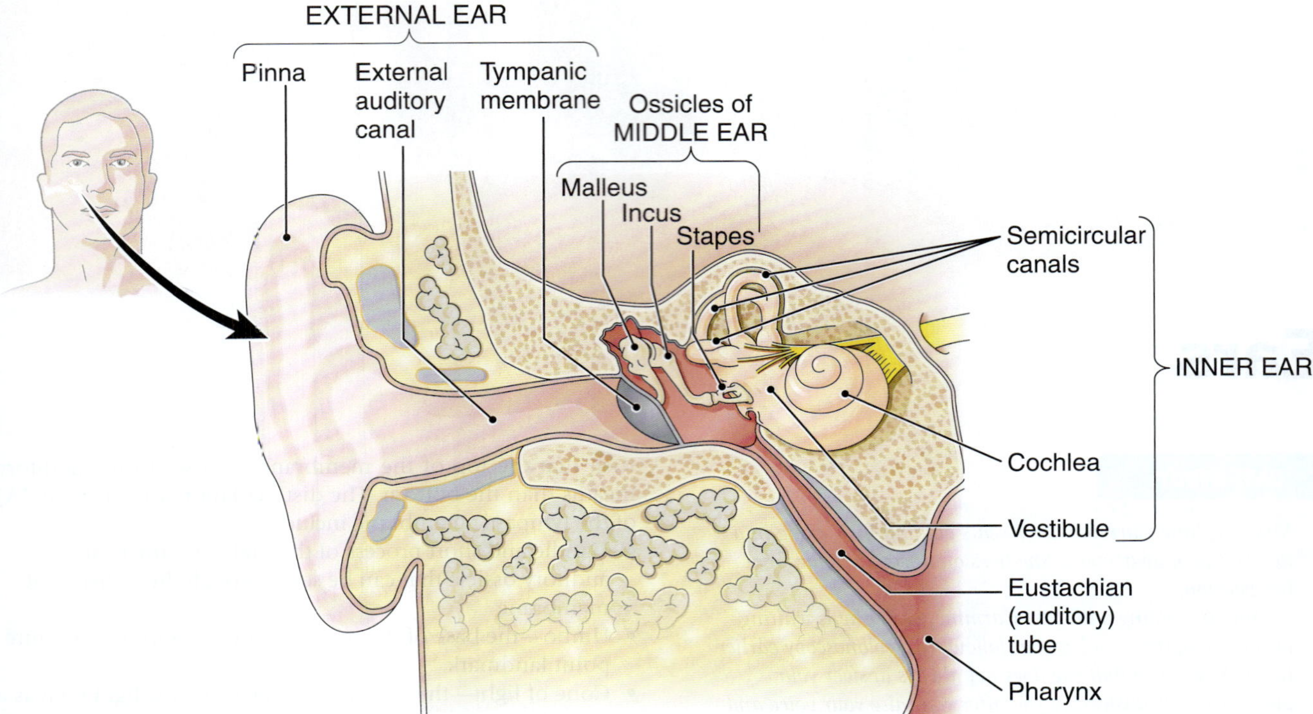

FIGURE 18-1 The ear. Structures in the external, middle and inner divisions are shown. (Cohen, B. J. & Hull, K. L. (2015). *Memmler's structure and function of the human body* [11th ed.]. Philadelphia: Lippincott Williams & Wilkins.)

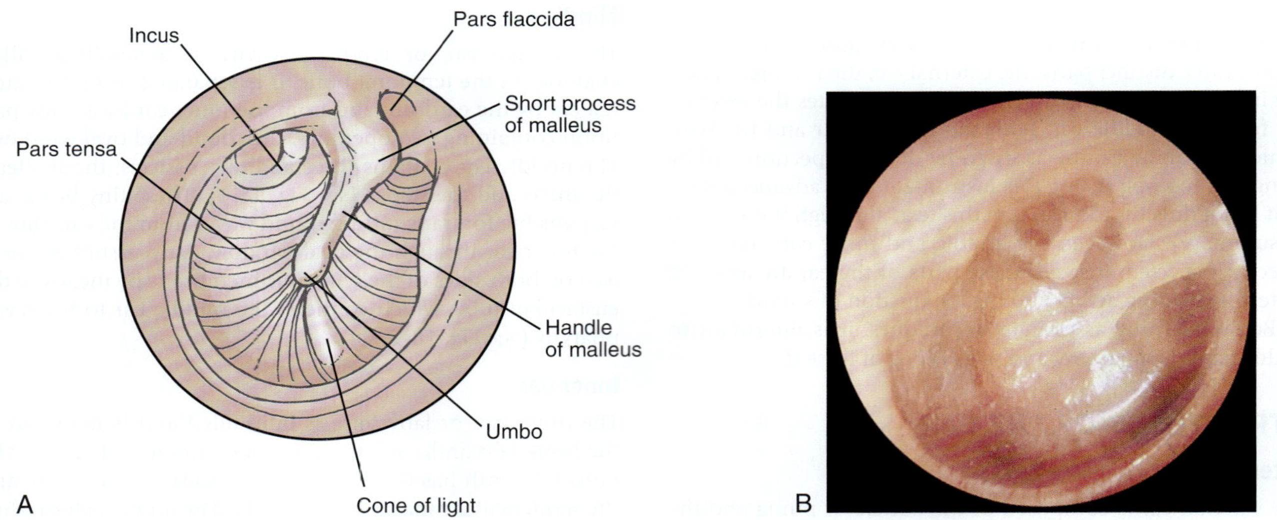

FIGURE 18-2 (A) Right tympanic membrane. **(B)** Normal otoscopic view of the right tympanic membrane. (Moore, K. L. & Agur, A. [2002]. *Essential clinical anatomy* [2nd ed.]. Philadelphia: Lippincott Williams & Wilkins.)

ossicles as the vibration of the eardrum causes the malleus, the incus and then the stapes to vibrate. As the stapes vibrate at the oval window, the sound waves are passed to the fluid in the inner ear. The movement of this fluid stimulates the hair cells of the spiral organ of Corti and initiates the nerve impulses that travel to the brain by way of the acoustic nerve.

The transmission of sound waves through the external ear and middle ear is referred to as conductive hearing and the transmission of sound waves in the inner ear is referred to as 'perceptive' or sensorineural hearing. Therefore, a conductive hearing loss would be related to a dysfunction of the external ear or middle ear (e.g. impacted cerumen, otitis media, foreign object, perforated eardrum, drainage in the middle ear or otosclerosis). A sensorineural hearing loss would be related to dysfunction of the inner ear (i.e. organ of Corti, cranial nerve VIII or temporal lobe of brain).

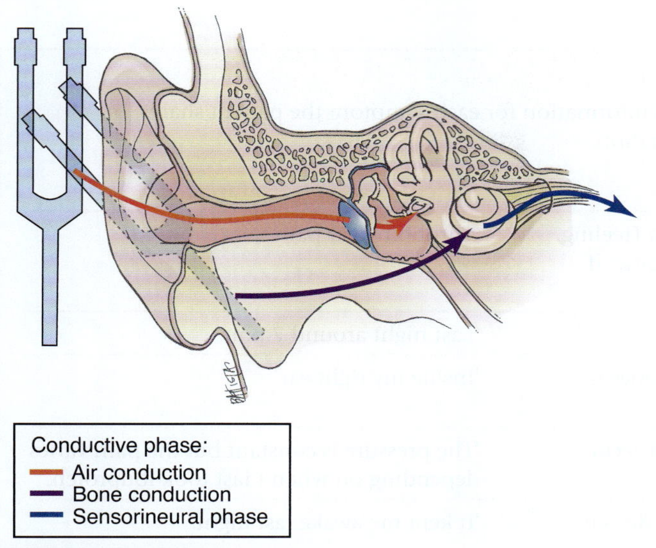

FIGURE 18-3 Pathways of hearing.

In addition to the usual pathway for sound vibrations detailed previously, the bones of the skull also conduct sound waves. This bone conduction, although less efficient, serves to augment the usual pathway of sound waves through air, bone and finally fluid (Fig. 18-3).

Health assessment

Beginning when the nurse first meets the patient, assessment of hearing provides important information about the patient's ability to interact with the environment. Changes in hearing are often gradual and go unrecognised by patients until a severe problem develops. Therefore, asking the patient specific questions about hearing may help in detecting disorders at an early stage. Thorough questioning of the patient specific to this area of health concern will also help in determining which examinations you decide to complete and what follow-up tests or referrals you think may be necessary.

COLLECTING SUBJECTIVE DATA: THE NURSING HEALTH HISTORY

First it is important to gather data from the patient about the current level of hearing and ear health as well as past and family health history problems related to the ear. During data collection, the examiner should be alert to signs of hearing loss such as inappropriate answers or frequent requests for repetition and so on. Collecting data concerning environmental influences on hearing and how these problems affect the patient's usual activities of daily living is also important. Answers to these types of questions help you to evaluate a patient's risk of hearing loss and, in turn, present ways that the patient may modify or lower the risk of ear and hearing problems.

History of present health concern

QUESTION	RATIONALE
Changes in hearing	
Describe any recent changes in your hearing.	A sudden decrease in ability to hear in one ear may be associated with otitis media. A patient reporting any sudden hearing loss should be referred to a doctor for evaluation. See Display 18-1—Ten ways to recognise hearing loss. **OLDER ADULT CONSIDERATIONS** **Presbycusis, a gradual hearing loss, is common after the age of 50 years.**
Are all sounds affected with this change or just some sounds?	Presbycusis often begins with a loss of the ability to hear high-frequency sounds.
Other symptoms	
Do you have any ear drainage? Describe the amount and any odour.	Drainage (otorrhoea) usually indicates infection. Purulent, bloody drainage suggests an infection of the external ear (external otitis). Purulent drainage associated with pain and a popping sensation is characteristic of otitis media with perforation of the tympanic membrane.
Do you have any ear pain? If so, do you have an accompanying sore throat, sinus infection or problem with your teeth or gums?	Earache (otalgia) can occur with ear infections, cerumen blockage, sinus infections or teeth and gum problems.
Do you experience any ringing or crackling in your ears?	Ringing in the ears (tinnitus) may be associated with excessive cerumen build-up, high blood pressure or certain ototoxic medications (such as gentamicin, neomycin, ethacrynic acid, frusemide, indomethacin or aspirin).

Continued on following page

COLDSPA

Example

Use the COLDSPA mnemonic as a guideline to collect needed information for each symptom the patient shares. In addition, the following questions help elicit important information.

Mnemonic	Question	Patient response example
Character	Describe the sign or symptom (feeling, appearance, sound, smell or taste, if applicable).	'Throbbing ear pain.'
Onset	When did it begin?	'Last night around 7 p.m.'
Location	Where is it? Does it radiate? Does it occur anywhere else?	'Inside my right ear.'
Duration	How long does it last? Does it recur?	'The pressure is constant but the pain varies depending on when I last took ibuprofen.'
Severity	How bad is it? or How much does it bother you?	'It kept me awake last night.'
Pattern	What makes it better or worse?	'I took an ibuprofen last night at around 8 p.m. and I woke up with the pain again at around 11 p.m. It hurts a lot when I cough.'
Associated factors/How it **A**ffects the patient	What other symptoms occur with it? How does it affect you?	'Everything sounds muffled—I can hardly hear. I had a cold about a week ago and it went away, but now I have this earache.'

DISPLAY 18-1 TEN WAYS TO RECOGNISE HEARING LOSS

The following questions will help you determine if you need to have your hearing evaluated by a medical professional.

Do you have a problem hearing over the telephone?
Yes ☐ No ☐

Do you have trouble following the conversation when two or more people are talking at the same time?
Yes ☐ No ☐

Do people complain that you turn the TV volume up too high?
Yes ☐ No ☐

Do you have to strain to understand conversation?
Yes ☐ No ☐

Do you have trouble hearing in a noisy background?
Yes ☐ No ☐

Do you find yourself asking people to repeat themselves?
Yes ☐ No ☐

Do many people you talk to seem to mumble (or not speak clearly)?
Yes ☐ No ☐

Do you misunderstand what others are saying and respond inappropriately?
Yes ☐ No ☐

Do you have trouble understanding the speech of women and children?
Yes ☐ No ☐

Do people get annoyed because you misunderstand what they say?
Yes ☐ No ☐

If you answered 'yes' to three or more of these questions, you may want to see an otolaryngologist (an ear, nose and throat specialist) or an audiologist for a hearing evaluation.

The material on this page is for general information only and is not intended for diagnostic or treatment purposes. A doctor or other health care professional must be consulted for diagnostic information and advice regarding treatment.

Excerpt from NIH Publication No. 01-4913. For more information, contact the NIDCD Information Clearinghouse.

History of present health concern (continued)

QUESTION	RATIONALE
Do you ever feel like you are spinning or that the room is spinning? Do you ever feel dizzy or unbalanced?	Vertigo (true spinning motion) may be associated with an inner ear problem. It is termed *subjective vertigo* when the patient feels that they are spinning around and *objective vertigo* when the patient feels that the room is spinning around them. It is important to distinguish vertigo from dizziness.

PROMOTE HEALTH | **OTITIS MEDIA**

OVERVIEW

Otitis media is an inflammation or infection of the middle ear, which often causes fluid to build up behind the ear drum. Otitis media often begins when a throat or respiratory viral infection spreads to the middle ear. Ear infections are often associated with dysfunction or swelling of the eustachian tube. By age 3, 75% of children will have had at least one episode of otitis media and many children will have many recurrent ear infections. The fact that children are more susceptible than adults to otitis media is due mostly to the shorter, straighter, narrower eustachian tubes of children.

Aboriginal and Torres Strait Islander children experience otitis media from a younger age, more frequently, for longer periods and with more complications than non-Aboriginal and Torres Strait Islander children (Jervis-Brady et al., 2014). The reported prevalence of otitis media in Aboriginal and Torres Strait Islander children ranges from 10% to 30%, and otitis media persists at higher rates later into childhood among this group (Jervis-Brady et al., 2014). This disease process has substantial long-term negative consequences on Aboriginal and Torres Strait Islander children's hearing, childhood speech and language development, and education outcomes (O'Conner et al., 2009), making early recognition and treatment a priority. It should also be recognised that public health programs directed towards prevention and treatment of otitis media would benefit all populations but probably most particularly Aboriginal and Torres Strait Islander Australians.

Risk factors

- Age (highest rate between 6 and 18 months old, but occur from 4 months to 4 years; rarely in adults)
- Group child care and increased exposure to respiratory pathogens
- Formula feeding
- Poor air quality (tobacco smoke and air pollution)
- Family history
- Ethnicity (Aboriginal or Torres Strait Islander peoples or Māori)
- Household overcrowding

Teach risk reduction tips

- Keep child away from sick children (limit time in group care).
- Protect child from second-hand smoke.
- Breastfeed baby for at least 6 months.
- Ask child's primary carer about preventive pneumococcal vaccine.

Past health history

QUESTION	RATIONALE
Have you ever had any problems with your ears such as infections, trauma or earaches?	A history of repeated infections can affect the tympanic membrane and hearing (see Promote health—Otitis media).
Describe any past treatments you have received for ear problems (medication, surgery, hearing aids). Were these successful? Were you satisfied?	Patient may be dissatisfied with past treatments for ear or hearing problems. **OLDER ADULT CONSIDERATIONS** **The older patient may have had a bad experience with certain hearing aids and may refuse to wear one. The patient may also associate a negative self-image with a hearing aid.**

Family history

QUESTION	RATIONALE
Is there a history of hearing loss in your family?	Age-related hearing loss tends to run in families.

Lifestyle and health practices

QUESTION	RATIONALE
Do you work or live in an area with frequent or continuous loud noise? How do you protect your ears from the noise?	Continuous loud noises (e.g. machinery, music, explosives) can cause a hearing loss unless the ears are protected with ear guards (see Promote health—Hearing loss).
Do you spend a lot of time swimming or in water? How do you protect your ears?	Swimmer's ear (infection of the ear canal) may be seen when contaminated water is left in the ear. Earplugs may help to keep water out and over-the-counter ear drops may be used to dry out water in the external canal.
Has your hearing loss affected your ability to care for yourself? To work?	Hearing loss or ear pain may interfere with the patient's ability to perform usual activities of daily living. Patients may not be able to drive, talk on the telephone or operate machinery safely because of poor hearing ability. The ability to perform in occupations that rely heavily on hearing, such as a receptionist or telephone operator, may be affected.

Continued on following page

Lifestyle and health practices (continued)

QUESTION	RATIONALE
Has your hearing loss affected your socialising with others?	Patients who have decreased hearing may withdraw, or become isolated or depressed because of the stress of verbal communication.
When was your last hearing examination?	Yearly hearing tests are recommended for patients who are exposed to loud noises for long periods. Knowing the date of the examination helps to determine recent changes.
How do you care for your ears? **SAFETY TIP** **Never insert anything into your ear canal, including cotton-tipped swabs, pens, hairpins and so on. Never use an 'ear candle' to remove cerumen (earwax). These are ineffective and may cause burns, obstruction of the ear canal or perforation of the tympanic membrane. Irrigation devices should be used only by health care professionals (American Academy of Otolaryngology—Head and Neck Surgery [AAO-HNS], 2012).**	Use of cotton wool buds inside the ear can cause ear wax to become impacted and cause ear damage.

PROMOTE HEALTH — HEARING LOSS

OVERVIEW

Hearing loss is a common problem today because of the effects of noise, disease, ageing, heredity and exposure to traumatic injury. There are three types of hearing loss: conductive, sensorineural and mixed. Conductive hearing loss results in sound not being conducted through the canal to the drum and ossicles in the middle ear. This affects the hearing of faint sounds. Sensorineural hearing loss occurs when there is damage to the cochlea of the inner ear and to the nerve pathways to the brain. This loss affects faint sounds and the ability to hear clearly and understand speech. Mixed hearing loss occurs when both middle ear and nerves are damaged. There are many descriptors of hearing loss, including degree and configuration. Genetic hearing loss occurs in about 1/1,000 births. Also of genetic origin is late onset hearing loss, which occurs with age (presbycusis) and affects 25% of persons between 65 and 75, and 75% of those age over 75 years. Causes of hearing loss include the gradual loss from noise over time, cerumen build-up, ear drum rupture, infections, tumours and damage to bones or nerves in ear.

Risk factors

- Age (greater than 65 years)
- Loud noises (above 85 decibels from tractors or farm machinery; recreation: firearms, motorcycles, loud music)
- Heredity
- Otitis media (especially if chronic or untreated)
- Particular medications (e.g. gentamicin, some chemotherapeutic drugs, high-dose aspirin, non-steroidal anti-inflammatory drugs, antimalaria drugs and loop diuretics)
- Some illnesses (with high temperatures, e.g. meningitis; viral infections, e.g. mumps, measles, chicken pox; brain diseases, e.g. multiple sclerosis, tumour, stroke)
- Child of mother who contracted rubella while pregnant

Teach risk reduction tips

- Use ear protection when working or spending time in noise levels above 85 decibels. Follow Standards Australia guidelines for time spent in high-noise environments.
- Have regular ear examinations, especially if spending time in noisy environments.
- Avoid medications associated with ototoxicity, if possible.
- Obtain treatment for otitis media; seek treatment for recurrent sinusitis, which can lead to otitis media.
- Have a sudden hearing loss, dizziness and tinnitus evaluated as soon as possible.

CASE STUDY

You decide to collect some subjective data around Mrs Carmino's hearing.

CRITICAL THINKING

1. What questions would you ask Mrs Carmino about her hearing?
2. Considering Mrs Carmino's hearing appears poor, would you ask questions about her history and lifestyle? Why or why not?

CHILD CASE STUDY

Otitis media

Lucy is a 16-month-old child brought into the emergency department late in the evening by her parents. They are concerned as they report that she has had a cold, a runny nose and fevers over the last few days but tonight became very distressed, crying and is able to sleep for only short periods in their arms. Lucy's parents think she is in pain. She hasn't eaten much in the last 24 hours and has been consuming only half the amount of fluids she would normally drink. She is sitting on her father's lap, makes eye contact with you and is alert.

CRITICAL THINKING

3. What information in the case would lead you to suspect otitis media could be the cause of Lucy's recent illness?
4. What questions would you ask to obtain further family history information from Lucy's parents to determine if Lucy has any of the risk factors that increase the likelihood she has otitis media?
5. What is the link between Lucy's poor oral intake and pain related to otitis media?

CLINICAL TIP

Child ear examination: **Children under approximately 5 years perceive ear examination as invasive and distressing. This is often due to the unusual sensation of the otoscope, localised tenderness if there is infection or inflammation present, and anxiety about what you are doing out of their field of vision. To conduct an examination of a child's ears, seat them on a parent's lap and ask the parent to gently restrain them in a huglike hold. This is best done by asking the parent to put one arm around the child's chest, their other hand over the child's forehead and hug the child against their body. This will steady the child and keep their head and torso still so they do not move suddenly while you examine their outer ear with the otoscope. Being gently restrained by a parent is not perceived as traumatic by the child and allows the examination to be conducted quickly with little pain or distress.**

Note: **See Figure 32-19 in Chapter 32 and note how the carer is gently holding the child for examination.**

COLLECTING OBJECTIVE DATA: PHYSICAL EXAMINATION

The purpose of the ear and hearing examination is to evaluate the condition of the external ear, the condition and patency of the ear canal, the status of the tympanic membrane, bone and air conduction of sound vibrations, hearing acuity and equilibrium. The external ear structures and ear canal are relatively easy to assess through inspection. Using the tuning fork to evaluate bone and air conduction is also a fairly simple procedure. However, as an advanced clinical skill, extensive practice and expertise are needed to use the otoscope correctly to examine the condition of the structures of the tympanic membrane (use of an otoscope is addressed as an overview within this text, not as a detailed clinical skill).

Preparing the patient

Make sure the patient is seated comfortably during the ear examination. This helps to promote the patient's participation, which is very important in this examination. In addition, the test should be explained thoroughly to guarantee accurate results. To ease any patient anxiety, explain in detail what you will be doing. Also answer any questions the patient may have.

As you prepare the patient for the ear examination, carefully note how the patient responds to your explanations. Does the patient appear to hear you well or does it seem he or she is straining to catch everything you say? Does the patient respond to you verbally or non-verbally or do you have to repeat what you say to get a response? This initial observation provides you with clues to the status of the patient's hearing.

Equipment

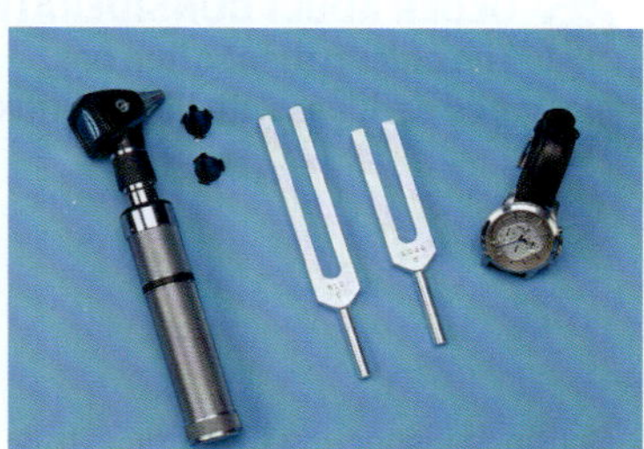

- Watch with a second-hand for Romberg test
- Tuning fork (512 Hz or 1,024 Hz)
- Otoscope (Equipment spotlight 18-1: Otoscope—this is frequently used in the advanced ear assessment)

Physical assessment

Before performing examination make sure to:

- Recognise the role of hearing in communication and adaptation to the environment particularly in regard to ageing
- Understand the usefulness and significance of basic hearing tests.

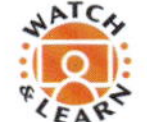

Physical assessment: Assessing the ears

EQUIPMENT SPOTLIGHT 18-1 OTOSCOPE

The otoscope is a penlight-type viewer used to visualise the tympanic membrane and external ear canal (refer to Fig. 18-1). In conjunction with a patient history, an otoscope is useful in the diagnosis of otitis media. The otoscope allows you to view the tympanic membrane, which is important as otitis media is an inflammation of the middle ear. In otitis media, decreased mobility and opacification of the tympanic membrane are present. In general, acute otitis media is diagnosed when the tympanic membrane is bulging, whereas otitis media with effusion is diagnosed when the tympanic membrane is in a neutral position or retracted. Mastery of otoscopic examination techniques, although necessary to accurately diagnose otitis media and differentiate its forms, is an advanced clinical skill (Shaikh et al., 2010).

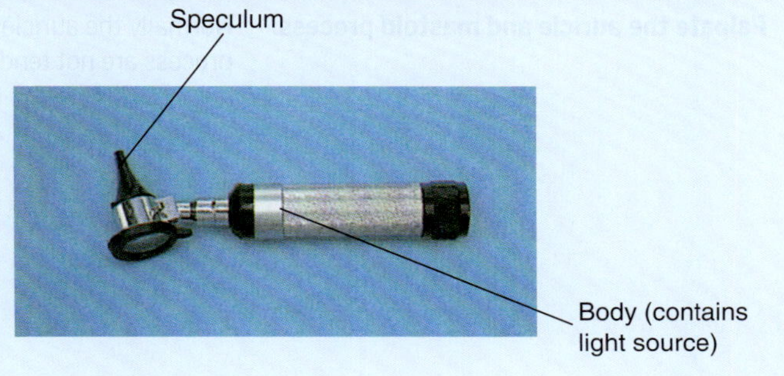

PHYSICAL ASSESSMENT

ASSESSMENT PROCEDURE	NORMAL FINDINGS	ABNORMAL FINDINGS
External ear structures		
INSPECTION AND PALPATION		
Inspect the auricle, tragus and lobule. Note size, shape and position (Fig. 18-4).	Ears are equal in size bilaterally (normally 4 to 10 cm). The auricle aligns with the corner of each eye and within a 10-degree angle of the vertical position. Earlobes may be free, attached or soldered (tightly attached to adjacent skin with no apparent lobe).	Ears are smaller than 4 cm or larger than 10 cm. Malaligned or low-set ears may be seen with genitourinary disorders or chromosomal defects.
CULTURAL CONSIDERATIONS **People have attached or free ear lobes related to their genetic ancestry. Either type, attached or free, is a normal finding.** **OLDER ADULT CONSIDERATIONS** **The older patient often has elongated earlobes with linear wrinkles.**	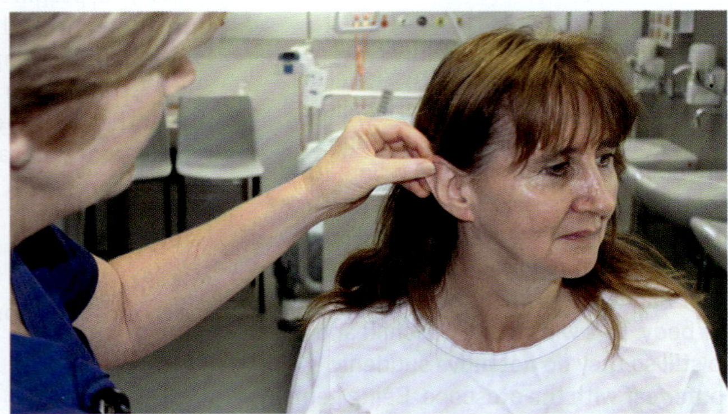 **FIGURE 18-4** Inspecting the external ear.	
Continue inspecting the auricle, tragus and lobule. Observe for lesions, discolourations and discharge. 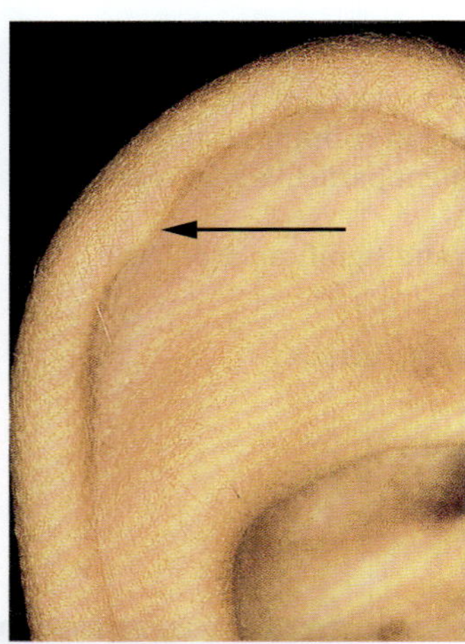 **FIGURE 18-5** Darwin tubercle.	The skin is smooth, with no lesions, lumps or nodules. Colour is consistent with facial colour. Darwin's tubercle, which is a clinically insignificant projection, may be seen on the auricle (Fig. 18-5). No discharge should be present.	Some abnormal findings suggest various disorders, including: • Enlarged preauricular and postauricular lymph nodes—infection • Tophi (non-tender, hard, cream-coloured nodules on the helix or antihelix, containing uric acid crystals)—gout • Blocked sebaceous glands—postauricular cysts • Ulcerated, crusted nodules that bleed—skin cancer (most often seen on the helix due to skin exposure) • Redness, swelling, scaling or itching—otitis externa • Pale blue ear colour—frostbite (Abnormal findings 18-1).
Palpate the auricle and mastoid process.	Normally the auricle, tragus and mastoid process are not tender.	A painful auricle or tragus is associated with otitis externa or a postauricular cyst. Tenderness over the mastoid process suggests mastoiditis. Tenderness behind the ear may occur with otitis media.

PHYSICAL ASSESSMENT (continued)

ASSESSMENT PROCEDURE	NORMAL FINDINGS	ABNORMAL FINDINGS
Internal ear: Otoscopic examination		
INSPECTION		
Inspect the external auditory canal. Use the otoscope (see Assessment guide 18-1). Note any discharge along with the colour and consistency of cerumen (earwax).	A small amount of odourless cerumen (earwax) is the only discharge normally present. Cerumen colour may be yellow, orange, red, brown, grey or black. Consistency may be soft, moist, dry, flaky or even hard. **CULTURAL CONSIDERATIONS** **The viscosity of cerumen is variable and is associated with a person's genetic background. Cerumen may be sticky and wet or flaky and dry. Both are normal findings.** **OLDER ADULT CONSIDERATIONS** **In some older patients, hard, dry cerumen tends to build up as cilia in the ear canal become more rigid. Coarse, thick, wirelike hair may grow at the ear canal entrance as well. This is an abnormal finding only if it impairs hearing.**	Abnormal findings associated with specific disorders include: • Foul-smelling, sticky, yellow discharge—otitis externa or impacted foreign body • Bloody, purulent discharge—otitis media with ruptured tympanic membrane • Blood or watery drainage (cerebrospinal fluid)—skull trauma (refer patient to doctor immediately) • Impacted cerumen blocking the view of the external ear canal—conductive hearing loss • Refer any patient with presence of foreign bodies such as bugs, plants or food to the health care practitioner for prompt removal to avoid swelling and infection. If the object in the ear is a button-type battery, medical attention is urgent as leaking chemicals can burn and damage the ear canal even in a short time such as 1 hour (Cunha, 2011).

Continued on following page

ASSESSMENT GUIDE 18-1 Otoscope

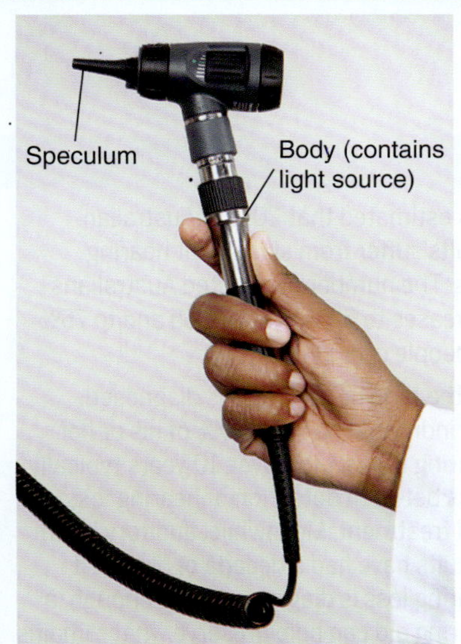

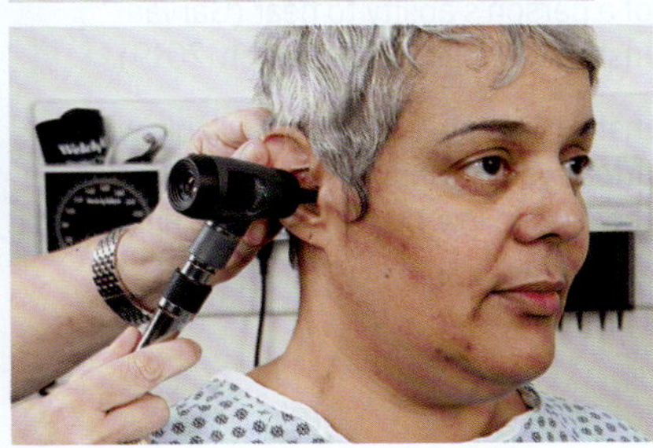

The otoscope is a penlight-type viewer used to visualise the eardrum and external ear canal. Some guidelines for using the otoscope effectively are:

1. Ask the patient to sit comfortably with the back straight and the head tilted slightly away from you towards his or her opposite shoulder.
2. Choose the largest speculum that fits comfortably into the patient's ear canal (usually 5 mm in the adult) and attach it to the otoscope. Holding the instrument in your dominant hand, turn the otoscope light to 'on'.
3. Use the thumb and fingers of your opposite hand to grasp the patient's auricle firmly but gently. Pull out, up and back to straighten the external auditory canal. Do not alter this positioning at any time during the otoscope examination.
4. Grasp the handle of the otoscope between your thumb and fingers and hold the instrument up or down.
5. Position the hand holding the otoscope against the patient's head or face. This position prevents forceful insertion of the instrument and helps to steady your hand throughout the examination, which is especially helpful if the patient makes any unexpected movements.
6. Insert the speculum gently down and forwards into the ear canal (approximately 13 mm). As you insert the otoscope, be careful not to touch either side of the inner portion of the canal wall. This area is bony and covered by a thin, sensitive layer of epithelium. Any pressure will cause the patient pain.
7. Move your head close to the otoscope and position your eye to look through the lens.

PHYSICAL ASSESSMENT (continued)

ASSESSMENT PROCEDURE	NORMAL FINDINGS	ABNORMAL FINDINGS
Hearing and equilibrium tests (continued)		
Observe the colour and consistency of the ear canal walls and inspect the character of any nodules.	The canal walls should be pink and smooth, without nodules.	Abnormal findings in the ear canal may include: • Reddened, swollen canals—otitis externa • Exostoses (non-malignant nodular swellings) • Polyps may block the view of the eardrum (Abnormal findings 18-2).
Inspect the tympanic membrane (eardrum). Note colour, shape, consistency and landmarks.	The tympanic membrane should be pearly, grey, shiny and translucent, with no bulging or retraction. It is slightly concave, smooth and intact. A cone-shaped reflection of the otoscope light is normally seen at 5 o'clock in the right ear and 7 o'clock in the left ear. The short process and handle of the malleus and the umbo are clearly visible (see Fig. 18-2A and B). **OLDER ADULT CONSIDERATIONS** **The older patient's eardrum may appear cloudy. The landmarks may be more prominent because of atrophy of the tympanic membrane associated with the normal process of ageing.**	Abnormal findings in the tympanic membrane may include: • Red, bulging eardrum and distorted, diminished or absent light reflex—acute otitis media • Yellowish, bulging membrane with bubbles behind—serous otitis media • Bluish or dark red colour—blood behind the eardrum from skull trauma • White spots—scarring from infection • Perforations—trauma from infection • Prominent landmarks—eardrum retraction from negative ear pressure resulting from an obstructed eustachian tube • Obscured or absent landmarks—eardrum thickening from chronic otitis media (Abnormal findings 18-2).
To evaluate the mobility of the tympanic membrane, perform *pneumatic otoscopy* by using an otoscope with bulb insufflators. Observe the position of the tympanic membrane when the bulb is inflated and again when the air is released.	The healthy membrane flutters when the bulb is inflated and returns to the resting position once the air released.	With otitis media, the membrane does not move or flutter when the bulb is inflated.
Hearing and equilibrium tests		
Display 18-2 describes hearing loss and testing.		It is estimated that 20% of Australian adults suffer from significant hearing loss. The number of affected Australians increases to 50% over age 65 and to 75% of people over age 70. By the time hearing loss is diagnosed, the individual has lost 60% of his or her hearing range. Moreover, 10 years typically pass between detection of hearing loss and treatment. Meanwhile, auditory brain circuits have had a decade of disuse. If hearing loss is diagnosed early enough, a hearing aid can help preserve what remains of a person's ability to hear (Garvan Institute of Medical Research, 2019).
Perform the whisper test by asking the patient to gently occlude the ear not being tested and rub the tragus with a finger in a circular motion. Start with testing the better hearing ear and then the poorer one. With your head half a metre away behind the patient (so the patient cannot see your lips move), whisper a two-syllable word such as 'popcorn' or 'football'.	Able to correctly repeat the two-syllable word as whispered.	Inability to repeat the two-syllable word after two tries indicates hearing loss and requires follow-up testing by an audiologist.

DISPLAY 18-2 HEARING LOSS AND TESTING

Sensorineural hearing and hearing loss

Actual hearing takes place when sound waves are channelled through the auditory canal, causing the tympanic membrane to vibrate. These vibrations are transmitted through the middle ear by the auditory ossicles to the inner ear, where they are converted into nerve impulses that travel to the brain for interpretation.

A sensorineural hearing loss results when damage is located in the inner ear. Conduction of sound waves is occurring through normal pathways, but the impaired inner ear cannot make the conversion into nerve impulses. Possible causes of sensorineural hearing loss are prolonged exposure to loud noises or using ototoxic medications.

OLDER ADULT CONSIDERATIONS

Presbycusis, a gradual sensorineural hearing loss due to degeneration of the cochlea or vestibulocochlear nerve, is common in older (over age 50) patients. The patient with presbycusis has difficulty hearing consonants and whispered words; this difficulty increases over time.

Conductive hearing and loss

Bone conduction occurs when the temporal bone vibrates with sound waves and the vibrations are picked up by the tympanic membrane or auditory ossicles. This type of conduction results in the perception of sound but is virtually ineffective for interpretation of sounds.

A conductive hearing loss occurs when something blocks or impairs the passage of vibrations from getting to the inner ear. Although a number of causes exist, cerumen build-up and fluid in the middle ear are the most common barriers to 'vibration' transmission.

OLDER ADULT CONSIDERATIONS

Conductive hearing impairment is not uncommon in the older patient due to an increased build-up of cerumen and atrophy or sclerosis of the tympanic membrane. A condition called otosclerosis often occurs with ageing as the auditory ossicles develop a spongy consistency that results in conductive hearing loss.

Hearing tests

The tests discussed in this chapter are performed to give the examiner a basic idea of whether the patient has hearing loss, what type (conduction or sensorineural) of hearing loss it might be and whether there is a problem with equilibrium. These tests present an opportunity to educate patients about risk factors for hearing loss. These tests are not completely accurate and do not provide the examiner with any exact percentage of hearing loss. Therefore, the patient should be referred to an audiologist for more accurate testing if a problem is suspected.

Auditory testing performed with a tuning fork is meant for screening only and should not be used for diagnostic purposes. Variations from expected findings in any tests using a tuning fork are simply an indication of the need for more elaborate testing and referral.

PHYSICAL ASSESSMENT (continued)

ASSESSMENT PROCEDURE	NORMAL FINDINGS	ABNORMAL FINDINGS
Ask the patient to repeat it back to you. If the response is incorrect the first time, whisper the word one more time. Identifying three out of six whispered words is considered passing the test. The whisper test has been studied in both paediatric and adult patients to evaluate hearing acuity and has been found to have a high sensitivity and specificity (Pirozzo et al., 2003).		
Perform Weber's test if the patient reports diminished or lost hearing in one ear. The test helps to evaluate the conduction of sound waves through bone to help distinguish between conductive hearing (sound waves transmitted by the external and middle ear) and sensorineural hearing (sound waves transmitted by the inner ear). Strike a tuning fork softly with the back of your hand and place it at the centre of the patient's head or forehead (Fig. 18-6). Centring is the important part. Ask whether the patient hears the sound better in one ear or the same in both ears.	Vibrations are heard equally well in both ears. No lateralisation of sound to either ear.	With *conductive hearing loss,* the patient reports lateralisation of sound to the poor ear—that is, the patient 'hears' the sounds in the poor ear. The good ear is distracted by background noise and conducted air, which the poor ear has trouble hearing. Thus, the poor ear receives most of the sound conducted by bone vibration. With *sensorineural hearing loss,* the patient reports lateralisation of sound to the good ear. This is because of limited perception of the sound due to nerve damage in the bad ear, making sound seem louder in the unaffected ear. With *conductive hearing loss,* bone conduction (BC) sound is heard longer than or as long as air conduction (AC) sound (BC ≥ AC).

Continued on following page

PHYSICAL ASSESSMENT (continued)

ASSESSMENT PROCEDURE	NORMAL FINDINGS	ABNORMAL FINDINGS
Hearing and equilibrium tests (continued)		
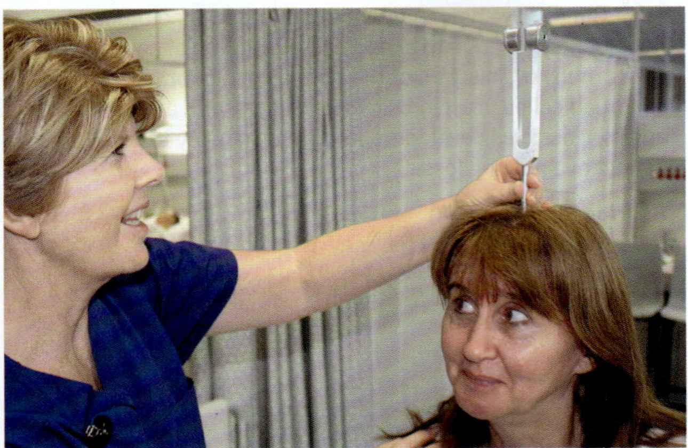 FIGURE 18-6 The Weber test assesses sound conducted via bone.		Conductive hearing loss occurs when sound is not conducted through the outer ear canal to the eardrum and ossicles of the middle ear. Possible causes include: fluid in middle ear, middle-ear infection (otitis media), allergies (serous otitis media), eustachian tube dysfunction, perforated eardrum, benign tumours, impacted cerumen, infection in the ear canal (external otitis) or presence of a foreign body (American Speech-Language-Hearing Association [ASHA], 2011a).
Perform the Rinne test. The Rinne test compares air and bone conduction sounds. Strike a tuning fork and place the base of the fork on the patient's mastoid process (Fig. 18-7A). Ask the patient to tell you when the sound is no longer heard. Move the prongs of the tuning fork to the front of the external auditory canal (Fig. 18-7B). Ask the patient to tell you if the sound is audible after the fork is moved.	Air conduction sound is normally heard longer than bone conduction sound (AC > BC).	With *sensorineural hearing loss,* air conduction sound is heard longer than bone conduction sound (AC > BC) if anything is heard at all. Sensorineural hearing loss occurs with damage to the inner ear (cochlea) or to the nerve pathways between the inner ear and the brain. This is the most common type of permanent hearing loss. It decreases one's ability to hear faint sounds. Even loud speech may be muffled. Causes include ototoxic drugs, genetic hearing loss, ageing, head trauma, malformation of the inner ear and loud noise exposure (ASHA, 2011b).

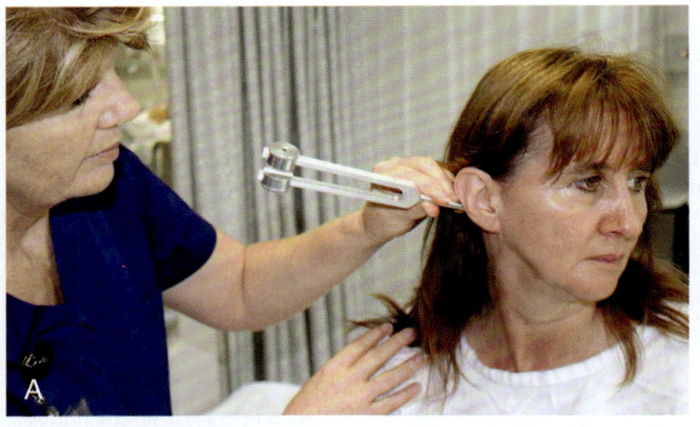

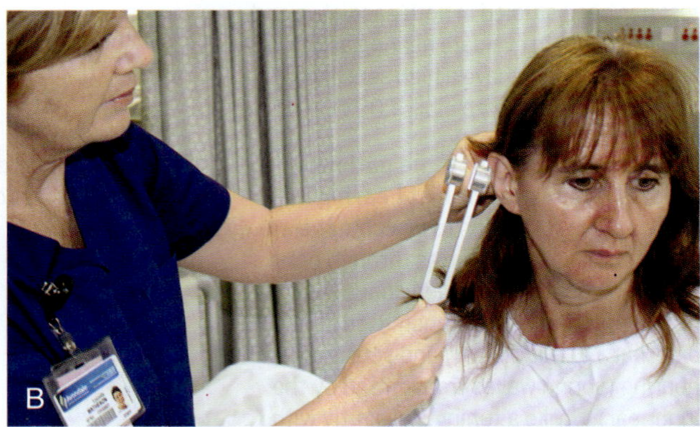

FIGURE 18-7 For the Rinne test, the tuning fork base is placed first on the mastoid process **(A)**, after which the prongs are moved to the front of the external auditory canal **(B)**.

ASSESSMENT PROCEDURE	NORMAL FINDINGS	ABNORMAL FINDINGS
Perform the Romberg test. This tests the patient's equilibrium. Ask the patient to stand with feet together, arms at sides and eyes open, then with the eyes closed. **SAFETY TIP** **When performing this test, put your arms around the patient without touching him or her to prevent falls.**	Patient maintains position for 20 seconds without swaying or with minimal swaying.	Patient moves feet apart to prevent falls or starts to fall from loss of balance. This may indicate a vestibular disorder.

ABNORMAL FINDINGS 18-1 Abnormalities of the external ear and ear canal

Many abnormalities may affect the external ear and ear canal; among them are infections and abnormal growths. Some are pictured below.

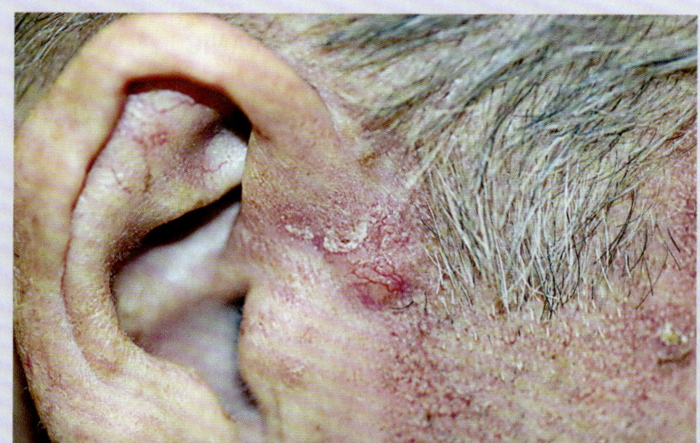

Malignant lesion.

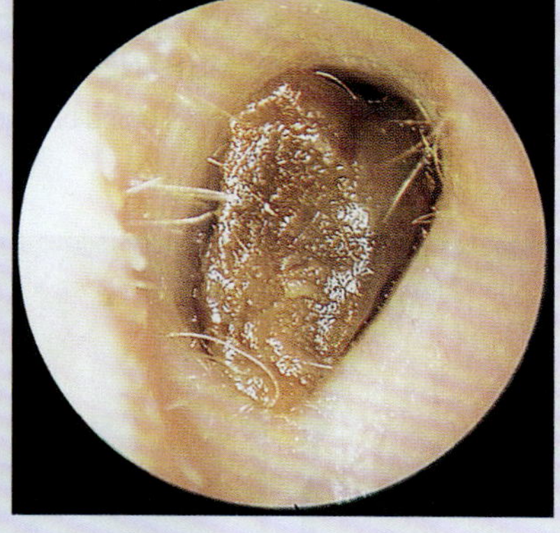

Build-up of cerumen in ear canal.

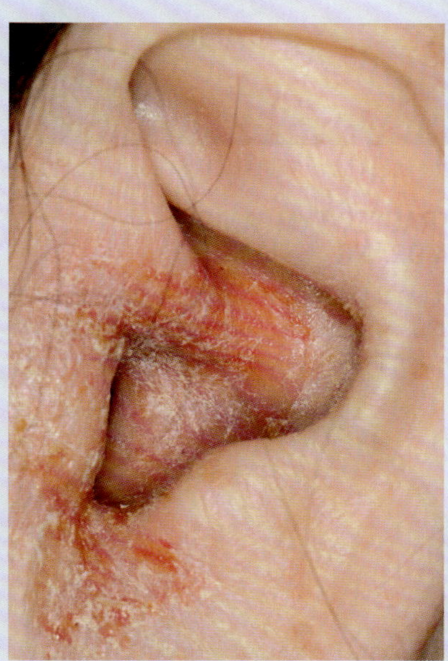

Otitis externa. (Dr. P. Marazzi/Science Photo Library.)

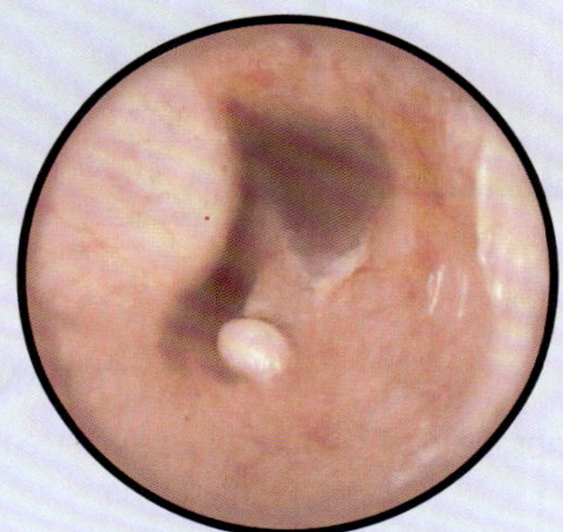

Polyp.

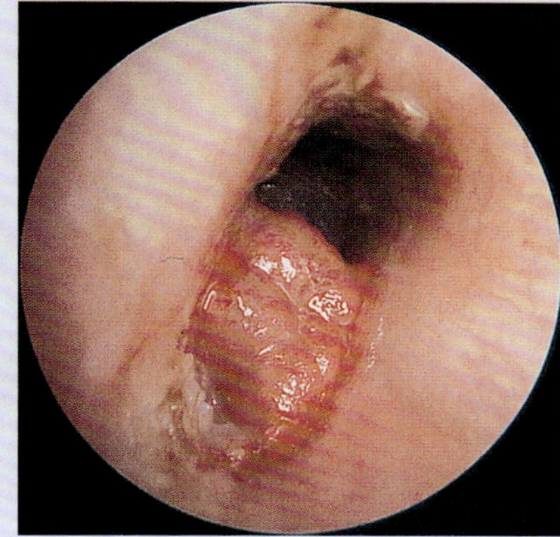

Exostosis.

ABNORMAL FINDINGS 18-2 Abnormalities of the tympanic membrane

The thin, drumlike structure of the tympanic membrane is essential for hearing. It is also essential for promoting equilibrium and barring infection. Damage to the membrane may have grave consequences.

ACUTE OTITIS MEDIA

Note the red, bulging membrane; decreased or absent light reflex.

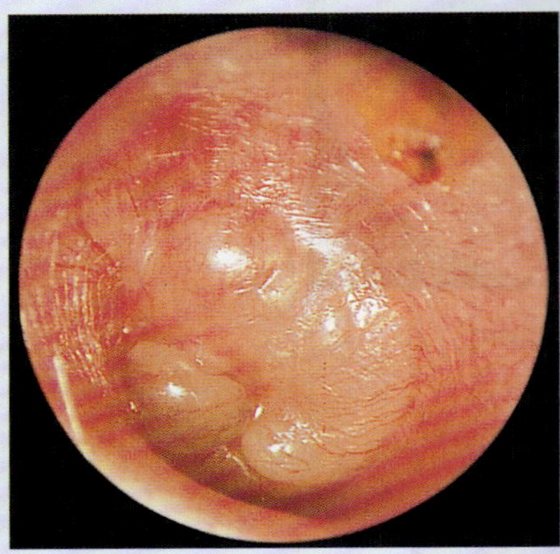

BLUE/DARK RED TYMPANIC MEMBRANE

Indicates blood behind eardrum due to trauma.

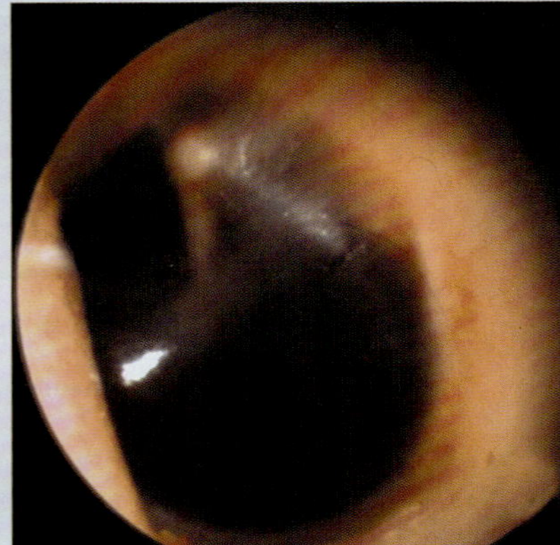

PERFORATED TYMPANIC MEMBRANE

Perforation results from rupture caused by increased pressure, usually from untreated infection or trauma.

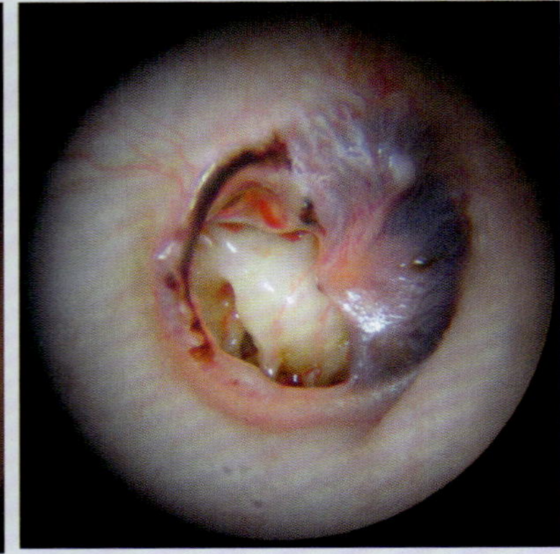

(Shutterstock.com/Mikhail V. Komarov.)

SEROUS OTITIS MEDIA

Note the yellowish, bulging membrane with bubbles behind it.

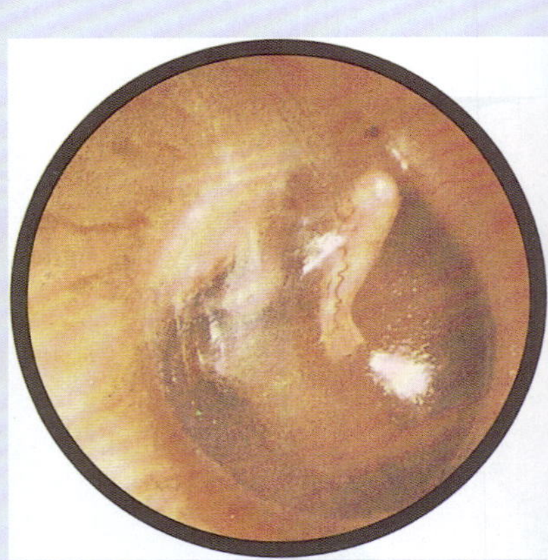

SCARRED TYMPANIC MEMBRANE

White spots and streaks indicate scarring from infections.

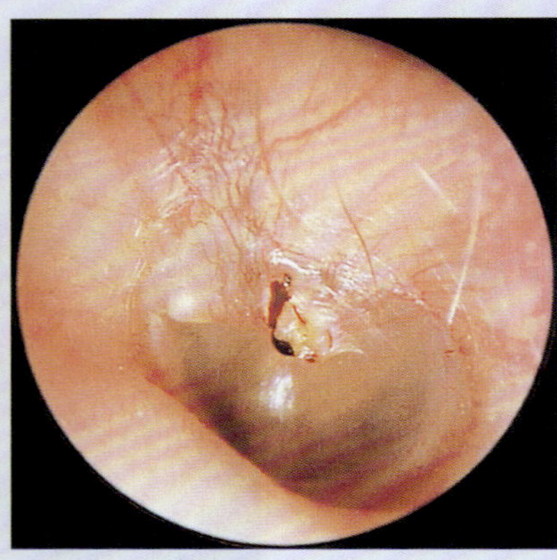

RETRACTED TYMPANIC MEMBRANE

Prominent landmarks are caused by negative ear pressure due to obstructed Eustachian tube or chronic otitis media.

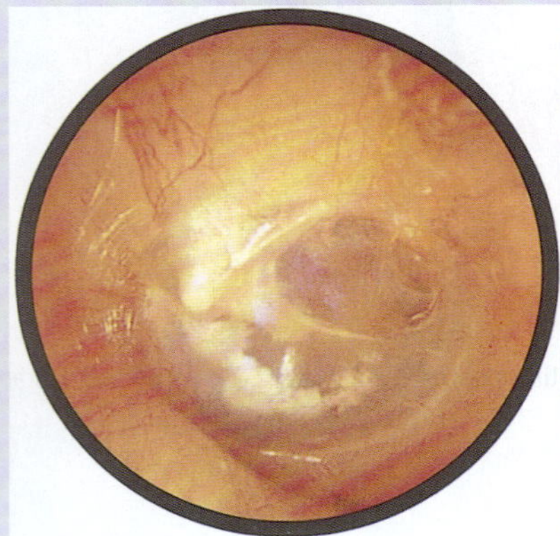

CRITICAL THINKING

6. Most health assessments are based around common sense. Prior to reading the following physical assessment section, what do you think would be the important things to assess or examine specific to a patient's ears and hearing? Considering this, how would you physically assess Mrs Carmino's ears and test her hearing?
7. Explain why, if you were to place a vibrating tuning fork against a patient's skull immediately behind the ear, the patient can perceive sound. If the patient can 'hear' the perceived sound of the tuning fork but not sounds such as a softly spoken word, why might this occur? Where would the problem with sound transmission lie? If you are not sure of the answer, revisit the 'Hearing' section at the front of this chapter and consider the information contained in Display 18-1.

CASE STUDY

You are concerned about Mrs Carmino's hearing and decide to check it with the whisper test. She asks you to repeat the word several times and finally tells you with annoyance in her voice, 'You just have to speak up if you expect people to hear you!' You decide to complete a Rinne test and find that her bone conduction is greater than her air conduction (BC > AC). When you question her about any hearing problems, she denies having any hearing loss. She says she has never had audiometric studies and that she can't afford them now. She also tells you, 'I never talk on the phone because my friends do not speak loudly enough.'

CRITICAL THINKING

8. If Mrs Carmino could hear the perceived sound of the vibrating tuning fork clearly, but not your whispered words, what would this tell you about her hearing problems?

VALIDATING AND DOCUMENTING FINDINGS

Validate the ear assessment data that you have collected. This is necessary to verify that the data are reliable and accurate. Document the assessment data following health care facility or agency policy.

The following subjective and objective data are included as examples you can follow in practising data collection and documentation.

After you have collected your assessment data, you will need to analyse the data using diagnostic reasoning skills. Refer to the discussion of the diagnostic reasoning process in Chapter 5.

Sample of subjective data

Patient denies recent changes in hearing. No drainage, pain or ringing. Has not experienced any spinning sensations. States history of one ear infection several years ago. Has had no surgery, does not use a hearing aid device. Denies frequent exposure to loud noises. Last hearing examination was 3 years ago.

Sample of objective data

Ears equal in size bilaterally, auricles aligned with the corner of each eye within a 10-degree angle of vertical position. Skin smooth, no lumps, lesions, nodules. No discharge. Non-tender on palpation. Small amount of moist yellow cerumen in external canal, no nodules present. Whisper test: Patient repeats two-syllable word. Weber's test: Hears vibration equally well in both ears. Rinne test: AC > BC. Romberg test: Maintains position for 10 seconds without swaying.

Analysis of data

DIAGNOSTIC REASONING: POSSIBLE CONCLUSIONS

After collecting subjective and objective data pertaining to the ears, identify abnormal findings and patient strengths. Then cluster the data to reveal any significant patterns or abnormalities. These data may be used to make clinical judgements about the status of the patient's ears.

Potential patient risks

- Risk of injury (related to hearing impairment)
- Risk of social (isolation related to hearing loss)

Potential patient problems

- Disturbed auditory perception (related to conductive or sensorineural hearing loss)
- Acute pain (related to infection of external or middle ear)
- Impaired social interaction (related to inability to interact effectively with others secondary to hearing loss)
- Disturbed body image (related to concern over appearance of hearing aids)

Selected collaborative problems

After grouping the data, it may become apparent that certain collaborative problems emerge. Remember that collaborative problems cannot be prevented by nursing interventions. However, these physiological complications of medical conditions can be detected and monitored by the nurse. In addition, the nurse can use doctor- and nurse-prescribed interventions to minimise the complications of these problems. The nurse may also have to refer the patient in such situations for further treatment of the problem. The following is a list of collaborative problems that may be identified when assessing the ear:

- Otitis media (acute, chronic or serous)
- Otitis externa
- Perforated tympanic membrane.

Medical problems

If, after grouping the data, it becomes apparent that the patient has signs and symptoms that may require medical diagnosis and treatment, referral to a primary care provider is necessary.

ONLINE RESOURCES

An extensive range of additional resources to enhance teaching and learning and to facilitate understanding may be found online at the text's accompanying website, located on thePoint at http://thepoint.lww.com. These include Watch and Learn videos, Concepts in Action animations, journal articles, case studies, discussion topics and quizzes.

Subscribers may also access Lippincott Procedures, an extensive online point-of-care procedure guide that provides reliable step-by-step instructions for more than 1700 procedures, including 450 evidence-based Australian procedures, and skills in a variety of speciality settings, together with a wealth of supporting information.

CASE STUDY

The case study demonstrates how to analyse ear assessment data for a specific patient. The exercises included in the ancillary product on thePoint that complements this text offer further opportunities to enhance your skills.

Mrs Josephine Carmino is 67 years old and lives alone in a two-bedroom apartment. She lives on a fixed income from her pension. You are talking with Mrs Carmino while she is waiting for her daughter to collect her following a colonoscopy earlier today. You notice that she does not always answer your questions, only answering you after you raise your voice and repeat the question. You also notice that Mrs Carmino talks very softly when she instigates the conversation. You decide to collect some subjective data around her hearing. You are concerned about Mrs Carmino's hearing and decide to check it with the whisper test. She asks you to repeat the word several times and finally tells you with annoyance in her voice, 'You just have to speak up if you expect people to hear you!' You decide to complete a Rinne test and find that her bone conduction is greater than her air conduction (BC > AC). When you question her about any hearing problems, she denies having any hearing loss. She says she has never had audiometric studies and that she can't afford them now. She also tells you, 'I never talk on the phone because my friends do not speak loudly enough.'

The following concept map illustrates the diagnostic reasoning process.

Applying COLDSPA

Applying COLDSPA for patient symptoms: 'Patient answers questions inappropriately and speaks very softly.'

Mnemonic	Question	Data provided	Missing data
Character	Describe the sign or symptom (feeling, appearance, sound, smell or taste, if applicable).	During routine check-up, patient answers questions inappropriately and speaks very softly	
Onset	When did it begin?	Denies hearing loss and has never had any audiometric studies.	When did you first notice your friends were not speaking loud enough on the phone?
Location	Where is it? Does it radiate? Does it occur anywhere else?		Test for conductive and sensory hearing loss in both ears.
Duration	How long does it last? Does it recur?	Asks examiner to repeat the whispered word several times	When do you find talking with others the most comfortable or beneficial to you?
Severity	How bad is it? or How much does it bother you?	Seems annoyed when unable to hear your questions	Do you find it easier to visit in a group or with just one other person?
Pattern	What makes it better or worse?	'You just have to speak up if you expect people to hear you!'	What is your preferred way of communicating with others?
Associated factors/How it Affects the patient	What other symptoms occur with it? How does it affect you?	'I never talk on the phone because my friends do not speak loudly enough.'	

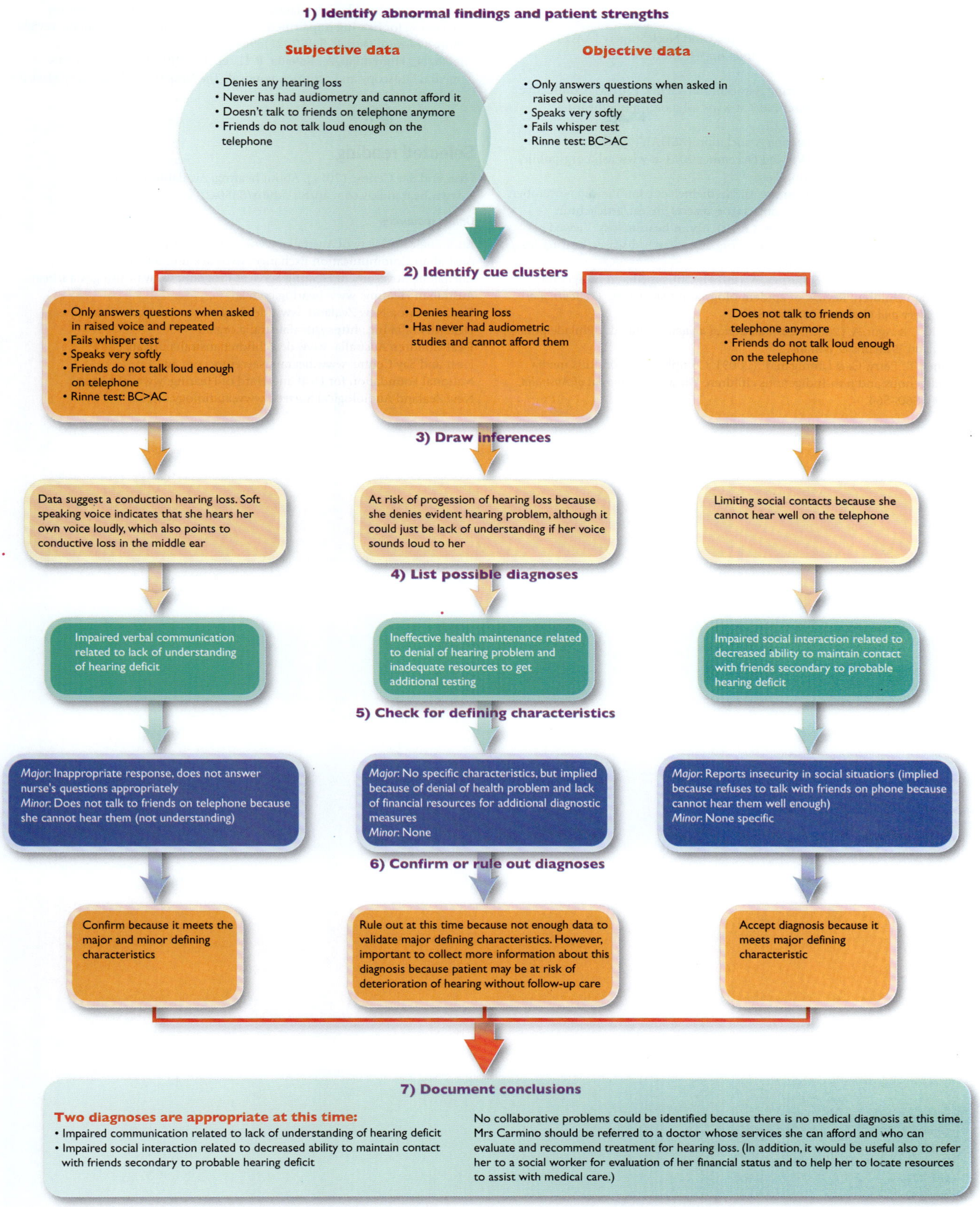

1) Identify abnormal findings and patient strengths
Subjective data
• Denies any hearing loss
• Never has had audiometry and cannot afford it
• Doesn't talk to friends on telephone anymore
• Friends do not talk loud enough on the telephone
Objective data
• Only answers questions when asked in raised voice and repeated
• Speaks very softly
• Fails whisper test
• Rinne test: BC>AC
2) Identify cue clusters
• Only answers questions when asked in raised voice and repeated
• Fails whisper test
• Speaks very softly
• Friends do not talk loud enough on telephone
• Rinne test: BC>AC
• Denies hearing loss
• Has never had audiometric studies and cannot afford them
• Does not talk to friends on telephone anymore
• Friends do not talk loud enough on the telephone
3) Draw inferences
Data suggest a conduction hearing loss. Soft speaking voice indicates that she hears her own voice loudly, which also points to conductive loss in the middle ear
At risk of progession of hearing loss because she denies evident hearing problem, although it could just be lack of understanding if her voice sounds loud to her
Limiting social contacts because she cannot hear well on the telephone
4) List possible diagnoses
Impaired verbal communication related to lack of understanding of hearing deficit
Ineffective health maintenance related to denial of hearing problem and inadequate resources to get additional testing
Impaired social interaction related to decreased ability to maintain contact with friends secondary to probable hearing deficit
5) Check for defining characteristics
Major: Inappropriate response, does not answer nurse's questions appropriately
Minor: Does not talk to friends on telephone because she cannot hear them (not understanding)
Major: No specific characteristics, but implied because of denial of health problem and lack of financial resources for additional diagnostic measures
Minor: None
Major: Reports insecurity in social situations (implied because refuses to talk with friends on phone because cannot hear them well enough)
Minor: None specific
6) Confirm or rule out diagnoses
Confirm because it meets the major and minor defining characteristics
Rule out at this time because not enough data to validate major defining characteristics. However, important to collect more information about this diagnosis because patient may be at risk of deterioration of hearing without follow-up care
Accept diagnosis because it meets major defining characteristic
7) Document conclusions
Two diagnoses are appropriate at this time:
• Impaired communication related to lack of understanding of hearing deficit
• Impaired social interaction related to decreased ability to maintain contact with friends secondary to probable hearing deficit
No collaborative problems could be identified because there is no medical diagnosis at this time. Mrs Carmino should be referred to a doctor whose services she can afford and who can evaluate and recommend treatment for hearing loss. (In addition, it would be useful also to refer her to a social worker for evaluation of her financial status and to help her to locate resources to assist with medical care.)

References

American Academy of Otolaryngology—Head and Neck Surgery (AAO-HNS). (2012). Earwax. Available at www.entnet.org/HealthInformation/earwax.Cfm.

American Speech-Language-Hearing Association (ASHA). (2011a). Conductive hearing loss. Viewed December 2013 at www.asha.org/public/hearing/Conductive-Hearing-Loss.

American Speech-Language-Hearing Association (ASHA). (2011b). Sensorineural hearing loss. Viewed December 2013 at www.asha.org/public/hearing/Sensorineural-Hearing-Loss.

Cunha, J. (2011). Foreign body in the ear. MedicineNet.com. Viewed November 2019 at www.medicinenet.com/objects_or_insects_in_ear/article.htm.

Garvan Institute of Medical Research. (2019). About hearing loss. Viewed November 2019 at https://www.garvan.org.au/research/diseases/hearing-loss/about#diagnosis-and-treatment.

Jervis-Brady, J., Sanchez, L. & Carney, A. (2014). Otitis media in Indigenous Australian children: Review of epidemiology and risk factors. *The Journal of Laryngology and Otology, 128*, S16–S17.

Moore, K. L. & Agur, A. (2002). *Essential clinical anatomy* (2nd ed.). Philadelphia: Lippincott Williams & Wilkins.

O'Conner, T., Perry, C. & Lannigan, F. (2009). Complications of otitis media in Indigenous and non-Indigenous children. *The Medical Journal of Australia, 2*(191), S60–S64.

Pirozzo, S., Papinczak, T. & Glasziou, P. (2003). Whispered voice test for screening for hearing impairment in adults and children: Systematic review. *British Medical Journal, 327*(7421), 967.

Shaikh, N., Hoberman, A., Kaleida, P. H., et al. (2010). Diagnosing otitis media: Otoscopy and cerumen removal. *The New England Journal of Medicine, 362*(20), e62.

Selected reading

Hear and Say Centre. (2019). About hearing. Available at https://www.hearandsay.com.au/for-adults/8350-2/.

Online resources

Audiological Society of Australia: www.audiology.asn.au
Australian Communication Exchange: www.aceinfo.net.au
Australian Government Hearing Services Program: www.health.gov.au/hear
Australian Hearing: www.hearing.com.au
Deaf Aotearoa New Zealand: www.deaf.org.nz
Deaf Australia Inc.: https://deafaustralia.org.au/
Deaf Children Australia: www.deafchildrenaustralia.org.au
Hear and Say Centre: www.hearandsaycentre.com.au
National Foundation for Deaf and Hard of Hearing: www.nfd.org.nz
New Zealand Audiological Society: www.audiology.org.nz

CHAPTER 19

Mouth, throat, nose and sinuses

CASE STUDY

Jonathon Miller is a 22-year-old university student who visits the emergency department in mid-June, complaining of severe throat pain ('like swallowing razor blades'), swollen lymph nodes, chills, fever, general fatigue and anorexia.

Structure and function

The mouth and throat make up the first part of the airway and digestive system and are responsible for receiving food (ingestion), taste, preparing food for digestion and aiding in speech. Cranial nerves V (trigeminal), VII (facial), IX (glossopharyngeal) and XII (hypoglossal) assist with some of these functions (the cranial nerves are discussed in Chap. 29). The nose and paranasal sinuses constitute the first part of the respiratory system and are responsible for receiving, filtering, warming and moistening air to be transported to the lungs. Receptors of cranial nerve I (olfactory) are also located in the nose. These receptors are related to the sense of smell.

MOUTH

The mouth or oral cavity is formed by the lips, cheeks, hard and soft palates, uvula and the tongue and its muscles (Fig. 19-1). The mouth is the beginning of the digestive tract, with the upper and lower lips forming the entrance to the mouth. The roof of the oral cavity is formed by the anterior hard palate and the posterior soft palate. An extension of the soft palate is the uvula, which hangs in the posterior midline of the oropharynx. During swallowing, the soft palate and uvula act as a protective gateway by closing off the nasopharynx and preventing food from entering the nasal cavity. The cheeks form the lateral walls of the mouth, whereas the tongue and its muscles form the floor of the mouth. The mandible (jaw bone) provides the structural support for the floor of the mouth.

Contained within the mouth are the tongue, teeth, gums and openings of the salivary glands (parotid, submandibular and sublingual). The tongue is a mass of muscle. It is attached to the hyoid bone and styloid process of the temporal bone and is connected to the floor of the mouth by a fold of tissue called the frenulum. The tongue assists with moving food, swallowing and speaking. The gums (gingiva) are covered by mucous membrane and normally hold 32 permanent teeth in the adult (Fig. 19-2). The top, visible, white enamelled part of each tooth is the crown. The portion of the tooth that is embedded in the gums is the root. The crown and root are connected by the region of the tooth referred to as the neck. Small bumps called papillae cover the dorsal surface of the tongue. Taste buds, scattered over the tongue's surface, carry sensory impulses to the brain. The three pairs of salivary glands secrete saliva (watery, serous fluid–containing salts, mucus and salivary amylase) into the mouth (Fig. 19-3). Saliva helps break down and lubricates food. Amylase digests carbohydrates. The parotid glands, located below and in front of the ears, empty through Stensen ducts, which are located inside the cheek across from the second upper molar. The submandibular glands, located in the lower jaw, open under the tongue on either side of the frenulum through openings called Wharton ducts. The sublingual glands, located under the tongue, open through several ducts located on the floor of the mouth.

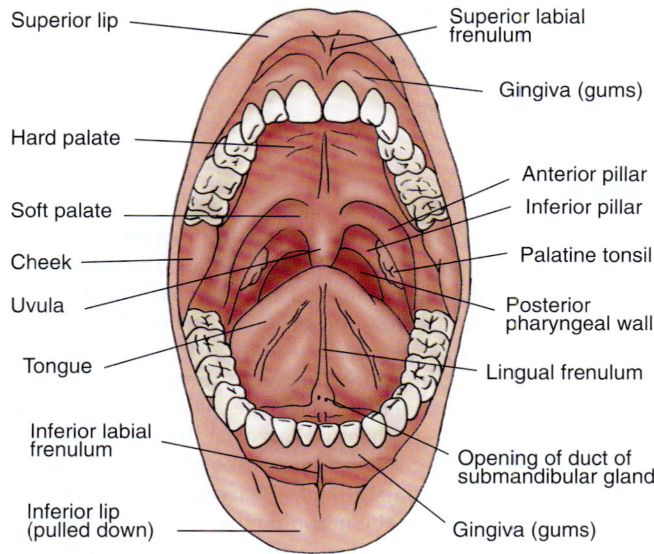

FIGURE 19-1 Structures of the mouth.

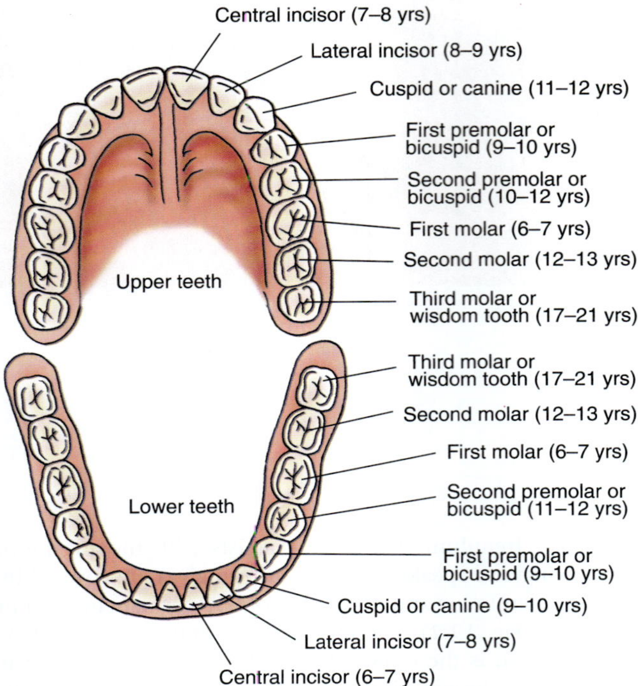

FIGURE 19-2 Teeth.

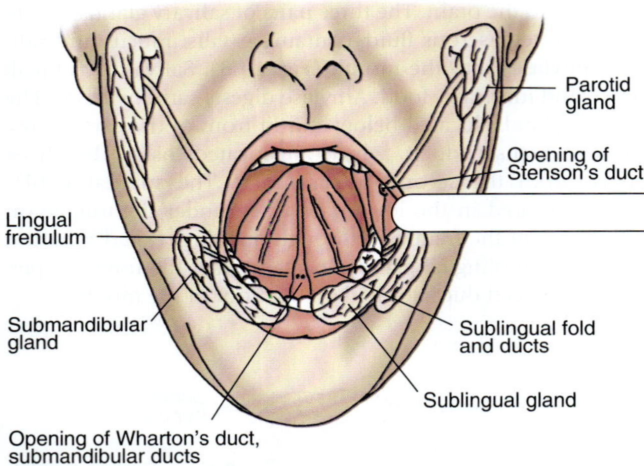

FIGURE 19-3 Salivary glands.

THROAT

The throat (pharynx), located behind the mouth and nose, serves as a muscular passage for food and air. The upper part of the throat is the nasopharynx. Below the nasopharynx lies the oropharynx and below the oropharynx lies the laryngopharynx. The soft palate, anterior and posterior pillars, and the uvula connect behind the tongue to form arches. Masses of lymphoid tissue referred to as the palatine tonsils are located on both sides of the oropharynx at the end of the soft palate between the anterior and posterior pillars. The lingual tonsils lie at the base of the tongue. Pharyngeal tonsils or adenoids are found high in the nasopharynx. Because tonsils are masses of lymphoid tissue, they help protect against infection (Fig. 19-4).

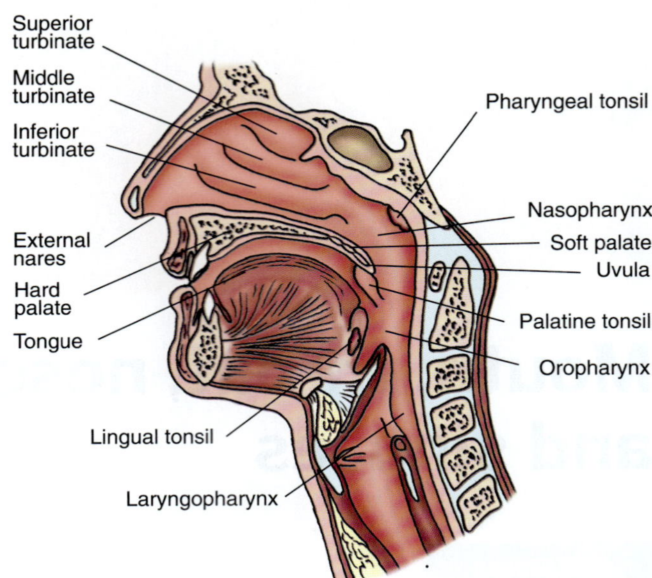

FIGURE 19-4 Nasal cavity and throat structures.

NOSE

The nose consists of an external portion covered with skin and an internal nasal cavity. It is composed of bone and cartilage and is lined with mucous membrane. The external nose consists of a bridge (upper portion), tip and two oval openings called nares. The nasal cavity is located between the roof of the mouth and the cranium. It extends from the anterior nares (nostrils) to the posterior nares, which open into the nasopharynx. The nasal septum separates the cavity into two halves. The front of the nasal septum contains a rich supply of blood vessels and is known as the Kiesselbach area. This is a common site for epistaxis.

The superior, middle and inferior turbinates are bony lobes, sometimes called conchae, that project from the lateral walls of the nasal cavity. These three turbinates warm, humidify and filter the air we breathe and serve to increase the surface area that is exposed to incoming air (see Fig. 19-4). As the person inspires air, nasal hairs (vibrissae) filter large particles from the air. Ciliated mucosal cells then capture and propel debris towards the throat, where it is swallowed. A meatus underlies each turbinate and receives drainage from the paranasal sinuses and the nasolacrimal duct. Receptors for the first cranial nerve (olfactory) are located in the upper part of the nasal cavity and septum.

SINUSES

Four pairs of *paranasal sinuses* (frontal, maxillary, ethmoidal and sphenoidal) are located in the skull (Fig. 19-5). These air-filled cavities decrease the weight of the skull and act as resonance chambers during speech. The paranasal sinuses are also lined with ciliated mucous membrane that traps debris and propels it towards the outside. The sinuses are often a primary site of infection because they can easily become blocked. The frontal sinuses (above the eyes) and the maxillary sinuses (in the upper jaw) are accessible to examination

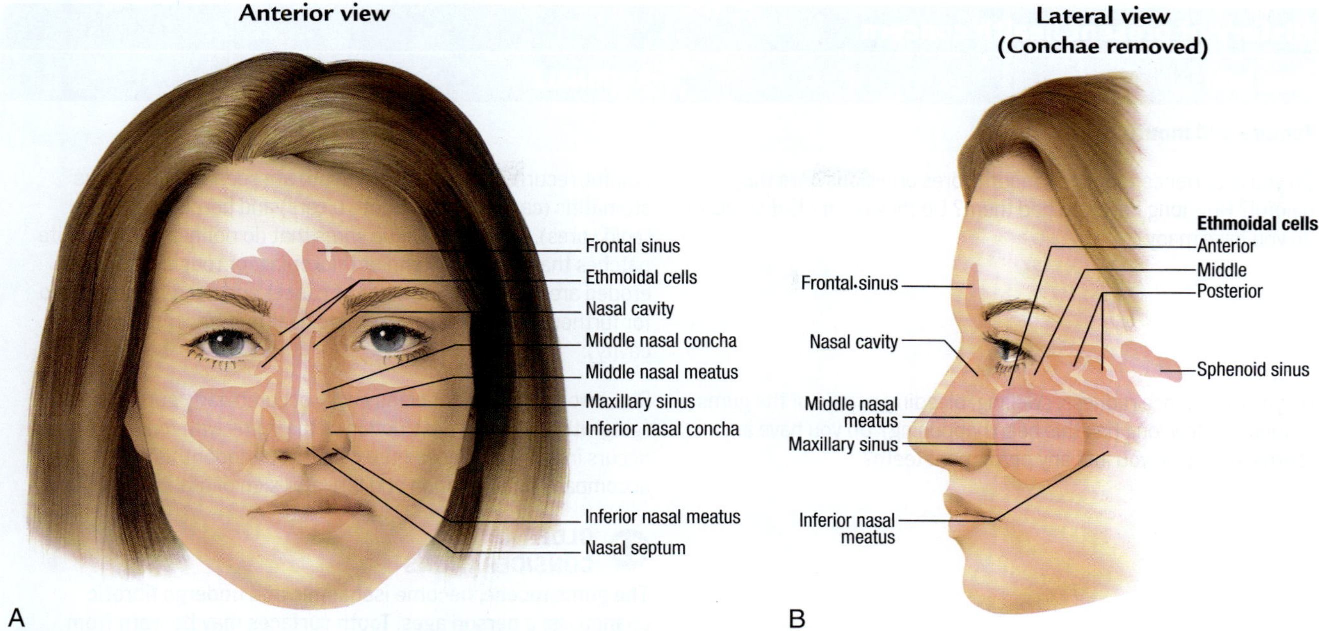

FIGURE 19-5 (A) Paranasal sinuses, anterior view. **(B)** Paranasal sinuses, lateral view. (Asset provided by Anatomical Chart Co.)

by the nurse. The ethmoidal sinuses and sphenoidal sinuses are smaller, located deeper in the skull and are not accessible for examination.

CASE STUDY

Mr Miller admitted that he had been studying 'day and night' for final exams and had 'only one more to go'. 'This is the third time I've had this problem this year,' he related. 'I didn't even bother coming in the first or second time. I just stayed in bed between classes and treated myself.'

Nursing assessment

COLLECTING SUBJECTIVE DATA: THE NURSING HEALTH HISTORY

Subjective data related to the mouth, throat, nose and sinus can aid in detecting diseases and abnormalities that may affect the patient's activities of daily living and in ensuring that the patient does not have any potential or actual problems that may lead to the airway being compromised (this may be evidenced by husky voice or stridor). Screening for cancer of the mouth, throat, nose and sinuses is an important area of this assessment. These cancers are highly preventable (see Promote health—Cancer of the oral cavity later in the chapter). Use of tobacco and heavy alcohol consumption increase a patient's risk of cancer. Data collected regarding the patient's risk factors may form the basis for preventive teaching.

Other problems may cause discomfort and loss of function and can lead to serious systemic disorders. For example, malnutrition may develop in a patient who cannot eat certain foods because of poorly fitting dentures. A patient with frequent sinus infections and headaches may have impaired concentration, which affects job or school performance.

This examination also allows the nurse to evaluate the patient's health practices. For example, improper use of nasal decongestants may explain recurrent sinus congestion, and infection and improper oral hygiene practices may cause tooth decay or gum disease. The nurse should provide teaching for a patient with these health practices.

CRITICAL THINKING

1. What additional information might you want to gather about Mr Miller's self-treatment?
2. Why might this be helpful in conducting your health history and examination?
3. What other questions might you need to ask Mr Miller about his history (other than his experience this year) for this type of problem?
4. Why might this be important information to gather?

History of present health concern	
QUESTION	**RATIONALE**
Tongue and mouth	
Do you experience tongue or mouth sores or lesions? Are they painful? How long have you had them? Do they recur? Is it single or do you have many?	Painful, recurrent ulcers in the mouth are seen with aphthous stomatitis (canker sores, mouth ulcers) and herpes simplex (cold sores). Mouth or tongue sores that do not heal; red or white patches that persist; a lump or thickening; or rough, crusty or eroded areas are warning signs of cancer and need to be referred for further evaluation (see Promote health—Cancer of the oral cavity).
Do you experience redness, swelling, bleeding or pain of the gums or mouth? How long has this been happening? Do you have any toothache? Have you lost any permanent teeth?	Red, swollen gums that bleed easily occur in early gum disease (gingivitis), whereas destruction of the gums with tooth loss occurs in more advanced gum disease (periodontitis). Pain can accompany inflammation and is a later sign of oral cancer. **OLDER ADULT CONSIDERATIONS** **The gums recede, become ischaemic and undergo fibrotic changes as a person ages. Tooth surfaces may be worn from prolonged use. These changes make the older patient more susceptible to periodontal disease and tooth loss.**
Nose and sinuses	
Do you have pain over your sinuses?	Sinusitis may cause pressure and pain over the sinuses (see Promote health—Sinusitis).
Do you experience epistaxis? How much bleeding? What colour is the blood?	Epistaxis may be seen with overuse of nasal sprays, excessively dry nasal mucosa, hypertension, leukaemia, thrombocytopenia and other blood disorders. A patient who experiences frequent nosebleeds should be referred for further evaluation.
Do you experience frequent clear or mucous drainage from your nose?	Thin, watery, clear nasal drainage (rhinorrhoea) can indicate a chronic allergy or, in a person with a past head injury, a cerebrospinal fluid leak. Mucous drainage, especially yellow, is typical of a cold, rhinitis or a sinus infection.
Can you breathe through both of your nostrils? Do you have a stuffy nose at times during the day or night?	Inability to breathe through both nostrils may indicate sinus congestion, obstruction or a deviated septum. Nasal congestion can interfere with daily activities or a restful sleep.
Do you have seasonal allergies, such as hay fever? Describe the timing of the allergies (e.g. spring, summer) and symptoms (e.g. sinus problems, runny nose or watery eyes).	Pollens cause seasonal rhinitis, whereas dust may cause rhinitis year round.
Have you experienced a change in your ability to smell or taste?	A decrease in the ability to smell may occur with upper respiratory infections, smoking, cocaine use or a neurological lesion or tumour in the frontal lobe of the brain or in the olfactory bulb or tract. A decreased ability to taste may be reported by patients with upper respiratory infections or lesions of the facial nerve (VII). Changes in perception of smell also occur from a zinc deficiency and from menopause in some women. **OLDER ADULT CONSIDERATIONS** **The ability to smell and taste decreases with age. Medications can also decrease sense of smell and taste in older people.**

History of present health concern (continued)

QUESTION	RATIONALE
Throat	
Do you have difficulty chewing or swallowing food? How long have you had this? Do you have any pain?	Dysphagia (difficulty swallowing) may be seen in oesophageal disorders, anxiety, poorly fitting dentures or a neurological disorder. Dysphagia increases the risk of aspiration, and patients with dysphagia may require consultation with a speech therapist. Difficulty chewing, swallowing or moving the tongue or jaws may be a late sign of oral cancer. Malocclusion may also cause difficulty chewing or swallowing.
Do you have a sore throat? How long have you had it? Describe. How often do you get sore throats?	Throat irritation and soreness are common with sinus drainage and may also occur with a viral or bacterial infection. A sore throat that persists without healing may signal throat cancer.
Do you experience hoarseness? How long?	Hoarseness is associated with upper respiratory infections, allergies, hypothyroidism, overuse of the voice, smoking or inhaling other irritants, and cancer of the larynx. If hoarseness lasts 2 weeks or longer, refer the patient for further evaluation.

Past health history

QUESTION	RATIONALE
Have you ever had any oral, nasal or sinus surgery?	Present symptoms may be related to past problems.
Do you have a history of sinus infections? Describe your symptoms. Do you use nasal sprays? (What type? How much? How often?)	Some patients are more susceptible to sinus infections, which tend to recur. Overuse of nasal sprays may cause nasal irritation, nosebleeds and rebound swelling.

Continued on following page

COLDSPA

Example

Use the COLDSPA mnemonic as a guideline to collect needed information for each symptom the patient shares. In addition, the following questions help elicit important information.

Mnemonic	Question	Patient response example
Character	Describe the sign or symptom (feeling, appearance, sound, smell or taste, if applicable).	'My throat is sore and it hurts to swallow.'
Onset	When did it begin?	'Last night.'
Location	Where is it? Does it radiate? Does it occur anywhere else?	'Just in my throat.'
Duration	How long does it last? Does it recur?	'The pain is constant, and getting worse.'
Severity	How bad is it? or How much does it bother you?	'I'm miserable.'
Pattern	What makes it better or worse?	'Ibuprofen helps some but it never goes away completely.'
Associated factors/How it Affects the patient	What other symptoms occur with it? How does it affect you?	'Headache, 38 °C fever, and my boyfriend says I have bad breath.'

PROMOTE HEALTH — CANCER OF THE ORAL CAVITY

OVERVIEW

More than 90% of oral cavity and oropharyngeal cancers are squamous cell cancers. Cancers develop in the lining, salivary glands, tonsils or base of the tongue, but only squamous cell cancers of the lips, oral and oropharyngeal cavity are discussed here. During 2016 in Australia and New Zealand, approximately 5,297 cases of lip, oral and oropharyngeal cavity cancer were diagnosed, making up approximately 2% to 3% of all cancer diagnoses. Rates in non-Aboriginal and Torres Strait Islander Australians were as much as 1.9 times higher, and Māori population incidence rates were slightly less than non-Māori population rates. Most cases (90%) occur in people who are heavy users of tobacco and alcohol and whose ages range in the 50s and 60s.

However, cases of oral cavity and tongue cancers are beginning to appear more frequently in people in their 30s and 40s. Incidence is higher in men but is increasing in women. People with oral and oropharyngeal cancer often have another cancer or develop one at a later time. Follow-up examinations and avoidance of risk factors are extremely important for these patients (Australian Institute of Health and Welfare, 2018; Cancer Council Australia, 2018; Ministry of Health New Zealand, 2016a).

Risk factors

- Tobacco use
- Alcohol consumption
- Combined tobacco and alcohol use
- Alcohol dependence accompanied with nutritional deficiencies
- Age over 40
- Male gender (twice as likely to affect males as females, but incidence is rising in females)
- Genetic predisposition, family history
- Occupation related to nickel refining, woodworking or textile fibres
- Diet low in fruits and vegetables; vitamin A deficiency
- Ultraviolet light exposure (especially the lips)
- Long-term irritation (i.e. poorly fitted dentures)

Possible risk factors

- Human papillomavirus) infection
- Immune system suppression
- Marijuana use
- Mouthwash

Teach risk reduction tips

- Stop smoking.
- Limit alcohol consumption.
- Eat a healthy, balanced diet.
- Take precautions when working in an environment where substances or particles could be inhaled.
- Avoid excessive exposure to ultraviolet light.
- Avoid sources of oral irritation.

PROMOTE HEALTH — SINUSITIS

OVERVIEW

Acute and chronic sinusitis is common in Australia: some 15% of the population suffer from sinusitis, an infection or inflammation of the sinuses. From 2017 to 2018, an estimated 2 million Australians (8.1% of the population) had chronic sinusitis (Australian Bureau of Statistics, 2018). Swelling in the sinuses or impaired function of the cilia, which normally move mucus out of the sinuses, cause sinusitis. Sinusitis is inflammation of the sinus cavity membranes; it may be an acute or chronic condition. Causes include allergic reactions to pollen, dust mites, moulds, airborne fungi and other substances; respiratory infections, nasal or sinus obstruction (anatomical or polyps); other diseases such as cystic fibrosis, HIV and other immunodeficiency diseases; facial trauma; changes in air pressure; overuse of decongestant sprays; smoking; swimming or diving; and presence of nasal polyps. Sinus infections (bacterial or viral) can also lead to chronic sinusitis.

Risk factors

- Poor hygiene, especially inadequate hand washing
- Chronic exposure to allergens
- Repeated upper respiratory illnesses
- Facial trauma
- Recurrent sinus infections
- Nasal polyps
- Overuse of decongestants
- Smoking
- Frequent swimming or diving
- Changes in air pressure (e.g. long air travel trips)

Teach risk reduction tips

- Maintain good hygiene, especially frequent and thorough hand washing.
- Maintain adequate fluid intake to keep nasal passages lubricated.
- Avoid cigarette smoking.
- Avoid polluted air.
- Avoid allergens when possible.
- Use a humidifier to increase moisture.
- Work with primary care provider to control allergies and cold symptoms.
- Keep immune system strong.

Family history

QUESTION	RATIONALE
Is there a history of mouth, throat, nose or sinus cancer in your family?	There is a genetic risk factor for mouth, throat, nose and sinus cancers.

Lifestyle and health practices

QUESTION	RATIONALE
Do you smoke? If so, how much? Are you interested in quitting this habit?	Cigarette, pipe and cigar smoking increase a person's risk of oral cancer. Tobacco use and heavy alcohol consumption are responsible for 75% of the oral cancers (Kamangar et al., 2009). Smoking a pipe is a risk factor for lip cancer. Patients who want to quit using tobacco may benefit from a referral to a smoking cessation program (see Promote health—Cancer of the oral cavity). (*Note:* The importation, distribution and use of smokeless tobacco has been banned in Australia and New Zealand since the late 1980s, but patients who may have used smokeless tobacco or chewing tobacco products before this time are at sufficiently higher risk of developing oral cancers than smokers (Madani et al., 2010), so consider asking about this if your patient was using tobacco products before the early 1990s.)
Do you drink alcohol? How much and how often?	Excessive use of alcohol increases a person's risk of oral cancer.
Do you grind your teeth?	Grinding the teeth (bruxism) may be a sign of stress or of slight malocclusion. The practice may also precipitate temporomandibular joint problems and pain.
Describe how you care for your teeth or dentures. How often do you brush and use dental floss? When was your last dental examination?	Proper brushing, flossing and oral hygiene can prevent dental cavities and gum disease. Regular dental checkups and screening can help to detect the early signs of gum disease and oral cancer, which promotes early treatment.
If the patient wears braces: How do you care for your braces? Do you avoid any specific types of foods? Describe your usual dietary intake for a day.	Patients with braces should avoid crunchy, sticky and chewy foods when wearing braces. These foods can damage the braces and the teeth. Poor nutrition also increases one's risk of oral cancers and gum disease.
OLDER ADULT CONSIDERATIONS If the patient wears dentures: How do your dentures fit?	Poorly fitting dentures may lead to poor eating habits, a reluctance to speak freely, and mouth sores or leucoplakia (thick white patches of cells). Leucoplakia is a precancerous condition.
Elderly patients and some patients with disabilities may have difficulty caring properly for teeth or dentures because of poor vision or impaired dexterity.	
Do you brush your tongue?	Cleaning the tongue is a way to prevent bad breath resulting from bacteria that accumulates on the posterior tongue.
How often are you in the sun? Do you use lip sunscreen products?	Exposure to the sun is the primary risk factor associated with lip cancer.

COLLECTING OBJECTIVE DATA: PHYSICAL EXAMINATION

Examination of the mouth and throat can help the nurse to detect abnormalities of the lips, gums, teeth, oral mucosa, tonsils and uvula. This examination also allows for early detection of oral cancer and infections. Examination of the nose and sinuses assists the nurse with detection of a deviated septum, patency of the nose and nasopharynx, and detection of sinus infection. In addition, assessment of the mouth, throat, nose and sinuses provides the nurse with clues to the patient's nutritional and respiratory status. The mouth and nose examination can be very useful to the nurse in many situations, both in the hospital and in the home. Detection of impaired oral mucous membranes or a poor dental condition may require a change in the patient's diet. Additional mouth care may be needed to facilitate ingestion of food or to prevent infection of the gums (gingivitis). Detection of nasal septal deviation may help the nurse to determine which nostril to use to insert a nasogastric tube or how to suction a patient. In addition, assessing for nasal obstruction may explain the reason for mouth breathing.

Assessment of the mouth, throat, nose and sinuses usually follows the examination of the head and neck. Techniques for this examination are fairly simple to perform. However, the nurse will continue to develop proficiency in interpreting findings with continued practice.

Preparing the patient

Have the patient assume a sitting position with the head erect. It is best if the patient's head is at your eye level. Explain the specific structures you will be examining, and ask the patient who wears dentures, a retainer or rubber bands on braces to remove them for an adequate oral examination. A patient wearing dentures may feel embarrassed and concerned about their appearance and about the possibility of breath odour on removing the dentures. A gentle, yet confident and matter-of-fact approach may help the patient to feel more at ease.

Equipment

- Gloves (wear gloves when examining any mucous membrane)
- Gauze squares
- Penlight
- Short, wide-tipped speculum attached to the head of an otoscope
- Tongue depressor
- Nasal speculum

Physical assessment

When preparing to examine the nose and mouth:

- Be able to identify and understand the relationship among the structures of the mouth and throat, nose and sinuses
- Know age-related changes of the oral cavity and nasal and sinus structures.
- Be aware of ethnocultural phenomena related to oral and nasal health.
- Refine your examination techniques.

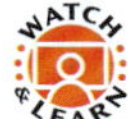
Assessing the nose and sinuses
Assessing the mouth and throat

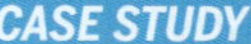

CASE STUDY

Upon examination, you note that Mr Miller's face and neck are flushed, with dark circles underlying his eyes. His vital signs are as follows: blood pressure 126/72 mmHg right arm, pulse 104, respirations 24 and oral temperature 39.6 °C. When inspecting his throat, you find erythema and oedema of the pharynx and uvula, with white patchy exudate on the tonsillar areas. Tonsils are 3+ and infected. Cervical and retropharyngeal lymph nodes are grossly palpable and very tender.

CRITICAL THINKING

5. Of the above findings, which do you think contribute towards generating a diagnosis for Mr Miller? Provide a justification for your decisions.
6. Some of Mr Miller's findings are within normal ranges. Should this be expected? If no aberration exists with particular findings, might this help in determining his problem? Justify your answer.

PHYSICAL ASSESSMENT

ASSESSMENT PROCEDURE	NORMAL FINDINGS	ABNORMAL FINDINGS
Mouth		
INSPECTION AND PALPATION		
Inspect the lips. Observe lip consistency and colour.	Lips are smooth and moist without lesions or swelling. Pink lips are normal in light-skinned patients as are bluish or freckled lips in some dark-skinned patients, especially those of Mediterranean descent. **CULTURAL CONSIDERATIONS** **Cleft lips, a birth abnormality where two parts of the lip do not fuse normally at birth, are seen more commonly in Asian-derived populations, with as many as 1 in 500 as opposed to 1 in 1,000 in European-derived populations (Dixon et al., 2011).**	Pallor around the lips (circumoral pallor) is seen in anaemia and shock. Bluish (cyanotic) lips may result from cold or hypoxia. Reddish lips are seen in patients with ketoacidosis, carbon monoxide poisoning and chronic obstructive pulmonary disease with polycythaemia. Swelling of the lips (oedema) is common in local or systemic allergic or anaphylactic reactions. Additional abnormal findings are pictured in Abnormal findings 19-1.
Inspect the teeth and gums. Ask the patient to open the mouth (Fig. 19-6). Note the number, colour, condition and alignment of the teeth.	Thirty-two pearly whitish teeth with smooth surfaces and edges. Upper molars should rest directly on the lower molars and the front upper incisors should slightly override the lower incisors. Some patients normally have only 28 teeth if the four wisdom teeth do not erupt. No repaired or decayed areas; no missing teeth or appliances.	Patients who smoke, drink large quantities of coffee or tea or have an excessive intake of fluoride may have yellow or brownish teeth. Use of some drugs while in utero or as a neonate may discolour teeth. Tooth decay (cavities) may appear as brown dots or cover more extensive areas of chewing surfaces. Missing teeth can affect chewing as well as self-image. A chalky white area in the

PHYSICAL ASSESSMENT (continued)

ASSESSMENT PROCEDURE	NORMAL FINDINGS	ABNORMAL FINDINGS
FIGURE 19-6 Inspecting the general condition of the teeth.		tooth surface is a cavity that will turn darker with time. Malocclusion of teeth is seen when upper or lower incisors protrude. Poor occlusion of teeth can affect chewing, wearing down of teeth, speech and self-image. White spots on teeth may result from antibiotic therapy.
Put on gloves and retract the patient's lips (Fig. 19-7) and cheeks to check gums for colour and consistency. 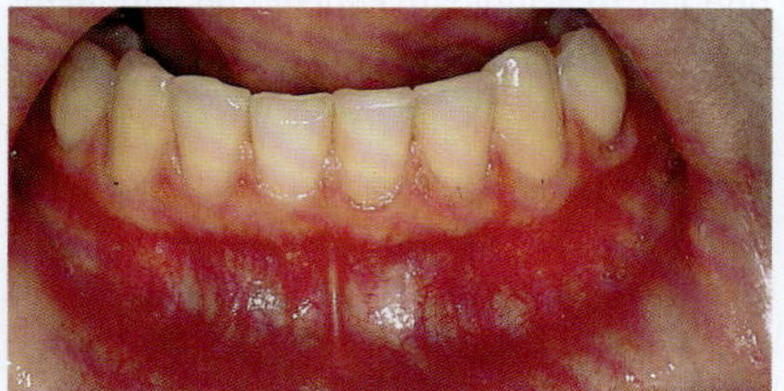 **FIGURE 19-7** Lower gingiva (gums).	**CULTURAL CONSIDERATIONS** **Compared with non-Aboriginal and Torres Strait Islander Australians, Aboriginal and Torres Strait Islander peoples are up to three times more likely to have untreated caries (Williams et al., 2011). Māori and Pasifika also report higher levels of untreated caries and missing teeth than the non-Māori population (Ministry of Health New Zealand, 2010b).**	Receding gums are abnormal in younger patients; in elderly patients, the teeth may appear longer because of age-related gingival recession, which is common. Red, swollen gums that bleed easily are seen in gingivitis, scurvy (vitamin C deficiency) and leukaemia. Receding red gums with loss of teeth are seen in periodontitis. Enlarged reddened gums (hyperplasia) that may cover some of the normally exposed teeth may be seen in pregnancy, puberty, leukaemia and use of some medications, such as phenytoin. A bluish-black or grey-white line along the gum line is seen in lead poisoning (see Abnormal findings 19-1).
Inspect the buccal mucosa. Use a penlight and tongue depressor to retract the lips and cheeks to check colour and consistency (Fig. 19-8). Also note Stensen ducts (parotid ducts) located on the buccal mucosa across from the second upper molars. 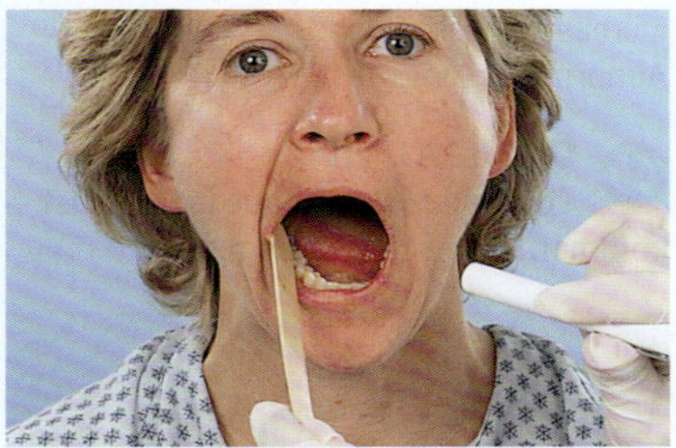 **FIGURE 19-8** Inspecting the buccal mucosa. (© B. Proud.)	It should appear pink in light-skinned patients; tissue pigmentation typically increases in dark-skinned patients. In both, tissue is smooth and moist without lesions. Stensen ducts are visible with flow of saliva and with no redness, swelling, pain or moistness in area. Fordyce spots or granules, yellowish-whitish raised spots, are normal ectopic sebaceous glands. **OLDER ADULT CONSIDERATIONS** **Oral mucosa is often drier and more fragile in the older patient because the epithelial lining of the salivary glands degenerates.**	Leucoplakia may be seen in chronic irritation and smoking. **CLINICAL TIP** **Smokers may also have a yellow-brown coating on the tongue, which is not leucoplakia.** Leucoplakia is a precancerous lesion, and the patient should be referred for evaluation. Whitish, curdlike patches that scrape off over reddened mucosa and bleed easily indicate 'thrush' (*Candida albicans*) infection. Koplik spots (tiny whitish spots that lie over reddened mucosa) are an early sign of the measles. Canker sores or mouth ulcers may be seen as many brown patches inside the cheeks of patients with adrenocortical insufficiency. See Abnormal findings 19-1.
Inspect and palpate the tongue. Ask patient to stick out the tongue. Inspect for colour, moisture, size and texture. Observe for fasciculations (fine tremors) and check for midline protrusion. Palpate any lesions present for induration (hardness).	Tongue should be pink, moist, a moderate size with papillae (little protuberances) present. A common variation is a fissured, topographic-maplike tongue, which is not unusual in older patients (Fig. 19-9). No lesions are present.	Among possible abnormalities are deep longitudinal *fissures* seen in dehydration; a *black tongue* indicative of bismuth (Pepto-Bismol) toxicity: *black, hairy tongue;* a smooth, reddish, shiny tongue without papillae indicative of niacin or vitamin B12 deficiencies, certain anaemias, and antineoplastic therapy (see Abnormal findings 19-1). An enlarged tongue suggests

Continued on following page

PHYSICAL ASSESSMENT (continued)

ASSESSMENT PROCEDURE	NORMAL FINDINGS	ABNORMAL FINDINGS
Mouth (continued)		
	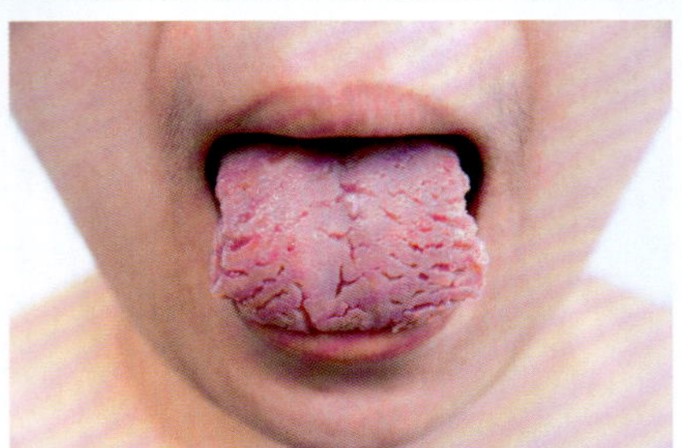 **FIGURE 19-9** Fissured tongue. (Shutterstock.com/photo one.)	hypothyroidism, acromegaly or Down syndrome, or angioneurotic oedema of anaphylaxis. A very small tongue suggests malnutrition. An atrophied tongue or fasciculations point to cranial nerve (hypoglossal, CN 12) damage.
Assess the ventral surface of the tongue. Ask the patient to touch the tongue to the roof of mouth, and use a penlight to inspect ventral surface of the tongue, frenulum and area under the tongue. Palpate the area (Fig. 19-10) if you see lesions, if the patient is over age 50 or if the patient uses tobacco or alcohol. Note any induration. Check also for a short frenulum that limits tongue motion (the origin of 'tongue-tied').	The tongue's ventral surface is smooth, shiny, pink or slightly pale with visible veins and no lesions. **OLDER ADULT CONSIDERATIONS** **The older patient may have varicose veins on the ventral surface of the tongue (Fig. 19-11).**	Leucoplakia, persistent lesions, ulcers or nodules may indicate cancer and should be referred. Induration increases the likelihood of cancer. **CLINICAL TIP** **The area underneath the tongue is the most common site of oral cancer.**
Inspect for Wharton ducts—openings from the submandibular salivary glands—located on either side of the frenulum on the floor of the mouth.	The frenulum is midline; Wharton ducts are visible with salivary flow or moistness in the area. The patient has no swelling, redness or pain.	Abnormal findings include lesions, ulcers, nodules or hypertrophied duct openings on either side of frenulum.
Observe the sides of the tongue; use a square gauze pad to hold the patient's tongue to each side (Fig. 19-12). Palpate any lesions, ulcers or nodules for induration.	No lesions, ulcers or nodules are apparent.	Canker sores or mouth ulcers may be seen on the sides of the tongue in patients receiving certain kinds of chemotherapy. Leucoplakia, persistent lesions, ulcers or nodules may indicate cancer and should be further evaluated medically. Induration increases the likelihood of cancer (see Abnormal findings 19-1). **CLINICAL TIP** **The side of the tongue is the most common site of tongue cancer.**
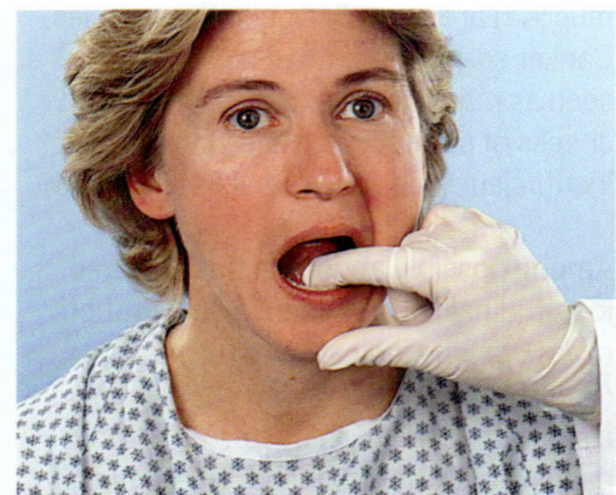 **FIGURE 19-10** Palpating the area under the tongue. (© B. Proud.)	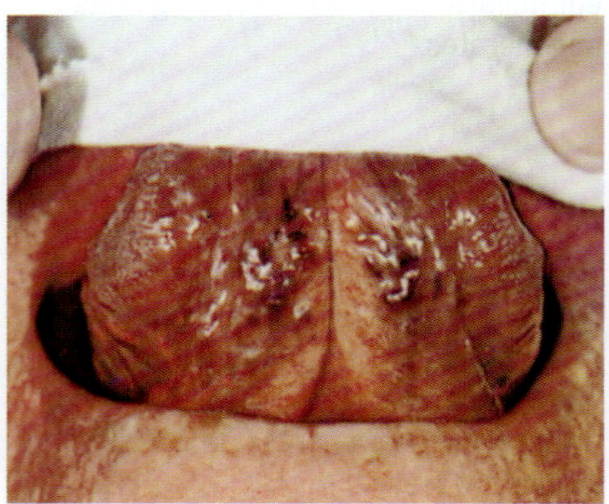 **FIGURE 19-11** Varicose veins on the ventral surface of the tongue.	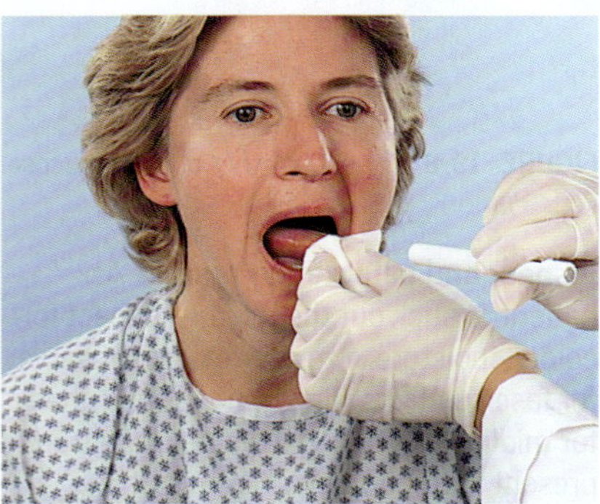 **FIGURE 19-12** Inspecting the side of the tongue. (© B. Proud.)

PHYSICAL ASSESSMENT (continued)

ASSESSMENT PROCEDURE	NORMAL FINDINGS	ABNORMAL FINDINGS
Check the strength of the tongue. Place your fingers on the external surface of the patient's cheek. Ask the patient to press the tongue's tip against the inside of the cheek to resist pressure from your fingers. Repeat on the opposite cheek.	The tongue offers strong resistance.	Decreased tongue strength may occur with a defect of the 12th cranial nerve—hypoglossal—or with a shortened frenulum that limits motion.
Check the anterior tongue's ability to taste by placing drops of sugar and salty water on the tip and sides of tongue with a tongue depressor.	The patient can distinguish between sweet and salty.	Loss of taste discrimination occurs with zinc deficiency, a seventh cranial nerve (facial) defect and certain medication use.
Inspect the hard (anterior) and soft (posterior) palates and uvula. Ask the patient to open the mouth wide while you use a penlight to look at the roof. Observe colour and integrity. 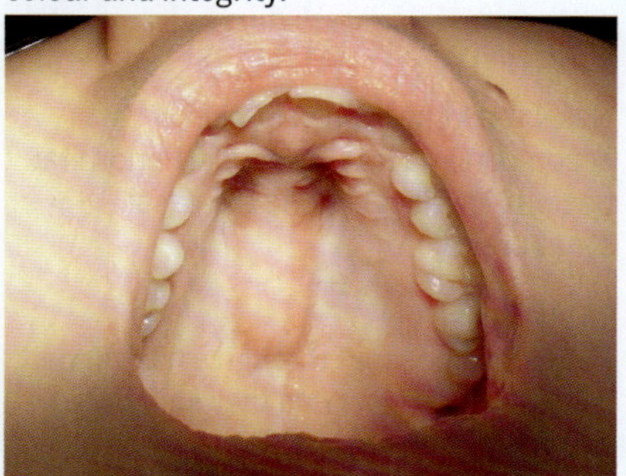 **FIGURE 19-13** Torus palatinus. (Wikimedia Commons. CC BY SA 3.0 Unported license. As at https://commons.wikimedia.org/wiki/File:Maxillary_tori.jpg [Accessed 9 April 2020].)	The hard palate is pale or whitish with firm, transverse rugae (wrinklelike folds).  **CULTURAL CONSIDERATIONS** **A bony protuberance in the midline of the hard palate, called a torus palatinus, is a normal variation seen more often in females, Inuit, Native Americans and Asians (Fig. 19-13).** Palatine tissues are intact; palate movable, spongy and smooth.	A candidal infection may appear as thick white plaques on the hard palate. Deep purple, raised or flat lesions may indicate a Kaposi sarcoma (seen in patients with acquired immunodeficiency syndrome; see Abnormal findings 19-1). A yellow tint to the hard palate may indicate jaundice because bilirubin adheres to elastic tissue (collagen). An opening in the hard palate is known as a cleft palate.
Note odour. While the mouth is wide open, note any unusual or foul odour.	No unusual or foul odour is noted.	Fruity or acetone breath is associated with diabetic ketoacidosis. An ammonia odour is often associated with kidney disease. Foul odours may indicate an oral or respiratory infection, or tooth decay. Alcohol or tobacco use may be identified by breath odour. Faecal breath odour occurs in bowel obstruction; sulfur odour (fetor hepaticus) occurs in end-stage liver disease.
Assess the uvula. Apply a tongue depressor to the tongue (halfway between the tip and back of the tongue) and shine a penlight into the patient's wide-open mouth (Fig. 19-14). Note the characteristics and positioning of the uvula. Ask the patient to say 'aaah' and watch for the uvula and soft palate to move. **CLINICAL TIP** **Depress the tongue slightly off centre to avoid eliciting the gag response.**	The uvula is a fleshy, solid structure that hangs freely in the midline. No redness of or exudate from uvula or soft palate. Midline elevation of uvula and symmetrical elevation of the soft palate. 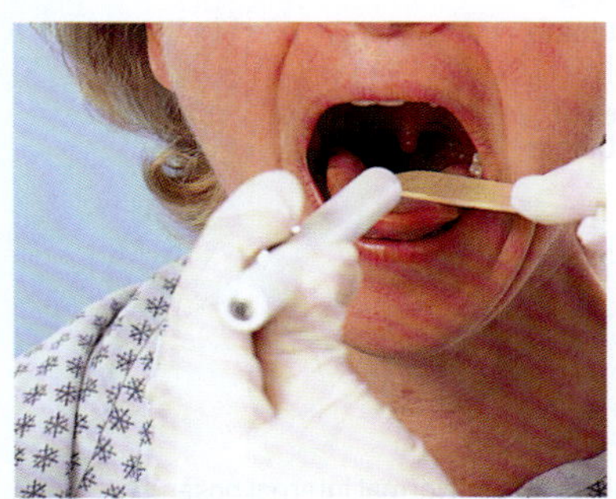 **FIGURE 19-14** Inspecting the uvula. (© B. Proud.)	A bifid uvula looks like it is split in two or partially severed. Patients with a bifid uvula may have a submucous cleft palate. Asymmetrical movement or loss of movement may occur after a cerebrovascular accident (stroke). Palate fails to rise and uvula deviates to normal side with cranial nerve X (vagus) paralysis.

Continued on following page

PHYSICAL ASSESSMENT (continued)

ASSESSMENT PROCEDURE	NORMAL FINDINGS	ABNORMAL FINDINGS
Mouth (continued)		
Inspect the tonsils. Using the tongue depressor to keep the mouth open wide, inspect the tonsils for colour, size and presence of exudate or lesions. Tonsils should be graded.	Tonsils may be present or absent. They are normally pink and symmetrical and may be enlarged to 1+ in healthy patients. No exudate, swelling or lesions should be present.	Tonsils are red, enlarged (to 21, 31 or 41), and covered with exudate in tonsillitis. Abnormal findings 19-2 depicts grading of tonsils. They also may be indurated with patches of white or yellow exudate.
Inspect the posterior pharyngeal wall. Keeping the tongue depressor in place, shine the penlight on the back of the throat. Observe the colour of the throat and note any exudate or lesions. Before inspecting the nose, discard gloves and perform hand hygiene.	Throat is normally pink without exudate or lesions. Atrophy of tonsils in adults is normal.	A bright-red throat with white or yellow exudate indicates pharyngitis. Yellowish mucus on throat may be seen with postnasal sinus drainage.
Nose		
INSPECTION AND PALPATION		
Inspect and palpate the external nose. Note nasal colour, shape, consistency and tenderness. Inspect external structures as well as periorbital area for swelling or oedema.	Colour is the same as the rest of the face; the nasal structure is smooth and symmetrical; the patient reports no tenderness.	Nasal tenderness on palpation accompanies a local infection. Periorbital oedema, swelling around the nasal structures.
Check patency of air flow through the nostrils by occluding one nostril at a time and asking patient to sniff. Inspect internal structures for swelling or oedema.	Patient is able to sniff through each nostril while other is occluded.	Patient cannot sniff through a nostril that is not occluded, nor can they sniff or blow air through the nostrils. This may be a sign of swelling, rhinitis or a foreign object obstructing the nostrils. A line across the tip of the nose just above the fleshy tip is common in patients with chronic allergies.
Inspect the internal nose. To inspect the internal nose, use an otoscope with a short wide-tip attachment (or you can also use a nasal speculum and penlight). Use your non-dominant hand to stabilise and gently tilt the patient's head back. Insert the short wide tip of the otoscope into the patient's nostril without touching the sensitive nasal septum (Fig. 19-15). Slowly 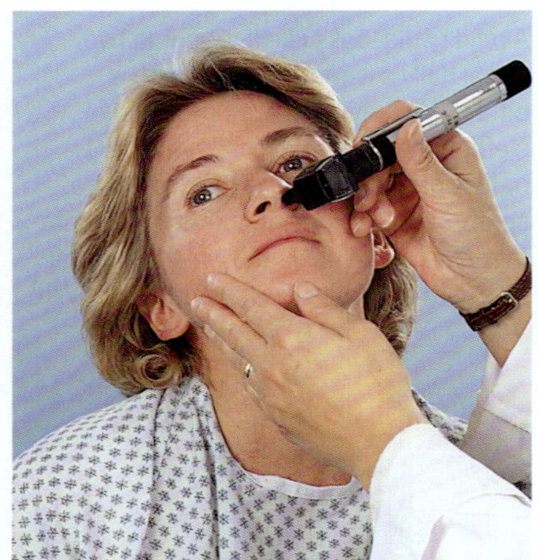 **FIGURE 19-15** Inspecting the internal nose using an otoscope and wide-tipped attachment. (© B. Proud.)	The nasal mucosa is dark pink, moist and free of exudate. The nasal septum is intact and free of ulcers or perforations. Turbinates are dark pink (redder than oral mucosa), moist and free of lesions (Fig. 19-16). The superior turbinate will not be visible from this point of view. A deviated septum may appear to be an overgrowth of tissue (Fig. 19-17). This is a normal finding as long as breathing is not obstructed. 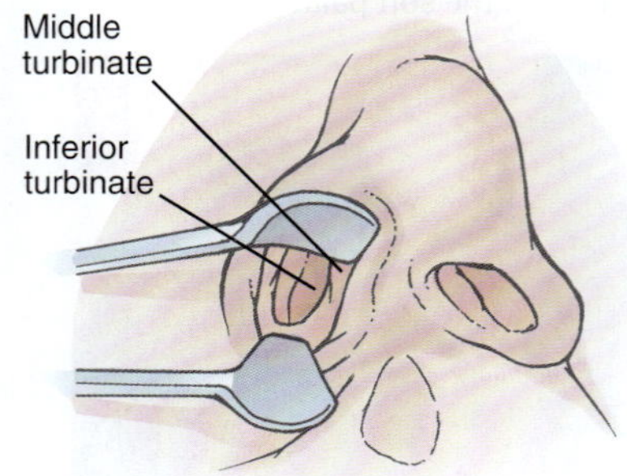 **FIGURE 19-16** Normal internal nose.	Nasal mucosa is swollen and pale pink or bluish grey in patients with allergies. Nasal mucosa is red and swollen with upper respiratory infection. Exudate is common with infection and may range from large amounts of watery discharge to thick yellow-green purulent discharge. Purulent nasal discharge is seen with acute bacterial rhinosinusitis. Bleeding (epistaxis) or crusting may be noted on lower anterior part of nasal septum with local irritation. Ulcers of the nasal mucosa or a perforated septum may be seen with use of cocaine, trauma, chronic 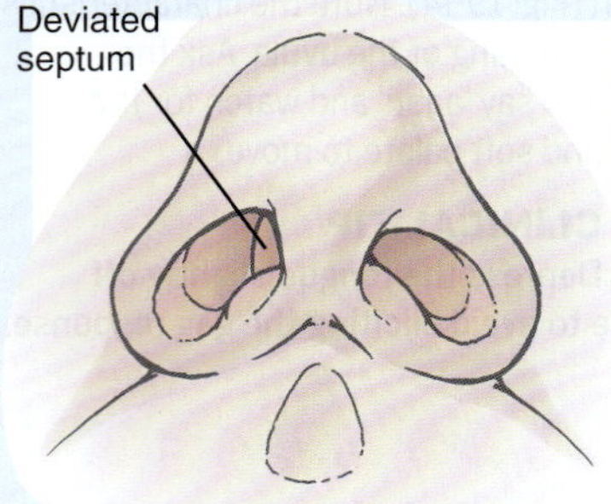 **FIGURE 19-17** Deviated septum.

PHYSICAL ASSESSMENT (continued)

ASSESSMENT PROCEDURE	NORMAL FINDINGS	ABNORMAL FINDINGS
direct the otoscope back and up to view the nasal mucosa, nasal septum, the inferior and middle turbinates, and the nasal passage (the narrow space between the septum and the turbinates). **CLINICAL TIP** **Position the otoscope's handle to the side to improve your view of the structures. If an otoscope is unavailable, use a penlight and hold the tip of the nose slightly up. A nasal speculum with a penlight also facilitates good visualisation.**		infection or chronic nose picking. Small, pale, round, firm overgrowths or masses on mucosa (polyps) are seen in patients with chronic allergies (see Abnormal findings 19-3).
Sinuses		
PALPATION		
Palpate the sinuses. When an infection is suspected, the nurse can examine the sinuses through palpation, percussion and transillumination. Palpate the frontal sinuses by using your thumbs to press up on the brow on each side of nose (Fig. 19-18).	Frontal and maxillary sinuses are non-tender to palpation, and no crepitus is evident.	Frontal or maxillary sinuses are tender to palpation in patients with allergies or acute bacterial rhinosinusitis. If the patient has a large amount of exudate, you may feel crepitus upon palpation over the maxillary sinuses.
Palpate the maxillary sinuses by pressing with thumbs up on the maxillary sinuses (Fig. 19-19).	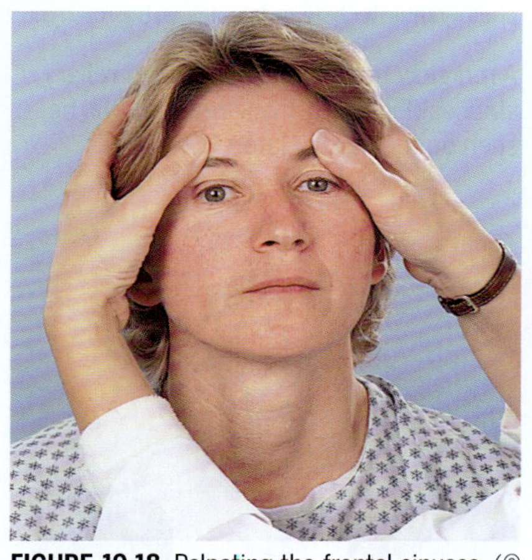 **FIGURE 19-18** Palpating the frontal sinuses. (© B. Proud.)	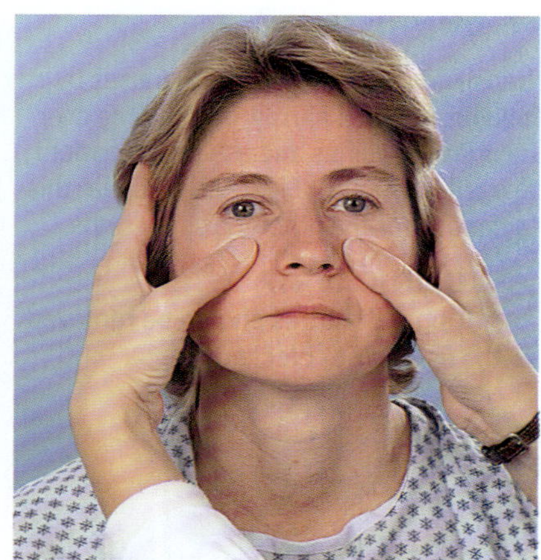 **FIGURE 19-19** Palpating the maxillary sinuses. (© B. Proud.)
PERCUSSION		
Percuss the sinuses. Lightly tap (percuss) over the frontal sinuses and over the maxillary sinuses for tenderness.	The sinuses are not tender on percussion.	The frontal and maxillary sinuses are tender upon percussion in patients with allergies or sinus infection.
TRANSILLUMINATION		
Transilluminate the sinuses. If sinus tenderness was detected during palpation and percussion, transillumination will let you see if the sinuses are filled with fluid or pus. Transilluminate the frontal sinuses by holding a strong, narrow light source snugly under the eyebrows (the room should be	A red glow transilluminates the frontal sinuses. This indicates a normal, air-filled sinus.	Absence of a red glow usually indicates a sinus filled with fluid or pus.

Continued on following page

PHYSICAL ASSESSMENT (continued)

ASSESSMENT PROCEDURE	NORMAL FINDINGS	ABNORMAL FINDINGS
Sinuses (continued)		
dark). Use your other hand to shield the light. Repeat this technique for the other frontal sinus. Figure 19-20 illustrates the technique.	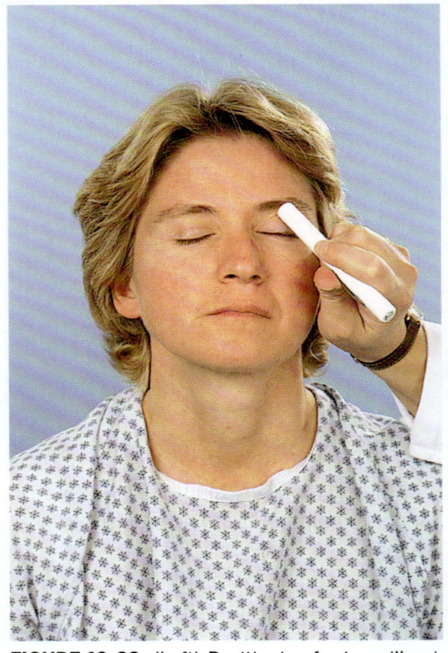	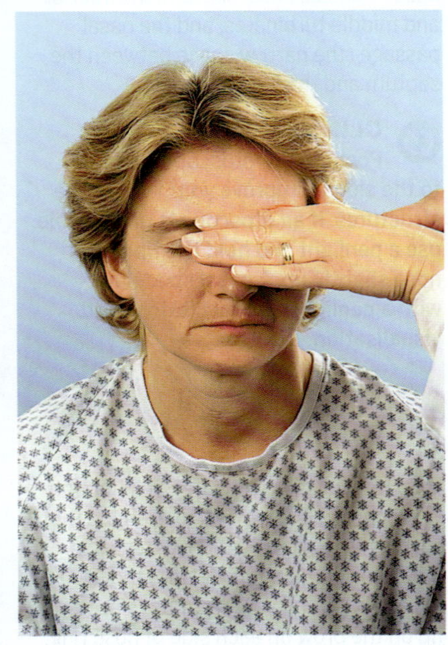
	FIGURE 19-20 (Left) Positioning for transillumination of frontal sinuses. (Right) Transillumination of frontal sinuses; note the red glow. (This photograph shows a lighted room because of a special photographic technique. In practice, the room must be dark to show the red glow. © B. Proud.)	
Transilluminate the maxillary sinuses by holding a strong, narrow light source over the maxillary sinus and asking the patient to open his mouth (Fig. 19-21). Repeat this technique for the other maxillary sinus. **CLINICAL TIP** **Upper dentures should be removed so the light is not blocked.**	A red glow transilluminates the maxillary sinuses (Fig. 19-22). The red glow will be seen on the hard palate. 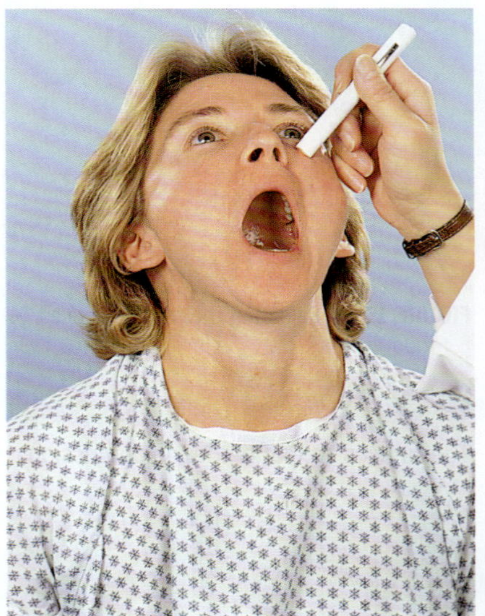 **FIGURE 19-21** Positioning for transillumination of maxillary sinuses. (© B. Proud.)	Absence of a red glow usually indicates a sinus filled with fluid, pus or thick mucus (from chronic sinusitis; see Promote health—Sinusitis). 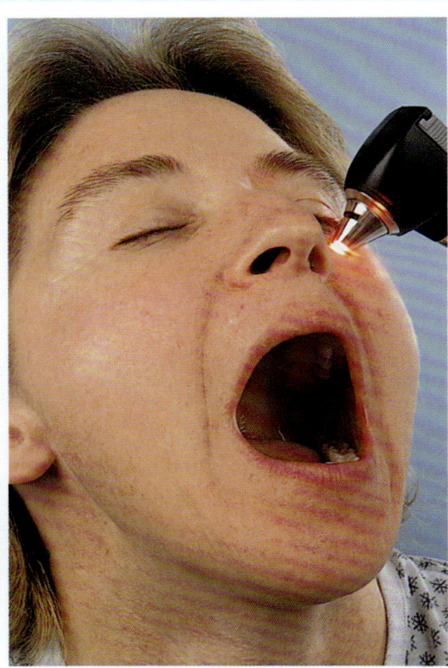 **FIGURE 19-22** Transillumination of maxillary sinuses; note the red glow. (This photograph shows a lighted room because of a special photographic technique. In practice, the room must be dark to show the red glow. © B. Proud.)

ABNORMAL FINDINGS 19-1 Abnormalities of the Mouth and Throat

This display depicts common abnormalities of the mouth and throat.

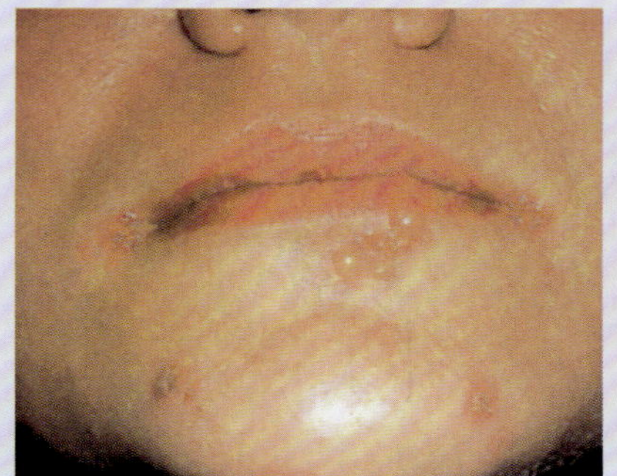
Herpes simplex type I

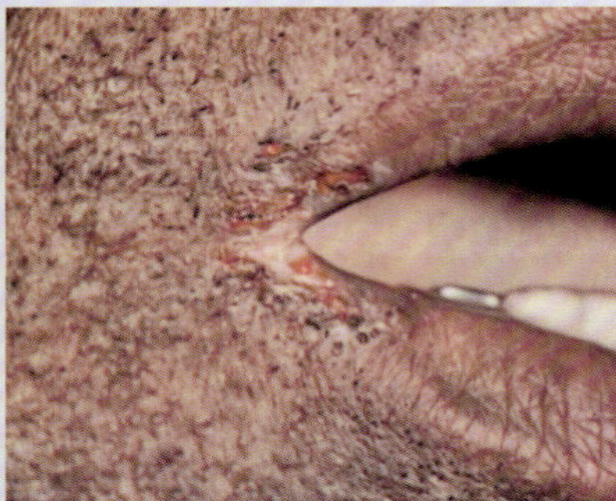
Cheilosis of lips.

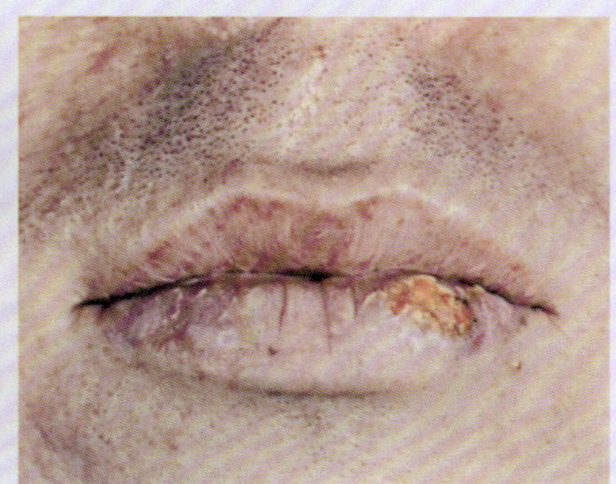
Carcinoma of lip

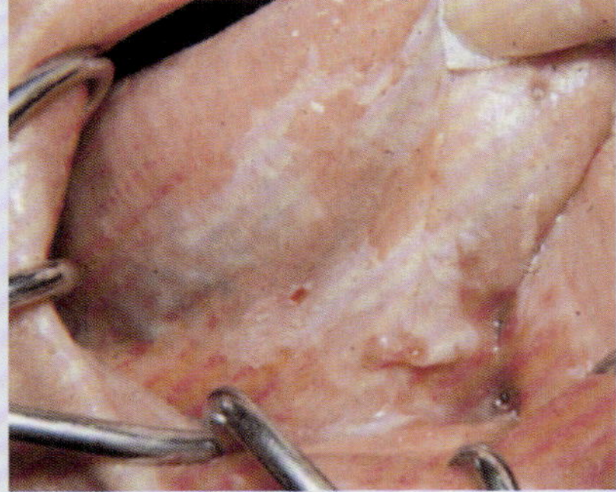
Leucoplakia (ventral surface)

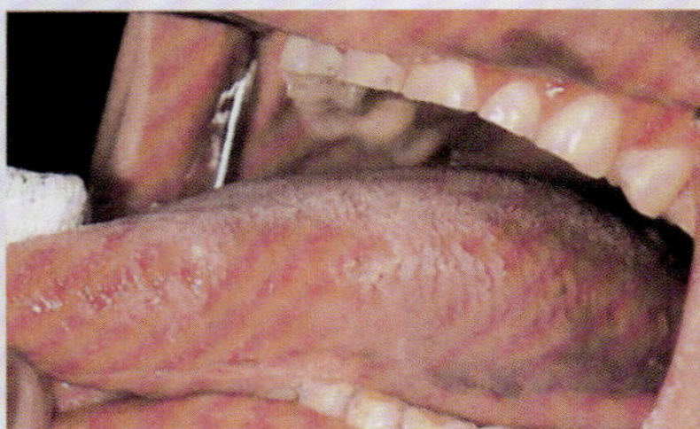
Hairy leucoplakia. (lateral surface)

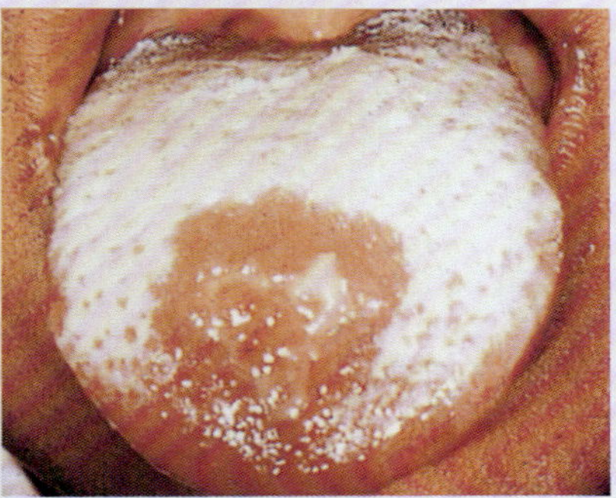
Candida albicans infection (thrush)

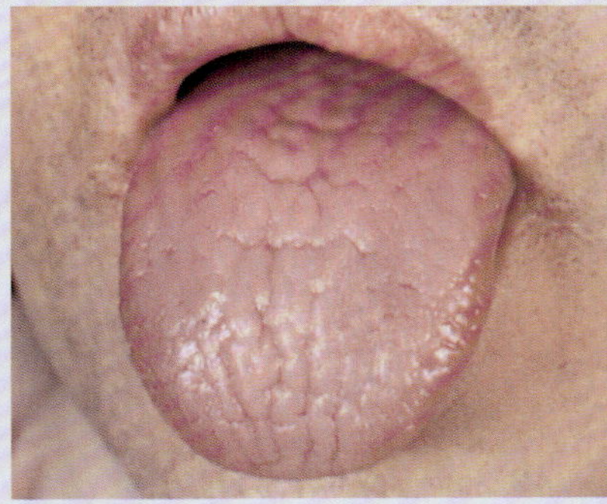
Smooth, reddish, shiny tongue without papillae due to vitamin B12 deficiency

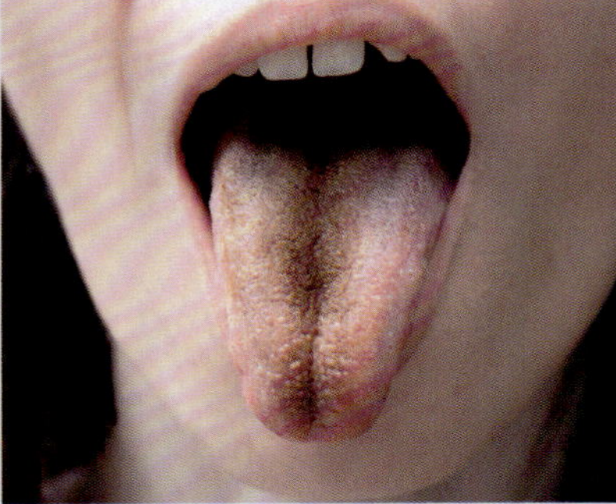
Black hairy tongue. (Shutterstock.com/sruilk.)

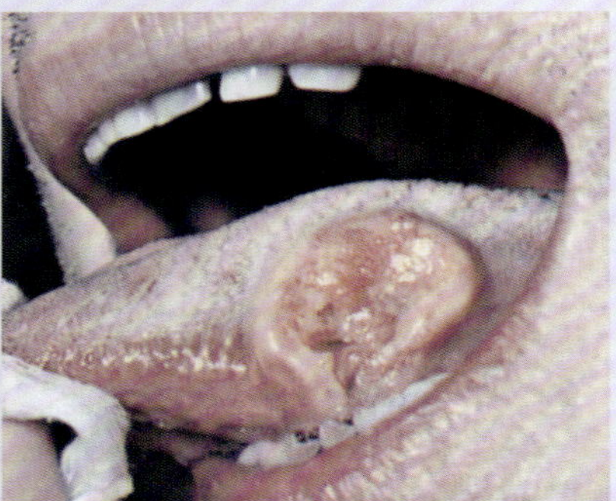
Carcinoma of tongue

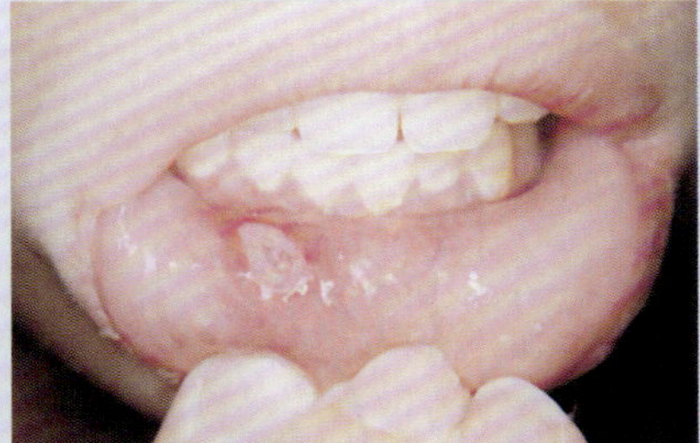
Canker sore or mouth ulcer

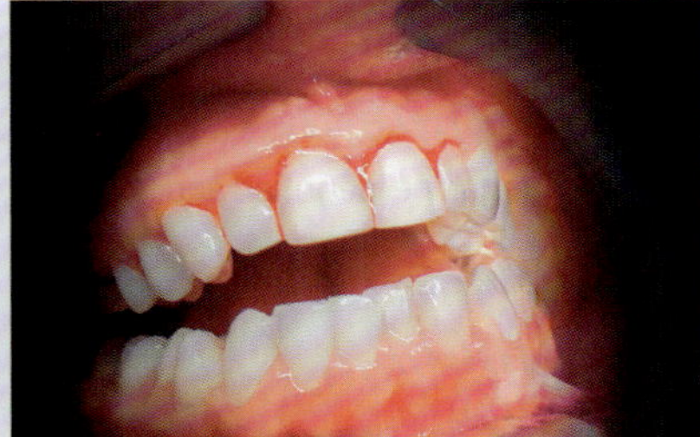
Gingivitis. (Shutterstock.com/Algirdas Gelazius.)

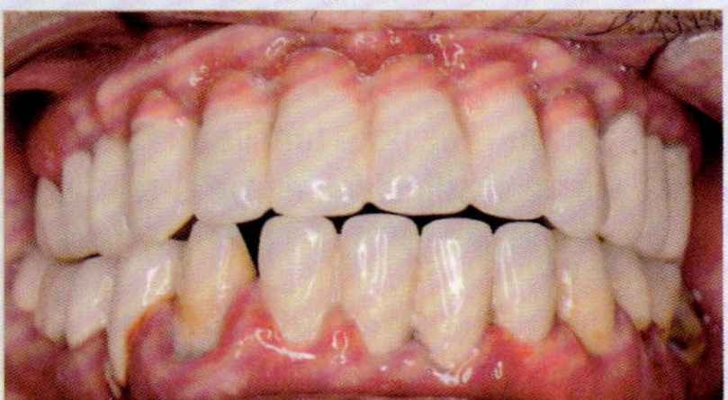
Receding gums (Shutterstock.com/Dirk Saegar.)

Continued on following page

ABNORMAL FINDINGS 19-1 Abnormalities of the Mouth and Throat (continued)

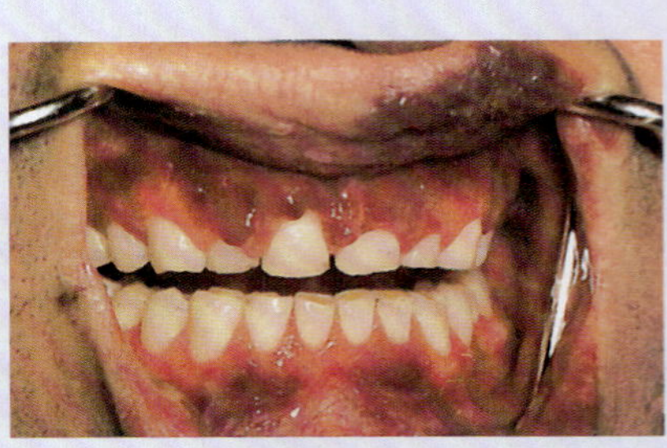

Kaposi sarcoma lesions

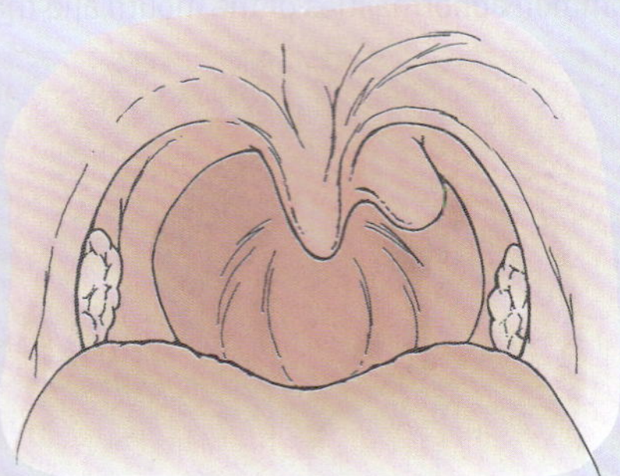

Bifid uvula.

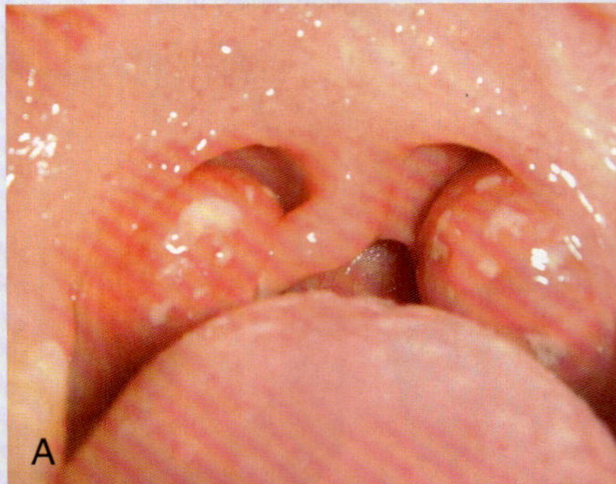

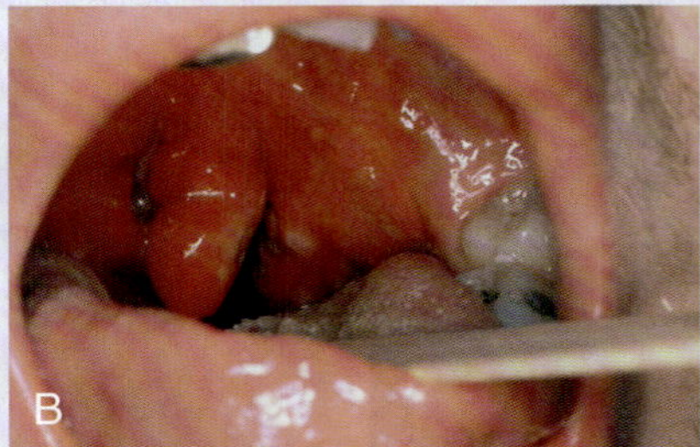

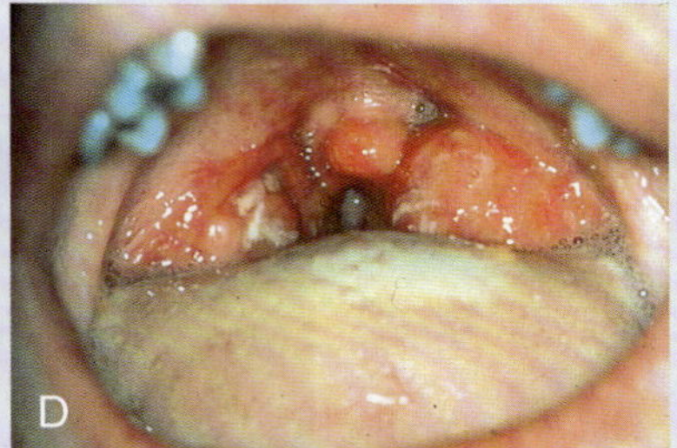

Acute tonsillitis and pharyngitis. (**A,** Wikimedia Commons/Pbeck.; **B,** St. Bartholomew's Hospital/Science Photo Library; **C,** Used with permission from Handler, S. D. & Myer, C. M. [1998]. *Atlas of ear, nose and throat disorders in children* [pp. 90, 91]. Ontario, Canada: BC Decker; **D,** From Bickley, L. [2003]. *Bates' guide to physical examination and history taking* [8th ed.]. Philadelphia: Lippincott Williams & Wilkins.)

ABNORMAL FINDINGS 19-2 Tonsillitis (Detecting and Grading)

In a patient who has both tonsils and a sore throat, tonsillitis can be identified and ranked with a grading scale from 1 to 4 as follows:

1+ Tonsils are visible.
2+ Tonsils are midway between tonsillar pillars and uvula.
3+ Tonsils touch the uvula.
4+ Tonsils touch each other.

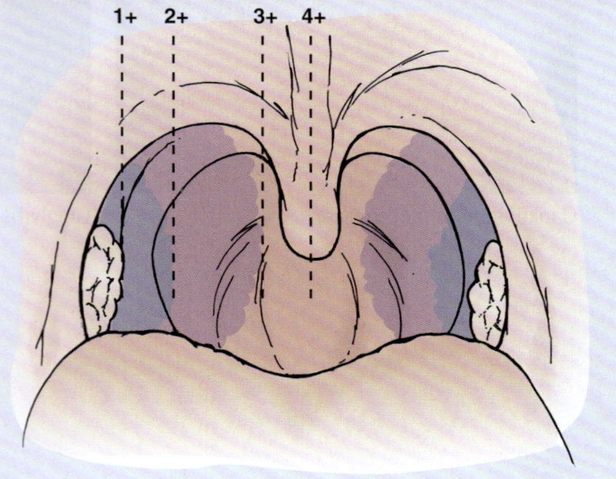

ABNORMAL FINDINGS 19-3 Abnormalities of the Nose

The following are common abnormalities of the nose.

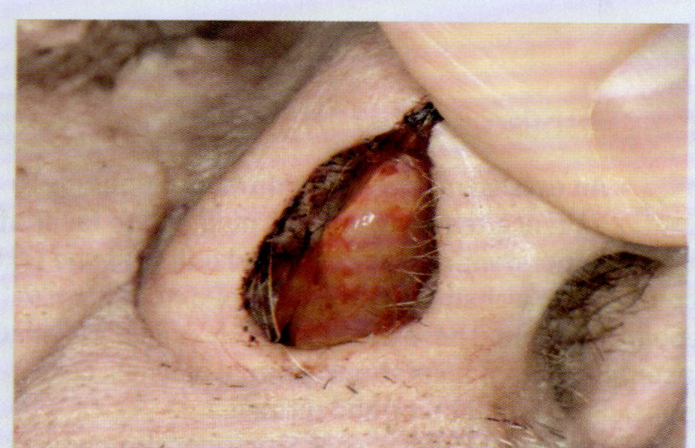

Nasal polyp. (Dr P. Marazzi/Science Photo Library.)

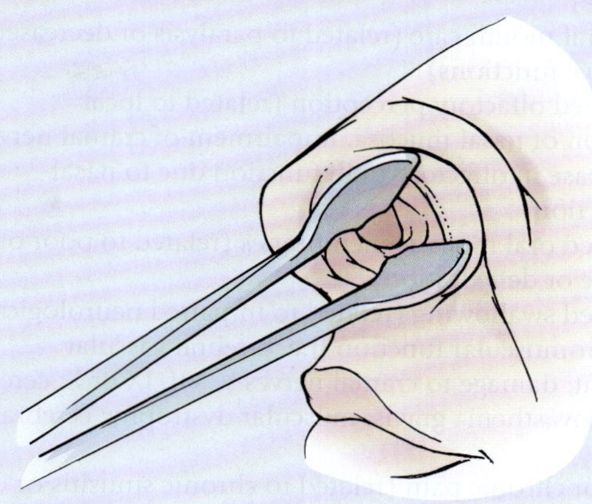

Perforated septum.

VALIDATING AND DOCUMENTING FINDINGS

Validate the mouth, throat, nose and sinus assessment data that you have collected. This is necessary to verify that the data are reliable and accurate. Document the assessment data following the health care facility or agency policy.

The following subjective and objective data samples do not relate specifically to Mr Miller and are included as examples you can follow in practising data collection and documentation for Mr Miller and other patients.

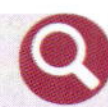

Sample of subjective data

Patient describes the condition of mouth, throat and nose as 'fine'. No history of past oral or nasal surgery. Has 32 permanent teeth. Had four teeth filled for cavities several years ago as a child. Brushes teeth twice a day and uses dental floss each evening. Occasional mild bleeding with flossing. Never needed braces. Receives regular dental checkups twice a year. Has occasional sinus headaches (one to two per year) and minor sore throats due to sinus drainage. Relieved with over-the-counter oral decongestants and paracetamol (Panadol). Nasal discharge clear to purulent occasionally. No oral or nasal lesions noted by patient. Does not smoke. No difficulty breathing through either nostril. Able to chew and swallow without difficulty. No oral or nasal pain or tenderness.

Sample of objective data

Lips pink, smooth and moist without lesions. Buccal mucosa pink, moist and without exudate. Parotid ducts visible with no redness or swelling. Moist bubbles are seen near ducts. Thirty-two white to yellowish teeth present. Gums pink without redness or swelling. Protrudes geographic tongue in midline with no tremors. Equal bilateral strength in tongue. Ventral surface of tongue smooth and shiny pink with small visible veins present. Frenulum in midline with visible submandibular ducts on each side. Torus palatinus visible on whitish hard palate. Soft palate smooth and pink. Midline and symmetrical elevation of uvula and soft palate with phonation. Tonsillar pillars pink and symmetrical. Tonsils absent.

Nose somewhat large but smooth and symmetrical. Able to sniff and blow through each nostril. Nasal septum slightly deviated to left but does not obstruct air flow. Inferior and middle turbinates dark pink, moist and free of lesions. No purulent drainage noted. Frontal and maxillary sinuses transilluminate and are non-tender to palpation and percussion.

After you have collected your assessment data, you will need to analyse the data using diagnostic reasoning skills. Refer to the discussion of the diagnostic reasoning process in Chapter 5.

Analysis of data

DIAGNOSTIC REASONING: POSSIBLE CONCLUSIONS

After collecting subjective and objective data pertaining to the mouth, throat, nose and sinuses, identify abnormal findings and patient strengths. Then cluster the data to reveal any significant patterns or abnormalities. These data may be used to make clinical judgements about the status of the patient's mouth, throat, nose and sinuses.

Potential patient risks

- Risk of aspiration (related to decreased or absent gag reflex)
- Risk of poor nutrition (related to poorly fitting dentures or gum disease)
- Risk of infection of gums (related to poor oral hygiene)
- Risk of injury to teeth and gums (related to participation in active sports and lack of knowledge of protective mouth gear)
- Risk of airway obstruction.

Potential patient problems

- Ineffective health maintenance (related to poor oral hygiene)
- Poor oral mouth care (related to paralysis or decreased cognitive functions)
- Disturbed olfactory perception (related to local irritation of nasal mucosa, impairment of cranial nerve I, decrease in olfactory bulb function due to nasal obstruction)
- Impaired oral mucous membranes (related to poor oral hygiene or dehydration)
- Impaired swallowing (related to impaired neurological or neuromuscular function [i.e. cerebral vascular accident; damage to cranial nerves V, VII, IX or X; cerebral palsy; myasthenia gravis; muscular dystrophy; cerebral palsy])
- Acute or chronic pain (related to chronic sinusitis or inflammation of oral mucous membranes [gingivitis, periodontitis, canker sores])
- Disturbed gustatory sensation (related to impairment of cranial nerve VII or IX, reduction of number of taste buds due to the ageing process)
- Poor nutrition (related to decreased appetite due to decreased sense of taste and smell and social isolation)

Selected collaborative problems

After grouping the data, certain collaborative problems may become apparent. Remember that collaborative problems cannot be prevented by nursing interventions. However, these physiological complications of medical conditions can be detected and monitored by the nurse. In addition, the nurse can use doctor- and nurse-prescribed interventions to minimise the complications of these problems. The nurse may also have to refer the patient in such situations for further treatment of the problem. The following is a list of collaborative problems that may be identified when assessing the mouth, throat, nose and sinuses.

- Epistaxis
- Airway compromise
- Sinus infection
- Stomatitis
- Gum infection (gingivitis, periodontitis)
- Oral lesions
- Laryngeal oedema.

Medical problems

If, after grouping the data, it becomes apparent that the patient has signs and symptoms that may require medical diagnosis and treatment, referral to a primary care provider is necessary.

ONLINE RESOURCES

An extensive range of additional resources to enhance teaching and learning and to facilitate understanding may be found online at the text's accompanying website, located on thePoint at http://thepoint.lww.com. These include Watch and Learn videos, Concepts in Action animations, journal articles, case studies, discussion topics and quizzes.

Subscribers may also access Lippincott Procedures, an extensive online point-of-care procedure guide that provides reliable step-by-step instructions for more than 1700 procedures, including 450 evidence-based Australian procedures, and skills in a variety of speciality settings, together with a wealth of supporting information.

SIMULATED LEARNING

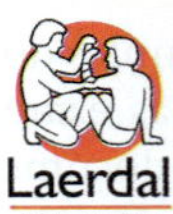

Having completed this chapter, explore the scenarios of Kenneth Bronson Part 1 and Part 2. Kenneth is a 27-year-old male with an acute strep throat. Incorporating the health assessment content in this chapter with your existing theoretical knowledge and clinical experience, progress through the simulation scenarios (this is best done in a small group). How would you manage Kenneth's care? When reflecting on your management of Kenneth, what do you think you did well and what do you think you can improve? Consider why you think this and also how you might manage a similar problem in the future.

CASE STUDY

The case study demonstrates how to analyse mouth, throat, nose and sinus assessment data for a specific patient. The exercises included in the ancillary product on thePoint that complements this text offer further opportunities to enhance your skills.

Jonathon Miller is a 22-year-old university student who visits the emergency department in mid-June, complaining of severe throat pain ('like swallowing razor blades'), swollen lymph nodes, chills, fever, general fatigue and anorexia. He admitted that he had been studying 'day and night' for final exams and had 'only one more to go'. 'This is the third time I've had this problem this year', he related. 'I didn't even bother coming in the first or second time. I just stayed in bed between classes and treated myself.'

Upon examination, you note that his face and neck are flushed, with dark circles underlying his eyes. His vital signs are as follows: blood pressure 126/72 mmHg right arm, pulse 104, respirations 24 and oral temperature 39.6 °C. When inspecting his throat, you find erythema and oedema of the pharynx and uvula, with white patchy exudate on the tonsillar areas. Tonsils are 3+ and infected. Cervical and retropharyngeal lymph nodes are grossly palpable and very tender.

The following concept map illustrates the diagnostic reasoning process.

Applying COLDSPA

Applying COLDSPA for patient symptoms: 'severe throat pain'.

Mnemonic	Question	Data provided	Missing data
Character	Describe the sign or symptom (feeling, appearance, sound, smell or taste, if applicable).	Severe throat pain	
Onset	When did it begin?		When did this pain first begin?
Location	Where is it? Does it radiate? Does it occur anywhere else?		Do you have any pain in your sinuses or neck?
Duration	How long does it last? Does it recur?	'Third time I have had this during the past year, but I have always just stayed in bed and treated it myself.'	
Severity	How bad is it? or How much does it bother you?	'Feels like I am swallowing razor blades.'	
Pattern	What makes it better or worse?		Have you tried anything that makes this better or worse?
Associated factors/How it Affects the patient	What other symptoms occur with it? How does it affect you?	'Swollen lymph nodes, chills, fever, fatigue and loss of appetite.'	

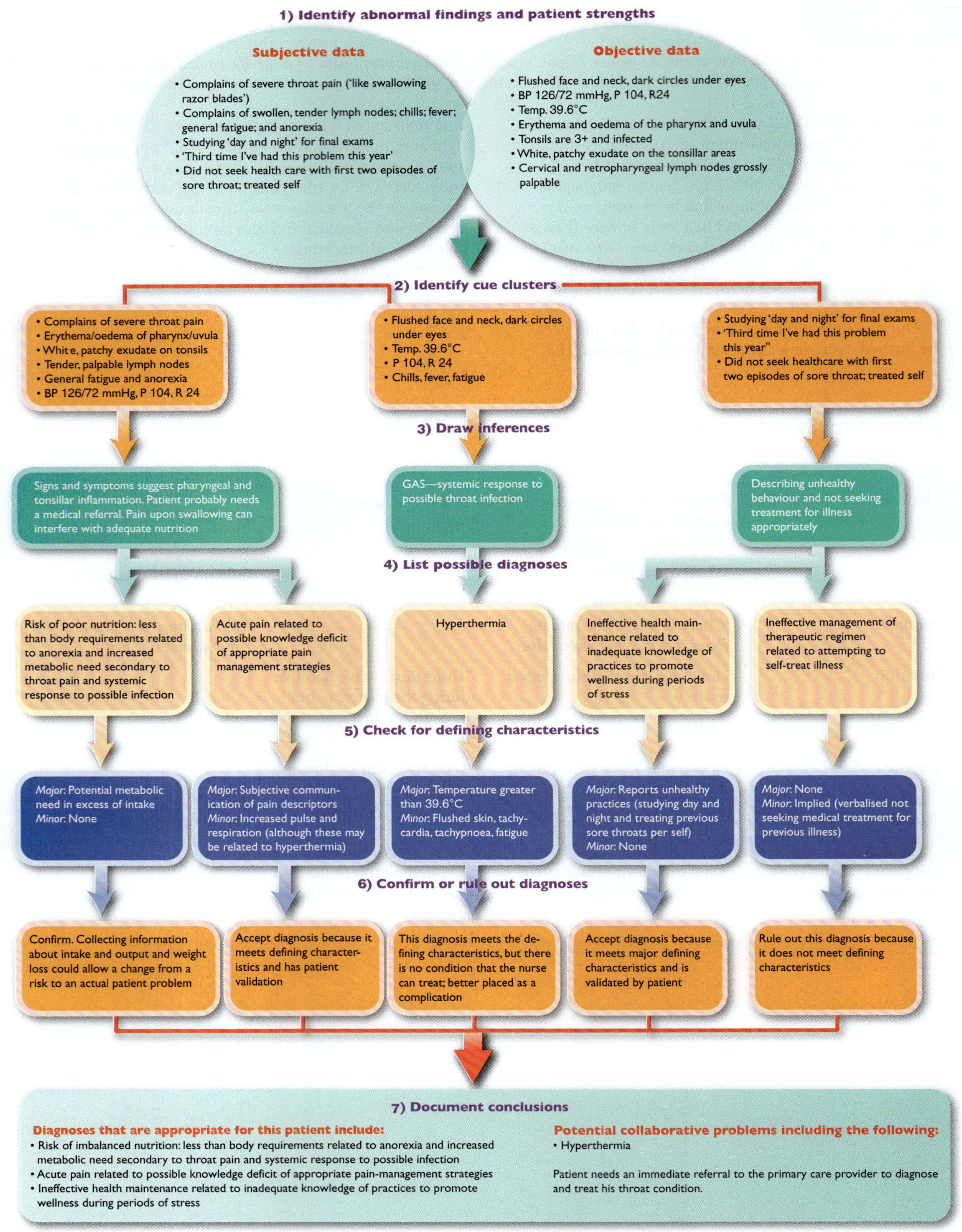

1) Identify abnormal findings and patient strengths

Subjective data

- Complains of severe throat pain ('like swallowing razor blades')
- Complains of swollen, tender lymph nodes; chills; fever; general fatigue; and anorexia
- Studying 'day and night' for final exams
- 'Third time I've had this problem this year'
- Did not seek health care with first two episodes of sore throat; treated self

Objective data

- Flushed face and neck, dark circles under eyes
- BP 126/72 mmHg, P 104, R24
- Temp. 39.6°C
- Erythema and oedema of the pharynx and uvula
- Tonsils are 3+ and infected
- White, patchy exudate on the tonsillar areas
- Cervical and retropharyngeal lymph nodes grossly palpable

2) Identify cue clusters

- Complains of severe throat pain
- Erythema/oedema of pharynx/uvula
- White, patchy exudate on tonsils
- Tender, palpable lymph nodes
- General fatigue and anorexia
- BP 126/72 mmHg, P 104, R 24

- Flushed face and neck, dark circles under eyes
- Temp. 39.6°C
- P 104, R 24
- Chills, fever, fatigue

- Studying 'day and night' for final exams
- 'Third time I've had this problem this year"
- Did not seek healthcare with first two episodes of sore throat; treated self

3) Draw inferences

Signs and symptoms suggest pharyngeal and tonsillar inflammation. Patient probably needs a medical referral. Pain upon swallowing can interfere with adequate nutrition

GAS—systemic response to possible throat infection

Describing unhealthy behaviour and not seeking treatment for illness appropriately

4) List possible diagnoses

Risk of poor nutrition: less than body requirements related to anorexia and increased metabolic need secondary to throat pain and systemic response to possible infection

Acute pain related to possible knowledge deficit of appropriate pain management strategies

Hyperthermia

Ineffective health maintenance related to inadequate knowledge of practices to promote wellness during periods of stress

Ineffective management of therapeutic regimen related to attempting to self-treat illness

5) Check for defining characteristics

Major: Potential metabolic need in excess of intake
Minor: None

Major: Subjective communication of pain descriptors
Minor: Increased pulse and respiration (although these may be related to hyperthermia)

Major: Temperature greater than 39.6°C
Minor: Flushed skin, tachycardia, tachypnoea, fatigue

Major: Reports unhealthy practices (studying day and night and treating previous sore throats per self)
Minor: None

Major: None
Minor: Implied (verbalised not seeking medical treatment for previous illness)

6) Confirm or rule out diagnoses

Confirm. Collecting information about intake and output and weight loss could allow a change from a risk to an actual patient problem

Accept diagnosis because it meets defining characteristics and has patient validation

This diagnosis meets the defining characteristics, but there is no condition that the nurse can treat; better placed as a complication

Accept diagnosis because it meets major defining characteristics and is validated by patient

Rule out this diagnosis because it does not meet defining characteristics

7) Document conclusions

Diagnoses that are appropriate for this patient include:

- Risk of imbalanced nutrition: less than body requirements related to anorexia and increased metabolic need secondary to throat pain and systemic response to possible infection
- Acute pain related to possible knowledge deficit of appropriate pain-management strategies
- Ineffective health maintenance related to inadequate knowledge of practices to promote wellness during periods of stress

Potential collaborative problems including the following:

- Hyperthermia

Patient needs an immediate referral to the primary care provider to diagnose and treat his throat condition.

References

Australian Bureau of Statistics. (2018). *National health survey: First results, 2017-18*. Canberra: Author. Cat. no. 4364.0.55.001.

Australian Institute of Health and Welfare (AIHW). (2018). Cancer data in Australia. Available at https://www.aihw.gov.au/reports/cancer/cancer-data-in-australia/contents/summary.

Bickley, L. (2003). *Bates' guide to physical examination and history taking* (8th ed.). Philadelphia: Lippincott Williams & Wilkins.

Brown, C. (2008). Chronic rhinosinusitis: 'It's my sinus, doc!'. *Australian Family Physician, 37*(4), 306–310.

Cancer Council Australia. (2018). Head and neck cancer. Viewed January 2019 at https://www.cancer.org.au/about-cancer/types-of-cancer/head-and-neck-cancer.html.

Dixon, M. J., Marazita, M. L., Beaty, T. H., et al. (2011). Cleft lip and palate: Understanding genetic and environmental influences. *Nature Reviews. Genetics, 12*(3), 167–178.

Handler, S. D. & Myer, C. M. (1998). *Atlas of ear, nose and throat disorders in children* (pp. 90–91). Ontario, Canada: BC Decker.

Kamangar, F., Chow, W. H., Abnet, C. C., et al. (2009). Environmental causes of oesophageal cancer. *Gastroenterology Clinics of North America, 38*(1), 25–57.

Madani, A. H., Jahromi, A. S., Dikshit, M., et al. (2010). Risk assessment of tobacco types and oral cancer. *American Journal of Pharmacology and Toxicology, 5*(1), 9–13.

Ministry of Health New Zealand. (2016a). Tables to accompany New cancer registrations 2016. Viewed January 2019 at https://www.health.govt.nz/publication/new-cancer-registrations-2016.

Ministry of Health New Zealand. (2010b). Our oral health: Key findings of the 2009 New Zealand Oral Health Survey. Viewed January 2019 at www.health.govt.nz/publication/our-oral-health-key-findings-2009-new-zealand-oral-health-survey.

Williams, S., Jamieson, L., MacRae, A., et al. (2011). Review of Indigenous oral health. Viewed January 2019 at https://healthinfonet.ecu.edu.au/key-resources/publications/20671/?title=Review%20of%20Indigenous%20oral%20health.

Selected reading

Australasian Society of Clinical Immunology and Allergy. (2015). Sinusitis and allergy. Available at https://www.allergy.org.au/images/pcc/ASCIA_PCC_Sinusitis_and_allergy_2015.pdf.

Online resources

Australian Cancer Research Foundation (ACRF): www.acrf.com.au

Australian Dental Association: www.ada.org.au

Australian and New Zealand Head & Neck Cancer Society: www.anzhncs.org

Australian Research Centre for Population Oral Health (ARCPOH): www.adelaide.edu.au/arcpoh

Cancer Council Australia: www.cancerorg.au

Cancer Society of New Zealand: www.cancernz.org.nz

New Zealand Dental Association: www.nzda.org.nz

CHAPTER 20

Thorax and lungs

CASE STUDY

George Burney is a 60-year-old retired Caucasian man. He was admitted to hospital 10 days ago following an episode of acute respiratory failure secondary to chronic obstructive pulmonary disease. You are caring for Mr Burney today.

Structure and function

The term thorax identifies the portion of the body extending from the base of the neck superiorly to the level of the diaphragm inferiorly. The lungs, the distal portion of the trachea and the bronchi are located in the thorax and constitute the lower respiratory system. The outer structure of the thorax is referred to as the thoracic cage; the thoracic cavity contains the respiratory components. A thorough assessment of the lower respiratory system focuses on the external chest as well as the respiratory components in the thoracic cavity.

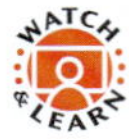

Anatomy review: Thorax

THORACIC CAGE

The thoracic cage is constructed of the sternum, 12 pairs of ribs, 12 thoracic vertebrae, muscles and cartilage. It provides support and protection for many important organs, including those of the lower respiratory system. Structures and landmarks of the anterior thoracic cage (Fig. 20-1) and the posterior thoracic cage (Fig. 20-2) are discussed below.

Sternum and clavicles

The sternum, or breastbone, lies in the centre of the chest anteriorly and is divided into three parts: the manubrium, the body, and the xiphoid process. In isolated circumstances the body of the sternum can also be referred to as the mesosternum when a practitioner wants to identify a precise point on the sternum (a sternebrae) where a particular rib originates—this is not common practice. The manubrium connects laterally with the clavicles and the first two pairs of ribs. The clavicles extend from the manubrium to the acromion of the scapula.

A U-shaped indentation located on the superior border of the manubrium is an important landmark known as the suprasternal notch. A few centimetres below the suprasternal notch, a bony ridge can be palpated at the point where the manubrium articulates with the body of the sternum. This landmark, often referred to as the *sternal angle* (or angle of Louis), is also the location of the second pair of ribs and becomes a reference point for counting ribs and intercostal spaces.

Ribs and thoracic vertebrae

The 12 pairs of ribs constitute the main structure of the thoracic cage. They are numbered superiorly to inferiorly, the uppermost pair being number one. Each pair of ribs has a corresponding pair of intercostal spaces located immediately inferior to it. Anteriorly the first seven pairs articulate with the sternum by way of costal cartilages. The first pair of ribs curves up immediately under the clavicles, so only a small portion of these ribs and the first interspaces are palpable. The second ribs and intercostal spaces are easily located adjacent to the sternal angle. Ribs two through to six are easy to count anteriorly because of their articulation with the sternal body.

The next four pairs of ribs (7 through to 10) connect to the cartilages of the pair lying superior to them rather than to the sternum (see Fig. 20-1). This configuration forms an angle between the right and left costal margins meeting at the level of the xiphoid process. This angle, commonly referred to as the *costal angle*, is an important landmark for assessment. It is normally less than 90 degrees but may be increased in instances of long-standing hyperinflation of the lungs, as in emphysema. The 11th and 12th pairs of ribs are called floating ribs because they do not connect to either the sternum or another pair of ribs anteriorly. Instead they are attached posteriorly to the vertebrae and their anterior tips are free and palpable (see Fig. 20-2).

The ribs are more difficult to palpate posteriorly. Each pair of ribs originate from their respective thoracic vertebra (hence, the 12th pair of ribs for example are attached to the 12th thoracic vertebrae). The spinous process of the seventh cervical vertebra (C7), also called the vertebra prominens, can be easily felt with the patient's neck flexed. The process immediately inferior to the vertebra prominens is the first thoracic vertebra, which is adjacent to the posterior aspect of the first rib.

CLINICAL TIP

When counting the spinous processes, it is helpful to know they align with their corresponding ribs only to the fourth thoracic vertebra (T4). After this, the spinous processes angle downwards from their own vertebral body and can be palpated over the vertebral body and rib below.

The lower tip of each scapula is at the level of the seventh or eighth rib when the patient's arms are at his or her side (see Fig. 20-2).

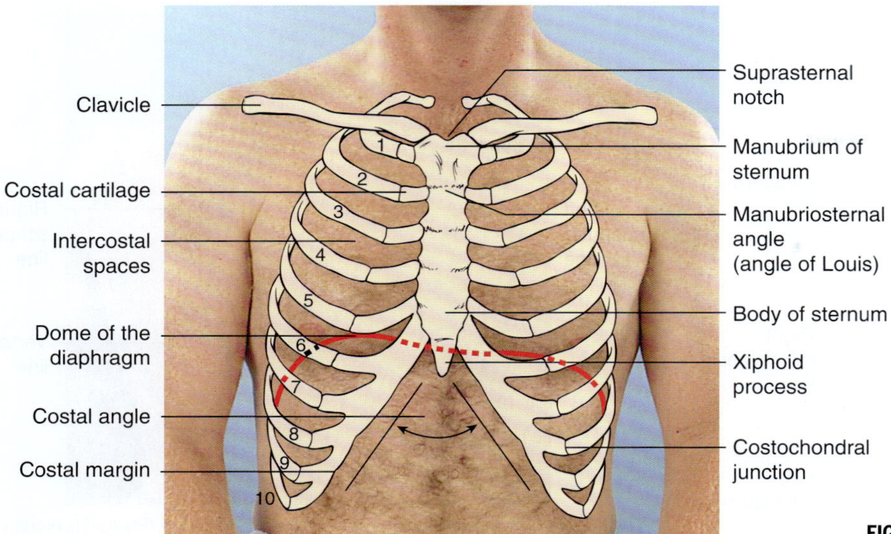

FIGURE 20-1 Anterior thoracic cage. (Photo © B. Proud.)

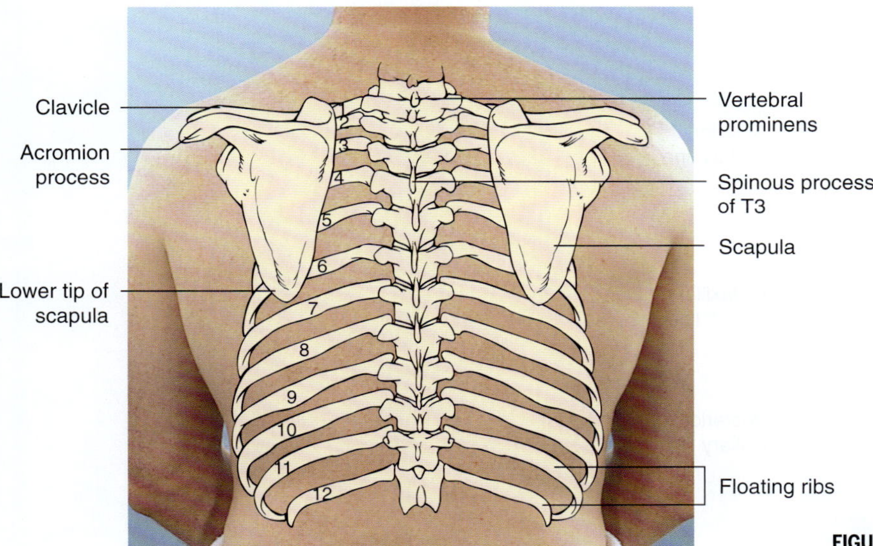

FIGURE 20-2 Posterior thoracic cage. (Photo © B. Proud.)

Vertical reference lines

By counting the ribs, an examiner can describe the location of a finding vertically. However, to describe a location around the circumference of the chest wall, the examiner uses imaginary lines running vertically on the chest wall. On the anterior chest, the vertical reference lines are the midsternal line and the right and left midclavicular lines (Fig. 20-3).

The vertical reference lines on the posterior thorax are the vertebral (or spinal) line and the right and left scapular lines, which extend through the inferior angle of the scapulae when the arms are at the patient's side (Fig. 20-4).

The lateral aspect of the thorax is divided into three parallel lines. The midaxillary line runs from the apex of the axillae to the level of the 12th rib. The anterior axillary line extends from the anterior axillary fold along the anterolateral aspect of the thorax, whereas the posterior axillary line runs from the posterior axillary fold down the posterolateral aspect of the chest wall (Fig. 20-5).

THORACIC CAVITY

The thoracic cavity consists of the mediastinum and the lungs. The mediastinum refers to a central area in the thoracic cavity that contains the trachea, oesophagus, heart and great vessels. These structures are discussed in separate chapters (Chaps 19 and 22). The lungs lie on each side of the mediastinum.

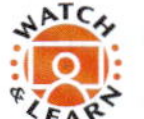

Anatomy review: Lungs

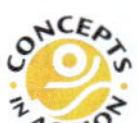

Respiratory: Gas exchange in alveoli

Lungs

The lungs are elastic structures that narrow as they ascend and are suspended within the thoracic cavity. The apex of each lung extends slightly above the clavicle; the base is at the level of the diaphragm. At the point of the midclavicular line on the

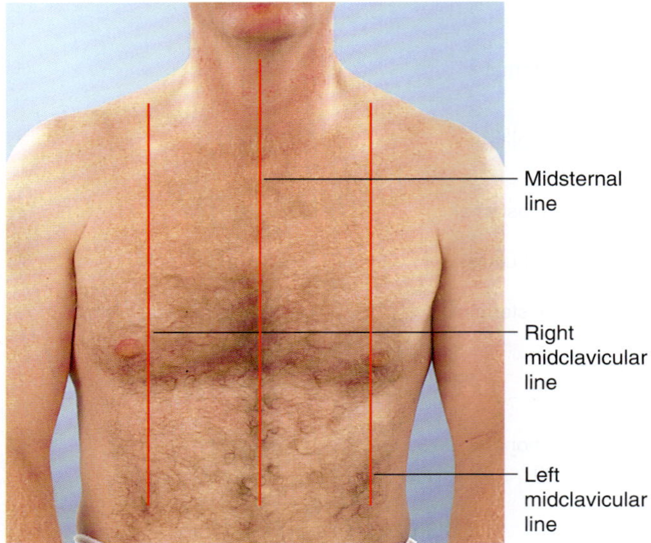

FIGURE 20-3 Anterior vertical lines (imaginary landmarks). (Photo © B. Proud.)

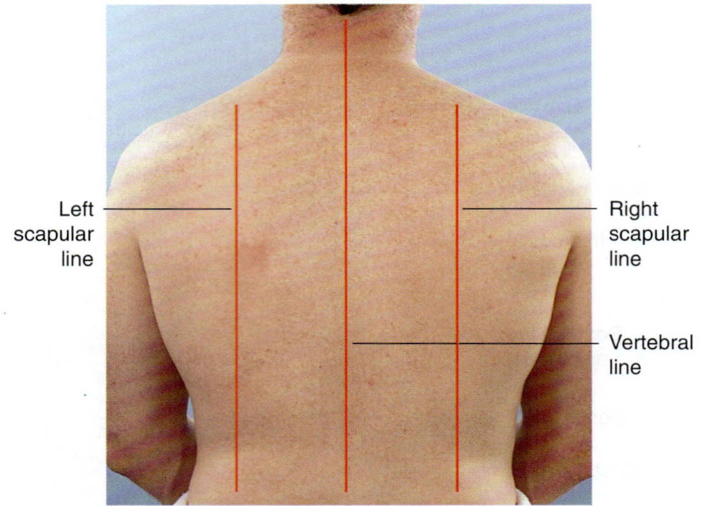

FIGURE 20-4 Posterior vertical lines (imaginary landmarks). (Photo © B. Proud.)

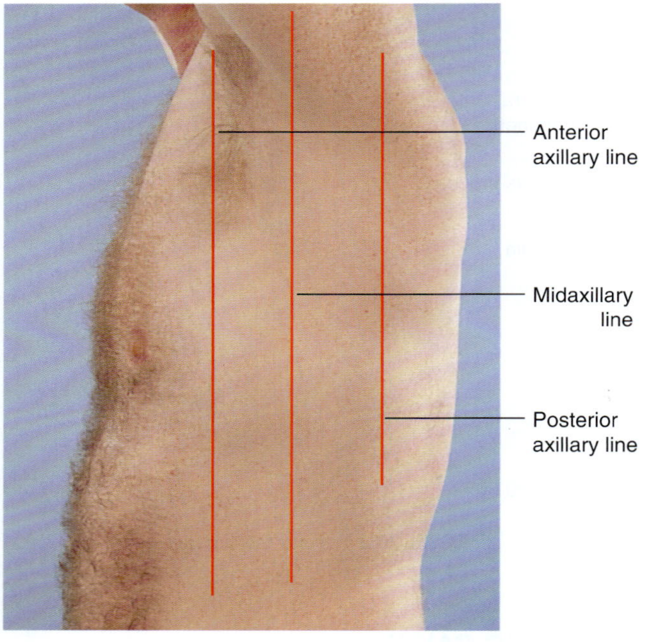

FIGURE 20-5 Lateral vertical lines (imaginary landmarks). (Photos © B. Proud.)

anterior surface of the thorax, the lung extends to approximately the sixth rib. Laterally lung tissue reaches the level of the 8th rib, and posteriorly the lung base lies at about the 10th rib (Fig. 20-6).

Although the lungs are paired, they are not completely symmetrical. Both are divided into lobes by fissures. The right lung is made up of three lobes, whereas the left lung contains only two lobes. Fissures separating the lobes run obliquely through the chest, making the lobes appear as diagonal sloping segments. Anteriorly the horizontal fissure separating the right upper lobe from the middle lobe extends from the fifth rib in the right midaxillary line to the third intercostal space or fourth rib at the right sternal border. Posteriorly oblique fissures extend on both right and left lungs from the level of T3 to the sixth rib at the midclavicular line.

During deep inspiration in the healthy adult, the lungs extend down to about the 8th intercostal space anteriorly and the 12th intercostal space posteriorly. During expiration, the lungs rise to the fifth or sixth intercostal space anteriorly and tenth posteriorly.

CLINICAL TIP

Remember that most lung tissue in the upper lobes of both lungs is located on the anterior surface of the chest. Similarly, the lower lobes of both lungs are primarily located towards the posterior surface of the chest wall. In addition, the right middle lobe of the lung does not extend to the posterior side of the thoracic wall and, thus, must be assessed from the anterior surface alone.

Pleural membranes

The thoracic cavity is lined by a thin, double-layered serous membrane, which is collectively referred to as the pleura (Fig. 20-7). The parietal pleura line the chest cavity, and the

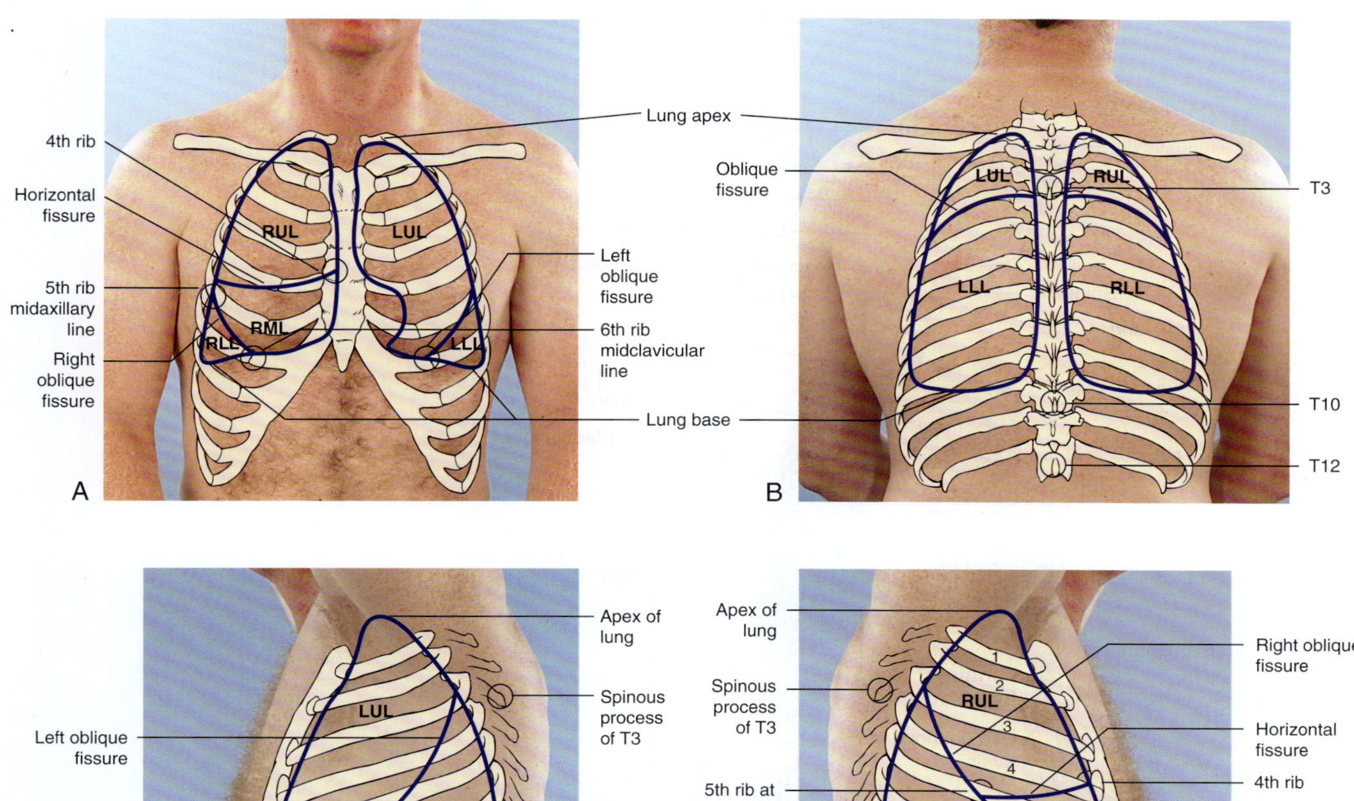

FIGURE 20-6 (A) Anterior view of lung position. **(B)** Posterior view of lung position. **(C)** Lateral view of left lung position. **(D)** Lateral view of right lung position. (Photos © B. Proud.)

visceral pleura cover the external surfaces of the lungs. The pleural space lies between the two pleural layers. In the healthy adult, the lubricating serous fluid between the layers allows movement of the visceral layer over the parietal layer during ventilation without friction. Because the pleural space is one of the physiological third spaces for body fluid storage, severe dehydration will reduce the volume of pleural fluid, resulting in the increased transmission of lung sounds and a possible friction rub.

Trachea and bronchi

The trachea is a flexible structure that lies anterior to the oesophagus. It begins at the level of the cricoid cartilage in the neck and is approximately 10 to 12 cm long in an adult (see Fig. 20-7). Approximately 16 to 20 C-shaped rings of hyaline cartilage compose the trachea; they help to maintain its shape and prevent its collapse during respiration.

CLINICAL TIP

No tracheal cartilage ring is complete—all are C-shaped. The only cartilage in the trachea to form a complete ring is the cricoid cartilage, which is attached to the first tracheal ring and to the bottom of the larynx. When a patient is unable to protect his or her airway (e.g. through oversedation), cricoid pressure is applied as the cricoid cartilage is the only complete ring of cartilage in the trachea. As a complete cartilage ring, the cricoid cartilage maintains patency of the airway despite pressure as it will not allow collapse and obstruction of the trachea. As anterior pressure is applied to the cricoid cartilage it also moves posteriorly and occludes the oesophagus to prevent the potential aspiration of stomach contents.

At the level of the sternal angle, the trachea bifurcates into the right and left main bronchi. Both bronchi are at an oblique position in the mediastinum and enter the lungs at the hilum. The right main bronchus is shorter and more vertical than the left main bronchus, making aspirated objects more likely to enter the right lung than the left (this is why, when you place patients in the recovery position, you place them on their left side and not on their right side).

The bronchi and trachea represent 'dead space' in the respiratory system, where air is transported but no gas exchange takes place. They function primarily as a passageway for both inspired and expired air. In addition, the trachea and bronchi

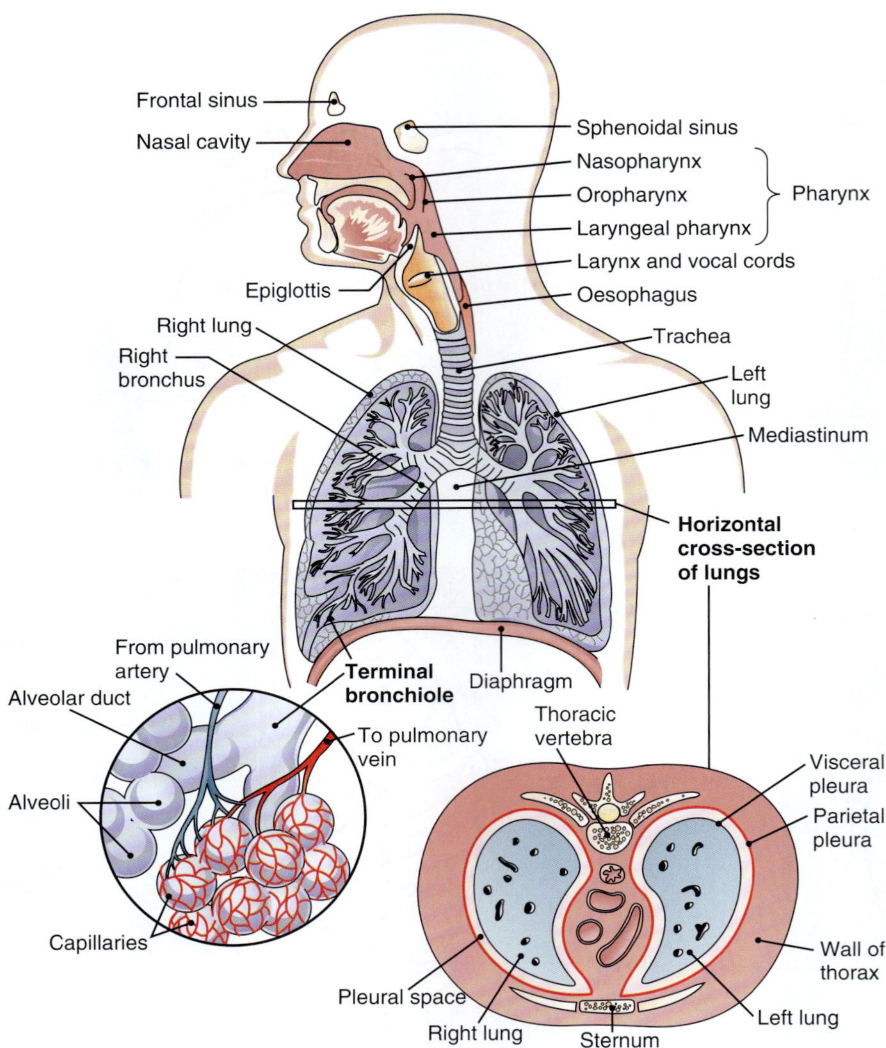

FIGURE 20-7 Major structures of the respiratory system.

are lined with mucous membranes containing cilia. These hairlike projections help sweep dust, foreign bodies and bacteria that have been trapped by the mucus towards the mouth for removal.

Inspired air travels through the trachea into the main bronchi and continues through the system. The bronchi repeatedly bifurcate into smaller passageways known as bronchioles. Eventually the bronchioles terminate at the alveolar ducts, and air is channelled into the alveolar sacs, which contain the alveoli (see Fig. 20-7). Alveolar sacs contain a number of alveoli in a cluster formation (resembling grapes), creating millions of interalveolar walls that serve to increase the surface area available for gas exchange.

MECHANICS OF BREATHING

The purpose of respiration is to maintain an adequate oxygen level in the blood to support cellular life in the body. By providing oxygen and eliminating carbon dioxide, respiration assists in the rapid compensation for metabolic acid–base defects; however, changes in the respiratory pattern can cause acid–base imbalances.

External respiration, or ventilation, is the mechanical act of breathing that is accomplished by expansion of the chest, both vertically and horizontally. *Vertical expansion* is accomplished through contraction of the diaphragm. *Horizontal expansion* occurs as intercostal muscles lift the sternum and elevate the ribs, resulting in an increase in anteroposterior diameter.

As a result of this enlargement of the chest cavity, a slight negative pressure is created in the lungs in relation to the atmospheric pressure, resulting in an inflow of air into the lungs as air moves from a higher pressure to a lower pressure. This process, called inspiration, is shown in Figure 20-8. Expiration is mostly passive in nature and occurs with relaxation of the intercostal muscles and the diaphragm. As the diaphragm relaxes, it assumes a domed shape. The resultant decrease in the size of the chest cavity creates a positive pressure, forcing air out of the lungs.

Breathing patterns change according to cellular demands—often without awareness on the part of the individual. Such involuntary control of respiration is the work of the medulla and pons located in the brainstem. The hypothalamus and the sympathetic nervous system also play a role in the involuntary control of respiration in response to emotional changes such as fear or excitement.

Hormonal regulation, changes in oxygen or carbon dioxide levels in the blood or changes in the hydrogen ion (pH) level can cause changes in breathing patterns. Under normal

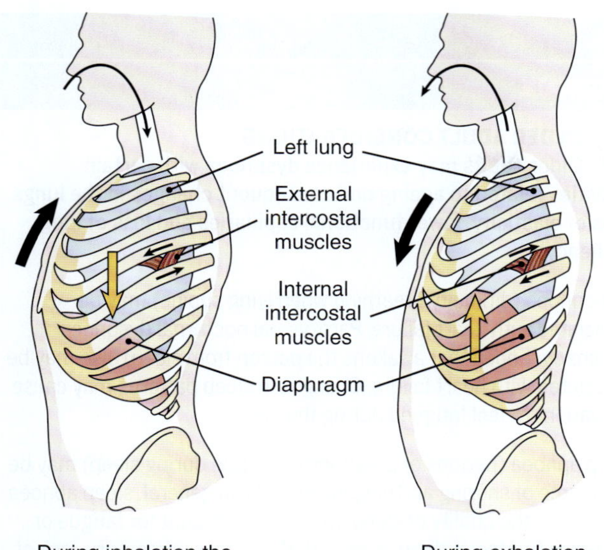

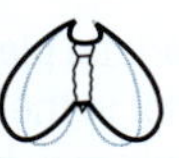

FIGURE 20-8 Mechanics of normal—not deep, not shallow—inspiration (left) and expiration (right).

circumstances, the strongest stimulus to breathe is an increase of carbon dioxide in the blood (*hypercapnia*). A decrease in oxygen (*hypoxaemia*) also increases respiration but is less effective than a rise in carbon dioxide levels.

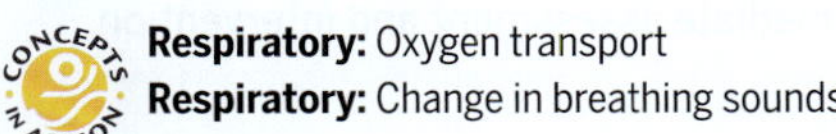

Respiratory: Oxygen transport
Respiratory: Change in breathing sounds

CASE STUDY

You are talking to Mr Burney before undertaking his clinical assessment. His eyes sparkling, he tells you he is feeling great and that he was able to walk to the toilet today without his oxygen. He uses oxygen at 2 L/minute when he exercises or walks outside the ward, and PRN [meaning 'as needed'] for shortness of breath. He reports a 'chronic cough, as usual'. He says he still has difficulty 'getting off a good cough' because 'I just don't have the energy anymore.'

CRITICAL THINKING

1. What further questions would you ask Mr Burney about his cough?
2. Considering Mr Burney's statement about his energy levels, what further questions would you ask him about his fatigue and lifestyle?

Health assessment

COLLECTING SUBJECTIVE DATA: THE NURSING HEALTH HISTORY

Subjective data related to the thoracic and lung assessment provide many clues to underlying respiratory problems and associated nursing diagnoses as well as clues to risk of developing lung disorders. Information about the patient's level of functioning is also important because certain respiratory problems greatly affect a person's ability to perform activities of daily living. When collecting subjective data, remember to follow up on the patient's related signs and symptoms to determine specific respiratory problems and associated nursing diagnoses.

Be careful to avoid judgemental approaches to poor health practices. Smoking, for example, has become a stigmatised addiction in our society. Avoid conveying feelings of intolerance when caring for a smoker with respiratory complaints. Based on the patient's readiness for teaching, the nurse may offer information about smoking cessation methods if this is something the patient is interested in. It is your responsibility to ensure the patient is able to make an informed decision—this might not necessarily be the decision you would personally make.

History of present health concern

QUESTION	RATIONALE
Difficulty breathing	
Do you ever experience difficulty breathing? Describe the difficulty.	Dyspnoea (difficulty breathing) can indicate a number of health problems, most of which are related to the respiratory system. Gradual onset of dyspnoea is usually indicative of lung changes such as emphysema, whereas sudden onset is associated with viral or bacterial infections.
Do you experience any other symptoms when you have difficulty breathing?	Associated symptoms provide clues to the underlying problem. Certain associated symptoms suggest problems in other body systems. For example, oedema or angina that occurs with dyspnoea may indicate a cardiovascular problem.

Continued on following page

History of present health concern (continued)

QUESTION	RATIONALE
Do you have difficulty breathing when you are resting or do any specific activities cause the difficulty?	**OLDER ADULT CONSIDERATIONS** **Older adults may experience dyspnoea with certain activities related to ageing and consequent changes in the lungs (loss of elasticity, fewer functional capillaries and loss of lung resiliency).**
Do you have difficulty breathing when you sleep? Do you use more than one pillow or elevate the head of the bed when you sleep?	Orthopnoea (difficulty breathing when lying supine) may be associated with heart failure. Paroxysmal nocturnal dyspnoea (severe dyspnoea that awakens the person from sleep) also may be associated with heart failure. Changes in sleep patterns may cause the patient to feel fatigued during the day.
Do you snore when you sleep? Have you been told that you stop breathing at night when you snore?	Sleep apnoea (periods of breathing cessation during sleep) may be the source of snoring and gasping sounds. In general, sleep apnoea diminishes the quality of sleep, which may account for fatigue or excessive tiredness, depression, irritability, loss of memory, lack of energy and a risk for vehicle and workplace accidents.
Chest pain	
Do you have chest pain? Is the pain associated with a cold, fever or deep breathing?	Pain-sensitive nerve endings are located in the parietal pleura, thoracic muscles and tracheobronchial tree but not in the lungs. Thus, chest pain associated with a pulmonary origin may be a late sign of pulmonary disease. **OLDER ADULT CONSIDERATIONS** **Chest pain related to pleuritis may be absent in older patients because of age-related alterations in pain perception.** **SAFETY TIP** **Immediately assess any reports of chest pain further to determine if it is due to cardiac ischaemia, which is a medical emergency requiring immediate assessment and intervention.**
Cough	
Do you have a cough? When and how often does it occur?	Continuous coughs are usually associated with acute infections, whereas those occurring only early in the morning are often associated with chronic bronchial inflammation or smoking. Coughs late in the evening may be the result of exposure to irritants during the day. Coughs occurring at night are often related to postnasal drip or sinusitis. **OLDER ADULT CONSIDERATIONS** **The ability to cough effectively may be decreased in the older patient because of weaker muscles and increased rigidity of the thoracic wall. Check the regular medications the patient is on—angiotensin-converting enzyme inhibitors may cause a persistent, ongoing cough.**
Do you produce any sputum when you cough? If so, what colour is the sputum? How much sputum do you cough up? Has this amount increased or decreased recently? Does the sputum have an odour?	Non-productive coughs are often associated with upper respiratory irritations and early congestive heart failure. White or mucoid sputum is often seen with common colds, viral infections or bronchitis. Yellow or green sputum is often associated with bacterial infections. Blood in the sputum (haemoptysis) is seen with more serious respiratory conditions. Rust-coloured sputum is associated with tuberculosis or pneumococcal pneumonia. Pink, frothy sputum may be indicative of pulmonary oedema. An increase in the amount of sputum is often seen in an increase in exposure to irritants, chronic bronchitis and pulmonary abscess. Patients with excessive, tenacious secretions may need instruction on controlled coughing and measures to reduce the viscosity of the secretions.

COLDSPA

Example for chest pain

Use the COLDSPA mnemonic as a guideline to collect needed information for each symptom the patient shares. In addition, the following questions help elicit important information.

Mnemonic	Question	Patient response example
Character	Describe the sign or symptom (feeling, appearance, sound, smell or taste, if applicable).	'I have pain in my chest when I cough or take a deep breath.'
Onset	When did it begin?	'About 6 days ago.'
Location	Where is it? Does it radiate? Does it occur anywhere else?	'It is on my right side.' *Patient points to right lower back side of chest.*
Duration	How long does it last? Does it recur?	'It hurts when I cough or take a deep breath.'
Severity	How bad is it? How much does it bother you?	'I can't sleep at night and have trouble going up stairs because I am short-winded.'
Pattern	What makes it better or worse?	'Mucomyst helps me to cough up phlegm but I still have the pain.'
Associated factors/How it **A**ffects the patient	What other symptoms occur with it? How does it affect you?	'I've had a 38.9 °C fever for the last 2 days. I am coughing up thick brown sputum. I smoke 1 pack a day but quit 2 days ago.'

History of present health concern (continued)

QUESTION	RATIONALE
Do you wheeze when you cough or when you are active?	Wheezing indicates narrowing of the airways due to spasm or obstruction. Wheezing is associated with congestive heart failure, asthma (reactive airway disease) or excessive secretions.
Gastrointestinal symptoms	
Do you have any gastrointestinal symptoms such as heartburn, frequent hiccups or chronic cough?	Studies have shown that patients with asthma often have gastro-oesophageal reflux disease (GORD) or are more susceptible to GORD.

Past health history

QUESTION	RATIONALE
Have you had prior respiratory problems?	A history of respiratory disease increases the risk of a recurrence. In addition, some respiratory diseases may imitate other disorders. For example, asthma symptoms may mimic symptoms commonly associated with emphysema or heart failure.
Have you ever had any thoracic surgery, biopsy or trauma?	Previous surgeries may alter the appearance of the thorax and cause changes in respiratory sounds. Trauma to the thorax can result in lung tissue changes.
Have you been tested for or diagnosed with allergies?	Many allergic responses are manifested with respiratory symptoms such as dyspnoea, cough or hoarseness. Patients may need education on controlling the amount of allergens in their environment.
Have you ever had a chest X-ray, tuberculosis (TB) skin test or influenza immunisation? Have you had any other pulmonary studies in the past?	Information on previous chest X-rays, TB skin tests, influenza immunisations and so forth is useful for comparison with current findings and gives information on self-care practices and possible teaching needs.
Have you recently travelled outside of Australia or New Zealand?	Travel to high-risk areas such as mainland China, Hong Kong, Hanoi (Vietnam), Taiwan, Singapore or Toronto (Canada) may have exposed the patient to severe acute respiratory syndrome.

Continued on following page

Family history

QUESTION	RATIONALE
Is there a history of lung disease in your family?	The development of lung cancer is thought to be partially based on genetics. A history of certain respiratory diseases (asthma, emphysema [see Promote health—Chronic obstructive pulmonary disease]) in a family may increase the risk for development of the disease. Exposure to viral or bacterial respiratory infections in the home increases the risk for development of these conditions. CONCEPTS IN ACTION **Respiratory:** Asthma
Did any family members in your home smoke when you were growing up?	Second-hand smoke puts individuals at risk of emphysema or lung cancer later in life.
Is there a history of other pulmonary illnesses or disorders in the family, e.g. asthma?	Some pulmonary disorders, such as asthma, tend to run in families.

Lifestyle and health practices

QUESTION	RATIONALE
Have you ever smoked cigarettes or other tobacco products? Do you currently smoke? At what age did you start? How much do you smoke and how much have you smoked in the past? What activities do you usually associate with smoking? Have you ever tried to quit?	Smoking is linked to a number of respiratory conditions, including lung cancer (see Promote health—Lung cancer). The number of years a person has smoked and the number of cigarettes per day influence the risk for development of smoking-related respiratory problems. Information on smoking behaviour and previous efforts to quit may be helpful later in identifying measures to assist with smoking cessation.
Are you exposed to any environmental conditions that affect your breathing? Where do you work? Are you around smokers?	Exposure to certain environmental inhalants can result in an increased incidence of certain respiratory conditions. Environmental irritants commonly associated with occupations include coal dust, insecticides, paint, pollution, asbestos fibres and the like.
Do you have difficulty performing your usual daily activities? Describe any difficulties.	Respiratory problems can negatively affect a person's ability to perform the usual activities of daily living.
Are you experiencing stress at this time? How does it affect your breathing?	Shortness of breath can be a manifestation of stress. Patient may need education about relaxation techniques.
Are you currently taking medications for breathing problems or other medications (prescription or over-the-counter) that affect your breathing? Do you use any other treatments at home for your respiratory problems?	Consider all medications when determining if respiratory problems could be attributed to adverse reactions. Certain medications, for example, beta-adrenergic antagonists (beta-blockers) such as atenolol or metoprolol and angiotensin-converting enzyme inhibitors such as enalapril or lisinopril are associated with the side effect of persistent cough. These medications are contraindicated with some respiratory problems such as asthma. If the patient is using oxygen or other respiratory therapy at home, it is important to evaluate knowledge of proper use and precautions as well as the patient's ability to afford the therapy.
Have you used any herbal medicines or alternative therapies to manage colds or other respiratory problems?	Many people use herbal therapies, such as echinacea, or alternative therapies, such as zinc lozenges, to decrease cold symptoms. Knowing what patients are using enables you to check for side effects or adverse interactions with prescribed medications.

PROMOTE HEALTH — CHRONIC OBSTRUCTIVE PULMONARY DISEASE

OVERVIEW

Chronic obstructive pulmonary disease (COPD) is used to describe several conditions that obstruct airflow to and from the alveoli. The two most common conditions are emphysema and chronic bronchitis. There are four stages (I to IV) of COPD, which rank the condition in terms of severity, with IV being the most severe. The Australian Institute of Health and Welfare (AIHW, 2019) highlighted the prevalence of COPD increases with age, mostly occurring in people aged 45 and over. One in 20 Australians aged 45 and over reported having COPD during the period from 2014 to 2015. In 2015, COPD was the fifth leading cause of death in Australia and ranked in the top three causes of total burden for those aged 65 to 74 and 75 to 84. In 2015, COPD was also the second highest ranked cause of total burden for men aged 75 to 84 (AIHW, 2016). COPD affects an estimated 8.8% of Aboriginal and Torres Strait Islander peoples aged 45 and over—approximately 10,300 people, based on self-reported data, although this is likely to be an underestimate. The prevalence of COPD (across all age groups) among Aboriginal and Torres Strait Islander peoples is 2.5 times as high as the prevalence for non-Aboriginal and Torres Strait Islander peoples after adjusting for differences in age structure (ABS, 2013).

In 2012, it was estimated that COPD affects 15% of the adult population over the age of 45 in New Zealand (Asthma Foundation, 2018). There have been no new studies of the incidence or prevalence of COPD since this report; however, based on data specific to hospital admissions related to COPD, in 2017, there were 44,002 New Zealanders reported to be living with COPD, for a total population prevalence of 0.95% (Telfar Barnard & Zhang, 2018). Age-standardised population prevalence was found to be highest for Māori, at 2.44%, followed by Pacific, at 2.19%, and trailed by non-Māori/Pacific/Asian peoples, at 0.77%. In the male population, age-standardised prevalence of COPD was 0.98%—this is 7.6% higher than the age-standardised prevalence of COPD in the female population (0.88%). In 2017, 96% of people with COPD were over the age of 45, giving a 2.2% prevalence of COPD-related hospitalisations in the above–45 age group (Telfar Barnard & Zhang, 2018).

Risk factors

According to Mayo Clinic (2019a), the risk factors associated with developing COPD are:

- Smoking cigarettes (however, only 20% to 30% of cigarette smokers develop COPD)
- Smoke exposure (cigar smoke, second-hand smoke and pipe smoke)
- People with asthma who smoke
- Air pollution
- Workplace exposure to dust, smoke or fumes from burning fuel
- Age 40 and above
- Alpha-1-antitrypsin deficiency (genetic variation responsible for 1% of COPD population).

Teach risk reduction tips

- Avoid smoking cigarettes or join a tobacco cessation program if you do smoke.
- Avoid passive smoke.
- Avoid respiratory illnesses (seek primary care advice regarding influenza vaccine).
- If exposed to occupational respiratory irritants, follow all preventive measures, such as wearing masks. Seek help to modify the environment, if possible, to make it less hazardous.
- Avoid cold, dry air; hot, humid air; or high altitudes when possible (especially prolonged exposure to these).
- Seek early diagnosis if symptoms develop so that treatment and further preventive strategies can be initiated.

PROMOTE HEALTH — LUNG CANCER

OVERVIEW

According to Cancer Council Australia (2019), cancer is a leading cause of death in Australia and New Zealand. Almost 50,000 deaths were estimated in Australia in 2019 that are attributed to cancer. In 2016 in New Zealand there were 24,218 new cases of cancer registered (New Zealand Ministry of Health, 2019).

One in two Australian men and women will be diagnosed with cancer before the age of 85. The most common forms of cancer in Australia are lung, prostate, breast, melanoma and colorectal cancer. These five cancers account for around 60% of all cancer diagnoses in Australia (Cancer Council Australia, 2019). Lung cancer is the leading cause of cancer death for both men and women in Australia and New Zealand largely because it is detected late (Cancer Council Australia, 2019; Ministry of Health, 2019).

In 2015, 11,788 new cases of lung cancer (including small cell and non-small cell lung cancers) were diagnosed in Australia. This accounts for close to 9% of all cancers diagnosed. The risk of being diagnosed with lung cancer in Australia by age 85 is 1 in 13 for men and 1 in 21 for women. In 2016, there were 8410 deaths caused by lung cancer in Australia. New Zealand recently evidenced a slight downward trend in newly diagnosed cases of lung cancer, partly due to a decrease in the number of Māori (both male and female) and non-Māori males presenting with lung cancer. Lung cancer accounts for nearly a third of all Māori cancer deaths, and 1- and 5-year survival rates remain poorer for Māori than for non-Māori. People who live in areas of high deprivation are also disproportionately affected by lung cancer, with men 3.2 times more likely to be diagnosed with lung cancer than men living in the least deprived areas (Ministry of Health, 2015).

Risk factors

- Cigarette smoking
- Genetic predisposition possibly associated with interaction of genetics and smoking
- Beta-carotene supplements, especially in the presence of heavy smoking, moderate alcohol intake
- Asbestos exposure
- Radon exposure
- Exposure to workplace pollutants—radioactive ores, mining chemicals (e.g. arsenic, vinyl chloride, nickel, coal, mustard gas, chloromethyl esters and fuels such as gasoline)
- Other environmental exposure—air pollution, passive tobacco smoke, marijuana smoking
- History of previous lung cancer, silicosis, berylliosis
- Recurring inflammation that leaves scars (e.g. tuberculosis, some types of pneumonia)
- Gender: women's lung cells may have a predisposition to lung cancer when exposed to tobacco smoke
- History of Hodgkin disease treated with chemotherapy, radiation or both
- Smokers who have been treated with chemotherapy or radiation
- Eating a poor diet with few fruits and vegetables

Teach risk reduction tips

- Do not start smoking or, if you do smoke, stop smoking.
- Join a smoking cessation program.
- Eat a healthy, low-cholesterol diet with adequate amounts of fruits and vegetables.
- If you smoke, avoid beta-carotene supplements or diet high in beta-carotene.
- Limit exposure to air pollution and harmful substances.
- Wear a mask when exposed to air pollution or dangerous airborne substances.

COLLECTING OBJECTIVE DATA: PHYSICAL EXAMINATION

Examination of the thorax and lungs begins when the nurse first meets the patient and observes any obvious breathing difficulties. However, complete examination of the thorax and lungs consists of inspection, palpation, percussion and auscultation of the posterior and anterior thorax, to evaluate functioning of the lungs. Inspection and palpation are simple skills to acquire; however, practice and experience are the best ways to become proficient with percussion and auscultation. It should also be remembered that a full set of vital signs, observation of a patient's behaviour and listening for any audible sounds (e.g. wheezing) will help to provide a background for the physical assessment of the thorax and lungs. **No assessment finding should ever be considered in isolation. Findings should also be considered within an individual patient's context.**

Preparing the patient

Have the patient remove all clothing from the waist up and put on an examination gown (if they are not already in hospital pyjamas). Examination of a female patient's chest may create anxiety because of embarrassment related to breast exposure. Explain that exposure of the entire chest is necessary during some parts of the examination and, to ease patient anxiety further, explain the procedures before initiating the examination.

For the beginning of the examination, ask the patient to sit in an upright position with their arms relaxed at their sides. Provide explanations during the examination as you perform the various assessment techniques. The patient should be encouraged to ask questions and to inform you of any discomfort or fatigue they experience during the examination. Try to make sure that the room temperature is comfortable for the patient.

Equipment

- Gloves (the wearing of gloves should be restricted to occasions where there is a specific need)
- Stethoscope (see Display 20-1)
- Light source
- Skin marker
- Metric ruler

Physical assessment

During examination of the patient, remember these key points:

- Provide privacy for the patient.
- Keep your hands warm to promote the patient's comfort during examination.
- Remain non-judgemental regarding the patient's habits and lifestyle, particularly about smoking. At the same time, educate and inform the patient about risks such as lung cancer and chronic obstructive pulmonary disease, which are related to such habits.
- When inspecting the chest, don't just observe for new or acute phenomena; be careful to observe for any old scarring or signs of past injury because this additional information will frequently inform a patient's presentation as much as acute observations.

CASE STUDY

Upon inspection, you note Mr Burney's facial colour and lips are ruddy, but his nail beds are pink. His breathing pattern is regular, unlaboured, but tachypnoeic at 28 respirations/minute, which he tells you is his usual rate. Examining his thorax, you note he is barrel-chested, with a transverse-to-lateral ratio of about 2.5 to 3. Although he is not using accessory muscles to breathe, you observe slight intercostal muscle bulging. His posture is rigidly upright in the chair. While auscultating Mr Burney's lungs, you note diminished breath sounds bilaterally in the lower lobes and a small, discrete area of coarse crackles in the upper portion of the left lower lobe. You also smell the odour of cigarettes on his breath and when you tell him you noticed the smell of cigarettes, he says, 'I didn't think one would hurt when I was outside.'

CRITICAL THINKING

3. Diminished breath sounds are not normal findings. Explain the implications for this finding for Mr Burney's respiratory function.
4. Describe the difference between coarse and fine crackles.

DISPLAY 20-1 USING A STETHOSCOPE

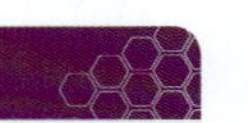

Stethoscope bell and diaphragm. Use the diaphragm of the stethoscope to detect high-pitched sounds. The diaphragm should be at least 3 cm wide for adults and smaller for children. Hold the diaphragm firmly against the body part being auscultated. Use the bell of the stethoscope to detect low-pitched sounds. Hold the bell lightly against the body part being auscultated. For the majority of the sounds you will auscultate, you will use the diaphragm of the stethoscope.

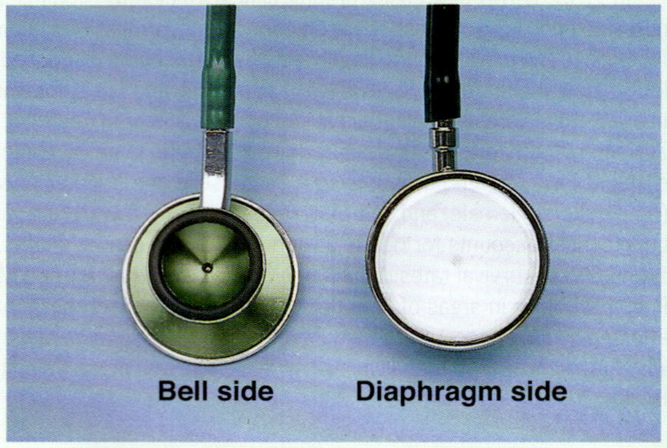

ANCILLARY HEALTH ASSESSMENTS

The specific focus of this text is physical health assessment of a patient. However, in many circumstances, additional assessment data can be gathered by the clinician with the use of specially designed equipment. For example, during assessment of a patient's thorax and lungs, it is often routine to record *oxygen saturations*. Additionally, in further assessing lung function, *spirometry* and *arterial blood gases* (ABGs) may be collected. To supplement the physical assessment data outlined in this chapter, Display 20-2 addresses oxygen saturations in detail. The subsequent two displays (Displays 20-3 and 20-4) provide a brief overview of spirometry and ABG. Because this text relates to physical health assessment, an overview only for both spirometry and arterial blood gases has been provided.

WATCH & LEARN

Assessing the posterior and lateral thorax
Assessing the anterior thorax
Anatomy review: Thorax
Anatomy review: Lungs
Thorax and lungs: Surveying the chest and respiration
Thorax and lungs: Examining the posterior thorax and lungs
Thorax and lungs: Normal and adventitious breath sounds
Thorax and lungs: Auscultation of the posterior thorax
Thorax and lungs: Examining the anterior thorax and lungs
Thorax and lungs: Auscultation of the anterior chest
Thorax and lungs: Summary

CRITICAL THINKING

Recalling our patient from the case study, Mr Burney, you are asked to measure Mr Burney's SpO_2 using a portable pulse oximeter as part of your clinical assessment.

5. What do you think his SpO_2 value would be? Why do you think this?
6. How would these data link to your physical assessment data collected on Mr Burney?
7. How would these data assist you in planning an intervention for Mr Burney?

DISPLAY 20-2 UNDERSTANDING OXYGEN SATURATION

Physiologically the oxyhaemoglobin dissociation curve reflects the affinity of oxygen to haemoglobin molecules. This curve represents a non-linear relationship between oxygen and haemoglobin molecules. Importantly, oxygen is transported in the body in two ways:

1. Between 97% and 99% of oxygen is bound to haemoglobin. Oxygen saturation refers to the percentage of haemoglobin molecules saturated with oxygen in arterial blood. This is most commonly measured by a portable pulse oximetry unit and the value derived is the SpO_2. The normal SpO_2 value is between 95% and 99% when the patient is breathing room air. The SpO_2 value only provides an estimate of the percentage of haemoglobin molecules saturated with oxygen—it does not reflect the amount of oxygen dissolved in the patient's plasma.
2. Between 1% and 3% of oxygen is carried around the body dissolved in plasma. This is measured by an *arterial blood gas*. This is referred to as the PaO_2 value. See Display 20-4.

Pulse oximetry is now a common adjunctive assessment tool used in most clinical settings. However, this standard tool does have some important limitations. Pulse oximetry measurement is:

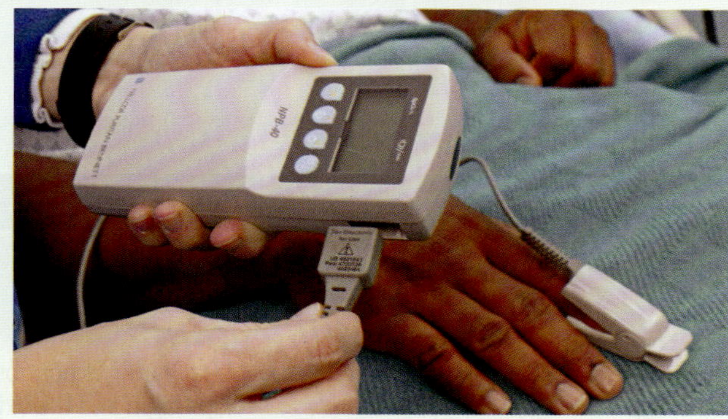

1. Most accurate when the SpO_2 is between 75% and 99%.
2. Less accurate when the patient has poor or weak pulses, vasoconstriction and other conditions such as anaemia or carboxyhaemoglobin.
3. Sensitive to motion artefact, external light interference and some intravenous dyes.

DISPLAY 20-3 SPIROMETRY EXPLAINED

Spirometry tests form an essential part of pulmonary assessment and pulmonary function tests, also called lung function tests. These are used to determine the patient's level of respiratory function, progression of respiratory disease and response to therapy. During lung function tests, the patient is either sitting upright or standing. The patient inhales deeply and exhales quickly and for as long as possible into tubing attached to the spirometer. The spirometer measures different lung volumes and capacities. Common bedside spirometry tests include assessment of forced expiratory volume in 1 second (FEV_1) and forced vital capacity (FVC), to evaluate the patient's respiratory status in response to treatment. The results of the test are compared with the predicted values that are calculated from the patient's age, size, weight, sex and ethnic group. The two curves shown after the test are the flow–volume curve and the volume–time loop.

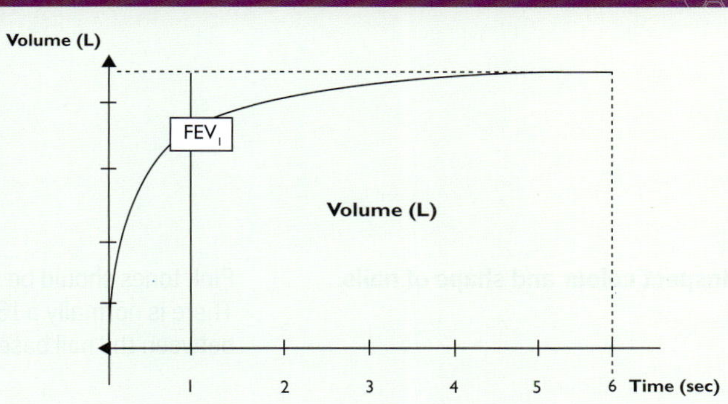

DISPLAY 20-4 ARTERIAL BLOOD GAS EXPLAINED

Table 20-1 Acid-based parameters for arterial blood gas studies

	Normal	Acid	Base
pH	7.35–7.45	<7.35	>7.45
$PaCO_2$	35–45 mmHg	>45 mmHg	<35 mmHg
HCO_3^-	21–28 mmol/L	<21 mmol/L	>28 mmol/L

Measuring arterial blood gases (ABGs) is a common laboratory test used to analyse how effectively the body is maintaining the pH with normal limits, through a series of chemical interactions, referred to as the *acid–base balance.* ABGs also form part of pulmonary function tests and measure a number of components (see Table 20-1).

The pH indicates a balance, acidaemia or alkalaemia, of the arterial blood. The $PaCO_2$ indicates the partial pressure (P) exerted on the arterial wall (a) by the molecule carbon dioxide (CO_2). The HCO_3^- level is the level of bicarbonate in arterial blood. An acid–base imbalance occurs when either the carbon dioxide or the bicarbonate levels are out of the normal ranges. For example:

- *Respiratory acidosis* is reflected by high $PaCO_2$ values and a fall in the pH level. Clinically this may be seen when a patient is hypoventilating.
- *Respiratory alkalosis* is reflected by low $PaCO_2$ values and an elevated pH value. Clinically this may be seen when a patient is hyperventilating.
- *Metabolic or non-respiratory acidosis* is characterised by a fall in the bicarbonate level and the pH level. Clinically this may be seen in a patient who has diarrhoea or diabetic ketoacidosis due to excess ketones.
- *Metabolic or non-respiratory alkalosis* is characterised by an elevated bicarbonate level and pH. Clinically this may be seen when a patient has loss of gastrointestinal fluids from vomiting or excessive nasogastric tube suction.

PHYSICAL ASSESSMENT

ASSESSMENT PROCEDURE	NORMAL FINDINGS	ABNORMAL FINDINGS
General		
INSPECTION		
Inspect for nasal flaring and pursed lip breathing.	Nasal flaring is not observed. Normally the diaphragm and the external intercostal muscles do most of the work of breathing. This is evidenced by outward expansion of the abdomen and lower ribs on inspiration and return to resting position on expiration.	Nasal flaring is seen with laboured respirations (especially in small children) and is indicative of hypoxia. Pursed lip breathing may be seen in asthma, emphysema or congestive heart failure (CHF) as a physiological response to help slow down expiration and keep alveoli open longer.
Observe colour of face, lips and chest.	The patient has evenly coloured skin tone without unusual or prominent discolouration.	Ruddy to purple complexion may be seen in patients with chronic obstructive pulmonary disease (COPD) or CHF as a result of polycythaemia. Cyanosis may be seen if patient is cold or hypoxic. **CULTURAL CONSIDERATIONS** **Cyanosis makes white skin appear blue-tinged, especially in the perioral, nailbed and conjunctival areas. Dark skin appears blue, dull and lifeless in the same areas.**
Inspect colour and shape of nails.	Pink tones should be seen in the nailbeds. There is normally a 160-degree angle between the nail base and the skin.	Pale or cyanotic nails may indicate hypoxia. Early clubbing (180-degree angle) and late clubbing (greater than a 180-degree angle) can occur from hypoxia.

PHYSICAL ASSESSMENT (continued)

ASSESSMENT PROCEDURE	NORMAL FINDINGS	ABNORMAL FINDINGS
Posterior thorax		
INSPECTION		
Inspect configuration. While the patient sits with their arms at their sides, stand behind them and observe the position of scapulae and the shape and configuration of the chest wall (Fig. 20-9). **CLINICAL TIP** **Some nurses prefer to inspect the entire thorax first, followed by palpation of the anterior and posterior thorax, then percussion and auscultation of the anterior and posterior thorax.**	Scapulae are symmetrical and non-protruding. Shoulders and scapulae are at equal horizontal positions. The ratio of anteroposterior to transverse diameter is 1:2. Spinous processes appear straight and thorax appears symmetrical with ribs sloping downwards at approximately a 45-degree angle in relation to the spine. **OLDER ADULT CONSIDERATIONS** **Kyphosis (an increased curve of the thoracic spine) is common in older patients (see Abnormal findings 20-1). It results from a loss of lung resiliency and a loss of skeletal muscle; it may be a normal finding.** **CULTURAL CONSIDERATIONS** **The size of the thorax, which affects pulmonary function, differs by race. Compared with Asians, adult Caucasians have a larger thorax and greater lung capacity (Overfield, 1995).**	Spinous processes that deviate laterally in the thoracic area may indicate scoliosis. Spinal configurations may have respiratory implications. Ribs appearing horizontal at an angle greater than 45 degrees with the spinal column are frequently the result of an increased ratio between the anteroposterior–transverse diameter (barrel chest). This condition is commonly the result of emphysema due to hyperinflation of the lungs. Abnormal findings 20-1 depicts various thoracic configurations.
Observe use of accessory muscles. Watch as the patient breathes and note use.	The patient does not use accessory (trapezius or shoulder) muscles to assist breathing. The diaphragm is the major muscle at work. This is evidenced by expansion of the lower chest during inspiration.	Trapezius, or shoulder, muscles are used to facilitate inspiration in cases of acute and chronic airway obstruction or atelectasis.
Inspect the patient's positioning. Note the patient's posture and his or her ability to support weight while breathing comfortably.	Patient should be sitting up and relaxed, breathing easily with arms at sides or in lap.	Patient leans forwards and uses arms to support weight and lift chest to increase breathing capacity, referred to as the *tripod position* (Fig. 20-10). This is often seen in COPD. See Promote health—Chronic obstructive pulmonary disease.

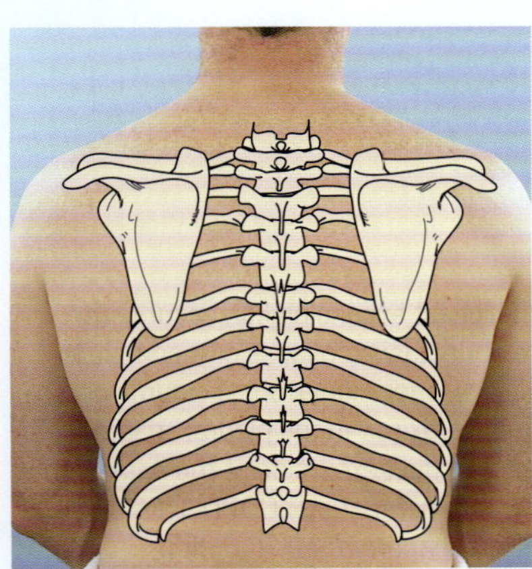

FIGURE 20-9 Observing the posterior thorax. (Photo © B. Proud.)

FIGURE 20-10 Tripod position.

Continued on following page

PHYSICAL ASSESSMENT (continued)

ASSESSMENT PROCEDURE	NORMAL FINDINGS	ABNORMAL FINDINGS
PALPATION		
Palpate for tenderness and sensation. Palpation may be performed with one or both hands; however, the sequence of palpation is established (Fig. 20-11). Use your fingers to palpate for tenderness, warmth, pain or other sensations. Start towards the midline at the level of the left scapula (over the apex of the left lung) and move your hand left to right, comparing findings bilaterally. Move systematically downwards and out to cover the lateral portions of the lungs at the bases.	Patient reports no tenderness, pain or unusual sensations. Temperature should be equal bilaterally. 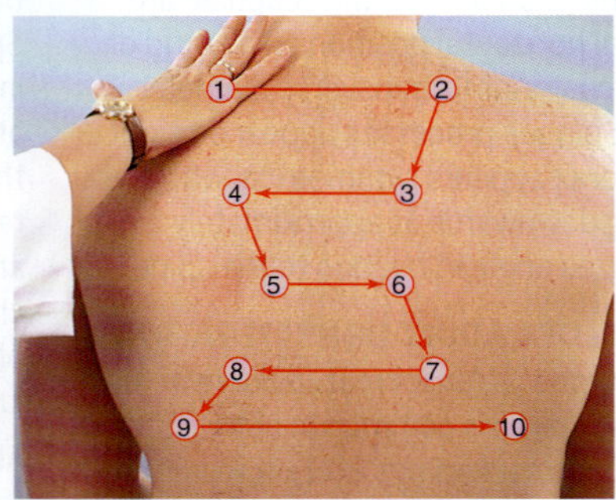 **FIGURE 20-11** Sequence for palpating the posterior thorax. (Photo © B. Proud.)	Tender or painful areas may indicate inflamed fibrous connective tissue. Pain over the intercostal spaces may be from inflamed pleurae. Pain over the ribs, especially at the costal chondral junctions, is a symptom of fractured ribs. Muscle soreness from exercise or the excessive work of breathing (as in acute respiratory infection) may be palpated as tenderness. Increased warmth may be related to local infection.
Palpate for crepitus. Crepitus, also called subcutaneous emphysema, is a crackling sensation (like bones or hairs rubbing against each other) that occurs when air passes through fluid or exudate. Use your fingers and follow the sequence in Figure 20-11 when palpating.	The examiner finds no palpable crepitus.	Crepitus can be palpated if air escapes from the lung or other airways into the subcutaneous tissue, as occurs after an open thoracic injury, around a chest tube or tracheostomy. It may also be palpated in areas of extreme congestion or consolidation. In such situations, mark margins and monitor to note any decrease or increase in the crepitant area.
Palpate surface characteristics. Put on gloves and use your fingers to palpate any lesions that you noticed during inspection. Also feel for any unusual masses.	Skin and subcutaneous tissue are free of lesions and masses.	Any unusual palpable mass should be evaluated further by a doctor or experienced nurse.
Palpate for fremitus. Following the above sequence, use the ball or ulnar edge of one hand to assess for fremitus (vibrations of air in the bronchial tubes transmitted to the chest wall). As you move your hand to each area, ask the patient to say 'ninety-nine'. Assess all areas for symmetry and intensity of vibration. **CLINICAL TIP** **The ball of the hand is best for assessing tactile fremitus because the area is especially sensitive to vibratory sensation.**	Fremitus is symmetrical and easily identified in the upper regions of the lungs. If fremitus is not palpable on either side, the patient may need to speak louder. A decrease in the intensity of fremitus is normal as the examiner moves towards the base of the lungs. However, fremitus should remain symmetrical for bilateral positions.	Unequal fremitus is usually the result of consolidation (which increases fremitus) or bronchial obstruction, air trapping in emphysema, pleural effusion or pneumothorax (which all decrease fremitus). Diminished fremitus even with a loud spoken voice may indicate an obstruction of the tracheobronchial tree.
Assess chest expansion. Place your hands on the posterior chest wall with your thumbs at the level of T9 or T10 and pressing together a small skin fold. As the patient takes a deep breath, observe the movement of your thumbs (Fig. 20-12).	When the patient takes a deep breath, the examiner's thumbs should move 5 to 10 cm apart symmetrically. **OLDER ADULT CONSIDERATIONS** **Because of calcification of the costal cartilages and loss of the accessory musculature, the older patient's thoracic expansion may be decreased although it should still be symmetrical.**	Unequal chest expansion can occur with severe atelectasis (collapse or incomplete expansion), pneumonia, chest trauma or pneumothorax (air in the pleural space). Decreased chest excursion at the base of the lungs is characteristic of COPD. This is due to decreased diaphragmatic function.

PHYSICAL ASSESSMENT (continued)

ASSESSMENT PROCEDURE	NORMAL FINDINGS	ABNORMAL FINDINGS
Posterior thorax (continued)		

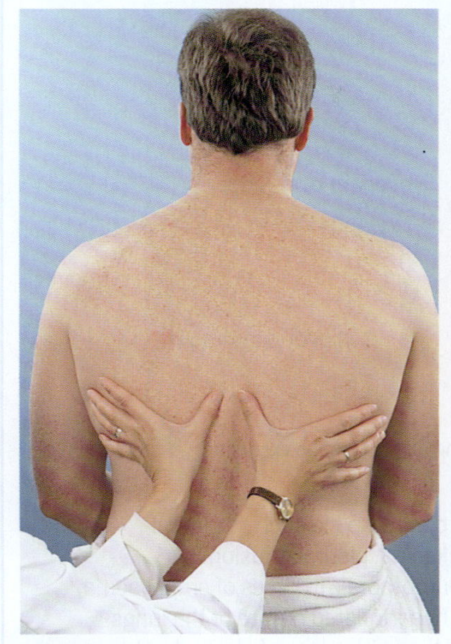

FIGURE 20-12 Starting position for assessing symmetry of chest expansion. (© B. Proud.)

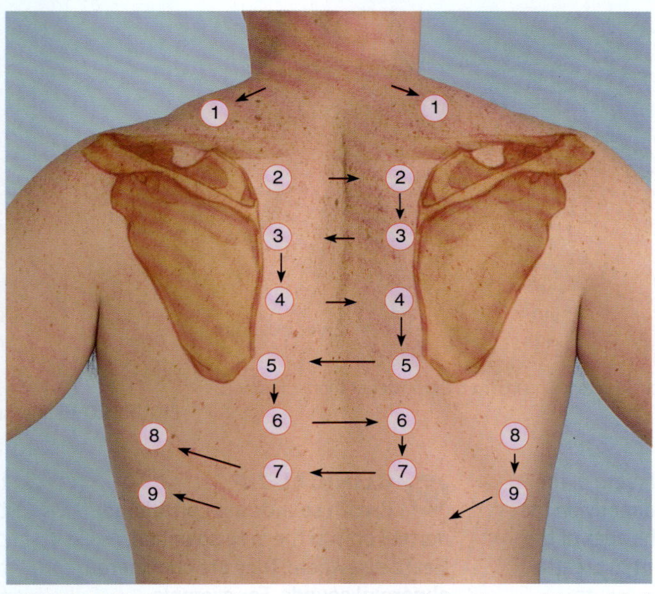

FIGURE 20-13 Sequence for percussing the posterior thorax. (Weber, J.R. & Kelley, J.H. [2017]. Health Assessment in Nursing, 6e, © Wolters Kluwer Health.)

PERCUSSION

ASSESSMENT PROCEDURE	NORMAL FINDINGS	ABNORMAL FINDINGS
Percuss for tone. Start at the apices of the scapulae and percuss across the tops of both shoulders. Then percuss the intercostal spaces across and down, comparing sides. Percuss to the lateral aspects at the bases of the lungs, comparing sides. Figure 20-13 depicts the sequence for percussion.	*Resonance* is the percussion tone elicited over normal lung tissue (Fig. 20-14). Percussion elicits flat tones over the scapula.	Hyper-resonance is elicited in cases of trapped air such as in emphysema or pneumothorax. Dullness is present when fluid or solid tissue replaces air in the lung or occupies the pleural space such as in lobar pneumonia, pleural effusion or tumour.
Percuss for diaphragmatic excursion. Ask the patient to *exhale* forcefully and hold the breath. Beginning at the scapular line (T7), percuss the intercostal spaces of the right posterior chest wall. Percuss downwards until the tone changes from resonance to dullness. Mark this level and allow the patient to breathe. Next ask the patient to *inhale* deeply and hold it. Percuss the intercostal spaces from the mark downwards until resonance changes to dullness. Mark the level and allow the patient to breathe. Measure the distance between the two marks (Fig. 20-15). Perform on both sides of the posterior thorax.	Excursion should be equal bilaterally and measure 3 to 5 cm in adults. The level of the diaphragm may be higher on the right because of the position of the liver. In well-conditioned patients, excursion can measure up to 7 or 8 cm.	Diaphragmatic descent may be limited by atelectasis of the lower lobes or by emphysema in which diaphragmatic movement and air trapping are minimal. The diaphragm remains in a low position on inspiration and expiration. Other possible causes for limited descent can be pain or abdominal changes such as extreme ascites, tumours or pregnancy. Uneven excursion may be seen with inflammation from unilateral pneumonia, damage to the phrenic nerve or splenomegaly.

AUSCULTATION

ASSESSMENT PROCEDURE	NORMAL FINDINGS	ABNORMAL FINDINGS
Auscultate for breath sounds. To best assess lung sounds, you will need to hear the sounds as directly as possible. Do not attempt to listen through clothing or a drape, which may produce additional sound or muffle lung sounds that exist.	Three types of normal breath sounds may be auscultated—bronchial, bronchovesicular and vesicular (Table 20-2).	Diminished or absent breath sounds often indicate that little or no air is moving in or out of the lung area being auscultated. This may indicate obstruction within the lungs as a result of secretions, mucus plug or a foreign object. It may also indicate abnormalities of

Continued on following page

PHYSICAL ASSESSMENT (continued)

ASSESSMENT PROCEDURE	NORMAL FINDINGS	ABNORMAL FINDINGS

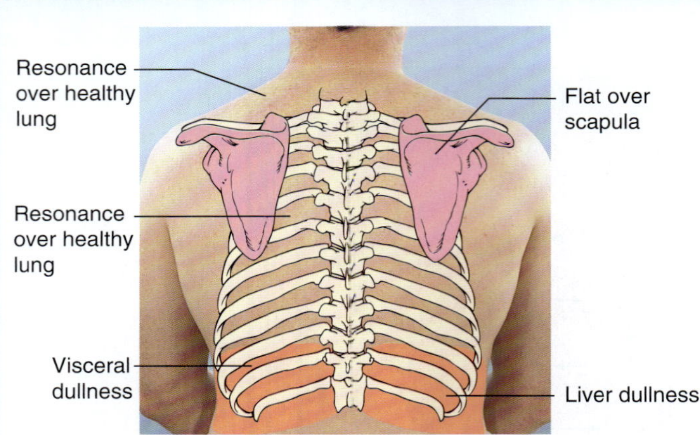

FIGURE 20-14 Normal percussion tones heard from the posterior thorax. (Photo © B. Proud.)

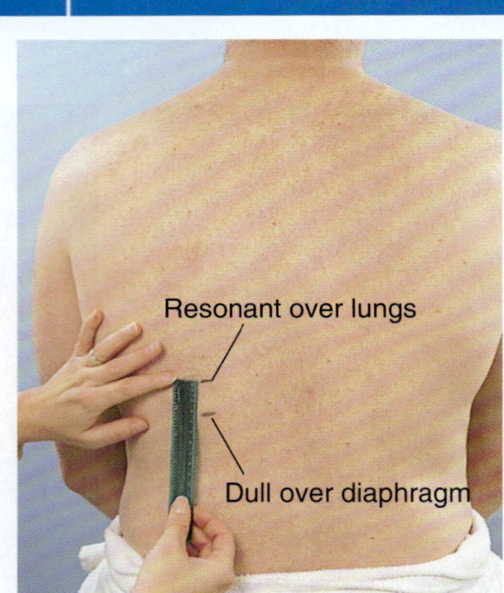

FIGURE 20-15 Measuring diaphragmatic excursion. (Photo © B. Proud.)

To begin, place the diaphragm of the stethoscope firmly and directly on the posterior chest wall at the apex of the lung at C7. Ask the patient to breathe deeply through his or her mouth for each area of auscultation (each placement of the stethoscope) in the auscultation sequence so you can best hear inspiratory and expiratory sounds. Be alert to the patient's comfort and offer times for rest and normal breathing if fatigue is becoming a problem.

OLDER ADULT CONSIDERATIONS

Deep breathing may be especially difficult for the older patient, who may fatigue easily. Thus offer rest as needed.

CLINICAL TIP

Breath sounds are considered normal only in the area specified. Heard elsewhere, they are considered abnormal sounds. For example, bronchial breath sounds are abnormal if heard over the peripheral lung fields.

Figure 20-16 depicts locations of normal breath sounds.

Sometimes breath sounds may be hard to hear with obese or heavily muscled patients due to increased distance to underlying lung tissue.

the pleural space such as pleural thickening, pleural effusion or pneumothorax. In cases of emphysema, the hyperinflated nature of the lungs, together with a loss of elasticity of lung tissue, may result in diminished inspiratory breath sounds. Increased (louder) breath sounds often occur when consolidation or compression results in a denser lung area that enhances the transmission of sound.

Table 20-2 Normal breath sounds

Type	Pitch	Quality	Amplitude	Duration	Location	Illustration
Bronchial	High	Harsh or hollow	Loud	Short during inspiration, long in expiration	Trachea and thorax	
Bronchovesicular	Moderate	Mixed	Moderate	Same during inspiration and expiration	Over the major bronchi—posterior: between the scapulae; anterior: around the upper sternum in the first and second intercostal spaces	
Vesicular	Low	Breezy	Soft	Long in inspiration, short in expiration	Peripheral lung fields	

PHYSICAL ASSESSMENT (continued)

ASSESSMENT PROCEDURE	NORMAL FINDINGS	ABNORMAL FINDINGS
Posterior thorax (continued)		
Auscultate from the apices of the lungs at C7 to the bases of the lungs at T10 and laterally from the axilla down to the seventh or eighth rib. Listen at each site for at least one complete respiratory cycle. Follow the auscultating sequence shown in Figure 20-17.	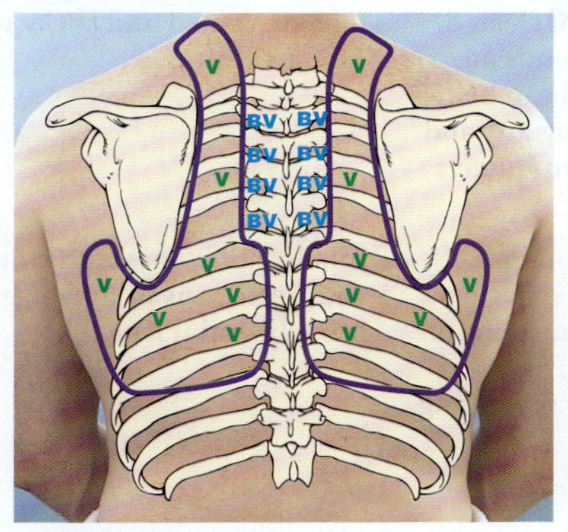 **FIGURE 20-16** Location of breath sounds for the posterior thorax. V, vesicular sounds; BV, bronchovesicular sounds. (Photo © B. Proud.)	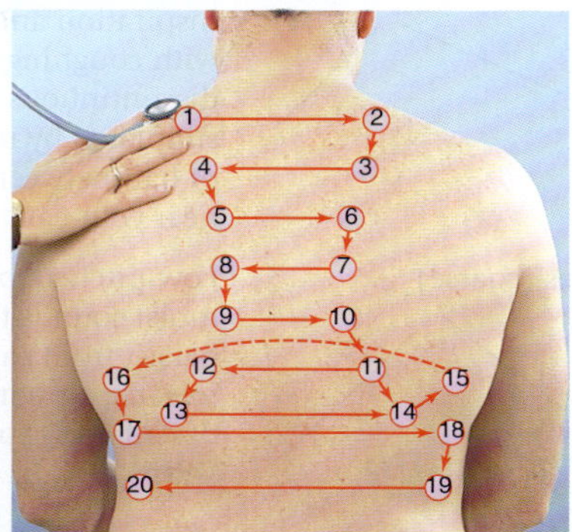 **FIGURE 20-17** Sequence for auscultating the posterior thorax. (Photo © B. Proud.)
Ausculate for adventitious sounds. Adventitious sounds are sounds added or superimposed over normal breath sounds and heard during auscultation. Be careful to note the location on the chest wall where adventitious sounds are heard as well as the location of such sounds within the respiratory cycle. **CLINICAL TIP** **If you hear an abnormal sound during auscultation, always have the patient cough, then listen again and note any change. Coughing may clear the lungs.**	No adventitious sounds, such as crackles (discrete and discontinuous sounds) or wheezes (musical and continuous), are auscultated.	Adventitious lung sounds, such as crackles (formerly called rales) and wheezes (formerly called rhonchi), are evident. See Table 20-3 for a complete description of each type of adventitious breath sound.
Auscultate voice sounds. ***Bronchophony:*** Ask the patient to repeat the phrase 'ninety-nine' while you auscultate the chest wall.	Voice transmission is soft, muffled and indistinct. The sound of the voice may be heard but the actual phrase cannot be distinguished.	The words are easily understood and louder over areas of increased density. This may indicate consolidation from pneumonia, atelectasis or tumour.
Egophony: Ask the patient to repeat the letter 'E' while you listen over the chest wall.	Voice transmission will be soft and muffled but the letter 'E' should be distinguishable.	Over areas of consolidation or compression, the sound is louder and sounds like 'A'.
Whispered pectoriloquy: Ask the patient to whisper the phrase 'one-two-three' while you auscultate the chest wall. **CLINICAL TIP** **While widely documented in textbooks, the practice of auscultating voice sounds is not common. It should be recognised that completing additional assessments such as these serve only to assist the examiner in distinguishing or confirming potential abnormalities. When patient assessment findings are normal, any additional tests such as these tend not to be completed.**	Transmission of sound is very faint and muffled. It may be inaudible.	Over areas of consolidation or compression, the sound is transmitted clearly and distinctly. In such areas, it sounds as if the patient is whispering directly into the stethoscope.

Continued on following page

Table 20-3 Adventitious breath sounds

Abnormal sound	Characteristics	Source	Associated conditions
Discontinuous sounds Crackles (fine)	High-pitched, short, popping sounds heard during inspiration and not cleared with coughing; sounds are discontinuous and can be simulated by rolling a strand of hair between your fingers near your ear.	Inhaled air suddenly opens the small deflated air passages that are coated and sticky with exudate.	Crackles occurring late in inspiration are associated with restrictive diseases such as pneumonia and congestive heart failure. Crackles occurring early in inspiration are associated with obstructive disorders such as bronchitis, asthma or emphysema.
Crackles (coarse)	Low-pitched, bubbling, moist sounds that may persist from early inspiration to early expiration; also described as softly separating Velcro.	Inhaled air comes into contact with secretions in the large bronchi and trachea.	May indicate pneumonia, pulmonary oedema or pulmonary fibrosis. 'Velcro rales' of pulmonary fibrosis are heard louder and closer to stethoscope, usually do not change location, and are more common in patients with long-term chronic obstructive pulmonary disease.
Continuous sounds Pleural friction rub	Low-pitched, dry, grating sound; sound is much like crackles, only more superficial and occurring during both inspiration and expiration.	Sound is the result of rubbing of two inflamed pleural surfaces.	Pleuritis
Wheeze (sibilant)	High-pitched, musical sounds heard primarily during expiration but may also be heard on inspiration.	Air passes through constricted passages (caused by swelling, secretions or tumour).	Sibilant wheezes are often heard in cases of acute asthma or chronic emphysema.
Wheeze (sonorous)	Low-pitched snoring or moaning sounds heard primarily during expiration but may be heard throughout the respiratory cycle. These wheezes may clear with coughing.	Same as sibilant wheeze. The pitch of the wheeze cannot be correlated to the size of the passageway that generates it.	Sonorous wheezes are often heard in cases of bronchitis or single obstructions and snoring before an episode of sleep apnoea. *Stridor* is a harsh honking wheeze with severe broncho-laryngospasm, such as occurs with croup.

PHYSICAL ASSESSMENT (continued)

ASSESSMENT PROCEDURE	NORMAL FINDINGS	ABNORMAL FINDINGS
Anterior thorax		
INSPECTION		
Inspect for shape and configuration. Have the patient sit with their arms at their sides. Stand in front of the patient and assess shape and configuration.	The anteroposterior diameter is less than the transverse diameter. The ratio of anteroposterior diameter to the transverse diameter is 1:2.	Anteroposterior equals transverse diameter, resulting in a barrel chest (see Abnormal findings 20-1). This is often seen in emphysema because of hyperinflation of the lungs.

PHYSICAL ASSESSMENT (continued)

ASSESSMENT PROCEDURE	NORMAL FINDINGS	ABNORMAL FINDINGS
Anterior thorax (continued)		
Inspect position of the sternum. Observe the sternum from an anterior and lateral viewpoint.	Sternum is positioned at midline and straight. **OLDER ADULT CONSIDERATIONS** **The sternum and ribs may be more prominent in the older patient because of loss of subcutaneous fat.**	*Pectus excavatum* is a markedly sunken sternum and adjacent cartilages (often referred to as funnel chest). It is a congenital malformation that seldom causes symptoms other than self-consciousness. *Pectus carinatum* is a forward protrusion of the sternum causing the adjacent ribs to slope backwards (often referred to as pigeon chest). (See Abnormal findings 20-1 for illustrations of both conditions.) Both conditions may restrict expansion of the lungs and decrease the lung capacity.
Watch for sternal retractions.	Retractions not observed.	Sternal retractions are noted with severely laboured breathing.
Inspect slope of the ribs. Assess the ribs from an anterior and lateral viewpoint.	Ribs slope downwards with symmetrical intercostal spaces. Costal angle is within 90 degrees.	Barrel-chest configuration results in a more horizontal position of the ribs and costal angle of more than 90 degrees. This often results from long-standing emphysema.
Observe quality and pattern of respiration. Note breathing characteristics as well as rate, rhythm and depth. Table 20-4 describes respiration patterns. **CLINICAL TIP** **When assessing respiratory patterns, it is more objective to describe the breathing pattern rather than just labelling the pattern.**	Respirations are relaxed, effortless and quiet. They are of a regular rhythm and normal depth at a rate of 10 to 20 per minute in adults. Tachypnoea and bradypnoea may be normal in some patients.	Laboured and noisy breathing is often seen with severe asthma or chronic bronchitis. Abnormal breathing patterns include tachypnoea, bradypnoea, hyperventilation, hypoventilation, Cheyne–Stokes respiration and Biot respiration.
Inspect the intercostal spaces. Ask the patient to breathe normally and observe the intercostal spaces.	No retractions or bulging of the intercostal spaces are noted.	Retraction of the intercostal spaces indicates an increased inspiratory effort. This may be the result of an obstruction of the respiratory tract or atelectasis. Bulging of the intercostal spaces indicates trapped air such as in emphysema or asthma.
Observe for use of accessory muscles. Ask the patient to breathe normally and observe for use of accessory muscles.	Use of accessory muscles (sternomastoid and rectus abdominis) is not seen with normal respiratory effort. After strenuous exercise or activity, individuals with normal respiratory status may use neck muscles for a short time to enhance breathing.	Neck muscles (sternomastoid, scalene and trapezius) are used to facilitate inspiration in cases of acute or chronic airway obstruction or atelectasis. The abdominal muscles and the internal intercostal muscles are used to facilitate expiration in COPD.
PALPATION		
Palpate for tenderness, sensation and surface masses. Use your fingers to palpate for tenderness and sensation. Start with your hand positioned over the left clavicle (over the apex of the left lung) and move your hand left to right, comparing findings bilaterally. Move your hand systematically downwards towards the midline at the level of the breasts and outwards at the base to include the lateral aspect of	No tenderness or pain is palpated over the lung area with respirations.	Tenderness over thoracic muscles can result from exercising (e.g. push ups and the like) especially in a previously sedentary patient.

Continued on following page

Table 20-4 Respiration patterns

Type	Description	Pattern	Clinical indication
Normal	12 to 20 per minute and regular		Normal breathing pattern
Tachypnoea	>24 per minute and shallow		May be a normal response to fever, anxiety or exercise Can occur with respiratory insufficiency, alkalosis, pneumonia or pleurisy
Bradypnoea	<10 per minute and regular		May be normal in well-conditioned athletes Can occur with medication-induced depression of the respiratory centre, diabetic coma, neurological damage
Hyperventilation	Increased rate and increased depth		Usually occurs with extreme exercise, fear or anxiety Kussmaul respirations are a type of hyperventilation associated with diabetic ketoacidosis. Other causes of hyperventilation include disorders of the central nervous system, an overdose of the drug salicylate or severe anxiety.
Hypoventilation	Decreased rate, decreased depth, irregular pattern		Usually associated with overdose of narcotics or anaesthetics
Cheyne–Stokes respiration	Regular pattern characterised by alternating periods of deep, rapid breathing followed by periods of apnoea		May result from severe congestive heart failure, drug overdose, increased intracranial pressure or renal failure May be noted in elderly persons during sleep, not related to any disease process
Biot respiration	Irregular pattern characterised by varying depths and rates of respirations followed by periods of apnoea		May be seen with meningitis or severe brain damage

PHYSICAL ASSESSMENT (continued)

ASSESSMENT PROCEDURE	NORMAL FINDINGS	ABNORMAL FINDINGS
the lung. The established sequence for palpating the anterior thorax (Fig. 20-18) serves as a guide for positioning your hands. **CLINICAL TIP** **Anterior thoracic palpation is best for assessing the right lung's middle lobe.**	**FIGURE 20-18** Sequence for palpating the anterior thorax. (Photo © B. Proud.)	

PHYSICAL ASSESSMENT (continued)

ASSESSMENT PROCEDURE	NORMAL FINDINGS	ABNORMAL FINDINGS
Anterior thorax (continued)		
Palpate for tenderness at costochondral junctions of ribs.	Palpation does not elicit tenderness.	**OLDER ADULT CONSIDERATIONS** **Tenderness or pain at the costochondral junction of the ribs is seen with fractures, especially in older patients with osteoporosis.**
Assess for crepitus as you would on the posterior thorax (described previously).	No crepitus is palpated.	In areas of extreme congestion or consolidation, crepitus may be palpated, particularly in patients with lung disease.
Also palpate for any surface masses or lesions.	No unusual surface masses or lesions are palpated.	Surface masses or lesions may indicate cysts or tumours.
Palpate for fremitus. Using the sequence for the anterior chest above, palpate for fremitus using the same technique as for the posterior thorax. **CLINICAL TIP** **When you assess for fremitus on the female patient, avoid palpating the breast. Breast tissue dampens the vibrations.**	Fremitus is symmetrical and easily identified in the upper regions of the lungs. A decreased intensity of fremitus is expected towards the base of the lungs; however, fremitus should be symmetrical bilaterally.	Diminished vibrations, even with a loud spoken voice, may indicate an obstruction of the tracheobronchial tree. Patients with emphysema may have considerably decreased fremitus as a result of air trapping.
Palpate anterior chest expansion. Place your hands on the patient's anterolateral wall with your thumbs along the costal margins and pointing towards the xiphoid process (Fig. 20-19). As the patient takes a deep breath, observe the movement of your thumbs.	Thumbs move outwards in a symmetrical fashion from the midline.	Unequal chest expansion can occur with severe atelectasis, pneumonia, chest trauma, pleural effusion or pneumothorax. Decreased chest excursion at the bases of the lungs is seen with COPD.
PERCUSSION		
Percuss for tone. Percuss the apices above the clavicles. Then percuss the intercostal spaces across and down, comparing sides (Fig. 20-20).	Resonance is the percussion tone elicited over normal lung tissue. Figure 20-21 depicts normal tones and their locations. Percussion elicits dullness over breast tissue, the heart and the liver. Tympany is detected over the stomach, and flatness is detected over the muscles and bones.	Hyper-resonance is elicited in cases of trapped air such as in emphysema or pneumothorax. Dullness may characterise areas of increased density such as consolidation, pleural effusion or tumour.

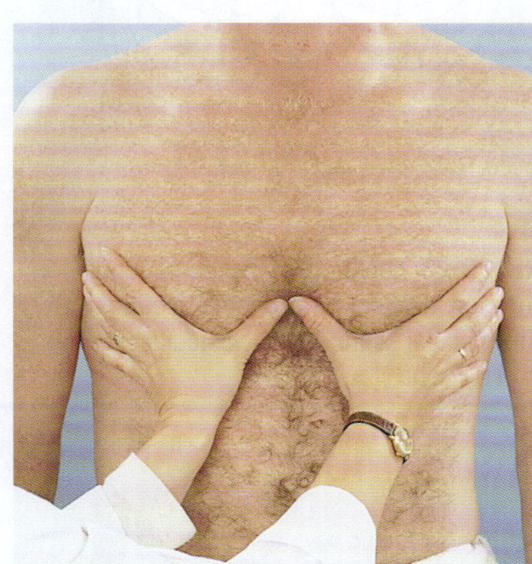

FIGURE 20-19 Palpating anterior chest expansion. (© B. Proud.)

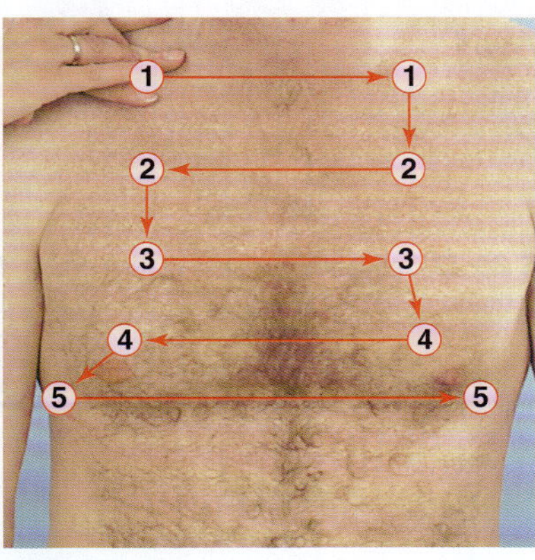

FIGURE 20-20 Sequence for percussing the anterior thorax. (Photo © B. Proud.)

Continued on following page

PHYSICAL ASSESSMENT (continued)

ASSESSMENT PROCEDURE	NORMAL FINDINGS	ABNORMAL FINDINGS

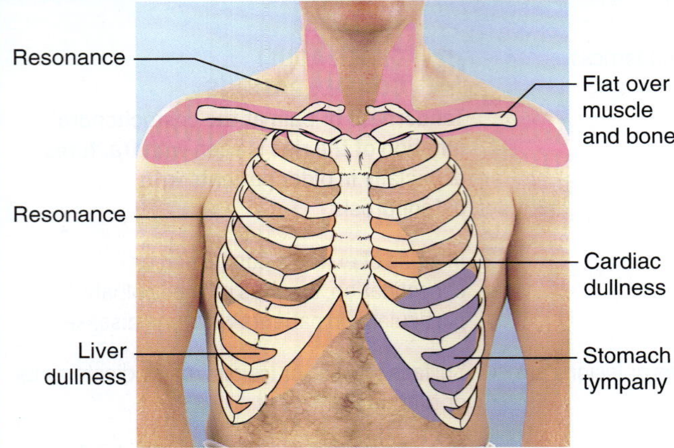

FIGURE 20-21 Normal percussion tones heard from the anterior thorax. (Photo © B. Proud.)

AUSCULTATION

ASSESSMENT PROCEDURE	NORMAL FINDINGS	ABNORMAL FINDINGS
Auscultate for anterior breath sounds, adventitious sounds and voice sounds. Place the diaphragm of the stethoscope firmly and directly on the anterior chest wall. Auscultate from the apices of the lungs slightly above the clavicles to the bases of the lungs at the sixth rib. Ask the patient to breathe deeply through the mouth to avoid transmission of sounds that may occur with nasal breathing. Be alert to the patient's comfort and offer times for rest and normal breathing if fatigue is becoming a problem, particularly for the older patient.	Figure 20-23 depicts locations for normal breath sounds. Refer to text in the posterior thorax section for normal voice sounds.	Refer to Table 20-2 for adventitious breath sounds. Refer to text in the posterior thorax section for normal voice sounds.

Listen at each site for at least one complete respiratory cycle. Follow the sequence for anterior auscultation shown in Figure 20-22.

CLINICAL TIP
Again, do not attempt to listen through clothing or other materials. However, if the patient has a large amount of hair on the chest, listening through a thin T-shirt can decrease extraneous sounds that may be misinterpreted as crackles.

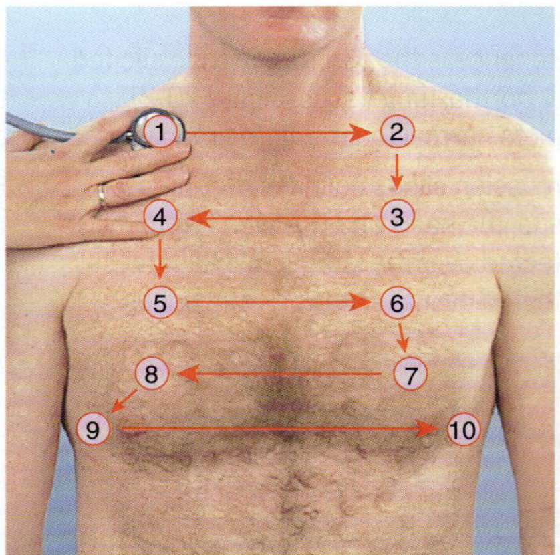

FIGURE 20-22 Sequence for auscultating the anterior thorax. (Photo © B. Proud.)

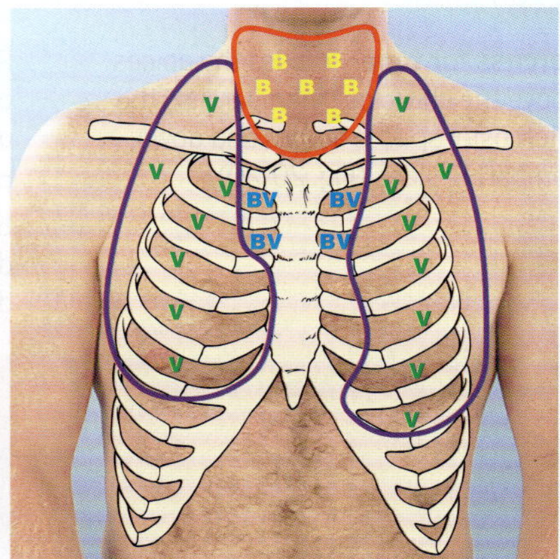

FIGURE 20-23 Location of breath sounds for the anterior thorax. B, bronchial sounds; BV, bronchovesicular sounds, V, vesicular sounds. (Photo © B. Proud.)

ABNORMAL FINDINGS 20-1 Thoracic deformities and configurations

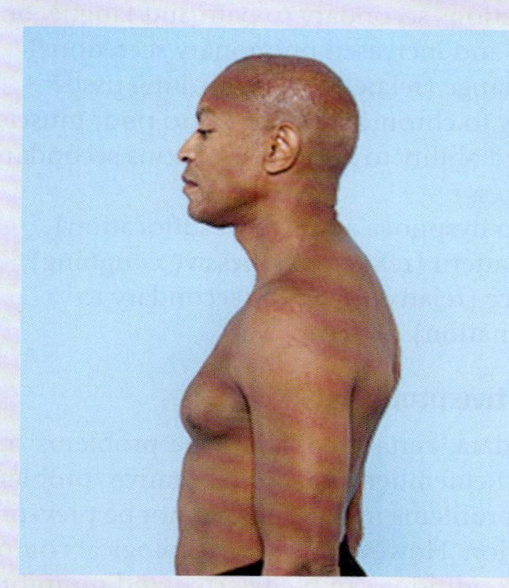

Normal chest configuration.

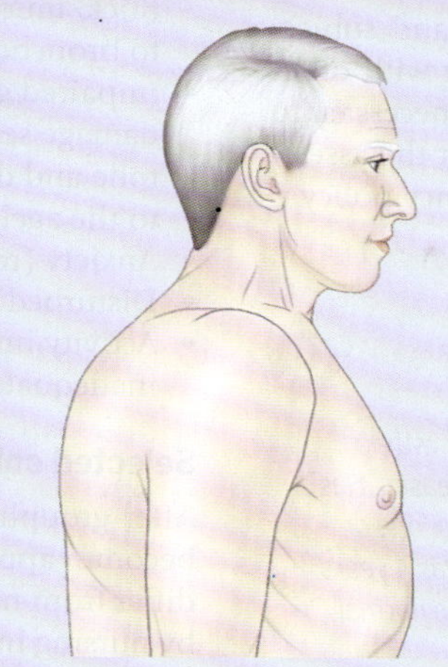

Barrel chest. (Farrell, M. & Dempsey, J. (2014) *Smeltzer & Bare's textbook of medical*-surgical nursing (3rd Australian and New Zealand ed.). Lippincott Williams & Wilkins.)

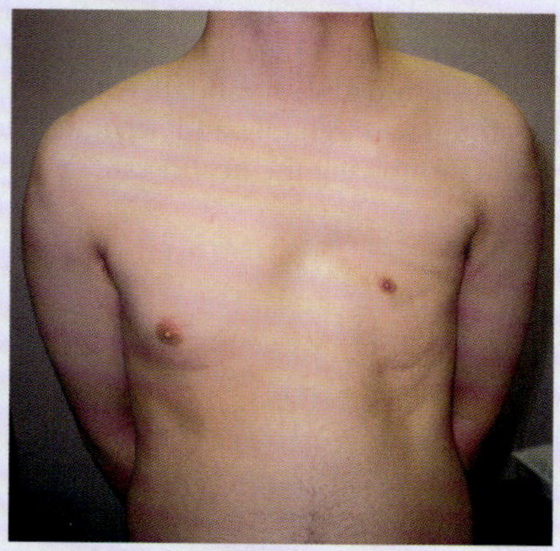

Pectus excavatum (funnel chest). (Berg, D. & Worzala K. [2006]. Atlas of adult physical diagnosis. Philadelphia: Lippincott Williams & Wilkins.)

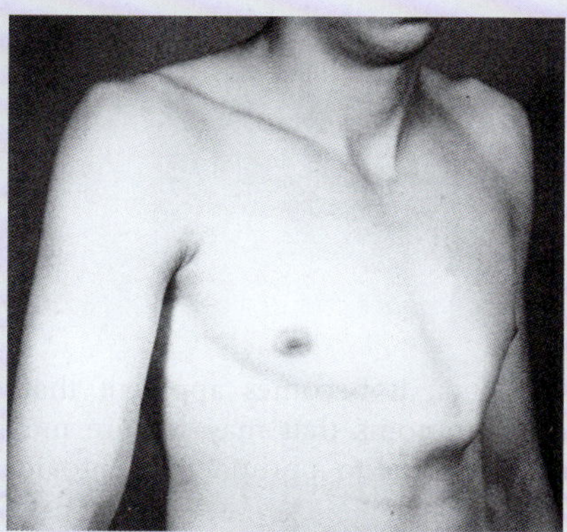

Pectus carinatum (pigeon chest). (Shamberger, R. C. [1994]. Chest wall deformities In Shields, T. W. [Ed.]. General thoracic surgery [4th ed., pp. 529–557]. Baltimore: Lippincott Williams & Wilkins.)

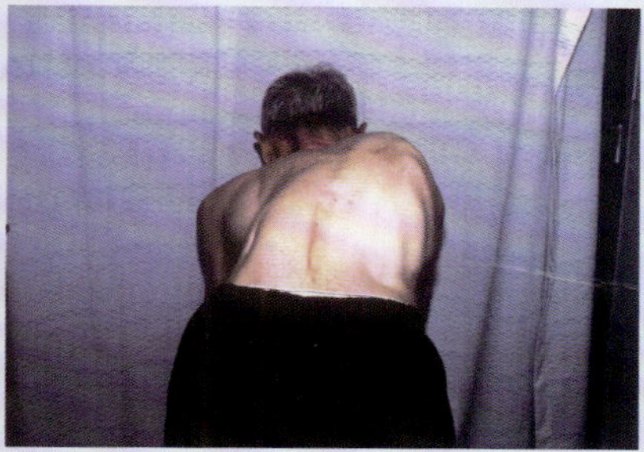

Scoliosis. (Berg, D. & Worzala, K. [2006]. Atlas of adult physical diagnosis. Philadelphia: Lippincott Williams & Wilkins.)

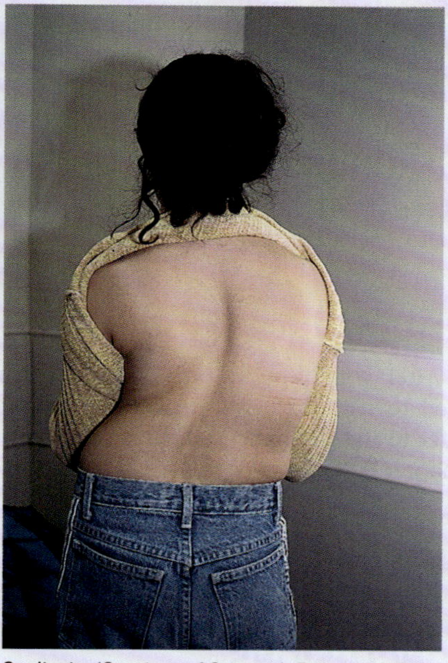

Scoliosis. (Courtesy of George A. Datto, III, MD.)

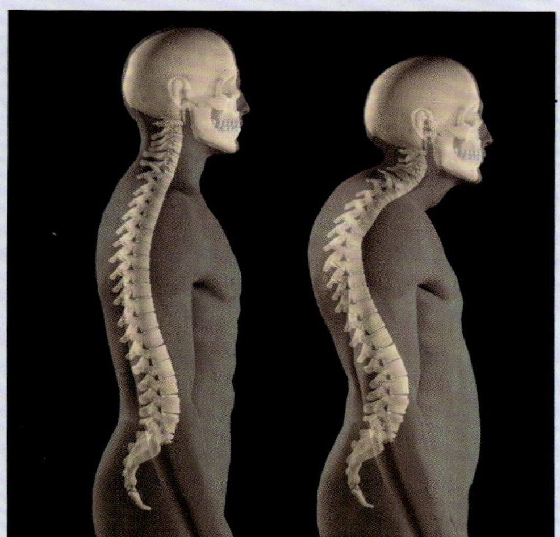

Kyphosis. LifeART image © 2014 Lippincott Williams & Wilkins. All rights reserved.

VALIDATING AND DOCUMENTING FINDINGS

If there are discrepancies between the objective and subjective data, or if abnormal findings are inconsistent with other data, you should always validate your data. This is necessary to verify all data are reliable and accurate. Document the assessment data following the health care facility or agency policy.

Sample of subjective data

No dyspnoea, cough or chest pain with breathing at rest or with activity. No past history or family history of respiratory diseases. Has never smoked and works in well-ventilated factory. Reports 'one or two' colds per year. No known allergies. Last chest X-ray was 4 years ago after 'minor' car accident. X-ray report at that time was normal.

Sample of objective data

Respirations 18 per minute, relaxed and even. Anteroposterior less than transverse diameter. Chest expansion symmetrical. No retracting or bulging of intercostal spaces. No pain or tenderness noted on palpation. Tactile fremitus symmetrical. Percussion tones resonant over all lung fields. Diaphragmatic excursion 4 cm and equal bilaterally. Vesicular breath sounds auscultated over lung fields. No adventitious sounds present.

After you have collected your assessment data, you will need to use diagnostic reasoning skills to analyse the data. Refer to the discussion of the diagnostic reasoning process in Chapter 5.

Analysis of data

DIAGNOSTIC REASONING: POSSIBLE CONCLUSIONS

After collecting subjective and objective data pertaining to the thorax and lung assessment, identify abnormal findings and patient strengths. Then cluster the data to reveal any significant patterns or abnormalities. These data may then be used to make clinical judgements about the status of the patient's thorax and lungs.

Potential patient risks

- Activity intolerance (related to imbalance between oxygen supply and demand)
- Imbalanced nutrition—less than body requirements (related to fatigue secondary to dyspnoea).

Potential patient problems

- Ineffective airway clearance (related to inability to clear thick, mucus secretions secondary to pain and fatigue, or to bronchospasm and increased pulmonary secretions)
- Impaired gas exchange (related to chronic lung tissue damage secondary to chronic smoking, or to poor muscle tone and decreased ability to remove secretions secondary to the ageing process)
- Anxiety (related to dyspnoea and fear of suffocation)
- Disturbed sleep pattern (related to excessive coughing)
- Activity intolerance (related to fatigue secondary to inadequate oxygenation)

Selected collaborative problems

After grouping the data, certain collaborative problems may become apparent. Remember that collaborative problems differ from nursing problems in that they cannot be prevented by nursing intervention. However, these physiological complications of medical conditions can be detected and monitored by the nurse. The following is a list of collaborative problems that may be identified:

- Atelectasis
- Pneumonia
- Chronic obstructive pulmonary disease
- Asthma
- Bronchitis
- Pleural effusion
- Pneumothorax
- Pulmonary oedema.

Medical problems

If, after grouping the data, it becomes apparent that the patient has signs and symptoms that may require medical diagnosis and treatment, referral to a primary care provider is necessary.

ONLINE RESOURCES

An extensive range of additional resources to enhance teaching and learning and to facilitate understanding may be found online at the text's accompanying website, located on thePoint at http://thepoint.lww.com. These include Watch and Learn videos, Concepts in Action animations, journal articles, case studies, discussion topics and quizzes.

Subscribers may also access Lippincott Procedures, an extensive online point-of-care procedure guide that provides reliable step-by-step instructions for more than 1700 procedures, including 450 evidence-based Australian procedures, and skills in a variety of speciality settings, together with a wealth of supporting information.

CASE STUDY

The case study demonstrates how to analyse thoracic and lung assessment data for a specific patient. The exercises included in the ancillary product on thePoint that complements this text offer further opportunities to enhance your skills.

George Burney is a 60-year-old retired Caucasian man. He was admitted to hospital 10 days ago following an episode of acute respiratory failure secondary to chronic obstructive pulmonary disease. You are caring for Mr Burney today.

You are talking to Mr Burney before undertaking his clinical assessment. His eyes sparkling, he tells you he is feeling great and that he was able to walk to the toilet today without his oxygen. He uses oxygen at 2 L/minute when he exercises or walks outside the ward, and PRN [meaning 'as needed'] for shortness of breath. He reports a 'chronic cough, as usual' but denies sputum production. He says he still has difficulty 'getting off a good cough' because 'I just don't have the energy anymore.'

Upon inspection, you note his facial colour and lips are ruddy, but his nail beds are pink. His breathing pattern is regular, unlaboured, but tachypnoeic at 28 respirations/minute, which he tells you is his usual rate. Examining his thorax, you note he is barrel-chested, with a transverse-to-lateral ratio of about 2.5 to 3. Although he is not using accessory muscles to breathe, you observe slight intercostal muscle bulging. His posture is rigidly upright in the chair. While auscultating his lungs, you note diminished breath sounds bilaterally in the lower lobes and a small, discrete area of coarse crackles in the upper portion of the left lower lobe. You also smell the odour of cigarettes on his breath and when you tell him you noticed the smell of cigarettes he says, 'I didn't think one would hurt when I was outside.'

The following concept map illustrates the diagnostic reasoning process.

Applying COLDSPA

Applying COLDSPA for patient symptoms: 'chronic cough'.

Mnemonic	Question	Data provided	Missing data
Character	Describe the sign or symptom (feeling, appearance, sound, smell or taste, if applicable).	'Chronic cough.'	
Onset	When did it begin?		When did you notice you could not bring up sputum when you cough?
Location	Where is it? Does it radiate? Does it occur anywhere else?		Do you have any chest pain?
Duration	How long does it last? Does it recur?		Are you short of breath when you walk or do other activities? How often do you use your oxygen?
Severity	How bad is it? or How much does it bother you?	'I am feeling great and I walked to the toilet today without my oxygen.'	
Pattern	What makes it better or worse?		What makes your shortness of breath and cough worse? Or better?'
Associated factors/How it Affects the patient	What other symptoms occur with it? How does it affect you?	Lacks energy to cough up any real sputum; smokes an occasional cigarette outside.	

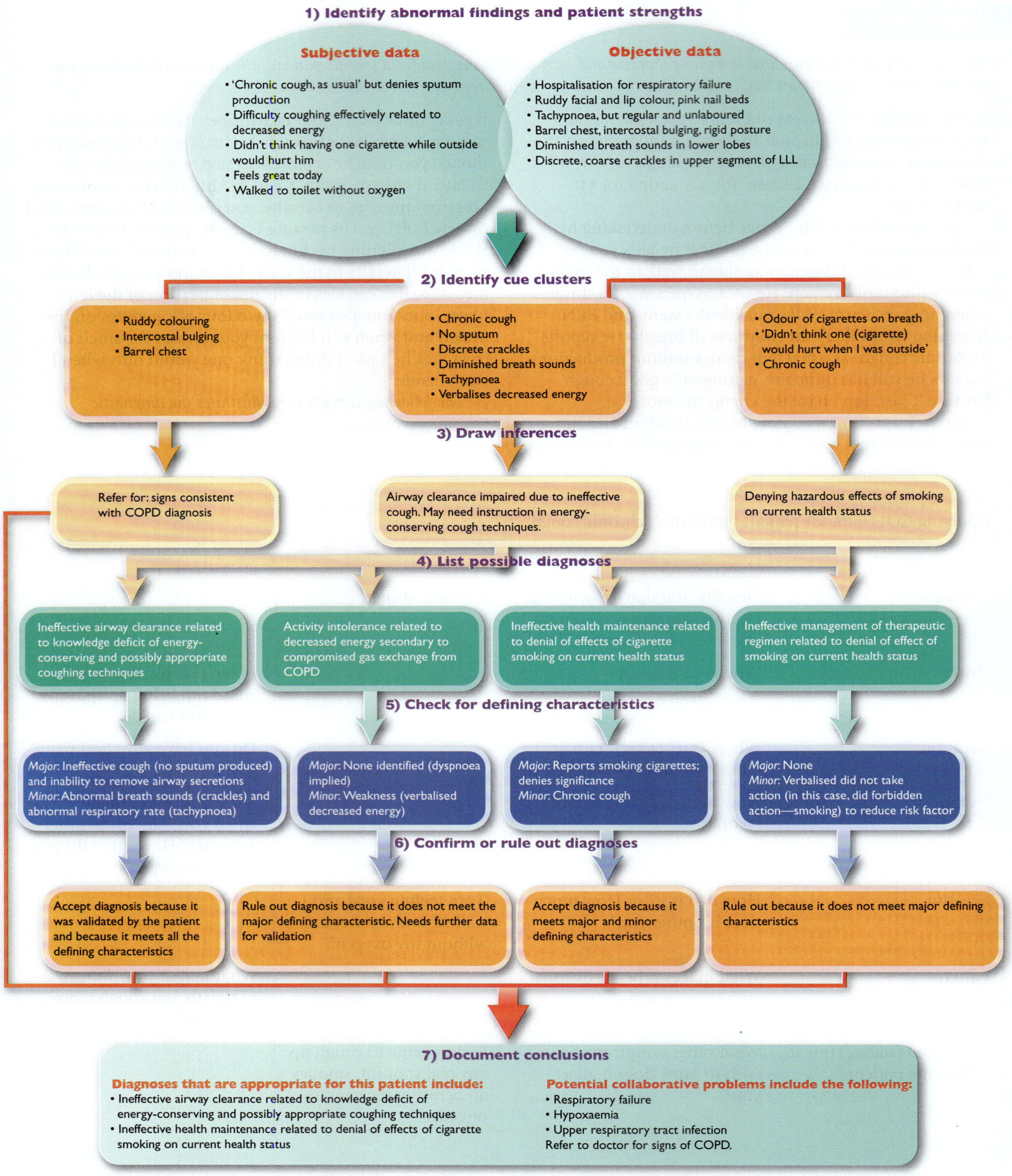

1) Identify abnormal findings and patient strengths

Subjective data

- 'Chronic cough, as usual' but denies sputum production
- Difficulty coughing effectively related to decreased energy
- Didn't think having one cigarette while outside would hurt him
- Feels great today
- Walked to toilet without oxygen

Objective data

- Hospitalisation for respiratory failure
- Ruddy facial and lip colour, pink nail beds
- Tachypnoea, but regular and unlaboured
- Barrel chest, intercostal bulging, rigid posture
- Diminished breath sounds in lower lobes
- Discrete, coarse crackles in upper segment of LLL

2) Identify cue clusters

- Ruddy colouring
- Intercostal bulging
- Barrel chest

- Chronic cough
- No sputum
- Discrete crackles
- Diminished breath sounds
- Tachypnoea
- Verbalises decreased energy

- Odour of cigarettes on breath
- 'Didn't think one (cigarette) would hurt when I was outside'
- Chronic cough

3) Draw inferences

Refer for: signs consistent with COPD diagnosis

Airway clearance impaired due to ineffective cough. May need instruction in energy-conserving cough techniques.

Denying hazardous effects of smoking on current health status

4) List possible diagnoses

Ineffective airway clearance related to knowledge deficit of energy-conserving and possibly appropriate coughing techniques

Activity intolerance related to decreased energy secondary to compromised gas exchange from COPD

Ineffective health maintenance related to denial of effects of cigarette smoking on current health status

Ineffective management of therapeutic regimen related to denial of effect of smoking on current health status

5) Check for defining characteristics

Major: Ineffective cough (no sputum produced) and inability to remove airway secretions
Minor: Abnormal breath sounds (crackles) and abnormal respiratory rate (tachypnoea)

Major: None identified (dyspnoea implied)
Minor: Weakness (verbalised decreased energy)

Major: Reports smoking cigarettes; denies significance
Minor: Chronic cough

Major: None
Minor: Verbalised did not take action (in this case, did forbidden action—smoking) to reduce risk factor

6) Confirm or rule out diagnoses

Accept diagnosis because it was validated by the patient and because it meets all the defining characteristics

Rule out diagnosis because it does not meet the major defining characteristic. Needs further data for validation

Accept diagnosis because it meets major and minor defining characteristics

Rule out because it does not meet major defining characteristics

7) Document conclusions

Diagnoses that are appropriate for this patient include:

- Ineffective airway clearance related to knowledge deficit of energy-conserving and possibly appropriate coughing techniques
- Ineffective health maintenance related to denial of effects of cigarette smoking on current health status

Potential collaborative problems include the following:

- Respiratory failure
- Hypoxaemia
- Upper respiratory tract infection

Refer to doctor for signs of COPD.

SIMULATED LEARNING

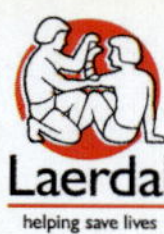

Having completed this chapter, explore the scenarios of Carl Shapiro Part 1 and Part 2, Jennifer Hoffman Part 1 and Part 2 and Vernon Watkins Part 1 and Part 2. Carl is a 54-year-old male presenting to the emergency department with a myocardial infarction. Jennifer is a 33-year-old asthmatic. Vernon is a 69-year-old man who is postoperative following a hemicolectomy and requires postoperative support. Incorporating the health assessment content in this chapter with your existing theoretical knowledge and clinical experience, progress through each simulation scenario (this is best done in a small group). How would you manage each patient's care? When reflecting on your management of each virtual patient, what do you think you did well and what do you think you can improve? Consider why you think this and how you might manage a similar problem in the future.

References

Australian Bureau of Statistics (ABS). (2013). Australian Aboriginal and Torres Strait Islander health survey: First results, Australia, 2012–13. ABS cat. no. 4727.0.55.001. Canberra: Australian Beaurea of Statistics.

Australian Institute of Health and Welfare (AIHW). (2016). Australian Burden of Disease Study: Impact and causes of illness and death in Australia 2011. Australian Burden of Disease Study series no. 3. BOD 4. Canberra: Author.

Australian Institute of Health and Welfare (AIHW). (2019). Chronic obstructive pulmonary disease. Canberra: Author. Viewed October 2019 at https://www.aihw.gov.au/reports/chronic-respiratory-conditions/copd/contents/copd.

Cancer Council Australia. (2019). Facts and figures. Canberra: Author. Viewed October 2019 at https://www.cancer.org.au/about-cancer/what-is-cancer/facts-and-figures.html.

Farrell, M. & Dempsey, J. (2017). *Smeltzer & Bare's textbook of medical-surgical nursing* (4th Australian and New Zealand ed.). Sydney: Lippincott Williams & Wilkins.

Mayo Clinic. (2019a). COPD definition. Viewed August 2019 at https://www.mayoclinic.org/diseases-conditions/copd/symptoms-causes/syc-20353679.

Ministry of Health. (2015). *Cancer patient survival 1994–2011*. Wellington: Ministry of Health.

New Zealand Ministry of Health. (2019). Cancer: Historical summary 1948–2016. Wellington: Author. Viewed October 2019 at https://www.health.govt.nz/publication/cancer-historical-summary-1948-2016.

Overfield, T. (1995). *Biological variation in health and illness: Race, age, and sex differences*. Menlo Park, CA: Addison-Wesley.

Shamberger, R. C. (1994). Chest wall deformities. In T. W. Shields (Ed). *General thoracic surgery* (4th ed., pp. 529–557). Baltimore: Lippincott Williams & Wilkins.

Telfar Barnard, L. & Zhang, J. (2018). The impact of respiratory disease in New Zealand: 2018 Update. Report for the Asthma and Respiratory Foundation of New Zealand: Wellington, New Zealand.

Selected readings

Andrews, J. (2019). Chest wall abnormalities. In R. Carachi & S. Doss (Eds). *Clinical embryology*. New York: Springer International Publishing.

Asthma Foundation. (2018). Respiratory disease in New Zealand. Wellington: Author. Viewed October 2019 at https://www.asthmafoundation.org.nz/resources/respiratory-disease-in-new-zealand.

Lopez, C. C., Macario, C. C., Trigo, J. M. M., et al. (2018). Comparison of the 2017 and 2015 global initiative for chronic obstructive lung disease reports. Impact on grouping and outcomes. *American Journal of Respiratory and Critical Care Medicine, 197*(4), 463–470.

Mayo Clinic. (2019b). Low down on lung cancer. Viewed August 2019 at www.xspeedtraining.com/2011/lowdown-on-lung-cancer.

Ministry of Health. (2014). *Cancer: New registrations and deaths 2011*. Wellington: Ministry of Health.

Online resources

Australian and New Zealand Guidelines for the Management of Chronic Obstructive Pulmonary Disease 2010: www.copdx.org.au
Australian Lung Foundation: www.lungfoundation.com.au
Cancer Control New Zealand: www.cancercontrolnz.govt.nz
Cancer Council Australia: www.cancer.org.au
Cancer Society of New Zealand: www.cancernz.org.nz
Mayo Clinic: https://www.mayoclinic.org/
Thoracic Society of Australia and New Zealand: www.thoracic.org.au

CHAPTER 21

Breasts and the lymphatic system

CASE STUDY

Nicole Barnes is a 42-year-old Aboriginal woman who is 2 days postoperative following an elective vaginal hysterectomy for the management of severe long-term endometriosis.

Structure and function

The **breasts** are paired mammary glands that lie over the muscles of the anterior chest wall, anterior to the pectoralis major and serratus anterior muscles. Depending on their size and shape, the breasts extend vertically from the second to the sixth rib and horizontally from the sternum to the midaxillary line (Fig. 21-1).

The male and female breasts are similar until puberty, when female breast tissue enlarges in response to the hormones oestrogen and progesterone released from the ovaries. The female breast is an accessory reproductive organ with two functions: to produce and store milk that provides nourishment for newborns and to aid in sexual stimulation. The male breasts have no functional capability.

For purposes of describing the location of assessment findings, the breasts are divided into four quadrants by drawing horizontal and vertical imaginary lines that intersect at the nipple.

The upper outer quadrant, extends into the axillary area and is referred to as the tail of Spence (Fig. 21-2). The upper quadrant is the most dense and where the highest frequency of breast tumours are located (Rummel et al., 2015). Lymph nodes are present in both male and female breasts. These structures drain lymph from the breasts to filter out microorganisms and return water and protein to the blood.

EXTERNAL ANATOMY

The skin of the breasts is smooth and varies in colour, depending on the patient's skin tones. The nipple, which is located in the centre of the breast, contains the tiny openings of the lactiferous ducts through which milk passes. The areola surrounds the nipple (generally 1 to 2 cm radius) and contains elevated sebaceous glands (Montgomery glands) that secrete a protective lipid substance during lactation. Hair follicles commonly appear around the areola. It is the smooth muscle fibres in the areola that cause the nipple to become more erect when stimulated through touch or cold temperature.

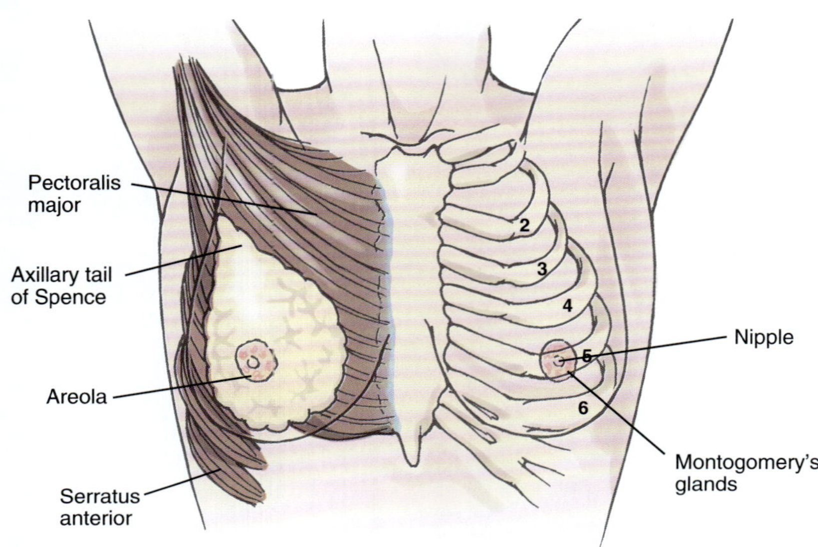

FIGURE 21-1 Anatomical breast landmarks and their position in the thorax.

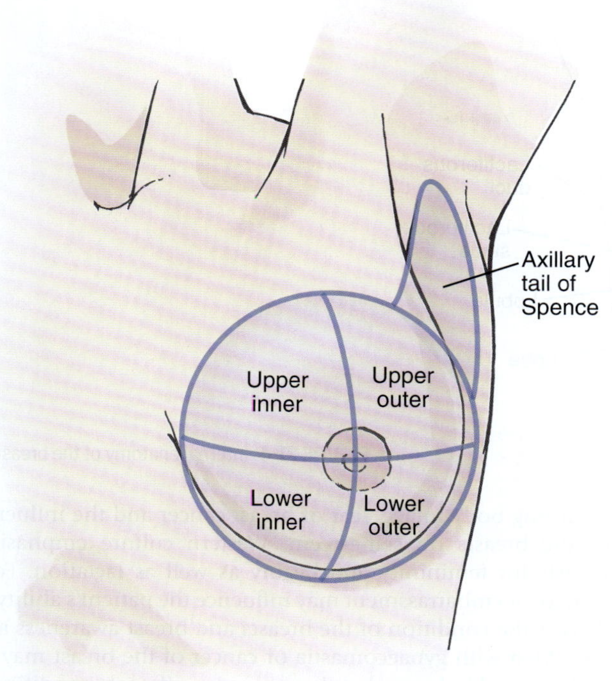

FIGURE 21-2 Breast quadrants. The upper outer quadrant is the area most targeted by breast cancer.

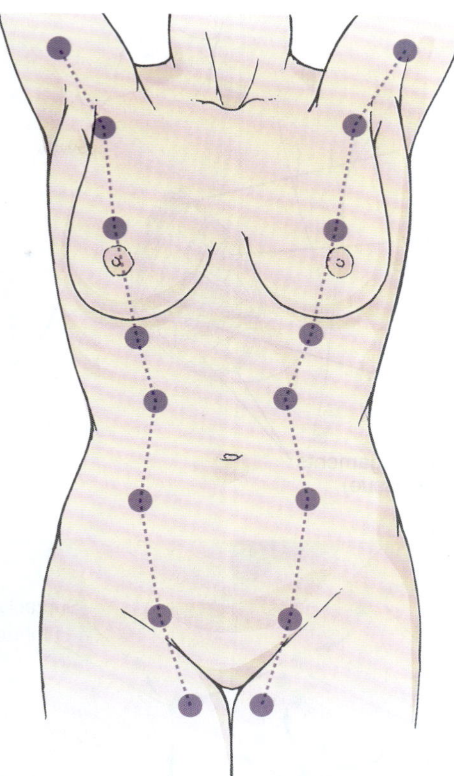

FIGURE 21-3 Supernumerary nipples along the 'milk line', which extends bilaterally from the axilla to the groin.

The nipple and areola typically have darker pigment than the surrounding breast. Their colour ranges from dark pink to dark brown, depending on the person's skin colour. The amount of pigmentation increases with pregnancy then decreases after lactation. However, it does not entirely return to its original colouration.

In some patients, supernumerary nipples or other breast tissue may appear along an area called the 'milk line' (Fig. 21-3). This milk line or ridge extends from each axilla to the groin area and appears during embryonic development. The line gradually atrophies and disappears as the person grows and develops.

INTERNAL ANATOMY

Female breasts consist of three types of tissue: glandular, fibrous and fatty (adipose) (Fig. 21-4). Glandular tissue constitutes the functional part of the breast, allowing for milk production. Glandular tissue is arranged in 15 to 20 lobes that radiate in a circular fashion from the nipple. Each lobe contains several lobules in which the secreting alveoli (acini cells) are embedded in grapelike clusters.

Mammary ducts from the alveoli converge into a single lactiferous duct that leaves each lobe and conveys milk to the nipple. The slight enlargement in each duct before it reaches the nipple is called the lactiferous sinus. The milk can be stored in the lactiferous sinus (or ampullae) until stimulated to be released from the nipple.

The fibrous tissue provides support for the glandular tissue, largely by way of bands called Cooper ligaments (suspensory ligaments). These ligaments run from the skin through the breast and attach to the deep fascia of the muscles of the anterior chest wall.

Fatty tissue is the third component of the breast. The glandular tissue is embedded in the fatty tissue. This subcutaneous and retromammary fat provides most of the substance to the breast and thus determines the size and shape of the breasts. The functional capability of the breast is not related to size but rather to the glandular tissue present. The amount of glandular, fibrous and fatty tissue varies according to various factors, including the patient's age, body build, nutritional status, hormonal cycle and whether she is pregnant or lactating.

This chapter covers the examination of the non-pregnant woman's breasts. Anatomical and physiological changes to the breast associated with pregnancy are covered in Chapter 31.

LYMPH NODES

The breast has extensive lymphatic drainage. The major axillary lymph nodes consist of the anterior (pectoral), posterior (subscapular), lateral (brachial) and central (midaxillary) nodes (Fig. 21-5). The anterior nodes drain the anterior chest wall and breasts. The posterior chest wall and part of the arms are drained by the posterior nodes.

The lateral nodes drain most of the arms, and the central nodes receive drainage from the anterior, posterior and lateral lymph nodes. A small proportion of the lymph also flows into the infraclavicular or supraclavicular lymph nodes or deeper into nodes within the chest or abdomen.

Health assessment

In Australia and New Zealand, breast awareness is now considered best practice, with regular *breast self-examination* (BSE)

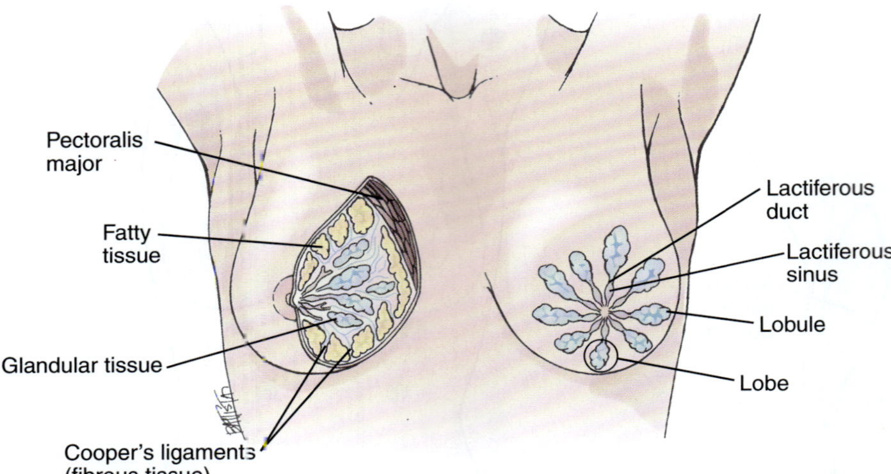

FIGURE 21-4 Internal anatomy of the breast.

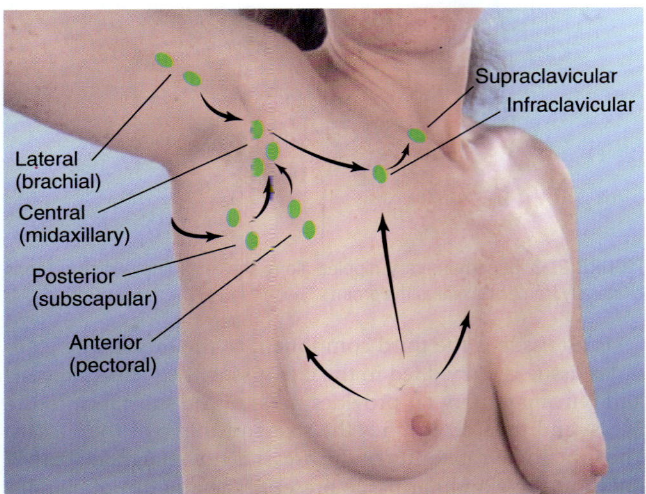

FIGURE 21-5 The lymph nodes drain impurities from the breasts (arrows show direction). (© B. Proud.)

no longer recommended (BreastScreen Aotearoa, 2018; Cancer Australia, 2019; Kosters & Gotzsche, 2008). A Cochrane review of breast self-examination studies by Kosters and Gotzsche (2008) found data that suggest screening through BSE had no beneficial effect, increasing harm instead in terms of higher numbers of benign lesions identified and an increased number of biopsies performed. Women are advised to be aware of the normal look and feel of their breasts and to report any changes to their doctor. *Clinical breast examination* (CBE) refers to examination of the breasts by a trained health professional and is usually undertaken when changes have been noted.

Clinical breast examination is an advanced clinical skill that will often be completed by Registered Nurses in specialty areas, but not by undergraduate nursing students. However, it is important that all nurses have an awareness of what is involved in CBE and BSE so that they can explain BSE to patients who wish to perform it themselves and clarify any problems they may have.

COLLECTING SUBJECTIVE DATA: THE NURSING HEALTH HISTORY

When interviewing patients—especially female patients—about their breasts, keep in mind that this topic may evoke a spate of emotions from the patient. Explore your own feelings regarding body image, fear of breast cancer and the influence of the breasts on self-esteem. Western culture emphasises breasts for femininity and beauty as well as lactation. Fear, anxiety or embarrassment may influence the patient's ability to discuss the condition of the breasts and breast awareness and BSE. Men with gynaecomastia or cancer of the breast may be embarrassed to have what they consider a 'female condition'.

This chapter covers the examination of the non-pregnant woman's breasts. Subjective data related to breast changes associated with pregnancy is covered in Chapter 31. Where the patient reports any symptom, you should explore this further by performing a symptom analysis using the following COLDSPA example as a guide.

CASE STUDY

Nicole tells you this procedure has made her think about her health and that she is now concerned about lumps and tenderness that occur in her breasts each month, just a few days before her menstrual period.

CRITICAL THINKING

1. Considering Nicole's history, would you ask her questions regarding her lifestyle and health history? Why or why not?
2. What questions would you ask Nicole regarding her knowledge of breast awareness?

CASE STUDY

In response to questioning, Nicole states she is a very 'heavy coffee drinker', is currently on Depo-Provera and is under a great deal of stress in her job and at home. When asked on her breast awareness, she is able to describe the normal look and feel of her breasts. When you question her about family history, she reports that her maternal aunt died of breast cancer. She wants to know if the lumps could be cancerous or what can be done to eliminate the breast problem. You suspect that she has fibrocystic changes characteristic of benign breast disease.

History of present health concerns

QUESTION	RATIONALE
Have you noticed any lumps or swelling in your breasts? If so, where? When did you first notice it? Has the lump grown or swelling increased? Is the lump or swelling associated with other problems? Does the lump or swelling change during your menstrual cycle? Have you noticed any lumps or swelling in the underarm area?	Lumps may be present with benign breast disease (fibrocystic breast disease), fibroadenomas or malignant tumours (see Promote health—Breast cancer). Any lumps should be assessed further, and the patient should be referred to a doctor. Premenstrual breast lumpiness and soreness that subside after the end of the menstrual cycle may indicate benign breast disease (fibrocystic breast disease).
Have you noticed any redness, warmth or dimpling of your breasts? Any rash on the breast, nipple or axillary area?	Redness and warmth indicate inflammation. A dimpling or retraction of the nipple or fibrous tissue may indicate breast cancer.
Have you noticed any change in the size or firmness of your breasts?	A recent increase in the size of one breast may indicate inflammation or abnormal growth. **OLDER ADULT CONSIDERATIONS** **The older patient may notice a decrease in the size and firmness of the breasts as she ages because of a decrease in oestrogen levels. Glandular tissue decreases whereas fatty tissue increases. A well-fitting supportive bra can reduce breast discomfort related to sagging breasts.**
Do you experience any pain in your breasts? If so, where? Does it occur at any specific time during your menstrual cycle? Is there a certain activity that seems to initiate the pain?	Pain and tenderness of the breasts are common in benign breast disease and just before and during menstruation. This is especially true for patients taking oral contraceptives. Breast pain can also be a late sign of breast cancer.
Do you have any discharge from the nipples? If so, describe its colour, consistency and odour, if any. When did it start? Which nipple has the discharge?	If the patient reports any blood or blood-tinged discharge, she should be referred to a doctor for further evaluation. Sometimes, a clear benign discharge may be manually expressed from a breast that is frequently stimulated. Certain medications (oral contraceptives, phenothiazines, steroids, digoxin and diuretics) are also associated with a clear discharge.

COLDSPA

Example for lump in breast

Use the COLDSPA mnemonic as a guideline to collect needed information for each symptom the patient shares. In addition, the following questions help elicit important information.

Mnemonic	Question	Patient response example
Character	Describe the sign or symptom (feeling, appearance, sound, smell or taste, if applicable).	'I found a lump in my left breast the size of a small coin.'
Onset	When did it begin?	'I just noticed it yesterday when I took a shower.'
Location	Where is it? Does it radiate? Does it occur anywhere else?	'It is in the left upper side of my left breast.'
Duration	How long does it last? Does it recur?	'It does not hurt.' 'I have not had it before'
Severity	How bad is it? or How much does it bother you?	'I am worried about what it might be because my mother had breast cancer.'
Pattern	What makes it better or worse?	'It seems to get bigger the more I feel it, but it does not go away.'
Associated factors/How it **A**ffects the patient	What other symptoms occur with it? How does it affect you?	'I try to work, but I just keep thinking about this lump in my breast.'

PROMOTE HEALTH | **BREAST CANCER**

OVERVIEW

In 2015, breast cancer was the most commonly diagnosed cancer and second most common cause of death from cancer among women in Australia (Cancer Australia, 2019). In New Zealand, breast cancer is the most common cancer and second most common cause of death from cancer among women, accounting for more than 600 deaths every year (NZMOH, 2018). Australia and New Zealand are in the top 10 countries in the world with the highest rate of breast cancer in women (World Cancer Research Fund International, 2018). However, early detection and treatment have resulted in increased survival rates. The number of newly diagnosed cases of breast cancer in Australia increased from 5,374 in 1982 to 17,004 in 2015 (Cancer Australia, 2019).

Breast cancer is the most commonly diagnosed cancer in Aboriginal and Torres Strait Islander women, accounting for 25% of all female cancers (Tapia et al., 2017). Aboriginal and Torres Strait Islander women are 20% less likely to be diagnosed with breast cancer compared with non-Aboriginal and Torres Strait Islander women (Australian Institute of Health and Welfare, 2017). In New Zealand, Māori women are reported as having one of the highest incidence of breast cancer in the world with poor survival compared with New Zealand European women (Lawrenson et al., 2016).

Risk factors (Cancer Australia, 2019)

- Gender (100 times more common in women)
- Age (risk increases with increasing age, especially after age 50 years)
- Place of residence (living in certain countries can increase risk of breat cancer)
- Remoteness of residence (living in an urbanised area compared with rural is associated with increased risk)
- Socio-economic status (living in a higher socio-economic area increases risk of breast cancer)
- Birthweight
- Height (being taller is associated with increased risk)
- Breast density (higher than average breast density is associated with an increased risk of breast cancer)
- Genetics (there are several genes in which mutations may be involved in the development of breast cancer, including *BRCA1* and *BRCA2*, *TP53*, *PTEN*, *CDH1* and *STK11*, and some rare moderate-risk gene mutations such as *PALB2*, *ATM* and *CHEK2*)
- Family history of breast cancer or ovarian cancer
- Certain benign breast conditions
- Lobular carcinoma in situ
- Ductal carcinoma in situ
- Previous chest radiation to treat cancer
- Early menarche and late age menopause
- Not having children
- First child born to mother over the age of 30
- Oral contraceptive use (oestrogen and progesterone)
- Hormone replacement therapy (oestogen and progesterone)
- Alcohol consumption
- Smoking

Risk reduction and health education

- Screening—promote the Australian Department of Health and New Zealand Ministry of Health recommendations for clinical evaluation and mammography.
- Alcohol—limit alcohol intake to a maximum of 1 standard drink a day.
- Body weight—promote a healthy body weight that is within a body mass index range of 18.5 to 25 kg/m^2, and have a waist circumference of below 80 cm (31.5 in.).
- Physical activity—promote at least 30 minutes of moderate-intensity physical activity every day.
- Menopausal hormone therapy (MHT)—promote regular review with general practitioner (GP) for women taking MHT.
- Breastfeeding—promote breastfeeding (the longer the duration of breastfeeding, the greater the benefits).
- Breast awareness—promote taking the time to know the normal look and feel of the breasts as part of the woman's daily routine (know the symptoms to look out for, and see the GP if any changes are found).

Past health history

QUESTION	RATIONALE
Have you had any prior breast disease? Have you ever had breast surgery, a breast biopsy, breast implants or breast trauma? If so, when did this occur? What was the result?	A personal history of breast cancer increases the risk of recurrence of cancer. Previous surgeries may alter the appearance of the breasts. Breast problems may occur with silicone breast implants. Trauma to the breasts from sports, accidents or physical abuse can result in breast tissue changes.
How old were you when you began to menstruate? Have you experienced menopause?	Early menses (before age 13) or delayed menopause (after age 52) increases the risk of breast cancer.
Have you given birth to any children? At what age did you have your first child?	The risk of breast cancer is greater for women who have never given birth or for those who had their first child after age 30.
When was the first and last day of your menstrual cycle?	This information will inform you if this is the optimal time to examine the breasts. Hormone-related swelling, breast tenderness and generalised lumpiness are reduced right after menstruation.

Family history

QUESTION	RATIONALE
Is there a history of breast cancer in your family? Who (sister, mother, maternal grandmother)?	A history of breast cancer in one's family increases one's risk for breast cancer.

Lifestyle and health practices

QUESTION	RATIONALE
Are you taking any hormones, contraceptives or antipsychotic agents?	Hormones and some antipsychotic agents can cause breast engorgement in women. Hormones and oral contraceptives also increase the risk of breast cancer. Haloperidol (Serenace), an antipsychotic drug, can cause galactorrhoea (persistent milk secretion whether or not the woman is breastfeeding) and lactation. This is also a side effect of medroxyprogesterone (Depo-Provera) injections.
Do you live or work in an area where you have excessive exposure to radiation, benzene or asbestos?	Exposure to these environmental hazards can increase the risk of breast cancer.
What is your typical daily diet?	A high-fat diet may increase the risk of breast cancer.
How much alcohol do you drink each day?	Alcohol intake exceeding two drinks per day has been associated with a higher risk of breast cancer.
How much coffee, tea, cola drinks (or other forms of caffeine) do you consume each day?	Caffeine can aggravate fibrocystic breast disease.
Do you engage in any type of regular exercise? If so, what type of bra do you wear when you exercise?	Breast tissue can lose its elasticity if vigorous exercise (i.e. running, aerobics) is performed without support for the breast. A well-fitting, supportive bra can also reduce discomfort in the breasts during exercise.
How important are your breasts to you in relation to a positive feeling about yourself and your physical appearance? Do you have any fears regarding breast disease?	The condition of the breasts may significantly influence how a woman feels about herself. Alterations in the breasts may threaten a woman's body image and feelings of self-worth, and men may be embarrassed to have enlarged breasts.
Are you aware of the normal look and feel of your breasts? Have you noted any changes in your breasts such as a lump, swelling, skin irritation or dimpling, nipple pain or retraction (turning inwards), redness or scaliness on nipple or breast skin, or discharge? If yes, have you reported this to your health care provider? **CLINICAL TIP** **Older patients and others who no longer menstruate may find it helpful to pick a set day of the month for BSE, a date they will remember each month such as the day of the month they were born.**	Women should be encouraged to be breast aware from the age of 20. Emphasise the importance of reporting any breast changes to a health professional. If a woman chooses to do BSE, instruct the woman on the proper technique (Self-assessment 21-1), allowing time for questions and review of her technique. The best time for BSE is right after menstruation or between the fourth and seventh day of the cycle if the cycle is regular. If the patient is on cyclic oestrogen therapy, she should examine her breasts on the last day the medicine is not being taken. It is important for women to know their breasts and report any breast changes promptly to their health care provider. Remember that most of the time breast changes are not cancer, but it is important to detect breast cancer early for effective treatment. Women who have had a breast lumpectomy, augmentation or breast reconstruction should be encouraged to perform BSE.
Have you ever had your breasts examined by a health professional? When was your last examination?	The New Zealand Breast Cancer Foundation and Cancer Australia recommend that a clinical breast examination is not best practice as a screening method for the early detection of breast cancer, and promote breast awareness. However, a clinical breast examination should be offered to women without symptoms who are concerned about breast cancer or who are symptomatic (BreastScreen Aotearoa, 2018; Cancer Australia, 2019).

Continued on following page

Lifestyle and health practices (continued)

QUESTION	RATIONALE
Have you ever had a mammogram? If so, when was your last one?	BreastScreen Aotearoa (2018) recommends a 2-yearly screening mammogram for New Zealand women aged 45 to 69. BreastScreen Australia (2015) recommends a 2-yearly screening mammogram for well women without symptoms who are aged 50 to 74, although women between the ages of 40 and 49, and those who are 75 years and older who have no breast cancer symptoms or signs, should talk with their doctor to see if they should attend free screening. Women at increased risk (e.g. family history, genetic tendency, past breast cancer) should talk to their doctor about the benefits and limitations of starting mammography screening earlier, having additional tests (i.e. breast ultrasound and magnetic resonance imaging) and having more frequent exams (BreastScreen Aotearoa, 2018).

COLLECTING OBJECTIVE DATA: PHYSICAL EXAMINATION

The purpose of breast assessment is to identify signs of breast disease and then to initiate early treatment. The incidence of breast cancer in women is rising, but early detection and treatment have resulted in increased survival rates. Breast cancer is the most common cancer among Australian and New Zealand women (BreastScreen Australia, 2020; BreastScreen Aotearoa, 2018; Cancer Australia, 2019).

Female breast examinations are often performed by the nurse before a mammogram, or by the gynaecologist or nurse practitioner before a routine pelvic examination. A breast examination should also be a routine part of the complete male assessment. However, the male breast examination is not as detailed as the female breast examination.

Keep in mind that breast palpation requires practice and skill because the consistency of the breasts varies widely from patient to patient. Some breasts are more difficult to palpate than others. For example, it is more difficult to palpate and inspect large, pendulous breasts to ensure adequate evaluation of all breast tissue. It may also be difficult to detect new lumps in women who have fibrocystic breast disease and who have granular, singular or multiple mobile, tender lumps in their breasts.

The actual hands-on physical examination of the breast may make the patient anxious. The patient may be embarrassed about exposing his or her breasts and may be anxious about what the assessment will reveal. Explain in detail what is happening throughout the assessment and answer any questions the patient might have. In addition, attempt to provide the patient with as much privacy as possible during the examination.

This chapter covers the examination of the non-pregnant woman's breasts. Objective data related to breast changes associated with pregnancy are covered in Chapter 31.

Preparing the patient

Prepare for the breast examination by having the patient sit in an upright position. Explain that it will be necessary to expose both breasts to compare them for symmetry during inspection. One breast may be draped while the other breast is palpated. Be sensitive to the fact that many women may feel embarrassed to have their breasts examined.

The breasts are first inspected in the sitting position while the patient is asked to hold their arms in different positions. The breasts are then palpated while the patient assumes a supine position.

The final part of the examination involves teaching patients breast awareness and, if requested, how to perform breast self-examination (BSE), asking them to demonstrate what they have learned. If the patient states that she or he already knows how to perform BSE, then ask the patient to demonstrate how this is done.

Equipment

- Centimetre ruler
- Small pillow
- Gloves
- Patient information handout for breast awareness

CRITICAL THINKING

3. Prior to reading the physical assessment section, what do you think are some of the important things you need to consider regarding cultural safety and competence?
4. Reread the section on lifestyle and health practices and consider the information contained in this section. What information do you think you can give Nicole regarding her lifestyle practices, given that she has a history of drinking large quantities of coffee?
5. What objective physical assessment technique could you perform on Nicole, and what would you look for?

CASE STUDY

On inspection of Nicole's breasts you notice that the breasts are bilaterally equal in size, with everted nipples. No dimpling, retraction or discharge is noted. You decide to inform the doctor of her concerns.

SELF-ASSESSMENT 21-1 BREAST SELF-EXAMINATION

sydney breast cancer foundation

3 STEP BREAST CHECK

1.

Step 1 THE SHOWER CHECK

Put your left hand behind your head. With the sensitive pads on your right fingers, use small circular movements to examine your left breast for anything unusual. At first feel lightly, checking for anything near the surface. Then press quite firmly, feeling for anything deeper. Continue around the breast, checking all areas. Also examine above your breast, up to the collarbone and out to the armpit. Then do the same for the right side.

2.

Step 2 THE BATHROOM MIRROR

After showering, place your hands at your sides and check your breasts in the mirror. Look for anything which is not normal for your breasts - changes in colour, size or shape, any dimpling of the skin or "pulling-in" of the nipple. Put your hands on your hips and push your shoulders forward to flex your chest muscles. Finally, raise your hands over your head and check for any changes.

3.

Step 3 CHECK LYING DOWN

Lie on your left side with your knees bent, roll your shoulders back so they are flat on the bed. Place your right arm under your head. Your breast should now be as flat as possible. Examine your right breast using the methods outlined in Step 1. Reverse procedure to check other breast.

Check your breasts at the same time each month, preferably 2-3 days after your period ends. If you no longer have periods, choose a regular day each month for breast examination.

The Breast Aware Message

Important! While all women should check their breasts regularly, self examination is in addition to, and NOT a substitute for a yearly breast examination by your GP and screening mammograms every two years.

Screening mammograms are available free of charge to every woman in Australia from age 40 by calling **Breast Screen Australia on 13 20 50.**

If you notice a change in your breasts, see your doctor immediately!

Women with a personal or family history of breast cancer may be at higher risk and should seek advice from their GP as soon as possible.

www.sbcf.org.au

sydney breast cancer foundation

Chris O'Brien Lifehouse

Be Breast Aware.

Raising the awareness of self-breast examination by women of all ages could increase the chance of early detection and diagnosis of breast cancer. Results have shown that early detection and diagnosis leads to an increase in survival rates among breast cancer patients.

SYDNEY BREAST CANCER FOUNDATION

The Sydney Breast Cancer Foundation at Chris O'Brien Lifehouse is dedicated to raising funds for research and treatment of breast cancer, raising awareness and supporting individuals and their families facing breast cancer.

We believe that all breast cancer patients deserve the best possible treatment and support and that increasing awareness is vital to beating the disease. Chris O'Brien Lifehouse is an integrated and patient-focused centre of excellence, offering everything a cancer patient needs in one place, including treatment, research, education, complementary therapies and psychosocial support.

One of our main goals is to increase awareness and early detection of breast cancer in order to improve survival rates for breast cancer patients.

This card is a small but powerful tool; Following its advice could save lives!

Since 1995 Sydney Breast Cancer Foundation has generated millions of dollars to support breast cancer patients and promote the "Breast Aware" message.

Help us continue this work

Chris O'Brien Lifehouse relies on donations and support from funds raised by the Sydney Breast Cancer Foundation for vital breast cancer treatment, research, patient education and specialised equipment.

To make a donation go to www.sbcf.org.au or call (02) 8514 0659.

www.sbcf.org.au

 Sydney Breast Cancer Foundation's mission is to improve early detection of breast cancer and the quality of life and survival rates of breast cancer patients. The Foundation raises funds for the Breast Unit at Chris O'Brien Lifehouse. You can donate to the foundation at https://www.sbcf.org.au/donate/.

Physical assessment

Key points for physical assessment include the following:

- Maintain privacy.
- Explain to the patient what the steps of the examination are and the rationale for each step.
- Warm your hands.
- Observe and inspect breast skin, areolas and nipples for size, shape, rashes, dimpling, swelling, discolouration, retraction, asymmetry and other unusual findings.
- Palpate breasts and axillary lymph nodes for swelling, lumps, masses, warmth or inflammation, tenderness and other abnormalities.
- Perform the physical assessment just as carefully on male patients..

PHYSICAL ASSESSMENT

ASSESSMENT PROCEDURE	NORMAL FINDINGS	ABNORMAL FINDINGS
Female breasts		
INSPECTION		
Inspect size and symmetry. Have the patient disrobe and sit with arms hanging freely (Fig. 21-6). Explain what you are observing to help ease patient anxiety.	Breasts can be a variety of sizes and are somewhat round and pendulous. One breast may normally be larger than the other. **OLDER ADULT CONSIDERATIONS** **The older patient often has more pendulous, less firm and saggy breasts.**	A recent increase in the size of one breast may indicate inflammation or an abnormal growth. A pigskinlike or orange-peel (*peau d'orange*) appearance results from oedema, which is seen in metastatic breast disease (Fig. 21-7). The oedema is caused by blocked lymphatic drainage.
Inspect colour and texture. Be sure to note patient's overall skin tone when inspecting the breast skin. Note any lesions.	Colour varies depending on the patient's skin tone. Texture is smooth with no oedema. Linear stretch marks may be seen during and after pregnancy or with significant weight gain or loss.	Redness is associated with breast inflammation.
Inspect superficial venous pattern. Observe visibility and pattern of breast veins.	Veins radiate either horizontally and towards the axilla (transverse) or vertically with a lateral flare (longitudinal). Veins are more prominent during pregnancy. **CULTURAL CONSIDERATIONS** **These two patterns are seen in varying proportions among different cultural groups. However, both patterns are normal and the transverse pattern predominates.**	A prominent venous pattern may occur as a result of increased circulation due to a malignancy. An asymmetrical venous pattern may be due to malignancy.
Inspect the areolas. Note the colour, size, shape and texture of the areolas of both breasts.	Areolas vary from dark pink to dark brown, depending on the patient's skin tones. They are round and may vary in size. Small Montgomery tubercles are present.	*Peau d'orange* skin, associated with carcinoma, may be first seen in the areola, whereas red, scaly, crusty areas are indicative of Paget's disease (Fig. 21-8).

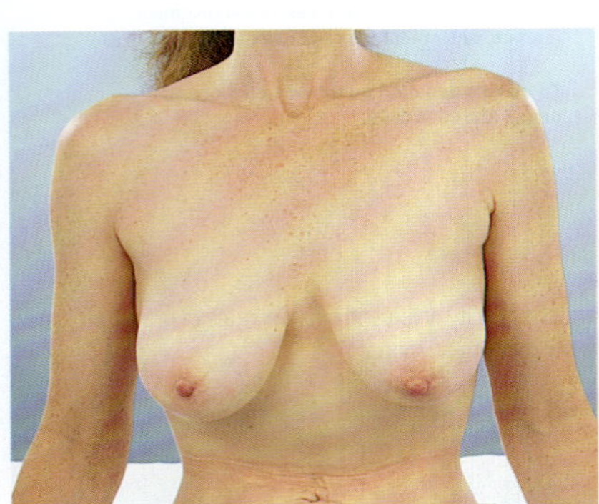

FIGURE 21-6 Patient should sit with arms hanging freely at sides during assessment of breast size and symmetry. (© B. Proud.)

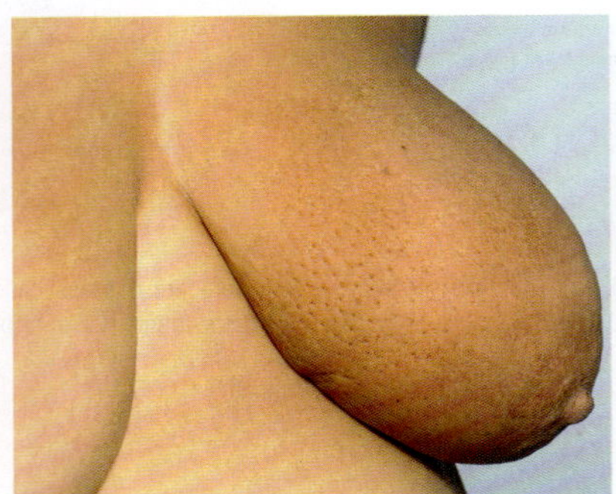

FIGURE 21-7 Resulting from oedema, an orange peel (*peau d'orange*) appearance of the breast is associated with cancer. (Alamy Stock Photo/ Mediscan.)

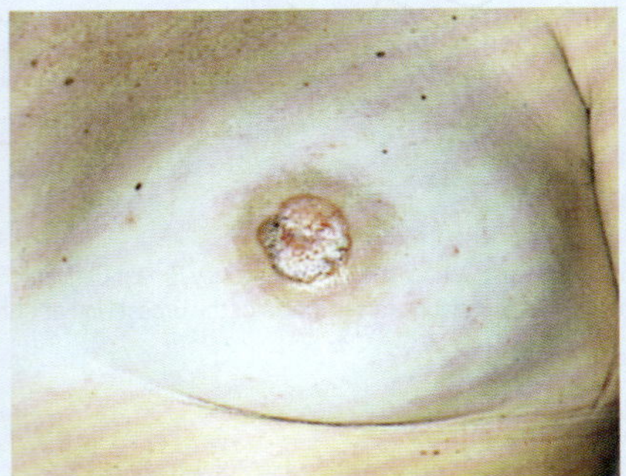

FIGURE 21-8 Paget disease is typified by a crusty, red scaliness of the nipple.

PHYSICAL ASSESSMENT (continued)

ASSESSMENT PROCEDURE	NORMAL FINDINGS	ABNORMAL FINDINGS
Female breasts (continued)		
Inspect the nipples. Note the size and direction of the nipples of both breasts. Also note any dryness, lesions, bleeding or discharge.	Nipples are nearly equal bilaterally in size and are in the same location on each breast. Nipples are usually everted, but they may be inverted or flat. Supernumerary nipples (Fig. 21-9) may appear along the embryonic 'milk line'. No discharge should be present. **OLDER ADULT CONSIDERATIONS** **The older patient may have smaller, flatter nipples that are less erectile on stimulation.**	A recently retracted nipple that was previously everted suggests malignancy (Fig. 21-10). Any type of spontaneous discharge should be referred for cytological study and further evaluation.

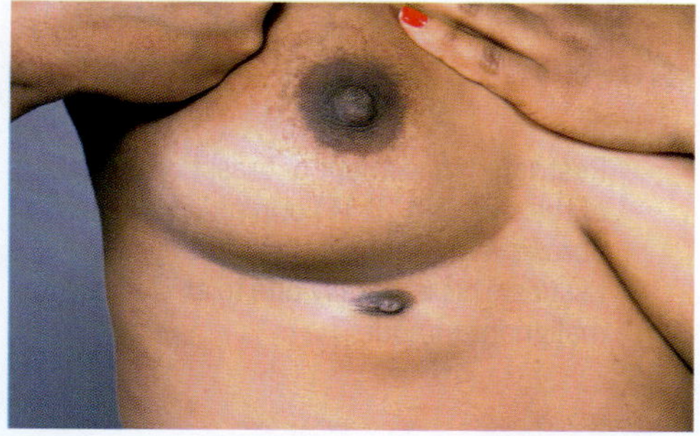

FIGURE 21-9 Supernumerary nipple (Mediscan/Alamy Stock Photo.)

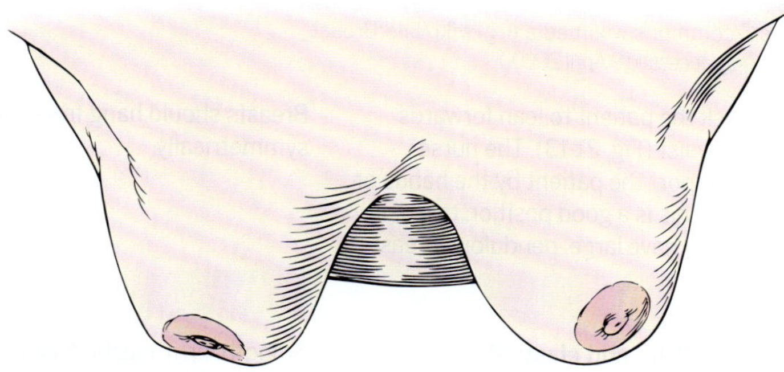

FIGURE 21-10 Retracted nipple.

ASSESSMENT PROCEDURE	NORMAL FINDINGS	ABNORMAL FINDINGS
Inspect for retraction and dimpling. To inspect the breasts accurately for retraction and dimpling, ask the patient to remain seated while performing several different manoeuvres. Ask the patient to raise her arms overhead (Fig. 21-11A); then press her hands against her hips (Fig. 21-11B). Next ask her to press her hands together (Fig. 21-11C). These actions contract the pectoral muscles.	The patient's breasts should rise symmetrically with no sign of dimpling or retraction.	Dimpling or retraction (Fig. 21-12) is usually caused by a malignant tumour that has fibrous strands attached to the breast tissue and the fascia of the muscles. As the muscle contracts, it draws the breast tissue and skin with it, causing dimpling or retraction.

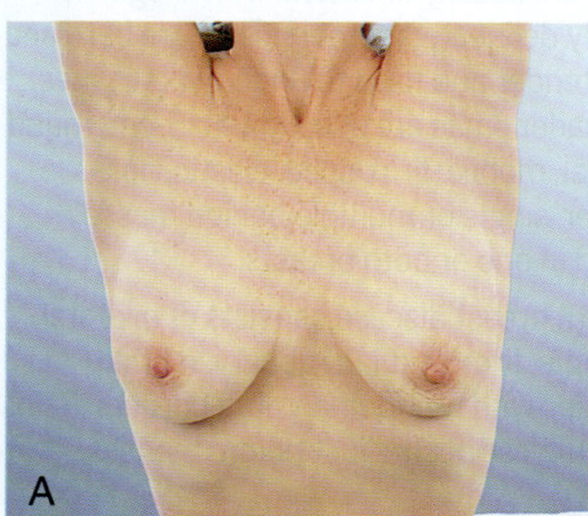

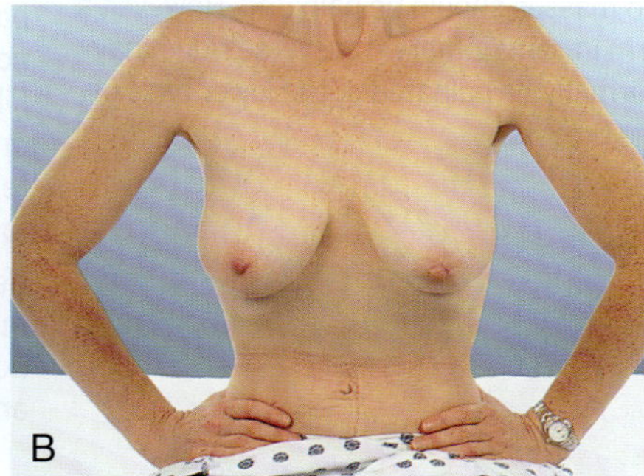

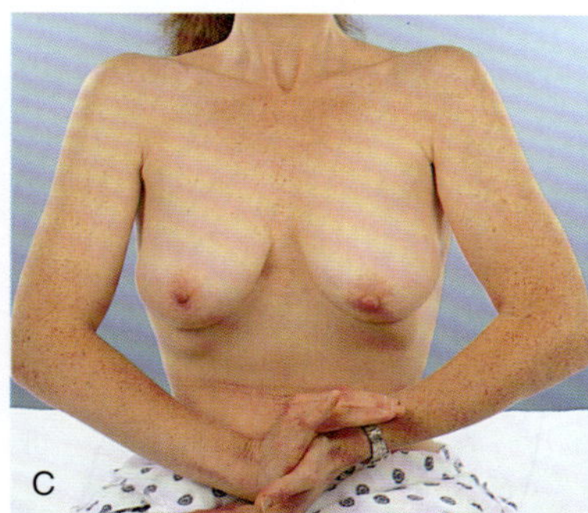

FIGURE 21-11 During assessment for retraction and dimpling, the patient first **(A)** raises her arms over her head , **(B)** lowers them and presses them against the hips and then **(C)** presses the hands together with the fingers of one hand pointing opposite to the fingers of the other hand. (© B. Proud.)

Continued on following page

PHYSICAL ASSESSMENT (continued)

ASSESSMENT PROCEDURE	NORMAL FINDINGS	ABNORMAL FINDINGS
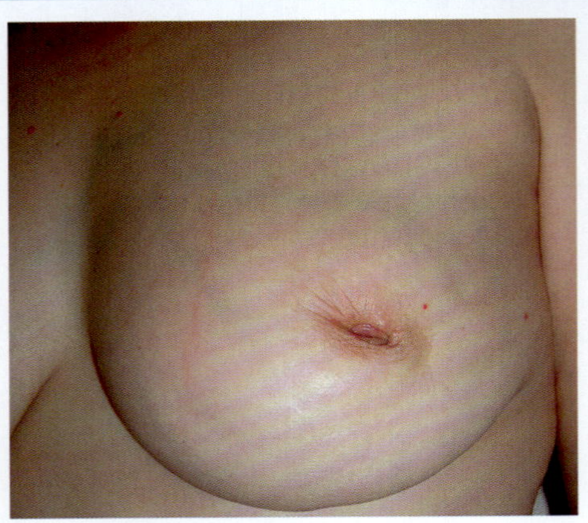 **FIGURE 21-12** Dimpling of the breast nipple (Wikimedia Commons/Hicet Nunc. CC BY SA 3.0 Unported License, https://commons.wikimedia.org/wiki/File:Breast_cancer.jpg, accessed 9 April 2020.)		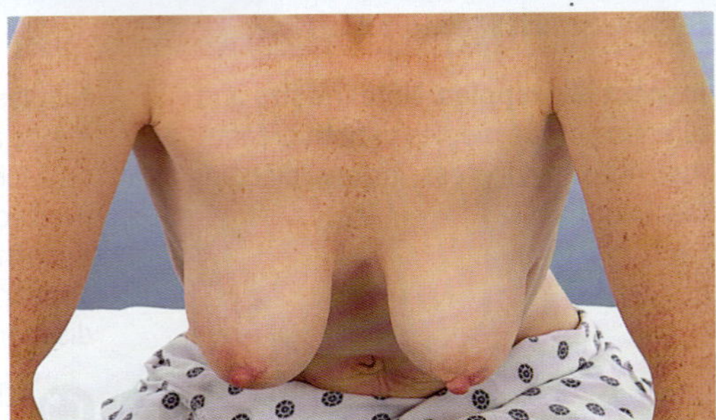 **FIGURE 21-13** Forward-leaning position for breast inspection. (© B. Proud.)
Finally ask the patient to lean forwards from the waist (Fig. 21-13). The nurse should support the patient by the hands or forearms. This is a good position to use in women who have large, pendulous breasts.	Breasts should hang freely and symmetrically.	Restricted movement of breast or retraction of the skin (Fig. 21-14) or nipple indicates fibrosis and fixation of the underlying tissues. This is usually due to an underlying malignant tumour.
PALPATION		
Palpate texture and elasticity. See Assessment tool 21-1 **Palpate tenderness and temperature.** See Assessment tool 21-1. **Palpate for masses.** Note location, size in centimetres, shape, mobility, consistency and tenderness (see Assessment tool 21-1). Also note the condition of the skin over the mass. If you detect any lump, refer the patient for further evaluation. 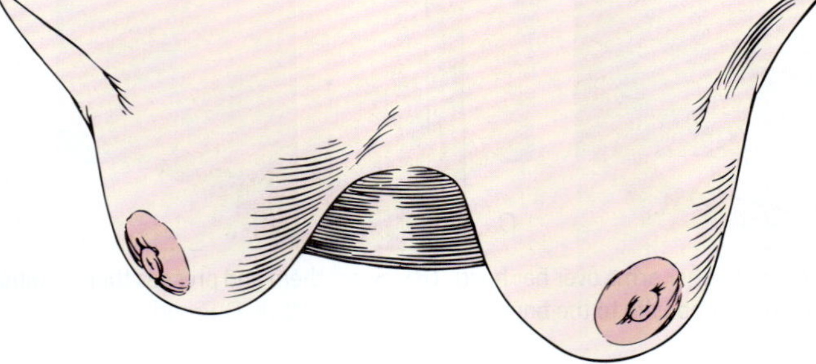 **FIGURE 21-14** Retracted breast tissue.	Smooth, firm, elastic tissue.  **OLDER ADULT CONSIDERATIONS** **The older patient's breasts may feel more granular and the inframammary ridge may be more easily palpated as it thickens.** A generalised increase in nodularity and tenderness may be a normal finding associated with the menstrual cycle or hormonal medications. Breasts should be a normal body temperature. No masses should be palpated. However, a firm inframammary transverse ridge may normally be palpated at the lower base of the breasts.	Thickening of the tissues may occur with an underlying malignant tumour. (See Abnormal findings 21-1.) Painful breasts may be indicative of benign breast disease but can also occur with a malignant tumour. The patient should be referred for further evaluation. Heat in the breasts of women who have not just given birth or who are not lactating indicates inflammation. Malignant tumours are most often found in the upper outer quadrant of the breast. They are usually unilateral with irregular, poorly delineated borders. They are hard and non-tender and fixed to underlying tissues. Fibroadenomas are usually 1- to 5-cm, round or oval, mobile, firm, solid, elastic, non-tender, single or multiple benign masses found in one or both breasts. Benign breast disease consists of bilateral, multiple, firm, regular, rubbery, mobile nodules with well-demarcated borders. Pain and fullness occurs just before menses.

Continued on page 390

ASSESSMENT TOOL 21-1 Guidelines for palpating the breasts

1. Ask the patient to lie down and to place overhead the arm on the same side as the breast being palpated. Place a small pillow or rolled towel under the breast being palpated.
2. Use the flat pads of three fingers to palpate the patient's breasts (A).

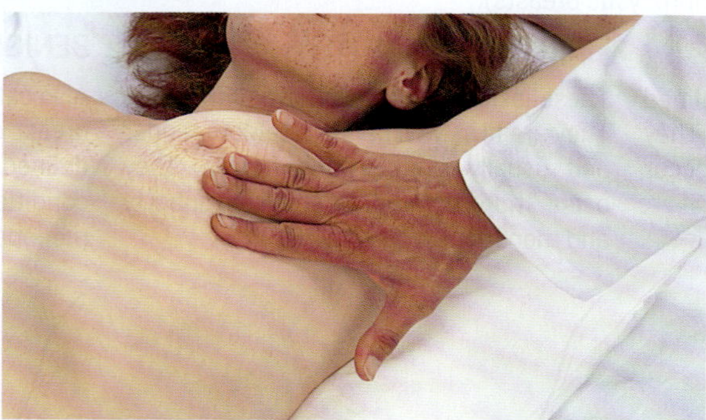

A

(© B. Proud.)

3. Palpate the breasts using one of three different patterns (B, C, and D). Choose one that is most comfortable for you, but be consistent and thorough with the method chosen.
4. Be sure to palpate every square centimetre of the breast, from the nipple and areola to the periphery of the breast tissue and up into the tail of Spence. Vary the levels of pressure as you palpate.
   Light—superficial
   Medium—mid-level tissue
   Firm—to the ribs

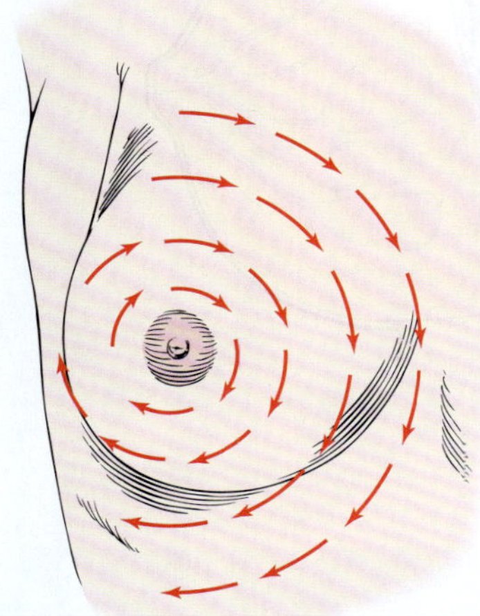

B Circular or clockwise.

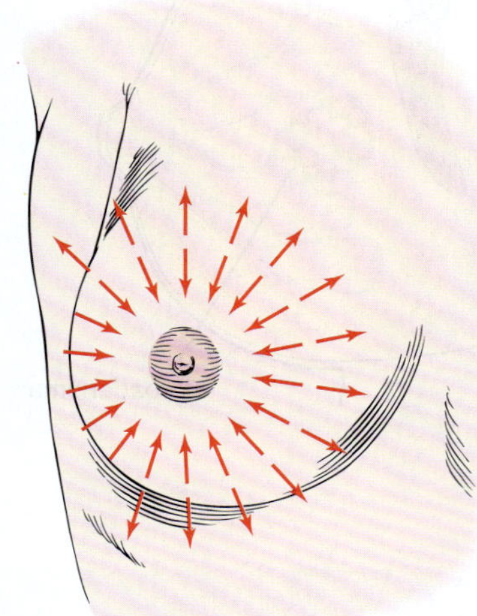

C Wedged.

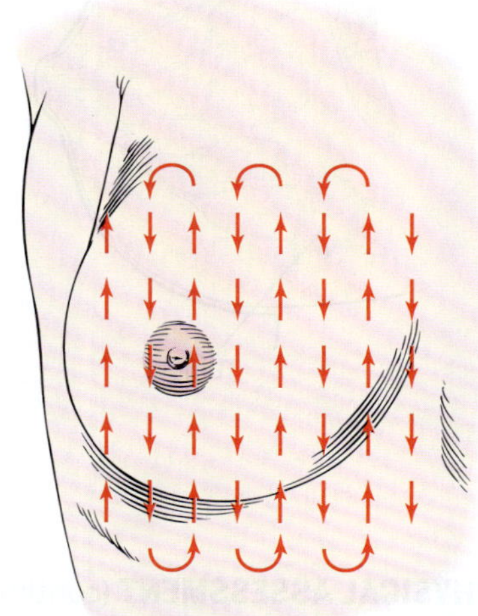

D Vertical strip.

5. Use the bimanual technique (E) if the patient has large breasts. Support the breast with your non-dominant hand and use your dominant hand to palpate.

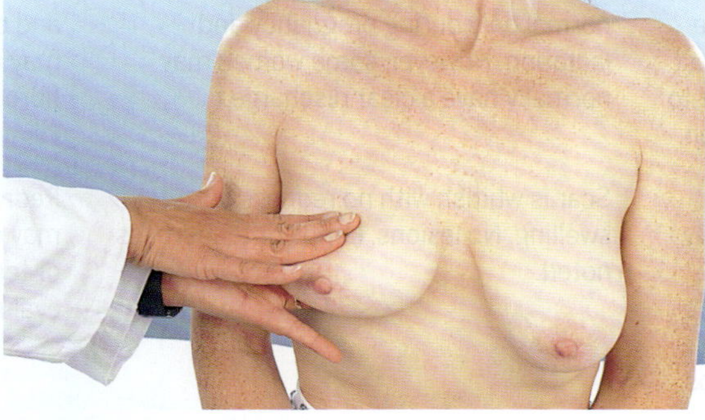

E Bimanual palpation.

(© B. Proud.)

ABNORMAL FINDINGS 21-1 Abnormalities noted on palpation of the breasts

Whereas some abnormalities of the breast are readily apparent, such as *peau d'orange* and Paget disease, some breast internal changes are detected only by palpation and mammography. The following illustrations represent breast abnormalities characteristic of tumours, fibroadenomas and benign disease (fibrocystic breasts).

CANCEROUS TUMOURS

These are irregular, firm, hard, not defined masses that may be fixed or mobile. They are not usually tender and usually occur after age 50.

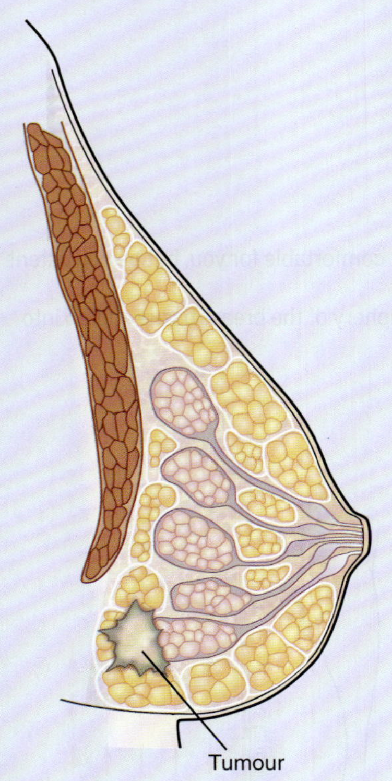

FIBROADENOMAS

These lesions are lobular, ovoid or round. They are firm, well defined, seldom tender and usually singular and mobile. They occur more commonly between puberty and menopause.

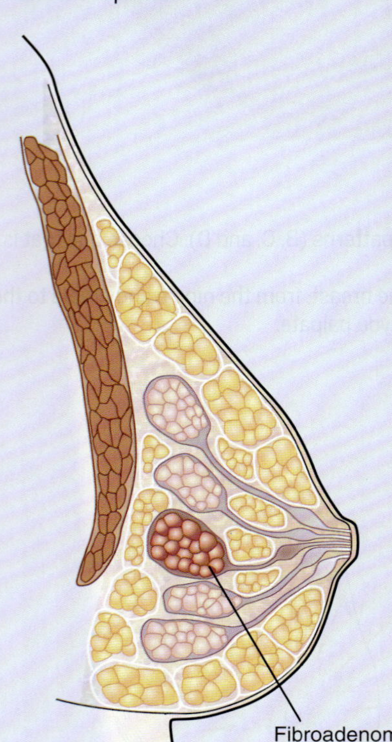

BENIGN BREAST DISEASE

Also called fibrocystic breast disease, benign breast disease is marked by round, elastic, defined, tender and mobile cysts. The condition is most common from age 30 to menopause, after which it decreases.

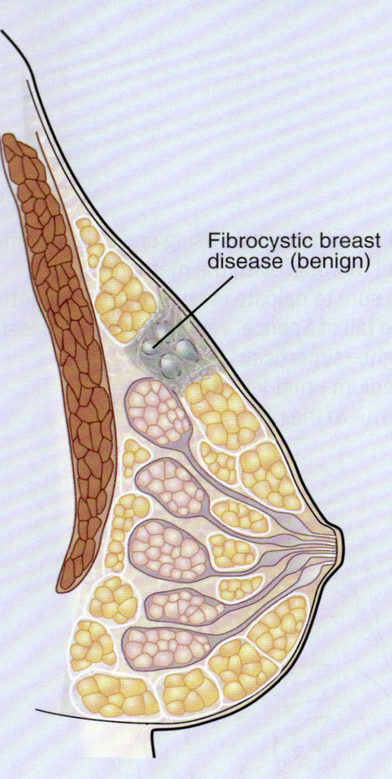

PHYSICAL ASSESSMENT (continued)

ASSESSMENT PROCEDURE	NORMAL FINDINGS	ABNORMAL FINDINGS
Palpate the nipples. Wear gloves to compress the nipple gently with your thumb and index finger (Fig. 21-15). Note any discharge. If spontaneous discharge occurs from the nipples, a specimen must be applied to a slide and the smear sent to the laboratory for cystological evaluation.	The nipple may become erect and the areola may pucker in response to stimulation. A milky discharge is usually normal only during pregnancy and lactation. However, some women may normally have a clear discharge.	Discharge may be seen in endocrine disorders and with certain medications (i.e. antihypertensives, tricyclic antidepressants and oestrogen). Discharge from one breast may indicate benign intraductal papilloma, fibrocystic disease or cancer of the breast.
Palpate mastectomy or lumpectomy site. If the patient has had a mastectomy or lumpectomy, it is still important to perform a thorough examination. Palpate the scar and any remaining breast or axillary tissue for redness, lesions, lumps, swelling or tenderness (Fig. 21-16).	Scar is whitish with no redness or swelling. No lesions, lumps or tenderness noted.	Redness and inflammation of the scar area may indicate infection. Any lesions, lumps or tenderness should be referred for further evaluation.

PHYSICAL ASSESSMENT (continued)

ASSESSMENT PROCEDURE	NORMAL FINDINGS	ABNORMAL FINDINGS
Female breasts (continued)		

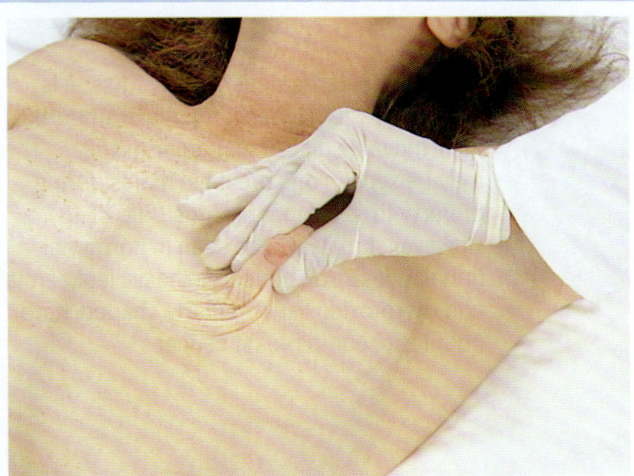

FIGURE 21-15 Palpating nipples for masses and discharge. (© B. Proud.)

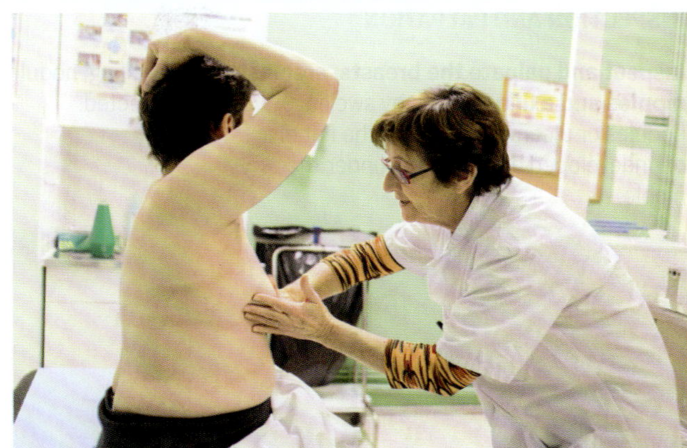

FIGURE 21-16 Palpating surgical site (Science Photo Library/Burger/Phanie.)

ASSESSMENT PROCEDURE	NORMAL FINDINGS	ABNORMAL FINDINGS
The axillae		
INSPECTION AND PALPATION		
Inspect and palpate the axillae. Ask the patient to sit up. Inspect the axillary skin for rashes or infection.	No rash or infection noted.	Redness and inflammation may be seen with infection of the sweat gland. Dark, velvety pigmentation of the axillae (acanthosis nigricans) may indicate an underlying malignancy.
Hold the patient's elbow with one hand and use the three fingerpads of your other hand to palpate firmly the axillary lymph nodes (Fig. 21-17).	No palpable nodes or one to two small (less than 1 cm), discrete, non-tender, movable nodes in the central area.	Enlarged (greater than 1 cm) lymph nodes may indicate infection of the hand or arm. Large nodes that are hard and fixed to the skin may indicate an underlying malignancy.
First palpate high into the axillae, moving downwards against the ribs to feel for the central nodes. Continue to move down the posterior axillae to feel for the posterior nodes. Use bimanual palpation to feel for the anterior axillary nodes. Finally palpate down the inner aspect of the upper arm. Ask the patient to demonstrate how she performs breast self-examination (BSE) if she chooses to receive feedback on her technique and method. This should be offered as an option and the patient's choice accepted. This time offers the nurse an opportunity to teach BSE. Give patients printed information (see Self-assessment 21-1).	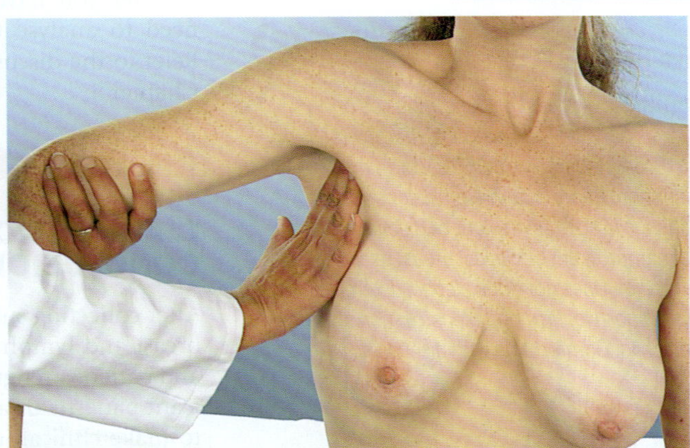 **FIGURE 21-17** Palpating the axillary lymph nodes. (© B. Proud.)	

Continued on following page

PHYSICAL ASSESSMENT (continued)

ASSESSMENT PROCEDURE	NORMAL FINDINGS	ABNORMAL FINDINGS
The male breasts		
INSPECTION AND PALPATION		
Inspect and palpate the breasts, areolas, nipples and axillae. Note any swelling, nodules or ulceration. Palpate the flat disc of undeveloped breast tissue under the nipple. 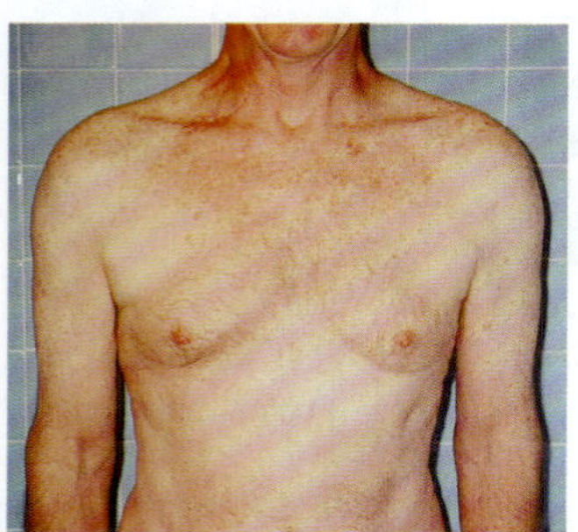 **FIGURE 21-18** Gynaecomastia.	No swelling, nodules or ulceration should be detected.	Soft, fatty enlargement of breast tissue is seen in obesity. Gynaecomastia, a smooth, firm, movable disc of glandular tissue, may be seen in one breast in males during puberty for a temporary time (Fig. 21-18). However, it may also be seen in hormonal imbalances, drug abuse, cirrhosis, leukaemia and thyrotoxicosis. Irregularly shaped, hard nodules occur in breast cancer.

VALIDATING AND DOCUMENTING FINDINGS

Validate the breast and lymph node assessment data you have collected. This is necessary to verify that the data are reliable and accurate. Document the assessment data following the health care facility or agency policy.

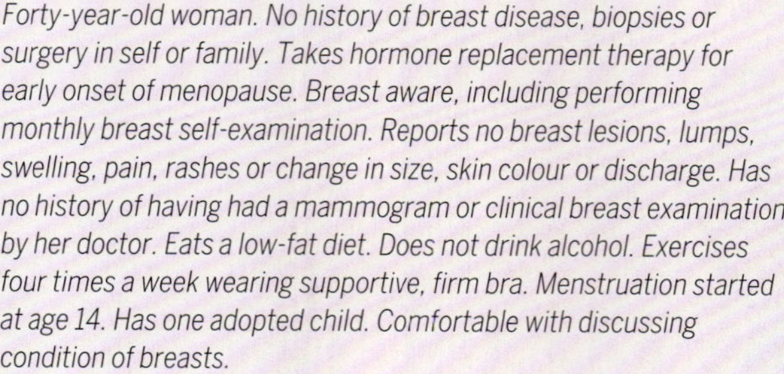

Sample of subjective data

Forty-year-old woman. No history of breast disease, biopsies or surgery in self or family. Takes hormone replacement therapy for early onset of menopause. Breast aware, including performing monthly breast self-examination. Reports no breast lesions, lumps, swelling, pain, rashes or change in size, skin colour or discharge. Has no history of having had a mammogram or clinical breast examination by her doctor. Eats a low-fat diet. Does not drink alcohol. Exercises four times a week wearing supportive, firm bra. Menstruation started at age 14. Has one adopted child. Comfortable with discussing condition of breasts.

Sample of objective data

Inspection

Bilateral breasts moderate in size, pendulous and symmetrical. Breast skin pale pink, with light-brown areola. Montgomery tubercles present. Nipples everted bilaterally. Free movement of breasts with position changes of arms and hands. No dimpling, retraction, lesions or inflammation noted. Axillae free of rashes or inflammation.

Palpation

No masses or tenderness palpated. Bilateral mammary ridge present. No discharge from nipples. Axillary (central, anterior or posterior) and lateral arm lymph nodes non-palpable. Demonstrates appropriate technique for breast self-examination.

After you have collected your assessment data, you will need to analyse the data using diagnostic reasoning skills. Refer to the discussion of the diagnostic reasoning process in Chapter 5.

Analysis of data

DIAGNOSTIC REASONING: POSSIBLE CONCLUSIONS

After collecting subjective and objective data pertaining to the breast and lymphatic assessment, identify abnormal findings and patient strengths. Then cluster the data to reveal any significant patterns or abnormalities. These data may then be used to make clinical judgements about the status of the patient's breasts and lymphatic health.

Potential patient risks

- Risk of ineffective management of therapeutic regimen (related to busy lifestyle and lack of knowledge of monthly breast awareness)

Potential patient problems

- Fear of breast cancer (related to increased risk factors)
- Ineffective individual coping (related to diagnoses of breast cancer)

- Disturbed body image (related to mastectomy)
- Anticipatory grieving (related to anticipation of poor outcome of breast biopsy)
- Ineffective management of therapeutic regimen (related to lack of knowledge about breast awareness)

Selected collaborative problems

After grouping the data, certain collaborative problems may become apparent. Remember that collaborative problems cannot be prevented or treated by nursing interventions alone. However, these physiological complications of medical conditions can be detected and monitored by the nurse. In addition, the nurse can use doctor- and nurse-prescribed interventions to minimise the complications of these problems. The nurse may also have to refer the patient in such situations for further treatment of the problem. The following is a list of collaborative problems that may be identified when obtaining a general impression:

- Infection (abscess)
- Haematoma
- Benign breast disease.

Medical problems

If, after grouping the data, it becomes apparent that the patient has signs and symptoms that may require medical diagnosis and treatment, referral to a primary care provider is necessary.

CASE STUDY

The case study demonstrates how to analyse breast and lymphatic assessment data for a specific patient. The critical thinking exercises included in the ancillary product on thePoint that complements this text also offer opportunities to analyse assessment data.

Nicole Barnes is a 42-year-old Aboriginal woman who is 2 days postoperative following an elective vaginal hysterectomy for the management of severe long-term endometriosis. She tells you this procedure has made her think about her health and that she is now concerned with lumps and tenderness that occur in her breasts each month, just a few days before her menstrual period. In response to questioning, she states she is a very 'heavy coffee drinker', is currently on Depo-Provera and is under a great deal of stress in her job and at home. When asked on her breast awareness, she is able to describe the normal look and feel of her breasts. When you question her about family history, she reports that her maternal aunt died of breast cancer. She wants to know if the lumps could be cancerous or what can be done to eliminate the breast problem. You suspect that she has fibrocystic changes characteristic of benign breast disease. On inspection of her breasts you notice that the breasts are bilaterally equal in size, with everted nipples. No dimpling, retraction or discharge is noted. You decide to inform the doctor of Nicole's concerns.

The following concept map illustrates the diagnostic reasoning process.

Applying COLDSPA

Applying COLDSPA for patient symptoms: 'lumps and tenderness in breasts each month'.

Mnemonic	Question	Data provided	Missing data
Character	Describe the sign or symptom (feeling, appearance, sound, smell or taste, if applicable).	'Lumps and tenderness in breasts.'	
Onset	When did it begin?	'Each month before menstrual period.'	
Location	Where is it? Does it radiate? Does it occur anywhere else?		Where are the lumps and tenderness? In both breasts or one breast? In one specific area or all over the breasts?
Duration	How long does it last? Does it recur?		How long do the tenderness and lumps last after they appear? Do they come and go or are they persistent?
Severity	How bad is it? or How much does it bother you?	'Can this be cancerous? What can I do to make this go away?'	
Pattern	What makes it better or worse?	Patient drinks a lot of coffee and has a lot of family- and work-related stress.	
Associated factors/How it **A**ffects the patient	What other symptoms occur with it? How does it affect you?	Patient's maternal aunt died of breast cancer.	

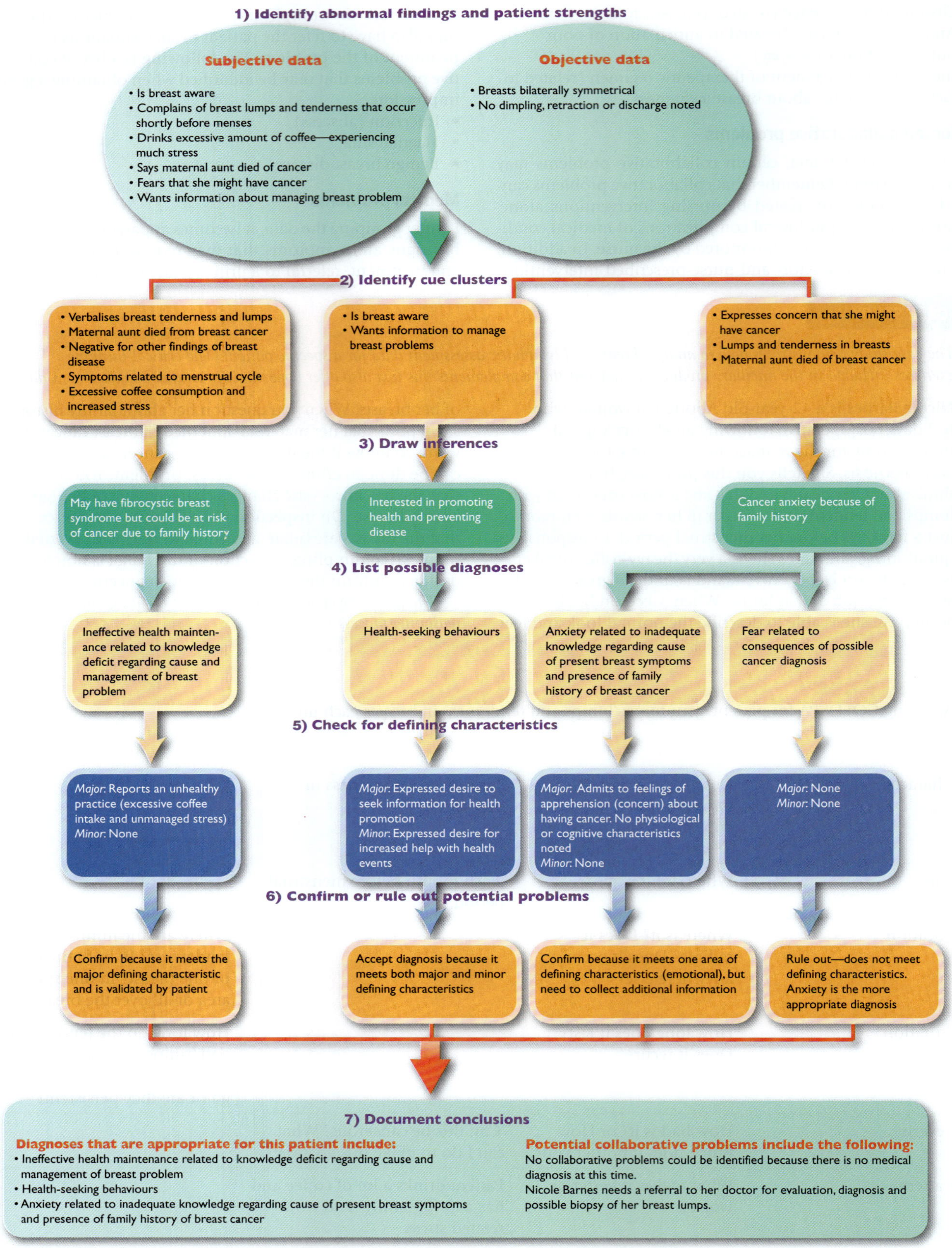

1) Identify abnormal findings and patient strengths

Subjective data

- Is breast aware
- Complains of breast lumps and tenderness that occur shortly before menses
- Drinks excessive amount of coffee—experiencing much stress
- Says maternal aunt died of cancer
- Fears that she might have cancer
- Wants information about managing breast problem

Objective data

- Breasts bilaterally symmetrical
- No dimpling, retraction or discharge noted

2) Identify cue clusters

- Verbalises breast tenderness and lumps
- Maternal aunt died from breast cancer
- Negative for other findings of breast disease
- Symptoms related to menstrual cycle
- Excessive coffee consumption and increased stress

- Is breast aware
- Wants information to manage breast problems

- Expresses concern that she might have cancer
- Lumps and tenderness in breasts
- Maternal aunt died of breast cancer

3) Draw inferences

May have fibrocystic breast syndrome but could be at risk of cancer due to family history

Interested in promoting health and preventing disease

Cancer anxiety because of family history

4) List possible diagnoses

Ineffective health maintenance related to knowledge deficit regarding cause and management of breast problem

Health-seeking behaviours

Anxiety related to inadequate knowledge regarding cause of present breast symptoms and presence of family history of breast cancer

Fear related to consequences of possible cancer diagnosis

5) Check for defining characteristics

Major: Reports an unhealthy practice (excessive coffee intake and unmanaged stress)
Minor: None

Major: Expressed desire to seek information for health promotion
Minor: Expressed desire for increased help with health events

Major: Admits to feelings of apprehension (concern) about having cancer. No physiological or cognitive characteristics noted
Minor: None

Major: None
Minor: None

6) Confirm or rule out potential problems

Confirm because it meets the major defining characteristic and is validated by patient

Accept diagnosis because it meets both major and minor defining characteristics

Confirm because it meets one area of defining characteristics (emotional), but need to collect additional information

Rule out—does not meet defining characteristics. Anxiety is the more appropriate diagnosis

7) Document conclusions

Diagnoses that are appropriate for this patient include:

- Ineffective health maintenance related to knowledge deficit regarding cause and management of breast problem
- Health-seeking behaviours
- Anxiety related to inadequate knowledge regarding cause of present breast symptoms and presence of family history of breast cancer

Potential collaborative problems include the following:

No collaborative problems could be identified because there is no medical diagnosis at this time.

Nicole Barnes needs a referral to her doctor for evaluation, diagnosis and possible biopsy of her breast lumps.

ONLINE RESOURCES

An extensive range of additional resources to enhance teaching and learning and to facilitate understanding may be found online at the text's accompanying website, located on thePoint at http://thepoint.lww.com. These include Watch and Learn videos, Concepts in Action animations, journal articles, case studies, discussion topics and quizzes.

Subscribers may also access Lippincott Procedures, an extensive online point-of-care procedure guide that provides reliable step-by-step instructions for more than 1700 procedures, including 450 evidence-based Australian procedures, and skills in a variety of speciality settings, together with a wealth of supporting information.

References

American Cancer Society (ACS). (2014). Breast cancer. Available at www.cancer.org/cancer/breastcancer/detailedguide/index.

Australian Institute of Health and Welfare (AIHW). (2017). Breast cancer in Australia: An overview. Available at https://www.aihw.gov.au/reports/cancer/breast-cancer-in-australia-an-overview/contents/table-of-contents.

BreastScreen Aotearoa. (2018). BreastScreen Aotearoa. Available at https://www.timetoscreen.nz/breast-screening/.

BreastScreen Australia. (2015). BreastScreen Australia Program. Available at http://www.cancerscreening.gov.au/internet/screening/publishing.nsf/Content/about-breast-screening.

BreastScreen Australia. (2020). About breast cancer. Available at http://www.cancerscreening.gov.au/internet/screening/publishing.nsf/Content/about-breast-cancer.

Cancer Australia. 2019. Breast cancer: The risk factors. Available at https://breastcancerriskfactors.gov.au/.

Kosters, J. P. & Gotzsche, P. C. (2008). Regular self-examination or clinical examination for early detection of breast cancer (Review). *The Cochrane Database of Systematic Reviews*, (3), doi:10.1002/14651858.CD003373.

Lawrenson, R., Seneviratne, S., Scott, N., et al. (2016). Breast cancer inequities between Māori and non-Māori women in Aotearoa/New Zealand. *European Journal of Cancer Care, 25*(2), 225–230.

Logan-Young, W. & Hoffman, N. Y. (1994). *Breast cancer: A practical guide to diagnosis*. Rochester, NY: Mt Hope Publishing.

New Zealand Breast Cancer Foundation (NZBCF). (2018). Early detection and screening. Available at www.nzbcf.org.nz/index.php/about-breast-cancer/early-detection-a-screening.

New Zealand Breast Cancer Foundation (NZBCF). (2018). What we do. Available at www.nzbcf.org.nz/what-we-do/breast-cancer-patient-registers.

New Zealand Ministry of Health. (2018). Breast cancer. Available at https://www.health.govt.nz/your-health/conditions-and-treatments/diseases-and-illnesses/breast-cancer.

Rummel, S., Hueman, M. T., Costantino, N., Shriver, C. D. & Ellsworth, R. E. (2015). Tumour location within the breast: Does tumour site have prognostic ability? *Ecancermedicalscience, 9*, 552. doi:10.3332/ecancer.2015.552Rummell.

Tapia, K., Garvey, G., Mc Entee, M., Rickard, M. & Brennan, P. (2017). Breast cancer in Australian indigenous women: Incidence, mortality, and risk factors. *Asian Pacific Journal of Cancer Prevention, 18*(4), 873–884.

World Cancer Research Fund International. (2018). Diet, nutrition, physical activity and breast cancer. Available at https://www.wcrf.org/sites/default/files/Breast-cancer-report.pdf.

Selected readings

Farrell, M. & Dempsey, J. (Eds). (2014). *Smeltzer & Bare's textbook of medical-surgical nursing* (3rd Australian & New Zealand ed.). Sydney: Lippincott Williams & Wilkins.

Haley, C. & Pillitteri, A. (2016). *Pillitteri's child and family health nursing in Australia and New Zealand* (2nd ed.). Philadelphia: Wolters Kluwer.

Promoting health websites—Breast cancer

Australian Indigenous *HealthInfoNet*, breast cancer: www.healthinfonet.ecu.edu.au/population-groups/women/publications/specific-topics/cancer/breast

Breast Cancer Network Australia: www.bcna.org.au

Breast Health Global Initiative: http://bhgi.org

BreastScreen Aotearoa: https://www.breastcancer.org.nz/aboutBC/detection/screening-tests/BSA

BreastScreenAustraliaProgram: https://www.health.gov.au/internet/screening/publishing.nsf/Content/breast-screening-1

Cancer Australia, breast cancer: http://canceraustralia.gov.au/affected-cancer/cancer-types/breast-cancer

Clinical Guidelines Network: www.cancer.org.au/health-professionals/clinical-guidelines-network

McGrath Foundation: www.mcgrathfoundation.com.au

Midwifery Council of New Zealand/Te Tatau o te Whare Kahu: www.midwiferycouncil.health.nz

National Breast Cancer Foundation, Australia: www.nbcf.org.au

New Zealand Breast Cancer Foundation (NZBCF): www.nzbcf.org.nz

Nursing and Midwifery Board of Australia (NMBA): www.nursingmidwiferyboard.gov.au

WebMD: www.webmd.com/breast-cancer

World Cancer Research Fund International: www.wcrf.org

CHAPTER 22

Heart and neck vessels

CASE STUDY

Malcolm Winchester is being admitted to the coronary care unit with a diagnosis of hypertension and angina. He is a tall, slender Caucasian man who looks younger than his stated age of 45. He appears to be in no acute distress. Mr Winchester says, 'I don't know why they brought me here—I guess my wife panicked and called 000. I have these pains all the time, but my doctor says they're from my high blood pressure. I'm not in any pain now.'

Mr Winchester's wife arrives, looking pale and anxious. 'I don't know what to do with him. I work so hard to keep him healthy, but he goes out to that fast-food place and eats hamburgers and chips. I'm so tired of dealing with him when he won't help himself.' Mr Winchester grins and says, 'That low-fat, low-salt diet my doctor put me on is impossible. There's nothing wrong with a little bit of indulgence every now and again.'

Structure and function

The cardiovascular system is a highly complex system that includes the heart and a closed system of blood vessels. To collect accurate data and correctly interpret those data, the examiner must have an understanding of the structure and function of the heart, the great vessels, the electrical conduction system of the heart, the cardiac cycle, the production of heart sounds, cardiac output and the neck vessels. This information helps the examiner to differentiate between normal and abnormal findings as they relate to the cardiovascular system.

HEART AND GREAT VESSELS

The heart is a hollow, muscular, four-chambered organ (left and right atria, and left and right ventricles) located in the middle of the thoracic cavity between the lungs in the space called the *mediastinum.* It is about the size of a clenched fist and weighs approximately 255 g in women and 310 g in men (this is a general weight based upon the average size of an individual; because women are generally smaller than men, their hearts frequently weigh less).

The heart extends vertically from the left second to the left fifth intercostal space and horizontally from the right edge of the sternum to the left midclavicular line. When anatomically identified, the top and bottom of the heart are the reverse of what you might think. The upper portion, near the left second intercostal space, is recognised anatomically as the *base,* whereas the lower portion, near the left fifth intercostal space and the left midclavicular line, is recognised as the *apex.* The anterior chest area that overlies the heart and great vessels is called the *praecordium* (Fig. 22-1). The right side of the heart pumps blood to the lungs for gas exchange (pulmonary circulation); the left side of the heart pumps blood to all other parts of the body (systemic circulation).

The large veins and arteries leading directly to and away from the heart are referred to as the great vessels. The superior and inferior vena cava return blood to the right atrium from the upper and lower torso, respectively. The pulmonary artery exits the right ventricle, bifurcates and carries blood to the lungs. The pulmonary veins (two from each lung) return oxygenated blood to the left atrium. The aorta transports oxygenated blood from the left ventricle to the body (Fig. 22-2).

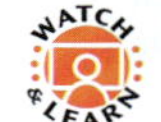

Anatomy review: Vascular structures of the neck
Anatomy review: Heart

Heart chambers and valves

The heart consists of four chambers: two upper chambers, the right and left atria, and two lower chambers, the right and left ventricles. The right and left sides of the heart are separated by a partition called the septum. The thin-walled atria receive

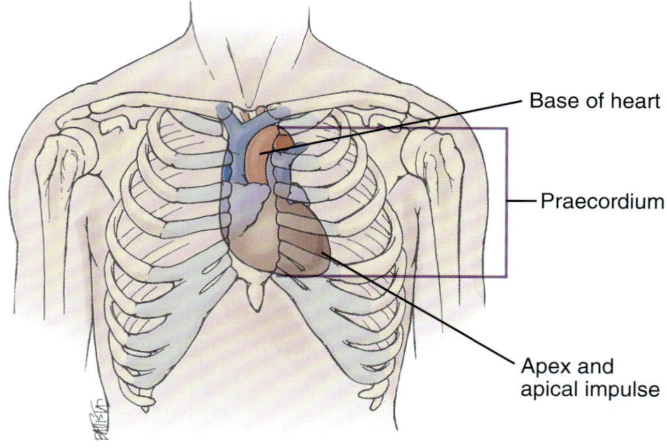

FIGURE 22-1 The heart and major blood vessels lie centrally in the chest behind the protective sternum.

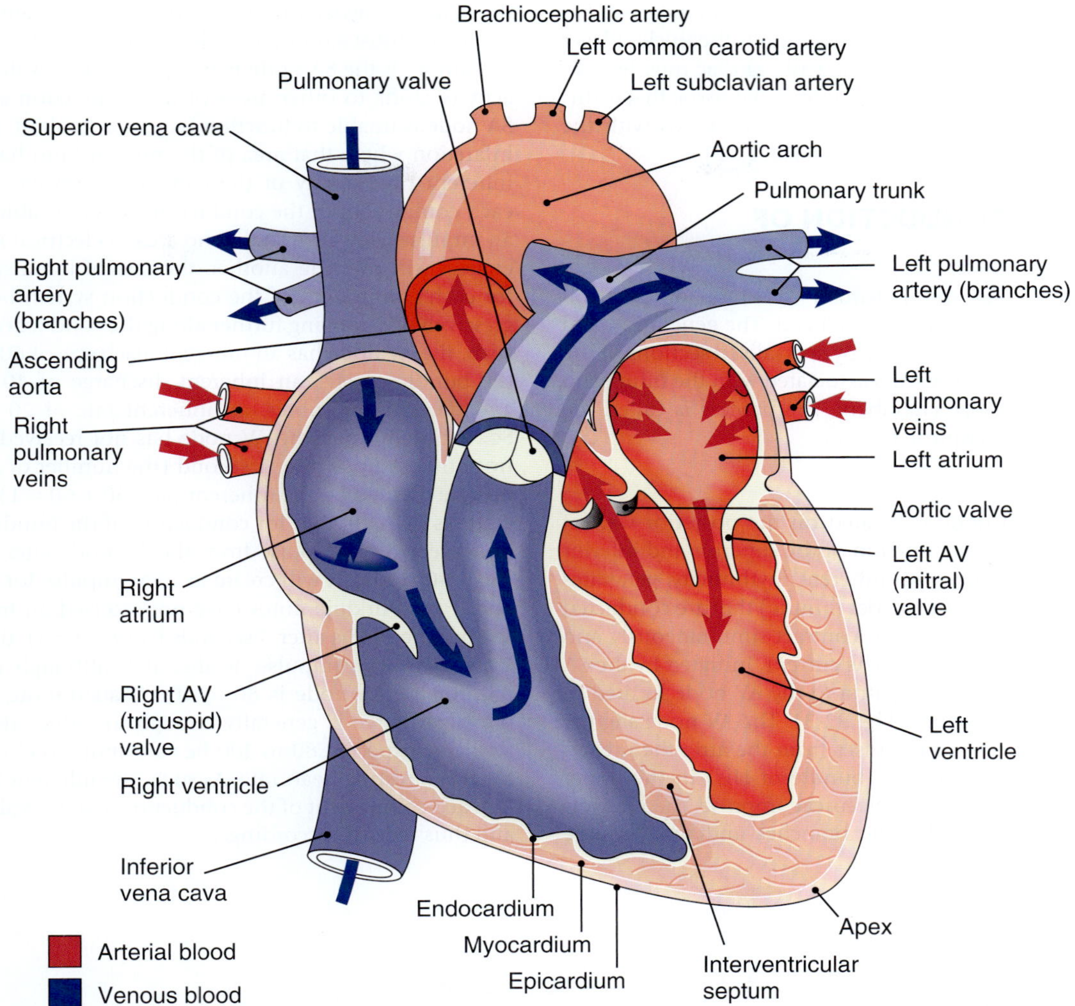

FIGURE 22-2 Heart chambers, valves and direction of circulatory flow. (Cohen, B. J. & Hull, K. L. (2015). *Memmler's structure and function of the human body* [11th ed.]. Philadelphia: Lippincott Williams & Wilkins.)

blood returning to the heart and pump blood into the ventricles. The thicker-walled ventricles pump blood out of the heart. The left ventricle is thicker and larger than the right ventricle because the left side of the heart's workload is greater.

The entrance and exit of each ventricle are protected by one-way valves that direct the flow of blood through the heart, ensuring it always moves forwards. The atrioventricular (AV) valves are located at the entrance into the ventricles. There are two AV valves: the tricuspid valve and the mitral (bicuspid) valve. The tricuspid valve is composed of three cusps or flaps and is located between the right atrium and the right ventricle; the mitral (bicuspid) valve is composed of two cusps or flaps and is located between the left atrium and the left ventricle. Collagen fibres, called chordae tendineae, anchor the AV valve flaps to papillary muscles within the ventricles.

Open AV valves allow blood to flow from the atria into the ventricles. However, as the pressure in the ventricles becomes greater than the pressure in the atria and the blood tries to move backwards, the AV valves close. This is particularly apparent as the ventricles begin to contract—the AV valves snap shut, preventing the regurgitation of blood into the atria. The valves are prevented from blowing open in the reverse direction (i.e. towards the atria) by their secure anchors to the papillary muscles of the ventricular wall. The semilunar valves (aortic and pulmonary valves) are located at the exit of each ventricle at the beginning of the great vessels. Each valve has three cusps or flaps that look like half-moons, hence the name 'semilunar'. There are two semilunar valves: the pulmonic valve is located at the entrance of the pulmonary artery as it exits the right ventricle, and the aortic valve is located at the beginning of the ascending aorta as it exits the left ventricle. These valves are open during ventricular contraction and close at the end of systole when the pressure in the arteries becomes greater than the pressure in the ventricles (i.e. blood will always try to move from an area of higher pressure to an area of lower pressure; valves stop the backward movement of blood as heart pressures change consequent to chamber contraction and ejection) (see Fig. 22-2).

Heart covering and walls

The pericardium is a tough, inextensible, loose-fitting, fibroserous sac that attaches to the great vessels and, thereby, surrounds the heart. A serous membrane lining, the parietal pericardium, secretes a small amount of pericardial fluid that allows for smooth, friction-free movement of the heart. This same type of serous membrane covers the outer surface of the heart and is known as the epicardium. The myocardium is the thickest layer of the heart and is made up of contractile cardiac muscle cells. The endocardium is a thin layer of endothelial tissue that forms the innermost layer of the heart and is continuous with the endothelial lining of blood vessels (see Fig. 22-2).

ELECTRICAL CONDUCTION OF THE HEART

Cardiac muscle cells spontaneously generate an electrical impulse and conduct it through the heart. The generation and conduction of electrical impulses by specialised sections of the myocardium regulate the events associated with the filling and emptying of the cardiac chambers. The process is called the cardiac cycle (see description below).

Pathways

The sinoatrial (SA) node is located on the posterior wall of the right atrium near the junction of the superior and inferior vena cava. The SA node, with inherent rhythmicity, generates impulses (at a rate of 80 to 100 per minute) that are conducted over both atria, causing them to contract simultaneously and eject blood into the ventricles. The current, initiated by the SA node, is conducted across the atria to the AV node located in the lower interatrial septum (Fig. 22-3). The AV node slightly delays incoming electrical impulses from the atria then relays the impulse to the AV bundle (bundle of His) in the upper interventricular septum. The electrical impulse then travels down the right and left bundle branches and the Purkinje fibres in the myocardium of both ventricles, causing them to contract almost simultaneously.

Although the SA node is the 'pacemaker of the heart', this activity shifts to other areas of the conduction system if the SA node is unable to function (e.g. as a result of a myocardial infarction where that area of the myocardium has died). The inherent rhythmicity of the conduction system ensures that each component of the conduction system is able to generate an impulse. However, so that no area of electrical impulse generation will override another, the rate of impulse generation for each component of the conduction system becomes progressively less moving further along the conduction system. As such, the AV node has an inherent discharge of 60 per minute, the bundle of His, an inherent discharge of 40 per minute and the Purkinje fibres, an inherent rate of 20 per minute. So, for example, if the AV node has not received an impulse from the SA node after 1 second (the number of seconds in a minute divided by the inherent rate: $60 \div 60 = 1$), it will generate its own impulse for conduction; if the bundle of His has not received an impulse from the AV node after 1.5 seconds ($60 \div 40 = 1.5$), it will create its own impulse for conduction; and if the Purkinje fibres have not received an impulse from the bundle of His after 3 seconds ($60 \div 20 = 3$), they will generate their own impulse. Realise that although the inherent rate for the SA node is 80 to 100 beats/minute, the tone of the vagal nerve is generally enough to reduce the heart rate from the expected 80 to 100 beats/minute to closer to 60 for a normal resting heart rate. As such, the inherent impulse rate for each component of the conduction system is also inhibited and thus reduced accordingly.

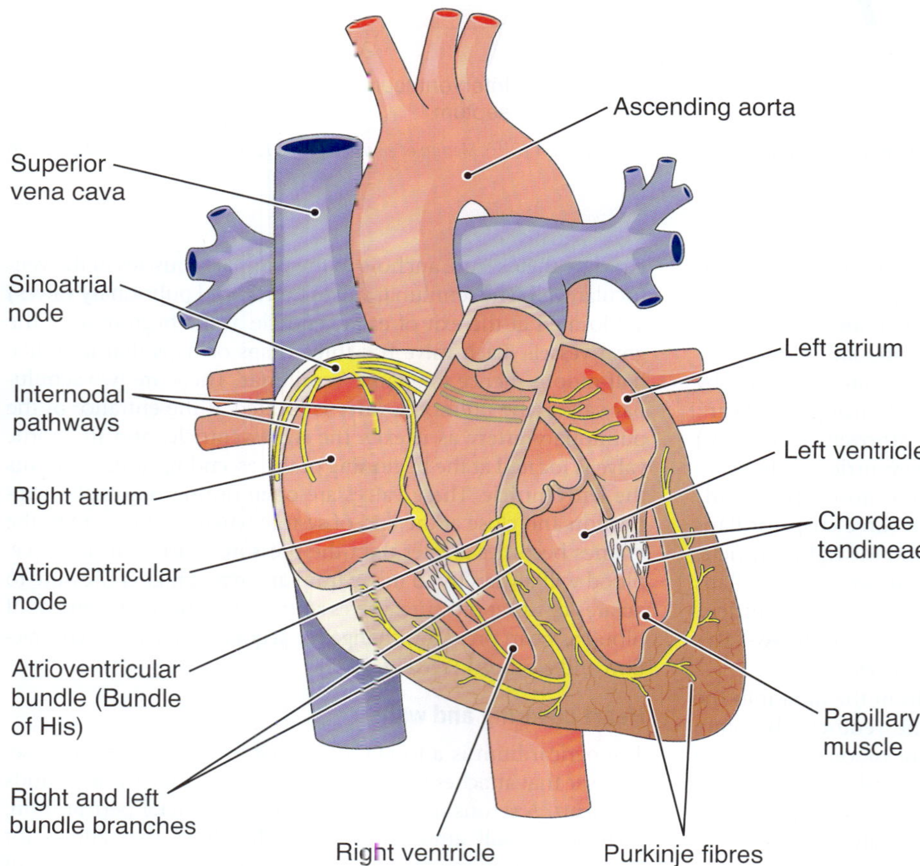

FIGURE 22-3 The electrical conduction system coordinates cardiac contraction. An initial impulse generated by the sinoatrial node follows the conduction pathways and is distributed throughout the heart. (Cohen, B. J. & Hull, K. L. (2015). *Memmler's structure and function of the human body* [11th ed.]. Philadelphia: Lippincott Williams & Wilkins.)

CLINICAL TIP

Each component of the cardiac conduction system has its own intrinsic rate. To ensure each does not override the other, these rates become progressively less when moving from the first point (the sinoatrial [SA] node) to the last point (the Purkinje fibres). When a patient has a low resting heart rate (less than 55 beats/minute), an assessment will sometimes reveal an occasional irregularity in the heart beat. If the atrioventricular (AV) node does not receive an impulse within the time frame of its intrinsic rate, it will generate its own impulse and this creates the irregular heart beat. This becomes more likely when the heart rate is reduced because the impulses the AV node is receiving from the SA node are fewer and further apart. Note that the parasympathetic action exerted on the heart through the vagal nerve, which reduces heart rate, is exerted globally across the heart. As such, all intrinsic rates within the cardiac conduction system are reduced and not every person with a low heart rate will exhibit an occasional irregularity.

Electrical activity

Electrical impulses, which are generated by the SA node and travel throughout the cardiac conduction circuit, can be detected on the surface of the skin. This electrical activity can be measured and recorded by electrocardiography (ECG), which records the depolarisation and repolarisation of the cardiac muscle. The phases of the ECG are known as P, Q, R, S and T. Display 22-1 describes the phases of the ECG.

THE CARDIAC CYCLE

The cardiac cycle refers to the filling and emptying of the heart's chambers. The cardiac cycle has two phases: diastole (relaxation of the ventricles, known as *filling*) and systole (contraction of the ventricles, known as *emptying*). Diastole endures for approximately two-thirds of the cardiac cycle and systole is the remaining one-third (Fig. 22-4).

CLINICAL TIP

When considering high blood pressure, a patient with a high diastolic pressure is of greater concern than a patient with a high systolic pressure. An increase in diastolic pressure will increase the mean vessel pressure twice as much as an increase in systolic pressure. Peak systolic pressure is achieved only for a very short period during cardiac ejection. Following this short-lived peak, vessel pressure is continually reducing until diastole is reached immediately prior to the following cardiac ejection. The average pressure in the arterial vessels is known as the mean arterial pressure (MAP). This is calculated by adding one systole with two diastoles and dividing by three (e.g. the MAP for a blood pressure of 120/80 mmHg would be 120 + [80 × 2] ÷ 3 = 93.3 mmHg).

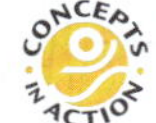

Cardiac: Cardiac cycle

Diastole

During ventricular diastole, the AV valves are open and the ventricles are relaxed. The pressure in the atria is higher than that of the ventricles as the ventricles have just ejected the majority of their volume and thus will start to passively fill from the atria. The early, rapid, passive filling of the ventricles is called early or protodiastolic filling. This is followed by a period of slow passive filling. Finally, near the end of ventricular diastole, the atria contract and complete the emptying of blood out of the upper chambers by propelling it into the ventricles. This final active filling phase is called presystole, atrial systole or sometimes the 'atrial kick'. This action raises left ventricular pressure.

CLINICAL TIP

If a patient's pulse is irregular, it is likely that the patient is in atrial fibrillation (AF), which means the atria are fibrillating or quivering and the atrial muscle is not contracting as a whole but rather as isolated parts. When a patient suffers from AF, the atria are unable to contract synchronously. Hence, the atria do

DISPLAY 22-1 PHASES OF THE ELECTROCARDIOGRAM

The phases of the electrocardiogram, which records depolarisation and repolarisation of the heart, are assigned letters: P, Q, R, S and T.

- **P wave:** Atrial depolarisation; conduction of the impulse throughout the atria.
- **PR interval:** Time from the beginning of the atrial depolarisation to the beginning of ventricular depolarisation, that is, from the beginning of the P wave to the beginning of the QRS complex.
- **QRS complex:** Ventricular depolarisation (also atrial repolarisation); conduction of the impulse throughout the ventricles, which then triggers contraction of the ventricles; measured from the beginning of the Q wave to the end of the S wave.
- **ST segment:** Period between ventricular depolarisation and the beginning of ventricular repolarisation.
- **T wave:** Ventricular repolarisation; the ventricles return to a resting state.
- **QT interval:** Total time for ventricular depolarisation and repolarisation, that is, from the beginning of the Q wave to the end of the T wave; the QT interval varies with heart rate.
- **U wave:** Rarely present; if it is present, it follows the T wave and represents the final phase of ventricular repolarisation.

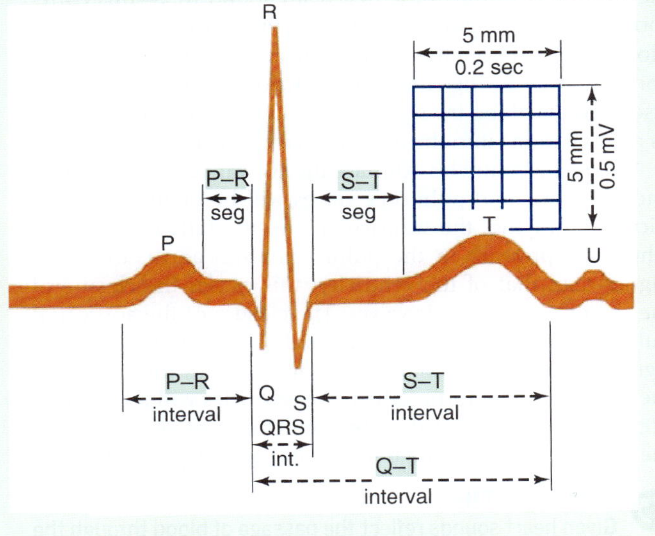

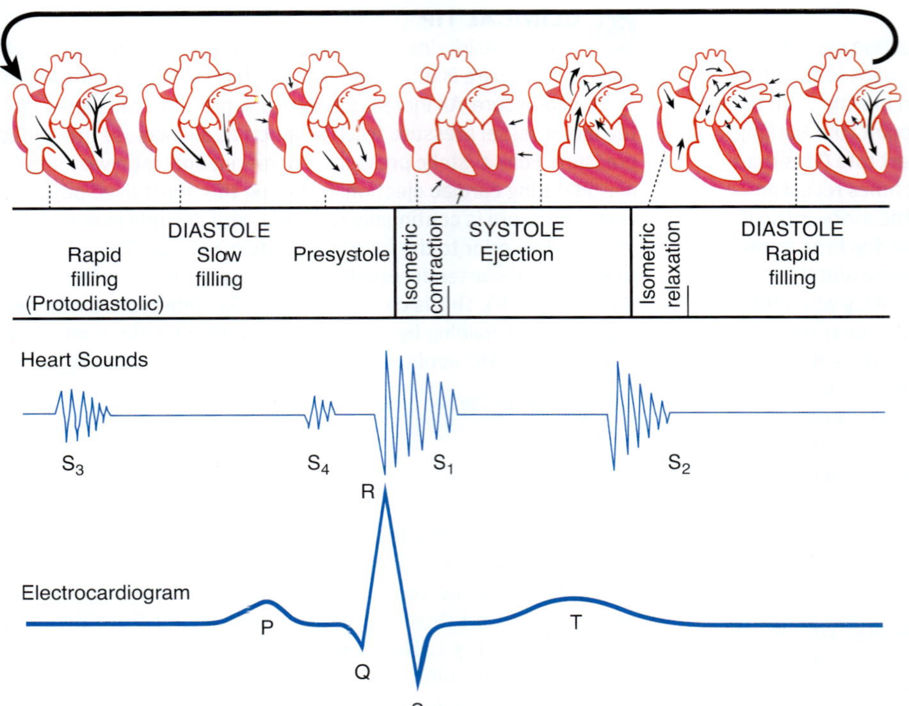

FIGURE 22-4 The cardiac cycle consists of filling and ejection. Heart sounds S_2, S_3 and S_4 are associated with diastole, whereas S_1 is associated with systole. Note S_1 and S_2 correspond to valvular closure, whereas S_3 and S_4 correspond to ventricular filling.

not eject as much blood to the ventricles as they normally would. Without this 'atrial kick', the ventricles fail to fill effectively and they in turn eject less blood when they contract. Owing to this decrease in cardiac output, a drop in blood pressure is sometimes seen.

Systole

The filling phases during diastole result in a large amount of blood in the ventricles, causing the pressure in the ventricles to become higher than the pressure in the atria. When the pressure in the ventricles becomes greater than the pressure in the atria, the AV valves (mitral and tricuspid) will shut. Closure of the AV valves produces the first heart sound (S_1)—this corresponds with the beginning of systole (the period of time where blood is ejected from the ventricles to enter the pulmonary and aortic arteries during cardiac contraction). This valve closure also prevents blood from flowing backwards (a process known as regurgitation) into the atria during ventricular contraction.

When the ventricles contract the AV valves will be closed and the aortic and pulmonic valves will be open. With ventricular emptying, the ventricular pressure falls to the point where the pressure in the pulmonary and aortic arteries is higher than that of the ventricles; this causes the closure of the pulmonic and aortic valves. The closure of the aortic and pulmonic valves produces the second heart sound (S_2), which signals the end of systole. Corresponding with the closure of the pulmonic and aortic valves, the ventricles will relax. Atrial pressure is now higher than the ventricular pressure, causing the AV valves to open and diastolic filling to begin again.

CLINICAL TIP

Given heart sounds reflect the passage of blood through the chambers in the heart and that heart sounds reflect the cessation of blood flow from one area to another, an understanding of the cardiac cycle helps you understand what is happening in the heart as you auscultate it.

CASE STUDY

Malcolm's physical assessment reveals a blood pressure of 210/110 mmHg right arm reclining and 200/108 mmHg left arm reclining; a pulse of 88 beats/minute, regular and strong; a respiratory rate of 16 breaths/minute, regular and moderately shallow; and a temperature of 36.5 °C. Malcolm's carotid pulse is 88 and strong; heart sounds S_1 and S_2 with no murmurs and clicks, but an S_4 is noted.

CRITICAL THINKING

1. Which of Malcolm's findings are abnormal?
2. Although it is likely considered that Malcolm's heart rate is within the normal range, would you expect a man as young as Malcolm to exhibit a heart rate of 88 beats/minute?
3. Does the heart rate affect blood pressure? Why or why not?
4. If S_1 reflects the closure of both AV valves, and S_2 reflects the closure of both ventricular valves, what might aberrations with these sounds identify?
5. An S_4 is an extra heart sound and does not reflect valvular closure. If heart sounds signify movement of blood within the heart, and an S_4 occurs immediately prior to S_1 (which notes closure of the AV valves), what might the S_4 signify?

HEART SOUNDS

Heart sounds are produced by the movement of blood in the heart. As blood normally flows silently through the heart, it is either the rapid cessation of blood movement or turbulent blood flow that is heard. Of these two sounds, the rapid cessation of blood flow is most easily auscultated. Given valvular closure causes the cessation of blood flow in the heart, the closure of the AV valves (S_1) and the closure of the ventricular valves (S_2) are the easiest heart sounds to auscultate. Occasionally, extra heart sounds and murmurs can be auscultated with a stethoscope over the praecordium (the area of the anterior chest overlying the heart and great vessels; see Spotlight technique 22-1). These sounds can be a result of problems with the cardiac valves (regurgitation or stenosis), or non-compliant or hypercompliant ventricles (where you can hear blood entering the ventricle). Extra heart sounds may also be heard as a result of the normal physiology of breathing and the pressure changes this causes within the thoracic cavity.

Normal heart sounds

Heart sounds may appear complicated, with clinicians referring to S_1, S_2, S_3, S_4 and murmurs. However, when recognised at a basic level, heart sounds can be easy to recognise. Normal heart sounds are often described as having a *lub-dub* sound. *Lub-dub* is the sound heard when placing a stethoscope on the patient's chest: *lub-dub*, pause, *lub-dub*, pause, *lub-dub*, pause.

Each *lub-dub* is reflective of one cardiac cycle. If we consider the flow of blood through the heart, it moves from the atria to the ventricle and then from the ventricle to the pulmonary and aortic arteries (great vessels). Given that it is the rapid cessation of blood flow that we can most easily auscultate, the first sound we hear (the *lub*) will coincide with the closure of the AV valves because once the majority of blood leaves the atria, the pressure in the ventricles becomes higher than that in the atria. As such, the blood will try to return to the atria and the AV valves will close, causing a rapid cessation in blood movement. The next occurrence is the contraction of the ventricles. Again, following substantial reduction in ventricular volume, pressure in the great vessels will be higher than that in the ventricles, causing blood to attempt to return; thus, closure of the ventricular valves occurs and the second heart sound can be heard (*dub*).

Heart sounds are described sequentially. Abbreviations are also used in their description. 'S' represents the word 'sound'. The heart sound sequence follows numerically, with the first sound represented as S_1, the second sound S_2, the third sound S_3 and the fourth sound S_4. Considering blood flow through the heart, the first sound in the sequence is the closure of the AV valves. Thus, the 'lub' sound is recognised as Sound 1 (S_1 or *lub*). Closure of the ventricular valves represents Sound 2 (S_2 or *dub*). S_3 and S_4 are classified as extra heart sounds because there are no further valves left to close in the passage of blood through the heart. S_3 and S_4 are discussed further under the heading 'Extra heart sounds'.

S_1 correlates with the beginning of systole (see Display 22-2 for more information about S_1 and variations of S_1). S_1 is usually heard as one sound but may be heard as two sounds. If heard as two sounds, the first component represents mitral valve closure, and the second component represents tricuspid closure. As both AV valves close almost simultaneously, the two sounds occur very close together and are frequently heard as a slightly longer S_1 sound rather than a 'split' S_1 sound. Mitral closure occurs first because of increased pressure on the left side of the heart and because of the route of myocardial depolarisation. Although S_1 may be heard over the entire praecordium, it is best heard where it originates at the apex of the heart (left midclavicular line, fifth intercostal space).

S_2 correlates with the beginning of diastole. As with S_1, S_2 is also usually heard as one sound but may be heard as two sounds. If S_2 is heard as two sounds, the first component represents aortic valve closure, and the second component represents pulmonic valve closure. Aortic valve closure occurs first because of increased pressure on the left side of the heart and because of the route of myocardial depolarisation. If S_2 is heard as two distinct sounds, it is called a split S_2. A splitting of S_2 may be exaggerated during inspiration and disappear during expiration (the increase in intrathoracic pressure during inspiration places greater pressure on the heart, causing the aortic valve to close slightly earlier than the pulmonic valve). S_2 is heard best at the base of the heart. See Display 22-3 for more information about variations of S_2.

Extra heart sounds

As heart sounds are described sequentially, S_3 and S_4 are heard after S_2. If heard, S_3 will occur immediately after S_2. S_4, however, if auscultated, occurs immediately prior to S_1. S_3 and S_4 are referred to as diastolic filling sounds or extra heart sounds, which result from ventricular vibration secondary to rapid ventricular filling. If present, S_3 can be heard early in diastole, immediately after S_2 (see Fig. 22-4). S_4 also results from ventricular vibration, but, contrary to S_3, the vibration is secondary to ventricular resistance (non-compliance) during atrial contraction (see Fig. 22-4). S_3 may be referred to as a ventricular gallop and S_4 as an atrial gallop.

Murmurs

Blood normally flows silently through the heart. There are conditions, however, that can create turbulent blood flow in which a swooshing or blowing sound may be auscultated over the praecordium. Conditions that contribute to turbulent blood flow include: (1) increased blood velocity; (2) structural valve defects; (3) valve malfunction; and (4) abnormal chamber openings (e.g. septal defect).

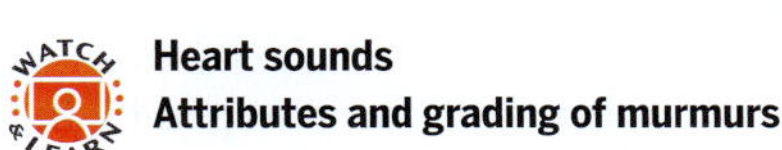

Heart sounds
Attributes and grading of murmurs

CLINICAL TIP

Heart sounds are numbered sequentially and can be used to identify movement of blood within the heart. When auscultating heart sounds, consider the movement of blood within the heart. The first occurrence is atrial contraction: atrial ejection of blood into the ventricles; final ventricular filling occurs (possible S4); atrial pressure becomes less than ventricular pressure; ventricular blood attempts to move from higher pressure to lower pressure and thus back into the atria, closing atrioventricular valves (S1). For ventricular contraction: ventricular ejection of blood into great vessels; ventricular pressure becomes less than great vessel pressure; blood in the great vessels attempts to move back into the ventricles, causing ventricular valve closure (S2); early ventricular filling from atria (possible S3).

DISPLAY 22-2 UNDERSTANDING NORMAL S_1 SOUNDS AND VARIATIONS

S_1, which is the first heart sound, is produced by atrioventricular closing. S_1 (the *lub* portion of *lub-dub*) correlates with the beginning of systole.

The intensity of S_1 depends on the position of the mitral valve at the start of systole, the structure of the valve leaflets and how quickly pressure rises in the ventricles. All of these factors influence the speed and amount of closure the valve experiences, which, in turn, determine the amount of sound produced.

CLINICAL TIP

Normal variations in S_1 are heard at the base and the apex of the heart. S_1 is softer at the base and louder at the apex of the heart. An S_1 may be split along the lower left sternal border, where the tricuspid component of the sound, usually too faint to be heard, can be auscultated. A split S_1 heard over the apex may be an S_4.

1st cardiac cycle | **Beginning of next cardiac cycle**

Accentuated S_1

An accentuated S_1 sound is louder than an S_2. This occurs when the mitral valve is wide open and closes quickly. Examples include:

- Hyperkinetic states in which blood velocity increases such as fever, anaemia and hyperthyroidism
- Mitral stenosis in which the leaflets are still mobile but increased ventricular pressure is needed to close the valve.

S_1 S_2 S_1

Diminished S_1

Sometimes the S_1 sound is softer than the S_2 sound. This occurs when the mitral valve is not fully open at the time of ventricular contraction and valve closing. Examples include:

- Delayed conduction from the atria to the ventricles as in first-degree heart block, which allows the mitral valve to drift closed before ventricular contraction closes it
- Mitral insufficiency, in which extreme calcification of the valve limits mobility
- Delayed or diminished ventricular contraction arising from forceful atrial contraction into a non-compliant ventricle, as in severe pulmonary or systemic hypertension.

S_1 S_2 S_1

Split S_1

As named, a split S_1 occurs as a split sound. This occurs when the left and right ventricles contract at different times (asynchronous ventricular contraction). Examples include:

- Conduction delaying the cardiac impulse to one of the ventricles, as in bundle branch block
- Ventricular ectopy in which the impulse starts in one ventricle, contracting it first, and then spreading to the second ventricle.

S_1 S_2 S_1

Varying S_1

A varying S_1 sound occurs when the mitral valve is in different positions when contraction occurs. Examples include:

- Rhythms in which the atria and ventricles are beating independently of each other
- Totally irregular rhythm, such as atrial fibrillation.

S_1 S_2 S_1 S_2

CARDIAC OUTPUT

Cardiac output (CO) is the amount of blood pumped by the ventricles during a given period of time (usually 1 minute). It is determined by the amount of blood ejected by the left ventricle, with each contraction—the stroke volume (SV)—multiplied by the heart rate (HR): SV × HR = CO. Normal adult cardiac output is between 3 and 5 L/min.

CRITICAL THINKING

6. The difference between 3 L/min and 5 L/min is quite large. Why would an average cardiac output vary as much as this? List six factors that would influence a person's cardiac output and provide a rationale for each.

Stroke volume

Stroke volume is the amount of blood pumped from the heart with each contraction (stroke volume from the left ventricle is usually 50 to 70 mL). Stroke volume is influenced by several factors:

- The degree of stretch of the heart muscle up to a critical point immediately prior to cardiac contraction (preload); the greater the preload, the greater the stroke volume. This holds true unless the heart muscle is stretched so much that it cannot contract effectively.
- The arterial pressure in the great vessels against which the heart muscle has to eject blood during contraction (afterload); an increased afterload results in decreased stroke volume.
- Synergy of contraction (i.e. uniform, synchronised contraction of the atria, followed by uniform synchronised contraction of the ventricles); conditions such as atrial fibrillation or complete heart block will cause an asynchronous contraction and decrease stroke volume.

DISPLAY 22-3 VARIATIONS IN S_2

The S_2 sound depends on the closure of the aortic and the pulmonic valves. Closure of the pulmonic valve is delayed by inspiration, resulting in a split S_2 sound. The components of the split sound are referred to as A_2 (aortic valve sound) and P_2 (pulmonic valve sound). If either sound is absent, no split sounds are heard. The A_2 sound is heard best over the second right intercostal space. P_2 is normally softer than A_2.

Accentuated S_2

An accentuated S_2 means that S_2 is louder than S_1. This occurs in conditions in which the aortic or pulmonic valve has a higher closing pressure.

Examples include:

- Increased pressure in the aorta from exercise, excitement or systemic hypertension (a booming S_2 is heard with systemic hypertension)
- Increased pressure in the pulmonary vasculature, which may occur with mitral stenosis or congestive heart failure
- Calcification of the semilunar valve in which the valve is still mobile, as in pulmonic or aortic stenosis.

Diminished S_2

A diminished S_2 means that S_2 is softer than S_1. This occurs in conditions in which the aortic or pulmonic valves have decreased mobility. Examples include:

- Decreased systemic blood pressure, which weakens the valves, as in shock
- Aortic or pulmonic stenosis in which the valves are thickened and calcified, with decreased mobility.

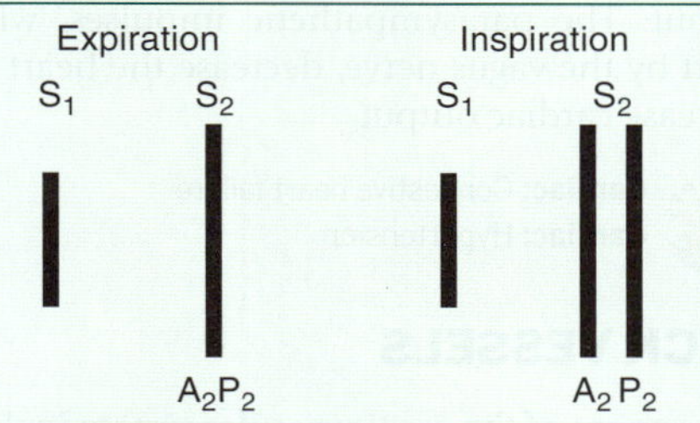

Normal (physiological) split S_2

A normal split S_2 can be heard over the second or third left intercostal space. It is usually heard best during inspiration and disappears during expiration. Over the aortic area and apex, the pulmonic component of S_2 is usually too faint to be heard and S_2 is a single sound resulting from aortic valve closure. In some patients, S_2 may not become single on expiration unless the patient sits up. Splitting that does not disappear during expiration is suggestive of heart disease.

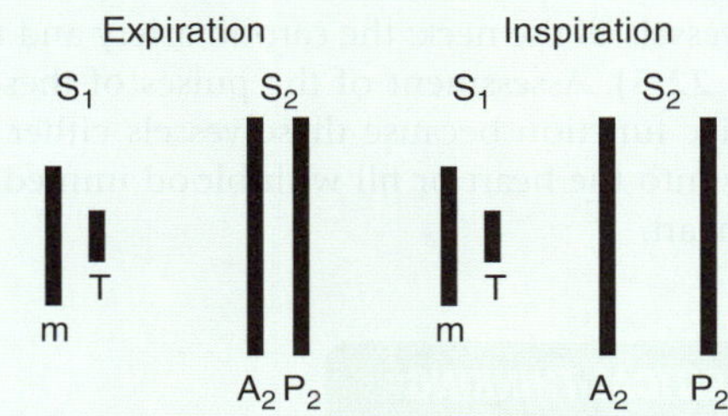

Wide split S_2

This is an increase in the usual splitting that persists throughout the entire respiratory cycle and widens on expiration. It occurs when there is delayed electrical activation of the right ventricle.

Example includes:

- Right bundle branch block, which delays pulmonic valve closing.

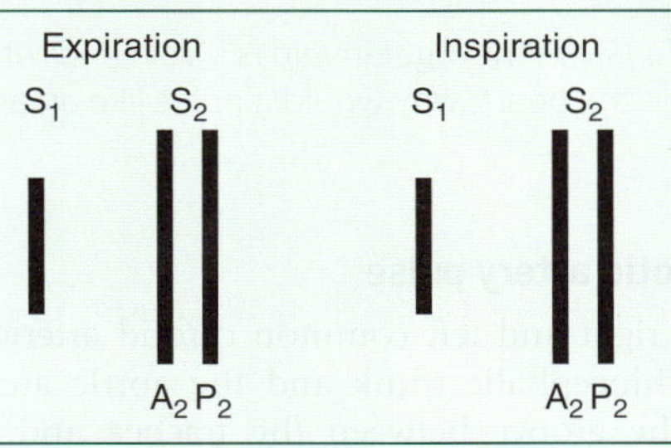

Fixed split S_2

This is a wide splitting that does not vary with respiration. It occurs when there is delayed closure of one of the valves. Examples include:

- Atrial septal defect and right ventricular failure, which delay pulmonic valve closing.

Expiration Inspiration

S_1 S_2 S_1 S_2

$A_2 P_2$ $A_2 P_2$

Reversed split S_2

This is a split S_2 that appears on expiration and disappears on inspiration—also known as paradoxical split. It occurs when closure of the aortic valve is abnormally delayed, causing A_2 to follow P_2 in expiration. Normal inspiratory delay of P_2 makes the split disappear during inspiration. Example includes:

- Left bundle branch block.

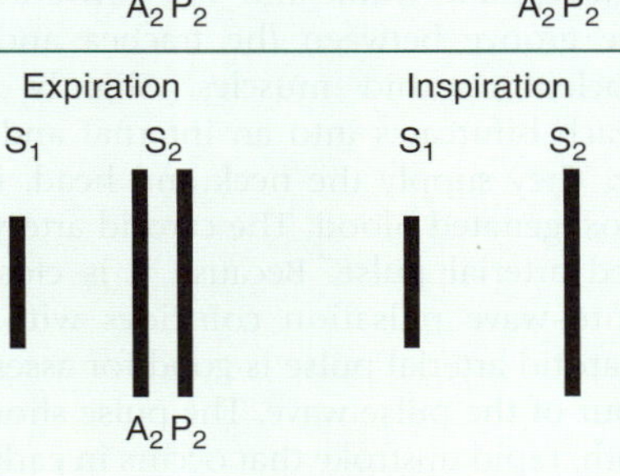

Continued on following page

DISPLAY 22-3 VARIATIONS IN S_2 (continued)

Accentuated A_2

An accentuated A_2 is loud over the right, second intercostal space. This occurs with increased pressure, as in systemic hypertension and aortic root dilation because of the closer position of the aortic valve to the chest wall.

Diminished A_2

A diminished A_2 is soft or absent over the right, second intercostal space. This occurs with immobility of the aortic valve in calcific aortic stenosis.

Accentuated P_2

An accentuated P_2 is louder than or equal to an A_2 sound. This occurs with pulmonary hypertension, dilated pulmonary artery and atrial septal defect. A wide split S_2, heard even at the apex, indicates an accentuated P_2.

Diminished P_2

A soft or absent P_2 sound occurs with an increased anteroposterior diameter of the chest (barrel chest), which is associated with ageing, pulmonic stenosis or chronic obstructive pulmonary disease.

- Compliance or suppleness and stretch of the ventricles; decreased compliance decreases stroke volume.
- Contractility or the force of myocardial contraction under given loading conditions; increased contractility increases stroke volume.

Although cardiac muscle has an innate pattern of contractility, cardiac activity is also mediated by the autonomic nervous system to respond to changing needs. The sympathetic impulses increase the heart rate and, therefore, cardiac output. The parasympathetic impulses, which travel to the heart by the vagus nerve, decrease the heart rate and therefore decrease cardiac output.

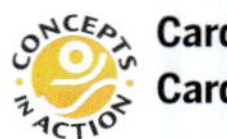

Cardiac: Congestive heart failure
Cardiac: Hypertension

NECK VESSELS

Assessment of the cardiovascular system includes evaluation of the vessels of the neck: the carotid artery and the jugular veins (Fig. 22-5). Assessment of the pulses of these vessels reflects cardiac function because these vessels either empty immediately into the heart or fill with blood immediately on exiting the heart.

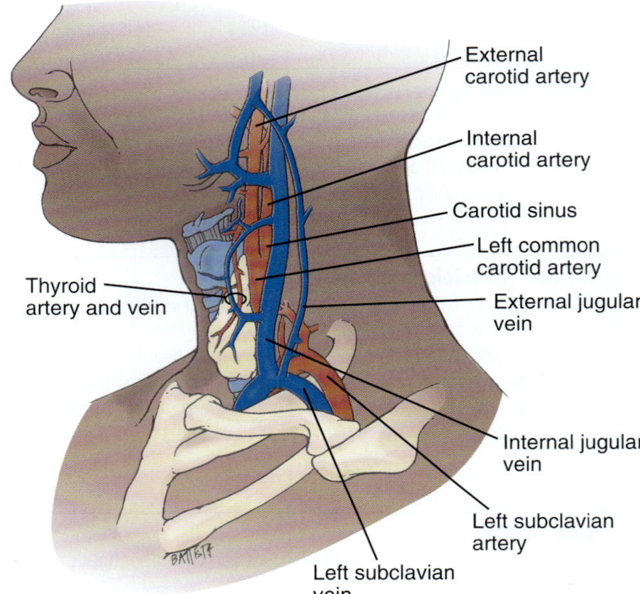

FIGURE 22-5 Major neck vessels, including the carotid arteries and jugular veins.

CRITICAL THINKING

7. Given the jugular vein is a vein and returns blood to the heart, why would it pulse like an artery?

Carotid artery pulse

The right and left common carotid arteries extend from the brachiocephalic trunk and the aortic arch and are located in the groove between the trachea and the right and left sternocleidomastoid muscles. Slightly below the mandible, each bifurcates into an internal and an external carotid artery. They supply the neck and head, including the brain, with oxygenated blood. The carotid artery pulse is a centrally located arterial pulse. Because it is close to the heart, the pressure–wave pulsation coincides with ventricular systole. The carotid arterial pulse is good for assessing amplitude and contour of the pulse wave. The pulse should normally have a smooth, rapid upstroke that occurs in early systole and a more gradual downstroke.

Jugular venous pressure

There are two sets of jugular veins: internal and external. The internal jugular veins lie deep and medial to the sternocleidomastoid muscle. The external jugular veins are more superficial; they lie laterally to the sternocleidomastoid muscle and above the clavicle. The jugular veins return blood to the heart from the head and neck by way of the superior vena cava.

As blood is returned to the heart via the jugular veins, assessment of the jugular venous pressure (JVP) is important for determining the haemodynamics of the right side of the heart. The jugular veins are inspected during cardiac assessment because they are proximal to the heart (approximately 10 cm from the right atria) and easily visualised on the lateral aspect of the neck. However, most importantly, the jugular veins empty into the superior vena cava, which in turn empties into the right atrium. Of all four jugular vessels (the right internal and external jugular veins, and the left internal and external jugular veins), the vessel with the most direct route to the heart is the right internal jugular vein. Consequently, although all jugular vessels can reflect cardiac function, the right internal jugular vein is the most accurate because of its anatomy.

The JVP reflects right atrial pressure (also known as the central venous pressure [CVP]). The CVP reflects both the body's fluid status (how well hydrated an individual is) and the degree of cardiac failure in a patient with right-sided heart failure or general heart failure. Because a patient with heart failure (right-sided or general) will have difficulty clearing blood from the right side of the heart, right-sided heart pressures will increase, making it more difficult for blood to enter the right atria. Consequently, blood entering the heart starts to back up and the JVP increases to a point where a pulse can be visualised. Generally, when a person is reasonably hydrated, there is a small amount of resistance to the blood as it enters the right side of the heart. This CVP (measured in either centimetres of water or millimetres of mercury) is approximately 0 to 6. Considering the heart and its proximal vessels are located within the thoracic cavity, they cannot be visualised. Furthermore, the vessels entering and leaving the heart cannot be visualised until they exit the thoracic cavity. Immediately superior to the clavicle is the first point where a jugular vessel can be inspected at its most proximal point to the heart. If a person is upright, this will be approximately 10 cm from the right atria and thus would reflect a CVP of 10 cm. As the person is moved to a more recumbent position, the vertical distance from the right atria to the jugular vessel will decrease and thus the JVP can be more easily visualised (e.g. if a person is lying flat the heart would be at the same level as the jugular vein and would thus reflect a CVP of 0 cm; as the person starts to move upright the heart becomes lower than the jugular vessels and a higher CVP is required for the pressure to be visualised in the jugular vessels) (Fig 22-6).

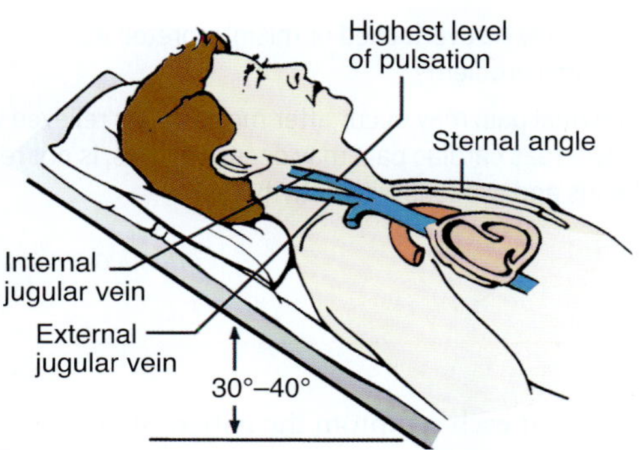

FIGURE 22-6 The jugular veins are the most proximal to the heart of all venous vasculature. The patient will be predominantly positioned in the semi-Fowler position for a chest assessment.

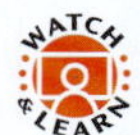

Estimating jugular venous pressure

CLINICAL TIP

The positioning of a patient (i.e. supine, semi-Fowler or Fowler) will impact greatly on whether the jugular venous pressure (JVP) can be visualised and the clinical significance of visualising a JVP. A significant JVP is when the jugular vein can be seen pulsing AND when the patient is in a semi-Fowler position or higher. The right internal jugular vein is most directly connected to the right atrium and provides the best assessment of pressure changes.

CASE STUDY

The evaluation of Malcolm's thorax reveals no heaves or visible pulsation. Neck veins are flat at an angle more than 45 degrees and no carotid bruits are noted. Skin is warm and dry, with pink nail beds. Pedal pulses are strong; 1+ ankle oedema is present.

CRITICAL THINKING

8. Why would Malcolm have these assessments completed?
9. If Malcolm had suffered a myocardial infarction, would you expect these assessments to differ? How and why?

Health assessment

COLLECTING SUBJECTIVE DATA: THE NURSING HEALTH HISTORY

Subjective data collected about the heart and neck vessels help the nurse to identify abnormal conditions that may affect the patient's ability to perform activities of daily living and to fulfil his or her role and responsibilities. Data collection also provides information on the patient's risk of cardiovascular disease and helps to identify areas where health education is needed. The patient may not be aware of the significant role that health promotion activities can play in preventing cardiovascular disease.

When compiling the nursing history of current complaints or symptoms, personal and family histories and lifestyle and health practices, remember to explore thoroughly the signs and symptoms the patient brings to your attention, either intentionally or inadvertently.

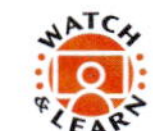

Health history taking

History of present health concern

QUESTION	RATIONALE
Chest pain and palpitations	
Do you experience chest pain? When did it start? Describe the type of pain, location, radiation, duration and how often you experience the pain. Rate the pain on a scale of 0 to 10, with 10 being the worst possible pain. Does activity make the pain worse? Did you have perspiration (diaphoresis) with the chest pain?	Chest pain can be cardiac, pulmonary, muscular or gastrointestinal in origin. Angina (cardiac chest pain) is usually described as a sensation of squeezing around the heart; a steady, severe pain; and a sense of pressure. It may radiate to the left shoulder and down the left arm or to the jaw. Diaphoresis and pain worsened by activity are usually related to cardiac chest pain.

Continued on following page

History of present health concern (continued)

QUESTION	RATIONALE
Do you experience palpitations?	Palpitations may occur with an abnormality of the heart's conduction system or during the heart's attempt to increase cardiac output by increasing the heart rate. Palpitations may cause the patient to feel anxious.
Other symptoms	
Do you tire easily? Do you experience fatigue? Describe when the fatigue started. Was it sudden or gradual? Do you notice it at any particular time of day?	Fatigue may result from compromised cardiac output. Fatigue related to decreased cardiac output is worse in the evening or as the day progresses.
Do you have difficulty breathing or shortness of breath (dyspnoea)?	Dyspnoea may result from congestive heart failure, pulmonary disorders, coronary artery disease, myocardial ischaemia or myocardial infarction. Dyspnoea may occur at rest, during sleep, or with mild, moderate or extreme exertion.
Do you wake up at night with an urgent need to urinate (nocturia)? How many times a night?	Increased renal perfusion during periods of rest or recumbency may cause nocturia. Decreased frequency may be related to decreased cardiac output.
Do you experience dizziness?	Dizziness may indicate decreased blood flow to the brain due to myocardial damage; however, there are several other causes for dizziness such as inner ear syndromes, decreased cerebral circulation and hypotension. Dizziness may put the patient at risk of falls.
Do you experience swelling (oedema) in your feet, ankles or legs?	Oedema of the lower extremities may occur as a result of heart failure.
Do you have frequent heart burn? When does it occur? What relieves it? How often do you experience it?	Cardiac pain may be overlooked or misinterpreted as gastrointestinal problems. Gastrointestinal pain may occur after meals and is relieved with antacids, whereas cardiac pain may occur anytime, is not relieved with antacids and worsens with activity.

Continued on following page

COLDSPA

Example for chest pain

Use the COLDSPA mnemonic as a guideline to collect needed information for each symptom the patient shares. In addition, the following questions help elicit important information.

Mnemonic	Question	Patient response example
Character	Describe the sign or symptom (feeling, appearance, sound, smell or taste, if applicable).	'Pressure, chest pain.'
Onset	When did it begin?	'Last night after dinner.'
Location	Where is it? Does it radiate? Does it occur anywhere else?	'Centre of chest and radiates down left arm.'
Duration	How long does it last? Does it recur?	'The pressure is constant, but the amount of pressure gets worse when I walk or move around.'
Severity	How bad is it? or How much does it bother you?	'It bothers me a lot and sometimes it really hurts a lot.'
Pattern	What makes it better or worse?	'It goes away a little when I sit down for a while.'
Associated factors/How it Affects the patient	What other symptoms occur with it? How does it affect you?	'Sometimes I feel lightheaded, sweaty and cold. It scares me because I can't do anything.'

Past health history

QUESTION	RATIONALE
Have you been diagnosed with a heart defect or a murmur?	Congenital or acquired defects affect the heart's ability to pump, decreasing the oxygen supply to the tissues.
Have you ever had rheumatic fever?	Approximately 40% of people with rheumatic fever develop rheumatic carditis. Rheumatic carditis develops after exposure to group A beta-haemolytic streptococci and results in inflammation of all layers of the heart, impairing contraction and valvular function.
Have you ever had heart surgery or cardiac balloon interventions?	Previous heart surgery may change the heart sounds heard during auscultation. Surgery and cardiac balloon interventions indicate prior cardiac compromise.
Have you ever had an electrocardiogram (ECG)? When was the last one performed? Do you know the results?	A prior ECG allows the health care team to evaluate for any changes in cardiac conduction or previous myocardial infarction.
Have you ever had a blood test called a lipid profile? Based on your last test, do you know what your cholesterol levels were?	Dyslipidaemia presents the greatest risk for developing coronary artery disease. Elevated cholesterol levels have been linked to the development of atherosclerosis (Joffres et al., 2013).
Do you take medications or use other treatments for heart disease? How often do you take them? Why do you take them?	Patients may have medications prescribed for heart disease but may not take them regularly. Patients may skip taking their diuretics because of having to urinate frequently. Beta-blockers may be omitted because of the adverse effects on sexual energy. Education about medications may be needed.
Do you monitor your own heart rate or blood pressure?	Self-monitoring of heart rate or blood pressure is recommended if the patient is taking cardiotonic or antihypertensive medications respectively. A demonstration is necessary to ensure appropriate technique.

Family history

QUESTION	RATIONALE
Is there a history of hypertension, myocardial infarction, coronary heart disease, elevated cholesterol levels or diabetes mellitus in your family?	A genetic predisposition to these risk factors increases a patient's chance of developing heart disease.

Lifestyle and health practices

QUESTION	RATIONALE
Do you smoke? How many packs of cigarettes per day and for how many years?	Cigarette smoking greatly increases the risk of heart disease (see Promote health—Coronary heart disease).
What type of stress do you have in your life? How do you cope with it?	Stress has been identified as a possible risk factor for heart disease.
Describe what you usually eat in a 24-hour period.	An elevated cholesterol level increases the chance of fatty plaque formation in the coronary vessels.
How much alcohol do you consume each day or each week?	Excessive intake of alcohol has been linked to hypertension. More than two drinks per day for men, or one for women, is associated with high blood pressure and other diseases (American Heart Association [AHA], 2017).
Do you exercise? What type of exercise and how often?	A sedentary lifestyle is a known modifiable risk factor contributing to heart disease. Aerobic exercise three times per week for 30 min is more beneficial than anaerobic exercise or sporadic exercise in preventing heart disease.

Continued on following page

Lifestyle and health practices (continued)

QUESTION	RATIONALE
Describe your daily activities. How are they different from your routine 5 or 10 years ago? Does fatigue, chest pain or shortness of breath limit your ability to perform daily activities? Describe. Are you able to care for yourself?	Heart disease may impede the ability to perform daily activities. Exertional dyspnoea or fatigue may indicate heart failure. An inability to complete activities of daily living may necessitate a referral for home care.
Has your heart disease had any effect on your sexual activity?	Many patients with heart disease are afraid that sexual activity will precipitate chest pain. If the patient can walk one block or climb two flights of stairs without experiencing symptoms, it is generally acceptable for the patient to engage in sexual intercourse. Glyceryl trinitrate can be taken before intercourse as a prophylactic for chest pain. In addition, the side-lying position for sexual intercourse may reduce the workload on the heart.
How many pillows do you use to sleep at night? Do you get up to urinate during the night? Do you feel rested in the morning?	If heart function is compromised, cardiac output to the kidneys is reduced during episodes of activity. At rest, cardiac output increases, as does glomerular filtration and urinary output. Orthopnoea (the inability to breathe while supine) and nocturia may indicate heart failure. In addition, these two conditions may also impede the ability to get adequate rest.
How important is having a healthy heart to your ability to feel good about yourself and your appearance? What fears about heart disease do you have?	A person's feeling of self-worth may depend on his or her ability to perform usual daily activities and fulfil his or her usual roles.

PROMOTE HEALTH — CORONARY HEART DISEASE

OVERVIEW

Coronary heart disease (CHD) is caused by atherosclerosis of the coronary arteries, which restricts blood flow to the coronary tissues. Too much pressure in the arteries makes the walls thick and stiff (arteriosclerosis, or hardening of the arteries). When the coronary arteries are affected, chest pain (angina) or heart attack (myocardial infarction) can occur. Signs and symptoms develop gradually and often do not appear until angina or a myocardial infarction occurs due to the formation of a blood clot resulting in an inadequate blood supply to the heart tissues. Atherosclerosis may begin as early as childhood and causes are still not clear. It is thought that damage to the inner layer of an artery begins the process. Risk factors may cause the damage or make it worse. The damage causes fatty deposits (plaques) made of cholesterol and other cellular waste products to accumulate and then harden. Thus, the space inside the artery is narrowed. Pieces of the fatty deposit may break off and enter the blood stream, and can cause a blood clot to form and further narrow the artery, leading to tissue damage such as a heart attack.

Age is a factor in cardiovascular disease. At younger ages, men face a greater risk of heart disease than women. On average, a first heart attack—the most common manifestation of this prevalent disease—strikes men at age 65. For women, the average age of a first heart attack is 72 (Harvard Health Publishing—Harvard Medical School, 2016). The World Health Organization (WHO, 2017) has reported that an estimated 17.9 million people died from cardiovascular diseases in 2016, representing 31% of all global deaths; of these deaths, 85% were due to heart attack and stroke. Cardiovascular diseases are the number one cause of death globally, with more people dying annually from cardiovascular diseases than any other cause.

In 2016, compared with non-Aboriginal and Torres Strait Islander peoples, Aboriginal and Torres Strait Islander Australians were 2 times as likely to have CHD; 2.4 times as likely to be hospitalised for CHD; 1.6 times as likely to die from CHD; and experiencing CHD at younger ages (in the 35 to 44 age group, 4.7 times as likely to report having CHD) (Australian Institute of Health and Welfare [AIHW], 2016).

From 2010 to 2012, the total cardiovascular disease mortality rate among Māori was more than twice as high as that among non-Māori (Ministry of Health, 2018).

Risk factors

- Age: Male over 45; female over 55 (postmenopausal or ovaries removed, and not using oestrogen replacement therapy)
- Family history, especially of aneurysm or early heart disease: father or brother diagnosed with CHD before age 55; mother or sister before age 65 (National Heart Lung and Blood Institute, 2019)
- The metabolic syndrome:
  - Abdominal obesity
  - Blood fat disorders: high triglycerides; low high-density lipoprotein (HDL) and high low-density lipoprotein (LDL)–cholesterol (total cholesterol above 200 mg/dL; HDL less than 40 mg/dL; LDL above 130 mg/dL)
  - High blood pressure
  - Insulin resistance or glucose intolerance (e.g. diabetes mellitus, especially non-insulin–dependent diabetes mellitus)
  - High fibrinogen or plasminogen activator inhibitor in blood
  - Low-grade infection or inflammation (e.g. elevated C-reactive protein in blood) (AHA, 2015)
- Body weight: overweight; upper body adiposity
- Smoking
- Sedentary lifestyle or limited physical activity
- Dietary intake low in antioxidants (especially fruit), high in saturated fat and low in fibre
- Excessive alcohol consumption (more than two drinks per day for men and one for women; leads to obesity, high blood pressure and other cardiac diseases) (AHA, 2015)
- Stress: psychological, emotional or physical stress; family relationship stresses; burnout; and daily hassles, especially in women (AHA, 2015).

PROMOTE HEALTH **CORONARY HEART DISEASE** (continued)

Teach risk reduction tips

- Stop smoking.
- Lower high blood cholesterol.
- Control high blood pressure.
- Maintain tight control of diabetes.
- Follow a regular exercise plan.
- Achieve and maintain your ideal body weight.
- Control stress and anger.
- Eat a diet low in saturated fat and cholesterol.

More detailed tips

- Seek help from smoking cessation groups to stop smoking.
- Undertake regular exercise such as brisk walking for at least 30 minutes a day.
- Eat a healthy diet: control portion size; eat more fruits and vegetables; select whole grains; limit unhealthy fats; choose low-fat protein sources; and reduce sodium in food (Mayo Clinic, 2019).
- If overweight, start a weight-reduction program.
- Reduce personal stress as much as possible. Try muscle relaxation and deep breathing. Seek help if necessary.
- Work with your health care provider to control high blood pressure, diabetes, blood glucose levels and other chronic diseases.
- Work with your health care provider to control elevated blood cholesterol.
- Know your family risk of atherosclerosis and CHD.
- If you drink alcohol, limit to one drink per day (women) or two drinks per day (men), especially of red wine. If you do not drink alcohol, do not start (AHA, 2015).
- Women: consult your primary care provider or your gynaecologist about the risk of taking postmenopausal hormone replacement.
- Learn about heart disease and the signs of heart attack:
    - Uncomfortable pressure, fullness, squeezing or pain in centre of chest that lasts more than a few minutes that may come and go
    - Pain spreading to shoulders, arms, neck, jaw or back
    - Chest discomfort with lightheadedness, fainting, sweating, nausea or shortness of breath
    - Women: shortness of breath, with or without chest discomfort
    - Women: extreme fatigue; sudden cold sweat.

COLLECTING OBJECTIVE DATA: PHYSICAL EXAMINATION

A major purpose of this examination is to identify any sign of heart disease and thereby initiate early referral and treatment.

Assessment of the heart and neck vessels is an essential part of the total cardiovascular examination. It is important to remember that additional data gathered during assessment of the blood pressure, skin, nails, head, thorax and lungs, and peripheral pulses all play a part in the complete cardiovascular assessment. These additional assessment areas are covered in Chapters 7, 15, 16, 20 and 23.

The part of the cardiovascular assessment covered in this chapter involves inspection, palpation and auscultation of the neck and anterior chest area (praecordium). Inspection is a fairly easy skill to acquire. However, auscultation requires considerable practice to develop expert proficiency. Novice practitioners may be able to recognise an abnormal heart sound but may have difficulty determining what and where it is exactly. Continued exposure and experience increase the practitioner's ability to determine the exact nature and characteristics of abnormal heart sounds. In addition, it may be difficult to palpate the apical impulse on many patients because the distance between the apex of the heart and the praecordium may be increased owing to a patient's obesity, barrel-shaped chest, large breasts or position. For this reason, palpation of the carotid artery should be considered. Heart and neck vessel assessment skills are useful to the nurse in all types of health care settings, including acute, clinical and home health care.

CLINICAL TIP
When performing a total body system examination (see Chap. 30), it is often convenient to assess the heart and neck vessels immediately after assessment of the thorax and lungs.

Preparing the patient

Prepare patients for the examination by explaining they will need to expose their anterior chest. Female patients may keep their breasts covered and may hold the left breast out of the way when necessary. Explain to the patient they will need to assume several different positions for a heart and neck examination.

Auscultation and palpation of the neck vessels, and inspection, palpation and auscultation of the praecordium are performed with the patient in the supine position, with the head elevated to about a 30-degree angle. The patient may be asked to assume a left lateral position if the examiner decides to palpate the apical impulse. In addition, the patient will be asked to assume a left lateral and a sitting-up and leaning-forward position so the examiner can auscultate for the presence of any abnormal heart sounds. As these positions change the pressure on the heart through moving the surrounding internal organs they may bring out an abnormal sound not detected with the patient in the supine position. Make sure you explain to the patient that you will be listening to the heart in a number of places and that this does not necessarily mean that anything is wrong. Provide the patient with as much modesty as possible during the examination; describe the steps of the examination and answer any questions the patient may have. These actions will help to ease any patient anxiety.

Equipment

- Stethoscope with a bell and diaphragm
- Small pillow
- Penlight or movable examination light
- Watch with a second hand
- Centimetre rulers (×2)

Physical assessment

Remember these key points during examination:

- Understand the anatomy and function of the heart and its major vessels to identify and interpret heart sounds and electrocardiograms accurately.
- Know normal variations of the cardiovascular system in the elderly patient.

Changes in the heart rate, the heart rhythm and pathological cardiac problems all alter heart sounds on auscultation. As mentioned earlier in this chapter, auscultation is a difficult skill to master and requires extensive practice. The following chapter content relating to auscultating heart sounds, although classified as advanced knowledge (and, as such, is advanced practice), is provided to assist as both a point of interest and potential problem-solving content if and when abnormal heart sounds are encountered. By no means is a novice practitioner expected to have a working knowledge of the following content.

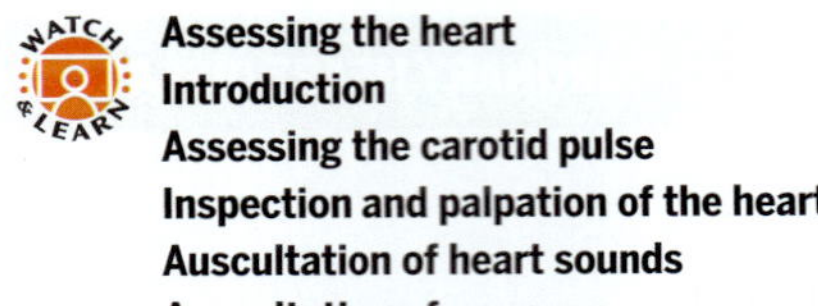

PHYSICAL ASSESSMENT

ASSESSMENT PROCEDURE	NORMAL FINDINGS	ABNORMAL FINDINGS
Neck vessels		
INSPECTION		
Observe the jugular venous pulse. Inspect the jugular venous pulse by standing on the right side of the patient. The patient should be in a supine position with the torso elevated 30 degrees to 45 degrees. Make sure the head and torso are on the same plane. Ask the patient to turn the head slightly to the left. Shine a tangential light source onto the neck to increase visualisation of pulsations as well as shadows. Next inspect the suprasternal notch or the area around the clavicles for pulsations of the internal jugular veins. **CLINICAL TIP** **Be careful not to confuse pulsations of the carotid arteries with pulsations of the internal jugular veins.**	The jugular venous pulse is not normally visible with the patient sitting upright. This position fully distends the vein, and pulsations may or may not be discernible.	Fully distended jugular veins with the patient's torso elevated more than 45 degrees indicate increased central venous pressure that may be the result of right ventricular failure, pulmonary hypertension, pulmonary emboli or cardiac tamponade.
Evaluate jugular venous pressure. Evaluate jugular venous pressure by watching for distension of the jugular vein. It is normal for the jugular veins to be visible when the patient is supine; to evaluate jugular vein distension, position the patient in a supine position with the head of the bed elevated 30 degrees, 45 degrees, 60 degrees and 90 degrees. At each increase of the elevation, have the patient's head turned slightly away from the side being evaluated. Using tangential lighting, observe for distension, protrusion or bulging. *Note:* It should be remembered when interpreting the jugular venous pressure that it is reflective of both right-sided heart failure or heart failure and central venous pressure. The normal range for central venous pressure is 0 to 6 (this is documented in either centimetres of water if measured externally, or millimetres of mercury if the measurement is taken using central venous pressure monitoring). As such, unless the jugular venous pressure can be visualised at a height greater than 6 cm than the sternal angle (the approximate point of entry to the right atria), it should be considered physiological.	The jugular vein should not be distended, bulging or protruding at 45 degrees or greater.	Distension, bulging or protrusion at 45 degrees, 60 degrees or 90 degrees may indicate right-sided heart failure. Document at which positions (45 degrees, 60 degrees or 90 degrees) you observe distension. Patients with obstructive pulmonary disease may have elevated venous pressure only during expiration. An inspiratory increase in venous pressure, called Kussmaul sign, may occur in patients with severe constrictive pericarditis.

PHYSICAL ASSESSMENT (continued)

ASSESSMENT PROCEDURE	NORMAL FINDINGS	ABNORMAL FINDINGS
Neck vessels (continued)		
AUSCULTATION AND PALPATION		
Auscultate the carotid arteries. Auscultate the carotid arteries if the patient is middle-aged or older or if you suspect cardiovascular disease. Place the bell of the stethoscope over the carotid artery and ask the patient to hold his or her breath for a moment so breath sounds do not conceal any vascular sounds (Fig. 22-7). **SAFETY TIP** **Always auscultate the carotid arteries before palpating because palpation may increase or slow the heart rate, therefore changing the strength of the carotid impulse heard.** **Palpate the carotid arteries.** Palpate each carotid artery alternately by placing the pads of the index and middle fingers medial to the sternocleidomastoid muscle on the neck (Fig. 22-8). Note the amplitude and contour of the pulse, elasticity of the artery and any thrills. **SAFETY TIP** **If you detect occlusion during auscultation, palpate very lightly to avoid blocking circulation or triggering vagal stimulation and bradycardia, hypotension or even cardiac arrest.** **SAFETY TIP** **Palpate the carotid arteries individually because bilateral palpation could result in reduced cerebral blood flow.** **OLDER ADULT CONSIDERATIONS** **Be cautious with older patients because atherosclerosis may have caused obstruction, and compression may impede or occlude circulation.**	No blowing or swishing or other sounds are heard. Pulses are equally strong; a 2+ or normal with no variation in strength from beat to beat. Contour is normally smooth and rapid on the upstroke and slower and less abrupt on the downstroke. Arteries are elastic and no thrills are noted. The strength of the pulse is evaluated on a scale from 0 to 4 as follows: **Pulse amplitude scale** 0 = Absent 1+ = Weak 2+ = Normal 3+ = Increased 4+ = Bounding	A bruit, a blowing or swishing sound caused by turbulent blood flow through a narrowed vessel is indicative of occlusive arterial disease. However, if the artery is more than two-thirds occluded, a bruit may not be heard. Pulse inequality may indicate arterial constriction or occlusion in one carotid. Weak pulses may indicate hypovolaemia, shock or decreased cardiac output. A bounding, firm pulse may indicate hypervolaemia or increased cardiac output. Variations in strength from beat to beat or with respiration are abnormal and may indicate a variety of problems (Display 22-4). A delayed upstroke may indicate aortic stenosis. Loss of elasticity may indicate arteriosclerosis. Thrills may indicate a narrowing of the artery.

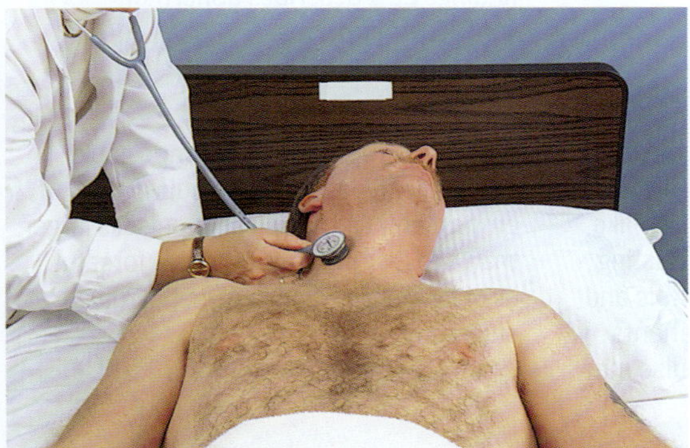

FIGURE 22-7 Auscultating the carotid artery. (© B. Proud.)

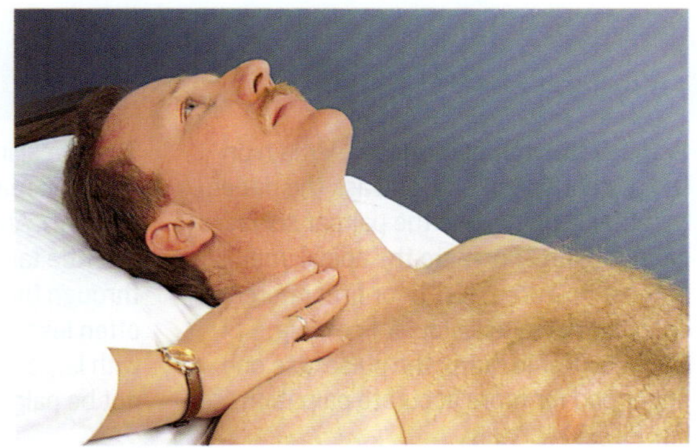

FIGURE 22-8 Palpating the carotid artery. (© B. Proud.)

Continued on following page

DISPLAY 22-4 ARTERIAL PULSE AND PRESSURE WAVES

A normal pulse, represented below, has a smooth, rounded wave with a notch on the descending slope. The pulse should feel strong and regular. The notch is not palpable. The pulse pressure (the difference between the systolic and diastolic pressure) is 30 to 40 mmHg. Pulse pressure may be measured in waveforms, which are produced when a pulmonary artery catheter is used to evaluate arterial pressure.

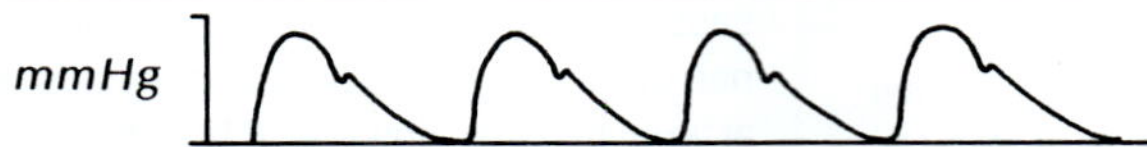

The arterial pressure waveform consists of five parts: Anacrotic limb, systolic peak, dicrotic limb, dicrotic notch and end diastole. The initial upstroke, or anacrotic limb, occurs as blood is rapidly ejected from the ventricle through the open aortic valve into the aorta. The anacrotic limb ends at the systolic peak, the waveform's highest point. Arterial pressure falls as the blood continues into the peripheral vessels and the waveform turns downwards, forming the dicrotic limb. When the pressure in the ventricle is less than the pressure in the aortic root, the aortic valve closes and a small notch (dicrotic notch) appears on the waveform. The closing of the aortic notch is the beginning of diastole. The pressure continues to fall in the aortic root until it reaches its lowest point, seen on the waveform as the diastolic peak.

Changes in circulation and heart rhythm affect the pulse and its waveform. Listed below are some of the variations you may find.

Small, weak pulse

Characteristics

- Diminished pulse pressure
- Weak and small on palpation
- Slow upstroke
- Prolonged systolic peak

Causes

- Conditions causing a decreased stroke volume
- Heart failure
- Hypovolaemia
- Severe aortic stenosis
- Conditions causing increased peripheral resistance
- Hypothermia
- Severe congestive heart failure

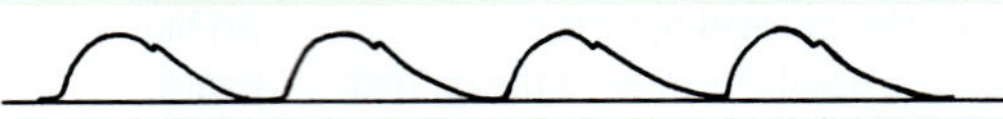

Large, bounding pulse

Characteristics

- Increased pulse pressure
- Strong and bounding on palpation
- Rapid rise and fall with a brief systolic peak

Causes

- Conditions that cause an increased stroke volume or decreased peripheral resistance
- Fever
- Anaemia
- Hyperthyroidism
- Aortic regurgitation
- Patent ductus arteriosus
- Conditions resulting in increased stroke volume due to decreased heart rate
- Bradycardia
- Complete heart block
- Conditions resulting in decreased compliance of the aortic walls
- Ageing
- Atherosclerosis

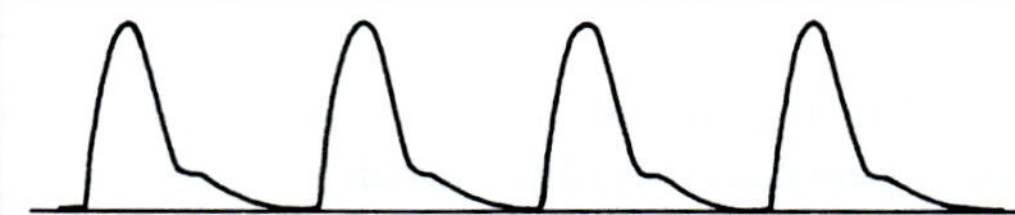

PHYSICAL ASSESSMENT (continued)

ASSESSMENT PROCEDURE	NORMAL FINDINGS	ABNORMAL FINDINGS
Heart (praecordium)		
INSPECTION		
Inspect pulsations. With the patient in the supine position with the head of the bed elevated between 30 degrees and 45 degrees, stand on the patient's right side and look for the apical impulse and any abnormal pulsations.	The apical impulse may or may not be visible. If apparent, it would be in the mitral area (left midclavicular line, fourth or fifth intercostal space). The apical impulse is a result of the left ventricle moving outwards during systole.	Pulsations, which may also be called heaves or lifts, other than the apical pulsation are considered abnormal and should be evaluated. A heave or lift may occur as a result of an enlarged ventricle from an overload of work. Abnormal findings 22-1 describes abnormal ventricular impulses.
PALPATION		
Palpate the apical impulse. Remain on the patient's right side and ask the patient to remain supine. Use the palmar surfaces of your hand to palpate the apical impulse in the mitral area (fourth or fifth intercostal space at the midclavicular line) (Fig. 22-9A). After locating the pulse, use one finger pad for more accurate palpation (see Fig. 22-9B).	The apical impulse is palpated in the mitral area and may be the size of a small coin (1 to 2 cm). Amplitude is usually small—like a gentle tap. The duration is brief, lasting through the first two-thirds of systole and often less. In obese patients or patients with large breasts, the apical impulse may not be palpable.	The apical impulse may be impossible to palpate in patients with pulmonary emphysema. If the apical impulse is larger than 1 to 2 cm, displaced, more forceful or of longer duration, suspect cardiac enlargement.

PHYSICAL ASSESSMENT (continued)

ASSESSMENT PROCEDURE	NORMAL FINDINGS	ABNORMAL FINDINGS
Heart (praecordium) (continued)		
CLINICAL TIP It is not always possible to palpate this pulsation. To maximise the chance of palpating the apical impulse, the heart should lie against the praecordium where you are attempting to palpate it. Position the patient upright and leaning forwards or in the left lateral position. Also, consider why you are palpating the apical impulse. Frequently there is no benefit to palpating the apical impulse when the carotid pulse can be more easily and less obtrusively palpated.	**OLDER ADULT CONSIDERATIONS** In older patients the apical impulse may be difficult to palpate because of increased anteroposterior chest diameter.	

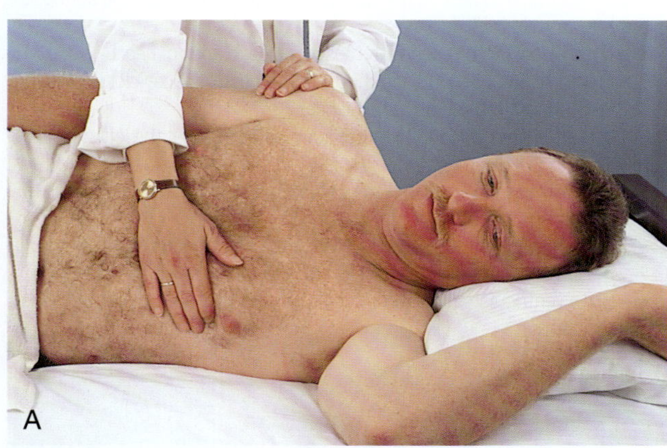

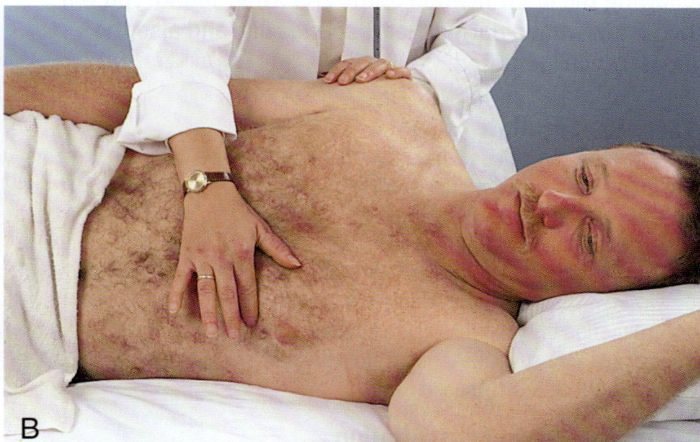

FIGURE 22-9 Locate the apical impulse with the palmar surface **(A)**, then palpate the apical impulse with the finger pad **(B)**. (© B. Proud)

ASSESSMENT PROCEDURE	NORMAL FINDINGS	ABNORMAL FINDINGS
Palpate for abnormal pulsations. Use your palmar surfaces to palpate the apex, left sternal border and base.	No pulsations or vibrations are palpated in the areas of the apex, left sternal border or base.	A thrill, which feels similar to a purring cat, or a pulsation is usually associated with a grade IV or higher murmur.
AUSCULTATION		
Auscultate heart rate and rhythm. Follow the guidelines given in Spotlight technique 22-1. Place the diaphragm of the stethoscope at the apex and listen closely to the rate and rhythm of the apical impulse.	Rate should be 60 to 100 beats/minute with regular rhythm. A regularly irregular rhythm, such as sinus arrhythmia when the heart rate increases with inspiration and decreases with expiration, may be normal in young adults.	Bradycardia (less than 60 beats/minute) or tachycardia (more than 100 beats/minute) may result in decreased cardiac output. Patients with irregular rhythms (i.e. premature atrial contraction or premature ventricular contractions) and irregular rhythms (i.e. atrial fibrillation and atrial flutter with varying block) should be referred for further evaluation. These types of irregular patterns may predispose the patient to decreased cardiac output, heart failure or emboli (see Abnormal findings 22-2).
If you detect an irregular rhythm, auscultate for a pulse rate deficit. This is done by palpating the radial pulse while you auscultate the apical pulse. Count for a full minute.	The radial and apical pulse rates should be identical.	A pulse deficit (difference between the apical and peripheral or radial pulses) may indicate atrial fibrillation, atrial flutter, premature ventricular contractions and varying degrees of heart block.

Continued on following page 415

SPOTLIGHT TECHNIQUE 22-1 AUSCULTATING HEART SOUNDS

Most nurses need many hours of practice in auscultating heart sounds to assess a patient's health status and interpret findings proficiently and confidently. Practitioners may be able to recognise an abnormal heart sound but may have difficulty determining what and where it is exactly. Continued exposure and experience increase one's ability to determine the exact nature and characteristics of abnormal heart sounds. An added difficulty involves palpation, particularly of the apical impulse in patients who are obese or barrel chested. These conditions increase the distance from the apex of the heart to the praecordium.

CLINICAL TIP

When you are on clinical placement, auscultate as many patients' hearts as you can. The more easily you can identify what a 'normal' heart sounds like, the easier it will become for you to identify an 'abnormal' sound. Although you will not likely recognise what the abnormal sound is, you will be able to identify that it shouldn't be there and notify the multidisciplinary team to investigate further. Additionally, following the identification of the abnormal sound, you will then know what a normal heart sounds like and also the anomaly you identified.

Where to auscultate

Heart sounds can be auscultated in the traditional five areas on the praecordium, which is the anterior surface of the body overlying the heart and great vessels. The traditional areas include the aortic area, the pulmonic area, Erb point, the tricuspid area and the mitral or apical area. The four valve areas do not reflect the anatomical location of the valves. Rather, they reflect the way in which heart sounds radiate to the chest wall. Sounds always travel in the direction of blood flow. For example, sounds that originate in the tricuspid valve are usually best heard along the left lower sternal border at the fourth or fifth intercostal space.

Traditional areas of auscultation

- Aortic area: Second intercostal space at the right sternal border—the base of the heart
- Pulmonic area: Second or third intercostal space at the left sternal border—the base of the heart
- Erb point: Third to fifth intercostal space at the left sternal border
- Tricuspid area: Fourth or fifth intercostal space at the left lower sternal border
- Mitral (apical): Fifth intercostal space near the left midclavicular line—the apex of the heart.

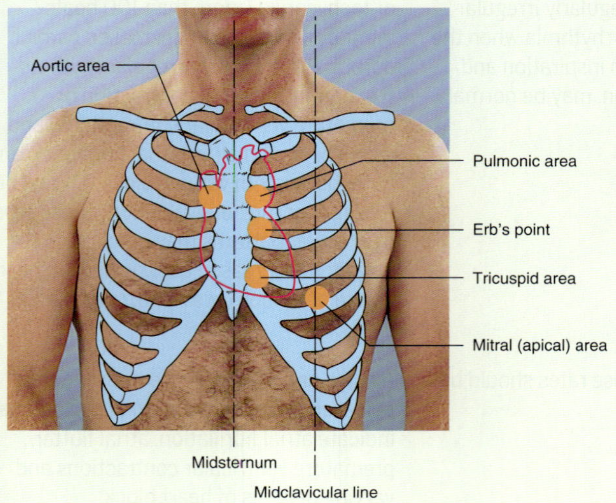

CLINICAL TIP

Closing your eyes reduces visual stimuli and distractions and may enhance your ability to concentrate on auditory stimuli.

Alternative areas of auscultation

In reality, the areas described above overlap extensively and sounds produced by the valves can be heard all over the praecordium. Therefore, it is important to listen to more than just five specific points on the praecordium. Keep the fact of overlap in mind and use the names of the chambers instead of Erb point, mitral and tricuspid areas when auscultating over the praecordium. 'Alternative' (versus the traditional) areas of auscultation overlap and are not as discrete as the traditional areas. The alternative areas are the aortic area, pulmonic area, left atrial area, right atrial area, left ventricular area and right ventricular area.

Cover the entire praecordium. As you auscultate in all areas, concentrate on systematically moving the stethoscope from left to right across the entire heart area from the base to the apex (top to bottom) or from the apex to the base (bottom to top).

- Aortic area: Right second intercostal space to apex of heart
- Pulmonic area: Second and third left intercostal spaces close to sternum but may be higher or lower
- Left atrial area: Second to fourth intercostal space at the left sternal border
- Right atrial area: Third to fifth intercostal space at the right sternal border
- Left ventricular area: Second to fifth intercostal spaces, extending from the left sternal border to the left midclavicular line
- Right ventricular area: Second to fifth intercostal spaces, centred over the sternum.

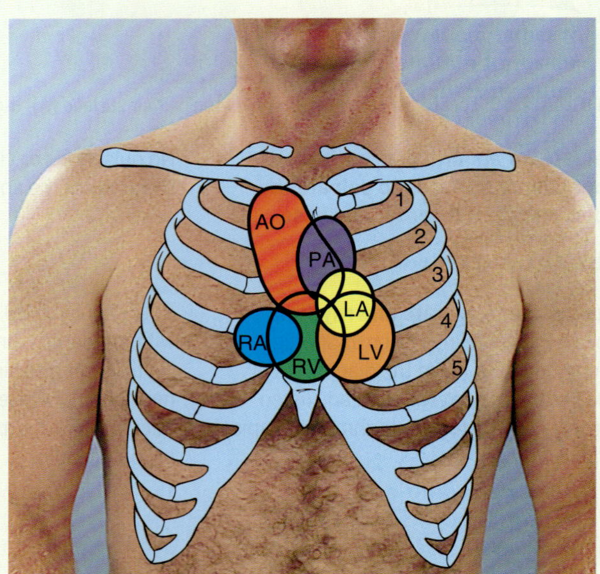

How to auscultate

Position yourself on the patient's right side (or left side if you are left-handed). The patient should be supine with the upper trunk elevated 30 degrees. Use the diaphragm of the stethoscope to auscultate all areas of the praecordium for high-pitched sounds. Use the bell of the stethoscope to detect (differentiate) low-pitched sounds or gallops. The diaphragm should be applied firmly to the chest, whereas the bell should be applied lightly.

SPOTLIGHT TECHNIQUE 22-1 AUSCULTATING HEART SOUNDS (continued)

Focus on one sound at a time as you auscultate each area of the praecordium. Start by listening to the heart's rate and rhythm. Then identify the first and second heart sounds, concentrate on each heart sound individually, listen for extra heart sounds, listen for murmurs and finally listen with the patient in different positions.

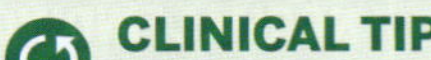

CLINICAL TIP

When using your stethoscope to auscultate the heart it should be remembered that the diaphragm is best for auscultating higher-pitched sounds, and the bell for lower-pitched sounds. As heart sounds are lower pitched, the bell is usually best for auscultating the heart.

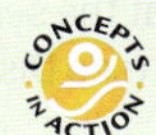

Cardiac: Myocardial blood flow

PHYSICAL ASSESSMENT (continued)

ASSESSMENT PROCEDURE	NORMAL FINDINGS	ABNORMAL FINDINGS
Heart (praecordium) (continued)		
Auscultate to identify S_1 and S_2. Auscultate the first heart sound (S_1 or 'lub') and the second heart sound (S_2 or 'dub'). Remember these two sounds make up the cardiac cycle of systole and diastole. S_1 starts systole, and S_2 starts diastole. The space, or systolic pause, between S_1 and S_2 is of short duration (thus S_1 and S_2 occur very close together), whereas the space, or diastolic pause, between S_2 and the start of another S_1 is of longer duration. 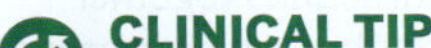 **CLINICAL TIP** **If you are experiencing difficulty differentiating S_1 from S_2, palpate the carotid pulse: the harsh sound that occurs with the carotid pulse is S_1 (Fig. 22-10).**	S_1 corresponds with each carotid pulsation and is loudest at the apex of the heart. S_2 immediately follows after S_1 and is loudest at the base of the heart. 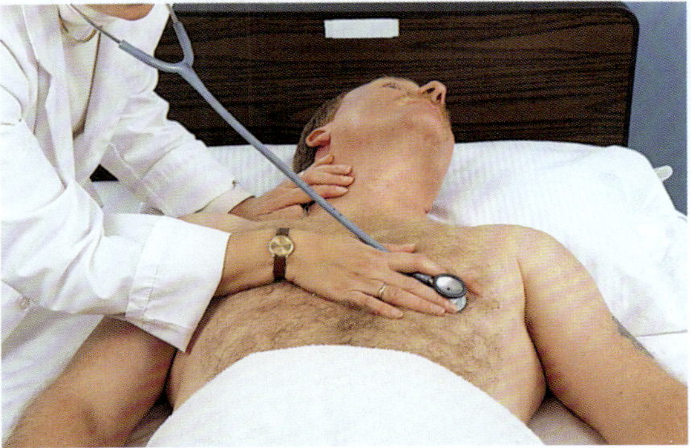 **FIGURE 22-10** Palpating the carotid pulse while auscultating S_1 and S_2. (© B. Proud.)	See Displays 22-2 and 22-3.
Listen to S_1. Use the diaphragm of the stethoscope to best hear S_1 (Fig. 22-11).	A distinct sound is heard in each area but is loudest at the apex. May become softer with inspiration. A split S_1 may be heard normally in young adults at the left lateral sternal border.	Accentuated, diminished, varying or split S_1 are all abnormal findings (see Display 22-2).

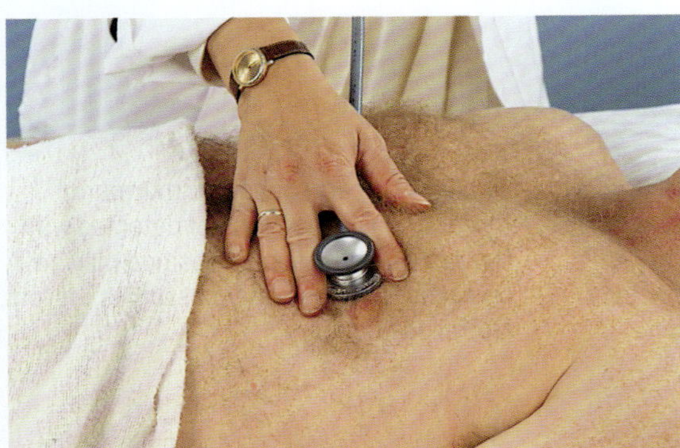

FIGURE 22-11 Auscultating S_1 (© B. Proud.)

Continued on following page

PHYSICAL ASSESSMENT (continued)

ASSESSMENT PROCEDURE	NORMAL FINDINGS	ABNORMAL FINDINGS
Listen to S_2. Use the diaphragm of the stethoscope. Ask the patient to breath regularly. **CLINICAL TIP** **Do not ask the patient to hold his or her breath. Breath holding will cause any normal or abnormal split to subside.**	Distinct sound is heard in each area but is loudest at the base. A split S_2 (into two distinct sounds of its components—A_2 and P_2) is normal and termed *physiological splitting.* It is usually heard late in inspiration at the second or third left interspaces (see Display 22-3).	Any split S_2 heard in expiration is abnormal. The abnormal split can be one of three types: wide, fixed or reversed.
Auscultate for extra heart sounds. Use the diaphragm first then the bell to auscultate over the entire heart area. Note the characteristics (e.g. location, timing) of any extra sound heard. Auscultate during the systolic pause (space heard between S_1 and S_2).	Normally no sounds are heard.	Ejection sounds or clicks (e.g. a midsystolic click associated with mitral valve prolapse). A friction rub may also be heard during the systolic pause. Abnormal findings 22-3 provides a full description of the extra heart sounds (normal and abnormal) of systole and diastole.
Auscultate during the diastolic pause (space heard between end of S_2 and the next S_1). **CLINICAL TIP** **While auscultating, keep in mind that development of a pathological S3 may be the earliest sign of heart failure.**	Normally no sounds are heard. A physiological S_3 heart sound is a benign finding commonly heard at the beginning of the diastolic pause in children, adolescents and young adults. It is rare after age 40. The physiological S_3 usually subsides upon standing or sitting up. A physiological S_4 heart sound may be heard near the end of diastole in well-conditioned athletes and in adults older than age 40 or 50 with no evidence of heart disease, especially after exercise.	A pathological S_3 (ventricular gallop) may be heard with ischaemic heart disease, hyperkinetic states (e.g. anaemia) or restrictive myocardial disease. A pathological S_4 (atrial gallop) towards the left side of the praecordium may be heard with coronary artery disease, hypertensive heart disease, cardiomyopathy and aortic stenosis. A pathological S_4 towards the right side of the praecordium may be heard with pulmonary hypertension and pulmonic stenosis. S_3 and S_4 pathological sounds together create a quadruple rhythm, which is called a *summation gallop.* Opening snaps occur early in diastole and indicate mitral valve stenosis. A friction rub may also be heard during the diastolic pause (see Abnormal findings 22-3).
Auscultate for murmurs. A murmur is a swishing sound caused by turbulent blood flow through the heart valves or great vessels. Auscultate for murmurs across the entire heart area. Use the diaphragm and the bell of the stethoscope in all areas of auscultation because murmurs have a variety of pitches. Also auscultate with the patient in different positions as described below because some murmurs occur or subside according to the patient's position.	Normally no murmurs are heard. However, innocent and physiological midsystolic murmurs may be present in a healthy heart.	Pathological midsystolic, pansystolic and diastolic murmurs. Abnormal findings 22-4 describes pathological murmurs.
Auscultate with the patient assuming other positions. Ask the patient to assume a left lateral position. Use the bell of the stethoscope and listen at the apex of the heart.	S_1 and S_2 heart sounds are normally present.	An S_3 or S_4 heart sound or a murmur of mitral stenosis that was not detected with the patient in the supine position may be revealed when the patient assumes the left lateral position.

PHYSICAL ASSESSMENT (continued)

ASSESSMENT PROCEDURE	NORMAL FINDINGS	ABNORMAL FINDINGS
Heart (praecordium) (continued)		
Ask the patient to sit up, lean forwards and exhale. Use the diaphragm of the stethoscope and listen over the apex and along the left sternal border (Fig. 22-12).	S_1 and S_2 heart sounds are normally present. 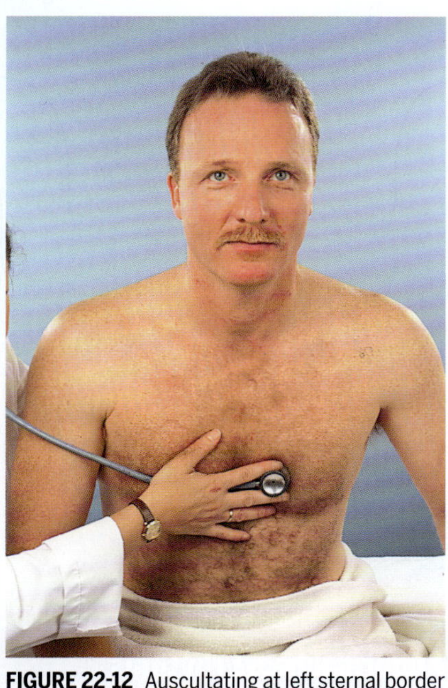 **FIGURE 22-12** Auscultating at left sternal border with patient sitting up, leaning forwards and exhaling. (© B. Proud.)	Murmur of aortic regurgitation may be detected when the patient assumes this position.

ABNORMAL FINDINGS 22-1 Ventricular impulses

Assessment of the chest may reveal abnormalities or variations of the ventricular impulse, signs of hypertension, hypertrophy, volume overload and pressure overload. Some of the abnormalities or variations include the following.

LIFT

A lift or heave appears as a diffuse 'lifting' at the left lower sternal border during systole; this is associated with right ventricular hypertrophy caused by pulmonic valve disease, pulmonic hypertension and chronic lung disease. When a lift or a heave is present, it is not uncommon to also see retraction at the apex which results from posterior rotation of the left ventricle due to an oversized right ventricle.

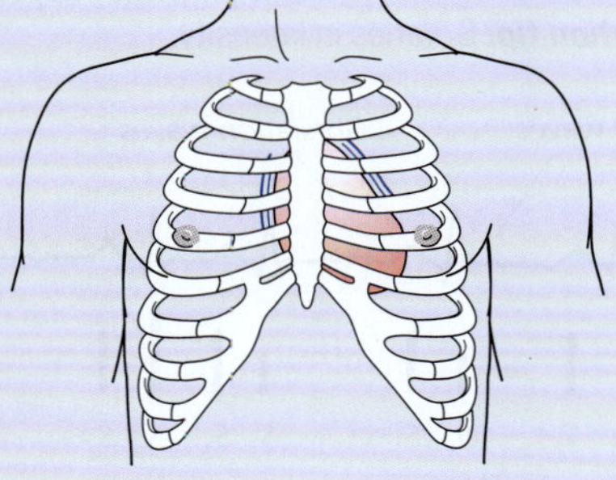

THRILL

A thrill is palpated over the second and third intercostal space; a thrill may indicate severe aortic stenosis and systemic hypertension. A thrill palpated over the second and third left intercostal spaces may indicate pulmonic stenosis and pulmonic hypertension.

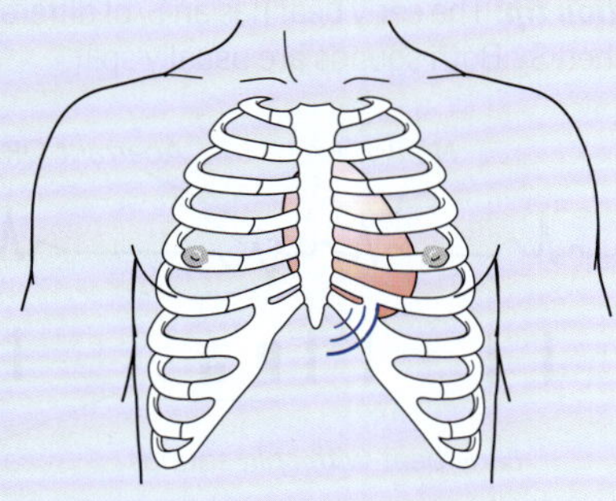

Continued on following page

ABNORMAL FINDINGS 22-1 Ventricular impulses (continued)

ACCENTUATED APICAL IMPULSE

A sign of pressure overload, the accentuated apical impulse has increased force and duration but is not usually displaced in left ventricular hypertrophy without dilation associated with aortic stenosis or systemic hypertension.

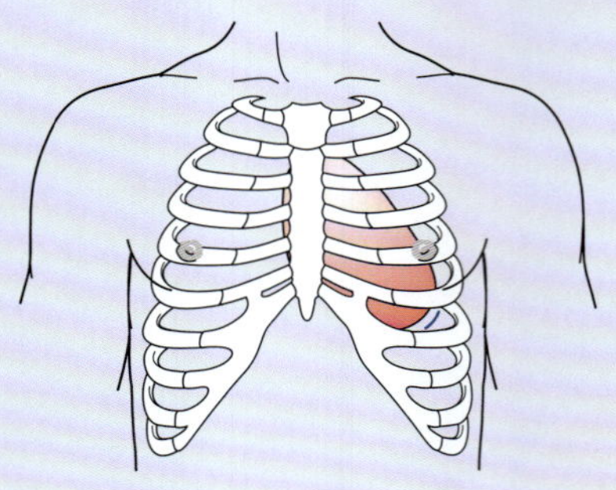

LATERALLY DISPLACED APICAL IMPULSE

A sign of volume overload, an apical impulse displaced laterally and found over a wider area is the result of ventricular hypertrophy and dilation associated with mitral regurgitation, aortic regurgitation or left-to-right shunts.

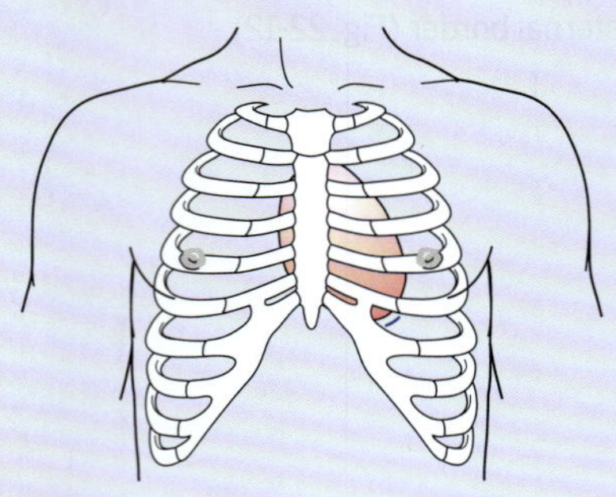

ABNORMAL FINDINGS 22-2 Abnormal heart rhythms

PREMATURE ATRIAL OR JUNCTIONAL CONTRACTIONS

These beats occur earlier than the next expected beat and are followed by a pause. The rhythm resumes with the next beat.

Auscultation tip: The early beat has an S_1 of different intensity and a diminished S_2. S_1 and S_2 are otherwise similar to normal beats.

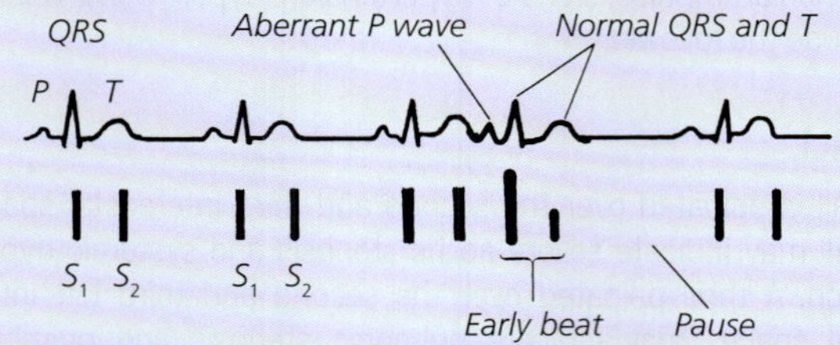

PREMATURE VENTRICULAR CONTRACTIONS

These beats occur earlier than the next expected beat and are followed by a pulse. The rhythm resumes with the next beat.

Auscultation tip: The early beat has an S_1 of different intensity and a diminished S_2. Both sounds are usually split.

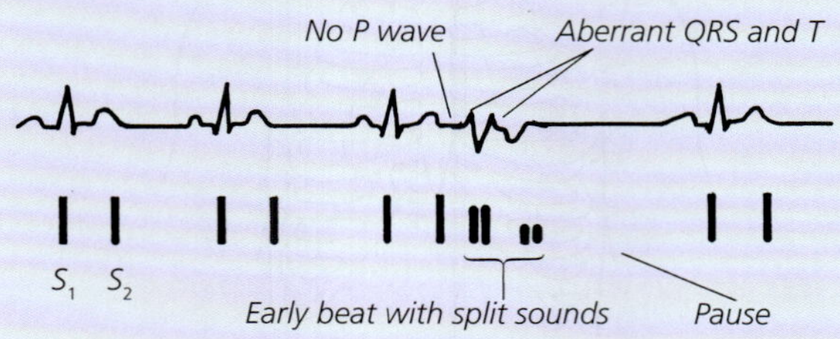

SINUS ARRHYTHMIA

With this dysrhythmia, the heart rate speeds up and slows down in a cycle, usually becoming faster with inhalation and slower with expiration.

Auscultation tip: S_1 and S_2 sounds are usually normal. The S_1 may vary with the heart rate.

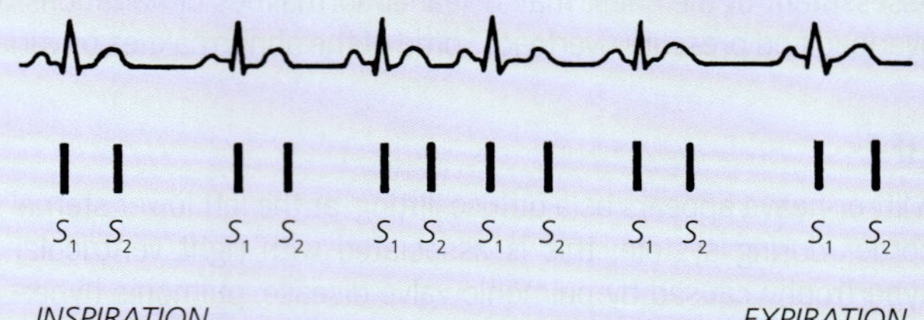

ATRIAL FIBRILLATION AND ATRIAL FLUTTER WITH VARYING VENTRICULAR RESPONSE

With this dysrhythmia, ventricular contraction occurs irregularly. At times, short runs of the irregular rhythm may appear regularly.

Auscultation tip: S_1 varies in intensity.

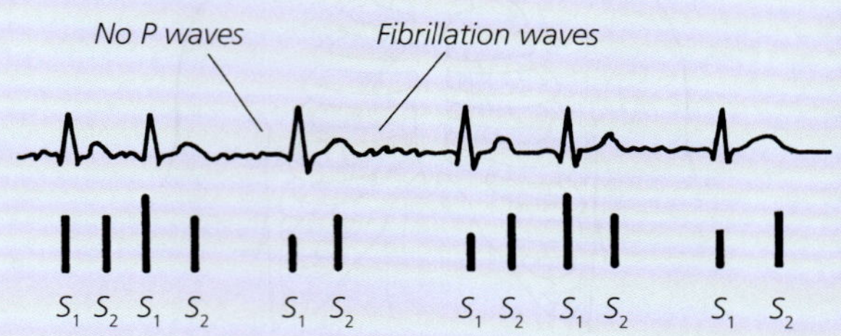

ABNORMAL FINDINGS 22-3 Extra heart sounds

Additional heart sounds can be classified by their timing in the cardiac cycle. The presence of the sound during systole or diastole helps in its identification. Some sounds extend into both systole and diastole.

EXTRA HEART SOUNDS DURING SYSTOLE—CLICKS

High-frequency sounds heard just after S_1 (ejection clicks) are produced by a functioning but diseased valve. Clicks can occur in early or mid-to-late systole and are best heard through the diaphragm of the stethoscope.

Aortic ejection click

Heard during early systole at the second right intercostal space and apex, the aortic ejection click occurs with the opening of the aortic valve and does not change with respiration.

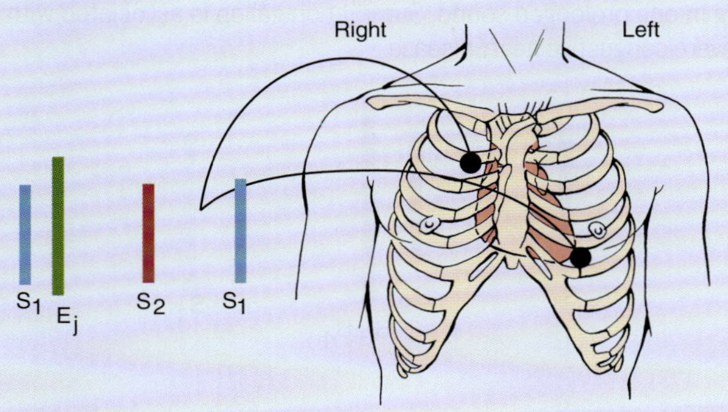

Pulmonic ejection click

Best heard at the second left intercostal space during early systole, the pulmonic ejection click often becomes softer with inspiration.

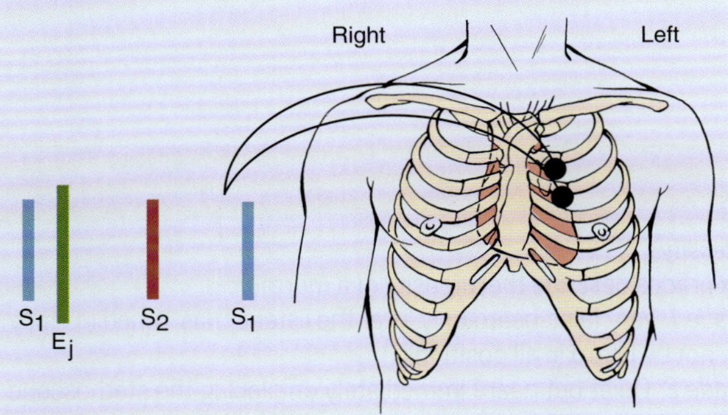

Midsystolic click

Heard in middle or late systole, a midsystolic click can be heard over the mitral or apical area and is the result of mitral valve leaflet prolapse during left ventricular emptying. A late systolic murmur typically follows, indicating mild mitral regurgitation.

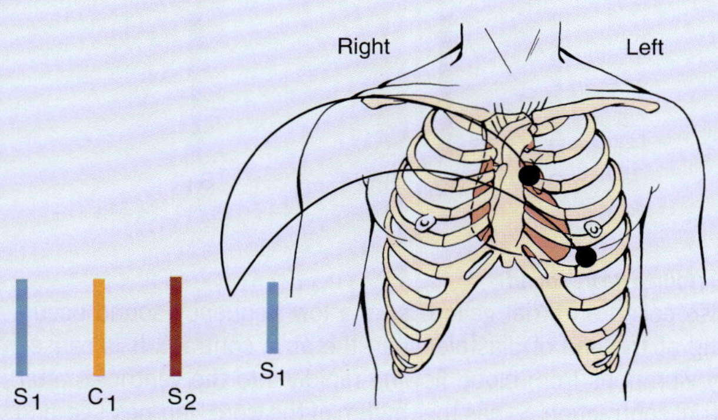

EXTRA HEART SOUNDS DURING DIASTOLE

Opening snap

Occurring in early diastole, an opening snap is heard with the opening of a stenotic or stiff mitral valve. Heard throughout the whole praecordium, it does not vary with respirations. Often mistaken for a split S_2 or an S_3, the opening snap occurs earlier in diastole and has a higher pitch than an S_3.

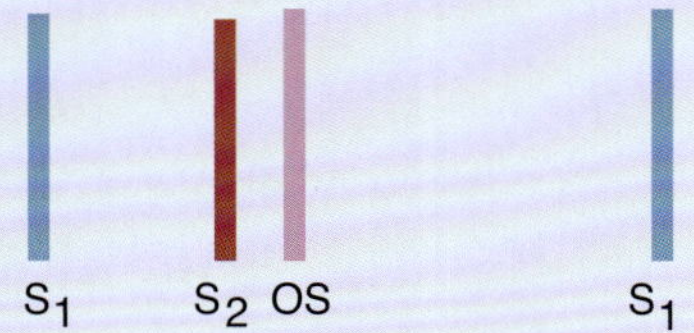

S_3 (third heart sound)

Also called a ventricular gallop, the S_3 has a low frequency and is heard best using the bell of the stethoscope at the apical area or lower right ventricular area of the chest with the patient in the left lateral position. The sound is often accentuated during inspiration and has the rhythm of the word 'Ken-tuc-ky'. S_3 is the result of vibrations caused by the blood hitting the ventricular wall during rapid ventricular filling.

Continued on following page

ABNORMAL FINDINGS 22-3 Extra heart sounds (continued)

The S_3 can be a normal finding in young children, people with a high cardiac output and the third trimester of pregnancy. It is rarely normal in people older than age 40 years and is usually associated with decreased myocardial contractility, myocardial failure, congestive heart failure and volume overload of the ventricle from valvular disease.

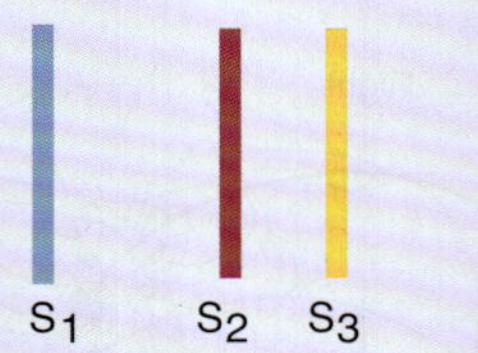

S_4 (fourth heart sound)

Also called an atrial gallop, S_4 is a low-frequency sound occurring at the end of diastole when the atria contract. It is caused by vibrations from blood flowing rapidly into the ventricles after atrial contraction. S_4 has the rhythm of the word 'Ten-nes-see' and may increase during inspiration. It is best heard with the bell of the stethoscope over the apical area with the patient in a supine or left lateral position and is never heard in the absence of atrial contraction.

The S_4 can be a normal sound in trained athletes and some older patients, especially after exercise. However, it is usually an abnormal finding and is associated with coronary artery disease, hypertension, aortic and pulmonic stenosis, and acute myocardial infarction.

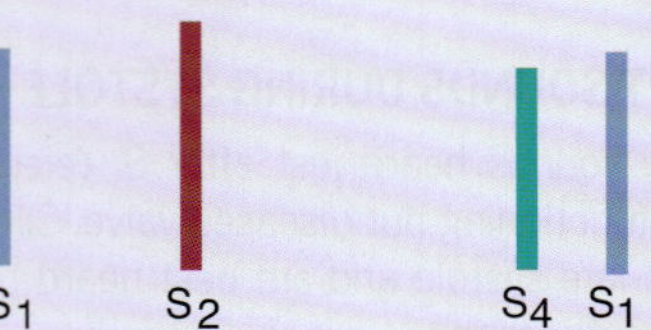

Summation gallop

The simultaneous occurrence of S_3 and S_4 is called a summation gallop. It is brought about by rapid heart rates in which diastolic filling time is shortened, moving S_3 and S_4 closer together, resulting in one prolonged sound. Summation gallop is associated with severe congestive heart disease.

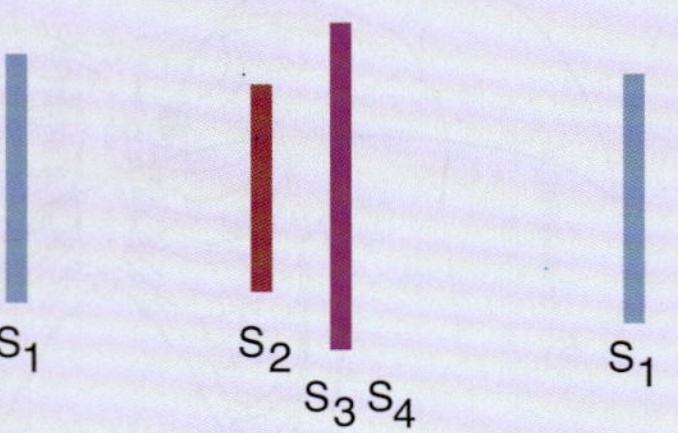

ABNORMAL FINDINGS 22-4 Heart murmurs

Heart murmurs are typically characterised by turbulent blood flow, which creates a swooshing or blowing sound over the praecordium. When listening to the heart, be alert for this turbulence and keep the characteristics of heart murmurs in mind.

CHARACTERISTICS

Heart murmurs are assessed according to various characteristics, which include timing, intensity, pitch, quality, shape or pattern, location, transmission, and ventilation and position.

Timing

A murmur can occur during systole or diastole. In addition to determining when it occurs, it is important to determine where it occurs, because a systolic murmur can be present in a healthy heart, whereas a diastolic murmur always indicates heart disease. Systolic murmurs can be divided into three categories: midsystolic, pansystolic and late systolic. Diastolic murmurs can be divided into three categories: early diastolic, mid-diastolic and late diastolic.

Intensity

Six grades describe the intensity of a murmur:

Grade 1: Very faint, heard only after the listener has 'tuned in'; may not be heard in all positions

Grade 2: Quiet but heard immediately on placing the stethoscope on the chest

Grade 3: Moderately loud

Grade 4: Loud

Grade 5: Very loud, may be heard with a stethoscope partly off the chest

Grade 6: May be heard with the stethoscope entirely off the chest.

Pitch

Murmurs can assume a high, medium or low pitch.

Quality

The sound murmurs make has been described as blowing, rushing, roaring, rumbling, harsh or musical.

ABNORMAL FINDINGS 22-4 Heart murmurs (continued)

Shape or pattern

The shape of a murmur is determined by its intensity from beginning to end. There are four different categories of shape: crescendo (growing louder), decrescendo (growing softer), crescendo–decrescendo (growing louder and then growing softer) and plateau (staying the same throughout).

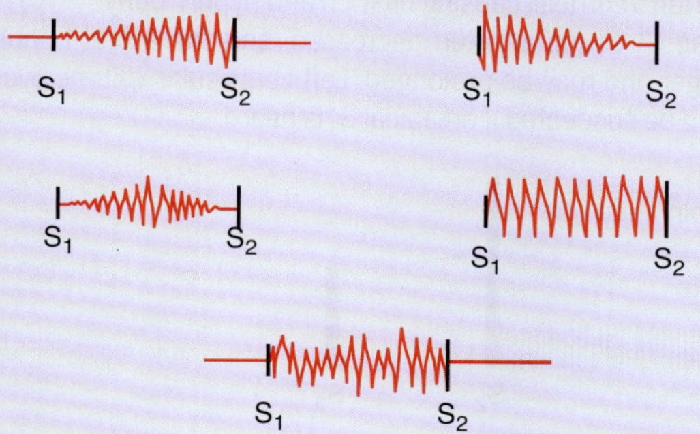

Location

Determine where you can best hear the murmur; this is the point where the murmur originates. Try to be as exact as possible in describing its location. Use the heart landmarks in your description (e.g. the second intercostal space at the left sternal border).

Transmission

The murmur may be felt in areas other than the point of origination. If you determine where the murmur transmits, you can determine the direction of blood flow and the intensity of the murmur.

Ventilation and position

Determine if the murmur is affected by inspiration, expiration or a change in body position.

MIDSYSTOLIC MURMURS

The most common type of heart murmurs, midsystolic murmurs occur during ventricular ejection and can be innocent, physiological or pathological. They have a crescendo–decrescendo shape and usually peak near midsystole and stop before S_2.

Innocent murmur

Not associated with any physical abnormality, innocent murmurs occur when the ejection of blood into the aorta is turbulent. Very common in children and young adults, they may also be heard in older people with no evidence of cardiovascular disease. A patient may have an innocent murmur and another kind of murmur.

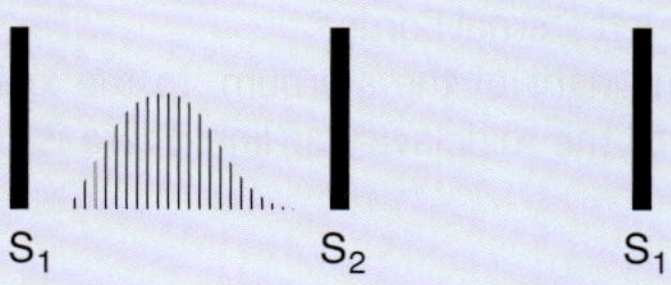

Location: Second to fourth left intercostal spaces between the left sternal border and the apex
Radiation: Little radiation
Intensity: Grade 1 to 2
Pitch: Medium
Quality: Variable
Position: Usually disappear when the patient sits

Physiological murmur

Caused by a temporary increase in blood flow, a physiological murmur can occur with anaemia, pregnancy, fever and hyperthyroidism.

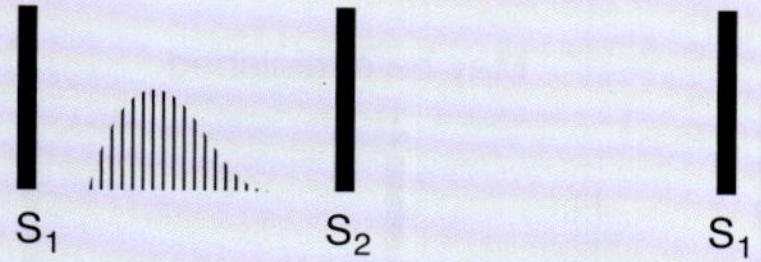

Location: Second to fourth left intercostal spaces between the left sternal border and the apex
Radiation: Little radiation
Intensity: Grade 1 to 2
Pitch: Medium
Quality: Harsh

Murmur of pulmonic stenosis

A pathological murmur, the murmur of pulmonic stenosis occurs from impeded flow across the pulmonic valve and increased right ventricular afterload. Often occurring as a congenital anomaly, the murmur is commonly found in children. Pathological changes in flow across the valve, as in atrial septal defect, may also mimic this condition.

With severe pulmonic stenosis, the S_2 is widely split and P_2 is diminished. An early pulmonic ejection sound is also common. A right-sided S_4 may also be present, and the right ventricular impulse is often stronger and may be prolonged.

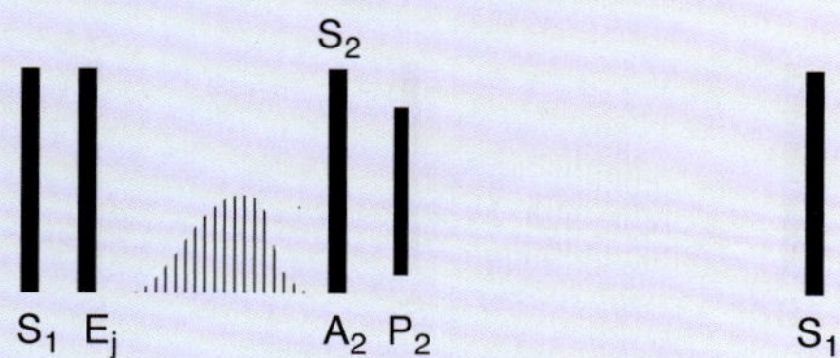

Location: Second and third intercostal spaces
Radiation: Towards the left shoulder and neck
Intensity: Soft to loud (may be associated with a thrill if loud)
Pitch: Medium
Quality: Harsh
Position: Loudest during inspiration

Continued on following page

ABNORMAL FINDINGS 22-4 Heart murmurs (continued)

Murmur of aortic stenosis

The murmur of aortic stenosis occurs when stenosis of the aortic valve impedes blood flow across the valve and increases left ventricular afterload. Aortic stenosis may result from a congenital anomaly, rheumatic disease or a degenerative process. Conditions that may mimic this murmur include aortic sclerosis, a bicuspid aortic valve, a dilated aorta or any condition that mimics the flow across the valve, such as aortic regurgitation.

If valvular disease is severe, A_2 may be delayed, resulting in an unsplit S_2 or a paradoxical split S_2. An S_4 may occur as a result of decreased left ventricular compliance. An aortic ejection sound, if present, suggests a congenital cause.

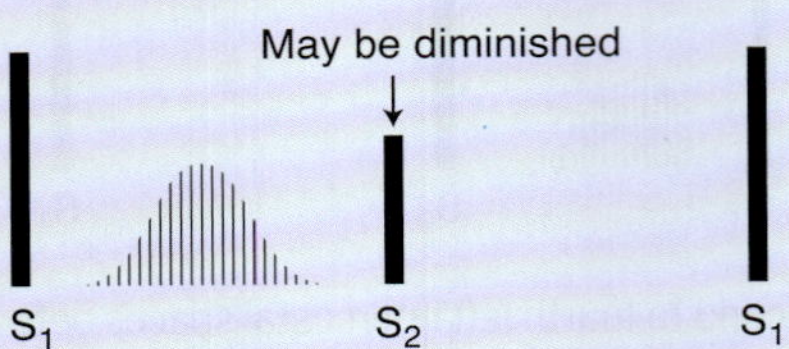

Location: Right second intercostal space
Radiation: May radiate to the neck and down the left sternal border to the apex
Intensity: Usually loud, with a thrill
Pitch: Medium
Quality: Harsh, may be musical at the apex
Position: Heard best with the patient sitting and leaning forwards, loudest during expiration

Murmur of hypertrophic cardiomyopathy

Caused by unusually rapid ejection of blood from the left ventricle during systole, the murmur of cardiac hypertrophy results from massive hypertrophy of the ventricular muscle. There may be a coexisting obstruction to blood flow. If there is an accompanying distortion of the mitral valve, mitral regurgitation may result. The patient may also have an S_3 and an S_4. There may be a sustained apical impulse with two palpable components.

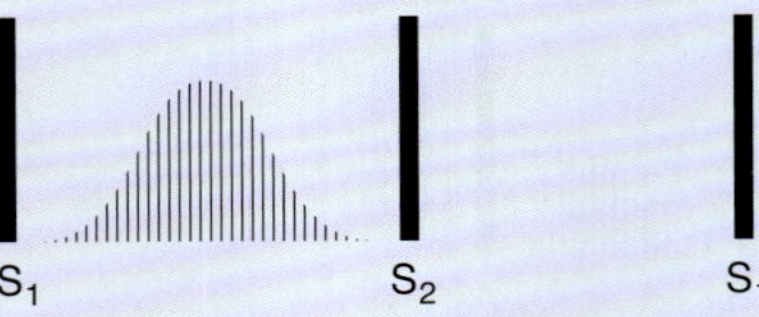

Location: Third and fourth left intercostal space, decreases with squatting, increases with straining down
Intensity: Variable
Pitch: Medium
Quality: Harsh

PANSYSTOLIC MURMURS

Occurring when blood flows from a chamber with high pressure to a chamber of low pressure through an orifice that should be closed, pansystolic murmurs are pathological. Also called *holosystolic murmurs*, these murmurs begin with S_1 and continue through systole to S_2.

Murmur of mitral regurgitation

Occurring when the mitral valve fails to close fully in systole, the murmur of mitral regurgitation is the result of blood flowing from the left ventricle back into the left atrium. Volume overload occurs in the left ventricle, causing dilation and hypertrophy.

The S_3 sound is often decreased, and the apical impulse is stronger and may be prolonged. Left ventricular volume overload should be suspected if an apical S_3 is heard.

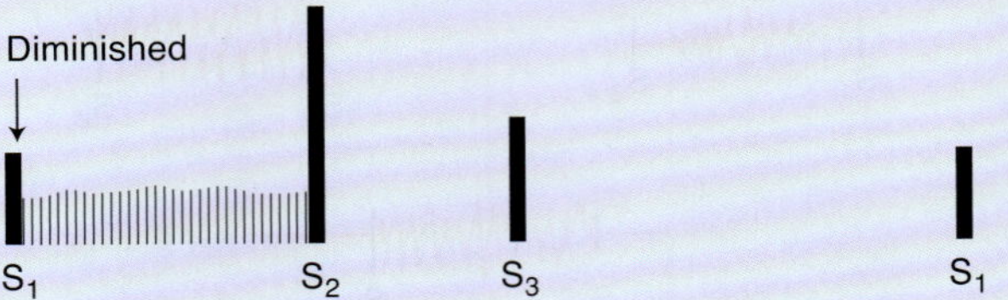

Location: Apex
Radiation: To the left axilla, less often to the left sternal border
Intensity: Soft to loud, an apical thrill is associated with loud murmurs
Pitch: Medium to high
Quality: Blowing
Position: Heard best with patient in the left lateral decubitus position; does not become louder with inspiration

Murmur of tricuspid regurgitation

Blood flowing from the right ventricle back into the right atrium over a tricuspid valve that has not fully closed causes the murmur of tricuspid regurgitation. Right ventricular failure with dilation is the most common cause and usually results from pulmonary hypertension or left ventricular failure.

With this murmur, the right ventricular impulse is stronger and may be prolonged. There may be an S_3 along the lower left sternal border and the jugular venous pressure is often elevated with visible *v* waves.

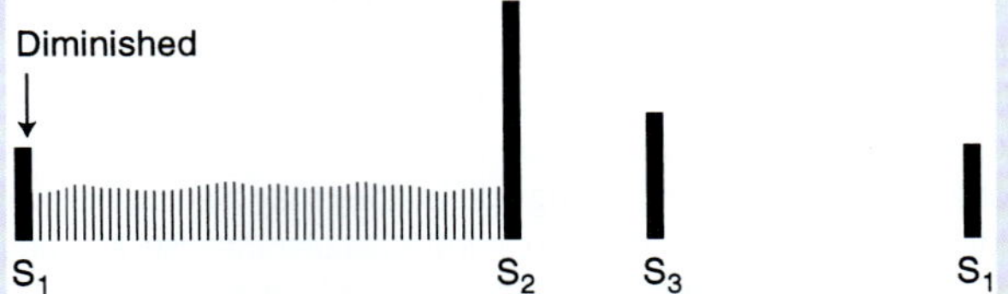

Location: Lower left sternal border
Radiation: To the right of the sternum, to the xiphoid area and sometimes to the midclavicular line; there is no radiation to the axilla
Intensity: Variable
Pitch: Medium to high
Quality: Blowing
Position: May increase slightly with inspiration

ABNORMAL FINDINGS 22-4 Heart murmurs (continued)

Ventricular septal defect

A congenital abnormality in which blood flows from the left ventricle into the right ventricle through a hole in the septum, a ventricular septal defect causes a loud murmur that obscures the A_2 sound. Other findings vary depending on the severity of the defect and any associated lesions.

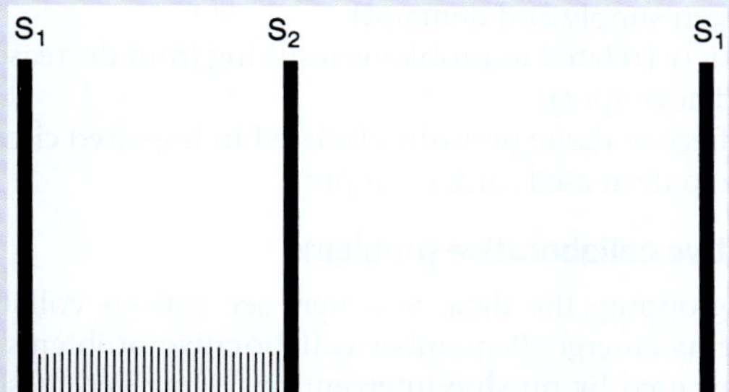

Location: Third, fourth and fifth left intercostal space
Radiation: Often wide
Intensity: Very loud, with a thrill
Pitch: High
Quality: Harsh
Position: Increase with exercise

DIASTOLIC MURMURS

Usually indicative of heart disease, diastolic murmurs occur in two types. Early decrescendo diastolic murmurs indicate flow through an incompetent semilunar valve, commonly the aortic valve. Rumbling diastolic murmurs in mid- or late diastole indicate valve stenosis, usually of the mitral valve.

Aortic regurgitation

Occurring when the leaflets of the aortic valve fail to close completely, the murmur of aortic regurgitation is the result of blood flowing from the aorta back into the left ventricle. This results in left ventricular volume overload. An ejection sound may also be present. Severe regurgitation should be suspected if an S_3 or S_4 is also present. The apical impulse becomes displaced downwards and laterally with a widened diameter and increased duration. As the pulse pressure increases, the arterial pulses are often large and bounding.

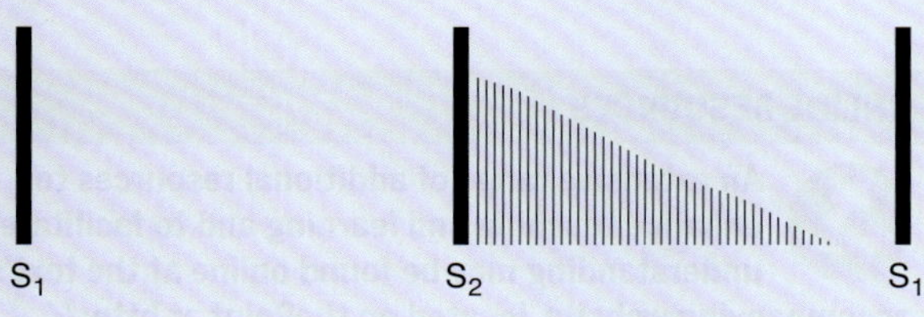

Location: Second to fourth left intercostal space
Radiation: May radiate to the apex or left sternal border
Intensity: Grade 1 to 3
Pitch: High
Quality: Blowing, sometime mistaken for breath sounds
Position: Heard best with the patient sitting, leaning forwards. Have the patient exhale and then hold his or her breath.

Murmur of mitral stenosis

The murmur of mitral stenosis is the result of blood flow across a diseased mitral valve. Thickened, stiff, distorted leaflets are usually the result of rheumatic fever. The murmur is loud during mid-diastole as the ventricle fills rapidly, grows quiet and becomes loud again immediately before systole, as the atria contract. In patients with atrial fibrillation, the second half of the murmur is absent because of the lack of atrial contraction.

The patient also has a loud S_1, which may be palpable at the apex. There is often an opening snap after S_2. P_2 becomes loud and the right ventricular impulse becomes palpable if pulmonary hypertension develops.

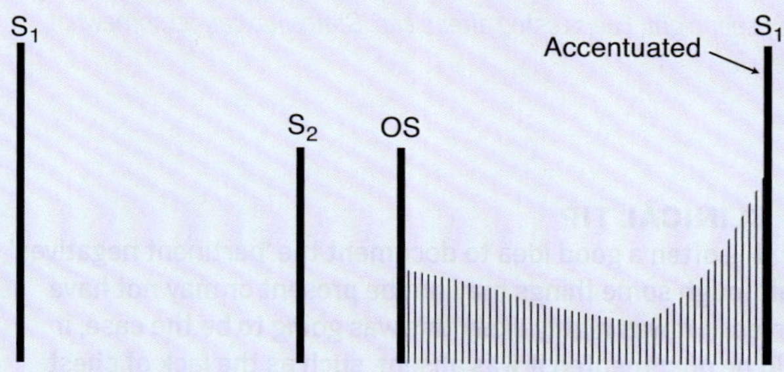

Location: Apex
Radiation: Little or none
Intensity: Grade 1 to 4
Pitch: Low
Quality: Rumbling
Position: Best heard with the bell exactly on the apex and the patient turned to a left lateral position. Mild exercise and listening during exhalation also make the murmur easier to hear.

Continued on following page

VALIDATING AND DOCUMENTING FINDINGS

Validate the heart and neck vessel assessment data that you have collected. This is necessary to verify that the data are reliable and accurate. Document the assessment data following the health care facility policy.

After you have collected your assessment data, you will need to analyse these data using diagnostic reasoning skills. Refer to the discussion of the diagnostic reasoning process in Chapter 5.

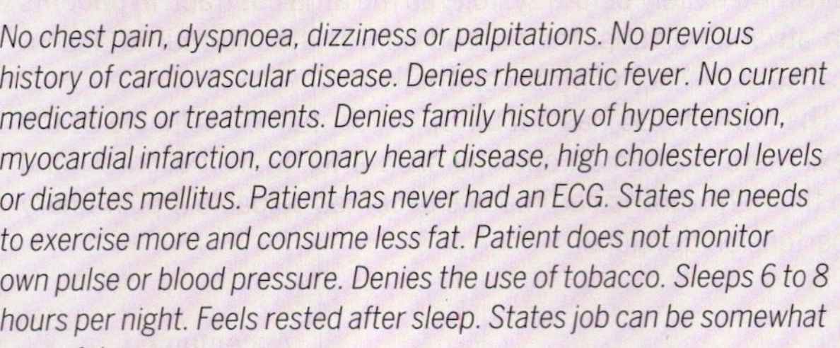

Sample of subjective data

No chest pain, dyspnoea, dizziness or palpitations. No previous history of cardiovascular disease. Denies rheumatic fever. No current medications or treatments. Denies family history of hypertension, myocardial infarction, coronary heart disease, high cholesterol levels or diabetes mellitus. Patient has never had an ECG. States he needs to exercise more and consume less fat. Patient does not monitor own pulse or blood pressure. Denies the use of tobacco. Sleeps 6 to 8 hours per night. Feels rested after sleep. States job can be somewhat stressful.

CLINICAL TIP

It is often a good idea to document the 'pertinent negatives' (i.e. although some things may not be present or may not have occurred, if it was highly likely this was going to be the case, it should be documented it was absent, such as the lack of chest pain, dyspnoea, dizziness or palpitations identified in the above sample subjective data.)

Sample of objective data

Carotid pulse equal bilaterally, 2+, elastic. No bruits auscultated over carotids. Jugular venous pulsation disappears when upright. JVP 2 cm—right internal jugular vein, patient 30 degrees, measured from sternal notch. No visible pulsations, heaves or lifts on praecordium. Heart rate auscultated, 70 beats/minute, regular rhythm; S_1 *heard best at apex;* S_2 *heard best at base. No* S_3 *or* S_4 *auscultated. No splitting of heart sounds, snaps, clicks or murmurs noted.*

Analysis of data

DIAGNOSTIC REASONING: POSSIBLE CONCLUSIONS

After collecting subjective and objective data pertaining to the heart and neck vessels, identify abnormal findings and patient strengths; cluster all data to reveal any significant patterns or abnormalities. These data may be used to make clinical judgements about the status of the patient's heart and neck vessels.

Potential patient risks

- Sexual dysfunction (related to misinformation or lack of knowledge regarding sexual activity and heart disease)

Potential patient problems

- Fatigue (related to decreased cardiac output)
- Activity intolerance (related to compromised oxygen transport secondary to heart failure)
- Acute cardiac pain (related to an inequality between oxygen supply and demand)
- Anxiety (related to problems resulting from decreased cardiac output)
- Ineffective tissue perfusion (related to impaired circulation due to decreased cardiac output)

Selective collaborative problems

After grouping the data, you may see various collaborative problems emerge. Remember collaborative problems cannot be prevented by nursing interventions. However, these physiological complications of medical conditions can be detected and monitored by the nurse. In addition, the nurse can use doctor- and nurse-prescribed interventions to minimise the complications of these problems. The nurse may also have to refer the patient in such situations for further treatment of the problem. The following is a list of collaborative problems that may be identified when assessing the heart and neck vessels:

- Decreased cardiac output
- Dysrhythmias
- Hypertension
- Congestive heart failure
- Angina
- Cerebrovascular accident
- Cerebral haemorrhage
- Renal failure.

Medical problems

Once the data are grouped, certain signs and symptoms may become evident and may require medical diagnosis and treatment. Notification of medical staff is required.

ONLINE RESOURCES

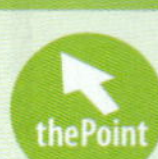

An extensive range of additional resources to enhance teaching and learning and to facilitate understanding may be found online at the text's accompanying website, located on thePoint at http://thepoint.lww.com. These include Watch and Learn videos, Concepts in Action animations, journal articles, case studies, discussion topics and quizzes.

Subscribers may also access Lippincott Procedures, an extensive online point-of-care procedure guide that provides reliable step-by-step instructions for more than 1700 procedures, including 450 evidence-based Australian procedures, and skills in a variety of speciality settings, together with a wealth of supporting information.

SIMULATED LEARNING

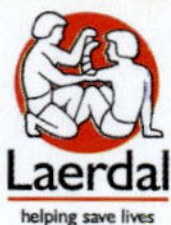

Having completed this chapter, explore the scenarios of Carl Shapiro Part 1 and Part 2. Carl is a 54-year-old male presenting to the emergency department with a myocardial infarction. Incorporating the health assessment content in this chapter with your existing theoretical knowledge and clinical experience, progress through the simulation scenarios (this is best done in a small group). How would you manage Carl's care? When reflecting on your management of Carl, what do you think you did well and what do you think you can improve? Consider why you think this and also how you might manage a similar problem in the future.

CASE STUDY

The case study demonstrates how to analyse heart and neck vessels assessment data for a specific patient. The exercises included in the ancillary product on thePoint that complements this text offer further opportunities to enhance your skills.

Malcolm Winchester is being admitted to the coronary care unit with a diagnosis of hypertension and angina. He is a tall, slender Caucasian man who looks younger than his stated age of 45. He appears to be in no acute distress. Mr Winchester says, 'I don't know why they brought me here—I guess my wife panicked and called 000. I have these pains all the time, but my doctor says they're from my high blood pressure. I'm not in any pain now.'

Mr Winchester's wife arrives, looking pale and anxious. 'I don't know what to do with him. I work so hard to keep him healthy, but he goes out to that fast food place and eats hamburgers and chips. I'm so tired of dealing with him when he won't help himself.' Mr Winchester grins and says, 'That low-fat, low-salt diet my doctor put me on is impossible. There's nothing wrong with a little bit of indulgence every now and again.'

Physical assessment reveals a blood pressure of 210/110 mmHg right arm reclining and 200/108 mmHg left arm reclining; a pulse of 88 beats/minute, regular and strong; a respiratory rate of 16 breaths/minute, regular and moderately shallow; and a temperature of 36.5 °C. His carotid pulse is also 88 beats/minute and strong; heart sounds: S_1 and S_2 with no murmurs and clicks, but an S_4 is noted. Evaluation of the thorax reveals no heaves or visible pulsation. Neck veins are flat at more than 45 degrees, and no carotid bruits are noted. Skin is warm and dry, with pink nail beds. Pedal pulses are strong; 1+ ankle oedema is present.

The following concept map illustrates the diagnostic reasoning process.

Applying COLDSPA

Applying COLDSPA for patient symptoms: 'high blood pressure/chest pain'.

Mnemonic	Question	Data provided	Missing data
Character	Describe the sign or symptom (feeling, appearance, sound, smell or taste, if applicable).	'I have these pains all the time; I'm not in any pain now.'	Describe how the pains feel to you.
Onset	When did it begin?		When did the chest pain first start this time?
Location	Where is it? Does it radiate? Does it occur anywhere else?		Point to where the pain was. Does it spread down your arm? To your back? Anywhere else?
Duration	How long does it last? Does it recur?		How long does the pain last when it occurs? How often does the pain recur?
Severity	How bad is it? or How much does it bother you?		Describe the intensity of the pain on a scale of 1 to 10 with 10 being the worst possible.
Pattern	What makes it better or worse?		What makes the chest pain come and go?
Associated factors/How it Affects the patient	What other symptoms occur with it? How does it affect you?	'My doctor said these pains were from my high blood pressure.'	When you have the chest pain, does it affect what you are doing?

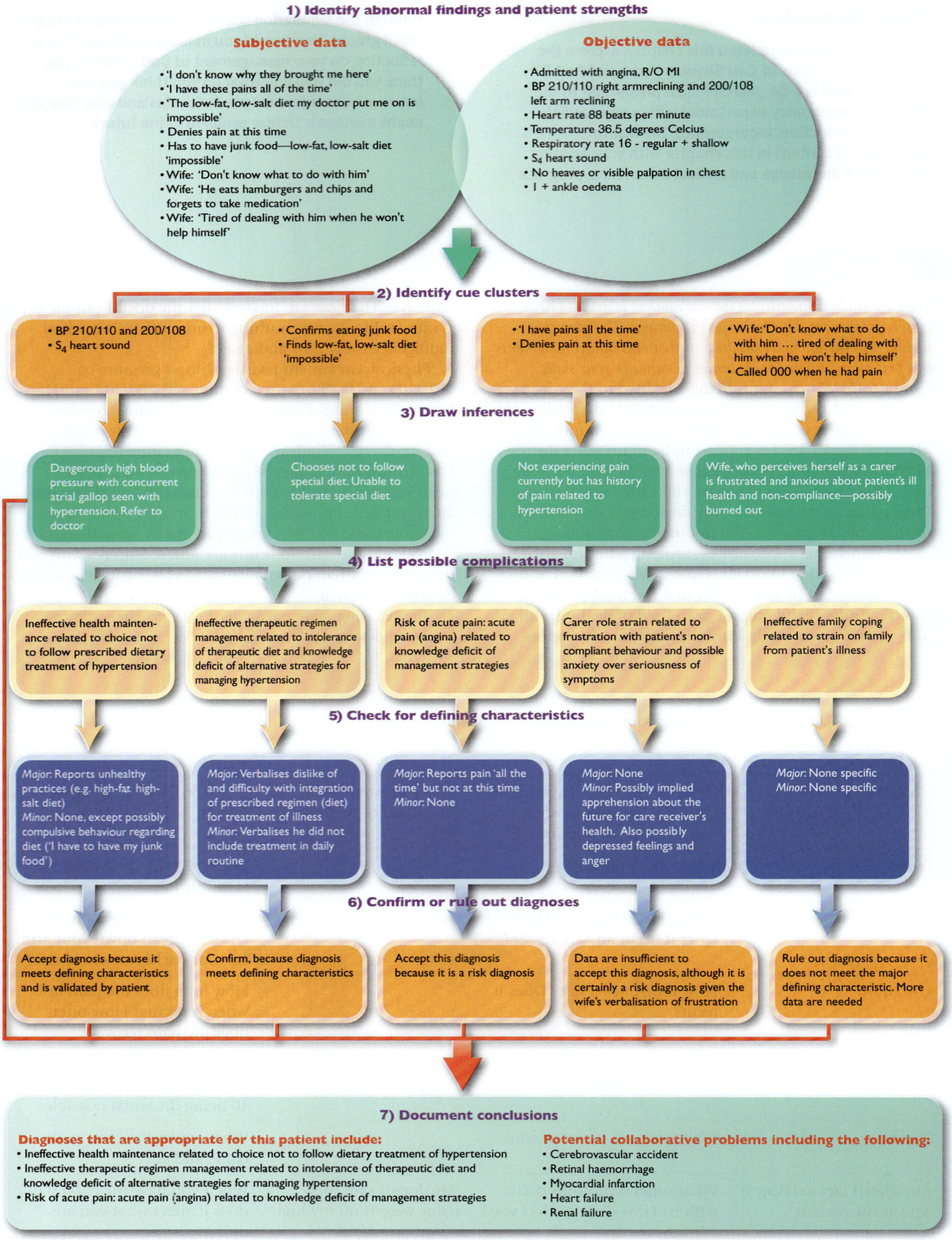

1) Identify abnormal findings and patient strengths

Subjective data

- 'I don't know why they brought me here'
- 'I have these pains all of the time'
- 'The low-fat, low-salt diet my doctor put me on is impossible'
- Denies pain at this time
- Has to have junk food—low-fat, low-salt diet 'impossible'
- Wife: 'Don't know what to do with him'
- Wife: 'He eats hamburgers and chips and forgets to take medication'
- Wife: 'Tired of dealing with him when he won't help himself'

Objective data

- Admitted with angina, R/O MI
- BP 210/110 right armreclining and 200/108 left arm reclining
- Heart rate 88 beats per minute
- Temperature 36.5 degrees Celcius
- Respiratory rate 16 - regular + shallow
- S_4 heart sound
- No heaves or visible palpation in chest
- 1 + ankle oedema

2) Identify cue clusters

- BP 210/110 and 200/108
- S_4 heart sound

- Confirms eating junk food
- Finds low-fat, low-salt diet 'impossible'

- 'I have pains all the time'
- Denies pain at this time

- Wife: 'Don't know what to do with him … tired of dealing with him when he won't help himself'
- Called 000 when he had pain

3) Draw inferences

Dangerously high blood pressure with concurrent atrial gallop seen with hypertension. Refer to doctor

Chooses not to follow special diet. Unable to tolerate special diet

Not experiencing pain currently but has history of pain related to hypertension

Wife, who perceives herself as a carer is frustrated and anxious about patient's ill health and non-compliance—possibly burned out

4) List possible complications

Ineffective health maintenance related to choice not to follow prescribed dietary treatment of hypertension

Ineffective therapeutic regimen management related to intolerance of therapeutic diet and knowledge deficit of alternative strategies for managing hypertension

Risk of acute pain: acute pain (angina) related to knowledge deficit of management strategies

Carer role strain related to frustration with patient's non-compliant behaviour and possible anxiety over seriousness of symptoms

Ineffective family coping related to strain on family from patient's illness

5) Check for defining characteristics

Major: Reports unhealthy practices (e.g. high-fat high-salt diet)
Minor: None, except possibly compulsive behaviour regarding diet ('I have to have my junk food')

Major: Verbalises dislike of and difficulty with integration of prescribed regimen (diet) for treatment of illness
Minor: Verbalises he did not include treatment in daily routine

Major: Reports pain 'all the time' but not at this time
Minor: None

Major: None
Minor: Possibly implied apprehension about the future for care receiver's health. Also possibly depressed feelings and anger

Major: None specific
Minor: None specific

6) Confirm or rule out diagnoses

Accept diagnosis because it meets defining characteristics and is validated by patient

Confirm, because diagnosis meets defining characteristics

Accept this diagnosis because it is a risk diagnosis

Data are insufficient to accept this diagnosis, although it is certainly a risk diagnosis given the wife's verbalisation of frustration

Rule out diagnosis because it does not meet the major defining characteristic. More data are needed

7) Document conclusions

Diagnoses that are appropriate for this patient include:

- Ineffective health maintenance related to choice not to follow dietary treatment of hypertension
- Ineffective therapeutic regimen management related to intolerance of therapeutic diet and knowledge deficit of alternative strategies for managing hypertension
- Risk of acute pain: acute pain (angina) related to knowledge deficit of management strategies

Potential collaborative problems including the following:

- Cerebrovascular accident
- Retinal haemorrhage
- Myocardial infarction
- Heart failure
- Renal failure

References

American Heart Association (AHA). (2015). Coronary artery disease: Coronary heart disease. Viewed September 2019 at https://www.heart.org/en/health-topics/consumer-healthcare/what-is-cardiovascular-disease/coronary-artery-disease.

American Heart Association (AHA). (2017). Know your risk factors for high blood pressure. Viewed September 2019 at https://www.heart.org/en/health-topics/high-blood-pressure/why-high-blood-pressure-is-a-silent-killer/know-your-risk-factors-for-high-blood-pressure.

Australian Institute of Health and Welfare (AIHW). (2016). Australia's Health 2016. Viewed September 2019 at https://www.aihw.gov.au/getmedia/2a44d779-bff1-4302-b129-f515e7b07842/ah16-3-5-coronary-heart-disease.pdf.aspx.

Cohen, B. J. & Hull, K. L. (2015). *Memmler's structure and function of the human body* (11th ed.). Philadelphia: Lippincott Williams & Wilkins.

Harvard Health Publishing—Harvard Medical School. (2016). The heart attack gender gap. Viewed September 2019 at https://www.health.harvard.edu/heart-health/the-heart-attack-gender-gap.

Joffres, M., Shields, M., Tremblay, M. S., et al. (2013). Dyslipidemia prevalence, treatment, control, and awareness. Canadian Health Measures Survey. *Canadian Journal of Public Health, 104*(3), 252–257.

Mayo Clinic. (2019). Heart-healthy diet: 8 steps to prevent heart disease. Viewed September 2019 at https://www.mayoclinic.org/diseases-conditions/heart-disease/in-depth/heart-healthy-diet/art-20047702.

Ministry of Health. (2018). Cardiovascular disease. Viewed September 2019 at https://www.health.govt.nz/our-work/populations/maori-health/tatau-kahukura-maori-health-statistics/nga-mana-hauora-tutohu-health-status-indicators/cardiovascular-disease.

National Heart Lung and Blood Institute. (2019). Ischemic heart disease. Viewed September 2019 at https://www.nhlbi.nih.gov/health-topics/ischemic-heart-disease.

World Health Organization (WHO). (2017). Cardiovascular diseases (CVDs). Viewed September 2019 at https://www.who.int/en/news-room/fact-sheets/detail/cardiovascular-diseases-(cvds).

Selected readings

Farrell, M. (Ed). (2016). *Smeltzer & Bare's textbook of medical-surgical nursing* (4th Australian & New Zealand ed.). Sydney: Lippincott Williams & Wilkins.

Hill, R., Hall, H. & Glew, P. J. (Eds). (2017). *Fundamentals of nursing and midwifery: A person-centred approach to care* (3rd Australian and New Zealand ed.). Sydney: Lippincott Williams & Wilkins.

Online resources

Australian Government's Eat for Health program: www.eatforhealth.gov.au

Australian Institute of Health and Welfare: https://www.aihw.gov.au/reports/heart-stroke-vascular-disease/cardiovascular-health-compendium/contents/how-many-australians-have-cardiovascular-disease

Cardiac Society of Australia and New Zealand: www.csanz.edu.au

Heart Foundation Australia: www.heartfoundation.org.au

Heart Foundation New Zealand: www.heartfoundation.org.nz

Mayo Clinic: https://www.mayoclinic.org/diseases-conditions/heart-disease/symptoms-causes/syc-20353118

New Zealand Ministry of Health: www.health.govt.nz

Nutrition Australia: www.nutritionaustralia.org

World Health Organization (WHO): www.who.int

World Heart Federation: www.worldheart.org

CHAPTER 23

Peripheral vascular system

CASE STUDY

Mr Marcus Andross is 78 years old and lives with his eldest daughter. Mr Andross has a 10-year history of severe chronic pain in his left hip due to osteoarthritis. Overtime his symptoms of joint swelling, decreased range of motion and joint stiffness in his hip have increased, and now he is longer able to mobilise. His doctor recommended a left total hip replacement, and he is now 4 days postoperative following his surgery. He has been assigned to you as one of your patients for the shift.

Structure and function

To perform a thorough peripheral vascular assessment, the nurse needs to understand the structure and function of the arteries and veins of the arms and legs, the lymphatic system and the capillaries. Equally important is an understanding of fluid exchange. The information provided on these pages can help you compile subjective and objective data related to the peripheral vascular system and differentiate normal vascular findings from normal variations and abnormalities.

ARTERIES

Arteries are the blood vessels that carry oxygenated, nutrient-rich blood from the heart to the capillaries. The arterial network is a high-pressure system. Blood is propelled under pressure from the left ventricle of the heart. Because of this high pressure, the arterial walls must be thick and strong; the arterial walls also contain elastic fibres so they can stretch. Figure 23-1 illustrates the layers and the relative thickness of the arterial walls. Each heartbeat forces blood through the arterial vessels under high pressure, creating a surge. This surge of blood is the arterial pulse. The pulse can be felt only by lightly compressing a superficial artery against an underlying bone. Many arteries are located in protected areas, far from the surface of the skin. Therefore, the arteries discussed in this chapter include only the major arteries of the arms and legs—the peripheral arteries—that are accessible to examination. The other major arteries accessible to examination—the temporal, carotid and aorta—are discussed in Chapters 16, 22 and 24, respectively.

Major arteries of the arm

The brachial artery is the major artery that supplies the arm. The brachial pulse can be palpated medial to the biceps tendon in and above the bend of the elbow. The brachial artery divides near the elbow to become the radial artery (extending down the thumb side of the arm) and the ulnar artery (extending down the little finger side of the arm). Both of these arteries provide blood to the hand. The radial pulse can be palpated on the lateral aspect of the wrist. The ulnar pulse, located on the medial aspect of the wrist, is a deeper pulse and may not be easily palpated. The radial and ulnar arteries join to form two arches just below their pulse sites. The superficial and deep palmar arches provide extra protection against arterial occlusion to the hands and fingers (Fig. 23-2).

Major arteries of the leg

The femoral artery is the major supplier of blood to the legs. Its pulse can be palpated just under the inguinal ligament. This artery travels down the front of the thigh then crosses to the back of the thigh, where it is termed the popliteal artery. The popliteal pulse can be palpated behind the knee. The popliteal artery divides below the knee into anterior and posterior branches. The anterior branch descends down the top of the foot, where it becomes the dorsalis pedis artery. Its pulse can be palpated on the great toe side of the top of the foot. The posterior branch is called the posterior tibial artery. The posterior tibial pulse can be palpated behind the medial malleolus of the ankle. The dorsalis pedis artery and posterior tibial artery form the dorsal arch, which, like the superficial and deep palmar arches of the hands, provides the feet and toes with extra protection from arterial occlusion (see Fig. 23-2). For a discussion of pulse measurement, see Assessment tool 23-2 later in the chapter.

VEINS

Veins are the blood vessels that carry deoxygenated, nutrient-depleted, waste-laden blood from the tissues back to the heart. The veins of the arms, upper trunk, head and neck carry blood to the superior vena cava, where it passes into the right atrium. Blood from the lower trunk and legs drains upwards into the inferior vena cava. The veins contain nearly 70% of the body's blood volume. Because blood in the veins is carried under much lower pressure than in the arteries, the vein walls

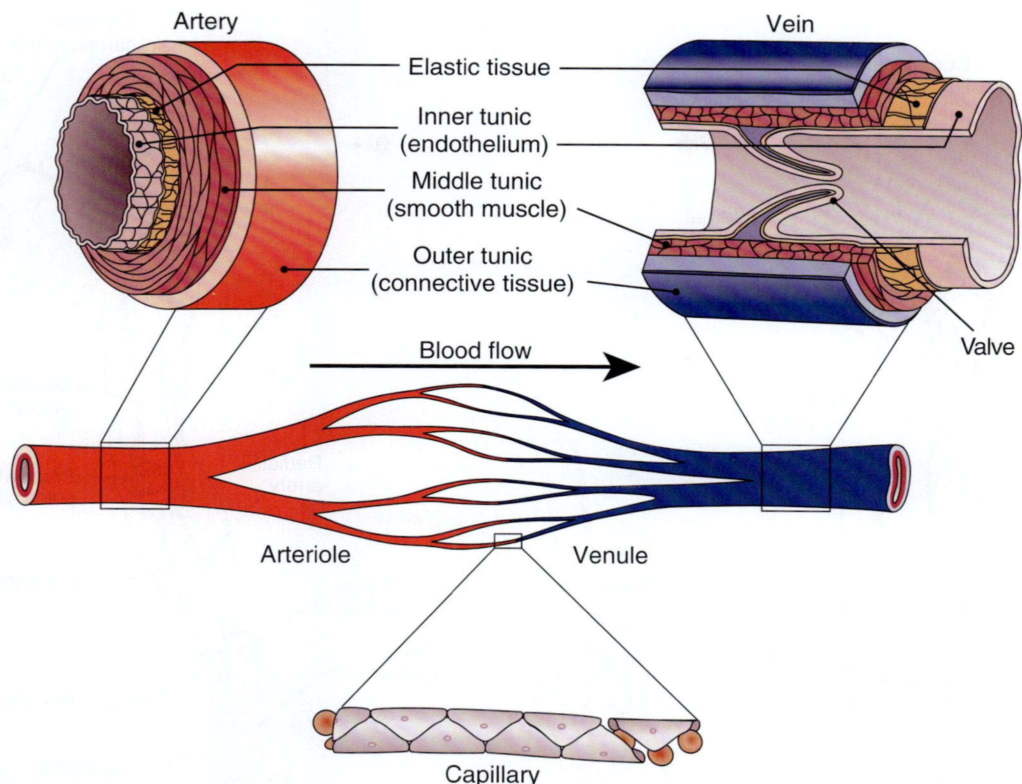

FIGURE 23-1 Blood vessel walls. Arterial walls are constructed to accommodate the high pulsing pressure of blood transported by the pumping heart, whereas venous walls are constructed with valves that promote the return of blood and prevent backflow. (Cohen, B. J. & Hull, K. L. (2015). *Memmler's structure and function of the human body* [11th ed.]. Philadelphia: Lippincott Williams & Wilkins.)

are much thinner (see Fig. 23-1). In addition, veins are larger in diameter than arteries and can expand if blood volume increases. This helps to reduce the workload on the heart.

This chapter focuses on those veins that are most susceptible to dysfunction: the three types of veins in the legs. Two other major veins that are important to assess—the internal and external jugular veins—are discussed in Chapter 22.

There are three types of veins: deep veins, superficial veins and perforator (or communicator) veins. The two deep veins in the leg are the femoral vein in the upper thigh and the popliteal vein located behind the knee. These veins account for about 90% of venous return from the lower extremities. The superficial veins are the great and small saphenous veins. The great saphenous vein is the longest of all veins and extends from the medial dorsal aspect of the foot, crosses over the medial malleolus and continues across the thigh to the medial aspect of the groin, where it joins the femoral vein. The small saphenous vein begins at the lateral dorsal aspect of the foot, travels up behind the lateral malleolus on the back of the leg and joins the popliteal vein. The perforator veins connect the superficial veins with the deep veins (Fig. 23-3).

Veins differ from arteries in that there is no force that propels forward blood flow; the venous system is a low-pressure system. This fact is of special concern in the veins of the leg. Blood from the legs and lower trunk must flow upwards with no help from the pumping action of the heart. Three mechanisms of venous function help to propel blood back to the heart.

The first mechanism has to do with the structure of the veins. Deep, superficial and perforator veins all contain one-way valves. These valves permit blood to pass through them on the way to the heart and then prevent blood from returning through them in the opposite direction. The second mechanism is muscular contraction. Skeletal muscles contract with movement and, in effect, squeeze blood towards the heart through the one-way valves. The third mechanism is the creation of a pressure gradient through the act of breathing. Inspiration decreases intrathoracic pressure while increasing abdominal pressure, thus producing a pressure gradient.

If there is a problem with any of these mechanisms, venous return is impeded and venous stasis results. Risk factors for venous stasis include long periods of standing still, sitting or lying down. Lack of muscular activity causes blood to pool in the legs, which, in turn, increases pressure in the veins. Other causes of venous stasis include varicose (tortuous and dilated) veins, which increase venous pressure. Damage to the vein wall can also contribute to venous stasis.

CAPILLARIES AND FLUID EXCHANGE

Capillaries are small blood vessels that form the connection between the arterioles and the venules and allow the circulatory system to maintain the vital equilibrium between the vascular and interstitial spaces. Oxygen, water and nutrients in the interstitial fluid are delivered by the arterial vessels to the microscopic capillaries (Fig. 23-4). Hydrostatic force (generated by the blood pressure) is the primary mechanism by which the interstitial fluid diffuses out of the capillaries and enters the tissue space. The interstitial fluid releases the oxygen, water and nutrients and picks up waste products such as carbon dioxide and other by-products of cellular metabolism. The fluid then re-enters the

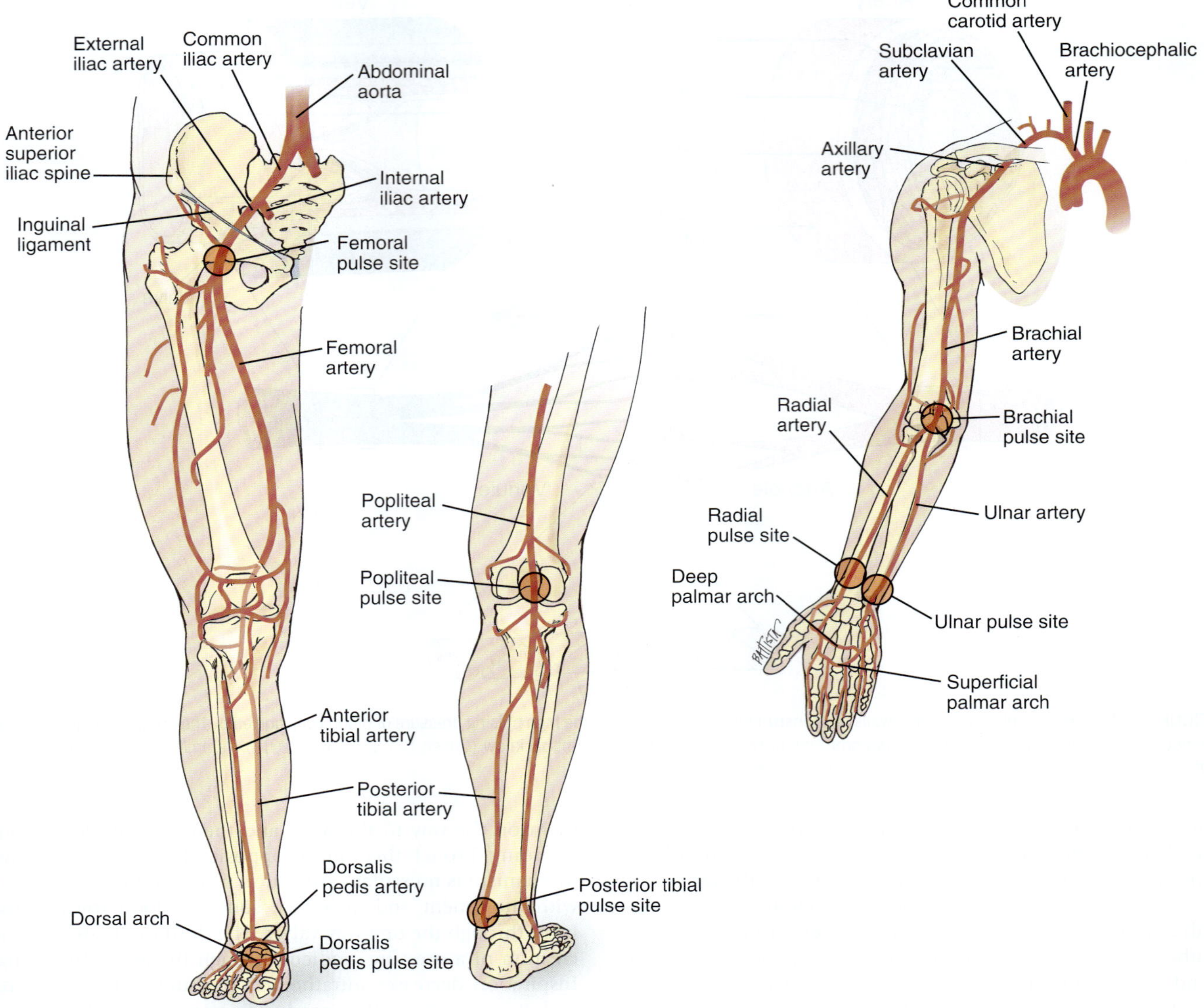

FIGURE 23-2 Major arteries of the arms and legs.

capillaries by osmotic pressure and is transported away from the tissues and interstitial spaces by venous circulation. As mentioned previously, the lymphatic capillaries function to remove any excess fluid left behind in the interstitial spaces. Thus, the capillary bed is very important in maintaining the equilibrium of interstitial fluid and preventing oedema.

THE LYMPHATIC SYSTEM

The lymphatic system, an integral and complementary component of the circulatory system, is a complex vascular system composed of lymphatic capillaries, lymphatic vessels and lymph nodes. Its primary function is to drain excess fluid and plasma proteins from bodily tissues and return them to the venous system. During circulation, more fluid leaves the capillaries than the veins can absorb. Draining excess fluid action prevents oedema, which is a build-up of fluid in the interstitial spaces. The fluids and proteins absorbed into the lymphatic vessels by the microscopic lymphatic capillaries become lymph. These capillaries join to form larger vessels that pass through filters known as lymph nodes, where microorganisms, foreign materials, dead blood cells and abnormal cells are trapped and destroyed. After the lymph is filtered, it travels to either the right lymphatic duct (which drains the upper right side of the body) or the thoracic duct (which drains the rest of the body) before travelling back into the venous system through the subclavian veins (Fig. 23-5).

This unique filtering feature of the lymph nodes allows the lymphatic system to perform a second function as a major part of the immune system defending the body against microorganisms. A third function of the lymphatic system is to absorb fats (lipids) from the small intestine into the bloodstream. Lymph nodes are somewhat circular or oval. Normally they vary from very small and non-palpable to 1 to 2 cm in diameter. Lymph nodes tend to be grouped together. They are both deep and superficial, and many are located near major joints. The superficial lymph nodes are the only lymph nodes accessible to examination. The cervical and axillary superficial lymph nodes are discussed in Chapters

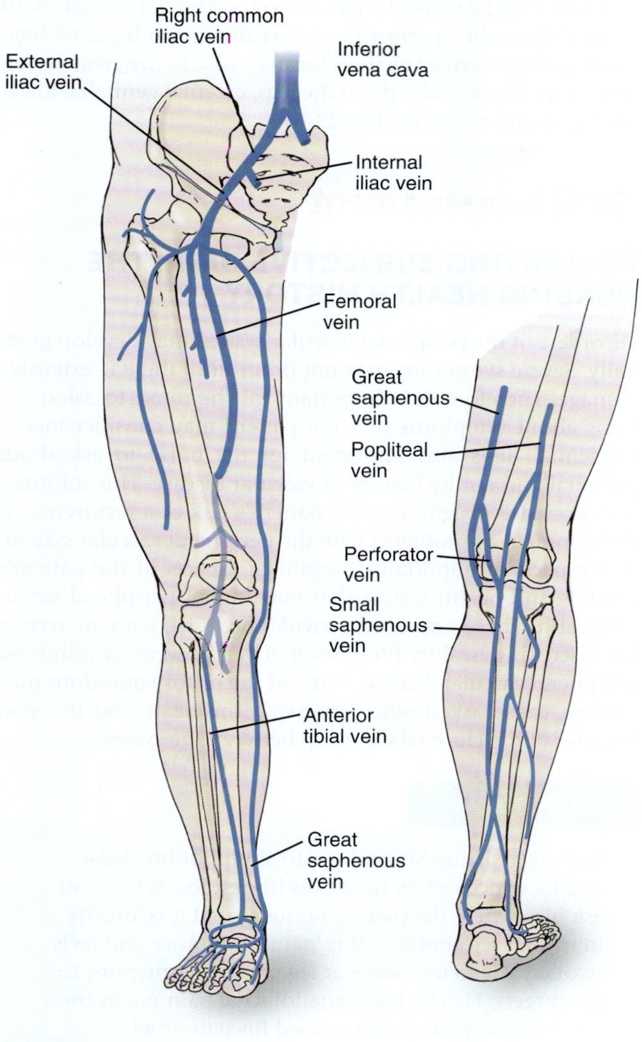

FIGURE 23-3 Major veins of the legs.

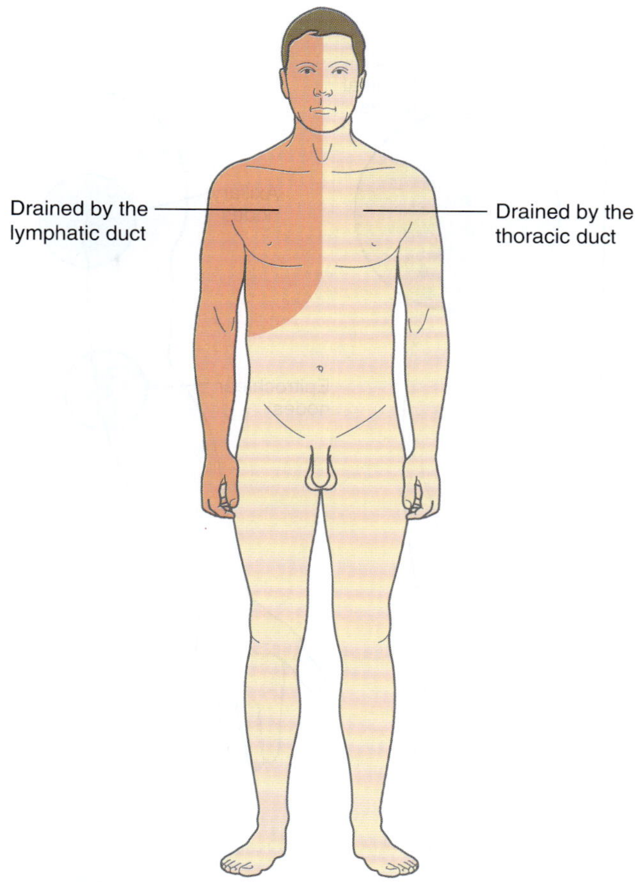

FIGURE 23-5 Lymphatic drainage.

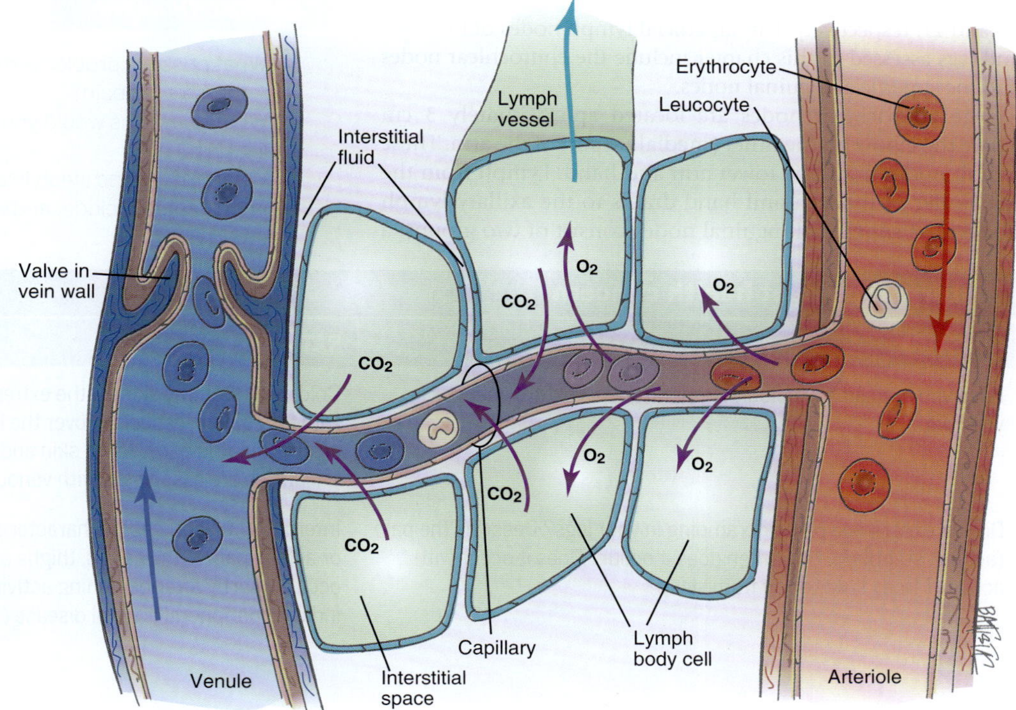

FIGURE 23-4 Normal capillary circulation ensures removal of excess fluid (oedema) from the interstitial spaces as well as delivery of oxygen (O_2) and removal of carbon dioxide (CO_2).

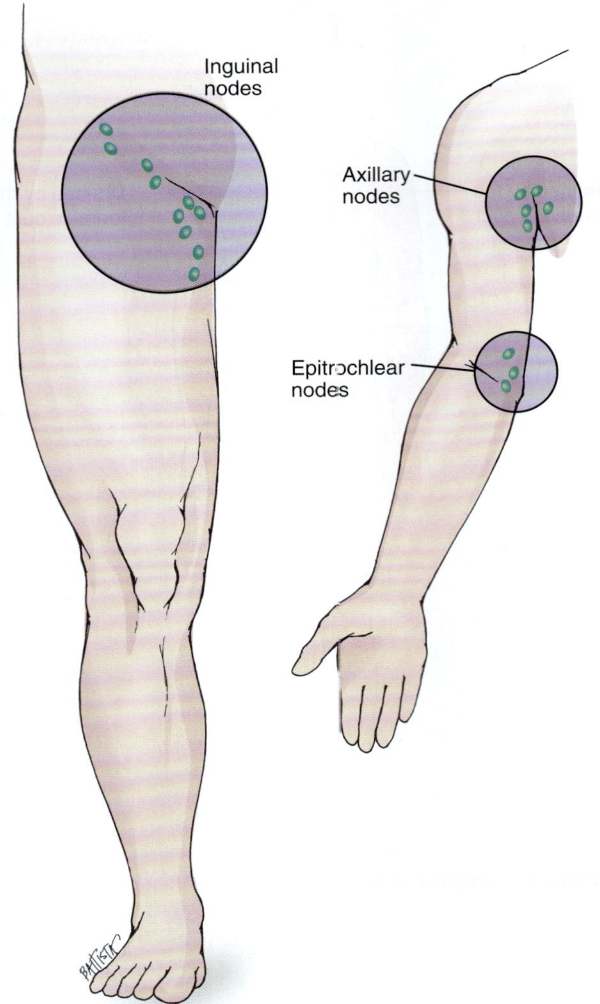

FIGURE 23-6 Superficial lymph nodes of the arms and legs.

16 and 21, respectively. The superficial lymph nodes of the arms and legs assessed in this chapter include the epitrochlear nodes and the superficial inguinal nodes.

The epitrochlear nodes are located approximately 3 cm above the elbow on the inner (medial) aspect of the arm. These lymph nodes drain the lower arm and hand. Lymph from the remainder of the arm and hand drains to the axillary lymph nodes. The superficial inguinal nodes consist of two groups: a horizontal and a vertical chain of nodes. The horizontal chain is located on the anterior thigh just under the inguinal ligament, and the vertical chain is located close to the great saphenous vein. These nodes drain the legs, external genitalia, lower abdomen and buttocks (Fig. 23-6).

Health assessment

COLLECTING SUBJECTIVE DATA: THE NURSING HEALTH HISTORY

Disorders of the peripheral vascular system may develop gradually. Severe symptoms may not occur until there is extensive damage. Therefore, it is important for the nurse to ask questions about symptoms that the patient may consider inconsequential. It is also important for the nurse to ask about personal and family history of vascular disease. This information provides insight into the patient's risk of a recurrence or development of problems with the peripheral vascular system. It is especially important to evaluate aspects of the patient's lifestyle and health factors that may impair peripheral vascular health. These questions provide the nurse with an avenue for discussing healthy lifestyles that can prevent or minimise peripheral vascular disease. Some of the history questions may overlap those asked when assessing the heart and the skin because of the close relationship between the systems.

CASE STUDY

You are assisting Mr Andross to sit up for breakfast, and he winces when he moves his left leg. When you ask him where the pain is, he states that it is 'mostly in my left leg' and that it is 'painful to move and feels swollen'. He denies knee or leg pain at home prior to his surgery. He last had Panadol forte pain medication 1 hour ago; it has not decreased his pain level.

CRITICAL THINKING

1. What possible problems may be causing Mr Andross's leg pain?
2. What questions would you ask Mr Andross about his leg pain?
3. What history and lifestyle questions would be important to include, and why?

History of present health concern

QUESTION	RATIONALE
Have you noticed any colour, temperature or texture changes in your skin?	Cold, pale, clammy skin on the extremities and thin, shiny skin with loss of hair, especially over the lower legs, are associated with arterial insufficiency. Warm skin and brown pigmentation around the ankles are associated with venous insufficiency.
Do you experience pain or cramping in your legs? Describe the pain (aching, stabbing). How often does it occur? Does it occur with activity? Does it wake you from sleep?	Intermittent claudication characterised by cramping, tired feeling or aching pain in the calves, thighs or buttocks and weakness that occurs shortly after beginning activity and is relieved with rest may indicate peripheral arterial disease (Schorr et al., 2017).

History of present health concern (continued)	
QUESTION	**RATIONALE**
	No intermittent claudication and pain relief when legs are elevated are associated with peripheral vascular disease (Wiltz-James & Foley, 2019). Leg pain that awakens a patient from sleep is often associated with advanced chronic arterial occlusive disease. However, the lack of pain may signal neuropathy in a diabetic patient. Reduced sensation or an absence of pain can result in a failure to recognise a problem or fully understand the problem's significance. **OLDER ADULT CONSIDERATIONS** **Older patients with arterial disease may not have the classic symptoms of intermittent claudication but may experience coldness, colour change, numbness and abnormal sensations.**
Do you have any leg veins that are ropelike, bulging or contorted?	Varicose veins are hereditary but may also develop from increased venous pressure and venous pooling (e.g. as happens during pregnancy). Standing in one place for long times also increases the risk for varicosities.
Do you have any sores or open wounds on your legs? Where are they located? Are they painful?	Ulcers associated with arterial disease are usually painful and are often located on the toes, foot or lateral ankle. Venous ulcers are usually painless and occur on the lower leg or medial ankle.
Do you have any swelling (oedema) in your legs or feet? At what time of day is swelling worst? Any pain with swelling?	Peripheral oedema (swelling) results from an obstruction of the lymphatic flow or from venous insufficiency from conditions such as incompetent valves. It may also occur with deep vein thrombosis. Unilateral calf pain and swelling are typical symptoms (see Promote health—Venous thromboembolism [VTE]). With leg or foot ulcers, oedema can reduce tissue perfusion and wound oxygenation.

Continued on following page

COLDSPA

Example for swelling in legs

Use the COLDSPA mnemonic as a guideline to collect needed information for each symptom the patient shares. In addition, the following questions help elicit important information.

Mnemonic	Question	Patient response example
Character	Describe the sign or symptom (feeling, appearance, sound, smell or taste, if applicable).	'I've gained 7 kilograms even though I've been eating about the same foods. I have swelling in my legs.'
Onset	When did it begin?	'About a week ago.' OR 'I have had this pain for years.'
Location	Where is it? Does it radiate? Does it occur anywhere else?	'It's mostly in my legs, ankles and feet. They seem heavy and puffy.'
Duration	How long does it last? Does it recur?	'Most of the time, though it does seem worse at the end of the day.'
Severity	How bad is it? or How much does it bother you?	'The swelling is getting worse"
Pattern	What makes it better or worse?	'It helps to lie down in the recliner and keep my feet up. The swelling is worse when I sit with my feet on the floor.'
Associated factors/How it **A**ffects the patient	What other symptoms occur with it? How does it affect you?	'The skin on my legs and feet feels so tight and now I can't wear anything but my old house shoes. I have to sit up at night in the recliner in order to breathe easier.'

PROMOTE HEALTH — VENOUS THROMBOEMBOLISM

OVERVIEW

Venous thromboembolism (VTE) is a disease process in which blood clots develop in the deep veins in the peripheral vascular system and the pulmonary system. Deep vein thrombosis (DVT) is a blood clot or thrombus in a deep vein. These clots can develop in the arm, lower leg, thigh or pelvis, but the thigh and pelvis are the more serious areas for clots because clots that develop here are more likely to dislodge and travel to the lungs, causing a potentially fatal pulmonary embolus (PE). About 1 in 1,000 of the population develops DVT each year, and 1 in 2,000 develops PE each year. Hospitalised patients are over 100 times more likely to develop a DVT or PE compared with the rest of the community (Australian Commission on Safety and Quality in Health Care [ACSQHC], 2019)

The morbidity associated with DVT is often under-recognised and includes serious long-term complications such as chronic oedema and pain, chronic venous insufficiency, recurrent venous ulceration and post-thrombotic syndrome. The risk factors and preventive strategies for VTE have been identified (ACSQHC, 2019). Risk factors are thought to be additive; thus, having more than one risk factor increases the risk of developing VTE.

Risk factors

- Any condition that increases blood clotting, including inherited conditions
- Major surgery or trauma
- Some cancers and cancer treatments
- Other vascular conditions such as varicose veins
- Sitting for long periods, such as in a car, aeroplane or office
- Pregnancy, especially the first 6 weeks after giving birth
- Age (the annual incidence of VTE rises with each decade over the age of 40)
- Marked obesity
- Oral contraceptive pills and oestrogen-containing hormone replacement therapy
- Previous VTE
- Medical condition associated with prolonged immobilisation (myocardial infarction, stroke, heart failure, active inflammatory conditions)

Teach risk reduction tips

- If sitting for long periods, stand up as often as possible or at least every hour. Exercise feet and lower leg muscles frequently.
- Get out of bed and walk as soon as possible after surgery or illness.
- Follow doctor's orders for taking clot preventing medicines if required for some surgeries and follow up with doctor as necessary. Report tenderness or pain, swelling, warmth or redness in calf or thigh.
- When travelling long distances, especially by plane:
  - Exercise leg muscles frequently in airport as well as on plane; curl and press toes down to improve circulation.
  - Wear compression stockings.
  - Avoid socks with tight elastic bands around tops.
  - Drink plenty of fluids to avoid dehydration.
  - Take aspirin if advised by doctor or not contraindicated by other medical conditions.
- On long car trips, stop every 2 hours to get out and walk around.

History of present health concern (continued)

QUESTION	RATIONALE
Do you have any swollen glands or lymph nodes? If so, do they feel tender, soft or hard?	Enlarged lymph nodes may indicate a local or systemic infection. **OLDER ADULT CONSIDERATIONS** **With ageing, lymphatic tissue is lost, resulting in smaller and fewer lymph nodes.**
For male patients: Have you experienced a change in your usual sexual activity? Describe.	Impotence may occur in patients with decreased blood flow or an occlusion of the blood vessels such as aortoiliac occlusion (Leriche syndrome). Men may be reluctant to report or discuss difficulties they have achieving or maintaining an erection.

Past health history

QUESTION	RATIONALE
Describe any problems you had in the past with the circulation in your arms and legs (e.g. blood clots, ulcers, coldness, hair loss, numbness, swelling or poor healing).	A history of peripheral vascular disease increases a person's risk for a recurrence. The following symptoms may signal peripheral arterial occlusive disease (Wiltz-James & Foley, 2019): an absence of a prior palpable pulse; cool, pale legs; thick and opaque or brittle nails; shiny, dry skin; leg ulcerations; and reduced hair growth (see Promote Health—Peripheral arterial disease). Following deep vein thrombosis, post-thrombotic syndrome leading to tissue damage may develop and persist indefinitely (Bhat et al., 2018).
Have you had any heart or blood vessel surgeries or treatments such as coronary artery bypass grafting, repair of an aneurysm or vein stripping?	Previous surgeries may alter the appearance of the skin and underlying tissues surrounding the blood vessels. Grafts for bypass surgeries are often taken from veins in the legs.

PROMOTE HEALTH — PERIPHERAL ARTERY DISEASE

OVERVIEW

According to Conte and Vale (2018), peripheral artery disease (PAD) is present in approximately 15% of adults in Australia. The disease prevalence increases with age and is associated with other diseases, such as diabetes. PAD is a major cause of impaired ambulation, lower-extremity wounds and amputations. The disease occurs when there is a reduced blood flow to the limbs, usually from atherosclerotic build-up in the vessels. Once the disease becomes symptomatic, the primary symptom is intermittent claudication (especially pain in the leg when walking, but may be pain in arms or legs with activity). Calf pain is the most common symptom, but other symptoms may include numbness, weakness, coldness, sores on toes, change in skin colour of legs, hair loss or slow growth on legs, shiny skin, slow-growing toenails, diminished pulses in legs and feet, and erectile dysfunction in men (Schorr et al., 2017; Wiltz-James & Foley, 2019). As noted by Wiltz-James and Foley (2019), PAD is usually an indication of more widespread atherosclerosis in other parts of the vascular system.

Routine screening for PAD using the ankle-brachial index or questionnaire is not currently recommended in Australia (Si et al., 2018) or New Zealand (Auckland Vascular Centre, 2019). Although screening has been recommended in other countries, it has not been shown to be of benefit in randomised controlled trials (Davies et al., 2017). Specific screening is reserved for at-risk populations such as people with diabetes (Barnes, 2018) or individuals with a high risk of developing cardiovascular disease.

Risk factors

Risk factors for lower-extremity PAD (Auckland Vascular Centre, 2019; Wiltz-James & Foley 2019) include:

- Age younger than 50 in people who have diabetes and one additional risk factor, such as smoking, dyslipidaemia, hypertension or hyperhomocystinaemia
- Ages 50 to 64 in people with a history of smoking or diabetes
- Age 65 or older—leg symptoms with exertion (suggesting claudication) or ischaemic rest pain
- Atherosclerotic coronary, carotid or renal artery disease
- Smoking, or history of smoking
- Diabetes
- Obesity (a body mass index over 30), reduced activity levels and sedentary lifestyle
- High blood pressure (140/90 mmHg or higher)
- High cholesterol (total blood cholesterol over 240 mg/dL, or 6.2 mmol/L)
- Family history of peripheral artery disease, heart disease or stroke
- Excess levels of homocysteine.

People who smoke or have diabetes have the greatest risk of developing PAD due to reduced blood flow.

Teach risk reduction tips ***(Wiltz-James & Foley, 2019)***

- Quit smoking if you are a smoker.
- If you have diabetes, keep your blood sugar in good control.
- Exercise regularly. Aim for 30 minutes at least three times a week after you have your doctor's OK.
- Lower your cholesterol and blood pressure levels, if necessary.
- Eat foods that are low in saturated fat.
- Maintain a healthy weight.

Family history

QUESTION	RATIONALE
Do you, or does your family, have a history of diabetes, hypertension, coronary heart disease, intermittent claudication or elevated cholesterol or triglyceride levels?	These disorders or abnormalities tend to be hereditary and cause damage to blood vessels. An essential aspect of treating peripheral vascular disease is to identify and then modify risk factors (Schorr et al., 2017).

Lifestyle and health practices

QUESTION	RATIONALE
Do you (or did you in the past) smoke cigarettes or use any other form of tobacco? How much and for how long? If you have used tobacco, are you willing to quit?	Smoking cigarettes (and using other forms of tobacco) significantly increases a person's risk of chronic arterial insufficiency. The risk increases according to the length of time a person smokes and the amount of tobacco smoked. If willing to quit smoking, provide resources to assist in quitting. If unwilling to quit, provide information and help identify barriers to quitting (www.quitnow.gov.au; cancer.org.au; www.quit.org.nz; smokefree.org.nz). Smoking cessation in middle age has the following benefits: reduced workload on the heart, improved respiratory function and reduced risk of lung cancer (Cohen-Mansfield, 2016).
Do you exercise regularly?	Regular exercise improves peripheral vascular circulation and decreases stress, pulse rate and blood pressure, thereby decreasing the risk of developing peripheral vascular disease.
For female patients: Are you on contraceptive (birth control) pills, injections or implants?	These contraceptives increase the risk of developing thrombophlebitis, Raynaud disease, hypertension and oedema.
Are you experiencing any stress in your life at this time?	Stress increases the heart rate and blood pressure and can contribute to vascular disease.
How have problems with your circulation (i.e. peripheral vascular system) affected your ability to function?	Discomfort or pain associated with chronic arterial disease and the aching heaviness associated with venous disease may limit a patient's ability to stand or walk for long periods. This, in turn, may affect job performance and the ability to care for a home and family or participate in social events.

Continued on following page

Lifestyle and health practices (continued)

QUESTION	RATIONALE
Do leg ulcers or varicose veins affect how you feel about yourself?	If patients perceive the appearance of their legs as disfiguring, their body image or feelings of self-worth may be negatively influenced.
Do you regularly take medications prescribed by your doctor to improve your circulation?	Antiplatelet drugs that inhibit platelet aggregation, such as dipyridamole or the group of drugs known as P2Y12 antagonists such as clopidogrel, prasugrel or ticagrelor may be prescribed to increase blood flow. Patients on this group of drugs need to be instructed to avoid grapefruit juice as this may increase bleeding. Aspirin also prevents blood clotting and is used to reduce the risks associated with peripheral vascular disease. Other drugs used for peripheral vascular disease include pentoxifylline, which reduces blood viscosity and improves blood flow, cilostazol, a vasodilator and antiplatelet, or oxerutins a drug that reduces oedema and capillary leakage. (See *Australian medicines handbook* for more information). Patients who fail to take their medications regularly are at risk of developing peripheral vascular problems. These patients require teaching about their medication and the importance of taking it regularly.
Do you wear compression stockings to treat varicose veins or prevent deep vein thrombosis?	Compression stockings help to reduce venous pooling and increase blood return to the heart.

COLLECTING OBJECTIVE DATA: PHYSICAL EXAMINATION

The purpose of the peripheral vascular assessment is to identify any signs or symptoms of peripheral vascular disease, including arterial insufficiency, venous insufficiency and lymphatic involvement. This is accomplished by performing an assessment first of the arms then the legs, concentrating on skin colour and temperature, major pulse sites and major groups of lymph nodes.

Examination of the peripheral vascular system is very useful in acute care, extended care and home health care settings. Early detection of peripheral vascular disease can prevent long-term complications. A complete peripheral vascular examination involves inspection, palpation and auscultation. In addition, several special assessment techniques should be performed on patients with suspected peripheral vascular problems.

The arms and legs should be closely compared bilaterally. Better objective data can be gained by assessing a particular feature on one extremity and then the other. For example, evaluate the strength of the dorsalis pedis pulse on the right foot and compare your findings with those of the left foot.

Obesity is on the increase, making it important to be aware of the effects of increased body mass index (BMI) on the ability to inspect and palpate the peripheral vascular system. Differentiating oedema from excess adipose tissue requires attention to specific details. In addition, in some patients increased BMI can affect both the ability to palpate lymph nodes and pulses and the interpretation of pulse strength. Doppler ultrasound devices can assist in pulse identification in the obese patient.

Preparing the patient

Have the patient wear an examination gown and sit upright on an examination table. Make sure the room is a comfortable temperature (about 22°C) without drafts. This helps to prevent vasodilation or vasoconstriction. Before you begin the assessment, inform the patient that it will be necessary to inspect and palpate all four extremities and that the groin will also need to be exposed for palpation of the inguinal lymph nodes and palpation and auscultation of the femoral arteries. Explain that the patient can sit for examination of the arms but will need to lie down for examination of the legs and groin, and will need to follow your directions for several special assessment techniques towards the end of the examination. As you perform the examination, explain in detail what you are doing and answer any questions the patient may have. This helps to ease any patient anxiety.

Equipment

- Tape measure
- Stethoscope
- Doppler ultrasound device
- Conductivity gel
- Tourniquet
- Gauze or tissue
- Waterproof pen
- Blood pressure cuff

Physical assessment

- Discuss risk factors for peripheral vascular disease with the patient.
- Accurately inspect the patient's arms and legs for oedema and venous patterning.
- Observe carefully for signs of arterial and venous insufficiency (skin colour, venous pattern, hair distribution, lesions or ulcers) and inadequate lymphatic drainage.
- Recognise characteristic clubbing.
- Palpate pulse points correctly.
- Use the Doppler ultrasound instrument correctly (Equipment spotlight 23-1).

EQUIPMENT SPOTLIGHT 23-1 HOW TO USE THE DOPPLER ULTRASOUND DEVICE

The Doppler ultrasound device transmits and receives ultrasound waves to evaluate blood flow. It works by transmitting ultra-high-frequency sound waves that strike red blood cells (RBCs) in an artery or vein. The rebounding ultrasound waves produce a whooshing sound when echoing from an artery and a non-pulsating rush when echoing from a vein. The strength of the sound is determined by the velocity of the RBCs. In partially occluded vessels, RBCs pass more slowly through the vessel, thus decreasing the sound. Fully occluded vessels produce no sound. The battery-operated hand-held Doppler device is used to:

- Assess unpalpable pulses in the extremities
- Determine the patency of arterial bypass grafts
- Assess tissue perfusion in an extremity.

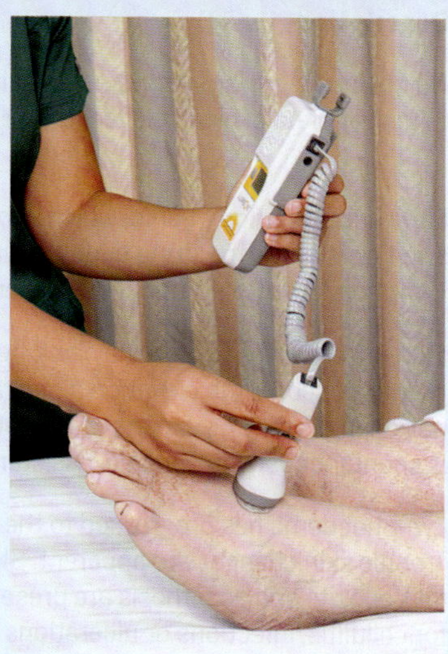

Operating the device

When assessing peripheral circulation with a Doppler ultrasound device, first inform the patient that the assessment is painless and non-invasive. Then the test can proceed as follows:

- Apply a fingertip-sized amount of lukewarm gel over the blood vessel to be assessed.
- At a 60- to 90-degree angle, lightly place the vascular probe at the top of the mound of gel.
- Listen for a whooshing (artery) or non-pulsating rushing (vein) sound.
- Clean the skin with a tissue.
- Clean the probe as recommended by the manufacturer.
- Mark the site with a permanent pen for easy reassessment.
- Record findings.

Improving results

- A warm extremity will increase signal strength.
- Place the tube or packet of gel in warm water before use because cold gel will promote vasoconstriction and make it more difficult to detect a signal.
- Avoid pressing the probe too snugly against the skin because this may obliterate the signal.

CASE STUDY

According to the medical notes, Mr Andross's surgery was uncomplicated. On his first day postoperative he was found to have an elevated temperature and symptoms of a chest infection. He is being treated for pneumonia with IV antibiotics. As a result of his condition he was not assisted to mobilise until 72 hours following his surgery. He states that he was up and walking frequently yesterday with the physiotherapist and when his daughter came to visit. He normally lives a sedentary lifestyle due to pain from the arthritis in his hip. His medical history includes diabetes, hypertension (he does not recall when it was first diagnosed) and family history of heart disease. He smoked one packet of cigarettes per day for 30 years but stopped 10 years ago. He normally uses a walking stick to get around. He has home care nurses visit him four times a week to help him shower, and his daughter does his cleaning, washing and shopping. He has had three admissions for uncontrolled diabetes about 10 years ago, but since his daughter started cooking and shopping for him, he has had stable blood sugar but remains on oral hypoglycaemic medications.

CRITICAL THINKING

4. Prior to reading the following physical assessment section, what do you think would be important to examine specific to a patient's peripheral vascular system? Considering this, what physical assessments would you conduct to help you determine the cause of Mr Andross's leg pain and swelling?
5. You are concerned that Mr Andross may have developed a deep vein thrombosis (DVT). What risk factors in his presentation predispose him to development of a DVT? Why is DVT a serious complication in a patient?
6. What physical assessment findings would you expect if Mr Andross has a DVT?

PHYSICAL ASSESSMENT

ASSESSMENT PROCEDURE	NORMAL FINDINGS	ABNORMAL FINDINGS
Arms		
INSPECTION		
Observe arm size and venous pattern; also look for oedema. If there is an observable difference, measure bilaterally the circumference of the arms at the same locations with each re-measurement and record findings in centimetres.	Arms are bilaterally symmetrical with minimal variation in size and shape. No oedema or prominent venous patterning.	Lymphoedema results from blocked lymphatic circulation, which may be caused by breast surgery. It usually affects one extremity, causing induration and non-pitting oedema. Prominent venous patterning with oedema may indicate venous obstruction. See Assessment tool 23-1.

Continued on following page

ASSESSMENT TOOL 23-1 Stages of lymphoedema

Grade	Description	Measurement
Stage 0 Absent	No obvious signs or symptoms. Impaired lymph drainage is sub-clinical. Latent or of no clinical relevance. Swelling is absent.	Oedema is not evident. Clinical detection does not occur until the normal interstitial volume increases by 30% or more.
Stage I Mild	Early accumulation of fluid, which subsides when limb is elevated. Some swelling is present. Pitting oedema may occur. Skin texture is smooth. Lymphoedema is spontaneously reversible.	<3 cm difference between extremities
Stage II Moderate	Skin tissue is firmer. Skin may look tight and shiny. Pitting oedema may or may not occur. Limb elevation alone rarely reduces swelling. Hair loss or nail changes may be experienced in an affected extremity. Lymphoedema is spontaneously irreversible. Assistance will be needed to reduce oedema.	3–5 cm difference between extremities
Stage III Severe	Lymphoedema has progressed to the elephantiasis stage. Pitting is absent Trophic skin changes are apparent. Skin is firm and thick. Hyperkeratosis, fat deposits and acanthosis are present. Skin folds develop. May be at risk for cellulitis, infections or ulcerations. An affected area may ooze fluid. Lymphoedema is irreversible. Elevation will not alleviate symptoms.	≥5 cm difference between extremities

From Arrivé et al., 2018.

PHYSICAL ASSESSMENT (continued)

ASSESSMENT PROCEDURE	NORMAL FINDINGS	ABNORMAL FINDINGS
CLINICAL TIP **Mark locations on arms with a permanent marker to ensure the exact same locations are used with each reassessment.**		
Observe colouration of the hands and arms (Fig. 23-7).	Colour varies depending on the patient's skin tone, although colour should be the same bilaterally (see Chap. 15 for more information).	Raynaud disease, a vascular disorder caused by vasoconstriction or vasospasm of the fingers or toes, is characterised by rapid changes of colour (pallor, cyanosis and redness), swelling, pain, numbness, tingling, burning, throbbing and coldness. The disorder commonly occurs bilaterally; symptoms last minutes to hours (Fig. 23-8).

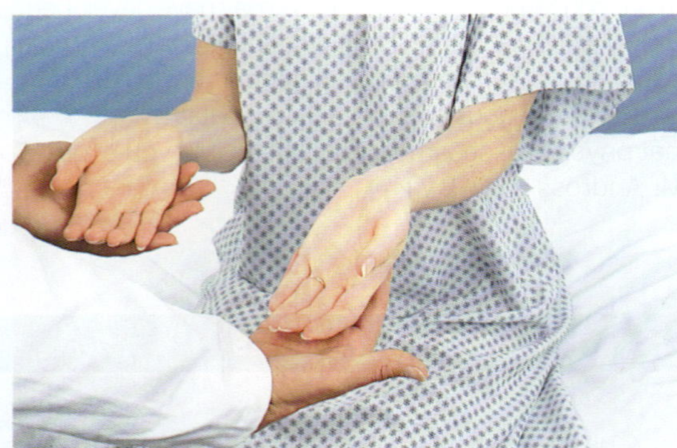

FIGURE 23-7 Inspecting colour related to circulation. (© B. Proud.)

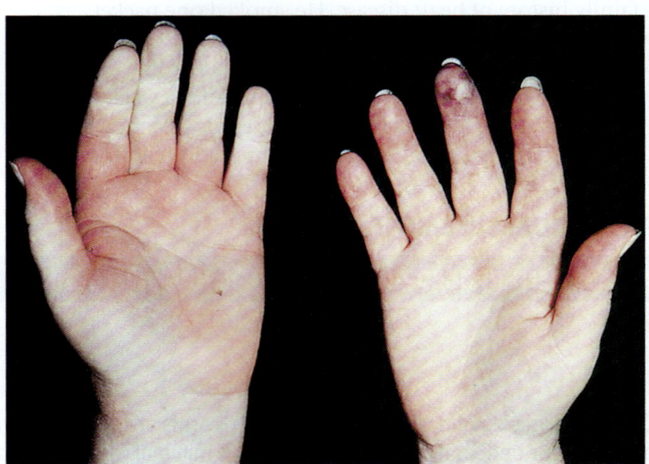

FIGURE 23-8 Hallmarks of Raynaud disease are colour changes. (With permission from Effeney, D. J. & Stoney, R. J. [1993]. *Wylie's atlas of vascular surgery: Disorders of the extremities.* Philadelphia: Lippincott Williams & Wilkins.)

PHYSICAL ASSESSMENT (continued)

ASSESSMENT PROCEDURE	NORMAL FINDINGS	ABNORMAL FINDINGS
PALPATION		
Palpate the patient's fingers, hands and arms, and note the temperature.	**Skin is warm to the touch bilaterally from fingertips to upper arms.**	**Cool extremities may be a sign of arterial insufficiency, reduced cardiac output or shock. A unilateral cold extremity can indicate arterial occlusion or localised trauma to an artery, whereas bilaterally cool extremities are a common sign in shock and specific conditions such as Raynaud disease.**
Palpate to assess capillary refill time. Compress the nailbed until it blanches. Release the pressure and calculate the time it takes for colour to return. This test indicates peripheral perfusion and reflects cardiac output. **CLINICAL TIP** **Inaccurate findings may result if the room is cool, if the patient has oedema or anaemia, or if the patient recently smoked a cigarette.**	Capillary beds refill (and, therefore, colour returns) in 2 seconds or less.	Capillary refill time exceeding 2 seconds may indicate vasoconstriction, decreased cardiac output, shock, arterial occlusion or hypothermia.
Palpate the radial pulse. Gently press the radial artery against the radius (Fig. 23-9). Note elasticity and strength. **CLINICAL TIP** **For difficult-to-palpate pulses, use a Doppler ultrasound device (Equipment spotlight 23-1).** FIGURE 23-9 Palpating the radial pulse. (© B. Proud.)	Radial pulses are bilaterally strong (3+). Artery walls have a resilient quality (bounce).	Increased radial pulse volume indicates a hyperkinetic state (4+ or bounding pulse) arising from a variety of conditions, including heavy exercise, pregnancy, anxiety, heart failure, hypertension, fever and atherosclerosis. Diminished (1+ or 2+) or absent (0) pulses suggest partial or complete arterial occlusion (more common in the legs than arms) as well as decreased blood pressure and other conditions causing reduced cardiac output such as hypovolaemic shock, aortic regurgitation, cardiac arrhythmias, severe sepsis and dehydration. (See Assessment tool 23-2.) Obliteration of the pulse may result from compression by external sources, as in compartment syndrome.
Palpate the ulnar pulses. Apply pressure with your first three fingertips to the medial aspects of the inner wrists. The ulnar pulses are not routinely assessed because they are located deeper than the radial pulses and are difficult to detect. Palpate the ulnar arteries if you suspect arterial insufficiency (Fig. 23-10).	The ulnar pulses may not be detectable.	Lack of resilience or inelasticity of the artery wall may indicate arteriosclerosis. The Allen test is an advanced clinical skill that can be used to evaluate patency of the radial and ulnar arteries. Blood flow to the hand is observed with first the radial and then the ulnar artery occluded. The Allen test is implemented when patency is questionable or before procedures such as a radial artery puncture.

Continued on following page

ASSESSMENT TOOL 23-2 Assessing pulse strength

Palpation of the pulses in the peripheral vascular examination is typically to assess amplitude or strength. Pulse amplitude is graded on a 0 to 4+ scale, with 4+ being the strongest. Elasticity of the artery wall may also be noted during the peripheral vascular examination, by palpating for a resilient (bouncy) quality rather than a more rigid arterial tone, whereas pulse rate and rhythm are best assessed during examination of the heart and neck vessels. (See Chap. 22.)

Pulse amplitude	
Pulse amplitude is typically graded as 0 to 4+:	
0 (absent pulse)	Pulse cannot be felt, even with the application of extreme pressure.
1+ (thready pulse)	Pulse is very difficult to feel, and applying slight pressure causes pulse to disappear.
2+ (weak pulse)	Pulse is stronger than a thready pulse, but applying light pressure causes pulse to disappear.
3+ (normal pulse)	Pulse is easily felt and requires moderate pressure to make it disappear.
4+ (bounding pulse)	Pulse is strong and does not disappear with moderate pressure.

Lynn, P. (2018). *Taylor's clinical nursing skills: A nursing process approach* (5th ed.). Wolters Kluwer/Lippincott Williams & Wilkins.

PHYSICAL ASSESSMENT (continued)

ASSESSMENT PROCEDURE	NORMAL FINDINGS	ABNORMAL FINDINGS

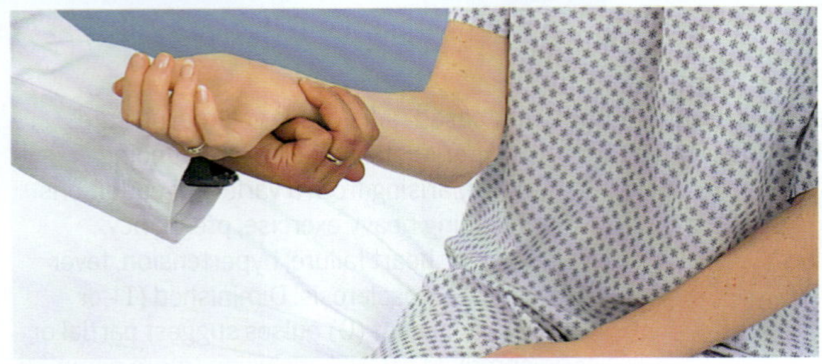
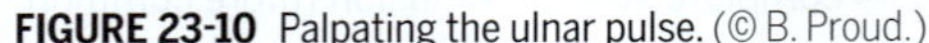

FIGURE 23-10 Palpating the ulnar pulse. (© B. Proud.)

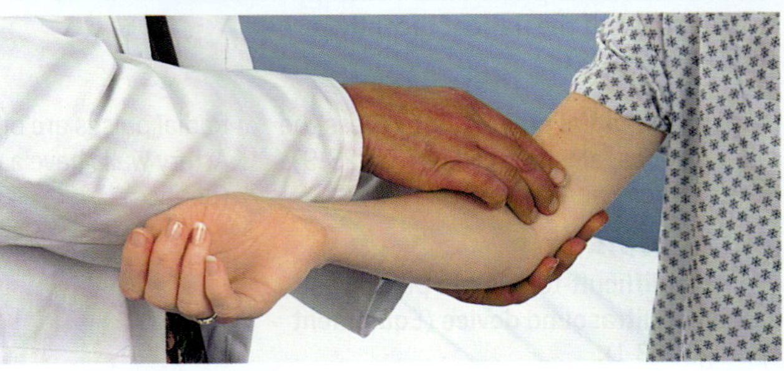

FIGURE 23-11 Palpating the brachial pulse. (© B. Proud.)

ASSESSMENT PROCEDURE	NORMAL FINDINGS	ABNORMAL FINDINGS
You can also palpate the brachial pulses if you suspect arterial insufficiency. Do this by placing the first three fingertips of each hand at the patient's right and left medial antecubital creases. Alternatively, palpate the brachial pulse in the groove between the biceps and triceps (Fig. 23-11).	Brachial pulses have equal strength bilaterally.	Brachial pulses are increased, diminished or absent.
Palpate the epitrochlear lymph nodes. Take the patient's left hand in your right hand as if you were shaking hands. Flex the patient's elbow about 90 degrees. Use your left hand to palpate behind the elbow in the groove between the biceps and triceps muscles (Fig. 23-12). If nodes are detected, evaluate for size, tenderness and consistency. Repeat palpation on the opposite arm.	Normally epitrochlear lymph nodes are not palpable.	Enlarged epitrochlear lymph nodes may indicate an infection in the hand or forearm, or they may occur with generalised lymphadenopathy. Enlarged lymph nodes may also occur because of a lesion in the area.

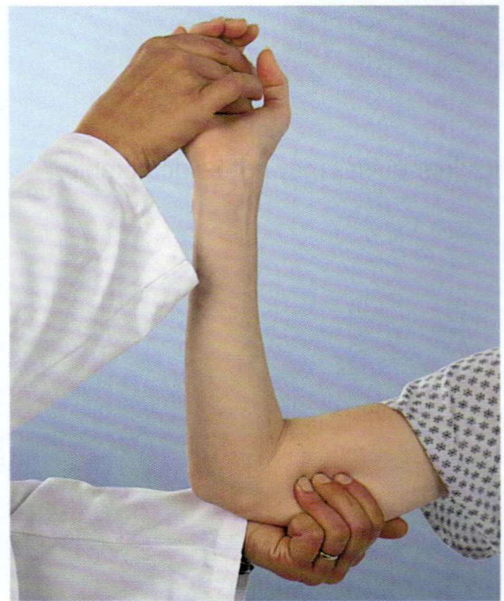

FIGURE 23-12 Palpating the epitrochlear lymph nodes located in the upper inside of the arm. (© B. Proud.)

PHYSICAL ASSESSMENT (continued)

ASSESSMENT PROCEDURE	NORMAL FINDINGS	ABNORMAL FINDINGS
Legs		
INSPECTION, PALPATION AND AUSCULTATION		
Ask the patient to lie supine. Then drape the groin area and place a pillow under the patient's head for comfort. Observe skin colour while inspecting both legs from the toes to the groin.	Pink colour for lighter-skinned patients and pink or red tones visible under darker-pigmented skin. There should be no changes in pigmentation.	Pallor, especially when elevated, and rubor, when dependent, suggests arterial insufficiency. Cyanosis when dependent suggests venous insufficiency. A rusty or brownish pigmentation around the ankles indicates chronic venous insufficiency. Unilateral pallor or rubor suggests arterial or venous occlusion, respectively.
Inspect distribution of hair.	Hair covers the skin on the legs and appears on the dorsal surface of the toes. It can be less abundant in some cultural groups and many women shave their leg hair. **OLDER ADULT CONSIDERATIONS** **Hair loss on the lower extremities occurs with ageing and is, therefore, not an absolute sign of arterial insufficiency in the older patient.**	Loss of hair on the legs suggests arterial insufficiency. Often thin, shiny skin is noted as well.
Inspect for lesions or ulcers. Arterial and venous insufficiency can cause lesions or ulcers in the lower extremities. Arterial and venous insufficiency is further assessed by noting change in colour with position change and determination of the ankle brachial pressure index.	Legs are free of lesions or ulcerations.	Ulcers with smooth, even margins that occur at pressure areas, such as the toes and lateral ankle, result from arterial insufficiency. Ulcers with irregular edges, bleeding and possible bacterial infection that occur on the medial ankle result from venous insufficiency (Abnormal findings 23-1).
Inspect for oedema. Inspect the legs for unilateral or bilateral oedema. Note veins, tendons and bony prominences. If the legs appear asymmetrical, use a tape measure to measure in four different areas: circumference at mid-thigh, largest circumference at the calf, smallest circumference above the ankle and across the forefoot. Compare both extremities at the same locations (Fig. 23-13).	Identical size and shape bilaterally; no swelling or atrophy.	Bilateral oedema may be detected by the absence of visible veins, tendons or bony prominences. Bilateral oedema usually indicates a systemic problem, such as congestive heart failure, or a local problem, such as lymphoedema (abnormal or blocked lymph vessels) or prolonged standing or sitting (orthostatic oedema). Unilateral oedema is characterised by a 1-cm difference in measurement at the ankles, or a 2-cm difference at the calf, and a swollen extremity. It is usually caused by venous stasis due to insufficiency or an obstruction such as deep vein thrombosis. It may also be caused by lymphoedema (Abnormal findings 23-2). A difference in measurement between legs may also be due to muscular atrophy. Muscular atrophy usually results from disuse due to stroke or from being in a cast for a prolonged time.

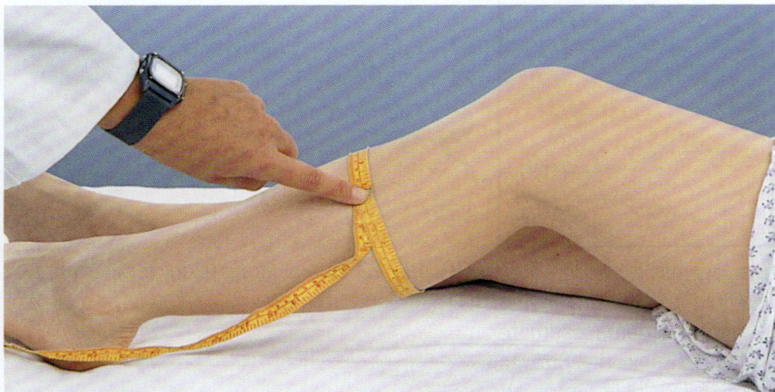

FIGURE 23-13 Measuring the calf circumference. (© B. Proud.)

Continued on following page

PHYSICAL ASSESSMENT (continued)

ASSESSMENT PROCEDURE	NORMAL FINDINGS	ABNORMAL FINDINGS
CLINICAL TIP **Taking a measurement in centimetres from the patella to the location to be measured can aid in getting the exact location on both legs. If additional readings are necessary, use a felt-tipped pen to ensure exact placement of the measuring tape.**		
Palpate oedema. If oedema is noted during inspection, palpate the area to determine if it is pitting or non-pitting (Abnormal findings 23-2). Press the oedematous area with the tips of your fingers, hold for a few seconds, then release. If the depression does not rapidly refill and the skin remains indented on release, pitting oedema is present.	No oedema (pitting or non-pitting) present in the legs.	Pitting oedema is associated with systemic problems, such as congestive heart failure or hepatic cirrhosis, and local causes such as venous stasis due to insufficiency or obstruction or prolonged standing or sitting (orthostatic oedema). A 1+ to 4+ scale is used to grade the severity of pitting oedema with 4+ being most severe (Fig. 23-14).
Palpate bilaterally for temperature of the feet and legs. Use the backs of your fingers. Compare your findings in the same areas bilaterally (Fig. 23-15). Note location of any changes in temperature.	Toes, feet and legs are equally warm bilaterally.	Generalised coolness in one leg or change in temperature from warm to cool as you move down the leg suggests arterial insufficiency. Increased warmth in the leg may be caused by superficial thrombophlebitis resulting from a secondary inflammation in the tissue around the vein. **CLINICAL TIP** **Bilateral coolness of the feet and legs suggests one of the following: The room is too cool or the patient may have recently smoked a cigarette, be anaemic or is anxious. All of these factors cause vasoconstriction, resulting in cool skin.**

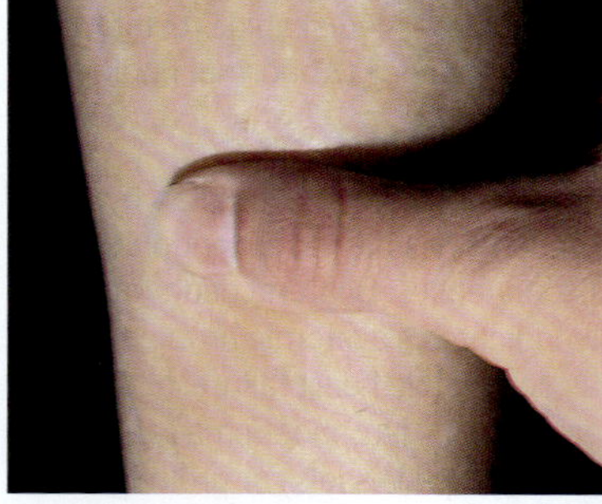

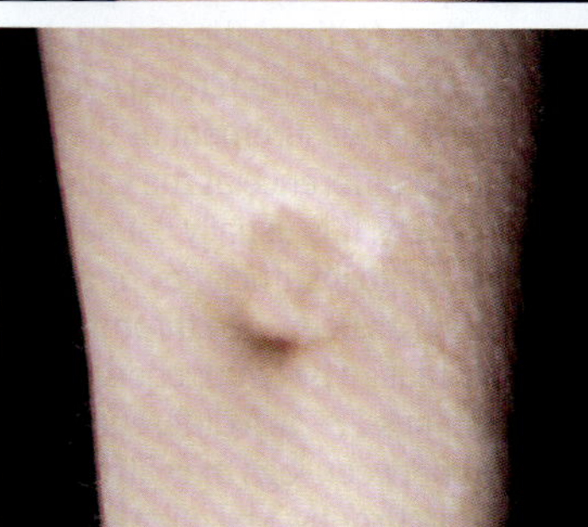

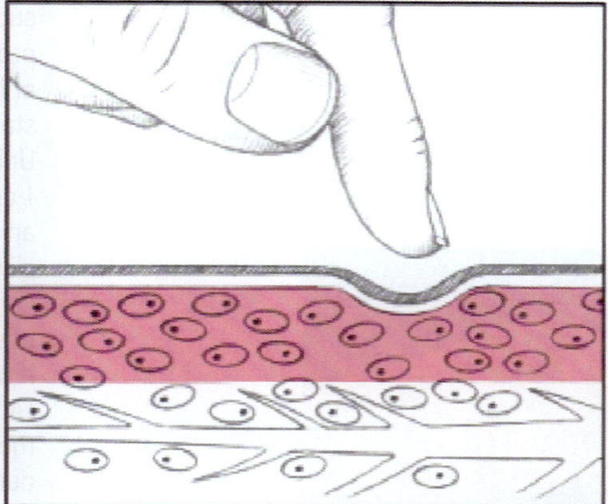

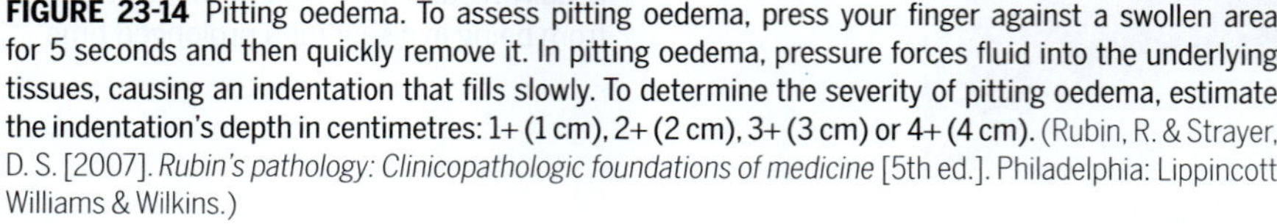
FIGURE 23-14 Pitting oedema. To assess pitting oedema, press your finger against a swollen area for 5 seconds and then quickly remove it. In pitting oedema, pressure forces fluid into the underlying tissues, causing an indentation that fills slowly. To determine the severity of pitting oedema, estimate the indentation's depth in centimetres: 1+ (1 cm), 2+ (2 cm), 3+ (3 cm) or 4+ (4 cm). (Rubin, R. & Strayer, D. S. [2007]. *Rubin's pathology: Clinicopathologic foundations of medicine* [5th ed.]. Philadelphia: Lippincott Williams & Wilkins.)

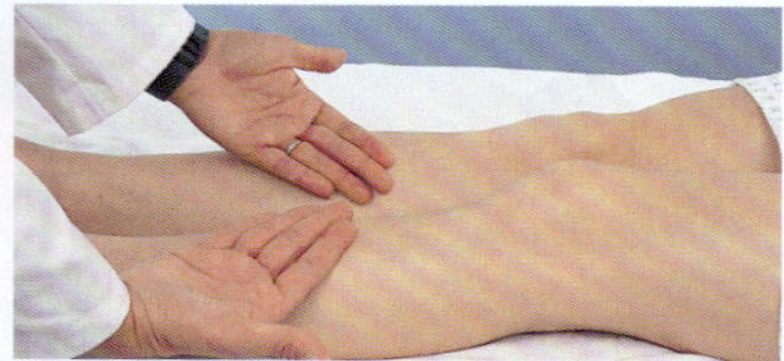

FIGURE 23-15 Palpating skin temperature. (© B. Proud.)

PHYSICAL ASSESSMENT (continued)

ASSESSMENT PROCEDURE	NORMAL FINDINGS	ABNORMAL FINDINGS
Legs (continued)		
Palpate the superficial inguinal lymph nodes. First, expose the patient's inguinal area, keeping the genitals draped. Feel over the upper medial thigh for the vertical and horizontal groups of superficial inguinal lymph nodes. If detected, determine size, mobility or tenderness. Repeat palpation on the opposite thigh.	Non-tender, movable lymph nodes up to 1 or even 2 cm are commonly palpated.	Lymph nodes larger than 2 cm with or without tenderness (lymphadenopathy) may be from a local infection or generalised lymphadenopathy. Fixed nodes may indicate malignancy.
Palpate the femoral pulses. Ask the patient to bend the knee and move it out to the side. Press deeply and slowly below and medial to the inguinal ligament. Use two hands if necessary. Release pressure until you feel the pulse. Repeat palpation on the opposite leg. Compare amplitude bilaterally (Fig. 23-16).	Femoral pulses strong and equal bilaterally. 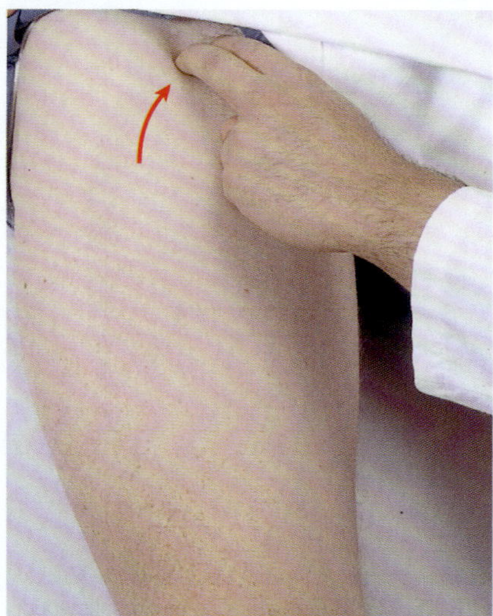 **FIGURE 23-16** Palpating the femoral pulses.	Weak or absent femoral pulses indicate partial or complete arterial occlusion.
Palpate the popliteal pulses. Ask the patient to raise (flex) the knee partially. Place your thumbs on the knee while positioning your fingers deep in the bend of the knee. Apply pressure to locate the pulse. It is usually detected lateral to the medial tendon (Fig. 23-17).	It is not unusual for the popliteal pulse to be difficult or impossible to detect, and yet for circulation to be normal.	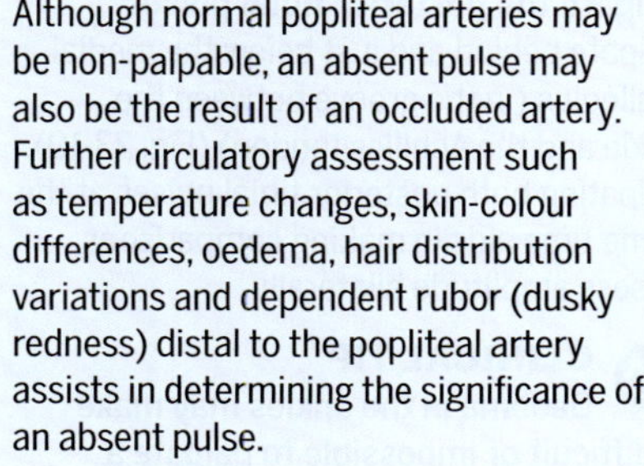 Although normal popliteal arteries may be non-palpable, an absent pulse may also be the result of an occluded artery. Further circulatory assessment such as temperature changes, skin-colour differences, oedema, hair distribution variations and dependent rubor (dusky redness) distal to the popliteal artery assists in determining the significance of an absent pulse.

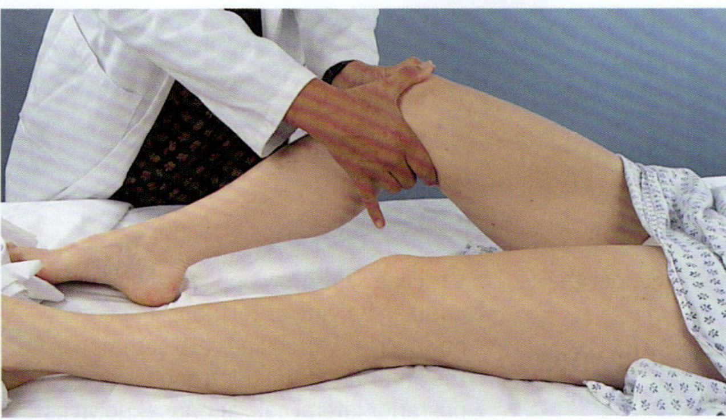

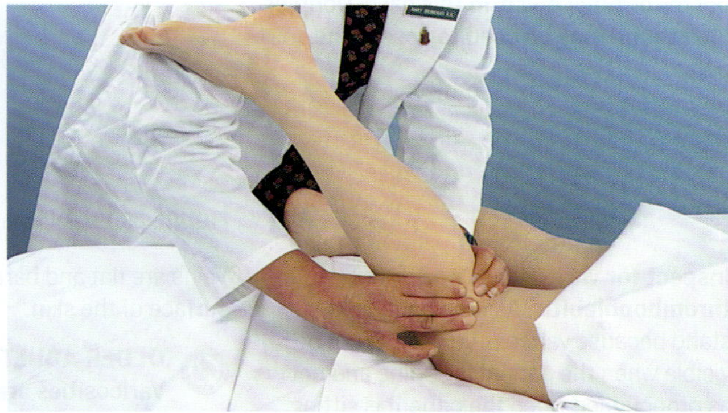

FIGURE 23-17 Palpating the popliteal pulse with the patient (left) supine and (right) prone. (© B. Proud.)

Continued on following page

PHYSICAL ASSESSMENT (continued)

ASSESSMENT PROCEDURE	NORMAL FINDINGS	ABNORMAL FINDINGS
CLINICAL TIP **If you cannot detect a pulse, try palpating with the patient in a prone position. Partially raise the leg and place your fingers deep in the bend of the knee. Repeat palpation in opposite leg and note amplitude bilaterally.**		
Palpate the dorsalis pedis pulses. Dorsiflex the patient's foot and apply light pressure lateral to and along the side of the extensor tendon of the big toe. The pulses of both feet may be assessed at the same time to aid in making comparisons. Assess amplitude bilaterally (Fig. 23-18). **CLINICAL TIP** **It may be difficult or impossible to palpate a pulse in an oedematous foot. A Doppler ultrasound device may be useful in this situation.**	Dorsalis pedis pulses are bilaterally strong. This pulse is congenitally absent in 5% to 10% of the population. 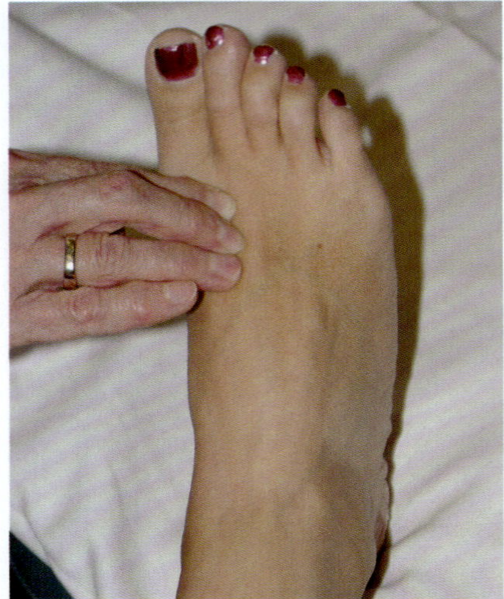 **FIGURE 23-18** Palpating the dorsalis pedis pulse.	A weak or absent pulse may indicate impaired arterial circulation. Further circulatory assessments (temperature and colour) are warranted to determine the significance of an absent pulse.
Palpate the posterior tibial pulses. Palpate behind and just below the medial malleolus (in the groove between the ankle and the Achilles tendon) (Fig. 23-19). Palpating both posterior tibial pulses at the same time aids in making comparisons. Assess amplitude bilaterally. **CLINICAL TIP** **Oedema in the ankles may make it difficult or impossible to palpate a posterior tibial pulse. In this case, Doppler ultrasound may be used to assess the pulse.**	The posterior tibial pulses should be strong bilaterally. However, in about 15% of healthy patients, the posterior tibial pulses are absent. 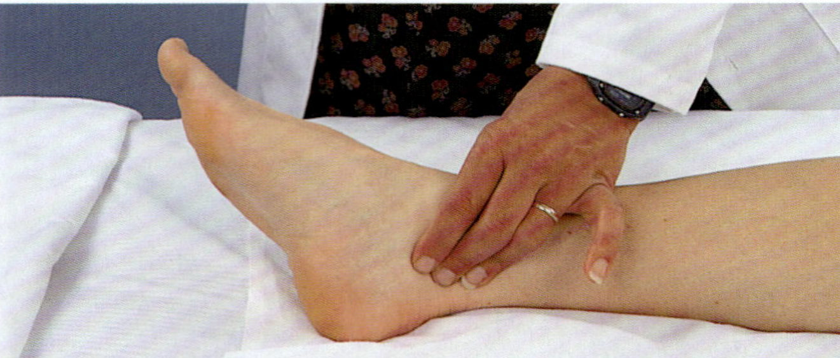 **FIGURE 23-19** Palpating the posterior tibial pulse. (© B. Proud.)	A weak or absent pulse indicates partial or complete arterial occlusion. In addition to a weak or absent pulse, a cool leg unilaterally, lack of hair and shiny skin on the leg suggest arterial occlusive disease (Wiltz-James & Foley, 2019).
Inspect for varicosities and thrombophlebitis. Ask the patient to stand because varicose veins may not be visible when the patient is supine and not as pronounced when the patient is sitting. As the patient is standing, inspect for superficial vein thrombophlebitis.	Veins are flat and barely seen under the surface of the skin. **OLDER ADULT CONSIDERATIONS** **Varicosities are common in the older patient.**	Varicose veins may appear as distended, nodular, bulging or tortuous, depending on severity. Varicosities are common in the anterior lateral thigh and lower leg, the posterior lateral calf, or anus (known as haemorrhoids). Varicose veins result

PHYSICAL ASSESSMENT (continued)

ASSESSMENT PROCEDURE	NORMAL FINDINGS	ABNORMAL FINDINGS
Legs (continued)		
To fully assess for a suspected phlebitis, palpate for tenderness. If superficial vein thrombophlebitis is present, note redness or discolouration on the skin surface over the vein.	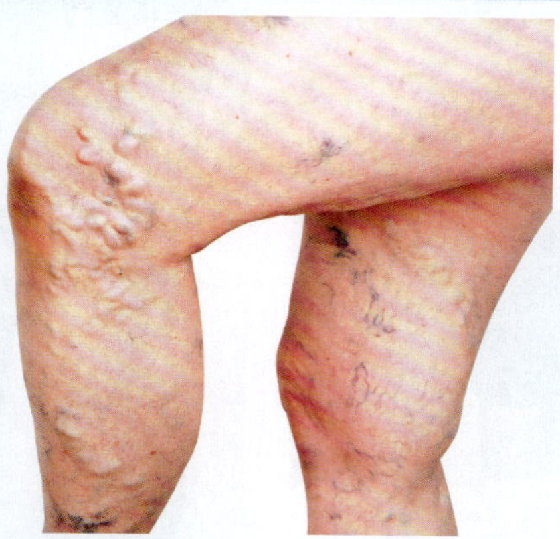 **FIGURE 23-20** Varicose veins. (Shutterstock.com/nixki.)	from incompetent valves in the veins, weak vein walls or an obstruction above the varicosity. Despite venous dilation, blood flow is decreased and venous pressure is increased. Superficial vein thrombophlebitis is marked by redness, thickening and tenderness along the vein. Aching or cramping may occur with walking or dorsiflexion of the foot. Swelling and inflammation are often noted (Fig. 23-20).
Special tests for arterial or venous insufficiency		
Perform position change test for arterial insufficiency. If pulses in the legs are weak, further assessment for arterial insufficiency is warranted. The patient should be in a supine position. Place one forearm under both of the patient's ankles and the other forearm underneath the knees. Raise the legs about 30 cm above the level of the heart. As you support the patient's legs, ask the patient to pump the feet up and down for about a minute to drain the legs of venous blood, leaving only arterial blood to colour the legs (Fig. 23-21a). At this point, ask the patient to sit up and dangle legs off the side of the examination table. Note the colour of both feet and the time it takes for colour to return (Fig. 23-21b). **CLINICAL TIP** **This assessment manoeuvre will not be accurate if the patient has peripheral vascular disease of the veins with incompetent valves.**	Feet pink to slightly pale in colour in the light-skinned patient with elevation. Inspect the soles in the dark-skinned patient, although it is more difficult to see subtle colour changes in darker skin. When the patient sits up and dangles the legs, a pinkish colour returns to the tips of the toes in 10 seconds or less. The superficial veins on top of the feet fill in 15 seconds or less. Normal responses with absent pulses suggest that an adequate collateral circulation has developed around an arterial occlusion.	Marked pallor with legs elevated is an indication of arterial insufficiency. Return of pink colour that takes longer than 10 seconds and superficial veins that take longer than 15 seconds to fill suggest arterial insufficiency. Persistent rubor (dusky redness) of toes and feet with legs dependent also suggests arterial insufficiency.

Continued on following page

PHYSICAL ASSESSMENT (continued)

ASSESSMENT PROCEDURE	NORMAL FINDINGS	ABNORMAL FINDINGS

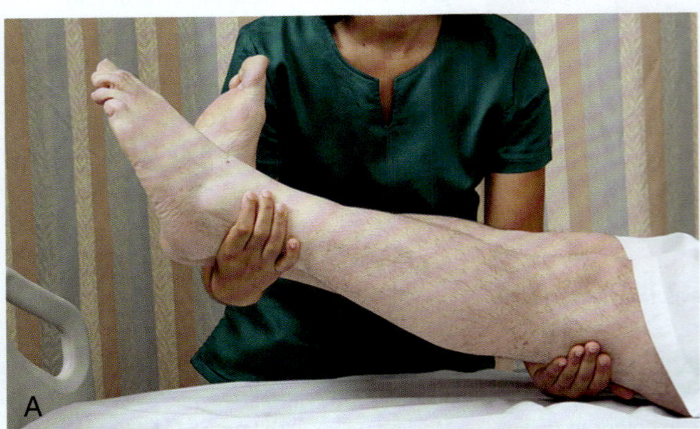
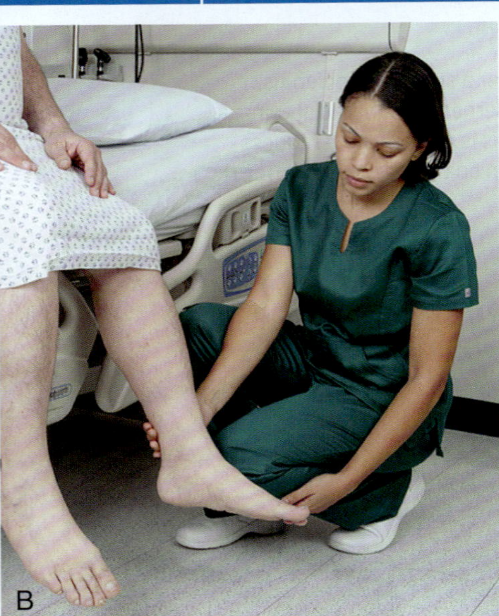

FIGURE 23-21 Testing for arterial insufficiency by elevating the legs **(A)**, followed by having client dangle the legs **(B)**.

Determine ankle-brachial pressure index (ABPI), also known as Ankle-Brachial Index (ABI). If the patient has symptoms of arterial occlusion, the ABPI should be used to compare the upper and lower limbs' systolic blood pressure (BP). The ABPI is the ratio of the ankle systolic BP to the arm (brachial) systolic BP. See Table 23-1. The ABPI is considered an accurate objective assessment for determining the degree of peripheral arterial disease. It detects decreased systolic pressure distal to the area of stenosis or arterial narrowing and allows the nurse to quantify this measurement. Use the following steps to measure ABPI:

- Have the patient rest in a supine position for at least 5 minutes.
- Apply the BP cuff to first one arm and then the other to determine the brachial pressure using the Doppler. First palpate the pulse and use the Doppler to hear the pulse. The 'whooshing' sound indicates the brachial pulse. Pressures in both arms are assessed because asymptomatic stenosis in the subclavian artery can produce an abnormally low reading and should not be used in the calculations. Record the *higher reading.*
- Apply the BP cuff to the right ankle, then palpate the posterior tibial pulse at the medial aspect of the ankle and the dorsalis pedis pulse on the dorsal aspect of the foot. Using the same Doppler

Generally the ankle pressure in a healthy person is the same or slightly higher than the brachial pressure, resulting in an ABPI of approximately 1, or no arterial insufficiency. Comparable findings between Doppler ultrasound and ABPI were noted in Ma et al.'s (2017) study.

In addition to the abnormal ABPI findings, reduced or absent pedal pulses, cool leg unilaterally, lack of hair and shiny skin on leg suggests peripheral arterial occlusive disease. People who smoke, are physically inactive, have a body mass index >30 or are hypertensive are more likely to have an abnormal ABPI, suggesting PAD (Woo et al., 2018).

Table 23-1	ABPI (ABI) guidelines
1.0–1.2 ABPI	Normal—no arterial insufficiency
0.8–1.0 ABPI	Mild insufficiency
0.5–0.8 ABPI	Moderate insufficiency
<0.5 ABPI	Severe insufficiency
<0.3 ABPI	Limb threatening

From Smith, S. F., Duell, D. J. & Martin, B. C (2011). Clinical nursing skills: Basic to advanced skills (8th ed.). Upper Saddle River, NJ: Pearson/Prentice Hall.
ABI, ankle-brachial index; ABPI, ankle-brachial pressure index.

PHYSICAL ASSESSMENT (continued)

ASSESSMENT PROCEDURE	NORMAL FINDINGS	ABNORMAL FINDINGS

Special tests for arterial or venous insufficiency (continued)

technique as in the arms, determine and record *both* systolic pressures. Repeat this procedure on the left ankle (Fig. 23-22). If you are unable to assess these pulses, use the peroneal artery (Fig. 23-23).

- ABPI calculation: Divide the higher ankle pressure for each foot by the higher brachial pressure. For example, you may have measured the highest brachial pulse as 160, the highest pulse in the right ankle as 80, and the highest pulse in the left ankle as 94. Dividing each by 160 (80/160 and 94/160) will result in a right ABPI of 0.5 and a left ABPI of 0.59.

CLINICAL TIP

- **Make sure to use a correctly sized BP cuff. The bladder of the cuff should be 20% wider than the diameter of the patient's limb.**
- **Document BP cuff sizes used on the nursing plan of care (e.g. '12-cm BP cuff used for brachial pressure: 10-cm BP cuff used for ankle pressure'). This minimises the risk of shift-to-shift discrepancies in ABPIs.**
- **Inflate the cuff enough to ensure complete closure of the artery. Inflation should be 20 to 30 mmHg beyond the point at which the last arterial signal was detected.**
- **Avoid deflating the cuff too rapidly. Instead, try to maintain a deflation rate of 2 to 4 mmHg for patients without arrhythmias and 2 mmHg or slower for patients with arrhythmias. Deflating the cuff more rapidly than that may cause you to miss the patient's highest pressure and record an erroneous (low) BP measurement.**
- **Be suspicious of arterial pressure recorded at less than 40 mmHg. This may mean that the venous signal was mistaken for the arterial signal. If you measure arterial pressure, which is normally 120 mmHg, at below 40 mmHg, ask a colleague to double check your findings before you record the arterial pressure.**
- **Suspect medial calcific sclerosis any time you calculate an ABPI of 1.3 or greater or measure ankle pressure at more than 300 mmHg. This condition is associated with diabetes mellitus, chronic renal failure and hyperparathyroidism. Medial calcific sclerosis produces falsely elevated ankle pressure by making the vessels non-compressible.**

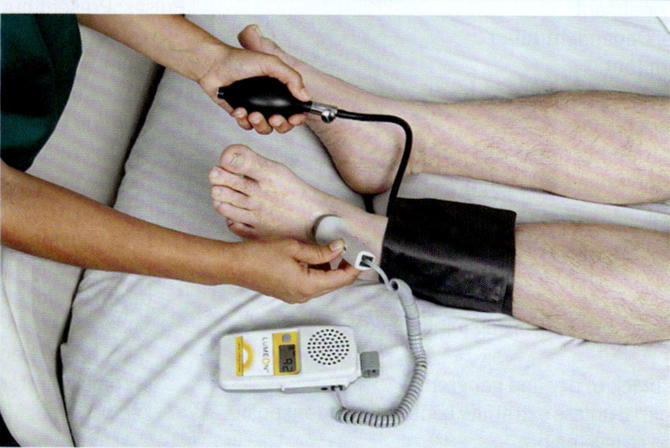

FIGURE 23-22 When measuring systolic pressure from the dorsalis pedis artery, apply the blood pressure cuff above the malleolus and the Doppler device at a 60- to 90-degree angle over the anterior tibial artery. Then move the device downwards along the length of the vessel.

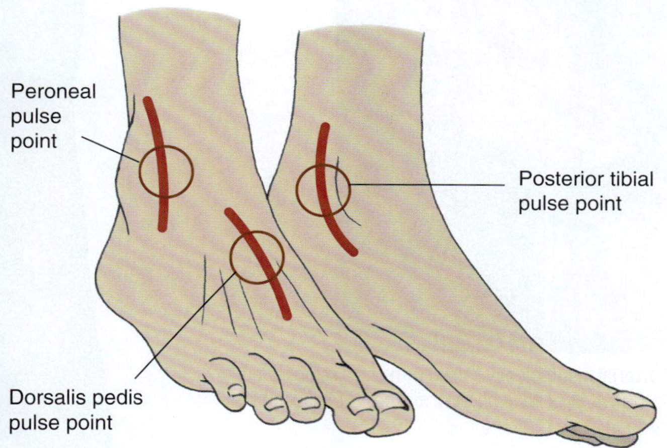

FIGURE 23-23 If you cannot measure pressure in the dorsalis pedis or posterior tibial artery, measure it in the peroneal artery. The blood pressure cuff can remain in place.

ABNORMAL FINDINGS 23-1 Characteristics of arterial and venous insufficiency

ARTERIAL INSUFFICIENCY

Pain: Intermittent claudication to sharp, unrelenting, constant
Pulses: Diminished or absent
Skin characteristics: Dependent rubor

- Elevation pallor of foot
- Dry, shiny skin
- Cool-to-cold temperature
- Loss of hair over toes and dorsum of foot
- Nails thickened and ridged

Ulcer characteristics:

- Location: Tips of toes, toe webs, heel or other pressure areas if confined to bed
- Pain: Very painful
- Depth of ulcer: Deep, often involving joint space
- Shape: Circular
- Ulcer base: Pale black to dry and gangrene
- Leg oedema: Minimal unless extremity kept in dependent position constantly to relieve pain

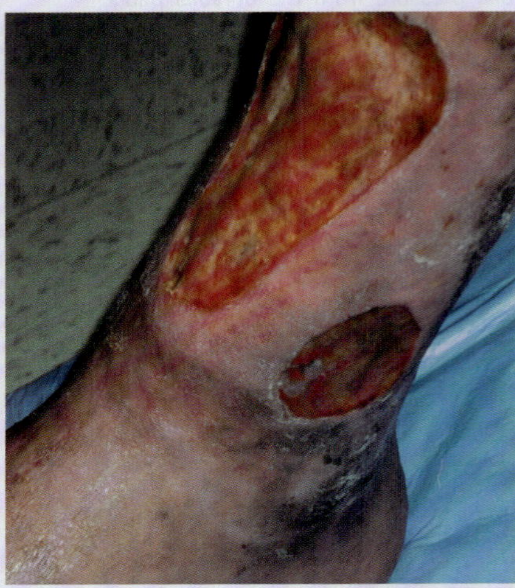

Characteristic ulcer of arterial insufficiency. (Used with permission from Berg, D. & Worzala, K. [2006]. *Atlas of adult physical diagnosis*. Philadelphia: Lippincott Williams & Wilkins.)

VENOUS INSUFFICIENCY

Pain: Aching, cramping
Pulses: Present but may be difficult to palpate through oedema
Skin characteristics:

- Pigmentation in gaiter area (area of medial and lateral malleolus)
- Skin thickened and tough
- May be reddish-blue
- Frequently associated with dermatitis

Ulcer characteristics:

- Location: Medial malleolus or anterior tibial area
- Pain: If superficial, minimal pain; but may be very painful
- Depth of ulcer: Superficial
- Shape: Irregular border
- Ulcer base: Granulation tissue—beefy-red to yellow fibrinous in chronic long-term ulcer
- Leg oedema: Moderate to severe

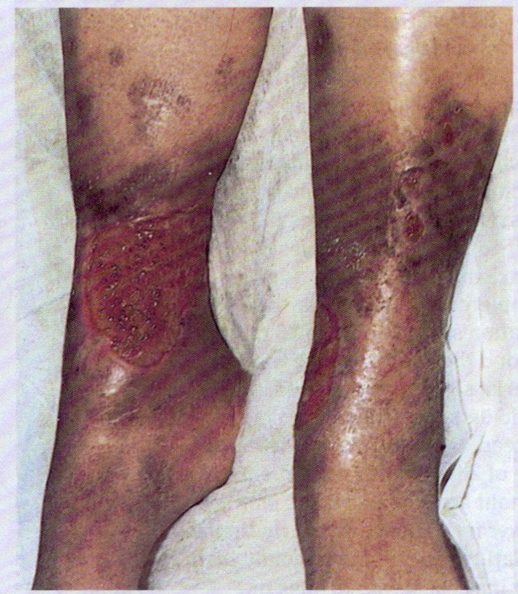

Characteristic ulcer of venous insufficiency. (Used with permission from Marks, R. [1987]. *Skin disease in old age*. Philadelphia: J. B. Lippincott.)

CASE STUDY

Your physical assessment reveals Mr Andross's left leg to be swollen from the mid-thigh down to the ankle. The circumference of his is left calf is 3 cm larger than the right; his skin is warm to touch and looks shiny; and his thigh is tender to palpation. There is bruising from his right lateral flank area extending down into the upper right buttock, the lateral side of the thigh and finishing behind the knee. A 12-cm surgical wound closed with clips on the lateral side of the upper thigh is dry, with no exudates or erythema at the wound site.

The dorsalis pedis pulse is palpable on both feet; the posterior tibial pulse is palpable on the right leg but not on the left because of oedema. Mr Andross denies numbness or tingling in either leg.

CRITICAL THINKING

7. Mr Andross is diagnosed with having a deep vein thrombosis. Which of the above data supports this diagnosis?

ABNORMAL FINDINGS 23-2 Types of peripheral oedema

OEDEMA ASSOCIATED WITH LYMPHOEDEMA

- Caused by abnormal or blocked lymph vessels
- Non-pitting
- Usually bilateral; may be unilateral
- No skin ulceration or pigmentation

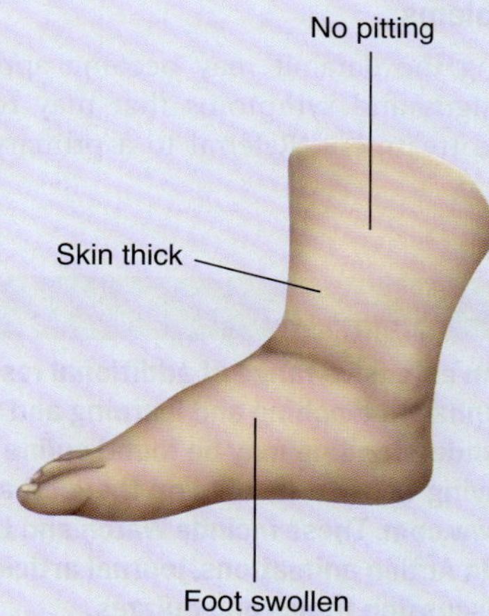

Swelling associated with lymphatic abnormality. (Bickley, L.S. [2007]. *Bates' Guide to Physical Examination and History Taking* [9th ed.], LWW.)

OEDEMA ASSOCIATED WITH CHRONIC VENOUS INSUFFICIENCY

- Caused by obstruction or insufficiency of deep veins
- Pitting, documented as:
  1+ = slight pitting
  2+ = deeper than 1+
  3+ = noticeably deep pit; extremity looks larger
  4+ = very deep pit; gross oedema in extremity
- Usually unilateral; may be bilateral
- Skin ulceration and pigmentation may be present

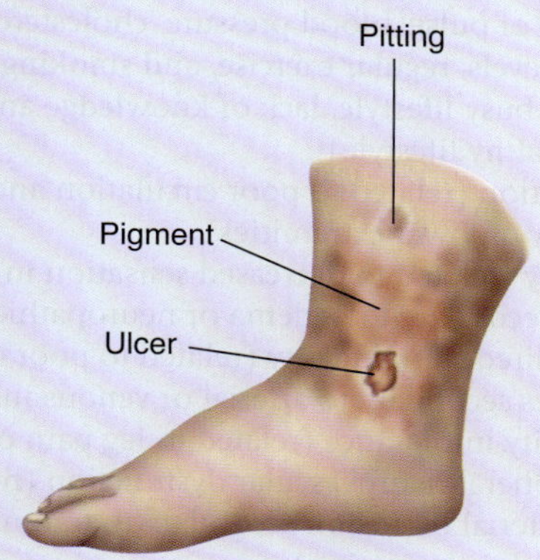

Oedema associated with chronic venous insufficiency. (Bickley, L.S. [2007]. *Bates' Guide to Physical Examination and History Taking* [9th ed.], LWW.)

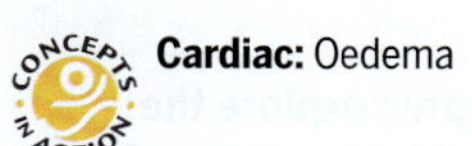
Cardiac: Oedema

VALIDATING AND DOCUMENTING FINDINGS

Validate the peripheral vascular assessment data you have collected. This is necessary to verify that the data are reliable and accurate. Document the assessment data following the health care facility or agency policy.

After you have collected your assessment data, you will need to analyse the data using diagnostic reasoning skills. Refer to the discussion of the diagnostic reasoning process in Chapter 5.

Sample of objective data

Arms are equal in size, no swelling, pinkish skin tone, no clubbing of fingertips, warm bilaterally. Capillary refill time less than 2 seconds, radial and brachial pulses 2+ bilaterally, no epitrochlear lymph nodes palpated. Legs are pink from toes to groin bilaterally, normal distribution of hair, no ulcers or oedema. Legs are warm bilaterally; 1-cm non-tender inguinal lymph nodes palpated; femoral, popliteal, dorsalis pedis and posterior tibial pulses 2+ bilaterally. No apparent varicosities or superficial thrombophlebitis.

Sample of subjective data

63-year-old woman reports 'pale' colour on her right foot and lower leg in comparison to her left leg. She states her right leg always feels cooler than her left; she reports no temperature changes to her arms. The patient complains of slight pins and needles in her right foot, however, no pain in her left leg; no open sores on legs, no adverse swelling of either arm or either leg. States no bulging veins, no swollen glands, no concerns with sexual activity, no past history of circulatory problems, no previous surgery on the veins or arteries. The patient explains that her mother died from a heart attack at age 60 years and her father died from complications of diabetes at age 70. Patient states she does not smoke, manages her stress well and exercises regularly.

Analysis of data

DIAGNOSTIC REASONING: POSSIBLE CONCLUSIONS

After collecting subjective and objective data pertaining to the peripheral vascular assessment, identify abnormal findings and patient strengths. Then cluster the data to reveal any significant patterns or abnormalities. These data may be used to make clinical judgements about the status of the patient's peripheral vascular system.

Potential patient risks

- Risk of ineffective therapeutic regimen management (monitoring of pulse, blood pressure, cholesterol and triglyceride levels, regular exercise, and smoking cessation) (related to a busy lifestyle, lack of knowledge and resources to follow healthy lifestyle)
- Risk of infection (related to poor circulation and impaired skin integrity of lower extremities)
- Risk of injury (related to decreased sensation in lower extremities secondary to oedema or neuropathies)
- Risk of impaired skin integrity (related to poor circulation to extremities secondary to arterial or venous insufficiency)
- Risk of activity intolerance (related to leg pain on walking)
- Risk of peripheral neurovascular dysfunction (related to venous or arterial occlusion secondary to trauma, surgery or mechanical compression)
- Risk of respiratory compromise secondary to development of deep vein thrombosis
- Risk of chronic venous insufficiency, pain and oedema (post-thrombotic syndrome) secondary to deep vein thrombosis

Potential patient problems

- Ineffective tissue perfusion (related to arterial insufficiency)
- Impaired skin integrity (related to arterial or venous insufficiency)
- Pain (related to arterial or venous insufficiency)
- Fear of loss of extremities (related to arterial insufficiency)
- Disturbed body image (related to leg ulcerations, oedema or varicosities)
- Fear of respiratory compromise and death (related to deep vein thrombosis)

Selected collaborative problems

After grouping the data, certain collaborative problems may become apparent. Remember that collaborative problems cannot be prevented through nursing interventions. However, these physiological complications of medical conditions can be detected and monitored by the nurse. In addition, the nurse can use doctor- and nurse-prescribed interventions to minimise the complications of these problems. The nurse may also have to refer the patient in such situations for further treatment of the problem. The following is a list of collaborative problems that may be identified when assessing the peripheral vascular system.

- Thromboembolic or deep vein thrombosis
- Arterial occlusion
- Peripheral vascular (arterial or venous) insufficiency
- Hypertension
- Ischaemic ulcers
- Gangrene
- Varicose veins.

Medical problems

After grouping the data, it may become apparent that the patient has signs and symptoms that may require medical diagnosis and treatment. Referral to a primary care provider is necessary.

ONLINE RESOURCES

An extensive range of additional resources to enhance teaching and learning and to facilitate understanding may be found online at the text's accompanying website, located on thePoint at http://thepoint.lww.com. These include Watch and Learn videos, Concepts in Action animations, journal articles, case studies, discussion topics and quizzes.

Subscribers may also access Lippincott Procedures, an extensive online point-of-care procedure guide that provides reliable step-by-step instructions for more than 1700 procedures, including 450 evidence-based Australian procedures, and skills in a variety of speciality settings, together with a wealth of supporting information.

SIMULATED LEARNING

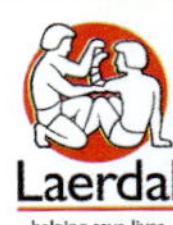

Having completed this chapter, explore the scenarios of Lloyd Bennett Part 1 and Part 2 and Marilyn Hughes Part 1 and Part 2. Lloyd is a 76-year-old male who is postoperative following a hip arthroplasty; he required a blood transfusion. Marilyn is a 45-year-old female who has broken her leg. Incorporating the health assessment content in this chapter with your existing theoretical knowledge and clinical experience, progress through each simulation scenario (this is best done in a small group). How would you manage each patient's care? When reflecting on your management of each virtual patient, what do you think you did well and what do you think you can improve? Consider why you think this and also how you might manage a similar problem in the future.

CASE STUDY

The case study demonstrates how to analyse peripheral vascular system assessment data for a specific patient. The exercises included in the ancillary product on thePoint that complements this text offer further opportunities to enhance your skills.

Mr Marcus Andross is 78 years old and lives with his eldest daughter. Mr Andross has a 10-year history of severe chronic pain in his left hip due to osteoarthritis. Overtime his symptoms of joint swelling, decreased range of motion and joint stiffness in his hip have increased, and now he is longer able to mobilise. His doctor recommended a left total hip replacement, and he is now 4 days postoperative following his surgery. He has been assigned to you as one of your patients for the shift.

You are assisting Mr Andross to sit up for breakfast, and he winces when he moves his left leg. When you ask him where the pain is, he states that it is 'mostly in my left leg' and that it is 'painful to move and feels swollen'. He denies knee or leg pain at home prior to his surgery. He last had Panadol forte pain medication 1 hour ago; it has not decreased his pain level.

According to the medical notes, Mr Adross's surgery was uncomplicated. On his first day postoperative he was found to have an elevated temperature and symptoms of a chest infection. He is being treated for pneumonia with IV antibiotics. As a result of his condition he was not assisted to mobilise until 72 hours following his surgery. He states that he was up and walking frequently yesterday with the physiotherapist and when his daughter came to visit. He normally lives a sedentary lifestyle due to pain from the arthritis in his hip. His medical history includes diabetes, hypertension (he does not recall when it was first diagnosed) and family history of heart disease. He smoked one packet of cigarettes per day for 30 years but stopped 10 year ago. He normally uses a walking stick to get around. He has home care nurses visit him four times a week to help him shower, and his daughter does his cleaning, washing and shopping. He has had three admissions for uncontrolled diabetes about 10 years ago, but since his daughter started cooking and shopping for him, he has had stable blood sugar but remains on oral hypoglycaemic medications.

Your physical assessment reveals Mr Andross's left leg to be swollen from the mid-thigh down to the ankle. The circumference of his is left calf is 3 cm larger than the right; his skin is warm to touch and looks shiny; and his thigh is tender to palpation. There is bruising from his right lateral flank area extending down into the upper right buttock, the lateral side of the thigh and finishing behind the knee. A 12-cm surgical wound closed with clips on the lateral side of the upper thigh is dry, with no exudates or erythema at the wound site. The dorsalis pedis pulse is palpable on both feet; the posterior tibial pulse is palpable on the right leg but not on the left because of oedema. Mr Andross denies numbness or tingling in either leg.

The following concept map illustrates the diagnostic reasoning process.

Applying COLDSPA

Applying COLDSPA for patient symptoms: 'Leg is painful to move and feels swollen.'

Mnemonic	Question	Data provided	Missing data
Character	Describe the sign or symptom (feeling, appearance, sound, smell or taste, if applicable).	Patient states that the pain is mostly in his left leg; his leg is painful to move and feels swollen.	Describe the pain or soreness in your leg. Is the pain different from the pain you experienced yesterday?
Onset	When did it begin?		When did you first notice the pain and swelling?
Location	Where is it? Does it radiate? Does it occur anywhere else?	Left leg swollen from mid-thigh to ankle. The left calf is 3 cm larger than left calf, skin is warm to touch, looks shiny and is tender to palpation.	Where is the pain specifically? Can you point to it? Does your pain radiate? Is there any pain elsewhere?
Duration	How long does it last? Does it recur?		Is the pain constant or intermittent?
Severity	How bad is it? or How much does it bother you?	Painful to move leg.	Rate your pain on a 10 point scale.

Continued on page 453

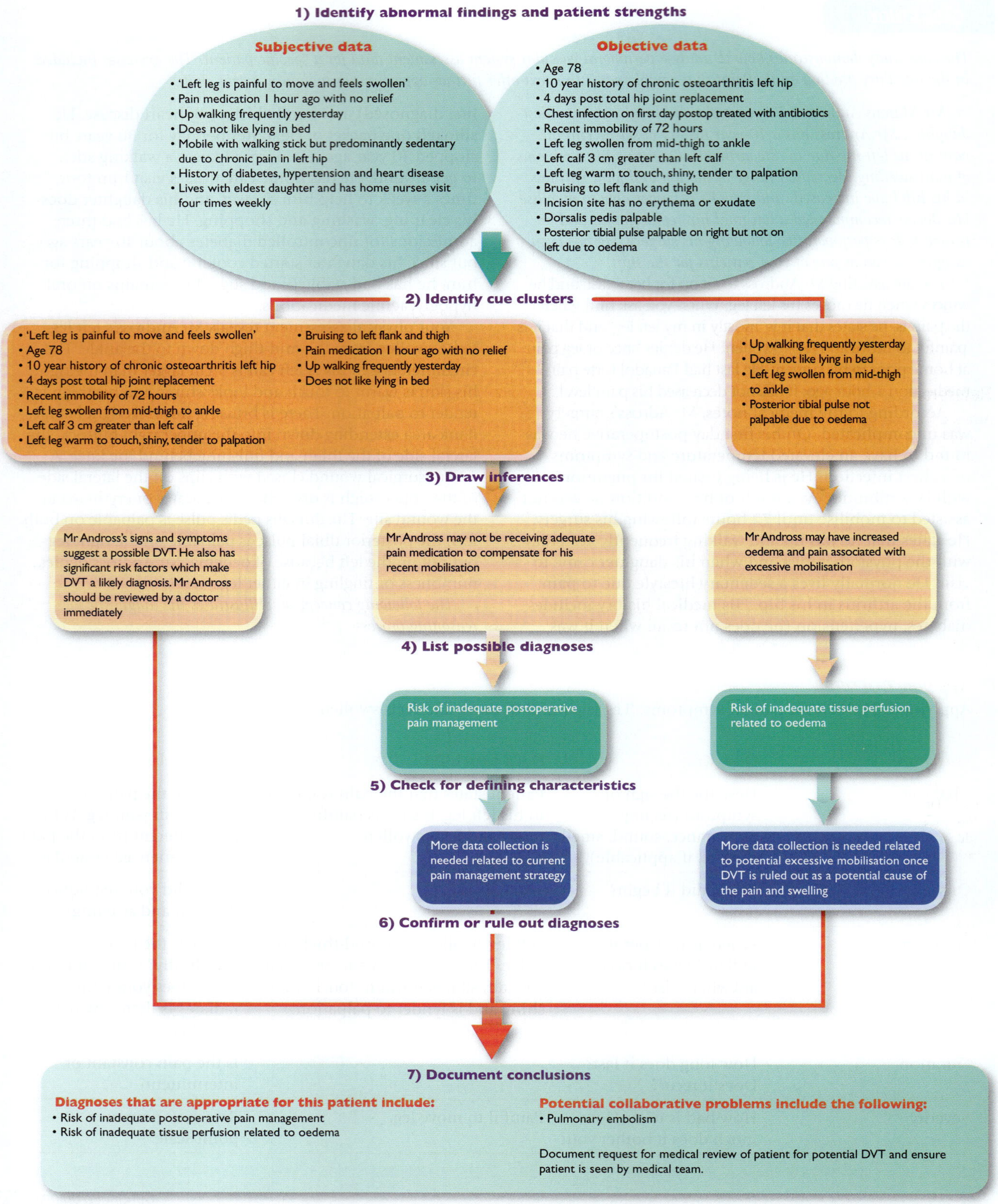

1) Identify abnormal findings and patient strengths

Subjective data

- 'Left leg is painful to move and feels swollen'
- Pain medication 1 hour ago with no relief
- Up walking frequently yesterday
- Does not like lying in bed
- Mobile with walking stick but predominantly sedentary due to chronic pain in left hip
- History of diabetes, hypertension and heart disease
- Lives with eldest daughter and has home nurses visit four times weekly

Objective data

- Age 78
- 10 year history of chronic osteoarthritis left hip
- 4 days post total hip joint replacement
- Chest infection on first day postop treated with antibiotics
- Recent immobility of 72 hours
- Left leg swollen from mid-thigh to ankle
- Left calf 3 cm greater than left calf
- Left leg warm to touch, shiny, tender to palpation
- Bruising to left flank and thigh
- Incision site has no erythema or exudate
- Dorsalis pedis palpable
- Posterior tibial pulse palpable on right but not on left due to oedema

2) Identify cue clusters

- 'Left leg is painful to move and feels swollen'
- Age 78
- 10 year history of chronic osteoarthritis left hip
- 4 days post total hip joint replacement
- Recent immobility of 72 hours
- Left leg swollen from mid-thigh to ankle
- Left calf 3 cm greater than left calf
- Left leg warm to touch, shiny, tender to palpation
- Bruising to left flank and thigh
- Pain medication 1 hour ago with no relief
- Up walking frequently yesterday
- Does not like lying in bed

- Up walking frequently yesterday
- Does not like lying in bed
- Left leg swollen from mid-thigh to ankle
- Posterior tibial pulse not palpable due to oedema

3) Draw inferences

Mr Andross's signs and symptoms suggest a possible DVT. He also has significant risk factors which make DVT a likely diagnosis. Mr Andross should be reviewed by a doctor immediately

Mr Andross may not be receiving adequate pain medication to compensate for his recent mobilisation

Mr Andross may have increased oedema and pain associated with excessive mobilisation

4) List possible diagnoses

Risk of inadequate postoperative pain management

Risk of inadequate tissue perfusion related to oedema

5) Check for defining characteristics

More data collection is needed related to current pain management strategy

More data collection is needed related to potential excessive mobilisation once DVT is ruled out as a potential cause of the pain and swelling

6) Confirm or rule out diagnoses

7) Document conclusions

Diagnoses that are appropriate for this patient include:

- Risk of inadequate postoperative pain management
- Risk of inadequate tissue perfusion related to oedema

Potential collaborative problems include the following:

- Pulmonary embolism

Document request for medical review of patient for potential DVT and ensure patient is seen by medical team.

Mnemonic	Question	Data provided	Missing data
Pattern	What makes it better or worse?	Movement makes it worse. Pain medication has not improved the pain.	How often are you taking pain medication? What is the type and dose of the pain medication? Is there anything else that makes the pain better?
Associated factors/How it Affects the patient	What other symptoms occur with it? How does it affect you?	Dorsalis pedis pulse is palpable; posterior tibial pulse is not palpable due to oedema. Denies numbness and tingling.	Describe your activity since your surgery. Do you have any other symptoms?

References

Arrivé, L., Derhy, S., Daham, B., et al. (2018). Primary lower limb lymphoedema classification with non-contrast MR lymphography. *European Radiology, 28*, 291–300. doi:10.1007/s00330-017-4948-z.

Auckland Vascular Centre. (2019). Peripհearl Artery Disease. Available at https://www.aucklandvascular.com/peripheral-arterial-disease-pad/.

Australian Commission on Safety and Quality in Health Care (ACSQHC). (2019). Venous thrombosis prevention clinical care standards. Available at https://www.safetyandquality.gov.au/our-work/clinical-care-standards/venous-thromboembolism-prevention-clinical-care-standard/.

Australian Medicines Handbook Pty Ltd. (2019). Adelaide.

Barnes, G. D. (2018). Screening for PAD and CVD risk with ABI: USPSTF Recommendations. *JAMA: The Journal of the American Medical Association, 320*, 177–183.

Berg, D. & Worzala, K. (2006). *Atlas of adult physical diagnosis*. Philadelphia: Lippincott Williams & Wilkins.

Bhat, M. N., Vadala, R., Rabindrarajan, E., et al. (2018). Curious case of acute unilateral deep vein thrombosis: May-Turner syndrome. *Indian Journal of Critical Care Medicine: Peer-Reviewed, Official Publication of Indian Society of Critical Care Medicine, 22*(7), 558–560. http://dx.doi.org.ezproxy.csu.edu.au/10.4103/ijccm.IJCCM_393_17.

Cohen, B. J. & Hull, K. L. (2015). *Memmler's structure and function of the human body* (11th ed.). Philadelphia: Lippincott Williams & Wilkins.

Cohen-Mansfield, J. (2016). Predictors of smoking cessation in old-old age. *Nicotine & Tobacco Research, 18*(7), 1675–1679. http://dx.doi.org.ezproxy.csu.edu.au/10.1093/ntr/ntw011.

Conte, S. M. & Vale, P. R. (2018). Peripheral arterial disease. *Heart, Lung and Circulation, 27*(4), 427–432. https://www.heartlungcirc.org/article/S1443-9506(17)31459-2/fulltext.

Davies, J. H., Richards, J., Conway, K., et al. (2017). Primary care screening for peripheral artery disease: a cross sectional observation study. *British Journal of General Practice, 67*(655), e103–e110. doi:10.3399/bjgp17X689137.

Effeney, D. J. & Stoney, R. J. (1993). *Wylie's atlas of vascular surgery: Disorders of the extremities*. Philadelphia: Lippincott Williams & Wilkins.

Lynn, P. (2018). *Taylor's clinical nursing skills: A nursing process approach* (5nd ed.). Wolters Kluwer/Lippincott Williams & Wilkins.

Ma, J., Liu, M., Chen, D., et al. (2017). The validity and reliability between automated oscillometric measurement of ankle brachial index and standard measurement by eco-Doppler in diabetic patients with or without diabetic foot. *International Journal of Endocrinology*, 1–6. http://dx.doi.org.ezproxy.csu.edu.au/10.1155/2017/2383651.

Marks, R. (1987). *Skin disease in old age*. Philadelphia: J. B. Lippincott.

Rubin, R. & Strayer, D. S. (2007). *Rubin's pathology: Clinicopathologic foundations of medicine* (5th ed.). Philadelphia: Lippincott Williams & Wilkins.

Schorr, E., Treat-Jacobson, D. & Lindquist, R. (2017). The relationship between peripheral artery disease symptomatology and ischaemia. *Nursing Research, 66*(5), 378–387. doi:10.1097/NNR.0000000000000230.

Si, S., Golledge, J., Norman, P., et al. (2018). Prevalence and outcomes of undiagnosed peripheral arterial disease high risk patients in Australia: An Australian REACH sub-study. *Heart, Lung and Circulation*, doi.org/10.1016/j.hlc.2018.04.292.

Smith, S. F., Duell, D. J. & Martin, B. C. (2011). *Clinical nursing skills: Basic to advanced skills* (8th ed.). Upper Saddle River, NJ: Pearson/Prentice Hall.

Wiltz-James, L. M. & Foley, J. (2019). Hospital discharge teaching for patients with peripheral vascular disease. *Critical Care Nursing Clinics of North America, 31*(1), 91–95. https://doi.org/10.1016/j.cnc.2018.11.003.

Woo, J., Chan, B. W. M. & Leung, J. (2018). Influence of dietary patterns and inflammatory markers on atherosclerosis using ankle brachial index as a surrogate. *The Journal of Nutrition, Health & Aging, 22*(5), 619–626. http://dx.doi.org.ezproxy.csu.edu.au/10.1007/s12603-018-1031-7.

Selected reading

Farrell, M. & Dempsey, J. (Eds). (2014). *Smeltzer & Bare's textbook of medical-surgical nursing* (3rd Australian & New Zealand ed.). Sydney: Lippincott Williams & Wilkins.

Online resources

Australasian Society of Thrombosis & Haemostasis: www.asth.org.au
Lymphoedema Association of Australia: http://lymphoedema.org.au
New Zealand Dermatological Society Incorporated: http://dermnetnz.org
New Zealand Wound Care Society: www.nzwcs.org.nz
Quitline Australia: www.quitnow.gov.au
Quitline New Zealand: www.quit.org.nz
Smokefree Nurses Aotearoa/New Zealand: www.smokefreenurses.org.nz
Smoking cessation training Australia: www.quit.org.au/resource-centre/training/training-for-health-professionals
Smoking cessation training New Zealand: www.heartfoundation.org.nz/programmes-resources/health-professionals/smoking-cessation-training

CHAPTER 24

Abdomen

CASE STUDY

Lottie Knowles is an 84-year-old resident of an aged-care facility. She has been admitted to the emergency department with a diagnosis of abdominal pain for investigation. She is alert and oriented and able to clearly describe her pain. She has no spouse or children and her closest relative is a niece who lives interstate.

Structure and function

The abdomen is bordered superiorly by the costal margins, inferiorly by the symphysis pubis and inguinal canals, and laterally by the flanks (Fig. 24-1). To perform an adequate assessment of the abdomen, the nurse needs to understand the anatomical divisions known as the abdominal quadrants, the abdominal wall muscles and the internal anatomy of the abdominal cavity.

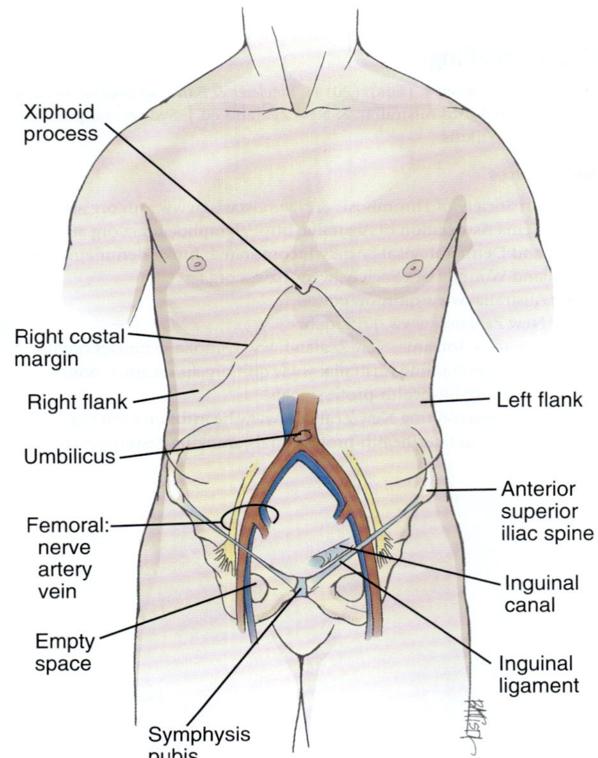

FIGURE 24-1 Landmarks of the abdomen.

THE ABDOMINAL QUADRANTS

For the purposes of examination, the abdomen can be described as having four quadrants termed the right upper quadrant (RUQ), the right lower quadrant (RLQ), the left lower quadrant (LLQ) and the left upper quadrant (LUQ). The quadrants are determined by an imaginary vertical line (midline) extending from the tip of the sternum (xiphoid) through the umbilicus to the symphysis pubis. This line is bisected perpendicularly by the lateral line, which runs through the umbilicus across the abdomen. Familiarisation with the organs and structures in each quadrant is essential to accurate data collection, interpretation and documentation of findings. Another, older method divides the abdomen into nine regions. Three of these regions are still commonly used to describe abdominal findings: epigastric, umbilical and hypogastric or suprapubic. Assessment tool 24-1 describes abdominal quadrants and regions.

ABDOMINAL WALL MUSCLES

The abdominal contents are enclosed externally by the abdominal wall musculature, which includes three layers of muscle extending from the back, around the flanks, to the front. The outermost layer is the external abdominal oblique; the middle layer is the internal abdominal oblique; and the innermost layer is the transverse abdominis (Fig. 24-2). Connective tissue from these muscles extends forwards to encase a vertical muscle of the anterior abdominal wall called the rectus abdominis. The fibres and connective tissue extensions of these muscles (aponeuroses) diverge in a characteristic plywoodlike pattern (several thin layers arranged at right angles to each other), which provides strength to the abdominal wall. The joining of these muscle fibres and aponeuroses at the midline of the abdomen forms a white line called the linea alba, which extends vertically from the xiphoid process of the sternum to the symphysis pubis. The abdominal wall muscles protect the internal organs and allow normal compression during functional activities such as coughing, sneezing, urination, defecation and childbirth.

ASSESSMENT TOOL 24-1 Locating abdominal structures by quadrants

Abdominal assessment findings are commonly allocated to the quadrant in which they are discovered, or their location may be described according to the nine abdominal regions that some practitioners may still use as reference marks. Quadrants and contents are listed here.

Right upper quadrant (RUQ)

Ascending and transverse colon
Duodenum
Gallbladder
Hepatic flexure of colon
Liver
Pancreas (head)
Pylorus (the small bowel—or ileum—traverses all quadrants)
Right adrenal gland
Right kidney (upper pole)
Right ureter

Right lower quadrant (RLQ)

Appendix
Ascending colon
Caecum
Right kidney (lower pole)
Right ovary and tube
Right ureter
Right spermatic cord

Left upper quadrant (LUQ)

Left adrenal gland
Left kidney (upper pole)
Left ureter
Pancreas (body and tail)
Spleen
Splenic flexure of colon
Stomach
Transverse descending colon

Left lower quadrant (LLQ)

Left kidney (lower pole)
Left ovary and tube
Left ureter
Left spermatic cord
Descending and sigmoid colon

Midline

Bladder
Uterus
Prostate gland

The older method of describing abdominal locations uses nine regions, pictured at right.

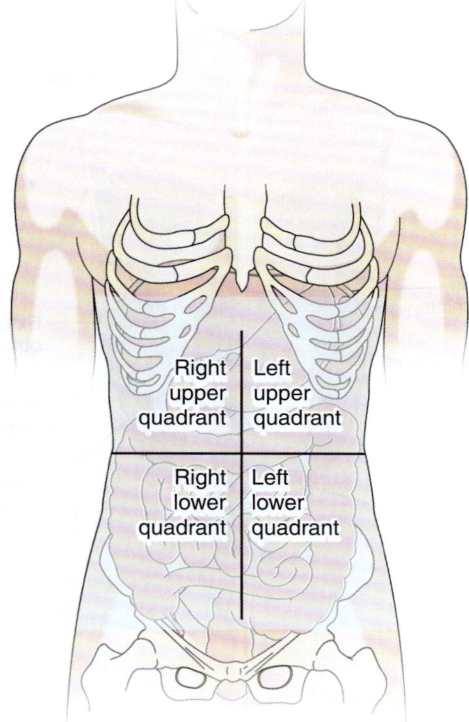

Abdominal quadrants.

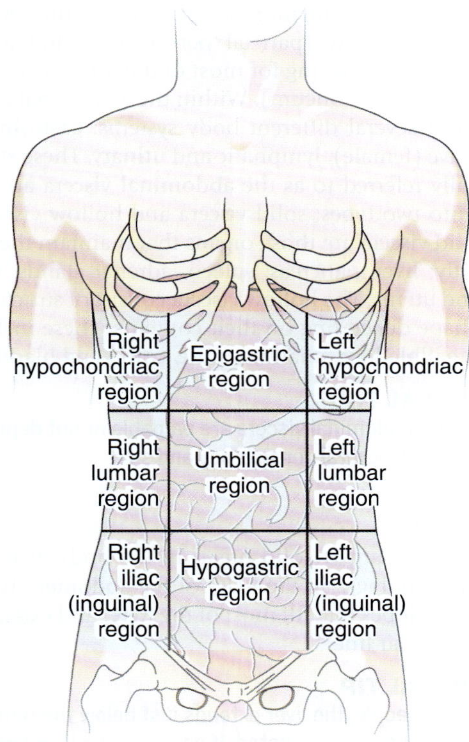

Abdominal regions.

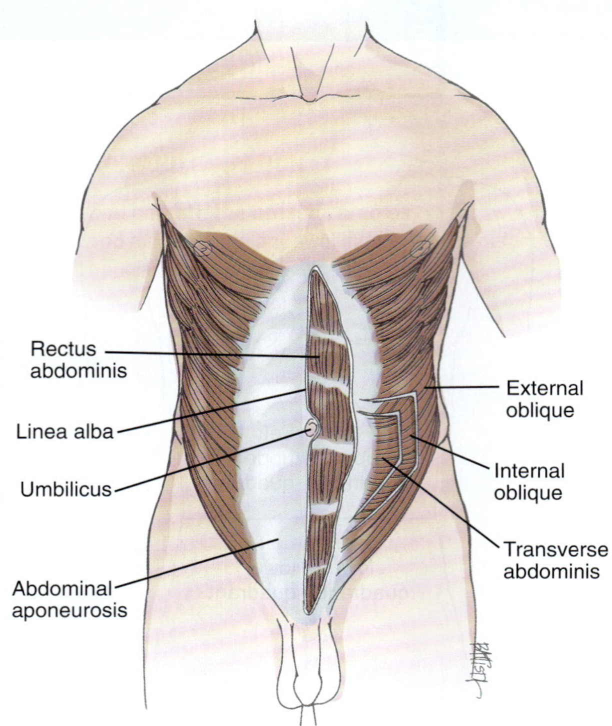

FIGURE 24-2 Abdominal wall muscles.

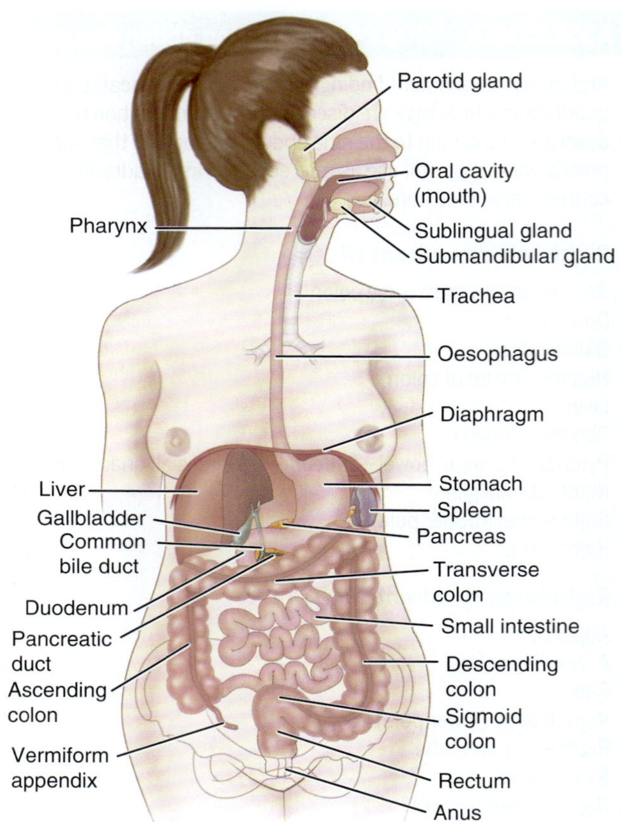

FIGURE 24-3 Abdominal viscera. (Farrell, M. & Dempsey, J. [Eds]. [2014]. *Smeltzer & Bare's textbook of medical-surgical nursing* [3rd Australian & New Zealand ed.]. Sydney: Lippincott Williams & Wilkins.)

INTERNAL ANATOMY

A thin, shiny, serous membrane called the peritoneum lines the abdominal cavity (parietal peritoneum) and also provides a protective covering for most of the internal abdominal organs (visceral peritoneum). Within the abdominal cavity are structures of several different body systems: gastrointestinal, reproductive (female), lymphatic and urinary. These structures are typically referred to as the abdominal viscera and can be divided into two types: solid viscera and hollow viscera (Fig. 24-3). Solid viscera are those organs that maintain their shape consistently: liver, pancreas, spleen, adrenal glands, kidneys, ovaries and uterus. The hollow viscera consist of structures that change shape depending on their contents. These include the stomach, gallbladder, small intestine, colon and bladder.

CLINICAL TIP
Whether abdominal viscera are palpable or not depends on their location, structural consistency and size.

Solid viscera

The liver is the largest solid organ in the body. It is located below the diaphragm in the RUQ of the abdomen. It is composed of four lobes that fill most of the RUQ and extend to the left midclavicular line.

CLINICAL TIP
In many people, the liver extends just below the right costal margin, where it may be palpated. If palpable, the liver has a soft consistency. The liver functions as an accessory digestive organ and has a variety of metabolic and regulatory functions as well, including glucose storage, formation of blood plasma proteins and clotting factors, urea synthesis, cholesterol production, bile formation, destruction of red blood cells, storage of iron and vitamins, and detoxification.

The pancreas, located mostly behind the stomach deep in the upper abdomen, is normally not palpable. It is a long gland extending across the abdomen from the RUQ to the LUQ. The pancreas has two functions: it is an endocrine gland, and it is an accessory organ of digestion.

The spleen is approximately 7 cm wide and is located above the left kidney just below the diaphragm at the level of the ninth, tenth and eleventh ribs. It is posterior to the left midaxillary line and posterior and lateral to the stomach. This soft, flat structure is normally not palpable. In some healthy patients, the lower tip can be felt below the left costal margin. The spleen functions primarily to filter the blood of cellular debris, to digest microorganisms and to return the breakdown products to the liver.

CLINICAL TIP
When the spleen enlarges, the lower tip extends down and towards the midline.

The kidneys are located high and deep under the diaphragm. These glandular, bean-shaped organs measuring approximately 10 × 5 × 2.5 cm are considered posterior organs and approximate with the level of the T12 to L3 vertebrae. The tops of both kidneys are protected by the posterior rib cage. Kidney tenderness is best assessed at the costovertebral angle (Fig. 24-4). The right kidney is positioned slightly lower because of

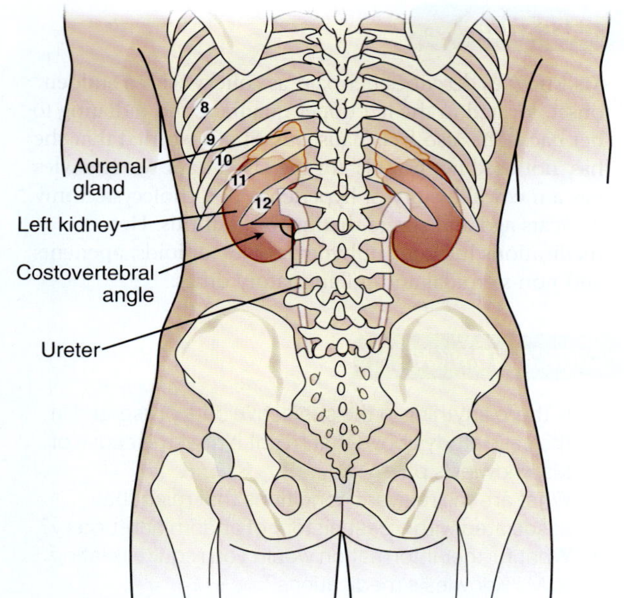

FIGURE 24-4 Position of the kidneys.

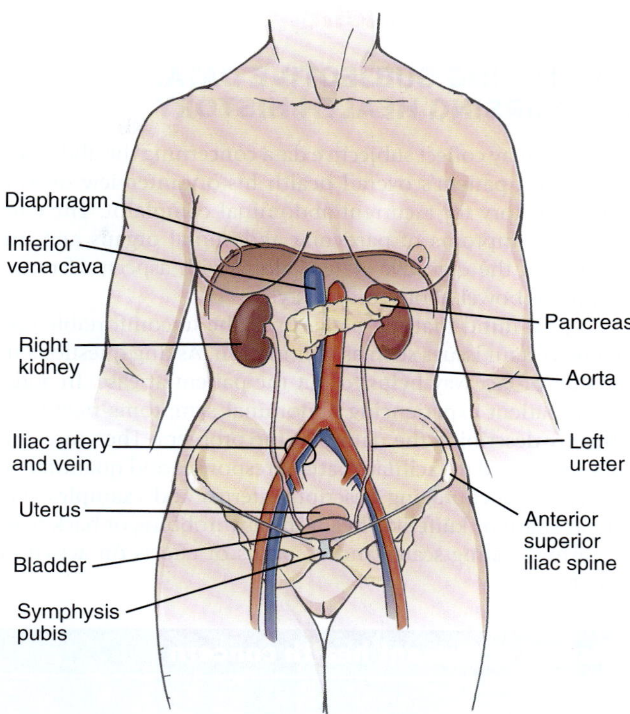

FIGURE 24-5 Abdominal and vascular structures (aorta and iliac artery and vein).

the position of the liver. Therefore, in some thin patients, the bottom portion of the right kidney may be palpated anteriorly. The primary function of the kidneys is filtration and elimination of metabolic waste products. However, the kidneys also play a role in blood pressure control and maintenance of water, salt and electrolyte balances. In addition, they function as endocrine glands by secreting hormones.

The ovaries are located in the RLQ and LLQ and are normally palpated only during a bimanual examination of the internal genitalia (see Chap. 25). The pregnant uterus may be palpated above the level of the symphysis pubis in the midline.

Hollow viscera

The abdominal cavity begins with the stomach. It is a distensible, flasklike organ located in the LUQ just below the diaphragm and between the liver and the spleen. The stomach is not usually palpable. The main function of the stomach is to store, churn and digest food.

The gallbladder, a muscular sac approximately 10 cm long, functions primarily to concentrate and store the bile needed to digest fat. It is located near the posterior surface of the liver lateral to the midclavicular line. It is not normally palpated because it is difficult to distinguish between the gallbladder and the liver.

The small intestine is actually the longest portion of the digestive tract (approximately 7 m long) but is named for its small diameter (approximately 2.5 cm). Two major functions of the small intestine are digestion and absorption of nutrients through millions of mucosal projections lining its walls. The small intestine, which lies coiled in all four quadrants of the abdomen, is not normally palpated.

The colon, or large intestine, has a wider diameter than the small intestine (approximately 6 cm) and is approximately 1.4 m long. It originates in the RLQ, where it attaches to the small intestine at the ileocaecal valve. The colon is composed of three major sections: ascending, transverse and descending. The ascending colon extends up along the right side of the abdomen. At the junction of the liver in the RUQ, it flexes at a right angle and becomes the transverse colon. The transverse colon runs across the upper abdomen. In the LUQ near the spleen, the colon forms another right angle then extends downwards along the left side of the abdomen as the descending colon. At this point, it curves in towards the midline to form the sigmoid colon in the LLQ. The sigmoid colon is often felt as a firm structure on palpation, whereas the caecum and ascending colon may feel softer. The transverse colon and the descending colon may also be felt on palpation.

The colon functions primarily to secrete large amounts of alkaline mucus to lubricate the intestine and neutralise acids formed by the intestinal bacteria. Water is also absorbed through the large intestine, leaving waste products to be eliminated in stool.

The urinary bladder, a distensible muscular sac located behind the pubic bone in the midline of the abdomen, functions as a temporary receptacle for urine. A bladder filled with urine may be palpated in the abdomen above the symphysis pubis.

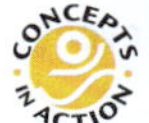

Digestive: Digestion of carbohydrates

Vascular structures

The abdominal organs are supplied with arterial blood by the abdominal aorta and its major branches (Fig. 24-5). Pulsations of the aorta are frequently visible and palpable midline in the upper abdomen. The aorta branches into the right and left iliac arteries just below the umbilicus. Pulsations of the right and left iliac arteries may be felt in the RLQ and LLQ.

Health assessment

COLLECTING SUBJECTIVE DATA: THE NURSING HEALTH HISTORY

The nurse may collect subjective data concerning the abdomen as part of a patient's overall health history interview or as a focused history for a current abdominal complaint. The data focus on symptoms of particular abdominal organs and the function of the digestive system along with aspects of nutrition, usual bowel habits and lifestyle.

Keep in mind that the patient may be uncomfortable discussing certain issues such as elimination. Asking questions in a matter-of-fact way helps to put the patient at ease. In addition, a patient experiencing abdominal symptoms may have difficulty describing the nature of the problem. Therefore, the nurse may need to facilitate patient responses and quantitative answers by encouraging descriptive terms and examples (i.e. pain as sharp or knifelike, headache as throbbing or back pain as searing), rating scales and accounts of effects on activities of daily living.

CASE STUDY

Ms Knowles describes her pain as colicky with a sudden onset, located in the left upper quadrant and radiating to her back. She also feels nauseous. She is worried that she has 'not used her bowels' for the last 4 days. Ms Knowles has a medical history of hypertension, a cholecystectomy 25 years ago and severe rheumatoid arthritis. Her medications include antihypertensives, opioids, aperients and non-steroidal anti-inflammatory drugs.

CRITICAL THINKING

1. Is there anything in the subjective data presented in the case study above that might hint at the cause of Ms Knowles's pain?
2. What are the relevant conditions that might be associated with a past history of abdominal surgery?
3. What further information would you require relating to Ms Knowles's medications?

History of present health concern

QUESTION	RATIONALE
Abdominal pain	
Are you experiencing abdominal pain?	Abdominal pain occurs when specific digestive organs or structures are affected by chemical or mechanical factors such as inflammation, infection, distension, stretching, pressure, obstruction or trauma.
How would you describe the pain? How bad is the pain (severity) on a scale of 1 to 10, with 10 being the worst?	The quality or character of the pain may suggest its origin (Display 24-1). The patient's perception of pain provides data on his or her response to and tolerance of pain. Sensitivity to pain varies greatly among individuals. (See Chapters 32 and 33 for a detailed coverage of child assessment.) Also refer to Chapter 8 for specifics around assessment of pain. **OLDER ADULT CONSIDERATIONS** **Sensitivity to pain may diminish with ageing. Therefore, elderly patients must be carefully assessed for acute abdominal conditions.**
How did (does) the pain begin?	The onset of pain is a diagnostic clue to its origin. For example, acute pancreatitis produces sudden onset of pain, whereas the pain of pancreatic cancer may be gradual or recurrent.
Where is the pain located? Does it move or has it changed from the original location?	Location helps to determine the pain source and whether it is primary or referred (see Display 24-1).
When does the pain occur (timing and relation to particular events such as eating, exercise, bedtime)?	Timing and the relationship of particular events may be a clue to the origin of pain (e.g. the pain of a duodenal ulcer may awaken the patient at night).
What seems to bring on the pain (precipitating factors), make it worse (exacerbating factors) or make it better (alleviating factors)?	Various factors can precipitate or exacerbate abdominal pain such as alcohol ingestion with pancreatitis or supine position with gastro-oesophageal reflux disease. Lifestyle and stress factors may be implicated in certain digestive disorders such as peptic ulcer disease. Alleviating factors, such as using antacids or histamine blockers, may be a clue to origin.

Continued on page 460

DISPLAY 24-1 MECHANISMS AND SOURCES OF ABDOMINAL PAIN

Patterns and referents of abdominal pain. (Cohen, B. J. & Hull, K. L. (2015). *Memmler's structure and function of the human body* [11th ed.]. Philadelphia: Lippincott Williams & Wilkins.)

Types of pain

Abdominal pain may be formally described as visceral, parietal or referred.

- *Visceral pain* occurs when hollow abdominal organs, such as the intestines, become distended or contract forcefully or when the capsules of solid organs such as the liver and spleen are stretched. Poorly defined or localised and intermittently timed, this type of pain is often characterised as dull, aching, burning, cramping or colicky.
- *Parietal pain* occurs when the parietal peritoneum becomes inflamed, as in appendicitis or peritonitis. This type of pain tends to localise more to the source and is characterised as more severe and steady.
- *Referred pain* occurs at distant sites that are innervated at approximately the same levels as the disrupted abdominal organ. This type of pain travels, or refers, from the primary site and becomes highly localised at the distant site. The accompanying illustrations show common clinical patterns and referents of pain.

Character of abdominal pain and implications

Dull, aching

Appendicitis
Acute hepatitis
Biliary colic
Cholecystitis
Cystitis
Dyspepsia
Glomerulonephritis
Incarcerated or strangulated hernia
Irritable bowel syndrome
Hepatocellular cancer
Pancreatitis
Pancreatic cancer
Perforated gastric or duodenal ulcer
Peritonitis
Peptic ulcer disease
Prostatitis

Burning, gnawing

Dyspepsia
Peptic ulcer disease
Cramping ('crampy')
Acute mechanical obstruction
Appendicitis
Colitis
Diverticulitis
Gastro-oesophageal reflux disease

Pressure

Benign prostatic hypertrophy
Prostate cancer
Prostatitis
Urinary retention

Colicky

Colon cancer

Sharp, knifelike

Splenic abscess
Splenic rupture
Renal colic
Renal tumour
Ureteral colic
Vascular liver tumour

Variable

Stomach cancer

History of present health concern (continued)

QUESTION	RATIONALE
Is the pain associated with any other symptoms such as nausea, vomiting, diarrhoea, constipation, gas, fever, weight loss, fatigue or yellowing of the eyes or skin?	Associated signs and symptoms may provide diagnostic evidence to support or rule out a particular origin of pain. For example, epigastric pain accompanied by tarry stools suggests a gastric or duodenal ulcer.
Indigestion	
Do you experience indigestion? Describe.	Indigestion (pyrosis), often described as heartburn, may be an indication of acute or chronic gastric disorders including hyperacidity, gastro-oesophageal reflux disease, peptic ulcer disease and stomach cancer. Take time to determine the patient's exact symptoms because many patients call burping, belching, bloating and nausea indigestion (see Promote health—Peptic ulcer disease).
Does anything in particular seem to cause or aggravate this condition?	Certain factors (e.g. food, drinks, alcohol, medications, stress) are known to increase gastric secretion and acidity and cause or aggravate indigestion.
Nausea and vomiting	
Do you experience nausea? Describe. Is it triggered by any particular activities, events or other factors?	Nausea may reflect gastric dysfunction and is also associated with many digestive disorders and diseases of the accessory organs, such as the liver and pancreas, as well as with renal failure and drug intolerance. Nausea may be precipitated by dietary intolerance, psychological triggers or menstruation. Nausea may also occur at particular times such as early in the day with some pregnant patients ('morning sickness'), after meals with gastric disorders or between meals with changes in blood glucose levels.

PROMOTE HEALTH — PEPTIC ULCER DISEASE

OVERVIEW

Peptic ulcers are eroded areas of the mucosa in the stomach or first part of the intestine. The location determines the name of the ulcer: gastric or duodenal. The ulcerated area results from wear and irritation and causes pain and/or bleeding. The mucous coating that normally protects the mucosa can be disrupted by bacteria such as *Helicobacter pylori* or by eroding medications such as non-steroidal anti-inflammatory medicines, allowing the digestive juices to erode the mucosa. Peptic ulcers can lead to perforation, obstruction or gastric cancer. The actual causes of ulcers remain elusive. Why some people who have *H. pylori* develop ulcers and others do not is unclear. Risk factors include those that actually cause ulcers and those that irritate the mucosal lining, allowing more likely infection with *H. pylori.*

Risk factors

- *H. pylori* infection
- Living in crowded, unsanitary conditions
- Taking non-steroidal anti-inflammatory or COX-2 inhibitor medications (corticosteroids, when used in combination with non-steroidal anti-inflammatory drugs, may increase the risk)
- Prior ulcer disease or family history of peptic ulcers
- Recent major surgery
- Zollinger-Ellison syndrome
- Recent severe injury or burn
- Head trauma
- Radiation therapy
- Congenital malformations of stomach or duodenum
- Some malignant diseases
- Age: duodenal for men; gastric for women
- Type O blood
- Stress not a cause but can exacerbate symptoms and prolong healing
- Possible risk factors: cigarette smoking, alcohol and acidic beverages (fruit juices, caffeine) increase irritation of stomach lining

Teach risk reduction tips

- Avoid contracting *H. pylori* if possible; wash hands, use gloves when in contact with another's body fluids.
- Stop smoking.
- Reduce or stop alcohol consumption.
- Reduce intake of acidic foods and drinks, and caffeine.
- Ask primary health care provider about protective medications if taking irritating medications such as non-steroidal anti-inflammatory medications.
- Consider stress management strategies.

History of present health concern (continued)

QUESTION	RATIONALE
Have you been vomiting? Describe the vomitus. Is it associated with any particular trigger factors?	Vomiting is associated with impaired gastric motility or reflex mechanisms. Description of vomitus (emesis) is a clue to the source. For example, bright haematemesis is seen with bleeding oesophageal varices and ulcers of the stomach or duodenum.  **SAFETY TIP** **Elderly or neuromuscular- or consciousness-impaired patients are at risk of lung aspiration with vomiting.**
Appetite	
Have you noticed a change in your appetite? Has this change affected how much you eat or your normal weight?	Loss of appetite (anorexia) is a general complaint often associated with digestive disorders, chronic syndromes, cancers and psychological disorders. Appetite changes should be carefully correlated with dietary history and weight monitoring. Significant appetite changes and food intake may adversely affect the patient's weight and put the patient at additional risk. 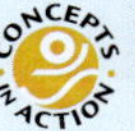 **OLDER ADULT CONSIDERATIONS** **Older patients may experience a decline in appetite from various factors such as altered metabolism, decreased taste sensation, decreased mobility and possibly depression. If appetite declines, the patient's risk of nutritional imbalance increases.** CONCEPTS IN ACTION **Digestive:** Metabolism of amino acids **Digestive:** General digestion
Bowel elimination	
Have you experienced a change in bowel elimination patterns? Describe.	Changes in bowel patterns must be compared with usual patterns for the patient. Normal frequency varies from two to three times per day to three times per week.
Do you have constipation? Describe. Do you have any accompanying symptoms?	Constipation is usually defined as a decrease in the frequency of bowel movements or the passage of hard and possibly painful stools. Signs and symptoms that accompany constipation may be a clue to the cause of constipation such as bleeding with malignancies or pencil-shaped stools with intestinal obstruction.
Have you experienced diarrhoea? Describe. Do you have any accompanying symptoms?	Diarrhoea is defined as frequency of bowel movements producing unformed or liquid stools. It is important to compare these stools with the patient's usual bowel patterns. Bloody and mucoid stools are associated with inflammatory bowel diseases (e.g. ulcerative colitis, Crohn disease); clay-coloured, fatty stools may be from malabsorption syndromes. Associated symptoms or signs may suggest the disorder's origin. For example, fever and chills may result from an infection or weight loss and fatigue may result from a chronic intestinal disorder or a cancer.  **OLDER ADULT CONSIDERATIONS** **Older patients are especially at risk of potential complications with diarrhoea, such as fluid volume deficit, dehydration, electrolyte and acid–base imbalances, because they have a higher fat-to-lean muscle ratio.**
Have you experienced any yellowing of your skin or whites of your eyes, itchy skin, dark urine (yellow-brown or tea-coloured) or clay-coloured stools?	These symptoms should be evaluated to rule out possible liver disease.

Continued on following page

COLDSPA

Example for abdominal pain

Use the COLDSPA mnemonic as a guideline to collect needed information for each symptom the patient shares. In addition, the following questions help elicit important information.

Mnemonic	Question	Patient response example
Character	Describe the sign or symptom (feeling, appearance, sound, smell or taste, if applicable).	'It started hurting all over and then got worse in my right side.'
Onset	When did it begin?	'Late last night'
Location	Where is it? Does it radiate? Does it occur anywhere else?	'On my right, lower part of my tummy'
Duration	How long does it last? Does it recur?	'It is continual. The pain will not let up.'
Severity	How bad is it? or How much does it bother you?	'It hurts so bad that I cannot focus on doing anything.'
Pattern	What makes it better or worse?	'It is getting worse. I tried some Mylanta but it did not help.'
Associated factors/How it Affects the patient	What other symptoms occur with it? How does it affect you?	'I feel like I am going to be sick. I can't move without it hurting, and I could not go to work this morning.'

Past health history

QUESTION	RATIONALE
Have you ever had any of the following gastrointestinal disorders: ulcers, gastro-oesophageal reflux, inflammatory or obstructive bowel disease, pancreatitis, gallbladder or liver disease, diverticulosis or appendicitis?	Presenting the patient with a list of the more common disorders may help the patient to identify any that they have or have had.
Have you had any urinary tract disease such as infections, kidney disease or nephritis, or kidney stones?	Urinary tract infections may become recurrent and chronic. Moreover, resistance to drugs used to treat infection must be evaluated. Chronic kidney infection may lead to permanent kidney damage. **OLDER ADULT CONSIDERATIONS** **Older patients are prone to urinary tract infections because the activity of protective bacteria in the urinary tract declines with age.**
Have you ever had viral hepatitis (type A, B or C)? Have you ever been exposed to viral hepatitis?	Various populations (e.g. school and healthcare personnel) are at increased risk of exposure to hepatitis viruses. Any type of viral hepatitis may cause liver damage.
Have you ever had abdominal surgery or trauma to the abdomen?	Prior abdominal surgery or trauma may cause abdominal adhesions, thereby predisposing the patient to future complications or disorders.
What prescription or over-the-counter medications do you take?	Medications may produce side effects that adversely affect the gastrointestinal tract. For example, aspirin, ibuprofen and steroids may cause gastric bleeding. Chronic use of antacids or histamine-2 blockers may mask the symptoms of more serious stomach disorders. Overuse of laxatives may decrease intestinal tone and promote dependency. High iron intake may lead to chronic constipation.

Family history

QUESTION	RATIONALE
Is there a history of any of the following diseases or disorders in your family: colon, stomach, pancreatic, liver, kidney or bladder cancer; liver disease; gallbladder disease; kidney disease?	Family history of certain disorders increases the patient's risk of those disorders. Genetic testing can now identify the risk for certain cancers (colon, pancreatic and prostate) and other diseases. Patient awareness of family history can serve as a motivation for health screening and positive health promotion behaviours.

Lifestyle and health practices

QUESTION	RATIONALE
Do you drink alcohol? How much? How often?	Alcohol ingestion can affect the gastrointestinal tract through immediate and long-term effects on such organs as the stomach, pancreas and liver. Alcohol-related disorders include gastritis, oesophageal varices, pancreatitis and liver cirrhosis.
What types of foods and how much food do you typically consume each day? How much non-caffeinated fluid do you consume each day? How much caffeine do you think you consume each day (e.g. in tea, coffee, chocolate and soft drinks)?	A baseline dietary and fluid survey helps to determine nutritional and fluid adequacy and risk factors for altered nutrition, constipation, diarrhoea and diseases such as cancer.
How much and how often do you exercise? Describe your activities during the day.	Regular exercise promotes peristalsis and thus regular bowel movements. In addition, exercise may help to reduce risk factors for various diseases such as cancer and hypertension (see Promote health—Bowel cancer).
What kinds of stress do you have in your life? How does it affect your eating or elimination habits?	Lifestyle and associated stress and psychological factors can affect gastrointestinal function through effects on secretion, tone and motility.
If you have a gastrointestinal disorder, how does it affect your lifestyle and how you feel about yourself?	Certain gastrointestinal disorders and their effects (e.g. weight loss) or treatment (e.g. drugs, surgery) may produce physiological or anatomical effects that affect the patient's perception of self, body image, social interaction and intimacy, and life goals and expectations.

PROMOTE HEALTH — BOWEL CANCER

OVERVIEW

In New Zealand, bowel cancer (colorectal cancer) is the most commonly diagnosed cancer and the second highest cause of cancer deaths (Healthcare Quality and Safety Commission New Zealand, 2017). It is the third most commonly diagnosed cancer in Australia and the most common cause of cancer death (Cancer Australia, 2019). Each year, more than 16,000 new cases are diagnosed in Australia, and in New Zealand the number is more than 3,000 (Cancer Australia, 2019; New Zealand Ministry of Health, 2018). In Australia, the risk of developing bowel cancer before the age of 85 is approximately 1 in 12 for men and 1 in 17 for women (Cancer Australia, 2019). People who are diagnosed in the early stage of bowel cancer have an 89% to 99% chance of surviving the disease (National Cancer Control Indicators, 2019).

Risk factors

- Age over 50 (most significant)
- Male gender
- Family history of bowel cancer or polyps
- Inflammatory bowel disease such as Crohn disease or ulcerative colitis
- Previous polyps (adenomas) in the bowel
- Obesity
- Some scientists believe a diet high in animal fats and low in fruit and vegetable fibre may increase the risk of developing bowel cancer

Teach risk reduction tips

- Stop smoking.
- Eat a healthy diet with fresh fruit and vegetables.
- Maintain a healthy body weight.

COLLECTING OBJECTIVE DATA: PHYSICAL EXAMINATION

The abdominal examination is performed for a variety of different reasons: to have a comprehensive health examination; to explore gastrointestinal complaints; to assess abdominal pain, tenderness or masses; or to monitor the patient postoperatively. Assessing the abdomen can be challenging, considering the number of organs of the digestive system and the need to distinguish the source of clinical signs and symptoms.

The sequence for assessment of the abdomen differs from the typical order of assessment. Auscultate after you inspect to avoid altering the patient's pattern of bowel sounds. Percussion then palpation follow auscultation. Adjust the bed level as necessary throughout the examination and approach the patient from the right side. Use tangential lighting, if available, for optimal visualisation of the abdomen.

You need to understand and anticipate various concerns of the patient by listening and observing closely for verbal and non-verbal cues. Commonly patients feel anxious and modest during the examination, possibly from anticipated discomfort or fear that the examiner will find something seriously wrong. As a result, the patient may tense the abdominal muscles, voluntarily guarding the area. Ease the patient's anxiety by explaining each aspect of the examination, answering any questions and draping the patient's genital area and breasts (in women) when these are not being examined.

Another potential factor to deal with is ticklishness. A ticklish patient has trouble lying still and relaxing during the hands-on parts of the examination. Try to combat this using a controlled hands-on technique and by placing the patient's hand under your own for a few moments at the beginning of palpation. Finally, warm hands are essential for the abdominal examination. Cold hands cause the patient to tense the abdominal muscles. Rubbing your hands together or holding them under warm water just before the hands-on examination may be helpful.

Preparing the patient

Ask the patient to empty the bladder before beginning the examination to eliminate bladder distension and interference with an accurate examination. Instruct the patient to undress and put on a gown. Help the patient to lie supine with the arms folded across the chest or resting by the sides (Fig. 24-6).

CLINICAL TIP
Raising arms above the head or folding them behind the head will tense the abdominal muscles.

A flat pillow may be placed under the patient's head for comfort. Slightly flex the patient's legs by placing a pillow or rolled blanket under the patient's knees to help relax the abdominal muscles. Drape the patient with sheets so the abdomen is visible from the lower rib cage to the pubic area.

Instruct the patient to breathe through the mouth and to take slow, deep breaths; this promotes relaxation. Before touching the abdomen, ask the patient about painful or tender areas. These areas should always be assessed at the end of the examination. Reassure the patient that you will forewarn them when you will examine these areas. Approach the patient with slow, gentle and fluid movements.

Equipment

- Small pillow or rolled blanket
- Ruler
- Stethoscope (warm the diaphragm and bell)
- Marking pen

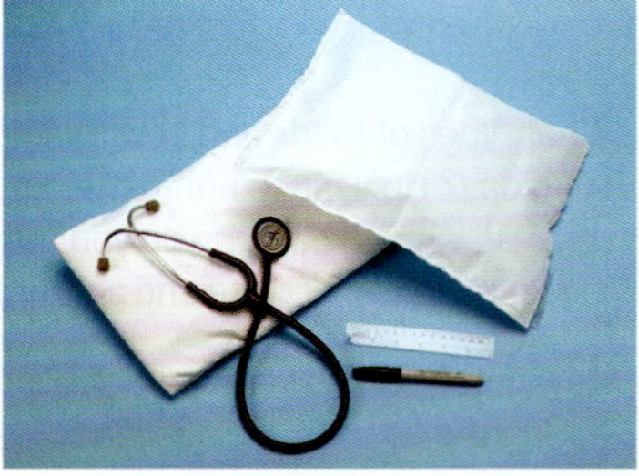

Physical assessment

The examination evaluates the following abdominal structures in the abdominal quadrants: skin, stomach, bowel, spleen, liver, kidneys, aorta and bladder. Remember to auscultate after inspection and before percussion and, finally, to palpate. Palpation is done last to avoid causing any muscle guarding associated with pain. Always palpate any identified tender areas last. Common abnormal findings include abdominal oedema, or swelling, signifying ascites; abdominal masses signifying abnormal growths or constipation; unusual pulsations such as those seen with an aneurysm of the abdominal aorta; and pain associated with appendicitis.

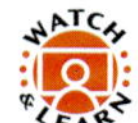

Physical assessment: Assessing the abdomen

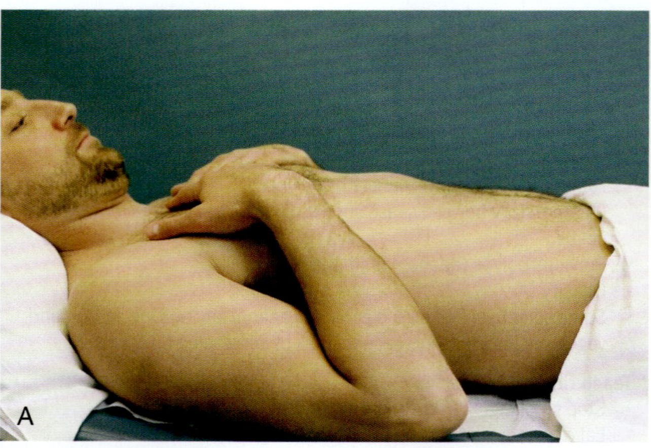

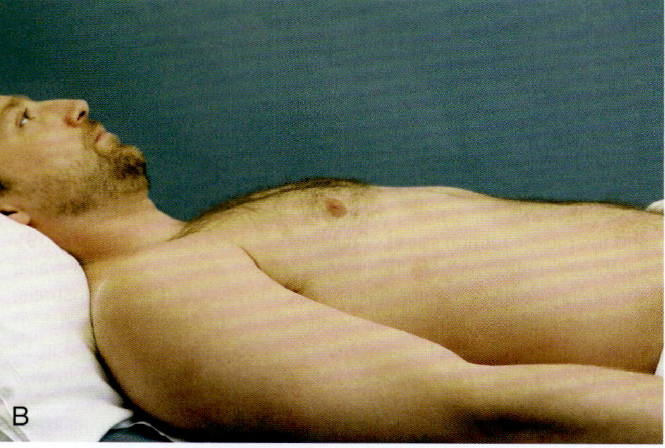

FIGURE 24-6 Two positions are appropriate for the abdominal assessment. The patient may lie supine with hands resting on the centre of the chest **(A)** or with arms resting comfortably at the sides **(B).** These positions best promote relaxation of the abdominal muscles. (© B. Proud.)

PHYSICAL ASSESSMENT

ASSESSMENT PROCEDURE	NORMAL FINDINGS	ABNORMAL FINDINGS
Inspection		
Observe the colouration of the skin.	Abdominal skin may be paler than the general skin tone because this skin is so seldom exposed to the natural elements.	Purple discolouration at the flanks (Grey Turner sign) indicates bleeding within the abdominal wall, possibly from trauma to the kidneys, pancreas or duodenum, or from pancreatitis. The yellow hue of jaundice may be more apparent on the abdomen. Pale, taut skin may be seen with ascites (significant abdominal swelling indicating fluid accumulation in the abdominal cavity). Redness may indicate inflammation. Bruises or areas of local discolouration are also abnormal.
Note the vascularity of the abdominal skin.	Scattered fine veins may be visible. Blood in the veins located above the umbilicus flows towards the head; blood in the veins located below the umbilicus flows towards the lower body. **OLDER ADULT CONSIDERATIONS** **Dilated superficial capillaries without a pattern may be seen in older patients. They are more visible in sunlight.**	Dilated veins may be seen with cirrhosis of the liver, obstruction of the inferior vena cava, portal hypertension or ascites. Dilated surface arterioles and capillaries with a central star (spider angioma) may be seen with liver disease or portal hypertension.
Note any striae.	Old, silvery, white striae or stretch marks from past pregnancies or weight gain are normal.	Dark bluish-pink striae are associated with Cushing syndrome. Striae may also be caused by ascites, which stretches the skin. Ascites usually results from liver failure or liver disease.
Inspect for scars. Ask about the source of a scar, and use a ruler to measure the scar's length. Document the location by quadrant and reference lines, shape, length and any specific characteristics (e.g. 3-cm vertical scar in RLQ 4 cm below the umbilicus and 5 cm left of the midline). With experience, many examiners can estimate the length of a scar visually without a ruler.	Pale, smooth, minimally raised old scars may be seen. **CLINICAL TIP** **Scarring should be an alert for possible internal adhesions.** **FIGURE 24-7** Keloid beyond the border of surgical scar.	Non-healing scars, redness, inflammation. Deep, irregular scars may result from burns. **CULTURAL CONSIDERATIONS** **Keloids (excess scar tissue) result from trauma or surgery and are more common in patients with dark skin (Fig. 24-7).**
Assess for lesions and rashes.	Abdomen is free of lesions or rashes. Flat or raised brown moles, however, are normal and may be apparent.	Changes in moles including size, colour and border symmetry. Any bleeding moles or petechiae (reddish or purple lesions) may also be abnormal (see Chap. 15).

Continued on following page

PHYSICAL ASSESSMENT (continued)

ASSESSMENT PROCEDURE	NORMAL FINDINGS	ABNORMAL FINDINGS
Inspect the umbilicus. Note the colour of the umbilical area.	Umbilical skin tones are similar to surrounding abdominal skin tones or even pinkish.	Bluish or purple discolouration around the umbilicus (Cullen sign) indicates intra-abdominal bleeding.
Observe umbilical location.	Umbilicus is midline at lateral line.	A deviated umbilicus may be caused by pressure from a mass, enlarged organs, hernia, fluid or scar tissue.
Assess contour of umbilicus.	It is recessed (inverted) or protruding no more than 0.5 cm and is round or conical.	An everted umbilicus is seen with abdominal distension (see Abnormal findings 24-1). An enlarged, everted umbilicus suggests umbilical hernia (see Abnormal findings 24-2).
Inspect abdominal contour. Look across the abdomen at eye level from the patient's side (Fig. 24-8), from behind the patient's head and from the foot of the bed. Measure abdominal girth as indicated (see Assessment tool 24-2). 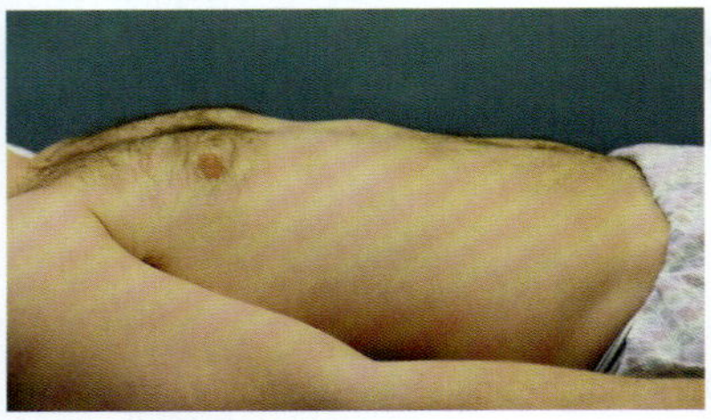 **FIGURE 24-8** View abdominal contour from the patient's side. Many abdomens are more or less flat; and many are round, scaphoid or distended. (© B. Proud.)	Abdomen is flat, rounded or scaphoid (usually seen in thin adults) (Fig. 24-9). Abdomen should be evenly rounded.	A generalised protuberant or distended abdomen may be due to obesity, air (gas) or fluid accumulation (see Abnormal findings 24-1). Distension below the umbilicus may be due to a full bladder, uterine enlargement or an ovarian tumour or cyst. Distension of the upper abdomen may be seen with masses of the pancreas or gastric dilation. **CLINICAL TIP** **The major causes of abdominal distension are sometimes referred to as the '6 Fs': Fat, faeces, fetus, fibroids, flatulence and fluid (Abnormal findings 24-1).** A scaphoid (sunken) abdomen may be seen with severe weight loss or cachexia related to starvation or terminal illness.

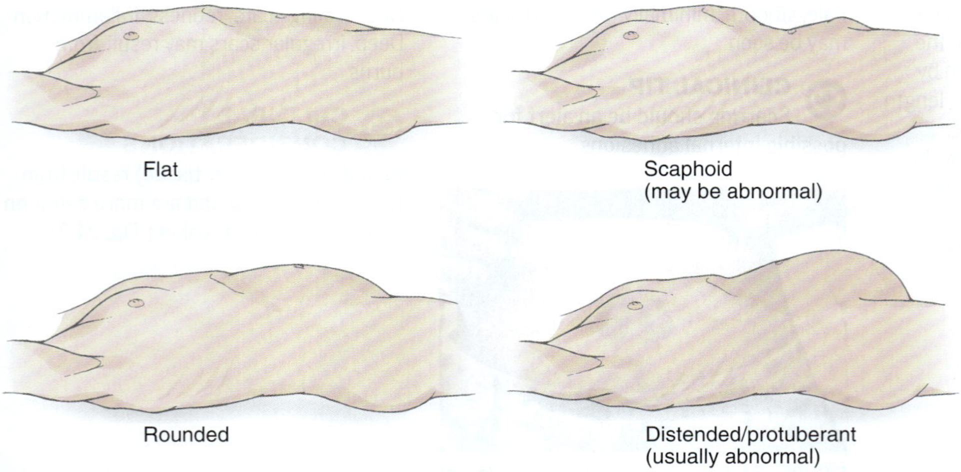

Flat

Scaphoid (may be abnormal)

Rounded

Distended/protuberant (usually abnormal)

FIGURE 24-9 Abdominal contours.

ASSESSMENT PROCEDURE	NORMAL FINDINGS	ABNORMAL FINDINGS
Assess abdominal symmetry. Look at the patient's abdomen as he or she lies in a relaxed supine position.	Abdomen is symmetrical.	Asymmetry may be seen with organ enlargement, large masses, hernia, diastasis recti or bowel obstruction.

ASSESSMENT TOOL 24-2 Measuring abdominal girth

In patients with abdominal distension, abdominal girth (circumference) should be assessed periodically (daily in hospital, during a doctor's office visit, with home nursing visits) to evaluate the progress or treatment of distension. Waist circumference measurement is also recommended in screening for cardiovascular risk factors.*

To facilitate accurate assessment and interpretation, the following guidelines are recommended:

1. Measure abdominal girth at the same time of day, ideally in the morning just after voiding, or at a designated time for bedridden patients or those with indwelling catheters.
2. The ideal position for the patient is standing; otherwise, the patient should be in the supine position. The patient's head may be slightly elevated (for orthopnoeic patients). The patient should be in the same position for all measurements.
3. Use a disposable or easily cleaned tape measure. If a tape measure is not available, use a strip of cloth or gauze, then measure the gauze with a cloth tape measure or ruler.
4. Place the tape measure behind the patient and measure at the umbilicus. **Use the umbilicus as a starting point when measuring abdominal girth, especially when distension is apparent.**
5. Record the distance in designated units (centimetres).
6. Take all future measurements from the same location. Marking the abdomen with a ballpoint pen can help you identify the measuring site. As a courtesy, explain the purpose of the marking pen and ask the patient not to wash the mark off until it is no longer needed.

*Central obesity is defined as a waist circumference greater than 102 cm in men and greater than 88 cm in women. These values are for people of European ancestry and vary for other ethnicities. Central obesity is correlated with metabolic syndrome and increased risk of coronary heart disease (Purnell, 2018).

PHYSICAL ASSESSMENT (continued)

ASSESSMENT PROCEDURE	NORMAL FINDINGS	ABNORMAL FINDINGS
Inspection (continued)		
To further assess the abdomen for herniation or diastasis recti or to differentiate a mass within the abdominal wall from one below it, ask the patient to raise the head.	Abdomen does not bulge when patient raises head.	A hernia (protrusion of the bowel through the abdominal wall) is seen as a bulging in the abdominal wall. Diastasis recti appears as a bulging between a vertical midline separation of the abdominis rectus muscles. This condition is of little significance. An incisional hernia may occur when a defect develops in the abdominal muscles because of a surgical incision. A mass within the abdominal wall is more prominent when the head is raised, whereas a mass below the abdominal wall is obscured (Abnormal findings 24-2).
Inspect abdominal movement when the patient breathes (respiratory movements).	Abdominal respiratory movement may be seen, especially in male patients.	Diminished abdominal respiration or change to thoracic breathing in male patients may reflect peritoneal irritation.
Observe aortic pulsations.	A slight pulsation of the abdominal aorta, which is visible in the epigastrium, extends full length in thin people.	Vigorous, wide, exaggerated pulsations may be seen with abdominal aortic aneurysm.
Observe for peristaltic waves.	Normally peristaltic waves are not seen, although they may be visible in very thin people as slight ripples on the abdominal wall.	Peristaltic waves are increased and progress in a ripplelike fashion from the LUQ to the RLQ with intestinal obstruction (especially small intestine). In addition, abdominal distension typically is present with intestinal wall obstruction.
Auscultation		
Auscultate for bowel sounds. Use the diaphragm of the stethoscope and make sure that it is warm before you place it on the patient's abdomen.	A series of intermittent, soft clicks and gurgles are heard at a rate of 5 to 30 per minute. Hyperactive bowel sounds that may be heard normally are the loud, prolonged gurgles characteristic of stomach growling. These hyperactive bowel sounds are called 'borborygmi.'	Hypoactive bowel sounds indicate diminished bowel motility. Common causes include abdominal surgery or late bowel obstruction.

Continued on following page

PHYSICAL ASSESSMENT (continued)

ASSESSMENT PROCEDURE	NORMAL FINDINGS	ABNORMAL FINDINGS
Apply light pressure or simply rest the stethoscope on a tender abdomen. Begin in the RLQ and proceed clockwise, covering all quadrants. **CLINICAL TIP** **Bowel sounds may be more active over the ileocecal valve in the RLQ.** Confirm bowel sounds in each quadrant. Listen for up to 5 minutes (minimum of 1 minute per quadrant) to confirm the absence of bowel sounds. **CLINICAL TIP** **Bowel sounds normally occur every 5 to 15 seconds. An easy way to remember is to equate one bowel sound to one breath sound.** Note the intensity, pitch and frequency of the sounds.	**CLINICAL TIP** **Postoperatively, bowel sounds resume gradually depending on the type of surgery. The small intestine functions normally in the first few hours postoperatively; stomach emptying takes 24 to 48 hours to recover; and the colon requires 3 to 5 days to recover propulsive activity.**	Hyperactive bowel sounds indicate increased bowel motility. Common causes include diarrhoea, gastroenteritis or early bowel obstruction. Decreased or absent bowel sounds signify the absence of bowel motility, which constitutes an emergency requiring immediate referral. Absent bowel sounds may be associated with peritonitis or paralytic ileus. High-pitched tinkling and rushes of high-pitched sounds with abdominal cramping usually indicate obstruction. **CLINICAL TIP** **The increasing pitch of bowel sounds is most diagnostic of obstruction because it signifies intestinal distension.**
Auscultate for vascular sounds. Use the bell of the stethoscope to listen for bruits (low-pitched, murmurlike sound) over the abdominal aorta and renal, iliac and femoral arteries (Fig. 24-10). **CLINICAL TIP** **Auscultating for vascular sounds is especially important if the patient has hypertension or if you suspect arterial insufficiency to the legs.**	Bruits are not normally heard over abdominal aorta or renal, iliac or femoral arteries. However, bruits confined to systole may be normal in some patients depending on other differentiating factors.	A bruit with both systolic and diastolic components occurs when blood flow in an artery is turbulent or obstructed. This usually indicates aneurysm or arterial stenosis. If the patient has hypertension and you auscultate a renal artery bruit with both systolic and diastolic components, suspect renal artery stenosis as the cause.

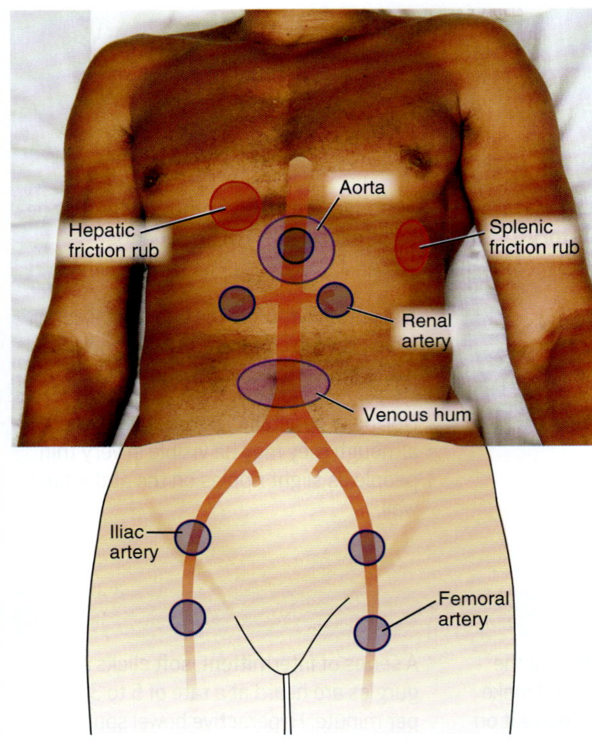

FIGURE 24-10 Vascular sounds and friction rubs can best be heard over these areas.

PHYSICAL ASSESSMENT (continued)

ASSESSMENT PROCEDURE	NORMAL FINDINGS	ABNORMAL FINDINGS
Auscultation (continued)		
Using the bell of the stethoscope, listen for a venous hum in the epigastric and umbilical areas.	Venous hum is not normally heard over the epigastric and umbilical areas.	Venous hums are rare. However, an accentuated venous hum heard in the epigastric or umbilical areas suggests increased collateral circulation between the portal and systemic venous systems, as in cirrhosis of the liver.
Auscultate for a friction rub over the liver and spleen. Listen over the right and left lower rib cage with the diaphragm of the stethoscope.	No friction rub over liver or spleen is present.	Friction rubs are rare. If heard, they have a high-pitched, rough, grating sound produced when the large surface area of the liver or spleen rubs the peritoneum. They are heard in association with respiration. A friction rub heard over the lower right costal area is associated with hepatic abscess or metastases. A rub heard at the anterior axillary line in the lower left costal area is associated with splenic infarction, abscess, infection or tumour.
Percussion		
Percuss for tone. Lightly and systematically percuss all quadrants. Two sequences are illustrated in Figure 24-11.	Generalised tympany predominates over the abdomen because of air in the stomach and intestines. Normal dullness is heard over the liver and spleen. Dullness may also be elicited over a non-evacuated descending colon (Fig. 24-12).	Accentuated tympany or hyperresonance is heard over a gaseous distended abdomen. An enlarged area of dullness is heard over an enlarged liver or spleen. Abnormal dullness is heard over a distended bladder, large masses or ascites. If you suspect ascites, perform the shifting dullness and fluid wave tests. These special techniques are described later in this chapter.

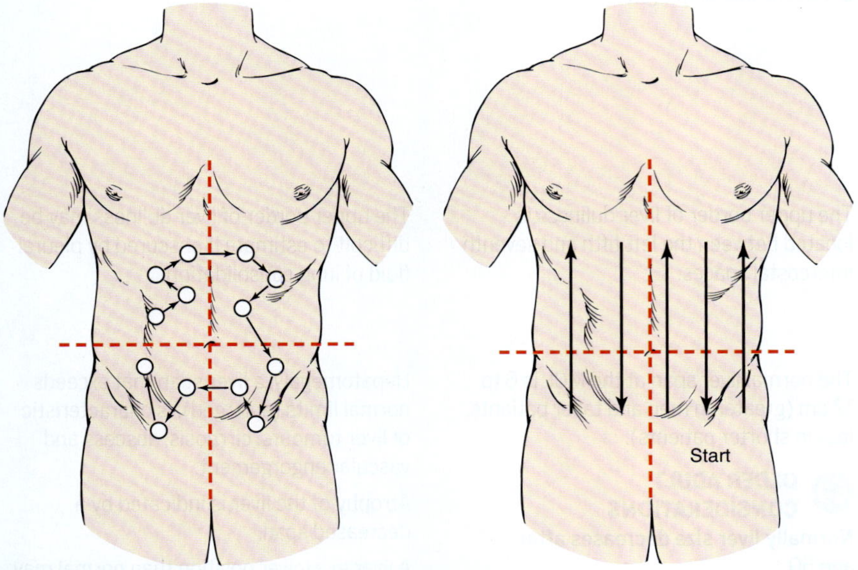

Start

FIGURE 24-11 Abdominal percussion sequences may proceed clockwise or up and down over the abdomen.

Continued on following page

PHYSICAL ASSESSMENT (continued)

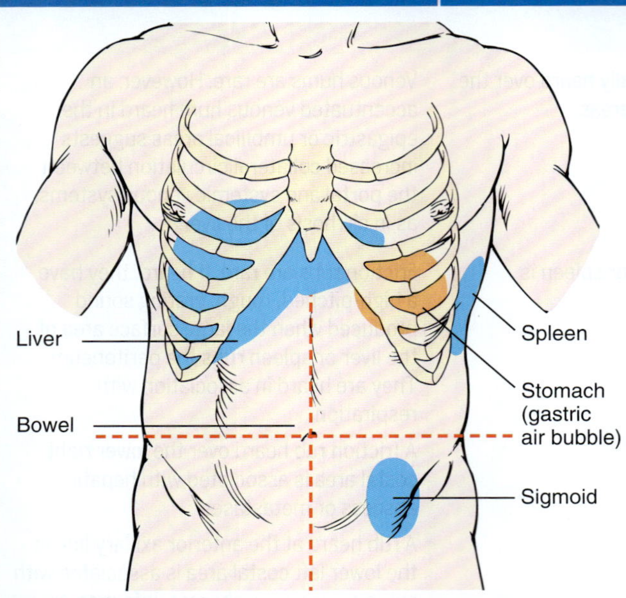

FIGURE 24-12 Normal percussion findings. Blue indicates dullness. Orange indicates tympany.

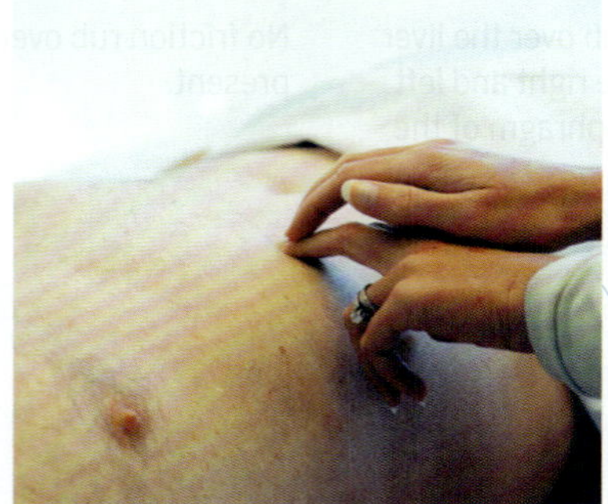

FIGURE 24-13 Begin liver percussion in the RLQ and percuss upwards towards the chest. (© B. Proud.)

ASSESSMENT PROCEDURE	NORMAL FINDINGS	ABNORMAL FINDINGS
Percuss the span or height of the liver by determining its lower and upper borders.	The lower border of liver dullness is located at the costal margin to 1 to 2 cm below.	**CLINICAL TIP** **If you cannot find the lower border of the liver, keep in mind that the lower border of liver dullness may be difficult to estimate when obscured by intestinal gas.**
To assess the lower border, begin in the RLQ at the midclavicular line (MCL) and percuss upwards (Fig. 24-13). Note the change from tympany to dullness. Mark this point: It is the lower border of liver dullness. To assess the descent of the liver, ask the patient to take a deep breath and hold; then repeat the procedure. Remind the patient to exhale after percussing.	On deep inspiration, the lower border of liver dullness may descend from 1 to 4 cm below the costal margin.	
To assess the upper border, percuss over the upper right chest at the MCL and percuss downwards, noting the change from lung resonance to liver dullness. Mark this point: It is the upper border of liver dullness.	The upper border of liver dullness is located between the left fifth and seventh intercostal spaces.	The upper border of liver dullness may be difficult to estimate if obscured by pleural fluid of lung consolidation.
Measure the distance between the two marks: this is the span of the liver (Fig. 24-14).	The normal liver span at the MCL is 6 to 12 cm (greater in men and taller patients, less in shorter patients).  **OLDER ADULT CONSIDERATIONS** **Normally liver size decreases after age 50.**	Hepatomegaly, a liver span that exceeds normal limits (enlarged), is characteristic of liver tumours, cirrhosis, abscess and vascular engorgement. Atrophy of the liver is indicated by a decreased span. A liver in a lower position than normal may be caused by emphysema, whereas a liver in a higher position than normal may be caused by an abdominal mass, ascites or a paralysed diaphragm. A liver in a lower or higher position should have a normal span (Abnormal findings 24-3).

PHYSICAL ASSESSMENT (continued)

ASSESSMENT PROCEDURE	NORMAL FINDINGS	ABNORMAL FINDINGS
Percussion (continued)		

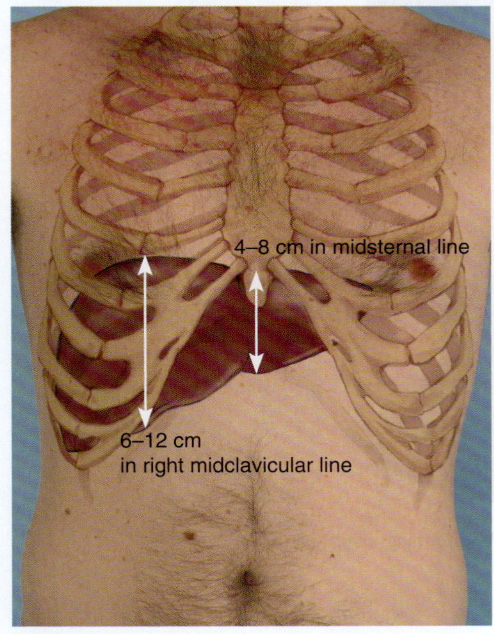

FIGURE 24-14 Normal liver span. (Rhoads, J. [2006]. *Advanced health assessment and diagnostic reasoning.* Philadelphia: Lippincott Williams & Wilkins.)

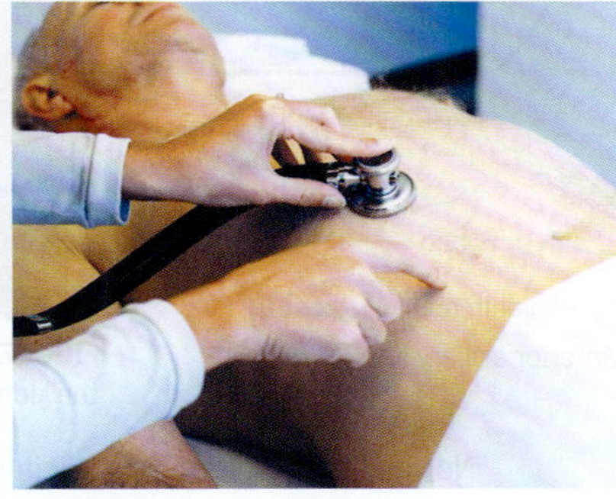

FIGURE 24-15 The scratch test. (© B. Proud.)

ASSESSMENT PROCEDURE	NORMAL FINDINGS	ABNORMAL FINDINGS
Repeat percussion of the liver at the midsternal line (MSL). If you cannot accurately percuss the liver borders, perform the scratch test (Fig. 24-15). Auscultate over the liver and, starting in the RLQ, scratch lightly over the abdomen, progressing upwards towards the liver.	The normal liver span at the MSL is 4 to 8 cm. The sound produced by scratching becomes more intense over the liver.	An enlarged liver may be roughly estimated (not accurately) when more intense sounds outline a liver span or borders outside the normal range.
Percuss the spleen. Begin posterior to the left midaxillary line (MAL), and percuss downwards, noting the change from lung resonance to splenic dullness. **CLINICAL TIP** **Results of splenic percussion may be obscured by air in the stomach or bowel.**	The spleen is an oval area of dullness approximately 7 cm wide near the left 10th rib and slightly posterior to the MAL.	Splenomegaly is characterised by an area of dullness greater than 7 cm wide. The enlargement may result from traumatic injury, portal hypertension or glandular fever.
A second method for detecting splenic enlargement is to percuss the last left interspace at the anterior axillary line (AAL) while the patient takes a deep breath (Fig. 24-16). **CLINICAL TIP** **Other sources of dullness (e.g. full stomach or faeces in the colon) must be ruled out before confirming splenomegaly.**	Normally tympany (or resonance) is heard at the last left interspace.	On inspiration, dullness at the last left interspace at the AAL suggests an enlarged spleen (see Abnormal findings 24-3).

Continued on following page

PHYSICAL ASSESSMENT (continued)

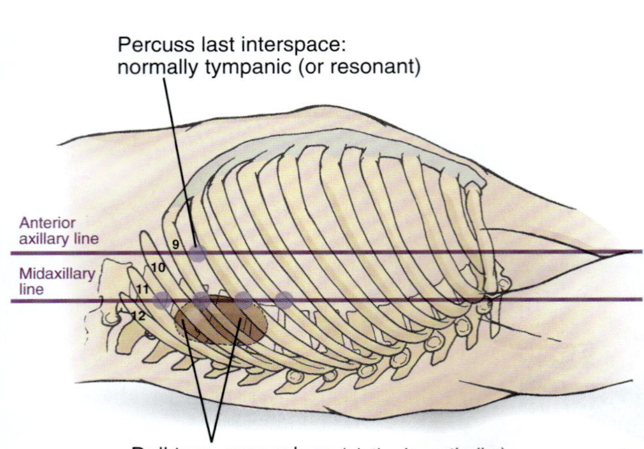

FIGURE 24-16 Last left interspace at the anterior axillary line.

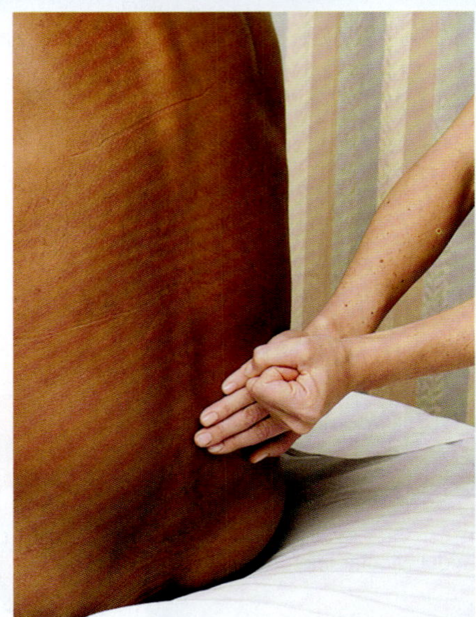

FIGURE 24-17 Performing blunt percussion over the kidney.

ASSESSMENT PROCEDURE	NORMAL FINDINGS	ABNORMAL FINDINGS
Perform blunt percussion on the liver and the kidneys. This is to assess for tenderness in difficult-to-palpate structures. Percuss the liver by placing your left hand flat against the lower right anterior rib cage. Use the ulnar side of your right fist to strike your left hand.	Normally no tenderness is elicited.	Tenderness elicited over the liver may be associated with inflammation or infection (e.g. hepatitis or cholecystitis).
Perform blunt percussion on the kidneys at the costovertebral angles (CVA) over the 12th rib (Fig. 24-17). **CLINICAL TIP** **This technique requires that the patient sit with his or her back to you. Therefore, it may be best to incorporate blunt percussion of the kidneys with your thoracic assessment because the patient will already be in this position.**	Normally no tenderness or pain is elicited or reported by the patient. The examiner senses only a dull thud.	Tenderness or sharp pain elicited over the CVA suggests kidney infection (pyelonephritis), renal calculi or hydronephrosis.
Palpation		
Perform light palpation. Display 24-2 provides considerations for palpation. Light palpation is used to identify areas of tenderness and muscular resistance. Using the fingertips, begin palpation in a non-tender quadrant, and compress to a depth of 1 cm in a dipping motion. Then gently lift the fingers and move to the next area (Fig. 24-18). To minimise the patient's voluntary guarding (a tensing or rigidity of the abdominal muscles usually involving the entire abdomen), see Display 24-2. Keep in mind that the rectus abdominis muscle relaxes on expiration.	Abdomen is non-tender and soft. There is no guarding.	Involuntary reflex guarding is serious and reflects peritoneal irritation. The abdomen is rigid and the rectus muscle fails to relax with palpation when the patient exhales. It can involve all or part of the abdomen but is usually seen on the side (i.e. right vs. left rather than upper or lower) because of nerve tract patterns. Right-sided guarding may be due to cholecystitis.

PHYSICAL ASSESSMENT (continued)

ASSESSMENT PROCEDURE	NORMAL FINDINGS	ABNORMAL FINDINGS
Palpation (continued)		

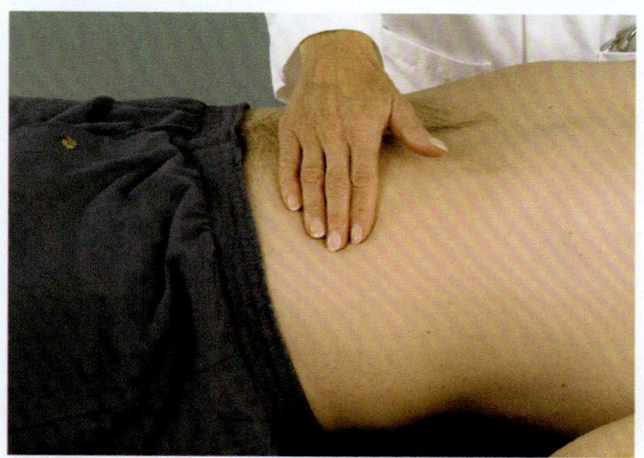

FIGURE 24-18 Performing light palpation. (Rhoads, J. [2006]. *Advanced health assessment and diagnostic reasoning.* Philadelphia: Lippincott Williams & Wilkins.)

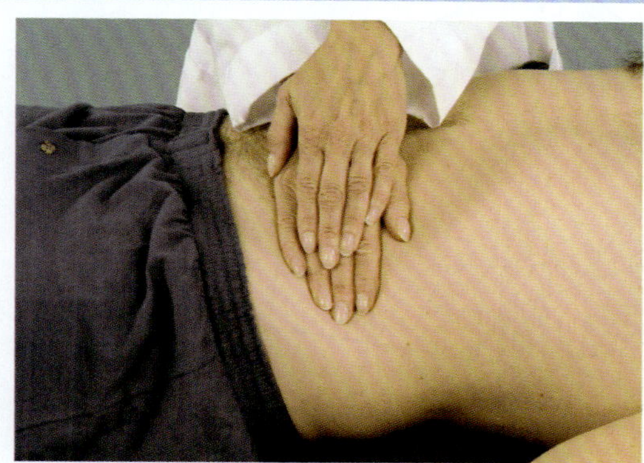

FIGURE 24-19 Performing deep bimanual palpation. (Rhoads, J. [2006]. *Advanced health assessment and diagnostic reasoning.* Philadelphia: Lippincott Williams & Wilkins.)

ASSESSMENT PROCEDURE	NORMAL FINDINGS	ABNORMAL FINDINGS
Deeply palpate all quadrants to delineate abdominal organs and detect subtle masses. Using the palmar surface of the fingers, compress to a maximum depth (5 to 6 cm). Perform bimanual palpation if you encounter resistance or to assess deeper structures (Fig. 24-19).	Normal (mild) tenderness is possible over the xiphoid, aorta, caecum, sigmoid colon and ovaries with deep palpation.	Severe tenderness or pain may be related to trauma, peritonitis, infection, tumours or enlarged or diseased organs.
Palpate for masses. Note their location, size (cm), shape, consistency, demarcation, pulsatility, tenderness and mobility. Do not confuse a mass with a normally palpated organ or structure (Fig. 24-20).	No palpable masses are present.	A mass detected in any quadrant may be due to a tumour, cyst, abscess, enlarged organ, aneurysm or adhesions.
Palpate the umbilicus and surrounding area for swellings, bulges or masses.	Umbilicus and surrounding area are free of swellings, bulges or masses.	A soft centre of the umbilicus can be a potential for herniation. Palpation of a hard nodule in or around the umbilicus may indicate metastatic nodes from an occult gastrointestinal cancer.
Palpate the aorta. Use your thumb and first finger or use two hands and palpate deeply in the epigastrium, slightly to the left of midline (Fig. 24-21). Assess the pulsation of the abdominal aorta.	The normal aorta is approximately 2.5 to 3.0 cm wide with a moderately strong and regular pulse. Possibly mild tenderness may be elicited.	A wide, bounding pulse may be felt with an abdominal aortic aneurysm. A prominent, laterally pulsating mass above the umbilicus with an accompanying audible bruit strongly suggests an aortic aneurysm (see Abnormal findings 24-3).

Continued on following page

DISPLAY 24-2 CONSIDERATIONS FOR PALPATING THE ABDOMEN

- Avoid touching tender or painful areas until last, and reassure the patient of your intentions.
- Perform light palpation before deep palpation to detect tenderness and superficial masses.
- Keep in mind that the normal abdomen may be tender, especially in the areas over the xiphoid process, liver, aorta, lower pole of the kidney, gas-filled caecum, sigmoid colon and ovaries.
- Overcome ticklishness and minimise voluntary guarding by asking the patient to perform self-palpation. Place your hands over the patient's. After a while, let your fingers glide slowly onto the abdomen while still resting mostly on the patient's fingers. The same can be done by using a warm stethoscope as a palpating instrument, again letting your fingers drift over the edge of the diaphragm and palpating without promoting a ticklish response.
- Work with the patient to promote relaxation and minimise voluntary guarding. Use the following techniques:
  - Place a pillow under the patient's knees.
  - Ask the patient to take slow, deep breaths through the mouth.
  - Apply light pressure over the patient's sternum with your left hand while palpating with the right. This encourages the patient to relax the abdominal muscles during breathing against sternal resistance.

PHYSICAL ASSESSMENT (continued)

ASSESSMENT PROCEDURE	NORMAL FINDINGS	ABNORMAL FINDINGS

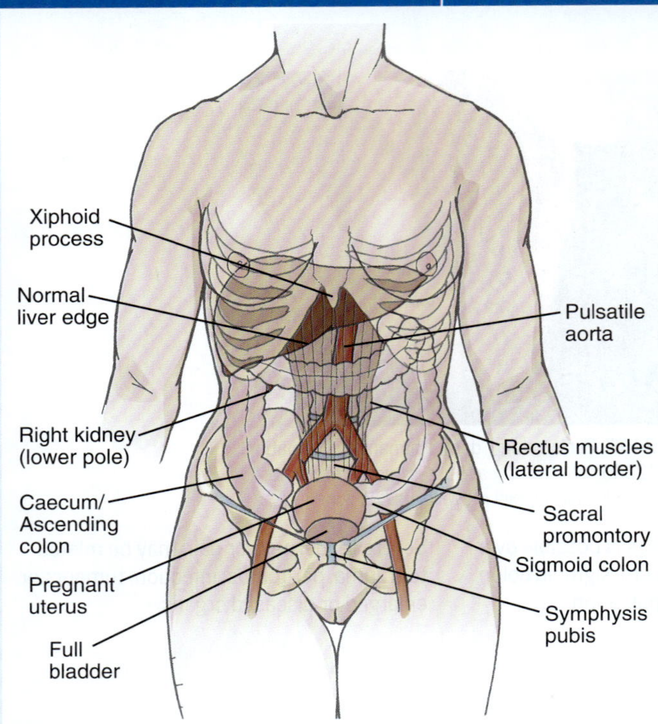

FIGURE 24-20 Normally palpable structures in the abdomen.

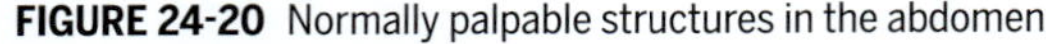

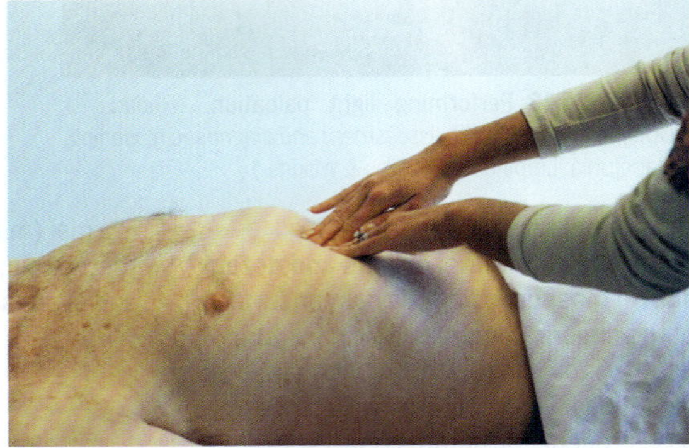

FIGURE 24-21 Palpating the aorta. (© B. Proud.)

OLDER ADULT CONSIDERATIONS

If the patient is older than age 50 or has hypertension, assess the width of the aorta.

CLINICAL TIP

Do not palpate a pulsating midline mass; it may be a dissecting aneurysm that can rupture from the pressure of palpation. Also avoid deep palpation over tender organs as in the case of polycystic kidneys, transplantation or suspected splenic trauma.

ASSESSMENT PROCEDURE	NORMAL FINDINGS	ABNORMAL FINDINGS
Palpate the liver. Note consistency and tenderness. To palpate bimanually, stand at the patient's right side and place your left hand under the patient's back at the level of the 11th to 12th ribs. Lay your right hand parallel to the right costal margin (your fingertips should point towards the patient's head). Ask the patient to inhale then compress upwards and inwards with your fingers (Fig. 24-22). To palpate by *hooking,* stand to the right of the patient's chest. Curl (hook) the fingers of both hands over the edge of the right costal margin. Ask the patient to take a deep breath and gently but firmly pull inwards and upwards with your fingers (Fig. 24-23).	The liver is not usually palpable, although it may be felt in some thin patients. If the lower edge is felt, it should be firm, smooth and even. Mild tenderness may be normal.	A hard, firm liver may indicate cancer. Nodularity may occur with tumours, metastatic cancer, late cirrhosis or syphilis. Tenderness may be from vascular engorgement (e.g. congestive heart failure), acute hepatitis or abscess. A liver more than 1 to 3 cm below the costal margin is considered enlarged (unless pressed down by the diaphragm). Enlargement may be due to hepatitis, liver tumours, cirrhosis or vascular engorgement.

PHYSICAL ASSESSMENT (continued)

ASSESSMENT PROCEDURE	NORMAL FINDINGS	ABNORMAL FINDINGS

Palpation (continued)

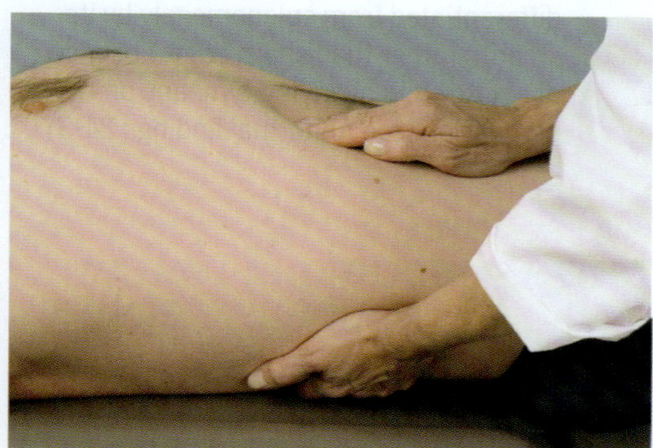

FIGURE 24-22 Bimanual technique for liver palpation.

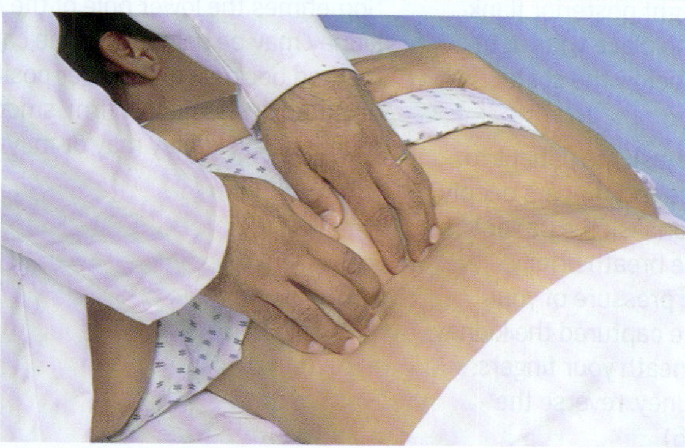

FIGURE 24-23 Hooking technique for liver palpation.

Palpate the spleen. Stand at the patient's right side, reach over the abdomen with your left arm and place your hand under the posterior lower ribs. Pull up gently.

Place your right hand below the left costal margin with the fingers pointing towards the patient's head. Ask the patient to inhale and press inwards and upwards as you provide support with your other hand (Fig. 24-24). Alternatively asking the patient to turn onto the right side may facilitate splenic palpation by moving the spleen downwards and forwards (Fig. 24-25). Document the size of the spleen in centimetres below the left costal margin. Also note consistency and tenderness.

CLINICAL TIP
Be sure to palpate with your fingers below the costal margin so you do not miss the lower edge of an enlarged spleen.

The spleen is seldom palpable at the left costal margin; rarely, the tip is palpable in the presence of a low, flat diaphragm (e.g. chronic obstructive lung disease) or with deep diaphragmatic descent on inspiration.

If the edge of the spleen can be palpated, it should be soft and non-tender.

A palpable spleen suggests enlargement (up to three times the normal size), which may result from trauma, glandular fever, chronic blood disorders or cancer. The splenic notch may be felt, which is an indication of splenic enlargement.

SAFETY TIP
Caution: To avoid traumatising and possibly rupturing the organ, be gentle when palpating an enlarged spleen.

The spleen feels soft with a rounded edge when it is enlarged from infection. It feels firm with a sharp edge when it is enlarged from chronic disease.

Tenderness accompanied by peritoneal inflammation or capsular stretching is associated with splenic enlargement.

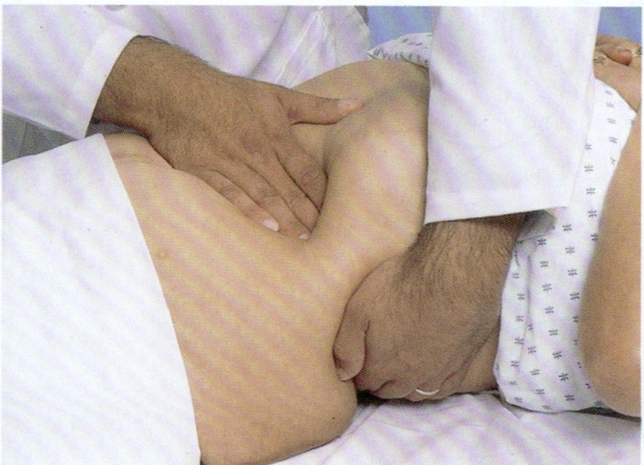

FIGURE 24-24 Palpating the spleen.

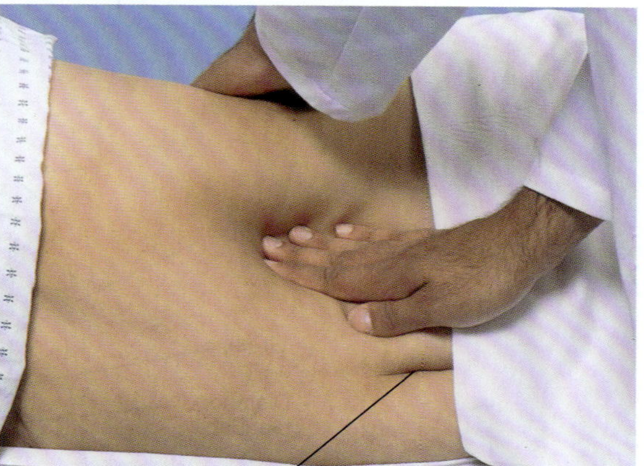

FIGURE 24-25 Palpating the spleen with the patient in side-lying position.

Continued on following page

PHYSICAL ASSESSMENT (continued)

ASSESSMENT PROCEDURE	NORMAL FINDINGS	ABNORMAL FINDINGS
Palpate the kidneys. To palpate the right kidney, support the right posterior flank with your left hand and place your right hand in the RUQ just below the costal margin at the MCL. To capture the kidney, ask the patient to inhale. Then compress your fingers deeply during peak inspiration. Ask the patient to exhale and hold the breath briefly. Gradually release the pressure of your right hand. If you have captured the kidney, you will feel it slip beneath your fingers. To palpate the left kidney, reverse the procedure (Fig. 24-26).	The kidneys are normally not palpable. Sometimes the lower pole of the right kidney may be palpable by the capture method because of its lower position. If palpated, it should feel firm, smooth and rounded. The kidney may or may not be slightly tender.	An enlarged kidney may be due to a cyst, tumour or hydronephrosis. It can be differentiated from splenomegaly by its smooth rather than sharp edge, absence of a notch and overlying tympany on percussion (see Abnormal findings 24-3).

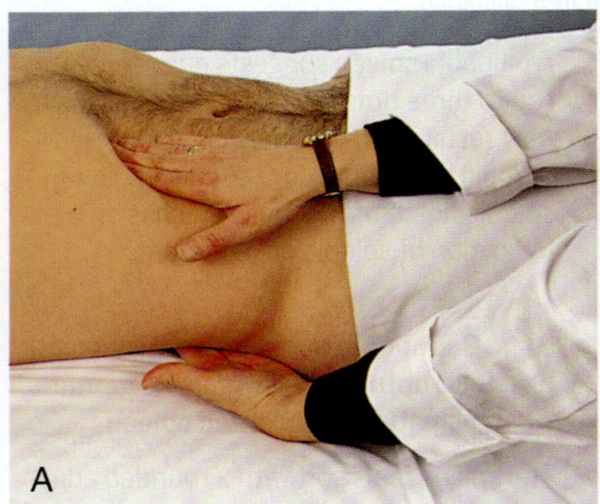

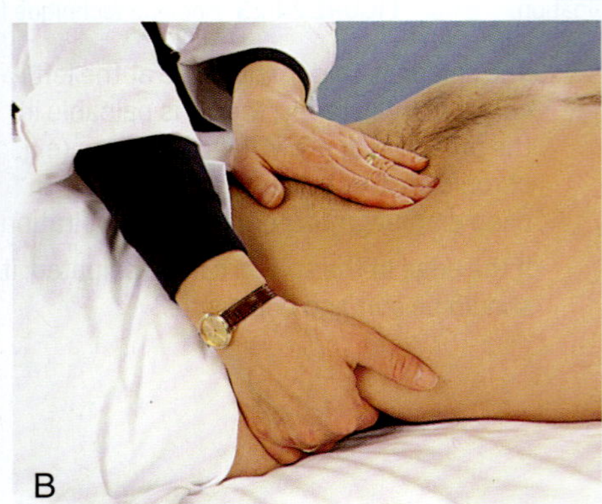

FIGURE 24-26 Palpating the right kidney **(A)** and the left kidney **(B).** (© B. Proud.)

ASSESSMENT PROCEDURE	NORMAL FINDINGS	ABNORMAL FINDINGS
Palpate the urinary bladder. Palpate for a distended bladder when the patient's history or other findings warrant (e.g. dull percussion noted over the symphysis pubis). Begin at the symphysis pubis and move upwards and outwards to estimate bladder borders (Fig. 24-27).	Normally the bladder is not palpable.	A distended bladder is palpated as a smooth, round and somewhat firm mass extending as far as the umbilicus. It may be further validated by dull percussion tones.

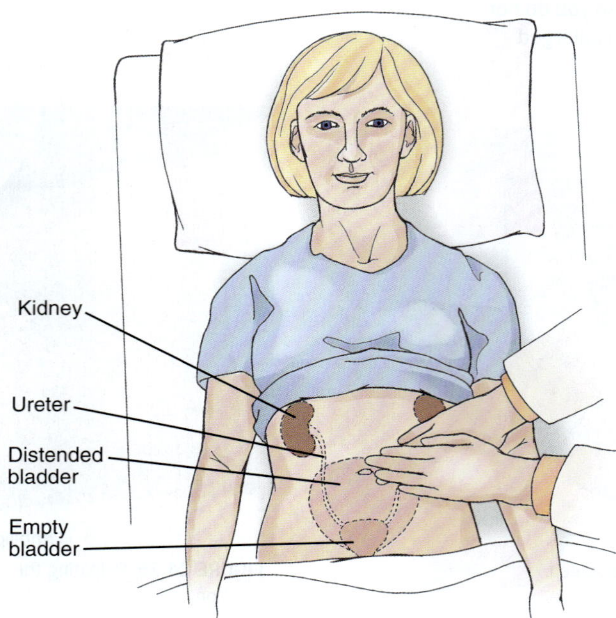

FIGURE 24-27 Palpating distended bladder (*larger dotted line is area of distension*).

PHYSICAL ASSESSMENT (continued)

ASSESSMENT PROCEDURE	NORMAL FINDINGS	ABNORMAL FINDINGS
Special abdominal tests		
TESTS FOR ASCITES		
Test for shifting dullness. If you suspect that the patient has ascites because of a distended abdomen or bulging flanks, perform this special percussion technique. The patient should remain supine. Percuss the flanks from the bed upward towards the umbilicus. Note the change from dullness to tympany and mark this point. Now help the patient turn onto their side. Percuss the abdomen from the bed upwards. Mark the level where dullness changes to tympany (Fig. 24-28).	The borders between tympany and dullness remain relatively constant throughout position changes.	When ascites is present and the patient is supine, the fluid assumes a dependent position and produces a dull percussion tone around the flanks. Air rises to the top and tympany is percussed around the umbilicus. When the patient turns onto one side and ascites is present, the fluid assumes a dependent position and air rises to the top. There is a marked increase in the height of the dullness. This test is not always reliable and definitive testing by ultrasound is necessary.

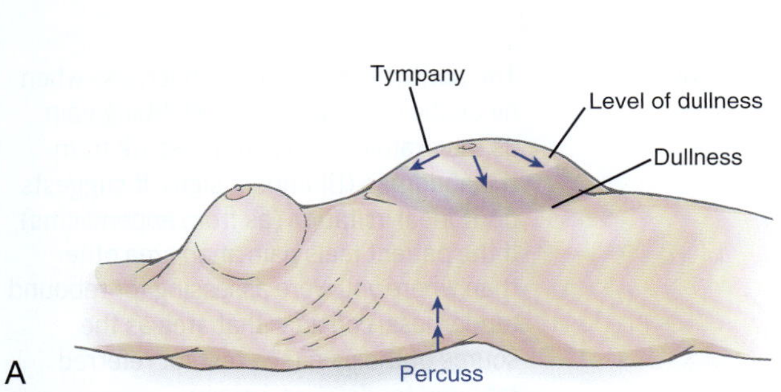

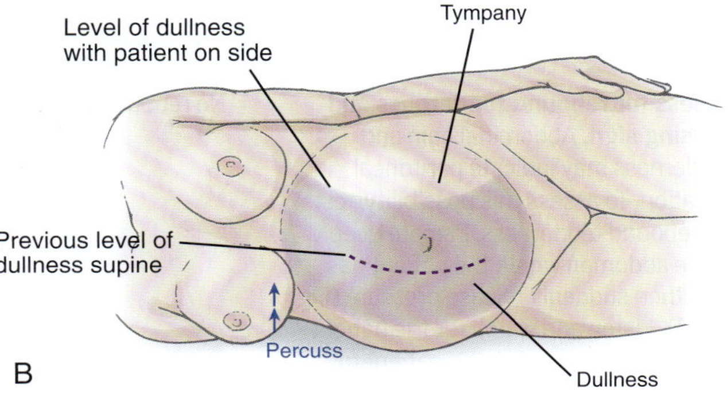

FIGURE 24-28 Percussing for level of dullness with patient supine **(A)** and lying on the side **(B).**

ASSESSMENT PROCEDURE	NORMAL FINDINGS	ABNORMAL FINDINGS
Perform the fluid wave test. A second special technique to detect ascites is the fluid wave test. The patient should remain supine. You will need assistance with this test. Ask the patient or an assistant to place the ulnar side of the hand and the lateral side of the forearm firmly along the midline of the abdomen. Firmly place the palmar surface of your fingers and hand against one side of the patient's abdomen. Use your other hand to tap the opposite side of the abdominal wall (Fig. 24-29).	No fluid wave is transmitted.	Movement of a fluid wave against the resting hand suggests large amounts of fluid are present (ascites). Because this test is not completely reliable, definitive testing by ultrasound is needed.
Use ballottement technique. Ballottement is a palpation technique performed to identify a mass or enlarged organ within an ascitic abdomen. Ballottement can be performed two different ways: single-handedly or bimanually (Fig. 24-30). *Single-handed method:* Using a tapping or bouncing motion of the fingerpads over the abdominal wall, feel for a floating mass. *Bimanual method:* Place one hand under the flank (receiving/feeling hand) and push the anterior abdominal wall with the other hand.	No palpable mass or masses are present.	In the patient with ascites, you can feel a freely movable mass moving upwards (floats). It can be felt at the fingertips. A floating mass can be palpated for size.

Continued on following page

PHYSICAL ASSESSMENT (continued)

ASSESSMENT PROCEDURE	NORMAL FINDINGS	ABNORMAL FINDINGS

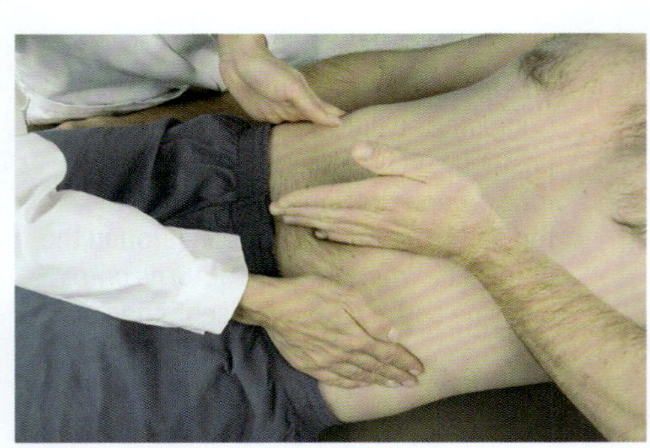

FIGURE 24-29 Performing the fluid wave test. (Rhoads, J. [2006]. *Advanced health assessment and diagnostic reasoning.* Philadelphia: Lippincott Williams & Wilkins.)

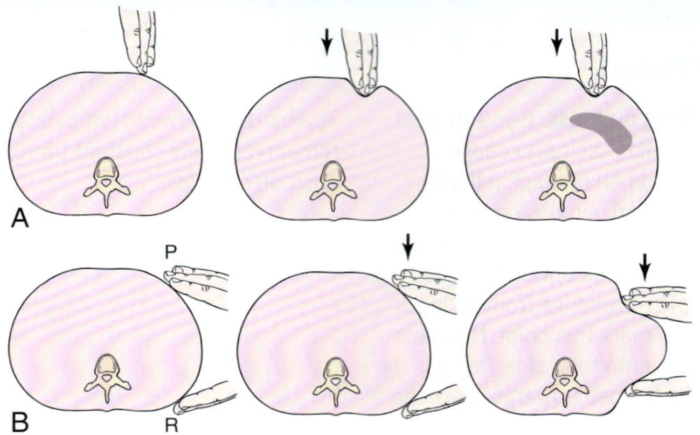

FIGURE 24-30 Performing ballottement with one hand **(A)** and bimanually **(B).**

TESTS FOR APPENDICITIS

ASSESSMENT PROCEDURE	NORMAL FINDINGS	ABNORMAL FINDINGS
Assess for rebound tenderness and Rovsing sign. Abdominal pain and tenderness may indicate peritoneal irritation. To assess this possibility, test for rebound tenderness. Palpate deeply in the abdomen where the patient has pain then suddenly release pressure (Fig. 24-31). Listen and watch for the patient's expression of pain. Ask the patient to describe which hurt more—the pressing in or the releasing—and where on the abdomen the pain occurred.	No rebound tenderness is present.	The patient has rebound tenderness when he or she perceives sharp, stabbing pain as the examiner releases pressure from the abdomen (Blumberg sign). It suggests peritoneal irritation (as from appendicitis). If the patient feels pain at an area other than where you were assessing for rebound tenderness, consider that area as the source of the pain (see test for referred rebound tenderness, below).

CLINICAL TIP

Test for rebound tenderness should always be performed at the end of the examination because a positive response produces pain and muscle spasm that can interfere with the remaining examination.

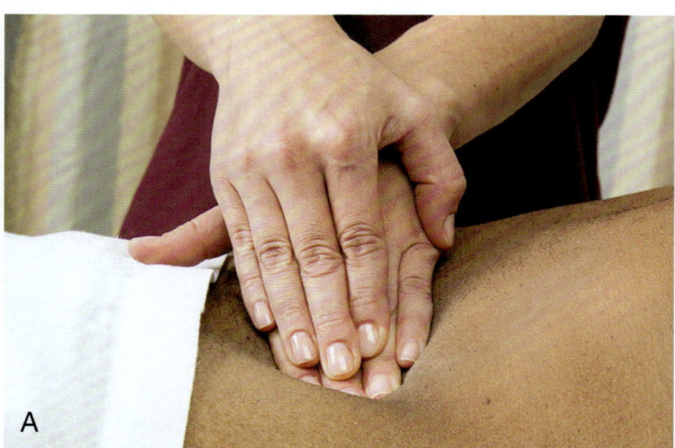

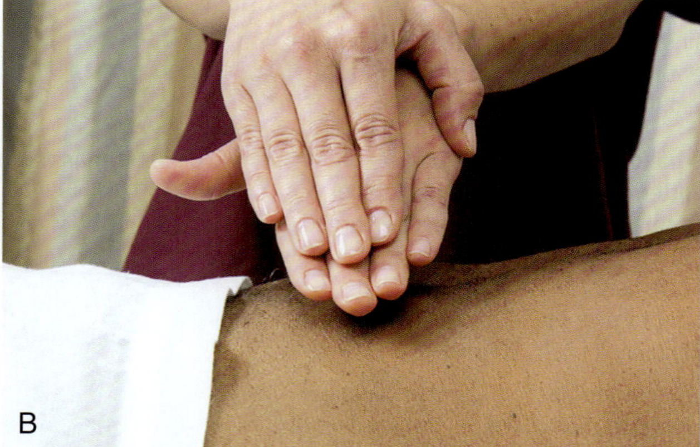

FIGURE 24-31 Assessing for rebound tenderness: palpating deeply **(A)**; releasing pressure rapidly **(B).**

PHYSICAL ASSESSMENT (continued)

ASSESSMENT PROCEDURE	NORMAL FINDINGS	ABNORMAL FINDINGS
Special abdominal tests (continued)		
Test for referred rebound tenderness. Palpate deeply in the LLQ and quickly release pressure.	No rebound pain is elicited.	Pain in the RLQ during pressure in the LLQ is a positive Rovsing sign. It suggests acute appendicitis. **SAFETY TIP** **Avoid continued palpation when test findings are positive for appendicitis because of the danger of rupturing the appendix.**
Assess for psoas sign. Raise the patient's right leg from the hip and place your hand on the lower thigh. Ask the patient to try to keep the leg elevated as you apply pressure downwards against the lower thigh (Fig. 24-32).	No abdominal pain is present.	Pain in the RLQ (psoas sign) is associated with irritation of the iliopsoas muscle due to an appendicitis (an inflamed appendix).
Assess for obturator sign. Support the patient's right knee and ankle. Flex the hip and knee and rotate the leg internally and externally (Fig. 24-33).	No abdominal pain is present.	Pain in the RLQ indicates irritation of the obturator muscle due to appendicitis or a perforated appendix.
Perform hypersensitivity test. Stroke the abdomen with a sharp object (e.g. broken cotton bud or tongue blade) or grasp a fold of skin with your thumb and index finger and quickly let go. Do this several times along the abdominal wall.	The patient feels no pain and no exaggerated sensation.	Pain or an exaggerated sensation felt in the RLQ is a positive skin hypersensitivity test and may indicate appendicitis.
TEST FOR CHOLECYSTITIS		
Assess RUQ pain or tenderness, which may signal cholecystitis (inflammation of the gallbladder). Press your fingertips under the liver border at the right costal margin and ask the patient to inhale deeply.	No increase in pain is present.	Accentuated sharp pain that causes the patient to hold his or her breath (inspiratory arrest) is a positive Murphy sign and is associated with acute cholecystitis.

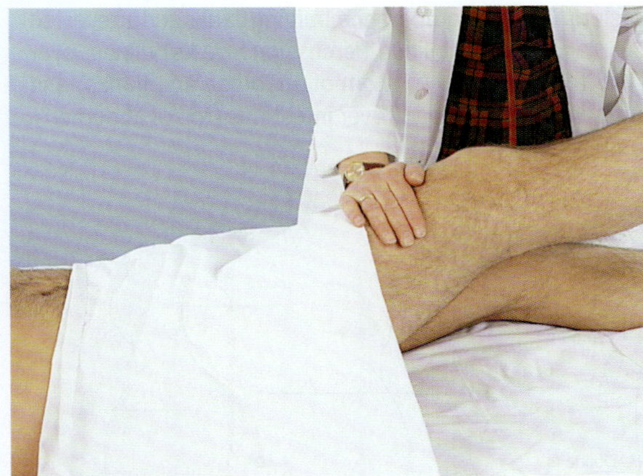

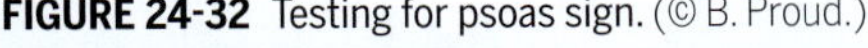

FIGURE 24-32 Testing for psoas sign. (© B. Proud.)

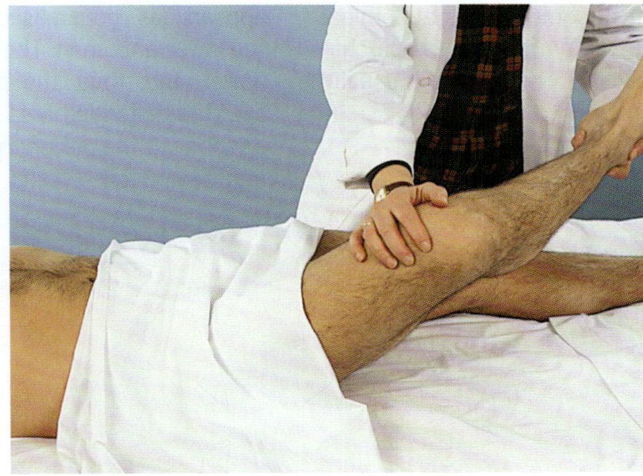

FIGURE 24-33 Testing for obturator sign. (© B. Proud.)

ABNORMAL FINDINGS 24-1 Abdominal distension

With the exception of pregnancy, abdominal distension is usually considered an abnormal finding. Percussion may help determine the cause.

PREGNANCY (NORMAL FINDING)

Pregnancy is included here so the examiner may differentiate it from abnormal findings.

It causes a generalised protuberant abdomen, protuberant umbilicus, a fetal heart beat that can be heard on auscultation, percussible tympany over the intestines and dullness over the uterus.

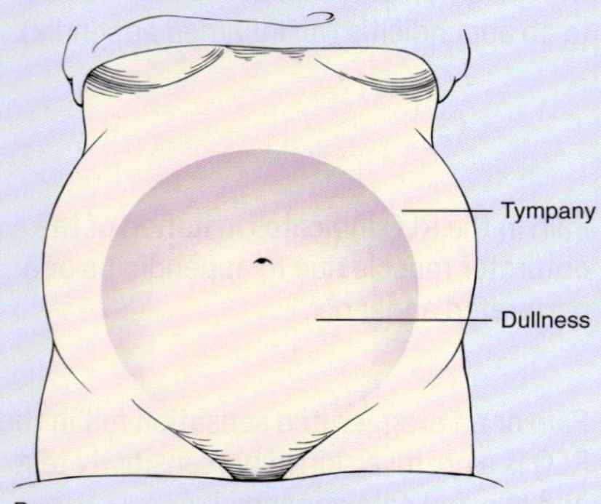

Pregnancy.

FAECES

Hard stools in the colon appear as a localised distension. Percussion over the area discloses dullness.

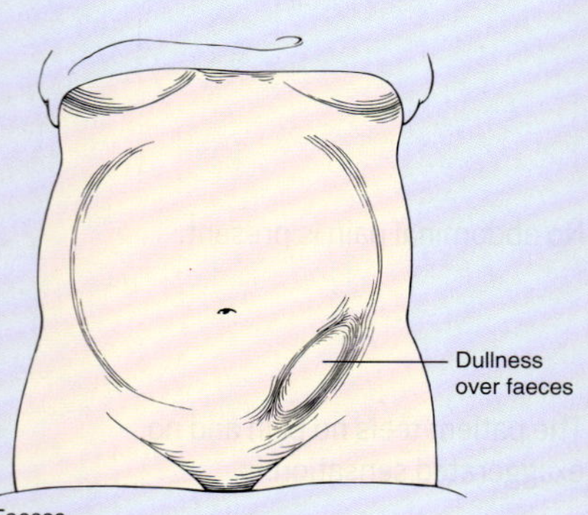

Faeces.

FLATUS

The abdomen distended with gas may appear as a generalised protuberance (as shown), or it may appear more localised. Tympany is the percussion tone over the area.

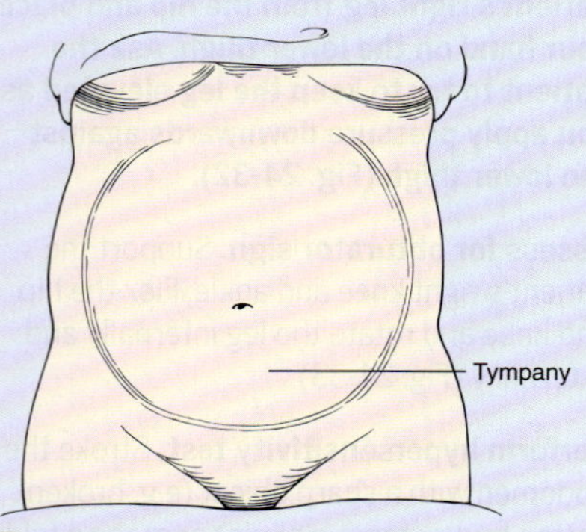

Flatus.

FAT

Obesity accounts for most uniformly protuberant abdomens. The abdominal wall is thick and tympany is the percussion tone elicited. The umbilicus usually appears sunken.

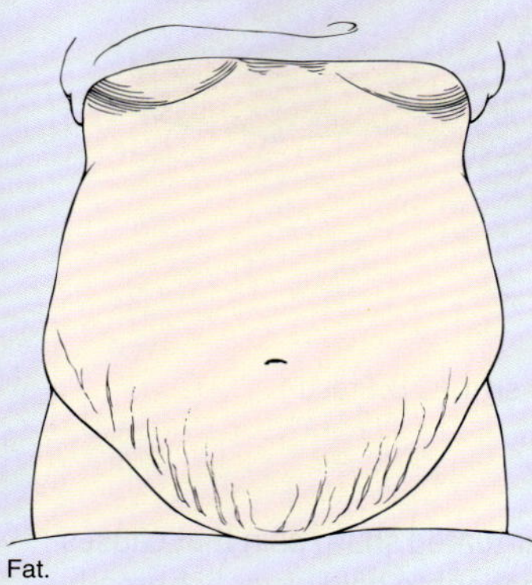

Fat.

FIBROIDS AND OTHER MASSES

A large ovarian cyst or fibroid tumour appears as generalised distension in the lower abdomen. The mass displaces bowel, and, thus, the percussion tone over the distended area is dullness with tympany at the periphery. The umbilicus may be everted.

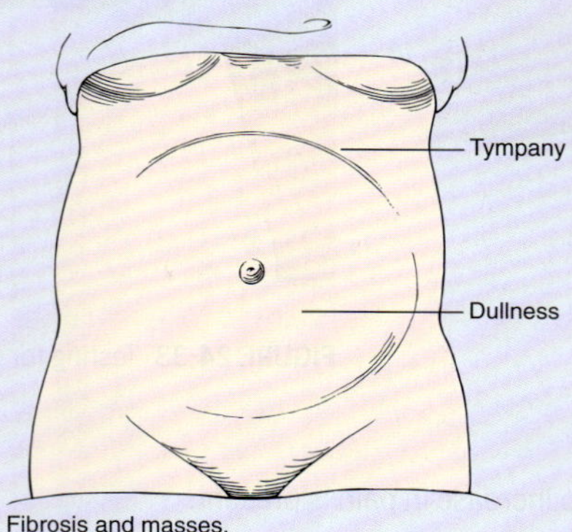

Fibrosis and masses.

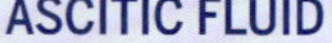

ASCITIC FLUID

Fluid in the abdomen causes generalised protuberance, bulging flanks and an everted umbilicus. Percussion reveals dullness over fluid (bottom of abdomen and flanks) and tympany over intestines (top of abdomen).

Tympany

Dullness

Bulging flank

Fluid.

ABNORMAL FINDINGS 24-2 Abdominal bulges

UMBILICAL HERNIA

An umbilical hernia results from the bowel protruding through a weakness in the umbilical ring. This condition occurs more frequently in infants, but it also occurs in adults.

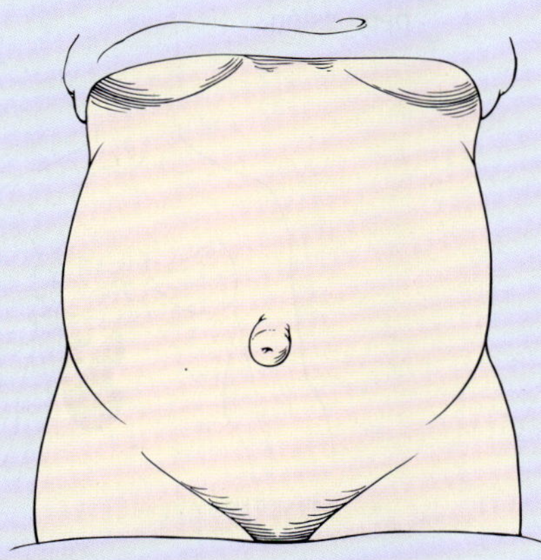

Umbilical hernia.

DIASTASIS RECTI

Diastasis recti occurs when bowel protrudes through a separation between the two rectus abdominis muscles. It appears as a midline ridge. The bulge may appear only when patient raises head or coughs. The condition is of little significance.

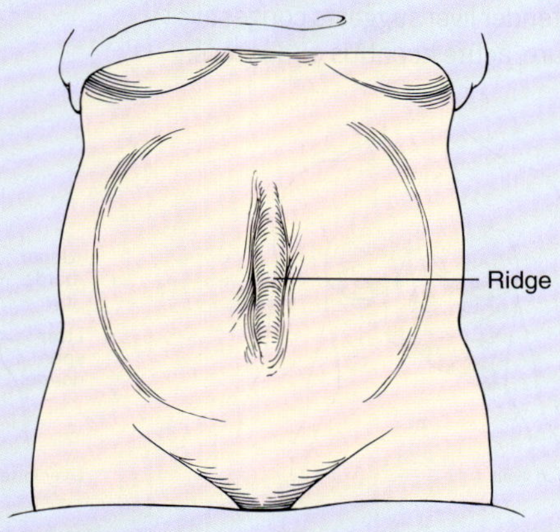

Diastasis recti.

EPIGASTRIC HERNIA

An epigastric hernia occurs when bowel protrudes through a weakness in the linea alba. The small bulge appears midline between the xiphoid process and the umbilicus. It may be discovered only on palpation.

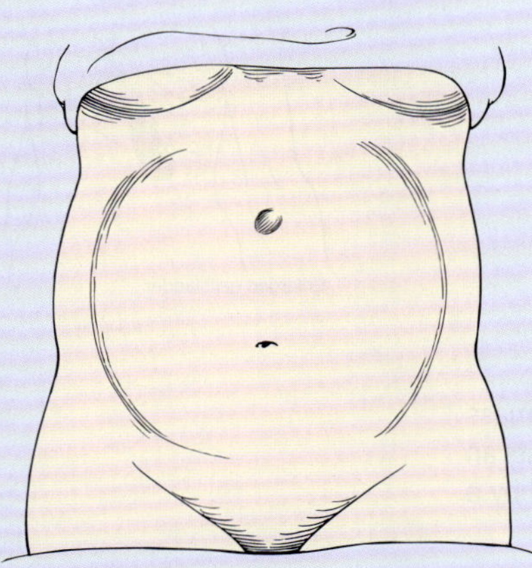

Epigastric hernia.

INCISIONAL HERNIA

An incisional hernia occurs when bowel protrudes through a defect or weakness resulting from a surgical incision. It appears as a bulge near a surgical scar on the abdomen.

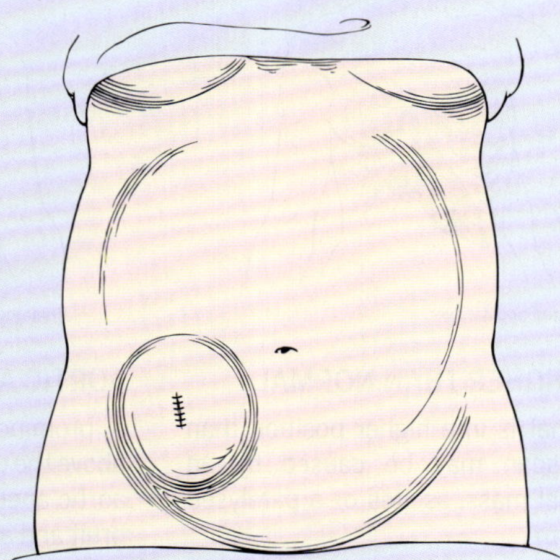

Incisional hernia.

ABNORMAL FINDINGS 24-3 Enlarged abdominal organs and other abnormalities

ENLARGED LIVER

An enlarged liver (hepatomegaly) is defined as a span greater than 12 cm at the midclavicular line and greater than 8 cm at the midsternal line. An enlarged non-tender liver suggests cirrhosis. An enlarged tender liver suggests congestive heart failure, acute hepatitis or abscess.

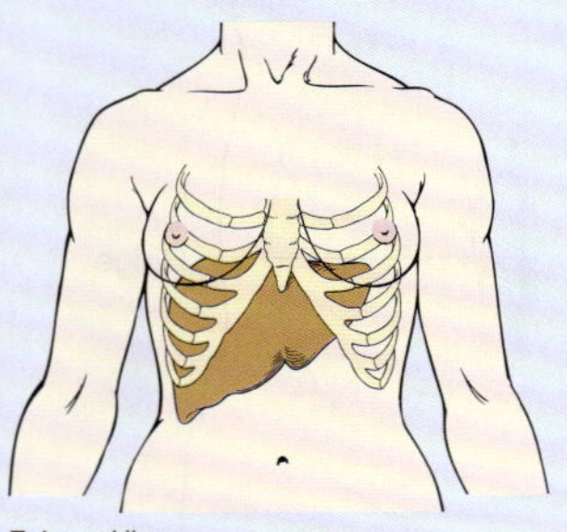

Enlarged liver.

LIVER LOWER THAN NORMAL

A liver in a lower position than normal with a normal span may be caused by emphysema because the diaphragm is low.

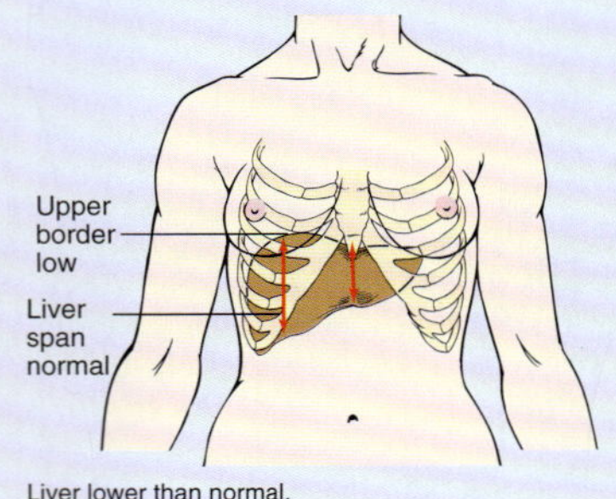

Liver lower than normal.

ENLARGED KIDNEY

An enlarged kidney may be due to a cyst, tumour or hydronephrosis. It may be differentiated from an enlarged spleen by its smooth rather than sharp edge, the absence of a notch and tympany on percussion.

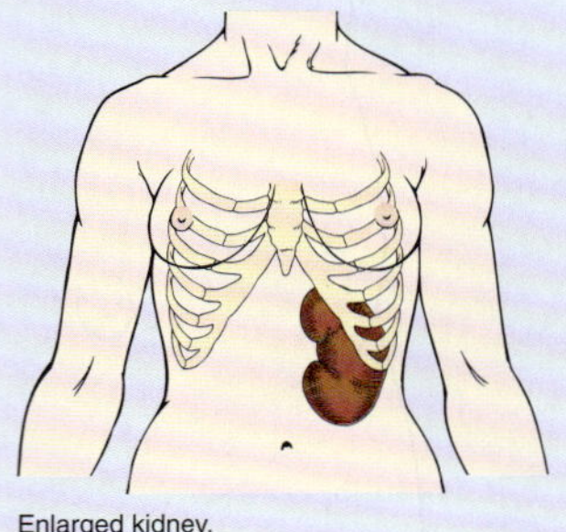

Enlarged kidney.

ENLARGED NODULAR LIVER

An enlarged firm, hard, nodular liver suggests cancer. Other causes may be late cirrhosis or syphilis.

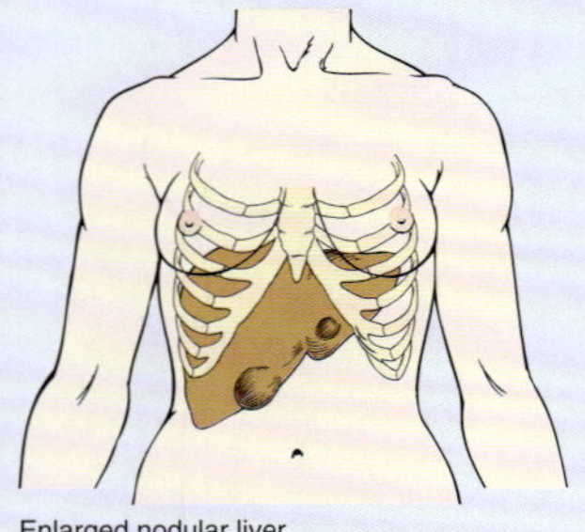

Enlarged nodular liver.

ENLARGED SPLEEN

An enlarged spleen (splenomegaly) is defined by an area of dullness exceeding 7 cm. When enlarged, the spleen progresses downwards and in towards the midline.

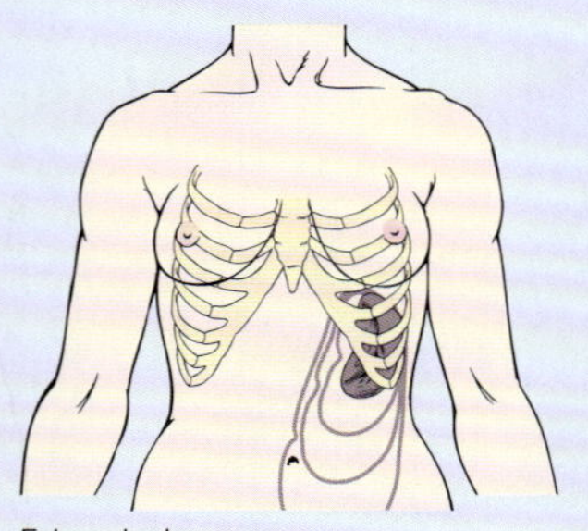

Enlarged spleen.

ENLARGED GALLBLADDER

An extremely tender, enlarged gallbladder suggests acute cholecystitis. A positive finding is Murphy sign (sharp pain that causes the patient to hold the breath).

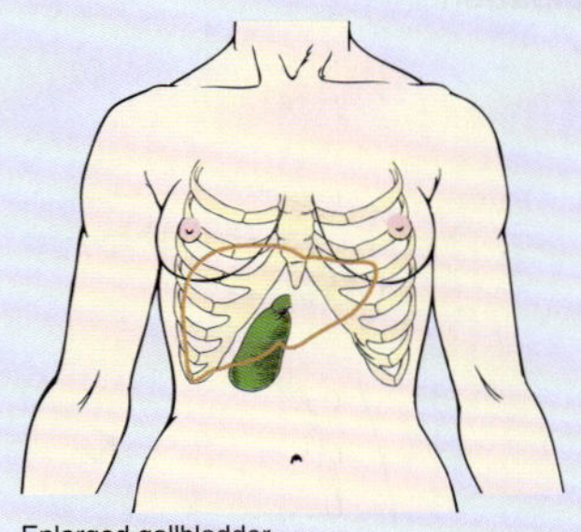

Enlarged gallbladder.

LIVER HIGHER THAN NORMAL

A liver that is in a higher position than normal span may be caused by an abdominal mass, ascites or a paralysed diaphragm.

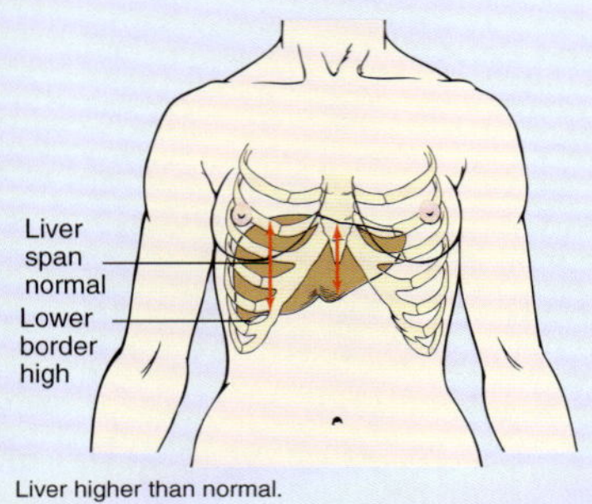

Liver higher than normal.

AORTIC ANEURYSM

A prominent, laterally pulsating mass above the umbilicus strongly suggests an aortic aneurysm. It is accompanied by a bruit and a wide, bounding pulse.

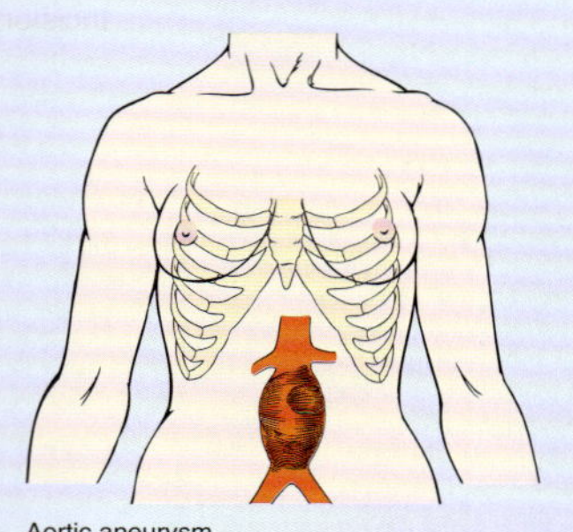

Aortic aneurysm.

VALIDATING AND DOCUMENTING FINDINGS

Validate the abdominal assessment data you have collected. This is necessary to verify that the data are reliable and accurate. Document the assessment data following the hospital policy.

After you have collected your assessment data, you will need to analyse the data using diagnostic reasoning skills. Refer to the discussion of the diagnostic reasoning process in Chapter 5.

Sample of subjective data

A 44-year-old male patient denies pain in the abdomen, indigestion, nausea, vomiting, constipation and diarrhoea. He says that he has had no change in his usual bowel habits and denies yellowing of skin, itching, dark urine or clay-coloured stools. He states that he has never had ulcers, gastro-oesophageal reflux, inflammatory or obstructive bowel disease, pancreatitis, gallbladder or liver disease, diverticular disease or appendicitis. He did have one urinary tract infection 3 years ago but has had no other problems since that time. He has never had viral hepatitis and denies known exposure. He denies abdominal surgery or trauma to the abdomen. He does not take prescribed or over-the-counter medications except for an occasional ibuprofen for headache. He denies any family history of colon, stomach, pancreatic, liver, kidney or bladder cancer; liver disease; gallbladder disease; or kidney disease. He tries to follow a low-fat, high-carbohydrate, moderated protein diet and drinks a lot of fluids daily. He has approximately 2 alcoholic drinks per week, runs 3 days a week and cycles 2 days a week. He reports a moderate amount of stress from work but copes with it through exercise and spending time with his wife and children.

Sample of objective data

Skin of abdomen is free of striae, scars, lesions and rashes. Umbilicus is midline and recessed with no bulging. Abdomen is flat and symmetrical with no bulges or lumps. No bulges noted when patient raises head. Slight respiratory movements and aortic pulsations noted. No peristaltic waves seen. Soft clicks and gurgles heard at a rate of 15 per minute. No bruits, venous hums or friction rubs auscultated.

Percussion reveals generalised tympany over all four quadrants with dullness over the liver, spleen and descending colon. Percussion of liver span reveals midclavicular line is 8 cm and midsternal line is 6 cm. Percussion over spleen discloses a dull oval area approximately 7 cm wide near the left 10th rib posterior to midaxillary. No tenderness elicited with blunt percussion over liver and kidneys. No tenderness or guarding in any quadrant with light palpation. Mild tenderness elicited over xiphoid, aorta, caecum and sigmoid colon with deep palpation. No masses palpated. Umbilicus and surrounding area free of masses, swelling and bulges. Aortic pulsation moderately strong, regular and approximately 3 cm wide. Liver, spleen, kidneys and urinary bladder not palpable. Test for shifting dullness reveals constant borders between tympany and dullness throughout position changes. No fluid wave transmitted during fluid wave test. No mass palpated during ballottement test. All test findings for appendicitis are negative, as is the test finding for cholecystitis.

CASE STUDY

Abdominal inspection for Ms Knowles reveals a pale, distended abdomen with a midline smooth minimally raised 8-cm scar. Auscultation findings include infrequent high-pitched bowel sounds in all quadrants except for the left lower quadrant. A faint low-pitched murmur is present over the epigastric region.

On percussion, the abdomen is mostly tympanic with mild dullness present in the left lower quadrant. Liver margins are normal. Because of abdominal tenderness, only light palpation is performed. A pulsating mass is palpable 5 cm above the umbilicus, and an 8-cm firm mass is present in the left lower quadrant.

CRITICAL THINKING

4. What are some of the possible implications of the abdominal scarring for Ms Knowles's current admission?
5. What might each of the two masses indicate?
6. What further assessment is required?

Analysis of data

DIAGNOSTIC REASONING: POSSIBLE CONCLUSIONS

After collecting subjective and objective data pertaining to the abdomen, identify abnormal findings and patient strengths. Then cluster the data to reveal any significant patterns or abnormalities. These data may be used to make clinical judgements about the status of the patient's abdomen.

Potential patient risks

- Risk of fluid volume deficit (related to excessive nausea and vomiting or diarrhoea)
- Risk of impaired skin integrity (related to fluid volume deficit secondary to decreased fluid intake, nausea, vomiting, diarrhoea, faecal or urinary incontinence or ostomy drainage)
- Risk of impaired oral mucous membranes (related to fluid volume deficit secondary to nausea, vomiting, diarrhoea or gastrointestinal intubation)
- Risk of urinary tract infection (related to urinary stasis and decreased fluid intake)
- Risk of inadequate nutrition (related to lack of dietary information or inadequate intake of nutrients secondary to values or religious beliefs or eating disorders)

Potential patient problems

- Inadequate nutrition (related to malabsorption, decreased appetite, frequent nausea and vomiting)
- Imbalanced nutrition: greater than body requirements (related to intake that exceeds kilojoule needs)
- Disturbed body image (related to change in abdominal appearance secondary to presence of stoma)

- Diarrhoea (related to malabsorption and chronic irritable bowel syndrome or medications)
- Constipation (related to decreased fluid intake, decreased dietary fibre, decreased physical activity, bed rest or medications)
- Bowel incontinence (related to muscular or neurological dysfunction secondary to age, disease or trauma)
- Disturbed self-concept (related to obesity and difficulty losing weight)
- Activity intolerance (related to faecal or urinary incontinence)
- Social isolation (related to anxiety and fear of faecal or urinary incontinence)
- Abdominal pain (referred, distension or surgical incision)
- Impaired urinary elimination (related to catheterisation secondary to obstruction, trauma, infection, neurological disorders or surgical intervention)
- Urinary retention (related to obstruction of part of the urinary tract or malfunctioning of drainage devices (catheters) and the need to learn bladder emptying techniques)
- Functional incontinence (related to age-related urgency and inability to reach the toilet in time secondary to decreased bladder tone and inability to recognise 'need-to-void cues')
- Stress incontinence (related to knowledge deficit of pelvic floor muscle exercises)
- Total incontinence (related to the need for a bladder retraining program)
- Urge incontinence (related to the need for knowledge of preventive measures secondary to infection, trauma or neurogenic problems)

Selected collaborative problems

After grouping the data, certain collaborative problems may emerge. Remember that collaborative problems cannot be prevented by nursing interventions. However, these physiological complications of medical conditions can be detected and monitored by the nurse. In addition, the nurse can use doctor- and nurse-prescribed interventions to minimise the complications of these problems. The nurse may also have to refer the patient in such situations for further treatment of the problem. The following is a list of collaborative problems that may be identified when assessing the abdomen:

- Peritonitis
- Ileus
- Afferent loop syndrome
- Early dumping syndrome
- Late dumping syndrome
- Malabsorption syndrome
- Intestinal bleeding
- Renal calculi
- Abscess formation
- Bowel obstruction
- Toxic megacolon
- Mesenteric thrombosis
- Obstruction of bile flow
- Fistula formation
- Hyponatraemia or hypernatraemia
- Hypokalaemia or hyperkalaemia
- Hypoglycaemia or hyperglycaemia
- Hypocalcaemia or hypercalcaemia
- Metabolic acidosis
- Uremic syndrome
- Stomal changes
- Urinary obstruction
- Hypertension
- Gastro-oesophageal reflux disease
- Peptic ulcer disease
- Hepatic failure
- Pancreatitis.

Medical problems

If, after grouping the data, it becomes apparent that the patient has signs and symptoms that may require medical diagnosis and treatment, referral to a primary care provider is necessary.

ONLINE RESOURCES

An extensive range of additional resources to enhance teaching and learning and to facilitate understanding may be found online at the text's accompanying website, located on thePoint at http://thepoint.lww.com. These include Watch and Learn videos, Concepts in Action animations, journal articles, case studies, discussion topics and quizzes.

Subscribers may also access Lippincott Procedures, an extensive online point-of-care procedure guide that provides reliable step-by-step instructions for more than 1700 procedures, including 450 evidence-based Australian procedures, and skills in a variety of speciality settings, together with a wealth of supporting information.

SIMULATED LEARNING

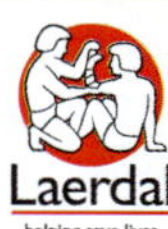

Having completed this chapter, explore the scenarios of Doris Bowman Part 1 and Part 2, Stan Checketts Part 1 and Part 2 and Vernon Watkins Part 1 and Part 2. Doris is a 39-year-old female who is postoperative following a total abdominal hysterectomy. Stan is a 64-year-old admitted with abdominal pain diagnosed as a bowel obstruction. Vernon is a 69-year-old man who is postoperative following a hemicolectomy and requires postoperative support. Incorporating the health assessment content in this chapter with your existing theoretical knowledge and clinical experience, progress through each simulation scenario (this is best done in a small group). How would you manage each patient's care? When reflecting on your management of each virtual patient, what do you think you did well and what do you think you can improve? Consider why you think this and also how you might manage a similar problem in the future.

CASE STUDY

The case study demonstrates how to analyse abdomen assessment data for a specific patient. The exercises included in the ancillary product on thePoint that complements this text offer further opportunities to enhance your skills.

Lottie Knowles is an 84-year-old resident of an aged-care facility. She has been admitted to the emergency department with a diagnosis of abdominal pain for investigation. She is alert and oriented and able to clearly describe her pain. She has no spouse or children and her closest relative is a niece who lives interstate.

Ms Knowles describes her pain as colicky with a sudden onset, located in the left upper quadrant and radiating to her back. She also feels nauseous. She is worried that she has 'not used her bowels' for the last 4 days. Ms Knowles has a past medical history of hypertension, a cholecystectomy 25 years ago and severe rheumatoid arthritis. Her medications include antihypertensives, opioids, aperients and non-steroidal anti-inflammatory drugs.

Abdominal inspection for Ms Knowles reveals a pale, distended abdomen with a midline smooth minimally raised 8-cm scar. Auscultation findings include infrequent high-pitched bowel sounds in all quadrants except for the left lower quadrant. A faint low-pitched murmur is present over the epigastric region.

On percussion, the abdomen is mostly tympanic with mild dullness present in the left lower quadrant. Liver margins are normal. Because of abdominal tenderness, only light palpation is performed. A pulsating mass is palpable 5 cm above the umbilicus and an 8-cm firm mass is present in the left lower quadrant.

The following concept map illustrates the diagnostic reasoning process.

Applying COLDSPA

Applying COLDSPA for patient symptoms: 'abdominal pain'.

Mnemonic	Question	Data provided	Missing data
Character	Describe the sign or symptom (feeling, appearance, sound, smell or taste, if applicable).	'Colicky pain.'	'Describe the pain.' Ensure the patient's definition of 'colicky' is the same as yours (sharp, cramping, specific pain).
Onset	When did it begin?	'Sudden onset.'	When did the 'sudden onset' occur? Specific time frame required.
Location	Where is it? Does it radiate? Does it occur anywhere else?	'Located in the left upper quadrant and radiating to her back.'	Is the pain constant or does it come and go? Does it vary in intensity? Have you eaten much in the last 5 days [to determine background behind lack of bowel movement]? What are your normal bowel habits?
Duration	How long does it last? Does it recur?	Has not moved bowels for 4 days.	
Severity	How bad is it? or How much does it bother you?		How would you rate the pain out of 10 (1 being no pain and 10 the worst pain imaginable)?
Pattern	What makes it better or worse?		Has the pain worsened since its onset or has the level of pain been consistent? Are there specific events that increase or reduce the pain?
Associated factors/How it Affects the patient	What other symptoms occur with it? How does it affect you?	Nausea.	Ask questions specific to nausea to see whether this appears to link to the colicky pain.

1) Identify abnormal findings and patient strengths

Subjective data

- Complains of sudden onset left upper quadrant colicky abdominal pain radiating to back
- Nausea
- Not used bowels for 4 days
- Reported history of hypertension, cholecystectomy, rheumatoid arthritis
- Prescribed medications: antihypertensives, opioids, aperients and NSAIDs

Objective data

- Alert and oriented
- Pale, distended abdomen with midline 8-cm scar
- Frequent high-pitched bowel sounds in all quadrants except left lower
- Faint low-pitched murmur present over epigastric region
- Abdomen mostly tympanic on percussion; mild dullness left lower quadrant
- Liver appears normal
- Pulsating mass palpable 5 cm superior to umbilicus
- 8-cm firm mass present in left lower quadrant

2) Identify cue clusters

- Sudden onset left upper quadrant colicky abdominal pain radiating to back
- Nausea
- No bowel motion for 4 days
- History of hypertension and rheumatoid arthritis
- Use of prescribed medications (possible liver dysfunction and consequent decreased drug metabolism related to age)

- Distended abdomen
- Absent bowel sounds left lower quadrant
- Low-pitched murmur over epigastric region
- Dullness over left lower quadrant
- Pulsating mass palpable 5 cm superior to umbilicus
- 8-cm firm mass present in left lower quadrant

3) Draw inferences

Patient may have a ruptured abdominal aortic aneurism (posterior rupture only as anterior would result in death; alternatively, the abdominal aorta may not yet have ruptured but may demonstrate acute dilation due to vessel weakness)

Patient is constipated

Patient has a paralytic ileus

4) List possible diagnoses

Abdominal aortic aneurism related to vessel weakness and ageing

Constipation related to increased abdominal pressure due to abdominal aortic aneurism

Paralytic ileus of unknown origin

5) Check for defining characteristics

Major: acute onset of pain, low-pitched murmur over epigastric region, pulsating midline mass, history of hypertension
Minor: constipation, nausea, distended abdomen

Major: decreased frequency, hard stool, abdominal distension, firm abdominal mass, absent bowel sounds (in many cases diminished not necessarily absent)
Minor: abdominal discomfort

Major: onset of acute colicky abdominal pain, absent bowel sounds
Minor: nausea

6) Confirm or rule out diagnoses

Confirm because meets both major and minor defining characteristics

Confirm because meets both major and minor defining characteristics

Rule out: while possible, unlikely due to presentation of pain (not sharp or severe enough to indicate ileus)

7) Document conclusions

Nursing diagnoses that are appropriate for this patient:

- Abdominal aortic aneurism related to weakening of vessel wall of the abdominal aorta (it is likely to have had either a posterior rupture or large and rapid dilation due to the acute onset of symptoms—most abdominal aortic aneurisms remain asymptomatic)
- Constipation related to increased abdominal pressure due to enlarged/ruptured abdominal aortic aneurism

References

Cancer Australia. (2019). Bowel cancer statistics. Viewed June 2019 at https://bowel-cancer.canceraustralia.gov.au/statistics.

Cohen, B. J. & Hull, K. L. (2015). *Memmler's structure and function of the human body* (11th ed.). Philadelphia: Lippincott Williams & Wilkins.

Farrell, M. (Ed). (2016). *Smeltzer & Bare's textbook of medical-surgical nursing* (4th Australian & New Zealand ed.). Sydney: Lippincott Williams & Wilkins.

Healthcare Quality and Safety Commission New Zealand. (2017). Bowel Cancer. Viewed June 2019 at https://www.hqsc.govt.nz/our-programmes/health-quality-evaluation/projects/atlas-of-healthcare-variation/bowel-cancer/.

National Cancer Control Indicators. (2019). Relative survival by stage at diagnosis (colorectal cancer). Available at https://ncci.canceraustralia.gov.au/outcomes/relative-survival-rate/relative-survival-stage-diagnosis-colorectal-cancer.

New Zealand Ministry of Health. (2018). Bowel cancer. Available at https://www.health.govt.nz/your-health/conditions-and-treatments/diseases-and-illnesses/bowel-cancer.

Purnell, J. Q. (2018). Definitions, classification, and epidemiology of obesity. In K. R. Feingold, B. Anawalt, A. Boyce, et al. (Eds). *Endotext*. South Dartmouth, MA: MDText.com, Inc. Available at https://www.ncbi.nlm.nih.gov/books/NBK279167/.

Rhoads, J. (2006). *Advanced health assessment and diagnostic reasoning*. Philadelphia: Lippincott Williams & Wilkins.

Selected readings

Felder, S., Margel, D., Murrell, Z., et al. (2014). Usefulness of bowel sound auscultation: A prospective evaluation. *Journal of Surgical Education, 71*(5), 768–773.

Jacob, L. (2017). Auscultation of bowel sounds in critical care: The role of the nurse. *British Journal of Nursing, 20*(17), 962–963.

Rabinowitz, S. S., Dean, E. & Roberts, K. E. (2017). Abdominal examination: Overview, preparation, technique. Medscape, Available at https://emedicine.medscape.com/article/1909183-overview.

Online resources

Australian Institute of Health and Welfare, Cancer in Australia 2019: www.aihw.gov.au/reports/cancer/cancer-in-australia-2019/related-material

Bowel Cancer New Zealand: bowelcancernz.org.nz

Cancer Council Australia: www.cancer.org.au/about-cancer/types-of-cancer/bowel-cancer

healthdirect: https://www.healthdirect.gov.au/obesity

New Zealand Ministry of Health, Bowel Cancer: www.health.govt.nz/your-health/conditions-and-treatments/diseases-and-illnesses/bowel-cancer

CHAPTER 25

Female genitalia

CASE STUDY

Melinda is a 22-year-old woman who has been admitted to a ward with suspected appendicitis. When asked about her medical history, she complains. 'I feel like I have the flu; no energy, a headache and fever.'

Structure and function

To perform an adequate assessment of the female genitalia, the nurse needs to have a thorough understanding of the structure and function of the female reproductive system. This will guide the physical examination and readily assist in identifying abnormalities. The female genitalia consist of external structures and internal structures.

EXTERNAL GENITALIA

The external genitalia include those structures that can be readily identified through inspection (Fig. 25-1). The area is sometimes referred to as the vulva or *pudendum* and extends from the mons pubis to the anal opening. The mons pubis is the fat pad located over the symphysis pubis. The normal adult mons pubis is covered with pubic hair in a triangular pattern. It functions to absorb force and to protect the symphysis pubis during coitus. The labia majora are two folds of skin that extend posteriorly and inferiorly from the mons pubis to the perineum. The skin folds are composed of adipose tissue, sebaceous glands and sweat glands. The outer surface of the labia majora is covered with pubic hair in the adult, whereas the inner surface is pink, smooth and moist.

Inside the labia majora are the thinner skin folds of the labia minora. These folds join anteriorly at the clitoris and form a *prepuce* or hood; posteriorly the two folds join to form the frenulum. Compared with the labia majora, the labia minora are hairless and usually darker pink. They contain numerous sebaceous glands that promote lubrication and maintain a moist environment in the vaginal area. The clitoris is located at the anterior end of the labia minora. It is a small, cylindrical mass of erectile tissue and nerves with three parts: the glans, the corpus and the crura. The glans is the visible rounded portion of the clitoris. The corpus is the body, and the crura are two bands of fibrous tissue that attach the clitoris to the pelvic bone. The clitoris is similar to the male penis and contains many blood vessels that become engorged during sexual arousal.

The skin folds of the labia majora and labia minora form a boat-shaped area or fossa called the vestibule. The vestibule contains several openings. Located between the clitoris and the vaginal orifice is the urethral meatus. The openings of Skene glands are located on either side of the urethral opening. They are usually not visible. These small glands are often referred to as the *lesser vestibular glands.* Skene glands secrete mucus that lubricates and maintains a moist vaginal environment.

Below the urethral meatus is the vaginal orifice. This is the external opening of the vagina and has either a slitlike or irregular circular structure, depending on the configuration of a hymen. The hymen is a fold of membranous tissue that covers part of the vagina. On either side of, and slightly posterior to, the vaginal orifice (between the vaginal orifice and the labia minora) are the openings to Bartholin glands. Through the openings, the glands secrete mucus, which lubricates the area during sexual intercourse. These small glands are often referred to as the *greater vestibular glands.* The glands and the openings are not visible to the naked eye.

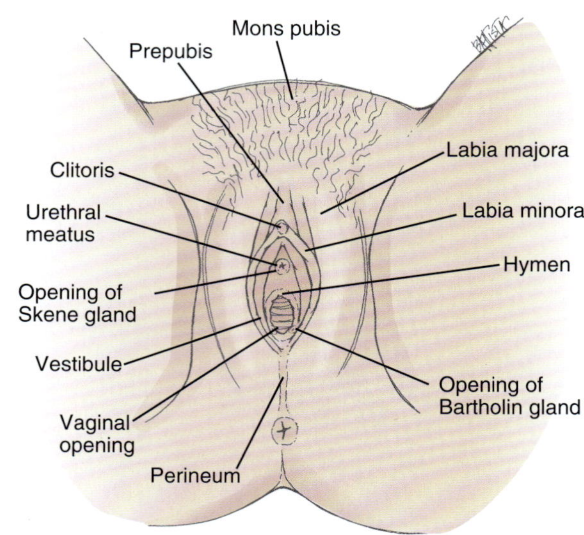

FIGURE 25-1 External genitalia.

INTERNAL GENITALIA

The internal genital structures function as the female reproductive organs (Fig. 25-2). They include the vagina, the uterus, the cervix, the fallopian tubes and the ovaries. The vagina, a muscular, tubular organ, extends up and slightly back towards the rectum from the vaginal orifice (external opening) to the cervix. It lies between the rectum posteriorly and the urethra and bladder anteriorly and is approximately 10 cm long. The vagina performs many functions. It allows the passage of menstrual flow, it receives the penis during sexual intercourse and it serves as the lower portion of the birth canal during delivery.

The vaginal wall comprises four layers. The outer layer is composed of pink squamous epithelium and connective tissue. It is under the direct influence of the hormone oestrogen and contains many mucus-producing cells. This outer layer of epithelium lies in transverse folds called rugae. These transverse folds allow the vagina to expand during intercourse; they also facilitate vaginal delivery of a fetus. The second layer is the submucosal layer. It contains blood vessels, nerves and lymphatic channels. The third layer is composed of smooth muscle, and the fourth layer consists of connective tissue and the vascular network. The normal vaginal environment is acidic (pH of 3.8 to 4.2). This environment is maintained because the vaginal flora is composed of Doderlein bacilli, and the bacilli act on glycogen to produce lactic acid. This acidic environment helps to prevent vaginal infection.

In the upper end of the vagina, the cervix dips down and forms a circular recess that gives rise to areas known as the anterior and posterior fornices. The cervix (or neck of the uterus) separates the upper end of the vagina from the isthmus of the uterus. The junction of the isthmus and the cervix forms the internal os, and the junction of the cervix and the vagina forms the external os or ectocervix. The 'os' refers to the opening in the centre of the cervix.

CLINICAL TIP

A woman who is nulliparous (i.e. a woman who has never been pregnant) has a small, round opening or os that appears as a depression on examination. A woman who has had her cervix dilated during childbirth has an external os that is slightly enlarged and irregular in shape.

The cervix is composed of smooth muscle, muscle fibres and connective tissue. Two types of epithelium cover the external os or ectocervix: pink squamous epithelium (which lines the vaginal walls) and red, rough-looking columnar epithelium (which lines the endocervical canal). The columnar epithelium may be visible around the os. The point where the two types of epithelium meet is called the *squamocolumnar junction*. The squamocolumnar junction migrates towards the cervical os with maturation or with increased oestrogen levels. This migration creates an area known as the transformation zone. The transformation zone is important for two reasons: (1) 90% of the neoplasms of the lower genital track originate in this area (i.e. squamous cell carinoma), so (2) this is the area from which cells are obtained for the cervical screening test to detect human papillomavirus, the virus that can lead to cellular changes of the cervix. The cervix functions to allow the entrance of sperm into the uterus and to allow the passage of menstrual flow. It also secretes mucus and prevents the entrance of vaginal bacteria. During childbirth, the cervix can stretch to allow the passage of the fetus.

The uterus is a pear-shaped muscular organ that has two components: the *corpus*, or body, and the *cervix*, or neck (discussed previously). The corpus of the uterus is divided into the fundus (upper portion), the body (central portion) and the isthmus (narrow lower portion). The uterus is usually situated in a forward position above the bladder at approximately a 45-degree angle to the vagina when a woman is standing (anteverted and anteflexed position). The normal-sized uterus

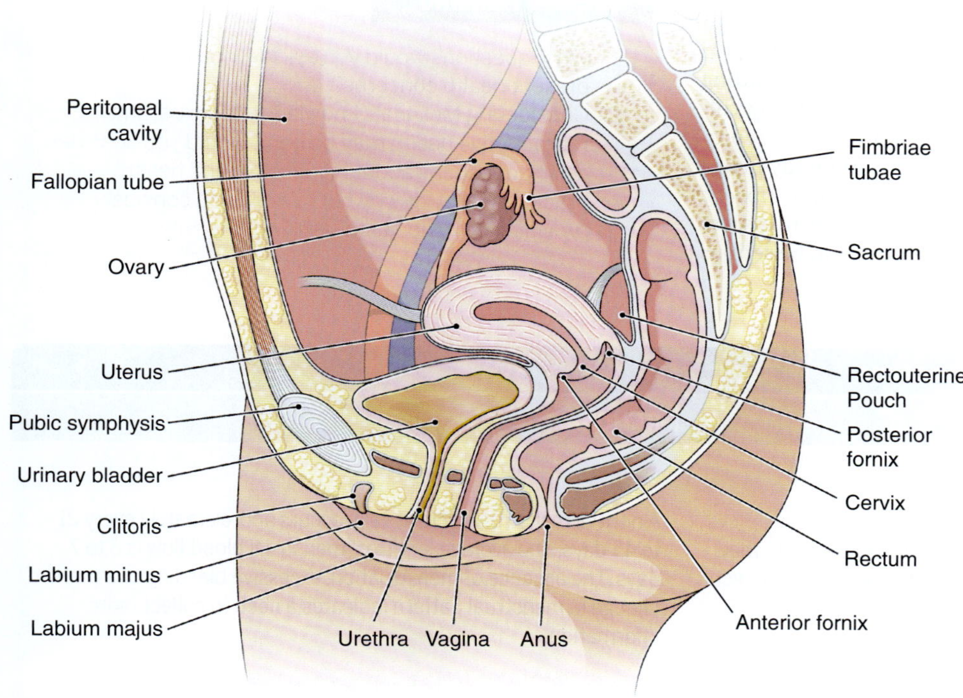

FIGURE 25-2 Female reproductive system (sagittal section). This view shows the relationship of the reproductive organs to each other and to other structures in the pelvic cavity. (Cohen, B. J. & Hull, K. L. (2015). *Memmler's structure and function of the human body* [11th ed.]. Philadelphia: Lippincott Williams & Wilkins.)

is approximately 7.5 cm long, 5 cm wide and 2.5 cm thick. The uterus is movable.

The endometrium, the myometrium and the *peritoneum* are the three layers of the uterine wall. The endometrium is the inner mucosal layer. The endometrium is composed of epithelium, connective tissue and a vascular network; the thickness of this tissue is influenced by oestrogen and progesterone. Uterine glands contained within the endometrium secrete an alkaline substance that keeps the uterine cavity moist. A portion of the endometrium sheds during menses and childbirth. The myometrium is the middle layer of the uterus. It is composed of three layers of smooth muscle fibres that surround blood vessels. This layer functions to expel the products of conception.

The peritoneum is the outer uterine layer that covers the uterus and separates it from the abdominal cavity. The peritoneum forms anterior and posterior pouches around the uterus. The posterior pouch is called the rectouterine pouch or the pouch of Douglas.

The ovaries are a pair of small, oval-shaped organs. Each is approximately 3 cm long, 2 cm wide and 1 cm deep; each is situated on a lateral aspect of the pelvic cavity. The ovaries are connected to the uterus by the ovarian ligament. The ovary functions to develop and release ova and to produce hormones such as oestrogen, progesterone and testosterone. The ovum travels from the ovary to the uterus through the fallopian tubes. These 8- to 12-cm long tubes begin near the ovaries and enter the uterus just beneath the fundus. The end of the tube near the ovary has fringelike extensions called fimbriae tubae. The ovaries, fallopian tubes and supporting ovarian ligaments are referred to as the adnexa (Latin for 'appendages').

Health assessment

COLLECTING SUBJECTIVE DATA: THE NURSING HEALTH HISTORY

When interview topics turn to sexual and reproductive health (i.e. the reproductive system and female genitalia), keep in mind the sensitivities of the patient and nurse regarding body image, fear of cancer, sexuality and the like. Many cultures tend to emphasise the importance of a woman's reproductive ability, thereby entwining self-esteem and body image with gender roles. Cultural and social norms, stigma, anxiety, embarrassment or fear may affect the patient's ability to discuss problems and ask questions. As some problems can be serious or even life-threatening, it is important to establish a trusting relationship with the patient because the information gathered during the subjective examination may suggest a problem or point to the possibility of a problem developing. Cancer of the cervix, for example, is associated with both morbidity and mortality but related risk factors are highly modifiable and cure rates are high in disease that is detected early.

When taking health histories, it is important to address the patient's potential concerns around privacy and confidentiality particularly as gathering information about sexuality and reproductive health can cause discomfort or embarrassment The nurse may choose to discuss any concerns the patient has regarding the consultation before attempting to gather data.

CULTURAL CONSIDERATIONS

Patients from some cultures (e.g. Islam) may accept subjective or physical assessment only by a female nurse, especially when genital and sexual issues are being addressed.

CASE STUDY

Melinda reports a recent outbreak of genital lesions after a sexual encounter 10 days ago (her 'first and only') with a new partner. She denies the use of any protection or birth control, stating, 'He refused to use anything and I didn't insist.' She denies any problems with her menstrual cycle, no previous sexual activity and no vaginal infections. 'I have always been healthy; I don't know why I behaved so stupidly and put my health at risk.'

CRITICAL THINKING

1. What questions would you ask Melinda about her present health concerns?
2. Considering Melinda's knowledge of sexual and reproductive health may be poor, would you consider asking questions about her lifestyle and health practices? Why or why not? Would you consider providing any education? Why or why not?

History of present health concerns

QUESTION	RATIONALE
Menstrual cycle	
What was the date of your last menstrual period? Do your menstrual cycles occur on a regular schedule? How long do they last? Describe the typical amount of blood flow you have with your periods. Any clotting?	A normal menstrual cycle usually occurs approximately every 21 to 45 days. The average length of menstrual blood flow is 3 to 7 days. The absence of menstruation, excessive bleeding or a marked change in menstrual pattern indicates a need to collect more information.

History of present health concerns (continued)

QUESTION	RATIONALE
What other symptoms do you experience before or during your period (cramps, bloating, moodiness, breast tenderness)?	Headache, weight gain, mood swings, abdominal cramping and bloating are common complaints before or during the menstrual period. Some women experience premenstrual syndrome, in which the symptoms become severe enough to impair the women's ability to function.
How old were you when you started your period?	In Australia the average age of menarche (i.e. the first menstruation, or period) is between 12 and 13 years. Menarche usually occurs a year or two following the appearance of other puberty-related changes such as breast development and pubic and underarm hair growth. Menarche is also related to size and weight. Girls with higher body mass index (BMI), who gain weight over time, or who are overweight during childhood are likely to have earlier menarche (Juul et al., 2017). *Note:* Menarche (beginning of menstruation) tends to begin earlier in women living in high-income countries and later in women who live in low- and middle- income countries (Sommer, 2013). Age at menarche ranges from 10 to 16 years, with earlier onset being associated with excess weight and shorter stature (Karapanou & Papadimitriou, 2010).
Have you stopped menstruating or have your periods become irregular? Do you have any spotting between periods? What symptoms have you experienced?	Irregularities or amenorrhoea may be due to pregnancy, lactation, depression, low body weight, excessive exercise, ovarian tumours, ovarian cysts, autoimmune disease, some medications or hormonal imbalances. Cessation of menstruation is termed *menopause;* see next rationale.
Menopause	
Are you still having periods? Have your periods changed?	Menopause is a normal physiological process that occurs naturally in most women between the ages of 45 and 60 years, with an average age of 51 (Royal Australian and New Zealand College of Obstetricians and Gynaecologists [RANZCOG], 2016). Menopause occurring before age 40 affects around 1% of women and is termed *premature menopause* (AMS, 2015); menopause between ages 40 and 45 is considered *early menopause* (Australasian Menopause Society [AMS], 2015); menopause occurring in women older than age 55 years is termed *delayed menopause.* Premature and delayed menopause may be due to genetic predisposition, an endocrine disorder or gynaecological dysfunction. Induced or surgical menopause occurs in women who have ovarian insufficiency or who have had their ovaries removed surgically. During the perimenopausal period, hormone levels may fluctuate, resulting in menstrual irregularities. Periods may be heavier or may become scant.
Are you experiencing any symptoms of menopause?	Vasomotor symptoms, or hot flushes and night sweats, are classical symptoms of menopause. Around half of menopausal women experience hot flushes and night sweats (Gartoulla et al., 2015). Sleep disturbance, mood changes, decreased appetite, vaginal dryness, spotting and irregular vaginal bleeding may also occur.
Are you on a hormone replacement therapy (HRT) regimen? If so, what type and dosage? Are you satisfied with HRT?	It is important to discuss and explain risks versus benefits of HRT.
Are you continuing to have any symptoms of menopause while taking HRT?	If vasomotor symptoms continue, the patient may need information to help reduce symptoms, HRT, or their HRT dosage adjusted.

Continued on following page

History of present health concerns (continued)

QUESTION	RATIONALE
What are your concerns about going through menopause?	Menopause is a normal stage in a woman's life. Some women have mixed feelings about experiencing menopause. Some may grieve their loss of childbearing capabilities, whereas others may welcome this new phase of life, as they feel relieved no longer having to be concerned about pregnancy.
Vaginal discharge, pain, masses	
Are you experiencing vaginal discharge that is unusual in terms of colour, amount or odour?	Vaginal discharge changes in colour and thickness throughout a woman's menstrual cycle though deviations in the amount, colour, smell or texture of the discharge may also represent an infection.
Do you experience pain or itching in your genital or groin area?	Complaints of pain in the area of the vulva, vagina, uterus, cervix or ovaries may indicate infection. Itching, irritation or burning may indicate infection or infestation. **OLDER ADULT CONSIDERATIONS** **The older patient is more susceptible to vaginal infection because of atrophy of the vaginal mucosa associated with ageing.**
Do you have any lumps, swelling or masses in your genital area?	These findings may indicate a blocked gland, infection, lymphoedema or cancer. Accompanying symptoms and past occurrences should be monitored for recurrence.
Urination	
Do you have any difficulty urinating? Do you have any burning or pain with urination? Has your urine changed colour or developed an odour? Have you noticed any blood in your urine?	Urinary frequency, burning or pain (dysuria) are signs of infection (urinary tract or sexually transmitted infection), whereas hesitancy or straining could indicate blockage. Change in colour and development of an abnormal odour could indicate infection.
Do you have difficulty controlling your urine?	Difficulty controlling urine (incontinence) may indicate urgency or stress incontinence. During sneezing or coughing, increased abdominal pressure causes spontaneous urination. **OLDER ADULT CONSIDERATIONS** **Urinary incontinence may develop in older women from muscle weakness or loss of urethral elasticity.**
Sexual dysfunction	
Do you have any problems with your sexual performance?	A broad opening question about sex allows the patient to focus the interview to areas where she has concerns. Some women have difficulty achieving orgasm and may believe there is something wrong with them.
Have you recently had a change in your sexual activity pattern or libido?	A change in sexual activity or libido needs to be investigated for the cause. A woman who is dissatisfied with her sexual performance may experience a decreased libido. **OLDER ADULT CONSIDERATIONS** **As women age, their oestrogen production decreases, causing atrophy of the vaginal mucosa. These women may need to use lubrication to increase comfort during intercourse. Women experiencing surgical menopause, symptoms of which occur more abruptly, may also benefit from lubrication.**
Do you experience (or have you experienced) problems with fertility?	Infertility is defined as unprotected sex for 1 year without pregnancy. Infertility effects around 15% of Australian couples, and of these, approximately 40% are related to female fertility factors (IVF Australia, 2011).

COLDSPA

Example

Use the COLDSPA mnemonic as a guideline to collect needed information for each symptom the patient shares. In addition, the following questions help elicit important information.

Mnemonic	Question	Patient response example
Character	Describe the sign or symptom (feeling, appearance, sound, smell or taste, if applicable).	'It burns when I urinate.'
Onset	When did it begin?	'Last night at about 11 p.m.'
Location	Where is it? Does it radiate? Does it occur anywhere else?	'The pain is right where my urine comes out. Sometimes it cramps right above my pubic area.'
Duration	How long does it last? Does it recur?	'It has not gone away since it started but it hurts even more when I go to the bathroom.'
Severity	How bad is it? or How much does it bother you?	'I can't do anything it hurts so bad.'
Pattern	What makes it better or worse?	'I went to the pharmacy last night and bought Ural and it gave me some relief.'
Associated factors/How it Affects the patient	What other symptoms occur with it? How does it affect you?	'There is blood in my urine now. I stayed home from work today because I feel terrible.'

Past health history

QUESTION	RATIONALE
Describe any prior gynaecological problems you have had and the results of any treatment.	Some problems, such as cancer, may recur. Prior problems directly affect the physical assessment.
When was your last pelvic examination by a health care provider? Was a cervical screening test performed? What was the result?	Pelvic and rectal examinations are used to detect masses, ovarian tenderness or organ enlargement. The cervical screening test screens for the human papillomavirus (HPV) infection, which is associated with the development of cervical cancer (see Promote health—Cervical cancer). The Australian Government recommends all women from age 25 who have had sex have a cervical screening test every 5 years, even if they are no longer having sex. Because the most common type of cervical cancer usually takes 10 or more years to develop, there is little advantage in having a cervical screening tests more frequently than is recommended (Australian Institute of Health and Welfare [AIHW], 2018a). General practitioners may recommend repeating the test in 12 months' time if HPV is detected , or if the woman experiences problems such as bleeding or pain after sex (AIHW, 2018a; see Display 25-1).
Have you ever been diagnosed with a sexually transmitted infection (STI)? If so, what? How was it treated?	STIs can increase the patient's risk of pelvic infections, which lead to scarring and adhesions on the fallopian tubes. Scarred fallopian tubes increase the risk of infertility and ectopic pregnancy.
Have you ever been pregnant? How many times? How many children do you have? Is there any chance that you might be pregnant now? Any miscarriages or abortions?	The female patient's ability to become pregnant and carry a fetus to term is important baseline information. It is important to know if the patient is pregnant in case medications or X-ray tests need to be prescribed.
Have you ever been diagnosed with diabetes?	Diabetes predisposes women to vaginal fungal infections.

PROMOTE HEALTH — CERVICAL CANCER

OVERVIEW

Despite advances in cervical cancer prevention and screening, cervical cancer continues to be a major health issue globally. In 2018, there were an estimated 570,000 cases of cervical cancer and 311,000 deaths from the disease worldwide, making cervical cancer the fourth most common cancer in women (after breast, colorectal and lung cancers) (Bray et al., 2018). However, cervical cancer rates vary dramatically across geographic regions. The highest incidence rates are reported in Eastern, Western and Southern Africa, Melanesia, Middle Africa, Southeast Asia and Eastern Europe, whereas the lowest rates are seen in Western Asia, Australia and New Zealand, North America and Western Europe (Bray et al., 2018).

In 2018, 930 Australian women were diagnosed with cervical cancer and 258 Australian women died from the disease (AIHW, 2018a). There are some variations in cervical cancer incidence and mortality by geographic region, with women living in rural and remote areas experiencing a greater mortality risk (AIHW, 2018b). Part of the variation can be attributed to the high cervical cancer rates among Aboriginal and Torres Strait Islander women. Between 2005 and 2009, Aboriginal and Torres Strait Islander women were twice as likely to develop cervical cancer and four times more likely to die from cervical cancer, when compared with non-Aboriginal and Torres Strait Islander women (AIHW, 2018c).

In New Zealand, an estimated 160 women will develop cervical cancer annually and 50 women die from the disease (New Zealand Ministry of Health, 2014). Again, some women are at greater risk than others of developing cervical cancer. For example, in New Zealand, women over age 40 who identify as Māori or Pasifika have higher rates of cervical cancer, and this is attributed to lower screening rates (National Screening Unit, 2012).

Cervical cancer is a slowly progressing condition beginning in the lining of the cervix wherein gradual changes lead to a precancerous state and then possibly to cancer. The cancer may be squamous cell carcinoma (80%) or adenocarcinoma (25%) or a few rarer types (Cancer Council Australia, 2018). Because early cervical cancers can usually be found by a cervical screening test and if detected early is often curable, routine screening is recommended. The new cervical screening test replaced the traditional Papanicolaou smear (Pap test). This more accurate and effective test is estimated to lower cervical cancer incidence and mortality by at least 20% (Lew et al., 2017).

According to the American Cancer Society (2019), most cervical cancers can be prevented. First, to prevent oncogenic human papillomavirus (HPV) infection, women should complete scheduled HPV vaccinations. Second, to prevent precancerous abnormalities, women can avoid risk factors (see Risk factors and Teach risk reduction tips). Third, to prevent invasive cancers, women should have a cervical screening test to detect HPV infection and precancerous abnormalities and thereby treat disease in the earliest stage possible.

RISK FACTORS

- HPV infection, the most important risk factor
- Failure to have regular cervical screening tests
- Cigarette smoking
- History of sexually transmitted infections
- Increasing age
- Daughter of a mother who took the drug diethylstilbestrol in early pregnancy to prevent miscarriage
- Immunosuppression

TEACH RISK REDUCTION TIPS

- Avoid exposure to HPV (of particular note, barrier contraceptives do not guarantee protection against HPV infection).
- Follow the National Cervical Screening Program guidelines for cervical screening and any recommended follow-up treatment (AIHW, 2019).
- Do not smoke cigarettes.
- Talk with health care provider about HPV vaccine.

DISPLAY 25-1 GUIDELINES FOR THE PREVENTION AND EARLY DETECTION OF CERVICAL CANCER

Cervical cancer is often associated with human papillomavirus (HPV) infection and as such is one of the most easily preventable and curable types of cancer (AIHW, 2019). Indeed, a significant proportion of cervical cancer can be prevented through vaccination against HPV. In 2006, the HPV vaccine was added to the Australian National Immunisation Program Schedule and is now provided to 12- to 13-year-old girls and boys in the first year of secondary school (AIHW, 2019). Women outside this age range may also benefit from vaccination if they haven't already been infected and there is a probability of future infection (Australian Government, Department of Health, 2017).

Screening is an effective way of detecting HPV and cervical abnormalities in the precancerous stages. All women who have ever had sexual intercourse (including those who no longer have sex or who have only ever had sex with another woman) and who are age 25 years and older should undergo cervical screening. The renewed National Cervical Screening Program guidelines, introduced in December 2017, includes the introduction of the cervical screening test, increasing the age at which screening starts from 18 years to 25 years (or 2 years after their last Pap test), offering screening to women from age 70 to 74 years and changing the frequency of tests from 2 to 5 years.

Another change to the National Cervical Screening Program guidelines is the introduction of self-collection of a vaginal sample for HPV testing. This screening is available for asymptomatic women aged 30 years or older who have declined to have a cervical sample collected by a clinician and are either (1) overdue for cervical screening by 2 years or longer (i.e. 4 years or more since their last Pap test, or 7 years or more since their last cervical screening test) or (2) have never screened.

Family history

QUESTION	RATIONALE
Is there a history of reproductive or genital cancer in your family? What type? How is the family member related to you?	Some cancers tend to occur in families. In such patients, the examination can focus on areas in which risk may be present.
Do you smoke?	Smoking and taking oral contraceptives increase the risk of cardiovascular problems. In addition, the risk of cervical cancer increases in patients who have human papillomavirus and who smoke.

Family history (continued)

QUESTION	RATIONALE
How many sexual partners do you have?	A patient who has multiple sexual partners increases her risk of contracting STIs. Refer to Promote health—Sexually transmitted infections (STIs) in Chapter 26 for information which you might consider providing a patient who is at risk of contracting an STI.
Do you use contraceptives? What kind? How often?	Minor side effects (e.g. weight gain, breast tenderness, headaches, nausea) might develop from oral contraceptives, but they usually subside after the third cycle. Major side effects, though rare, include thromboembolic disorders, cerebrovascular accident and myocardial infarction. Failure to use a barrier-type of contraceptive (male or female condom) may increase the risk of STIs including human immunodeficiency virus (HIV) infection. Failure to use any type of contraceptive increases the risk of becoming pregnant.
Have genital problems affected the way in which you normally function?	Diseases or disorders of the genitalia may cause pain, discomfort and bleeding that affect a patient's ability to work, to perform normal household duties or to care for family. In addition, normal sexual activity may be affected because of pain, embarrassment or decreased libido. Oral contraceptives increase the glycogen content of vaginal secretions, which increases the risk of vaginal fungal infections.
What is your sexual orientation?	An awareness of the patient's sexual orientation allows the examiner to focus the examination. If the patient identifies as lesbian or bisexual, she may have some specific health concerns related to her sexual behaviour. Women who have sex with women may engage in a range of sexual activities from vaginal fingering and cunnilingus, to use of vibrators and dildos and safer sex information to be tailored to meet the needs of the individual patient (Schick et al., 2012).
Do you feel comfortable communicating with your partner about your sexual likes and dislikes?	Sexual relationships are enhanced through open communication. Lack of open communication can cause problems with relationships or lead to feelings of guilt and depression.
Do you have any fears related to sex? Can you identify any stress in your current relationship that relates to sex?	Fear can inhibit performance and decrease sexual satisfaction. Stress can prevent satisfactory sex role performance.
Do you have concerns about fertility? If you have trouble with fertility, how has this affected your relationship with your partner or family?	Women often feel responsible for infertility and need to discuss their feelings. Concerns about fertility can increase stress. Problems with fertility can have a negative impact on relationships with the partner and can cause tension within a family, especially when other women in the family have children.
Do you perform monthly genital self-examinations?	Each female patient should be aware of the need for monthly genital self-examination and its importance in early diagnosis and treatment of problems.
How do you feel about going through menopause?	Menopause is a normal development of ageing. However, in some women the process induces fear, anxiety or even grief. The nurse can assist the patient to resolve some of these feelings.
Do you take oestrogen replacement therapy?	Oestrogen sometimes alleviates the symptoms of menopause. However, oestrogen has been linked to some types of cancer (i.e. breast, endometrial) and, in increasing the glycogen content in vaginal secretions, predisposes patients to yeast infections.
Have you ever been tested for HIV? What was the result? Why were you tested?	HIV increases the patient's risk of any other infection. A high-risk exposure may require serial testing.

Continued on following page

Family history (continued)

QUESTION	RATIONALE
What do you know about toxic shock syndrome?	Toxic shock syndrome is a life-threatening infection that can be prevented by frequently changing tampons.
What do you know about STIs and their prevention?	The patient's knowledge of STIs and prevention provides a basis for health education in this area.
Do you wear cotton underwear and avoid tight jeans?	Cotton allows air to circulate. Nylon and tight-fitting jeans create a moist environment, which promotes fungal infections.
After a bowel movement or urination, do you wipe from front to back?	The vaginal and urethral openings are close to the anus and are easily contaminated by *Escherichia coli* and other bacteria if care is not taken to wipe from front to back.
Do you douche frequently?	Frequent douching changes the natural flora of the vagina, predisposing the vagina to yeast infections.

COLLECTING OBJECTIVE DATA: PHYSICAL EXAMINATION

It should be recognised that collecting objective data specific to female genitalia requires advanced knowledge or specialist practice skills. The scope of a beginning practitioner will be limited primarily to observation and external palpation. However, the following section outlines both beginning practitioner skills and some advanced practice skills. A working knowledge of some of the more common female genitalia assessments will assist beginning practitioners in determining the scope of the subjective history they should be recording as well as recommendations that may be required following the completion of both their subjective and objective assessments.

The physical examination of the female genitalia may create patient anxiety. The patient may be very embarrassed about exposing her genitalia and nervous that an infection or disorder will be discovered. Nurses need to ensure they explain in detail what they will be doing throughout the examination and explain the significance of each portion of the examination. Encourage the patient to ask questions. Begin by sitting or standing at the end of the examination table and draping the patient so only the vulva is exposed. This helps to preserve the patient's modesty. The nurse should shine the light source so it illuminates the genital area, allowing the nurse to see all structures clearly.

Preparing the patient

When the patient arrives for the examination, ask her to urinate before the examination so she does not experience bladder discomfort. If a urine sample (either first catch or mid-stream, depending on the clinical history) is indicated, provide a container. If the patient is menstruating and has a tampon in place, ask her to leave the tampon in to collect the urine specimen but remove it prior to returning to the examination room. When the patient is back in the examining room, ask her to remove her underwear, get onto the examination table and use the sheet provided to cover herself. The nurse should maintain privacy by leaving the room while the patient changes or ensuring the curtains are closed.

After the patient has changed, the nurse should position the patient in a supine position. The patient should move their feet up towards their pelvis and abduct both legs. This will allow the nurse to visualise the perineum easily (stirrups are rarely used). Ask the patient not to put her hands over her head because this tightens the abdominal muscles. She should relax her arms at her sides. If possible, elevate the patient's head and shoulders. This allows the nurse to maintain eye contact with the patient during the examination and enables the patient to see what the nurse is doing.

Equipment

Some pieces of equipment used in examinations are:

- Light
- Water-soluble lubricant
- Cotton-tipped applicators
- Swabs and cervical sampler for specimen collection
- ThinPrep® or other liquid-based cytology collection solution
- Disposable gloves
- pH paper
- Sanitary pads.

CASE STUDY

Melinda's lesions present as vesicles and ulcerations on the external genitalia, labia and mons, with a few vesicles extending into the perianal area. The rest of the perineal and pelvic examination is negative. Some enlarged, tender lymph nodes are noted in the inguinal areas bilaterally. Melinda's temperature by oral route is 38.1 °C. When questioned, she confirms that she has a great deal of pain in the vaginal area and 'urinating hurts a lot'.

CRITICAL THINKING

3. What additional questions would you ask Melinda following your physical examination?
4. What do you think might be wrong with Melinda? (See note below.)

Note on critical thinking question 4

Critical thinking question 4 is complex. Being able to state 'It is likely that Melinda has genital herpes' is only part of the answer. Health assessment is not about always having the right answer (or having an answer at all); it is about gathering accurate information and drawing as many inferences from that information as you can (this will depend on both your knowledge and experience).

As such, firstly, the important information is that Melinda appears to have an infection that has resulted from genital lesions. Using a problem-solving approach, you can determine this because she is febrile and, importantly, her lymph nodes are inflamed in the inguinal areas, suggesting the infection to be at this site. Secondly, the lesions are troubling Melinda because when she urinates, it is painful. This would suggest the urine is running over the lesions and causing them to sting. It would be important then to examine for signs of dehydration because Melinda may be drinking less to urinate less frequently. Thirdly, the lesions are limited to her perineum and this would suggest (given her history of recent unprotected intercourse) that it is likely Melinda has acquired a sexually transmitted infection.

Physical assessment

During the examination of the patient, remember these key points:

- Respect the patient's privacy.
- Observe standard precautions.
- Tell your patient what you are about to do and what she should expect to feel.
- Be sure equipment is between room and body temperature.
- Inspect and palpate female external and internal structures correctly.
- Use examination and laboratory equipment properly.
- Recognise the difference between common variations and abnormal findings.

PHYSICAL ASSESSMENT

ASSESSMENT PROCEDURE	NORMAL FINDINGS	ABNORMAL FINDINGS
External genitalia		
INSPECTION		
Inspect the mons pubis. Wash your hands and put on gloves. As you begin the examination, note the distribution of pubic hair. Also, be alert for signs of infestation.	Pubic hair is distributed in an inverted triangular pattern and there are no signs of infestation.  **OLDER ADULT CONSIDERATIONS** **Older patients may have grey, thinning pubic hair.** Some patients shave or pluck the pubic hair. Piercings of the mons pubis are for aesthetics and do not enhance sexual pleasure.	Absence of pubic hair in the adult patient is abnormal. Lice or nits (eggs) at the base of the pubic hairs indicate infestation with pediculosis pubis. This condition, commonly referred to as 'crabs', is most often transmitted by sexual contact.
Observe and palpate the inguinal lymph nodes.	There should be no enlargement or swelling of the lymph nodes.	Enlarged inguinal nodes may indicate a vaginal infection or may be the result of irritation from shaving pubic hairs.
Inspect the labia majora and perineum. Observe the labia majora and perineum for lesions, swelling and excoriation (Fig. 25-3). Keep in mind the woman's childbearing status during inspection. For example, the labia of a woman who has not delivered offspring vaginally will meet in the middle. The labia of a woman who has delivered vaginally will not meet in the middle and may appear shrivelled.	The labia majora are equal in size and free of lesions, swelling and excoriation. A healed tear or episiotomy scar may be visible on the perineum if the patient has given birth. The perineum should be smooth. **CULTURAL CONSIDERATIONS** **In pubertal rites in some cultures, the clitoris is surgically removed, and the labia are sutured, leaving only a small opening for menstrual flow. Once married, the woman undergoes surgery to reopen the labia.** It is increasingly common to find piercings of the labia majora and minora. Depending on placement, these may enhance sexual pleasure.	Lesions may be from an infectious disease such as herpes or syphilis (see Abnormal findings 25-1). Excoriation and swelling may be from scratching or self-treatment of the lesions. All lesions must be evaluated, and the patient referred for treatment. 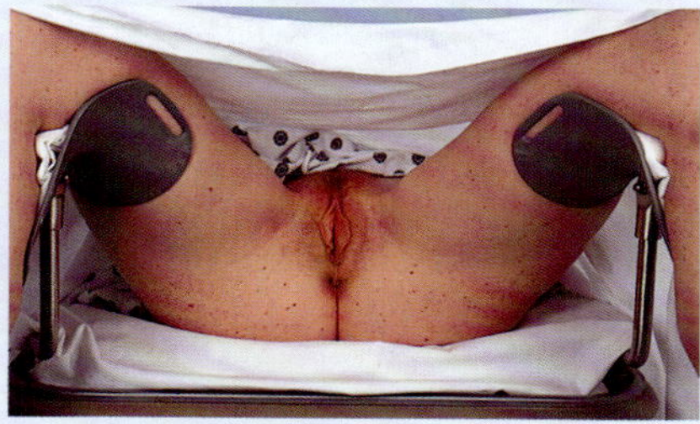 **FIGURE 25-3** Inspecting the pubic hair, labia majora and perineum. (*Note:* stirrups are not always used for clinical examinations.) (© B. Proud.)

Continued on following page

PHYSICAL ASSESSMENT (continued)

ASSESSMENT PROCEDURE	NORMAL FINDINGS	ABNORMAL FINDINGS
Inspect the labia minora, clitoris, urethral meatus and vaginal opening. Use your gloved hand to separate the labia majora and inspect for lesions, excoriation, swelling or discharge (Fig. 25-4). 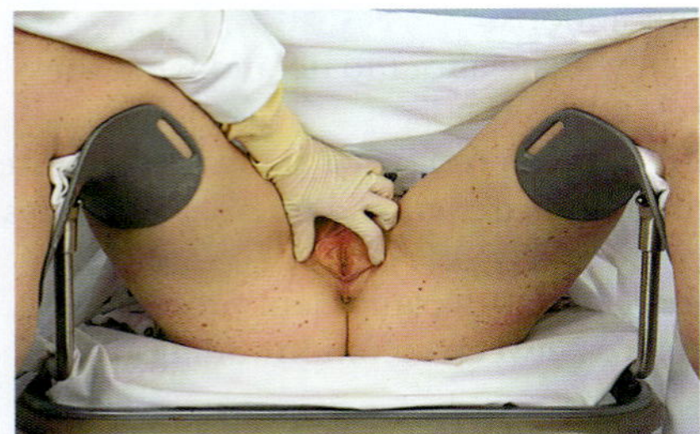 **FIGURE 25-4** Inspecting the labia minora, clitoris, urethral orifice and vaginal opening. (© B. Proud.)	The labia minora appear symmetrical, dark-pink and moist. The clitoris is a small mound of erectile tissue, sensitive to touch. The normal size of the clitoris varies. The urethral meatus is small and slit like. The vaginal opening is positioned below the urethral meatus. Its size depends on sexual activity or vaginal delivery; it may be covered partially or completely by a hymen.	Asymmetrical labia may indicate abscess. Lesions, swelling, bulging in the vaginal opening and discharge are abnormal findings (see Abnormal findings 25-1). Excoriation may result from the patient scratching or self-treating a perineal irritation.
PALPATION		
Palpate Bartholin glands. If the patient has labial swelling or a history of it, palpate the Bartholin glands for swelling, tenderness and discharge (Fig. 25-5). Place your index finger in the vaginal opening and your thumb on the labia majora. With a gentle pinching motion, palpate from the inferior portion of the posterior labia majora to the anterior portion. Repeat on the opposite side. **Palpate the urethra.** If the patient reports urethral symptoms or urethritis, or if you suspect inflammation of Skene glands, insert your gloved index finger into the superior portion of the vagina and milk the urethra from the inside, pushing up and out (Fig. 25-7).	Bartholin glands are usually soft, non-tender, and drainage free. No drainage should be noted from the urethral meatus. The area is normally soft and non-tender.	Swelling, pain and discharge may result from infection and abscess (Fig. 25-6). If you detect a discharge, obtain a specimen to send to the laboratory for culture. Drainage from the urethra indicates possible urethritis. Any discharge should be cultured. Urethritis may occur with infection with *Neisseria gonorrhoeae* or *Chlamydia trachomatis*.
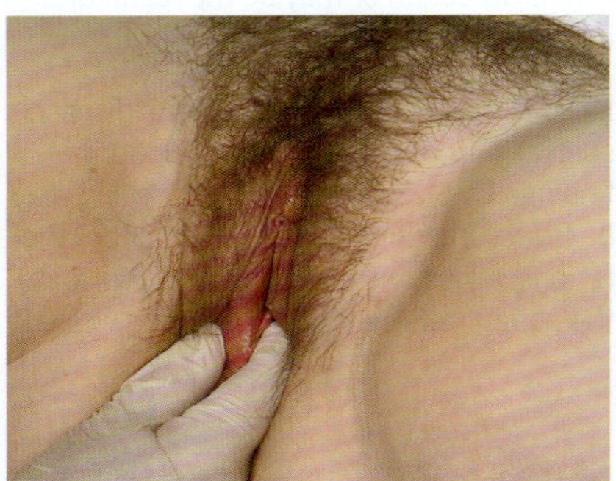 **FIGURE 25-5** Technique for palpating Bartholin glands. (Rhoads, J. [2006]. *Advanced health assessment and diagnostic reasoning*. Philadelphia: Lippincott Williams & Wilkins.)	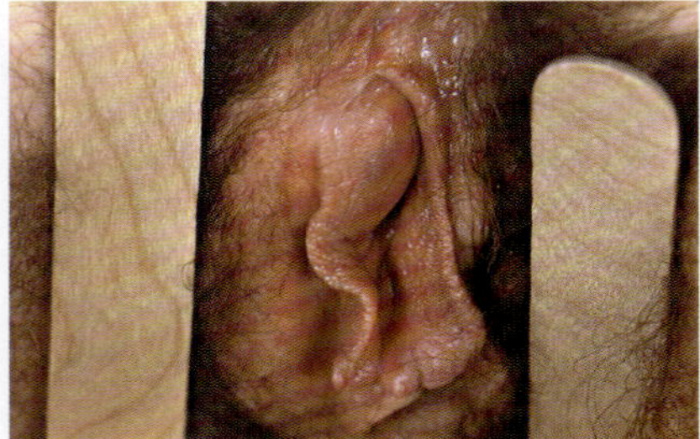 **FIGURE 25-6** Abscess of a Bartholin gland, a painful condition and common sign of *Neisseria gonorrhoeae* infection. (CDC/Public Health Image Library.)	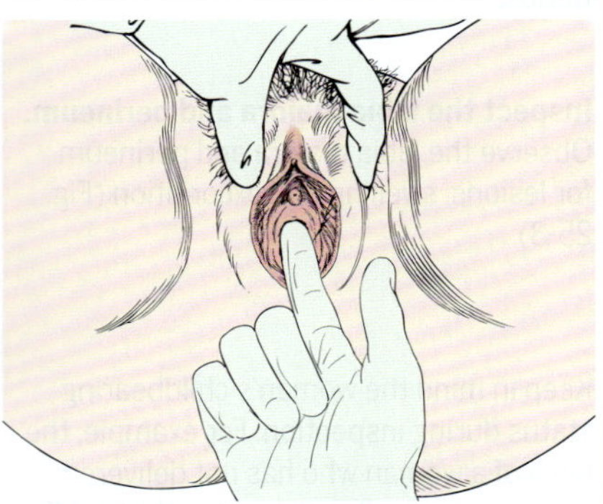 **FIGURE 25-7** Milking the urethra.

PHYSICAL ASSESSMENT (continued)

ASSESSMENT PROCEDURE	NORMAL FINDINGS	ABNORMAL FINDINGS
Internal genitalia		
INSPECTION		
Inspect the size of the vaginal opening and the angle of the vagina. Insert your gloved index finger into the vagina, noting the size of the opening. Then attempt to touch the cervix. This will help you establish the size of the speculum you need to use for the examination and the angle at which to insert it. Next while maintaining tension, gently pull the labia majora outwards. Note hymenal configuration and transections or injury.	The normal vaginal opening varies in size according to the patient's age, sexual history and whether she has given birth vaginally. The vagina is typically tilted posteriorly at a 45-degree angle.	Any loss of hymenal tissue between the 3 o'clock position and the 9 o'clock position indicates trauma (penetration by digits, penis or foreign objects) in children. See Chapter 33 for more information about sexual abuse in children. This finding is not as relevant in adults.
Inspect the vaginal musculature. Keep your index finger inserted in the patient's vaginal opening. Ask the patient to squeeze around your finger.	The patient should be able to squeeze around the examiner's finger. Typically, the nulliparous woman can squeeze tighter than the multiparous woman.	Absent or decreased ability to squeeze the examiner's finger indicates decreased muscle tone. Decreased tone may decrease sexual satisfaction.
Use your middle and index fingers to separate the labia minora. Ask the patient to bear down.	No bulging and no urinary discharge.	Bulging of the anterior wall may indicate a cystocele. Bulging of the posterior wall may indicate a rectocele. If the cervix or uterus protrudes down, the patient may have uterine prolapse (see Abnormal findings 25-1). If urine leaks out, the patient may have stress incontinence.
Inspect the cervix. Follow the guidelines for using a speculum in Equipment spotlight 25-1. With the speculum inserted in position to visualise the cervix, observe cervical colour, size and position.	The surface of the cervix is normally smooth, pink and even. Normally, it is midline in position and projects 1 to 3 cm into the vagina. See Common variations 25-1.	In a non-pregnant woman, a bluish cervix may indicate cyanosis; in a non-menopausal woman, a pale cervix may indicate anaemia. Redness may be from inflammation.
Also observe the surface and the appearance of the os. Look for discharge and lesions as well.	The cervical os normally appears as a small, round opening in nulliparous women and appears slitlike in parous women (Fig. 25-8). 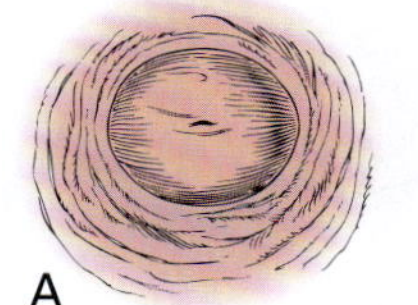 **FIGURE 25-8** The cervical os: **(A)** in nulliparous women; **(B)** in parous women.	Cervical enlargement or projection into the vagina more than 3 cm may be from prolapse or tumour, and further evaluation is needed.
After inspecting the cervix, obtain specimens for the cervical screening test and, if indicated, specimens to identify possible STIs. Follow the procedure presented in Assessment tool 25-1.	Cervical secretions are normally clear or white and without unpleasant odour. Secretions may vary according to timing within the menstrual cycle. In pregnant patients, the cervix appears blue (Chadwick sign).	Asymmetrical, reddened areas, strawberry spots and white patches are also abnormal, as is coloured, malodorous or irritating discharge; a specimen should be obtained for culture. Cervical lesions may result from polyps, cancer or infection.

Continued on following page

PHYSICAL ASSESSMENT (continued)

ASSESSMENT PROCEDURE	NORMAL FINDINGS	ABNORMAL FINDINGS
	 **OLDER ADULT CONSIDERATIONS** **In older women, the cervix appears pale after menopause.**	
Inspect the vagina. Unlock the speculum and slowly rotate and remove it. Inspect the vagina as you remove the speculum. Note the vaginal colour, surface, consistency and any discharge. If you are preparing a wet mount slide, use a cotton swab to collect the specimen of vaginal secretions from the anterior vaginal fornix or the lateral vaginal walls before you collect the specimens for the Pap or other test. Avoid the posterior fornix, which is contaminated with cervical secretions. Use part of the wet mount sample to test the pH of the vaginal secretions.	The vagina should appear pink, moist, smooth, and free of lesions and irritation. It should also be free of any coloured, malodorous discharge.	Reddened areas, lesions and coloured, malodorous discharge are abnormal and may indicate vaginal infections, STIs or cancer (Abnormal findings 25-2 and 25-3). Altered pH may indicate infection.
Bimanual evaluation		
PALPATION		
Palpate the vaginal walls. Tell the patient that you are going to do an internal examination and explain its purpose. Apply water-soluble lubricant to the gloved index and middle fingers of your dominant hand. Then stand and approach the patient at the correct angle. Placing your non-dominant hand on the patient's lower abdomen, insert your index and middle fingers into the vaginal opening. Apply pressure to the posterior wall and wait for the vaginal opening to relax before palpating the vaginal walls for texture and tenderness (Fig. 25-9).	The vaginal wall should feel smooth, and the patient should not report any tenderness. 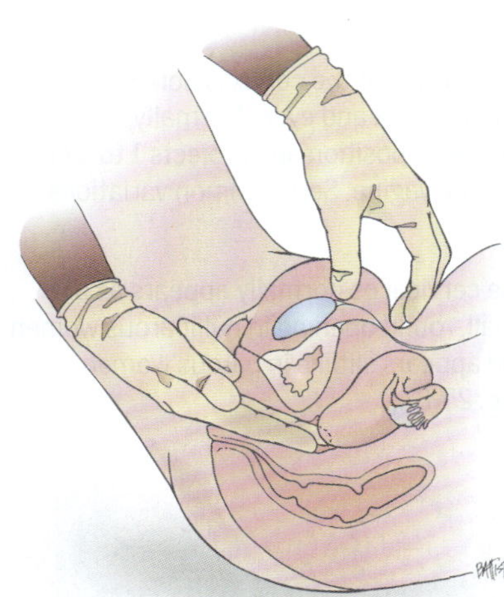 **FIGURE 25-9** Palpating the vaginal walls.	Tenderness or lesions may indicate infection. 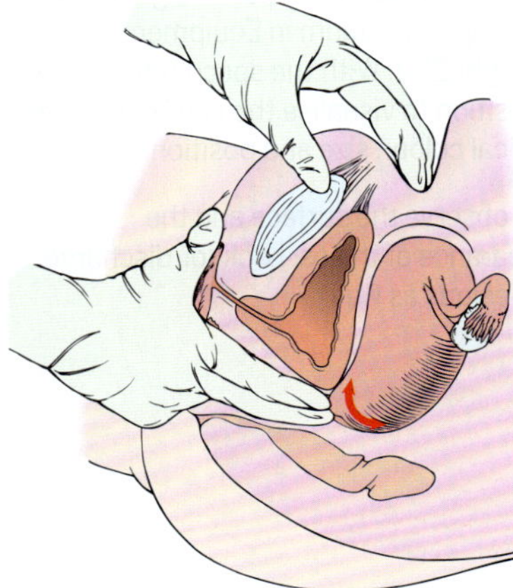 **FIGURE 25-10** Palpating the uterus, bimanual examination.
Palpate the cervix. Advance your fingers until they touch the cervix and run fingers around the circumference. Palpate for: • Contour • Consistency • Mobility • Tenderness.	The cervix should feel firm and soft (like the tip of your nose). It is rounded and can be moved somewhat from side to side without eliciting tenderness.	A hard, immobile cervix may indicate cancer. Pain with movement of the cervix may indicate infection.

PHYSICAL ASSESSMENT (continued)

ASSESSMENT PROCEDURE	NORMAL FINDINGS	ABNORMAL FINDINGS
Bimanual evaluation (continued)		
Palpate the uterus. Move your fingers intravaginally into the opening above the cervix and gently press the hand resting on the abdomen downwards, squeezing the uterus between the two hands (Fig. 25-10). Note uterine size, position, shape and consistency.	The fundus, the large upper end of the uterus, is normally round, firm and smooth. In most women, it is at the level of the pubis; the cervix is aimed posteriorly (anteverted position). However, several other positions are considered normal (Common variations 25-1).	An enlarged uterus above the level of the pubis is abnormal; an irregular shape suggests abnormalities such as myomas (fibroid tumours) or endometriosis (Abnormal findings 25-3).
Attempt to bounce the uterus between your two hands to assess mobility and tenderness.	The normal uterus moves freely and is not tender.	A fixed or tender uterus may indicate fibroids, infection or masses (see Abnormal findings 25-4).
Palpate the ovaries. Slide your intravaginal fingers towards the left ovary in the left lateral fornix and place your abdominal hand on the left lower abdominal quadrant. Press your abdominal hand towards your intravaginal fingers and attempt to palpate the ovary (Fig. 25-11)	Ovaries are approximately 3 × 2 × 1 cm (or the size of a walnut) and almond-shaped. 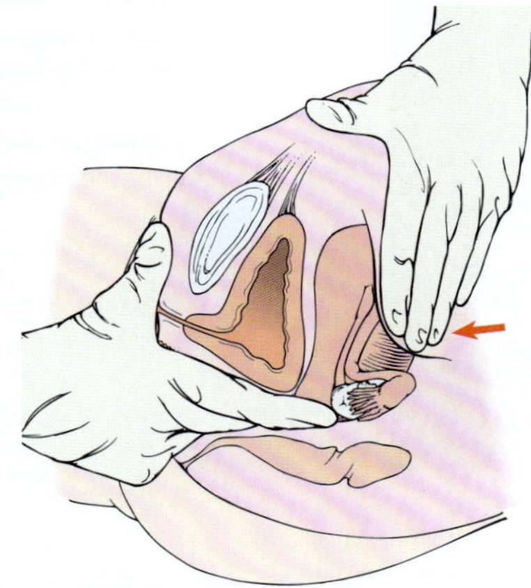 **FIGURE 25-11** Palpating the ovaries.	Enlarged size, masses, immobility and extreme tenderness are abnormal and should be evaluated (Abnormal findings 25-4).
Slide your intravaginal fingers to the right lateral fornix and attempt to palpate the right ovary. Note size, shape, consistency, mobility and tenderness.	Ovaries are firm, smooth, mobile and somewhat tender on palpation. **CLINICAL TIP** **It is normal for the ovaries to be difficult or impossible to palpate in obese women, in postmenopausal women because the ovaries atrophy, or in women who are tense during the examination.**	Ovaries that are palpable 3 to 5 years after menopause are also abnormal.
Withdraw your intravaginal hand and inspect the glove for secretions.	A clear, minimal amount of drainage appearing on the glove from the vagina is normal.	Large amounts of colourful, frothy or malodorous secretions are abnormal.

EQUIPMENT SPOTLIGHT 25-1 GUIDELINES FOR USING A SPECULUM

Speculum examinations are often performed as part of a vaginal examination and are generally done by a doctor, a nurse practitioner or an advanced practice nurse. The technique for performing a speculum examination and obtaining specimens is outlined below:

1. Before using the speculum, choose the instrument that is the correct size for the patient. Vaginal speculums come in two basic types:
   - *Graves speculum*—appropriate for most adult women and available in various lengths and widths.
   - *Pederson speculum*—appropriate for adolescent women and some postmenopausal women who have a narrow vaginal orifice. Speculums can be metal with a thumb screw that is tightened to lock the blades in place or plastic with a clip that is locked to keep the blades in place. (Plastic speculums are shown in Fig. A.)

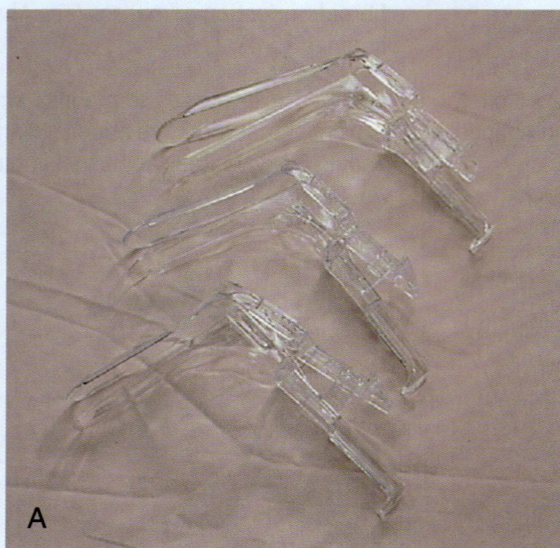
A

2. Encourage the patient to take deep breaths and to maintain her feet bent up towards her buttocks with her knees resting in an open, relaxed fashion.
3. Place two fingers of your non-dominant hand against the posterior vaginal wall and wait for relaxation to occur.
4. Insert the fingers of your non-dominant hand about 2.5 cm into the vagina and spread them slightly while pushing down against the posterior vagina.
5. Lubricate the blades of the speculum with warm tap water. Do not use commercial lubricants on the speculum. Lubricants are typically bacteriostatic and will alter vaginal pH and the cell specimens collected for cytological, bacterial and viral analysis.
6. Hold the speculum with two fingers around the blades and the thumb under the screw or lock. This is important for keeping the blades closed. Position the speculum so the blades are vertical.
7. Insert the speculum between your fingers into the posterior portion of the vaginal orifice at a 45-degree angle downwards. When the blades pass your fingers inside the vagina, rotate the closed speculum so the blades are in a horizontal position (Fig. B).

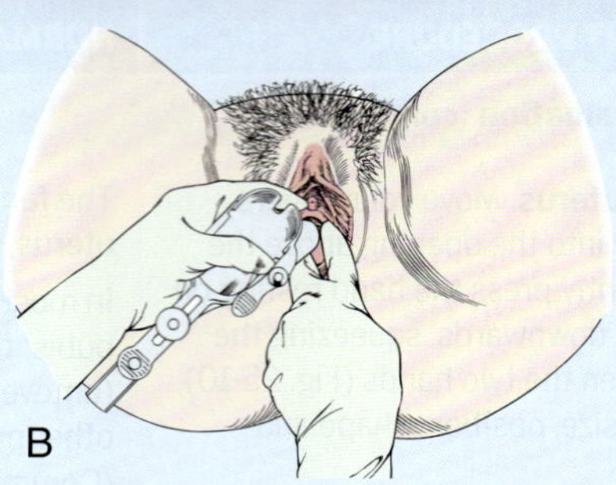
B

CLINICAL TIP

Be careful during the speculum insertion not to pinch the labia or pull the pubic hair. If the vaginal orifice seems tight or you are having trouble inserting the speculum, ask the patient to bear down. This may help relax the muscles of the perineum and promote opening.

8. Continue inserting the speculum until the base touches the fingertips inside the vagina.
9. Remove the fingers of your non-dominant hand from the patient's posterior vagina and press handles together (Fig. C) to open blades and allow visualisation of the cervix. Secure the speculum in place by tightening the thumb screw or locking the plastic clip (Fig. D).

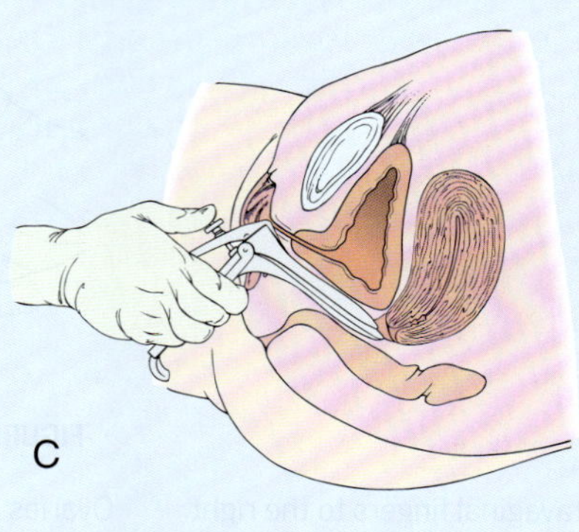
C

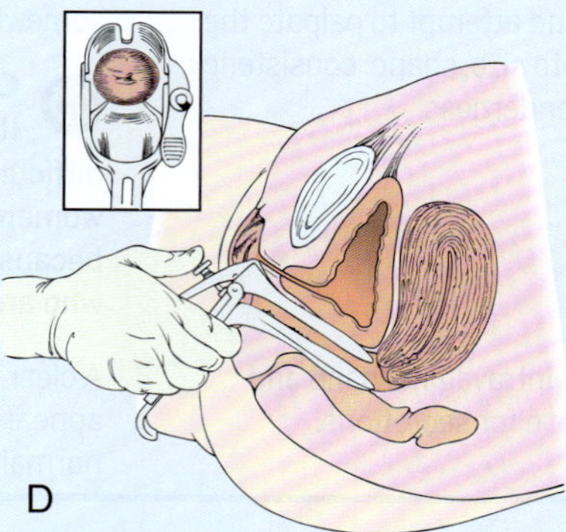
D

10. Various laboratory tests can be performed to detect infections and abnormalities of the vagina and cervix. The type of specimens collected will depend on the patient's reasons for presentation, clinical signs and symptoms, and the patient's clinical history.

ASSESSMENT TOOL 25-1 Obtaining tissue specimens for analysis

Various laboratory tests are based on an analysis of cells obtained from tissue specimens and prepared on culture media or on slides for microscopic examination. For women especially, such tests are lifesaving tools that can detect disease in early treatable stages. Some methods for obtaining tissue specimens follow:

Cervical screening test—Obtaining a specimen

The procedure for gathering the cervical cells is performed on non-pregnant patients using a cervical brush.

1. Insert the central bristles of the cervical brush into the endocervical canal ensuring the shorter bristles contact the exocervix (Fig. A).
2. Gently push and rotate the brush in a full circle five times, collecting cell specimens from the squamocolumnar junction and the cervical surface.
3. Withdraw the cervical brush.
4. Swish the brush in the preservative solution by pushing the brush into the bottom of the vial 10 times, forcing the bristles apart. Swirl the brush to further release material.
5. Discard the cervical brush.
6. Tighten the cap on the preservative and record the patient's name and date on the vial.
7. Send solution to the laboratory.

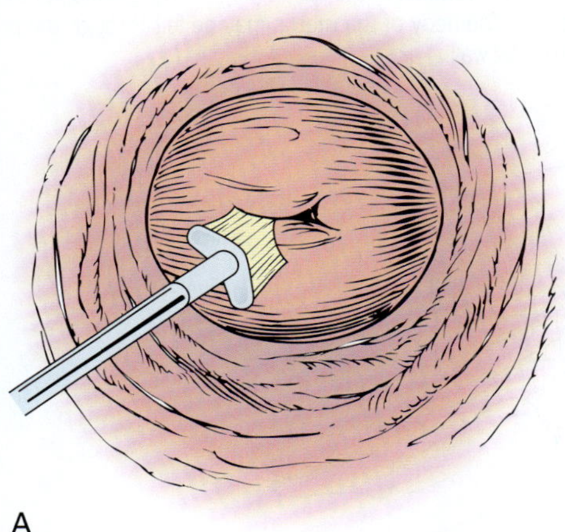

A

Vaginal specimen

Swabs of vaginal secretions are collected from the posterior fornix. Vaginal swabs can detect several infections, including *Trichomoniasis vaginalis*, *Candida albicans* and *Bacterial vaginosis*.

1. Insert the applicator into the vagina and rotate it against the vaginal wall, anterior and lateral to the cervix (Fig. B).
2. Withdraw the applicator.
3. Place swab into tube containing gel transport media.

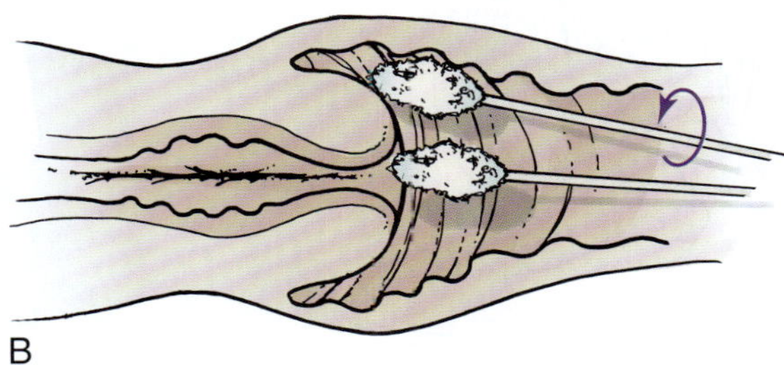

B

Note: Do not swab below the cervix, but to the side and above.

Culture specimens: Gonorrhoea and *Chlamydia*

The test for gonorrhoea or *Chlamydia* have recently changed. The polymerase chain reaction (PCR) is now best practice and has replaced routine slides and cultures. The PCR test is a highly sensitive test and can be used in a variety of settings as it does not require transport medium or refrigeration. The swab is obtained if the patient is symptomatic or has been at risk of acquiring a sexually transmitted infection. The exact procedures for gathering and preparing the specimens vary according to each laboratory's policy. General guidelines are provided below:

1. Use a separate swab to remove cervical mucus and discard.
2. Insert a cotton-tipped applicator into the cervical os and rotate it in a full circle.
3. Withdraw the applicator.
4. Place the swab into the collection tube.

Note: Women who do not need, or who refuse, to have a pelvic examination as part of their clinic consultation may be screened for *Chlamydia* and gonorrhoea by providing a self-collected vaginal swab. The clinician will need to instruct the patient on the technique for self-collection.

COMMON VARIATIONS 25-1 POSITIONS OF THE UTERUS

Anteverted

Figure A shows the most typical anteverted position of the uterus. The cervix is pointed posteriorly, and the body of the uterus is at the level of the pubis over the bladder.

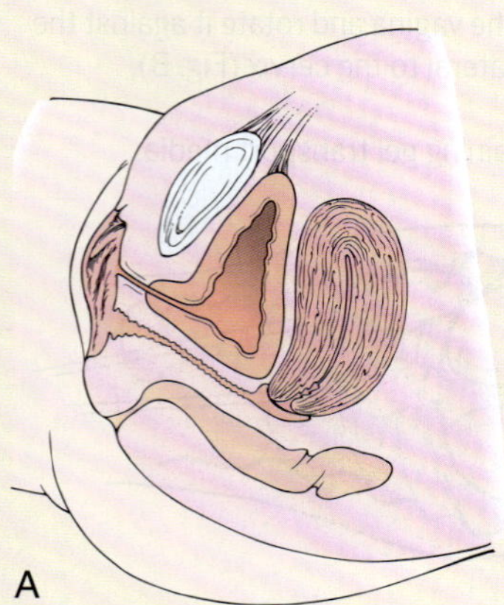

A

Midposition

This is a normal variation (Fig. B). The cervix is pointed slightly more anterior (compared with the anteverted position), and the body of the uterus is positioned more posterior than the anteverted position, midway between the bladder and the rectum. It may be difficult to palpate the body through the abdominal and rectal walls with the uterus in this position.

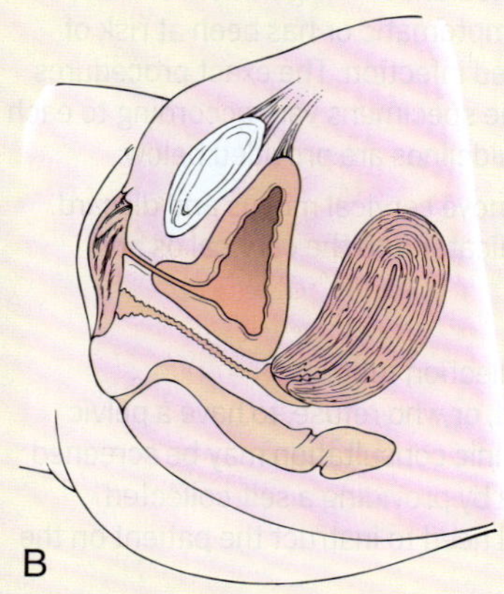

B

Anteflexed

Anteflexion is a normal variation that consists of the uterine body flexed anteriorly in relation to the cervix (Fig. C). The position of the cervix remains normal.

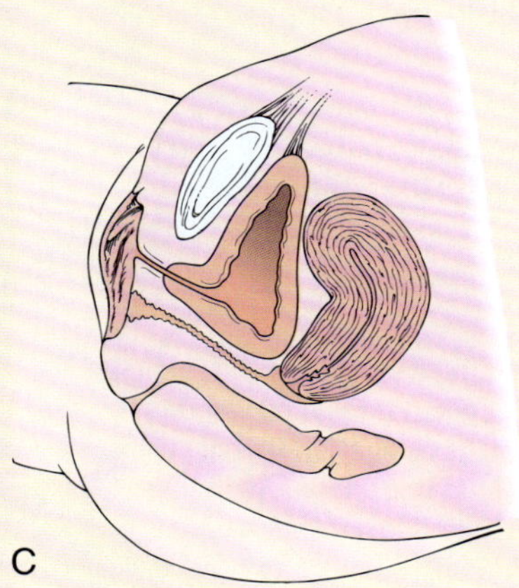

C

Retroverted uterus

Retroversion is a normal variation that consists of the cervix and body of the uterus tilting backwards (Fig. D). The uterine wall may not be palpable through the abdominal wall or the rectal wall in moderate retroversion. However, if the uterus is prominently retroverted, the wall may be felt through the posterior fornix or the rectal wall.

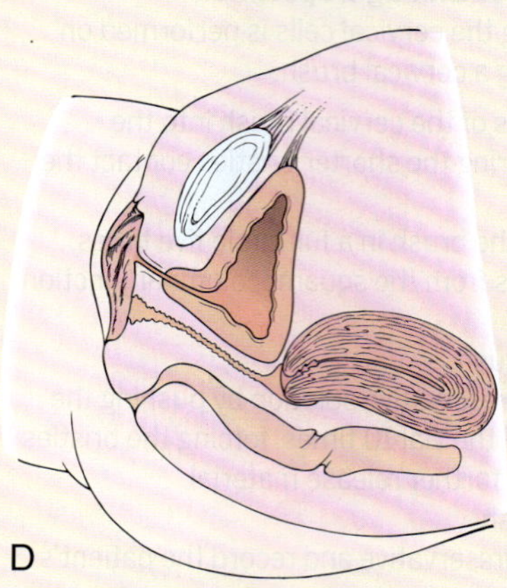

D

Retroflexed uterus

Retroflexion is a normal variation that consists of the uterine body being flexed posteriorly in relation to the cervix (Fig. E). The position of the cervix remains normal. The body of the uterus may be felt through the posterior fornix or the rectal wall.

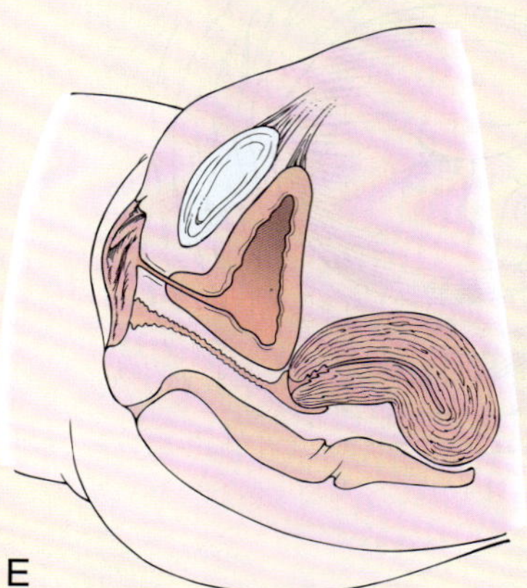

E

ABNORMAL FINDINGS 25-1 Abnormalities of the external genitalia and vaginal opening

When assessing the female genitalia, the nurse will see various abnormal lesions on the external genitalia as well as abnormal bulging in the vaginal opening. Some common findings appear below.

SYPHILITIC CHANCRE

Syphilitic chancres often first appear on the perianal area as silvery white papules that become superficial red ulcers. Syphilitic chancres are painless. They are sexually transmitted and usually develop at the site of initial contact with the infecting organism.

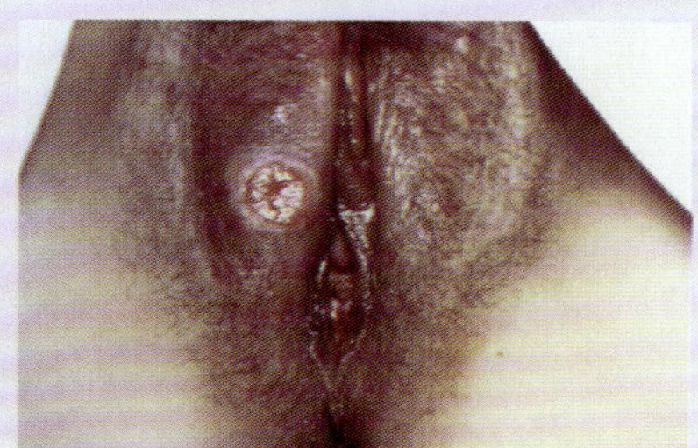

Syphilitic chancre. (CDC/Public Health Image Library.)

GENITAL HERPES SIMPLEX

The initial outbreak of herpes may have many small, painful ulcers with erythematous base. Recurrent herpes lesions are usually not as extensive.

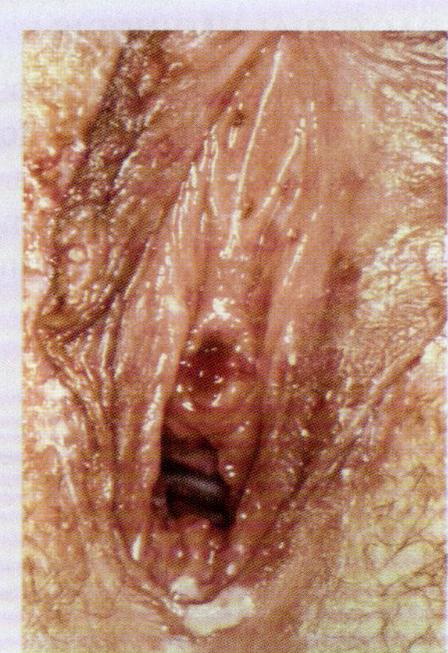

Genital herpes simplex, type II. (CDC/ Public Health Image Library.)

RECTOCELE

A rectocele is a bulging in the posterior vaginal wall caused by weakening of the pelvic musculature. Part of the rectum covered by the vaginal mucosa protrudes into the vagina.

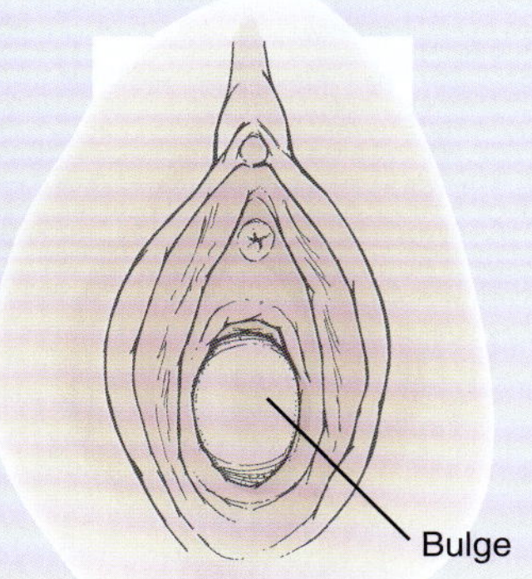

Rectocele.

GENITAL WARTS

Genital warts, caused by the human papillomavirus, are moist, fleshy lesions on the labia and within the vestibule. They are painless and believed to be sexually transmitted.

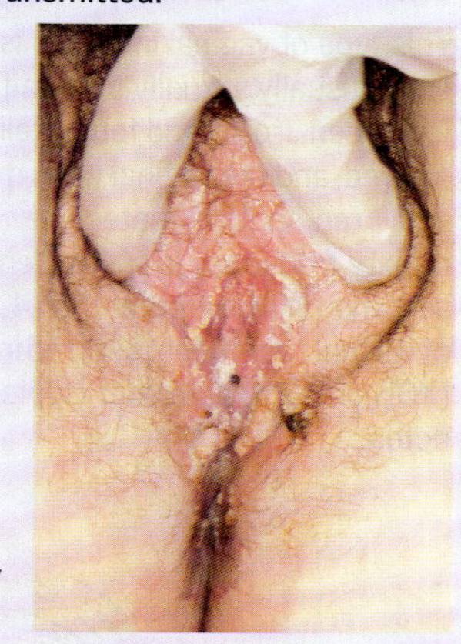

Genital warts. (Science Photo Library/ Alamy Stock Photo.)

CYSTOCELE

A cystocele is a bulging in the anterior vaginal wall caused by thickening of the pelvic musculature. As a result, the bladder, covered by vaginal mucosa, prolapses into the vagina.

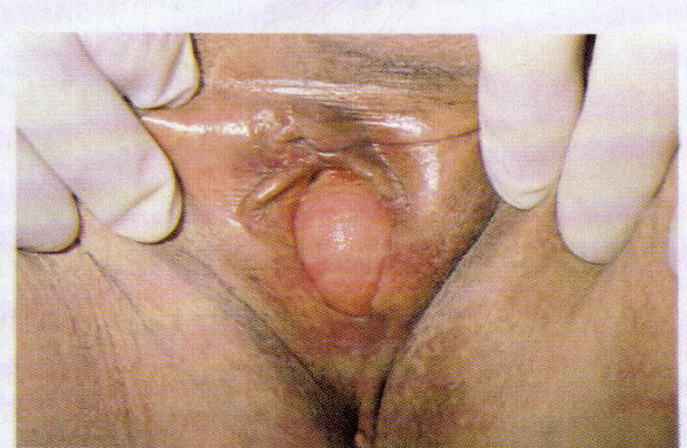

Cystocele. (Alamy Stock Photo/Science Photo Library.)

UTERINE PROLAPSE

Uterine prolapse occurs when the uterus protrudes into the vagina. It is graded according to how far it protrudes into the vagina. In first-degree prolapse, the cervix is seen at the vaginal opening; in second-degree prolapse the uterus bulges outside of vaginal openings; in third-degree prolapse, the uterus bulges completely out of the vagina.

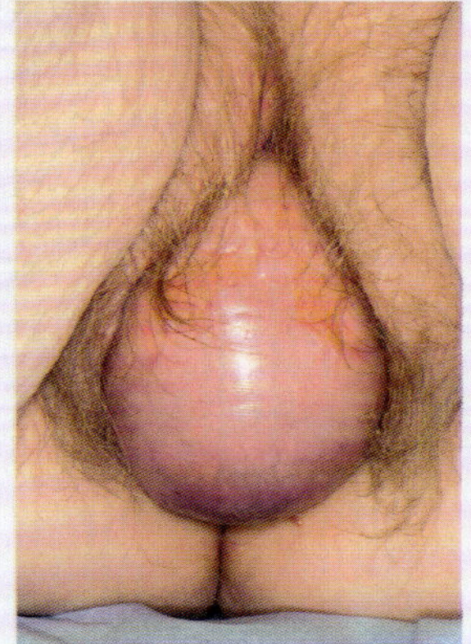

Prolapsed uterus. (Alamy Stock Photo/Science Photo Library.)

ABNORMAL FINDINGS 25-2 Vaginitis

In assessing female genitalia, the nurse may suspect vaginal infection from signs such as redness or lack of colour, unusual discharge and secretions, reported itching and other typical symptoms of the kinds of vaginitis discussed below.

TRICHOMONAS VAGINITIS (TRICHOMONIASIS)

This type of vaginal infection is caused by a protozoan organism and is usually sexually transmitted. The discharge is typically yellow-green, frothy and foul smelling. The labia may appear swollen and red, and the vaginal walls may be red, rough and covered with small red spots or petechiae. This infection causes itching and urinary frequency in the patient. Upon testing, the pH of vaginal secretion will be greater than 4.5 (usually 7.0 or more). If a sample of vaginal secretions is stirred into a potassium hydroxide solution (KOH prep), a foul odour (typically known as a '+' amine) may be noted.

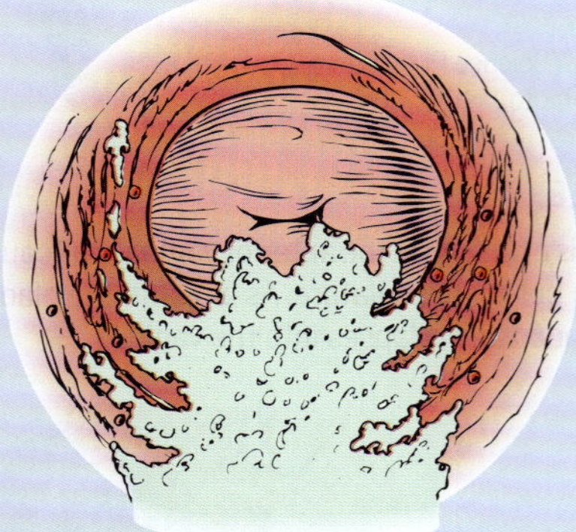

CANDIDAL VAGINITIS (MONILIASIS)

This infection is caused by the overgrowth of yeast in the vagina. It causes a thick, white, cheesy discharge. The labia may be inflamed and swollen. The vaginal mucosa may be reddened and typically contains patches of the discharge. This infection causes intense itching and discomfort.

The pH of vaginal secretions will be less than 4.5; amine (vaginal secretions in KOH) is negative.

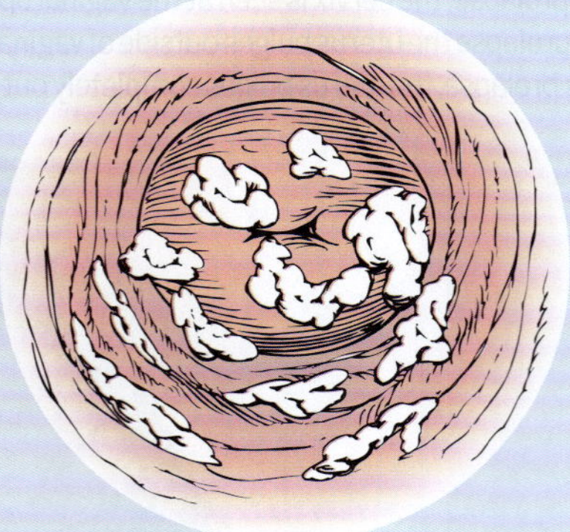

ATROPHIC VAGINITIS

Atrophic vaginitis occurs after menopause when oestrogen production is low. The discharge produced may be blood tinged and is usually minimal. The labia and vaginal mucosa appear atrophic. The vaginal mucosa is typically pale, dry and contains areas of abrasion that bleed easily. Atrophic vaginitis causes itching, burning, dryness and painful urination.

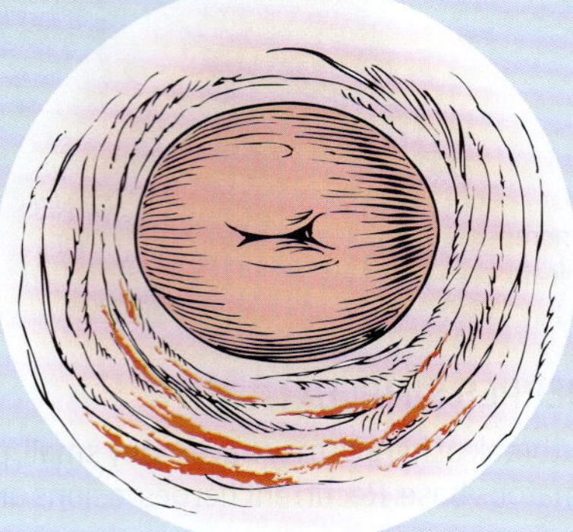

BACTERIAL VAGINOSIS

The cause of bacterial vaginosis is unknown (possibly anaerobic bacteria), but it is thought to be sexually transmitted. The discharge is thin and grey-white, has a positive amine (fishy smell), and coats the vaginal walls and ectocervix. The labia and vaginal walls usually appear normal and pH is greater than 4.5 (5.5 to 6.0).

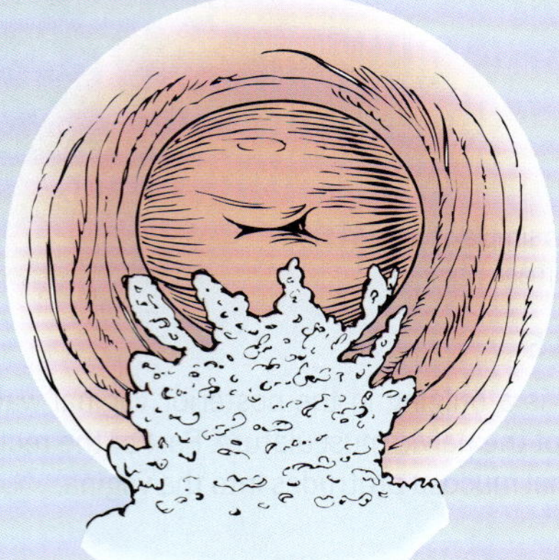

ABNORMAL FINDINGS 25-3 Uterine Enlargement

NORMAL ENLARGEMENT: PREGNANCY

The only uterine enlargement that is normal results from pregnancy and fetal growth. In such cases, the isthmus feels soft (Hegar sign) on palpation, and the fundus and isthmus are compressible at between 10 and 12 weeks of pregnancy.

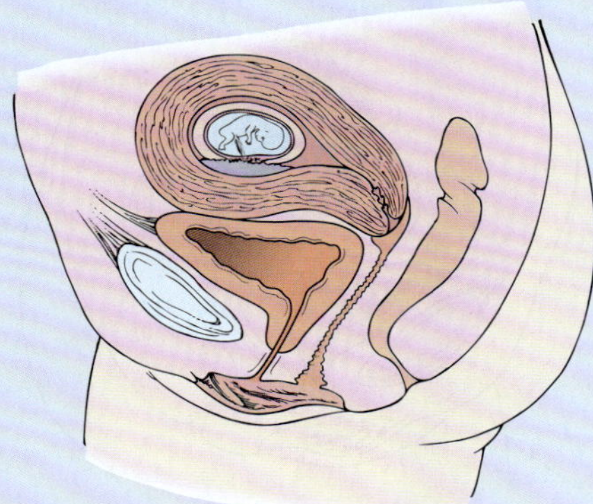

UTERINE FIBROIDS (MYOMAS)

Uterine fibroid tumours are common and benign. They are irregular, firm nodules that are continuous with the uterine surface. They may occur as one or many and may grow quite large. The uterus will be irregularly enlarged, firm and mobile.

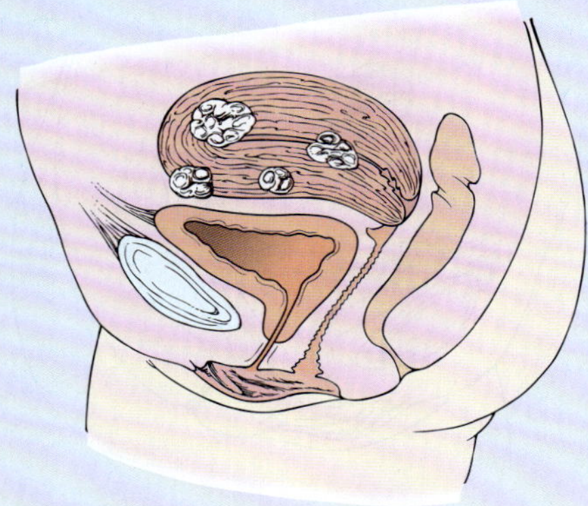

UTERINE CANCER (CANCER OF THE ENDOMETRIUM)

The uterus may be enlarged with a malignant mass. Irregular bleeding, bleeding between periods or postmenopausal bleeding may be the first sign of a problem.

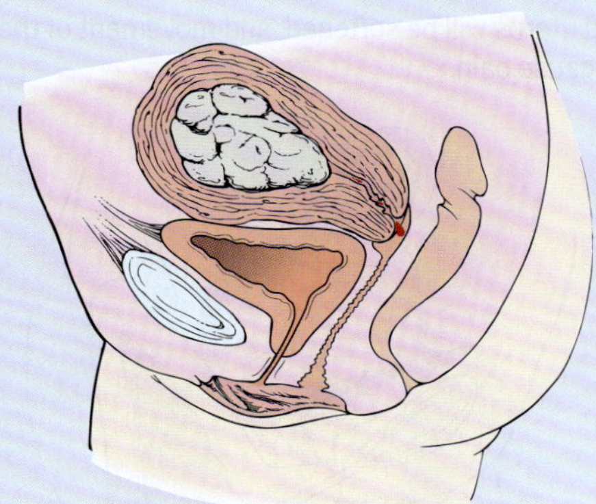

ENDOMETRIOSIS

In endometriosis, the uterus is fixed and tender. Growths of endometrial tissue are usually present throughout the pelvic area and may be felt as firm, nodular masses. Pelvic pain and irregular bleeding are common.

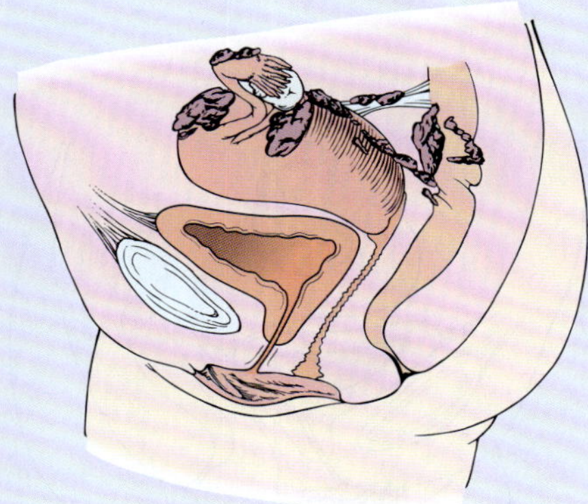

ABNORMAL FINDINGS 25-4 Adnexal Masses

PELVIC INFECTION

Pelvic infections are typically caused by infection of the fallopian tubes (salpingitis) or fallopian tubes and ovaries (salpingo-oophoritis) with a sexually transmitted infection (i.e. gonorrhoea, *Chlamydia*). It causes extremely tender and painful bilateral adnexal masses (positive chandelier sign).

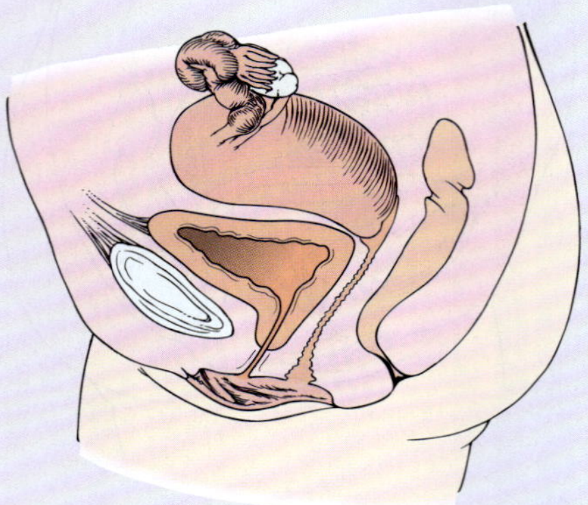

OVARIAN CYST

Ovarian cysts are benign masses on the ovary. They are usually smooth, mobile, round, compressible and non-tender.

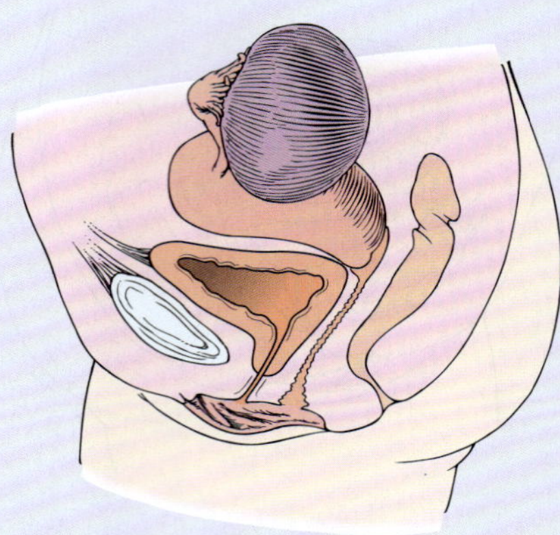

OVARIAN CANCER

Masses that are cancerous are usually solid, irregular, non-tender and fixed.

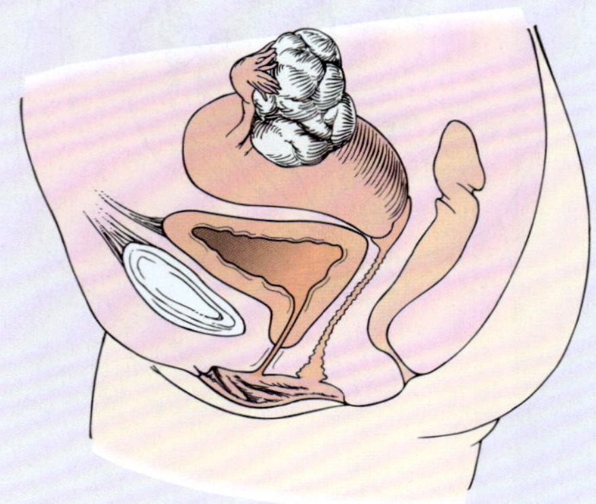

ECTOPIC PREGNANCY

Ectopic pregnancy occurs when a fertilised egg attaches to the fallopian tube and begins developing instead of continuing its journey to the uterus for development. A solid, mobile, tender and unilateral adnexal mass may be palpated if tenderness allows. The cervix and uterus will be softened, and movement of these structures will cause pain.

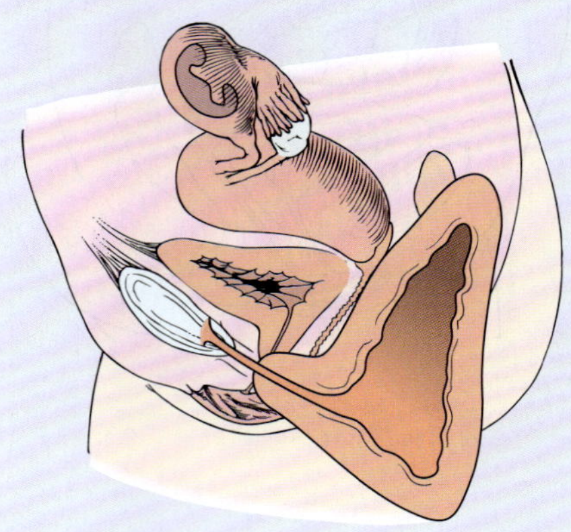

CRITICAL THINKING

5. After reading the physical examination section, which additional physical assessments might be worth considering for Melinda? Why or why not would you consider these?

VALIDATING AND DOCUMENTING FINDINGS

Validate the assessment data you have collected relating to the female genitalia. This is necessary to verify that the data are reliable and accurate. Document the assessment data following the hospital policy.

After you have collected your assessment data, you will need to analyse the data using diagnostic reasoning skills. Refer to the discussion of the diagnostic reasoning process in Chapter 5.

Sample of subjective data

Patient states regular 28-day menstrual cycle. Last menstrual period occurred 2 weeks ago, beginning on the 10th and ending on the 13th. Experiences bloating and mild cramping with period. No mid-cycle spotting, bleeding after sexual intercourse, vaginal discharge, pain, itching in genitalia, lumps, swelling or masses. No difficulty urinating or controlling urine. Denies problems with sexual performance, change in sexual patterns or decrease in sexual desire. No problems with fertility. No prior gynaecological problems.

Last pelvic examination and Pap test 1 year ago, with normal results. Denies history of sexually transmitted infections. Gravida 2, para 1 *[Latin terminology meaning two pregnancies, one delivery; i.e. the patient may be currently pregnant or may have had one miscarriage]. No family history of reproductive or gynaecological cancer. Patient states she does not smoke, is married has not had other partners since meeting her husband and uses condoms for birth control. She is comfortable discussing sexual issues with her husband. Performs vulvar self-examinations and only wears tampons during heavy flow and changes them every few hours.*

Sample of objective data

Palpation of inguinal lymph nodes shows no enlargement or tenderness. Inspection discloses normal hair distribution, no lesions, masses or swelling. Labia majora pink, smooth and free of lesions, excoriation and swelling. Labia minora dark pink, moist and free of lesions, excoriation, swelling and discharge. No bulging at vaginal orifice. No discharge from urethral opening.

Cervix slightly anterior, pink, smooth, slitlike os, mobile, non-tender and firm without lesions or discharge. Vaginal walls smooth and pink.

Palpation indicates firm fundus located anteriorly at level of symphysis pubis, without tenderness, lesions or nodules. Smooth, firm, almond-shaped, mobile ovaries approximately 3 cm in size, palpated bilaterally, no excessive tenderness or masses noted. No malodorous, coloured vaginal discharge on gloved fingers. Routine cervical screening test performed.

Analysis of data

DIAGNOSTIC REASONING: POSSIBLE CONCLUSIONS

After collecting subjective and objective data pertaining to the female genitalia, identify abnormal findings and patient strengths. Then cluster the data to reveal any significant patterns or abnormalities. These data may be used to make clinical judgements about the status of the patient's genitalia.

Potential patient risks

- Ineffective therapeutic regimen management (related to lack of knowledge of the importance of the examination)
- Infection (related to unprotected sexual intercourse)
- Disturbed body image (related to perceived effects on feminine role and sexuality).

Potential patient problems

- Fear of ovarian cancer (related to high incidence of risk factors)
- Ineffective sexuality pattern (related to decreased libido or perceptions of effects of surgery on sexual functioning and attractiveness)
- Ineffective therapeutic regimen management (related to lack of knowledge of external genitalia self-examination)
- Dysuria (related to infection)
- Anticipatory grieving (related to impending loss of reproductive organs secondary to gynaecological surgery)
- Acute pain (related to surgical incision)
- Dyspareunia (painful intercourse; related to inadequate vaginal lubrication).

Selected collaborative problems

After grouping the data, certain collaborative problems may become apparent. Remember that collaborative problems differ from nursing diagnoses in that they cannot be prevented by nursing interventions. However, these physiological complications of medical conditions can be detected and monitored by the nurse. In addition, the nurse can use doctor- and nurse-prescribed interventions to minimise the complications posed by these problems. The nurse may also have to refer the patient in such situations for further treatment of the problem. The following is a list of collaborative problems that may be identified when assessing the female genitalia:

- Candidiasis
- Trichomoniasis
- Gonorrhoea
- Syphilis
- *Chlamydia*
- Pelvic infection (or pelvic inflammatory disease)
- Infertility
- Pregnancy
- Urinary incontinence
- Ovarian nodule
- Abnormal cervical screening result
- Vaginal bleeding
- Retained foreign body (e.g. tampon, sponge)
- Dermatological condition (e.g. lichen sclerosis)
- Genital ulcerative disease or conditions (e.g. Donovanosis, herpes simplex virus, lymphogranuloma venereum).

Medical problems

After grouping the data, the patient's signs and symptoms may clearly require medical diagnosis and treatment. Referral to a primary care provider is necessary, for example, for uterine fibroids.

ONLINE RESOURCES

An extensive range of additional resources to enhance teaching and learning and to facilitate understanding may be found online at the text's accompanying website, located on thePoint at http://thepoint.lww.com. These include Watch and Learn videos, Concepts in Action animations, journal articles, case studies, discussion topics and quizzes.

Subscribers may also access Lippincott Procedures, an extensive online point-of-care procedure guide that provides reliable step-by-step instructions for more than 1700 procedures, including 450 evidence-based Australian procedures, and skills in a variety of speciality settings, together with a wealth of supporting information.

CASE STUDY

The case study demonstrates how to analyse female genitalia assessment data for a specific patient. The exercises included in the ancillary product on thePoint that complements this text offer further opportunities to enhance your skills.

Melinda is a 22-year-old woman who has been admitted to a ward with appendicitis. When about her history, she complains 'I feel like I have the flu; no energy, a headache and fever.' She reports a recent outbreak of genital lesions after a sexual encounter 10 days ago (her 'first and only') with a new partner. She denies the use of any protection or birth control, stating, 'He refused to use anything and I didn't insist.' She denies any problems with her menstrual cycle, no previous sexual activity and no vaginal infections. 'I have always been healthy; I don't know why I behaved so stupidly and put my health at risk.' Melinda's lesions present as vesicles and ulcerations on the external genitalia, labia and mons, with a few vesicles extending into the perianal area. The rest of the perineal and pelvic examination is negative. Some enlarged, tender lymph nodes are noted in the inguinal areas bilaterally. Melinda's temperature by oral route is 38.1 °C. When questioned, she confirms that she has a great deal of pain in the vaginal area and 'urinating hurts a lot'.

The following concept map illustrates the diagnostic reasoning process.

Applying COLDSPA

Applying COLDSPA for patient symptoms: 'flu-like symptoms'.

Mnemonic	Question	Data provided	Missing data
Character	Describe the sign or symptom (feeling, appearance, sound, smell or taste, if applicable).	'I feel like I have the flu; headache, no energy, and fever.' Also reports recent outbreak of genital lesions and painful urination.	
Onset	When did it begin?	'Had unsafe sex 10 days ago.'	When did flulike symptoms begin? When did painful urination begin?
Location	Where is it? Does it radiate? Does it occur anywhere else?		Describe your headaches.
Duration	How long does it last? Does it recur?		Do your headaches come and go? Does it hurt to urinate every time?
Severity	How bad is it? or How much does it bother you?		Do you know what your temperature has been?
Pattern	What makes it better or worse?		Have you taken anything to relieve these symptoms? What aggravates your symptoms?
Associated factors/How it **A**ffects the patient	What other symptoms occur with it? How does it affect you?	Recent outbreak of genital herpes, pain in vaginal area and hurts a lot when she urinates.	Have your symptoms restricted you from any activities that you normally perform?

1) Identify abnormal findings and patient strengths

Subjective data

- Flu-like symptoms: fatigue, headache, fever
- Recent outbreak of genital lesions after unprotected sex
- 'First and on ly'
- 'He refused to use anything, and I didn't insist'
- Denies previous sexual activity or gynaecological problems
- 'Always been healthy'
- 'I don't know why I behaved so stupidly and put my health at risk'
- Pain in vaginal area
- 'Urinating hurts a lot'

Objective data

- Admitted to hospital with appendicitis. During history, relevant sexual and reproductive health information was provided
- Vesicles and ulcerations on the external genitalia, labia and mons
- Few vesicles extending into the perianal area
- Rest of perineal and pelvic examination negative
- Enlarged, tender inguinal lymph nodes
- Oral temperature 38.1°C

2) Identify cue clusters

- Flu-like symptoms: fatigue, headache, fever
- Recent outbreak of genital lesions after unprotected sex
- Pain in vaginal area
- 'Urinating hurts a lot'
- Vesicles and ulcerations on the external genitalia, labia and mons
- Few vesicles extending into the perianal area
- Rest of perineal and pelvic examination normal
- Enlarged, tender inguinal lymph nodes
- Oral temperature 38.1°C

- Vesicles and ulcerative lesions on labia, mons and perianal area
- Reports much pain in vaginal area
- 'Urinating hurts a lot'
- 'I don't know why I behaved so stupidly and put my health at risk'

- Inpatient. Relevant sexual and reproductive health information provided during clinical history
- Came to nurse-managed clinic for help
- Recent outbreak of genital lesions after unprotected sex
- 'First and only'
- 'He refused to use anything and I didn't insist'
- Denies previous sexual activity or gynaecological problems
- 'Always been healthy'
- 'I don't know why I behaved so stupidly and put my health at risk'

3) Draw inferences

Data strongly suggest a STI. The nurse should obtain a specimen for culture of the lesions to assist in the medical diagnosis and refer the patient to the doctor. Collaborative problems should also be identified

Open, ulcerated lesions in this region can result in severe pain that can persist for weeks until lesions heal. In addition, the patient displays some degree of self-anger and blame, which can increase the pain because of increased emotional response to the situation

Patient's first sexual experience resulted in a probable STI; she appears to be experiencing negative feelings about her judgement and lack of assertiveness. Displays self-blame for her illness. She did seek help as soon as symptoms became apparent

4) List possible diagnoses

4) List possible diagnoses	5) Check for defining characteristics	6) Confirm or rule out diagnoses
Acute pain related to knowledge deficit of pain management strategies	*Major:* Communication of pain descriptors	Confirm because it meets the major defining characteristics
Acute pain related to possible excessive emotional response secondary to self-anger or blame	*Major:* Communication of pain descriptors self-focusing statement	This also meets the defining characteristics; however, the care for this patient might be better focused under a different diagnosis, such as situational low self-esteem
Situational low self-esteem related to perceived lack of assertiveness in protecting health	*Major:* None identified	Rule out, not specific enough
Situational low self-esteem related to unknown factors or changes occurring in present life situation	*Major:* Episodic occurrence of negative self-appraisal *Minor:* Self-negating verbalisations, expressions of shame/guilt (implied)	Confirm, but collect more data as to why she chose a relative stranger for a first sexual experience and why she was non-assertive regarding health protection
Health-seeking behaviours	*Major:* None—sought help for symptoms of illness *Minor:* Inferred desire for increased control of health	Rule out because patient sought illness management rather than health promotion at this time

7) Document conclusions

The diagnoses that are appropriate for this patient include:

- Acute pain related to knowledge deficit of pain management strategies
- Situational low self-esteem related to unknown factors or changes occurring in present life situation.

In addition, an identified potential complication could be urinary retention (secondary to dysuria)

- Likely sexually transmitted infection (STI)

Melinda should be referred to a doctor for diagnosis and treatment of her genital lesions

References

American Cancer Society. (2019). Can cervical cancer be prevented? The American Cancer Society Medical and Editorial Team, New York. Viewed October 2019 at https://www.cancer.org/cancer/cervical-cancer/causes-risks-prevention/prevention.html.

Australian Government, Department of Health. (2017). Evaluation of the national HPV program. Canberra: Author. Viewed October 2019 at https://www.health.gov.au/news/evaluation-of-the-national-hpv-program.

Australasian Menopause Society (AMS). (2015). *Spontaneous premature ovarian insufficiency*. Melbourne: Author.

Australian Institute of Health and Welfare (AIHW). (2018a). *Cervical screening in Australia 2018*. Canberra: Author.

Australian Institute of Health and Welfare (AIHW). (2018b). *Cancer incidence and mortality in Australia by small geographic areas*. Canberra: Author.

Australian Institute of Health and Welfare (AIHW). (2018c). *Cancer in Aboriginal & Torres Strait Islander people of Australia*. Canberra: Author.

Australian Institute of Health and Welfare. (2019). Cancer in Australia 2019. Viewed July 2019 at www.aihw.gov.au/reports/cancer/cancer-in-australia-2019/data.

Bray, F., Ferlay, J., Soerjomataram, I., et al. (2018). Global cancer statistics 2018: GLOBOCAN estimates of incidence and mortality worldwide for 36 cancers in 185 countries. *CA: A Cancer Journal for Clinicians, 68*(6), 394–424. doi:10.3322/caac.21492.

Cancer Council Australia. (2018). *Cervical Cancer Screening Guidelines Working Party. National Cervical Screening Program: Guidelines for the management of screen-detected abnormalities, screening in specific populations and investigation of abnormal vaginal bleeding*. Sydney: Author.

Cohen, B. J. & Hull, K. L. (2015). *Memmler's structure and function of the human body* (11th ed.). Philadelphia: Lippincott Williams & Wilkins.

Gartoulla, P., Bell, R. J., Worsley, R., et al. (2015). Moderate-severely bothersome vasomotor symptoms are associated with lowered psychological general wellbeing in women at midlife. *Maturitas, 81*(4), 487–492. https://doi.org/10.1016/j.maturitas.2015.06.004.

IVF Australia. (2011). *Female infertility & assisted reproductive technology (ART)*. Sydney: Author.

Juul, F., Chang, V. W., Brar, P., et al. (2017). Birth weight, early life weight gain and age at menarche: A systematic review of longitudinal studies. *Obesity Reviews : An Official Journal of the International Association for the Study of Obesity, 18*(11), 1272–1288. doi:10.1111/obr.12587.

Karapanou, O. & Papadimitriou, A. (2010). Determinants of menarche. *Reproductive Biology and Endocrinology, 8*, 115. doi:10.1186/1477-7827-8-115.

Lew, J.-B., Simms, K. T., Smith, M. A., et al. (2017). Primary HPV testing versus cytology-based cervical screening in women in Australia vaccinated for HPV and unvaccinated: Effectiveness and economic assessment for the National Cervical Screening Program. *The Lancet. Public Health, 2*(2), e96–e107. doi:10.1016/S2468-2667(17)30007-5.

National Screening Unit, New Zealand. (2012). Cervical cancer in New Zealand. Viewed October 2013 at www.nsu.govt.nz/current-nsu-programmes/1228.aspx.

New Zealand Ministry of Health. (2014). Cervical cancer. Viewed February 2019 at https://www.health.govt.nz/your-health/conditions-and-treatments/diseases-and-illnesses/cervical-cancer.

Royal Australian and New Zealand College of Obstetricians and Gynaecologists (RANZCOG). (2016). *Menopause*. Melbourne: Author.

Schick, V., Rosenberger, J. G., Herbenick, D., et al. (2012). Sexual behaviour and risk reduction strategies among a multinational sample of women who have sex with women. *Sexually Transmitted Infections, 88*(6), 407. doi:10.1136/sextrans-2011-050404.

Sommer, M. (2013). Menarche: A missing indicator in population health from low-income countries. *Public Health Reports, 128*(5), 399–401. doi:10.1177/003335491312800511.

ThinPrep® PapTest™. (2004). Quick Reference Guide: Broom-Like Device Protocol and Endocervical Brush/Spatula Protocol. Viewed January 2014 at www.thinprep.com/pdfs/pap_quick_reference.pdf.

Selected reading

Brotherton, J. M. L., Tabrizi, S. N., Phillips, S., et al. (2017). Looking beyond human papillomavirus (HPV) genotype 16 and 18: Defining HPV genotype distribution in cervical cancers in Australia prior to vaccination. *International Journal of Cancer, 141*(8), 1576–1584. doi:10.1002/ijc.30871.

Online resources

Auckland Sexual Health Service: www.ashs.org.nz

Australian Government Department of Health, Cancer Screening: www.cancerscreening.gov.au

Australian Institute of Health and Welfare (cancer rates): https://www.aihw.gov.au/reports/cancer/cancer-data-in-australia/contents/summary

Australian Women's Health Nurses Association: www.womenshealthnurses.asn.au

Cancer Council Australia: www.cancer.org.au

Cancer Society of New Zealand: www.cancernz.org.nz

Immunise Australia Program: www.immunise.health.gov.au

New Zealand Immunisation Schedule: www.health.govt.nz/our-work/preventative-health-wellness/immunisation

New Zealand National Screening Unit: www.nsu.govt.nz

New Zealand Sexual Health Society: www.nzshs.org

Queensland Health, Australian Government (fact sheets on sexual and reproductive health): www.health.qld.gov.au/sexhealth

Sexual Health and Family Planning Australia: www.shfpa.org.au

CHAPTER 26

Male genitalia

CASE STUDY

Joshua is a 22-year-old electrician. One of Joshua's work colleagues told him there were some sexually transmitted infections that you didn't know you had and that they could cause infertility. As he is sexually active, Joshua was keen to find out more about what he could do to protect himself and presented to a sexual health clinic. He met with, and was examined by, a registered nurse.

Structure and function

To assess the male genitalia, a basic understanding of normal structure and function is necessary because it helps to guide the physical examination and readily assists the examiner in identifying abnormalities.

Male genitalia are classified as external structures and internal structures. (*Note:* Glandular structures accessory to the male genital organs—the prostate, the seminal vesicles and Cowper [bulbourethral] glands—are discussed in Chap. 27.) In addition to an understanding of the male genital structures, the nurse needs to be familiar with the inguinal (or groin) structures because hernias are common in this area.

EXTERNAL GENITALIA

Penis

The external genitalia consist of the penis and the scrotum (Fig. 26-1). The penis is the male reproductive organ. Attached to the pubic arch by ligaments, the penis is freely movable. The shaft of the penis is composed of three cylindrical masses of vascular erectile tissue that are bound together by fibrous tissue—two *corpora cavernosa* on the dorsal side and the *corpus spongiosum* on the ventral side. The corpus spongiosum extends distally to form the acorn-shaped glans. The base of the glans, or *corona,* is somewhat larger than the shaft of the penis. If the man has not been circumcised, the glans is covered by a hood-like fold of skin called the *foreskin* or *prepuce.* In the centre of the corpus spongiosum is the urethra, which travels through the shaft and opens as a slit at the tip of the glans as the *urethral meatus*. A fold of foreskin that extends ventrally from the urethral meatus is called the *frenulum*. The penis has a role in both reproduction and urination.

Scrotum

The scrotum is a thin-walled sac that is suspended below the pubic bone, posterior to the penis. This darkly pigmented structure contains sweat and sebaceous glands and consists of folds of skin (rugae) and the cremaster muscle. The scrotum functions as a protective covering for the testes, epididymis and vas deferens (or ductus deferens) and helps to maintain the cooler-than-body temperature necessary for production of sperm (less than 37°C). The scrotum can maintain temperature control because the cremaster muscle is sensitive to changes in temperature. The muscle contracts when too cold, raising the scrotum and testes upwards towards the body for warmth (cremasteric reflex). This accounts for the wrinkled appearance of the scrotal skin. When the temperature is warm, the muscle relaxes, lowering the scrotum and testes away from the heat of the body. When the cremaster muscle relaxes, the scrotal skin appears smooth.

INTERNAL GENITALIA

Testes

Internally the scrotal sac is divided into two portions by a septum, each portion containing one testis (testicle; see Fig. 26-1). The testes are a pair of ovoid organs, similar to the ovaries in the woman, that are approximately 3.7 to 5 cm long, 2.5 cm wide and 2.5 cm wide. Each testis is covered by a serous membrane called the tunica vaginalis, which separates the testis from the scrotal wall. The tunica vaginalis is double-layered and lubricated to protect the testes from injury. The function of the testis is to produce spermatozoa and the male sex hormone testosterone.

Spermatic cord

The testes are suspended in the scrotum by a spermatic cord. The spermatic cord contains blood vessels, lymphatic vessels, nerves and the vas deferens, which transports spermatozoa away from the testis. The spermatic cord on the left side is usually longer; thus the left testis hangs lower than the right testis.

The epididymis is a comma-shaped, coiled tubular structure that curves up over the upper and posterior surface of the testis.

CLINICAL TIP

Although the epididymis is usually over the posterior surface of the testes, in about 6% to 7% of the male population it is located anteriorly.

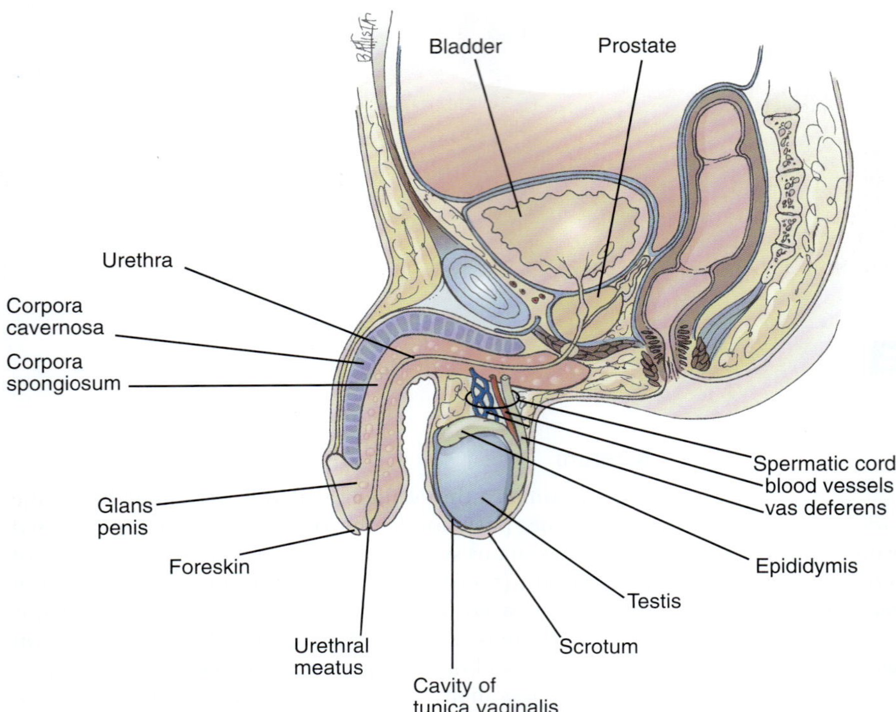

FIGURE 26-1 External and internal male genitalia.

It is within the epididymis that the spermatozoa mature. The vas deferens is a firm, muscular tube that is continuous with the lower portion of the epididymis (see Fig. 26-1). It travels up within the spermatic cord through the inguinal canal into the abdominal cavity. At this point, it separates from the spermatic cord and curves behind the bladder. It joins with the duct of the seminal vesicle and forms the ejaculatory duct. Finally, the ejaculatory duct empties into the urethra within the prostate gland.

The vas deferens provides the passage for transporting sperm from the testes to the urethra for ejaculation. Along the way, secretions from the vas deferens, seminal vesicles, prostate gland and Cowper or bulbourethral glands mix with the sperm and form semen.

INGUINAL AREA

When assessing the male genitalia, the nurse needs to be familiar with structures of the inguinal or groin area because hernias (protrusion of loops of bowel through weak areas of the musculature) are common in this location (Fig. 26-2). The inguinal area is contained between the anterior superior iliac spine laterally and the symphysis pubis medially.

Running diagonally between these two landmarks, just above and parallel with the inguinal ligament, is the *inguinal canal.* The inguinal canal is a tubelike structure (4 to 5 cm long in an adult) through which the vas deferens travels as it passes through the lower abdomen.

The external inguinal ring is the exterior opening of the inguinal canal and can be palpated above and lateral to the symphysis pubis. It feels triangular and slitlike. The internal inguinal ring is the internal opening of the inguinal canal. It is located 1 to 2 cm above the midpoint of the inguinal ligament and cannot be palpated. The *femoral canal* is another potential spot for a hernia. The femoral canal is located posterior to the inguinal canal and medial to and running parallel with the femoral artery and vein.

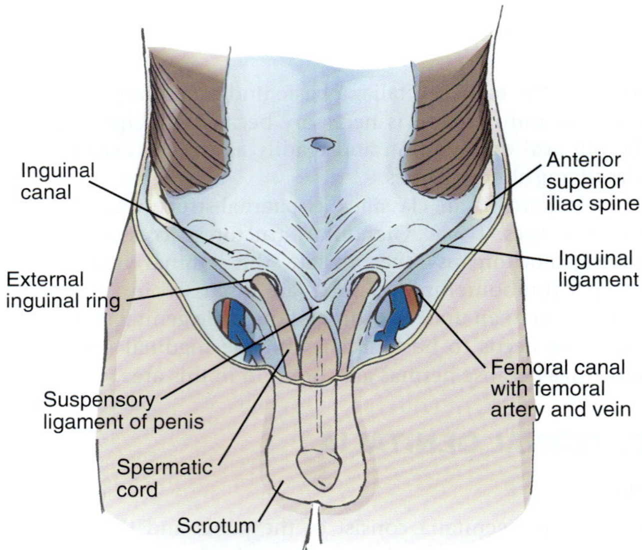

FIGURE 26-2 Inguinal area.

Health assessment

COLLECTING SUBJECTIVE DATA: THE NURSING HEALTH HISTORY

When interviewing the male patient for information regarding his genitalia, keep in mind that this may be a very sensitive topic for the patient and for the examiner as well. Moreover, the examiner should be aware of the patient's own feelings about body image, fear of cancer and sexuality.

Western culture emphasises the importance of the male sexual function. Self-esteem and body image are entwined with the male sex role. Anxiety, embarrassment and fear may influence the patient's ability to discuss problems and ask questions. A trusting relationship is the key to a successful interview. Keep in mind that serious or life-threatening problems may be present. Testicular cancer, for example, carries a high mortality rate, especially if not detected early. The information gathered during this portion of the health history assessment provides a basis for teaching the patient about important health screening issues such as testicular self-examination. Additionally symptoms that the patient reports, or hints at, need to be explored in some depth with a symptom analysis.

CASE STUDY

The nurse's questioning revealed the patient's urinary and sexual function was normal. Joshua reported he was not aware of any fertility problems but noted he had a history of a right inguinal hernia 4 years ago that was surgically repaired with no complications.

CRITICAL THINKING

1. What symptoms would you expect Joshua to have described when he was diagnosed with an inguinal hernia?
2. While undertaking this current health assessment, what subjective and objective evidence would identify Joshua as having had a past inguinal hernia and repair?

History of present health concern

QUESTION	RATIONALE
Pain	
Do you have pain in your penis, scrotum, testes or groin?	Complaints of pain in these areas may indicate a hernia or an infective or inflammatory process, such as epididymitis.
Lesions	
Have you noticed any lesions on your penis or genital area? If so, do the lesions itch, burn or sting? Please describe the lesions.	Lesions may be a sign of a sexually transmitted infection (STI) or cancer.
Discharge	
Have you noticed any discharge from your penis? If so, how much? What colour is it? What type of odour does it have?	Discharge may indicate an infection.
Lumps, swelling, masses	
Do you have any lumps, swelling or masses in your scrotum, genital or groin area? Have you noticed a change in the size of the scrotum or testes?	These findings may indicate infection, hernia or cancer. **OLDER ADULT CONSIDERATIONS** **Enlargement of the scrotum may indicate hydrocoele, haematocoele, hernia or cancer; the scrotum also enlarges with ageing.**
Do you have a heavy, dragging feeling in your scrotum?	A testicular tumour or scrotal hernia may cause a feeling of heaviness in the scrotum.
Urination	
Do you experience difficulty urinating (i.e. urgency, hesitancy, frequency, or difficulty starting or maintaining a stream)? How many times do you urinate during the night?	Difficulty urinating may indicate an infection or blockage including prostatic enlargement. Urinating more than one time during the night may indicate prostate abnormalities. Excessive intake of fluids may also cause nocturia.

Continued on following page

History of present health concerns (continued)

QUESTION	RATIONALE
Have you noticed any change in the colour, odour or amount of your urine?	Changes in urine colour or odour may indicate an infection. Blood in the urine (haematuria) should be referred for medical investigation because this may indicate infection, benign prostatic hypertrophy or cancer. A decrease in amount of voided urine may indicate prostate enlargement or kidney problems.
Do you experience any pain or burning when you urinate?	Painful urination may be a sign of urinary tract infection, prostatitis or STI.
Do you ever experience urinary incontinence or dribbling?	Incontinence may occur after prostatectomy. Dribbling may be a sign of overflow incontinence.
Sexual dysfunction	
Have you recently had a change in your pattern of sexual activity or sexual desire (libido)?	A change in sexual activity or sexual desire needs to be investigated to determine the cause.
Do you have difficulty attaining or maintaining an erection? Do you have any problem with ejaculation? Do you have pain with ejaculation?	Erectile dysfunction occurs frequently in adult males and may be attributed to various factors or disorders (e.g. alcohol use, diabetes, depression, antihypertensive medications). Pain with ejaculation may indicate epididymitis. **OLDER ADULT CONSIDERATIONS** **Erectile dysfunction increases in frequency with age.**
Do you have or have you had any trouble with fertility?	About 20% of all infertility experienced by couples is due to male infertility (Andrology Australia, 2019).

COLDSPA

Example for frequent urination

Use the COLDSPA mnemonic as a guideline to collect needed information for each symptom the patient shares. In addition, the following questions help elicit important information.

Mnemonic	Question	Patient response example
Character	Describe the sign or symptom (feeling, appearance, sound, smell or taste, if applicable).	'I have to get up a lot at night to urinate. I do not feel like I am emptying my bladder all the way and I have to go again about an hour later.'
Onset	When did it begin?	'Gradually over the last couple of months. But it is getting worse now.'
Location	Where is it? Does it radiate? Does it occur anywhere else?	(No information given)
Duration	How long does it last? Does it recur?	'It happens every night. I get up 3 to 4 times a night.'
Severity	How bad is it? or How much does it bother you?	'My wife can't sleep at night because my getting up disturbs her. I do not want to live with this the rest of my life.'
Pattern	What makes it better or worse?	'It is worse if I drink at bedtime; nothing makes it better.'
Associated factors/How it Affects the patient	What other symptoms occur with it? How does it affect you?	'I have to strain sometimes to get my urine out and my stream is weak.'

Past health history

QUESTION	RATIONALE
Describe any prior medical problems you have had, how they were treated, and the results.	Prior problems directly affect the physical assessment findings. For example, if cancer was present in the past, it may recur. Diabetes may cause impotence.
Do you regularly examine your testicles for lumps or changes?	According to the Cancer Council Australia (2019), testicular cancer is the second most common cause of cancer in young men (ages 18 to 39) Screening for this disease is simple and free—testicular self-examination (TSE). TSE is described in the following Promote health box and outlined in Self-assessment 26-1.
Have you ever been tested for human immunodeficiency virus (HIV), human papillomavirus, herpes simplex, chlamydia, gonorrhoea or trichomoniasis? What were the results? Why were you tested?	HIV increases the patient's risk for other infections. A high-risk exposure may require serial testing. See the accompanying Promote health box for further information on HIV and acquired immunodeficiency syndrome.

Continued on following page

PROMOTE HEALTH — TESTICULAR CANCER

OVERVIEW

Testicular cancer is a condition where the cells within the testis grow and divide abnormally and a tumour grows in the testis. A cancer will usually appear as a painless lump in a testis. If medical attention is sought as soon as a lump, swelling or pain in a testis is noticed, this cancer can remain localised (contained within the testis). However, if left unattended, it typically spreads via the blood or lymphatic system to other major organs such as the lungs. Although testicular cancer is a relatively new disease, in 2019 there were an estimated 852 new cases diagnosed in Australia, accounting for 1.1% of all new cancers in men (Australian Government, Cancer Australia, 2019). In Australia it is the second most common cancer in young men age 18 to 39, and in New Zealand it is the most common cancer in young men age 15 to 35 years, with about 130 New Zealand men diagnosed annually (Australian Government, Cancer Australia, 2019; Testicular Cancer NZ, 2019.)

All testicular cancers can be treated and, if discovered early and with the right treatment, over 98% of those diagnosed have a survival rate in excess of 5 years. The early detection of testicular cancer can lessen the toxic side effects of the treatments used (Andrology Australia, 2019).

RISK FACTORS

As the causes of testicular cancer are largely not known, there are no known ways to prevent it. There is no evidence of a link between injury or sporting strains, lifestyle (e.g. smoking, diet) or sexual activity with testicular cancer. An injury to the groin area may sometimes prompt men to check or notice a problem with the testes that needs further investigation by a health professional (Andrology Australia, 2019).

TEACH RISK REDUCTION TIPS

A testicular self-examination involves feeling the testes, one at a time, using fingers and thumb. It is a simple process to teach and should take men only a few minutes to perform (see Self-assessment 26-1). The objective of TSE is for men to be aware of the normal shape and feel of their testicles and report any abnormalities (Andrology Australia, 2019).

SELF-ASSESSMENT 26-1 TESTICULAR SELF-EXAMINATION

Testicular self-examination (TSE) should be performed once a month; it is neither difficult nor time consuming. A convenient time is often after a warm bath or shower when the scrotum is more relaxed.

1. Stand in front of a mirror and check for scrotal swelling.
2. Use both hands to palpate the testis; the normal testicle is smooth and uniform in consistency.
3. With the index and middle fingers under the testis and the thumb on top, roll the testis gently in a horizontal plane between the thumb and fingers (A).
4. Feel for any evidence of a small lump or abnormality.
5. Follow the same procedure and palpate upwards along the testis (B).
6. Locate the epididymis (C), a cord-like structure on the top and back of the testicle that stores and transports sperm.
7. Repeat the examination for the other testis. It is normal to find that one testis is larger than the other.
8. If you find any evidence of a small, pea-like lump, consult your doctor. It may be due to an infection or a tumour growth.

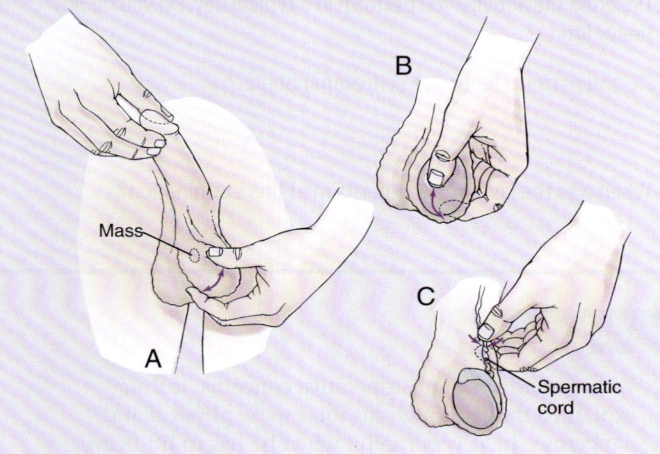

Family history

QUESTION	RATIONALE
Is there a history of cancer in your family? What type and which family member(s)?	Cancers of the prostate and testes have a familial tendency.

Lifestyle and health practices

QUESTION	RATIONALE
How many sexual partners do you have?	A patient with multiple sexual partners increases his risk of contracting a sexually transmitted infection (STI) or human immunodeficiency virus (HIV).
What kind of birth control method do you use, if any?	Vasectomy for permanent birth control results in a decreased amount of ejaculate, which concerns some men. Vasectomy affords no protection from STIs. The only type of temporary birth control method for men is the male condom. Failure to use condoms increases the patient's risk of contracting and transmitting STIs and HIV and increases the female partner's risk of becoming pregnant.
Are you satisfied with your current level of activity and sexual functioning?	Pain or heaviness due to hernias may limit the ability to work or perform regular exercise. Infection may limit a patient's ability to engage in sexual activity. An erectile dysfunction impedes sexual intercourse. Incontinence may affect the patient's ability to work or engage in social activities.
Do you have concerns about fertility? If you experience fertility troubles, how has this affected your relationship?	Concerns about fertility can increase stress and can have a negative impact on relationships.
What is your sexual preference?	An awareness of the patient's sexual preference allows the examiner to focus the examination. Acceptance of a patient's sexual preference helps to put the patient at ease. Therefore, the patient will be more likely to talk about his special health issues or fears.
Do you have any fears related to sex? Can you identify any stress in your current relationship that relates to sex?	Fear can cause inhibition and decrease sexual satisfaction. Stress can prevent satisfactory sexual performance.
Do you feel comfortable communicating with your partner about your sexual likes and dislikes?	Lack of open communication can cause problems with relationships and lead to feelings of guilt and depression.
What do you know about STIs and their prevention?	The patient's knowledge of STIs and their prevention provides a basis for health education in this area.
Are you currently exposed to chemicals or radiation? Have you been exposed in the past?	Exposure to radiation and certain chemicals increases the risk of developing cancer.
Describe the activity you perform in a typical day. Do you do any heavy lifting?	Strenuous activity and heavy lifting may predispose the patient to development of an inguinal hernia.
Do you perform testicular self-examinations?	Male patients who do not perform testicular self-examinations need to be informed about the connection between self-examination and early interventions for abnormalities.
When was the last time you performed this examination?	Male patients should be aware of the need for a monthly testicular self-examination and its importance in the early diagnosis and treatment of testicular cancer.

CASE STUDY

When asked about postoperative concerns, Joshua explained that although his job can be physical and dangerous, he is very careful when he has to lift heavy items; however, he requested further information on the risk that lifting heavy objects posed. Joshua also confided that although he performed testicular self-examinations, he had questions about his technique and the value of performing the examinations.

The nurse was able to determine that Joshua had no physical problems with his genitalia. The nurse created a safe environment and used good clear communication, which allowed Joshua to give an honest detailed medical and sexual history. Joshua was then able to confide that he had questions about his postoperative concerns regarding lifting. He was also able to seek clarification on performing testicular self-examination. Clear communication allowed the nurse to provide the patient with the help he required.

CRITICAL THINKING

3. How would you physically examine Joshua for an inguinal hernia?
4. What physical signs are you looking for?
5. What are some problems you might anticipate in performing this physical examination on Joshua?

PROMOTE HEALTH — HEALTH PROMOTION AND DISEASE PREVENTION: HIV/AIDS

OVERVIEW

Acquired immunodeficiency syndrome (AIDS) is a disease caused by the human immunodeficiency virus (HIV), which is transmitted from person to person via exchange of body fluids, usually through sexual transmission, but also through contact with infected blood (e.g. blood transfusions, infected needles); by mother to child during pregnancy, childbirth or breastfeeding; by intravenous drug users; and other mechanisms of body fluid transfer. The highest incidence of HIV still occurs in men who have sex with men (MSM), followed by intravenous drug users.

HIV damages the immune system by destroying CD4 (helper T cells) white blood cells and prevents the body from defending itself against other organisms. The time from infection with HIV to developing AIDS may be years. At present there is no cure for AIDS, but medications help to suppress the virus in most people who have access to these expensive treatments.

The World Health Organization (WHO, 2019) reports that at the end of 2018 there were 37.9 million people globally living with HIV, with 1.8 million new cases of HIV detected in the same year, representing 0.25 per 1,000 people. Of those living with HIV, 62% were receiving antiretroviral treatment as of 2018, equating to 23.3 million people globally.

In Australia there were 27,545 people living with HIV at the end of 2017 (AFAO, 2019). In New Zealand few people are infected with HIV. According to New Zealand AIDS Foundation (2019), approximately 3,500 New Zealanders are living with HIV, with 178 new diagnosis made in 2018.

The Australian Federation of AIDS Organisation (AFAO, 2019) reports that 63% of HIV/AIDS cases reported in 2017 were as a result of sexual contact between men. Nurses are often reluctant to discuss sexually related behaviours with adult males, but to do so is a necessary professional role and vital to good history taking.

Screening

Although there is no formal screening protocol in Australia, testing may be indicated in a number of contexts in Australia through the use of the National HIV testing policy (2017), such as a clinical suspicion of HIV infection. These clinical suspicions include opportunistic infection (including tuberculosis); HIV-linked malignancy; symptoms and signs consistent with primary HIV infection (e.g. mononucleosis-like syndrome); other HIV indicator conditions (e.g. immune thrombocytopenia); diagnosis of a condition with shared transmission route; sexually transmitted infection (STI); hepatitis B or C; reported high-risk exposure; unprotected sexual intercourse with a partner whose HIV status is unknown; and reported reuse of equipment used for skin penetration (ASHM, 2019)

In December 2012, Australia approved its first HIV rapid test. Also known as HIV Point of Care Testing (PoCT), the HIV rapid test is now a mainstay of practice within sexual health clinics. PoCT allows for on-the-spot HIV screening with results available in 10 to 20 minutes. It provides faster results than traditional testing and enables tests to be conducted outside of a laboratory setting. It is hoped that, by removing the need to wait or return to the doctor for a result, PoCT may increase the uptake and frequency of HIV testing in individuals at high risk by making tests easier, faster and more convenient (AFAO, 2019). However, it should be noted that a 'reactive' result on a PoCT is not a diagnosis of HIV; confirmation is always required by laboratory testing (AFAO, 2019).

Risk factors

Because HIV is preventable, knowing risks and practising risk-reducing behaviours will help to stem the epidemic of this infection. Risks include:

- Having unprotected sex (especially male-on-male anal intercourse)
- Having another STI
- Using intravenous drugs, especially sharing needles
- Uncircumcised male
- Fetus of HIV-positive mother
- Mother-to-infant transmission during pregnancy or delivery
- Exchange of blood or body fluids through blood transfusions, needle sticks, breastfeeding by HIV-infected mother, body piercing with non-sterilised instruments.

Teach risk reduction techniques

Use precautions to decrease transfer of body fluids:

- Avoid unprotected sex (use a new condom every time you have sex) or practise sexual abstinence.
- Avoid having multiple sex partners.
- Avoid anal sex.
- Avoid intravenous drug use.
- Avoid mixing sex and alcohol or drugs.
- If you take medications requiring needle use, use a new, sterile needle each time.
- Consider circumcision, if lifestyle is risky.
- Follow guidelines for handling body secretions, objects that touch bodily secretions or contaminated items.
- Openly discuss HIV risk behaviour history with partner and use above precautions.

If you already have HIV or AIDS:

- Eat a healthy, well-rounded diet.
- Avoid food and drink that may easily transmit foodborne illness (e.g. raw eggs, unpasteurised dairy products, raw seafood, undercooked meat).
- Get immunisations against other illnesses if allowed by doctor.
- Be aware that companion animals may harbour parasites that can cause infections.
- Tell your sex partner right away if you are HIV positive.
- If pregnant, seek medical care right away.
- Seek support from support group to deal with your emotions.
- Obtain and stay on antiretroviral protocol, if available.

COLLECTING OBJECTIVE DATA: PHYSICAL EXAMINATION

The purpose of examining the male genitalia is to detect abnormalities that may range from life-threatening diseases to painful conditions that interfere with normal function. Abnormalities should be detected as early as possible so the patient can be referred for further testing or treatment. The physical assessment is also a good time to allow the patient to demonstrate the proper techniques for testicular self-examination and to provide teaching if necessary.

The hands-on physical examination of the male genitalia may create anxiety, embarrassment and nervousness about exposing the genitals and about what might be discovered. Ease patient anxiety by explaining in detail what is going to occur and the significance of each portion of the examination while you are performing it. Also attempt to expose only those areas necessary at that point in the examination. This will help preserve the patient's modesty. It is helpful to encourage the patient to ask questions during the examination.

CLINICAL TIP

Nurses and the patient are often worried that the male patient will have an erection during the hands-on examination. Usually the patient is too nervous for this to occur. If it does occur, reassure the patient that it is not unusual and continue the examination in an unhurried and unflappable manner.

Preparing the patient

Before the examination, instruct the patient to empty his bladder so he will be comfortable. If a urine specimen is necessary, provide the patient with a container. If the patient is not wearing an examination gown for a total physical examination, provide a drape and ask him to lower his pants and underwear. Explain to the patient that he will be asked to stand (if able) for most of the examination.

Equipment

- Chair or stool
- Gown
- Disposable gloves
- Penlight (for possible transillumination)
- Stethoscope (for possible auscultation)

Physical assessment

During the examination of the patient, remember these key points:

- Wear disposable gloves.
- Preserve the patient's privacy.
- Inspect and palpate the penis, scrotum and inguinal area for inflammation, infestations, rashes, lesions and lumps.
- During the testicular examination, describe the importance of testicular self-examination and explain how to perform the examination as you are performing it.

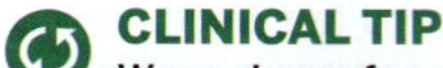

Wear gloves for every step of the male genitalia examination.

CLINICAL TIP

The use of a chaperone is a requirement in most Australian and New Zealand health settings to protect the interests of both the patient and the attending clinician throughout and post an intimate assessment.

PHYSICAL ASSESSMENT

ASSESSMENT PROCEDURE	NORMAL FINDINGS	ABNORMAL FINDINGS
Penis		
INSPECTION AND PALPATION		
Inspect the base of the penis and pubic hair. Sit on a stool with the patient facing you and standing (Fig. 26-3). Ask the patient to raise his gown or drape. Note pubic hair growth pattern and any excoriation, erythema or infestation at the base of the penis and within the pubic hair. 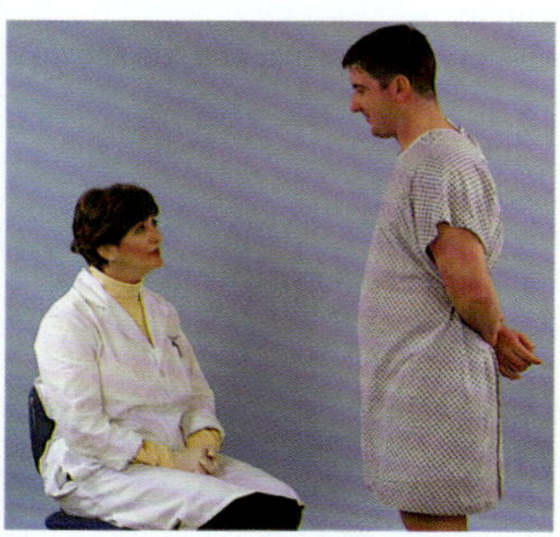 **FIGURE 26-3** In positioning the male patient for a genital examination, the nurse sits and the patient stands. (© B. Proud.)	Pubic hair is coarser than scalp hair. The normal pubic hair pattern in adults is hair covering the entire groin area, extending to the medial thighs and up the abdomen towards the umbilicus. The base of the penis and the pubic hair are free of excoriation, erythema and infestation (Fig. 26-4; Table 26-1). 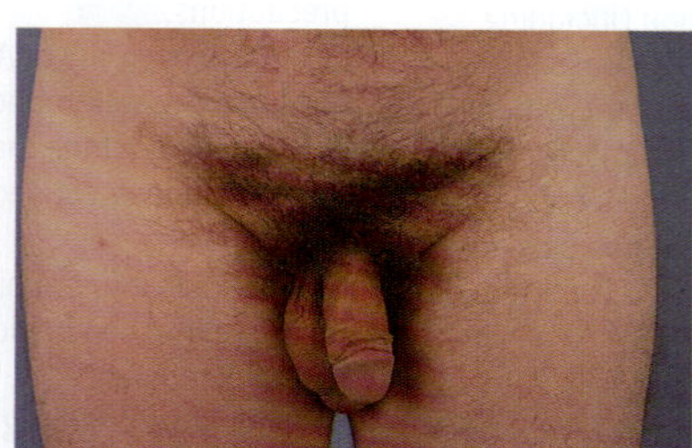 **FIGURE 26-4** Normal appearance of external male genitalia. (© B. Proud.)	Absence or scarcity of pubic hair may be seen in patients receiving chemotherapy. Lice or nit (eggs) infestation at the base of the penis or pubic hair is known as pediculosis pubis. This is commonly referred to as 'crabs'. 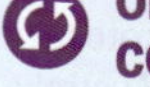 **OLDER ADULT CONSIDERATIONS** **Pubic hair may be grey and sparse in elderly patients. In addition, the penis becomes smaller and the testes hang lower in the scrotum in elderly patients.**

Table 26-1 Tanner sexual maturity rating for boys

Stage	Pubic hair	Penis	Testes and scrotum
1 (preadolescent)	None, except for fine body hair	Same size and proportions as in childhood	Same size and proportion as in childhood
2	Sparse growth, slightly curly	Slight or no enlargement	Both larger, reddened, exhibiting textural changes
3	Darker, coarse, curly, sparse hair over symphysis pubis	Larger, longer	Further enlargement
4	Coarse, curly hair that does not extend to medial thighs	Increased length and width, development of glans	Further enlargement and scrotal skin darkens
5	Adult hair in texture and quantity extends to medial aspect of thighs	Adult size and shape	Adult size and shape

Adapted from Tanner, J. M. (1962). *Growth at adolescence* (2nd ed.). Oxford: Blackwell Scientific Publications.

PHYSICAL ASSESSMENT (continued)

ASSESSMENT PROCEDURE	NORMAL FINDINGS	ABNORMAL FINDINGS
Inspect the skin of the shaft. Observe for rashes, lesions or lumps.	The skin of the penis is wrinkled and hairless and is normally free of rashes, lesions or lumps. Genital piercing is becoming more common, and nurses may see male patients with one or more piercings of the penis. **CULTURAL CONSIDERATIONS** **Pubertal rites in some Aboriginal and Torres Strait Islander cultures include slitting the penile shaft, leaving an opening that may result in disfigurement extending the entire length of the shaft (Schiegel & Barry, 2017).**	Rashes, lesions or lumps may indicate sexually transmitted infection (STI) or cancer (see Promote health—Sexually transmitted infections and Abnormal findings 26-1). Drainage around piercings indicates infection.
Palpate the shaft. Palpate any abnormalities noted during inspection. Also note any hardened or tender areas.	The penis in a non-erect state is usually soft, flaccid and non-tender.	Hardness along the ventral surface may indicate cancer or a urethral stricture. Tenderness may indicate inflammation or infection.
Inspect the foreskin. Observe for colour, location and integrity of the foreskin in uncircumcised men.	The foreskin, which covers the glans in an uncircumcised male patient, is intact and uniform in colour with the penis.	Discolouration of the foreskin may indicate scarring or infection.
Inspect the glans. Observe for size, shape and lesions or redness.	The glans size and shape vary, appearing rounded, broad or even pointed. The surface of the glans is normally smooth and free of lesions and redness.	Chancres (red, oval ulcerations) from syphilis, venereal warts and pimplelike lesions from herpes are sometimes detected on the glans.
If the patient is not circumcised, ask him to retract his foreskin (if the patient is unable to do so, the nurse may retract it) to allow observation of the glans. This may be painful.	The foreskin retracts easily. A small amount of whitish material, called smegma, normally accumulates under the foreskin.	A tight foreskin that cannot be retracted is called *phimosis.* A foreskin that once retracted cannot be returned to cover the glans is called *paraphimosis.* Chancres (red, oval ulcerations) from syphilis and venereal warts are sometimes detected under the foreskin (see Abnormal findings 26-1).
Note the location of the urinary meatus on the glans	The urinary meatus is slitlike and normally found in the centre of the glans. **CULTURAL CONSIDERATIONS** **If pubertal mutilation has occurred, actual discharge of urine and semen will occur at the location of the shaft opening.**	*Hypospadias* is displacement of the urinary meatus to the ventral surface of the penis. *Epispadias* is displacement of the urinary meatus to the dorsal surface of the penis (see Abnormal findings 26-1).

Continued on following page

PROMOTE HEALTH — SEXUALLY TRANSMITTED INFECTIONS

Sexually transmitted infections (STIs) include:

- Bacterial vaginosis
- Balanitis
- Chlamydia
- Crab louse (pubic lice)
- Genital warts
- Gonorrhoea
- Hepatitis B
- Herpes
- Human immunodeficiency virus
- Molluscum contagiosum
- Non-specific urethritis
- Scabies
- Syphilis
- Thrush (candidiasis)
- Trichomoniasis.

Some common signs of STIs are:

- Unusual discharge from the penis or vagina
- Rashes, blisters, lumps or sores in the genital area (or sometimes in the mouth, if sexual activity was oral)
- Lower abdominal pain
- Dysuria.

However, many STIs either don't exhibit symptoms or exhibit symptoms only some of the time, even though the infection is still there. It is important to realise that an individual might not always be aware he has an infection.

WAYS TO AVOID AN STI

- Have a 'healthy attitude' towards sex—always practise safer sex and get tested if anything interrupts safe practices.
- Understand that condoms will provide only some protection from most STIs: the male condom covers only part of the genitals and thus might not cover all of the infected area and infections (e.g. herpes, crabs and genital warts will spread through skin-to-skin contact).
- Choose not to have sex at all (i.e. abstain); however, this is not realistic for some people.
- Partners should talk honestly with each other about their sexual history and practices, and share information about their sexual activities.
- Partners could get tested together, to make it a supportive and honest process.
- If a decision has been made to have sex without protecting against STIs, make sure both partners have had recent STI tests and that both partners do not have unsafe sex with others.
- Remember to use a form of contraception if pregnancy is not sought.

STI TESTING

- Some STIs have no symptoms (e.g. chlamydia), whereas others may cause a discharge from the penis or vagina, a sore, a lump or an itch.
- Many STIs are easy to treat early, but if left for a long time they can be more difficult to treat.
- If left untreated, some STIs can make women and men infertile.
- Knowingly passing on an STI to a partner without their knowledge is an unnecessary, selfish and disrespectful thing to do.

Adapted from ASHA. (2019). *Australian STI management guidelines for use in primary care.* Viewed July 2019 at http://www.sti.guidelines.org.au/.

PHYSICAL ASSESSMENT (continued)

ASSESSMENT PROCEDURE	NORMAL FINDINGS	ABNORMAL FINDINGS
Palpate the urethral discharge. Gently squeeze the glans between your index finger and thumb (Fig. 26-5). 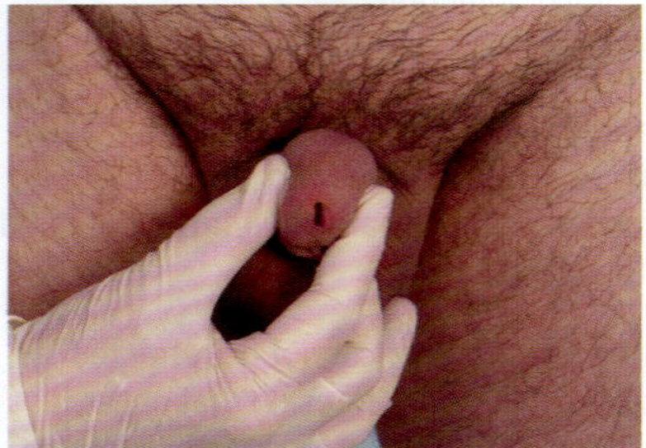 **FIGURE 26-5** Palpating for urethral discharge. (© B. Proud.)	The urinary meatus is normally free of discharge.	A yellow discharge is usually associated with gonorrhoea. A clear or white discharge is usually associated with urethritis. All discharge should be cultured.
Scrotum		
INSPECTION		
Inspect the size, shape and position. Ask the patient to hold his penis out of the way. Observe for swelling, lump or bulges.	The scrotum varies in size (according to temperature) and shape. The scrotal sac hangs below or at the level of the penis. The left side of the scrotal sac usually hangs lower than the right side.	An enlarged scrotal sac may result from fluid (hydrocoele), blood (haematocoele), bowel (hernia) or tumour (cancer) (see Abnormal findings 26-2).

PHYSICAL ASSESSMENT (continued)

ASSESSMENT PROCEDURE	NORMAL FINDINGS	ABNORMAL FINDINGS
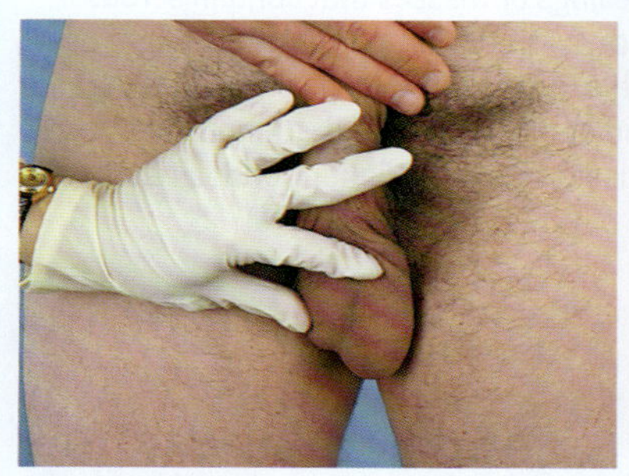 **FIGURE 26-6** When inspecting the scrotal skin, have the patient hold the penis aside while the nurse inspects. (© B. Proud.)	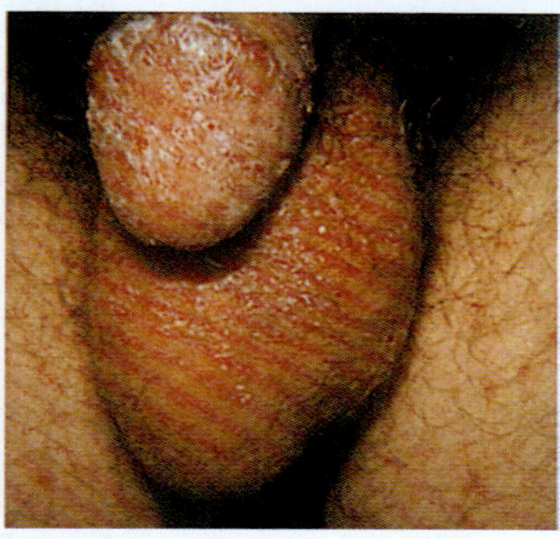 **FIGURE 26-7** Inflammation of the penis and scrotum may be seen in Reiter syndrome, and idiopathic inflammatory disorder affecting the skin, joints and mucous membranes. (With permission from Goodheart, H. P. [1999]. *A photoguide of common skin disorders*. Baltimore: Lippincott Williams & Wilkins.)	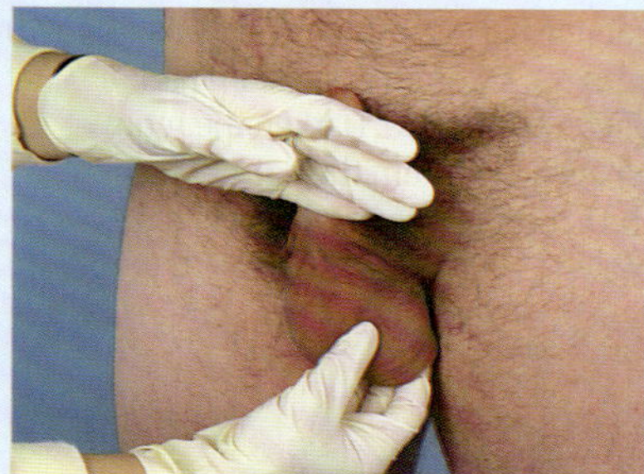 **FIGURE 26-8** Palpating the scrotal contents. (© B. Proud.)
Inspect the scrotal skin. Observe colour, integrity and lesions or rashes. To perform an accurate inspection, you must spread out the scrotal folds (rugae) of skin (Fig. 26-6). Lift the scrotal sac to inspect the posterior skin.	Scrotal skin is thin and rugated (crinkled) with little hair dispersion. Its colour is slightly darker than that of the penis. Lesions and rashes are not normally present. However, sebaceous cysts (small, yellowish, firm, non-tender, benign nodules) are a normal finding.	Rashes, lesions and inflammation are abnormal findings (Fig. 26-7).
PALPATION		
Palpate the scrotal contents. Palpate each *testis* and *epididymis* between your thumb and first two fingers (Fig. 26-8). Note size, shape, consistency, nodules and tenderness. **CLINICAL TIP** **Do not apply too much pressure to the testes because this will cause pain.**	Testes are ovoid, approximately 3.5 to 5 cm long, 2.5 cm wide and 2.5 cm deep, and equal bilaterally in size and shape. They are smooth, firm, rubbery, mobile, free of nodules and rather tender to pressure. The epididymis is non-tender, smooth and softer than the testes. **OLDER ADULT CONSIDERATIONS** **Testes do not get smaller with normal ageing although they may decrease in size with long-term illness.**	Absence of a testis suggests *cryptorchidism* (an undescended testicle). Painless nodules may indicate cancer. Tenderness and swelling may indicate acute orchitis, torsion of the spermatic cord, a strangulated hernia or epididymitis (see Abnormal findings 26-2). If the patient has epididymitis, passive elevation of the testes may relieve the scrotal pain (Prehn sign). If the patient has a strangulated hernia, the patient should be referred immediately to a surgeon and prepared for surgery.
Palpate each *spermatic cord* and vas deferens from the epididymis to the inguinal ring. The spermatic cord will lie between your thumb and finger (Fig. 26-9). Note any nodules, swelling or tenderness. 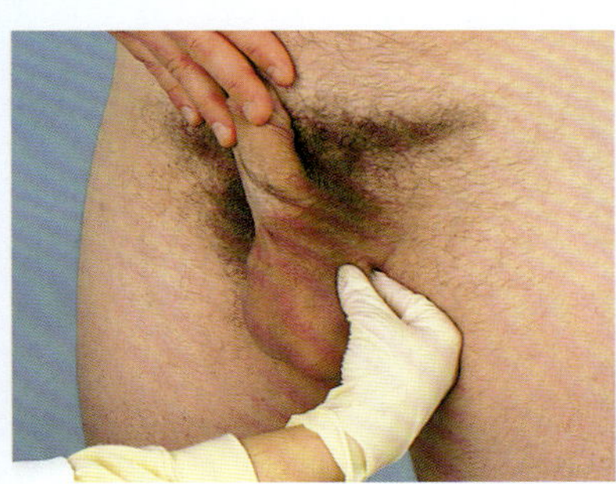	The spermatic cord and vas deferens should feel uniform on both sides. The cord is smooth, non-tender and ropelike. **FIGURE 26-9** When palpating the spermatic cord, have the patient hold the penis aside. (© B. Proud.)	Palpable, tortuous veins suggest varicocele. A beaded or thickened cord indicates infection or cysts. If you palpate a scrotal mass, have the patient lie down. The mass may return to the abdomen by itself. If it does not, place your fingers above the scrotal mass. If you can get your fingers above the mass, suspect hydrocoele (see Abnormal findings 26-2). Cyst suggests hydrocoele of the spermatic cord.

Continued on following page

PHYSICAL ASSESSMENT (continued)

ASSESSMENT PROCEDURE	NORMAL FINDINGS	ABNORMAL FINDINGS
TRANSILLUMINATION		
Transilluminate the scrotal contents. If an abnormal mass or swelling was noted in the scrotum, transillumination should be performed. Darken the room and shine a light from the back of the scrotum through the mass. Look for a red glow.	Normally scrotal contents do not transilluminate.	Swellings or masses that contain serous fluid—hydrocoele, spermatocele—light up with a red glow. Swellings or masses that are solid or filled with blood—tumour, hernias or varicocele—do not light up with a red glow.
Inguinal area		
INSPECTION		
Inspect for inguinal and femoral hernia. Inspect the inguinal and femoral areas for bulges. Ask the patient to turn his head and cough or to bear down as if having a bowel movement, and continue to inspect the areas.	The inguinal and femoral areas are normally free from bulges.	Bulges that appear at the external inguinal ring or at the femoral canal when the patient bears down may signal a hernia (see Abnormal findings 26-3).
PALPATION		
Palpate for inguinal hernia and inguinal nodes. Ask the patient to shift his weight to the left for palpation of the right inguinal canal, and vice versa. Place your right index finger into the patient's right scrotum and press upwards, invaginating the loose folds of skin (Fig. 26-10). Palpate up the spermatic cord until you reach the triangular, slitlike opening of the external inguinal ring. Try to push your finger through the opening and, if possible, continue palpating up the inguinal canal. When your finger is in the canal or at the external inguinal ring, ask the patient to bear down or cough. Feel for any bulges against your finger. Then repeat the procedure on the opposite side.	Bulging or masses are not normally palpated. 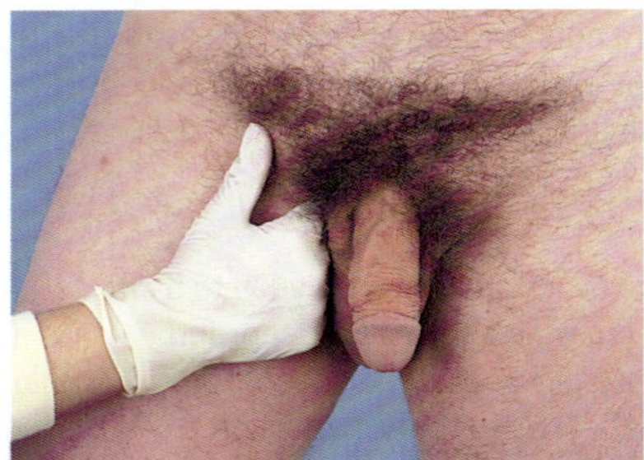 **FIGURE 26-10** Palpating for an inguinal hernia. (© B. Proud.)	A bulge or mass may indicate a hernia.
Palpate inguinal lymph nodes. If nodes are palpable, note size, consistency, mobility or tenderness.	No enlargement or tenderness is normal.	Enlarged or tender nodes may indicate an inflammatory process or lesion on the penis or scrotum.
Palpate for femoral hernia. Palpate on the front of the thigh in the femoral canal area (Fig. 26-11). Ask the patient to bear down or cough. Feel for bulges. Repeat on the opposite thigh.	Bulges or masses are not normally palpated. 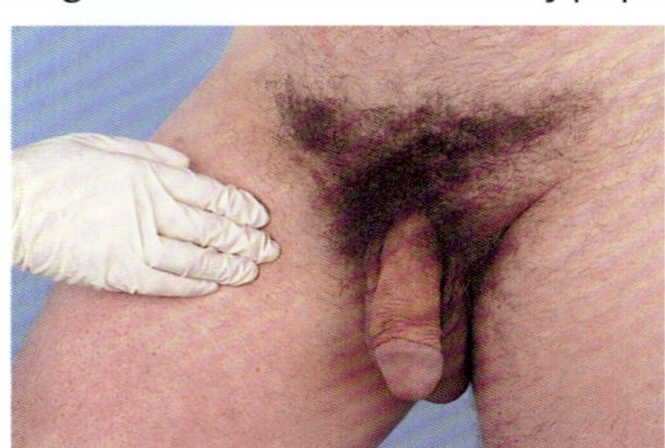 **FIGURE 26-11** Palpating for a femoral hernia. (© B. Proud.)	A bulge or mass may be from a hernia.

PHYSICAL ASSESSMENT (continued)

ASSESSMENT PROCEDURE	NORMAL FINDINGS	ABNORMAL FINDINGS
Inspect and palpate for scrotal hernia. If you discovered a mass during inspection and palpation of the scrotum and you suspect it may be a hernia, ask the patient to lie down; note whether the bulge disappears. If the bulge remains, auscultate it for bowel sounds. Finally, gently palpate the mass and try to push it upwards into the abdomen. **CLINICAL TIP** **If the patient complains of extreme tenderness or nausea, do not try to push the mass up into the abdomen.**	If the bulge disappears, no scrotal hernia is present, but the mass may result from something else and the patient should be referred for further evaluation. A mass on or around the scrotum should be considered malignant until testing proves otherwise.	If the bulge disappears when the patient lies down, a scrotal hernia is present. Bowel sounds auscultated over the mass indicate the presence of bowel and thus a scrotal hernia. If you cannot push the mass into the abdomen, suspect an *incarcerated hernia.* A hernia is *strangulated* when its blood supply is cut off. The patient typically complains of extreme tenderness and nausea (see Abnormal findings 26-3).

ABNORMAL FINDINGS 26-1 Abnormalities of the penis

SYPHILITIC CHANCRE

- Initially a small, silvery-white papule that develops a red oval ulceration.
- Painless.
- A sign of primary syphilis (a sexually transmitted infection) that spontaneously regresses.
- May be misdiagnosed as herpes.

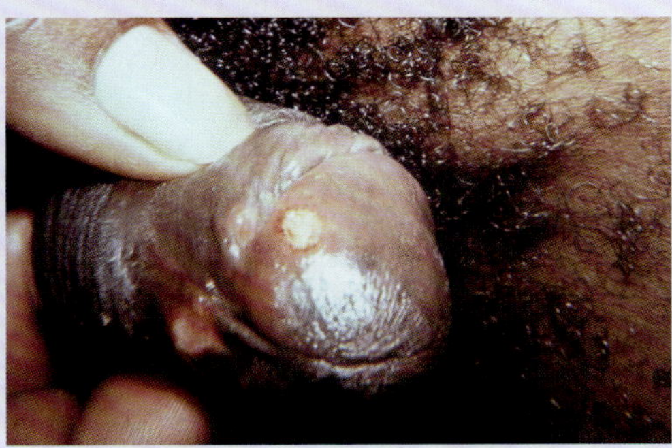

Syphilitic chancre. (CDC/Public Health Image Library.)

HERPES PROGENITALIS

- Clusters of pimple-like, clear vesicles that erupt and become ulcers.
- Painful.
- Initial lesions of this STI, typically caused by HSV-1 or HSV-2, disappear, and the infection remains dormant for varying periods of time. Recurrences can be frequent or minimally episodic.

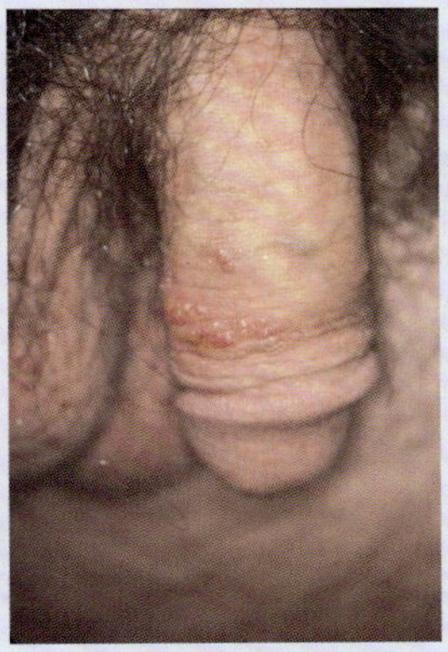

Herpes progenitalis. (CDC/Public Health Image Library.)

GENITAL WARTS

- Single or multiple, moist, fleshy papules.
- Painless.
- STI caused by the human papillomavirus.

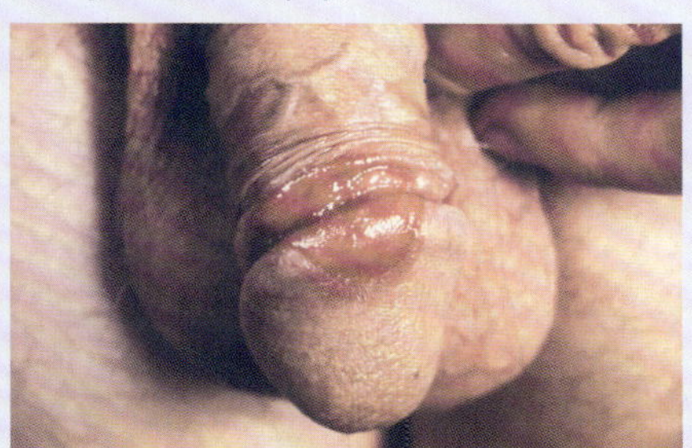

Genital warts. (CDC/Public Health Image Library.)

CANCER OF THE GLANS PENIS

- Appears as hardened nodule or ulcer on the glans.
- Painless.
- Occurs primarily in uncircumcised men.

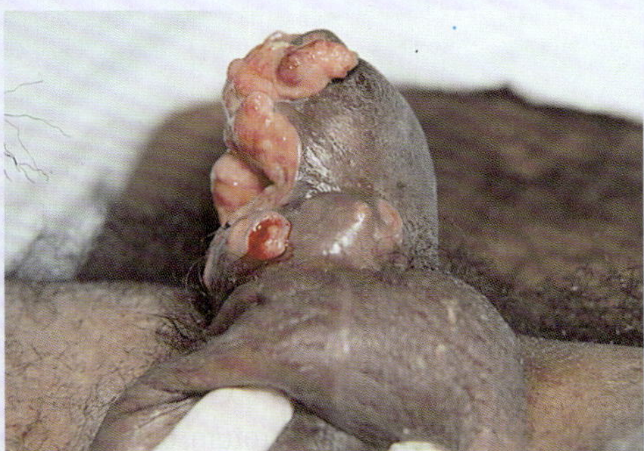

Genital warts.

Continued on following page

ABNORMAL FINDINGS 26-1 Abnormalities of the penis (continued)

PHIMOSIS

Foreskin is so tight that it cannot be retracted over the glans.

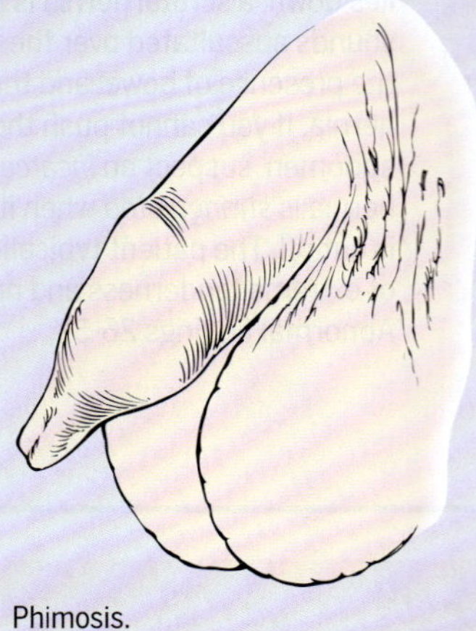

Phimosis.

PARAPHIMOSIS

Foreskin is so tight that, once retracted, it cannot be returned back over the glans.

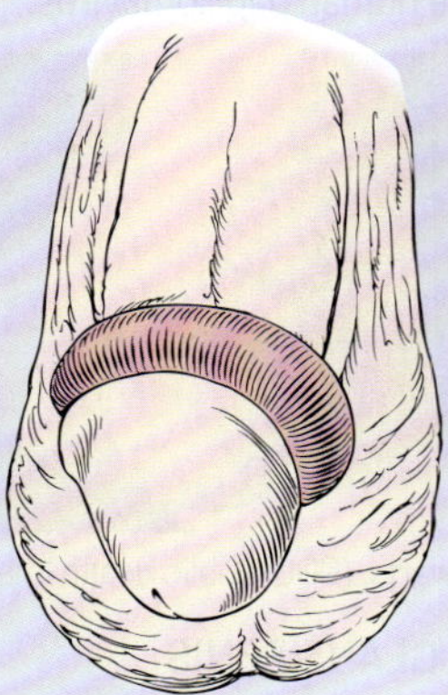

Paraphimosis.

HYPOSPADIAS

- Urethral meatus is located underneath the glans (ventral side).
- This condition is a congenital defect.
- A groove extends from the meatus to the normal location of the urethral meatus.

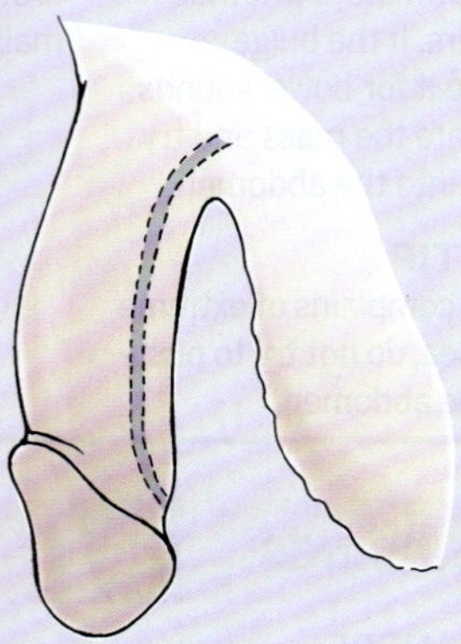

Hypospadias.

EPISPADIAS

- The urethral meatus is located on the top of the glans (dorsal side); occurs rarely.
- This condition is a congenital defect.

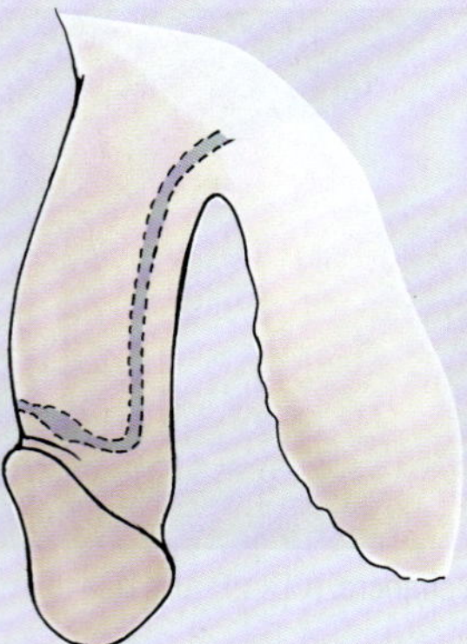

Epispadias.

ABNORMAL FINDINGS 26-2 Abnormalities of the scrotum

Although some scrotal abnormalities can be seen by visual inspection, most must be palpated. Some common abnormalities are described below.

HYDROCOELE

- Collection of serous fluid in the scrotum, outside the testes within the tunica vaginalis.
- Appears as swelling in the scrotum and is usually painless.
- Usually the examiner can get fingers above this mass during palpation.
- Will transilluminate (if there is blood in the scrotum, it will not transilluminate and is called a 'haematocoele').

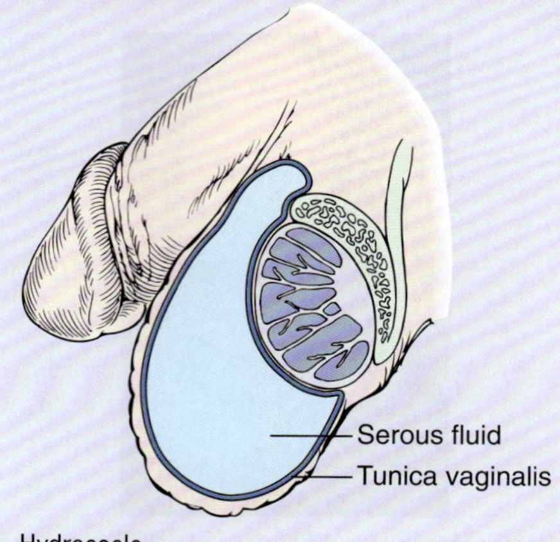

Hydrocoele.

ABNORMAL FINDINGS 26-2 Abnormalities of the scrotum (continued)

SCROTAL HERNIA

- A loop of bowel protrudes into the scrotum to create what is known as an indirect inguinal hernia.
- Hernia appears as swelling in the scrotum.
- Palpable as a soft mass and fingers cannot get above the mass.

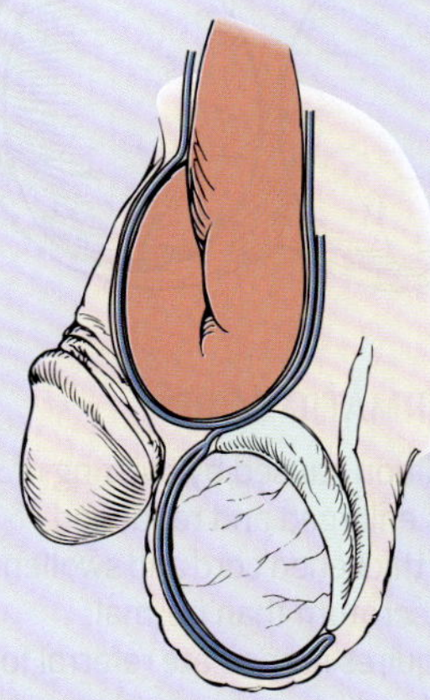

Scrotal hernia.

TESTICULAR TUMOUR

- Initially a small, firm, non-tender nodule on the testis.
- As the tumour grows, the scrotum appears enlarged and the patient complains of a heavy feeling.
- When palpated, the testis feels enlarged and smooth—tumour replaces testis.
- Will not transilluminate.

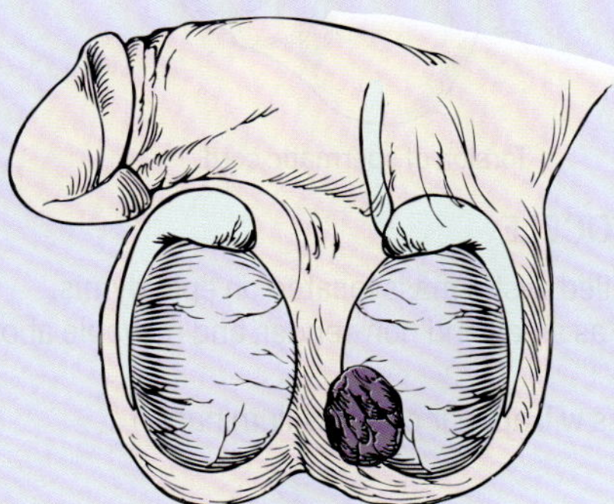

Testicular tumour (A) early

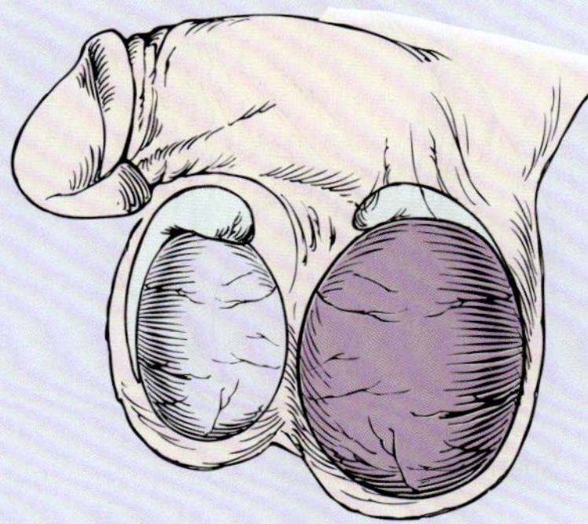

Testicular tumour (B) late

SMALL TESTES

- Small (less than 3.5 cm long), soft testes indicate atrophy. Atrophy may result from cirrhosis, hypopituitarism, oestrogen administration or extended illness, or the disorder may occur after orchitis.
- Small (less than 2 cm long), firm testes may indicate Klinefelter syndrome.

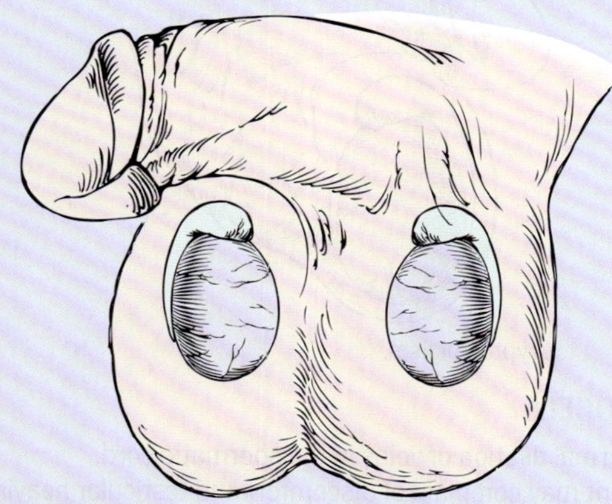

Small testes.

EPIDIDYMITIS

- Infection of the epididymis.
- Patient usually complains of sudden pain.
- Scrotum appears enlarged, reddened and swollen; tender epididymis is palpated.
- Usually associated with prostatitis or bacterial infection.

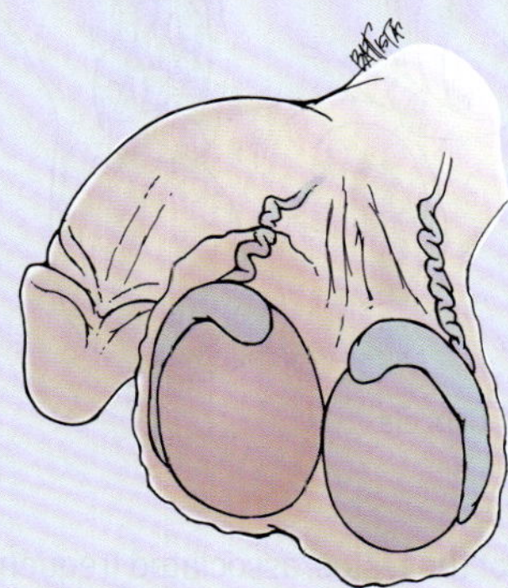

Epididymitis.

Continued on following page

ABNORMAL FINDINGS 26-2 Abnormalities of the scrotum (continued)

CRYPTORCHIDISM

- Failure of one or both testicles to descend into scrotum.
- Scrotum appears undeveloped and testis cannot be palpated.
- Causes increased risk of testicular cancer.

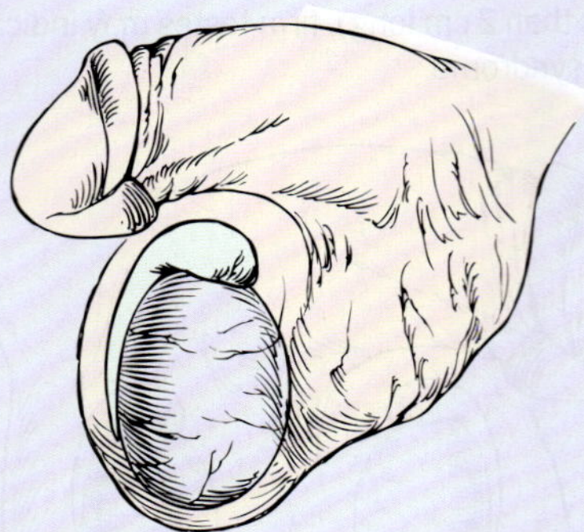

Cryptorchidism.

VARICOCELE

- Abnormal dilation of veins in the spermatic cord.
- Patient may complain of discomfort and testicular heaviness.
- Tortuous veins are palpable and feel like a soft, irregular mass or 'a bag of worms', which collapses when the patient is supine.
- Infertility may be associated with this condition.

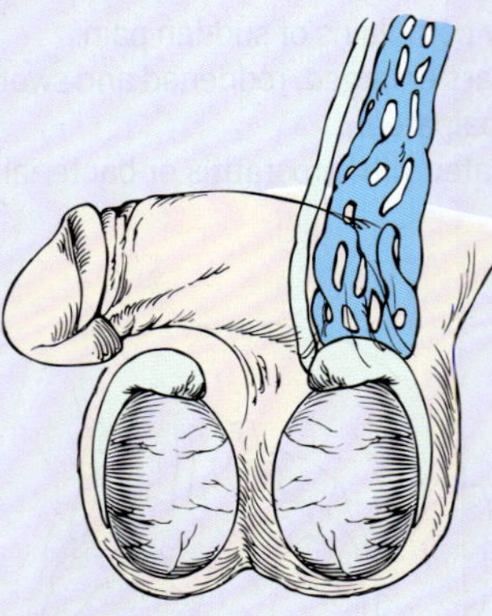

Varicocele.

ORCHITIS

- Inflammation of the testes, associated frequently with mumps.
- Patient complains of pain, heaviness and fever.
- Scrotum appears enlarged and reddened.
- Swollen, tender testis is palpated. The nurse may have difficulty differentiating between testis and epididymis.

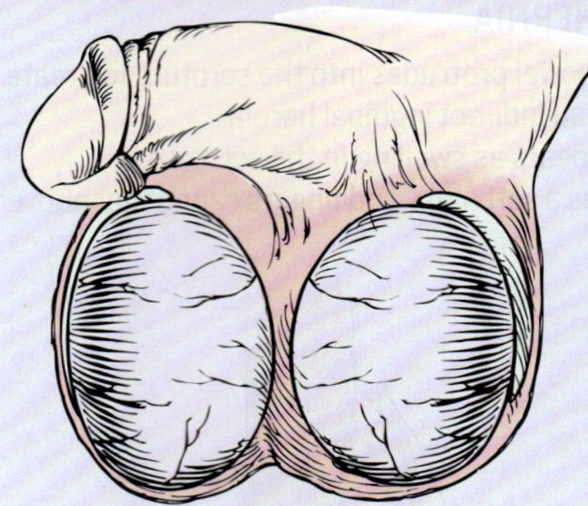

Orchitis.

TORSION OF SPERMATIC CORD

- Very painful condition caused by twisting of spermatic cord.
- Scrotum appears enlarged and reddened.
- Palpation reveals thickened cord and swollen, tender testis that may be higher in scrotum than normal.
- This condition requires immediate referral for surgery because circulation is obstructed.

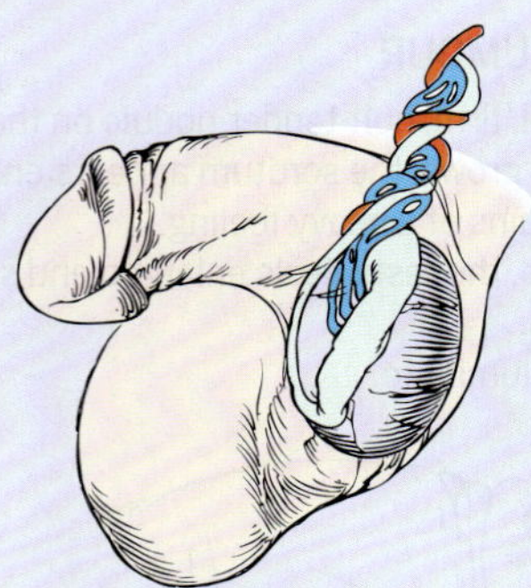

Torsion of spermatic cord.

SPERMATOCELE

- Sperm-filled cystic mass located on epididymis.
- Palpable as small and non-tender, and movable above the testis.
- This mass will appear on transillumination.

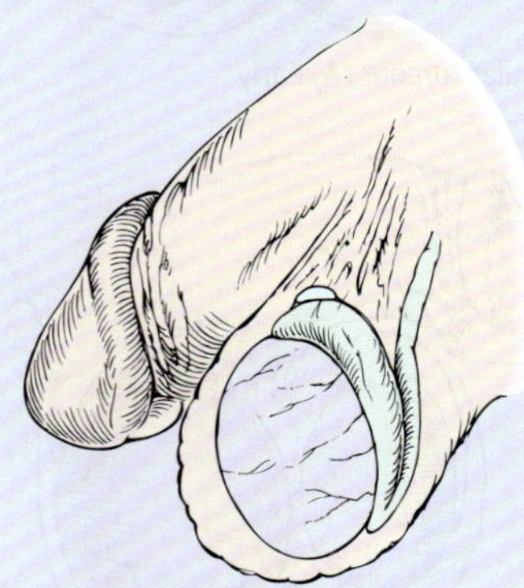

Spermatocele.

ABNORMAL FINDINGS 26-3 Inguinal and femoral hernias

INDIRECT INGUINAL HERNIA

- Bowel herniates through internal inguinal ring and remains in the inguinal canal or travels down into the scrotum (scrotal hernia).
- This is the most common type of hernia.
- It may occur in adults but is more frequent in children.

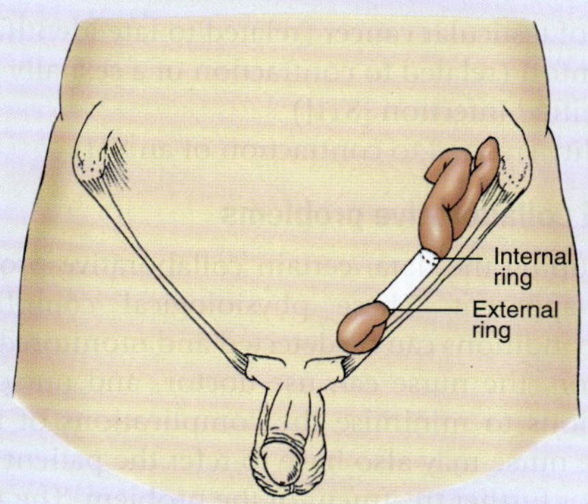

Indirect inguinal hernia.

DIRECT INGUINAL HERNIA

- Bowel herniates from behind and through the external inguinal ring. It rarely travels down into the scrotum.
- This type of hernia is less common than an indirect hernia.
- It occurs mostly in adult men older than age 40.

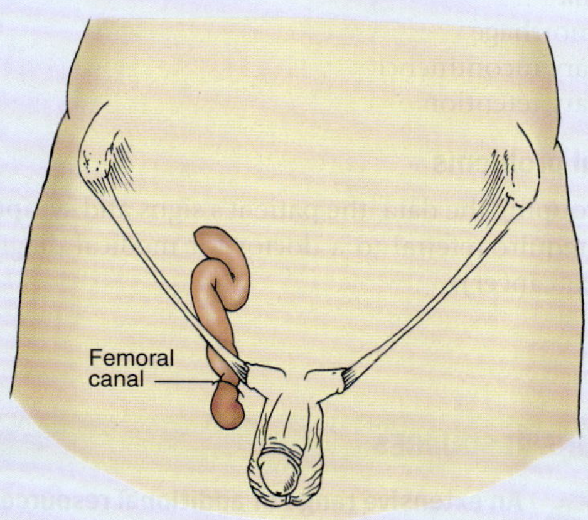

Femoral hernia.

FEMORAL HERNIA

- Bowel herniates through the femoral ring and canal. It never travels into the scrotum, and the inguinal canal is empty.
- This is the least common type of hernia.
- It occurs mostly in women.

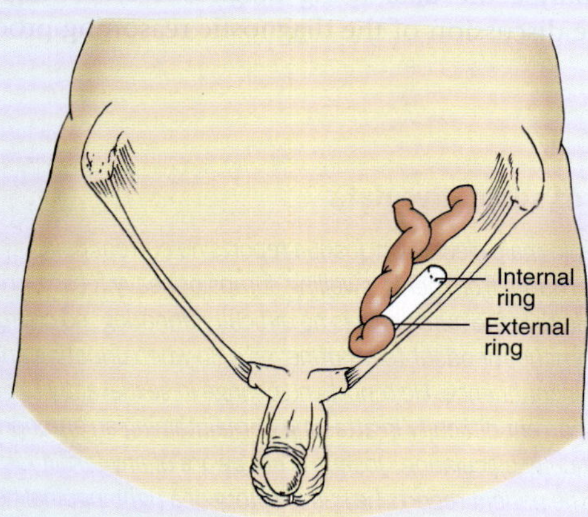

Direct inguinal hernia.

VALIDATING AND DOCUMENTING FINDINGS

Validate the male genitalia assessment data that you have collected. This is necessary to verify that the data are reliable and accurate. Document the assessment data in accord with the hospital or clinic policy.

After you have collected your assessment data, you will need to analyse the data using diagnostic reasoning skills. Refer to the discussion of the diagnostic reasoning process in Chapter 5.

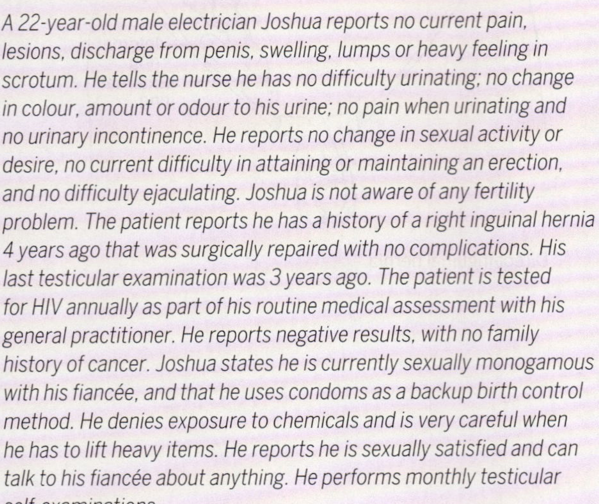

Sample of subjective data

A 22-year-old male electrician Joshua reports no current pain, lesions, discharge from penis, swelling, lumps or heavy feeling in scrotum. He tells the nurse he has no difficulty urinating; no change in colour, amount or odour to his urine; no pain when urinating and no urinary incontinence. He reports no change in sexual activity or desire, no current difficulty in attaining or maintaining an erection, and no difficulty ejaculating. Joshua is not aware of any fertility problem. The patient reports he has a history of a right inguinal hernia 4 years ago that was surgically repaired with no complications. His last testicular examination was 3 years ago. The patient is tested for HIV annually as part of his routine medical assessment with his general practitioner. He reports negative results, with no family history of cancer. Joshua states he is currently sexually monogamous with his fiancée, and that he uses condoms as a backup birth control method. He denies exposure to chemicals and is very careful when he has to lift heavy items. He reports he is sexually satisfied and can talk to his fiancée about anything. He performs monthly testicular self-examinations.

Sample of objective data

Pubic hair growth pattern is normal for adult male; pubic hair and base of penis are free of excoriation and infestation. Circumcised penis is free of rashes, lesions and lumps and is soft, flaccid and non-tender on palpation. Glans is rounded and free of lesions; urinary meatus is centrally located on glans; no discharge is palpated from urinary meatus. No masses or swelling noted in scrotum, and left side hangs slightly lower than right side. Skin is free of lesions and appears rugated and darkly pigmented. Two descended testes palpated. No swelling, tenderness or masses palpated along the testicle, epididymis or spermatic cord on either side. No bulges or masses palpated in inguinal or femoral canal.

Analysis of data

DIAGNOSTIC REASONING: POSSIBLE CONCLUSIONS

After collecting subjective and objective data pertaining to the male genitalia, identify abnormal findings and patient strengths. Then cluster the data to reveal any significant patterns or abnormalities. These data may then be used to make clinical judgements about the status of the male patient's genitalia.

Potential patient risks

- Not undertaking monthly testicular self-examinations (related to lack of knowledge of the importance of this procedure)
- Infection (related to unprotected sexual intercourse)

Potential patient problems

- Onset of testicular cancer (related to late identification)
- Discomfort (related to contraction of a sexually transmitted infection [STI])
- Infertility (related to contraction of an STI)

Selected collaborative problems

After grouping the data, certain collaborative problems may become apparent. These physiological complications of medical conditions can be detected and monitored by a nurse. In addition, the nurse can use doctor- and nurse-prescribed interventions to minimise the complications of these problems. The nurse may also have to refer the patient in such situations for further treatment of the problem. The following is a list of collaborative problems that may be identified when assessing the male genitalia:

- Gonorrhoea
- Syphilis
- Genital warts
- Erectile dysfunction
- Inability to ejaculate
- Hernia
- Haemorrhage
- Urinary incontinence
- Urinary retention.

Medical problems

After grouping the data, the patient's signs and symptoms may clearly require referral to a doctor for medical diagnoses (i.e. testicular cancer).

ONLINE RESOURCES

An extensive range of additional resources to enhance teaching and learning and to facilitate understanding may be found online at the text's accompanying website, located on thePoint at http://thepoint.lww.com. These include Watch and Learn videos, Concepts in Action animations, journal articles, case studies, discussion topics and quizzes.

Subscribers may also access Lippincott Procedures, an extensive online point-of-care procedure guide that provides reliable step-by-step instructions for more than 1700 procedures, including 450 evidence-based Australian procedures, and skills in a variety of speciality settings, together with a wealth of supporting information.

CASE STUDY

The case study demonstrates how to analyse male genitalia assessment data for a specific patient. It also demonstrates that often completion of a sound patient examination combined with the provision of clear patient education yields nothing to follow-up.

Joshua is a 22-year-old electrician. One of Joshua's work colleagues told him there were some sexually transmitted infections that you didn't know you had and that they could cause infertility. As he is sexually active, Joshua was keen to find out more about what he could do to protect himself and presented to a sexual health clinic. He met with, and was examined by a registered nurse.

The nurse's questioning revealed the patient's urinary and sexual function was normal. Joshua reported he was not aware of any fertility problems, but noted he had a history of a right inguinal hernia 4 years ago that was surgically repaired with no complications. When asked about postoperative concerns, Joshua explained that although his job can be physical and dangerous, he is very careful when he has to lift heavy items; however, he requested further information about the risk that lifting heavy objects posed. Joshua also confided that although he performed testicular self-examinations, he had questions about his technique and the value of performing the examinations.

The nurse was able to determine that Joshua had no physical problems with his genitalia. The nurse created a safe environment and used good clear communication, which allowed Joshua to give an honest detailed medical and sexual history. Joshua was then able to confide that he had questions regarding his postoperative concerns regarding lifting. He was also able to seek clarification on performing testicular self-examination. Clear communication allowed the nurse to provide the patient with the help he required.

Note: There is no COLDSPA or concept map for Joshua as his case has been provided as an example of a well patient; thus, further examination is not required in this instance.

References

Andrology Australia (Healthy Male). (2019). Testicular cancer. Viewed July 2019 at http://www.healthymale.org.au/mens-health/testicular-cancer.

ASHM. (2019). Testing portal, ASHM national HIV testing policy. Viewed July 2019 at http://testingportal.ashm.org.au/images/HIV_Testing_Policy_Feb_2017.pdf

Australian Government, Cancer Australia. (2019). Cancer statistics. Canberra: Author. View October 2019 at https://canceraustralia.gov.au/affected-cancer/cancer-statistics.

Australian Sexual Health Alliance (ASHA). (2019). Australian STI management guidelines for use in primary care, Viewed July 2019 at http://www.sti.guidelines.org.au/.

Australian Federation of AIDS Organisations (AFAO). (2019). HIV in Australia 2019. Viewed July 2019 at https://www.afao.org.au/wp-content/uploads/2018/12/HIV-in-Australia-2019_No-Bleed.pdf.

Cancer Council Australia. (2019) Testicular cancer. Viewed July 2019 at www.cancer.org.au/about-cancer/types-of-cancer/testicular-cancer.html.

Goodheart, H. P. (1999). *A photoguide of common skin disorders*. Baltimore: Lippincott Williams & Wilkins.

Schiegel, A. & Barry, H. (2017). Pain fear and circumcision in boy's adolescent initiation ceremonies. *Cross-Cultural Research, 51*(5), 435–463.

Tanner, J. M. (1962). *Growth at adolescence* (2nd ed.). Oxford: Blackwell Scientific Publications.

Testicular Cancer NZ. (2019). About testicular cancer. Viewed July 2019 at https://testicular.org.nz/about-testicular-cancer/.

WHO. (2019). HIV/AIDS. Viewed July 2019 at https://www.who.int/hiv/data/en/.

New Zealand AIDS Foundation. (2019). HIV in New Zealand. Viewed July 2019 at https://www.nzaf.org.nz/hiv-aids-stis/hiv-aids/hiv-in-new-zealand/.

Smith, Z. L., Werntz, R. P. & Eggener, S. E. (2018). Testicular cancer: Epidemiology, diagnosis and management. *The Medical Clinics of North America, 102*(2), 251–264.

Wilkinson, L. A., Pedrana, E. A., et al. (2016). The impact of a social marketing campaign on HIV and sexually transmissible infection testing among men who have sex with men in Australia. *Sexually Transmitted Diseases, 43*(1), 49–56.

Wu, C. & Jarvi, K. (2018). Chronic scrotal pain. *Current Urology Reports, 19*(8), 1–8.

Online resources

Andrology Australia (Healthy Male) (Monash University Centre of Excellence): www.andrologyaustralia.org

Auckland Sexual Health Service: www.ashs.org.nz

Australian Government Department of Health, cancer screening: www.cancerscreening.gov.au

Australian Institute of Health and Welfare, cancer rates: www.aihw.gov.au

Australian Sexual Health Alliance: www.sti.guidelines.org.au

Cancer Council Australia: www.cancer.org.au

Cancer Society of New Zealand: www.cancernz.org.nz

Health*direct*: www.healthdirect.gov.au

Mens Health Australia: www.menshealthaustralia.net

New Zealand National Screening Unit: www.nsu.govt.nz

New Zealand Sexual Health Society: www.nzshs.org

Testicular Cancer NZ: www.testicular.org.nz

Selected readings

Jefferies, M. T., Cox, A. C., et al. (2015). The management of acute testicular pain in children and adolescents. *British Medical Journal, 350*, 1–8.

CHAPTER 27

Anus, rectum and prostate

CASE STUDY

George Kowalsky, a 42-year-old male, is seeking advice from the local community health clinic because he has been 'bleeding from his rectum' and has pain and pressure in the rectal area. Mr Kowalsky is the head accountant and tax consultant for a high-profile company. He is currently preparing for the annual audit and reports to the nurse that he is 'very uptight'.

Structure and function

ANUS AND RECTUM

The anal canal is the final segment of the digestive system; it begins at the anal sphincter and ends at the anorectal junction (Fig. 27-1). It measures from 2.5 to 4 cm long. It is lined with skin that contains no hair or sebaceous glands but does contain many somatic sensory nerves, making it susceptible to painful stimuli. The anal opening or anal verge can be distinguished from the perianal skin by its hairless moist appearance. The anal verge extends interiorly, overlying the external anal sphincter.

Within the anus are the two sphincters that normally hold the anal canal closed except when passing gas and faeces. The external sphincter is composed of skeletal muscle and is under voluntary control. The internal sphincter is composed of smooth muscle and is under involuntary control by the autonomic nervous system. Dividing the two sphincters is the palpable intersphincteric groove. The anal canal proceeds upward towards the umbilicus. Just above the internal sphincter is the anorectal junction (also known as the pectinate line, mucocutaneous junction or dentate line), the dividing point of the anal canal and the rectum. The rectum is lined with folds of mucosa, known as the columns of Morgagni. The anorectal junction is not palpable, but may be visualised during internal examination. The folds contain a network of arteries, veins and visceral nerves. Between the columns are recessed areas known as anal crypts; there are 8 to 12 anal crypts and 5 to 8 papillae. If the veins in these folds undergo chronic pressure, they may become engorged with blood, forming haemorrhoids.

The rectum is the lowest portion of the large intestine and is approximately 12 cm long, extending from the end of the

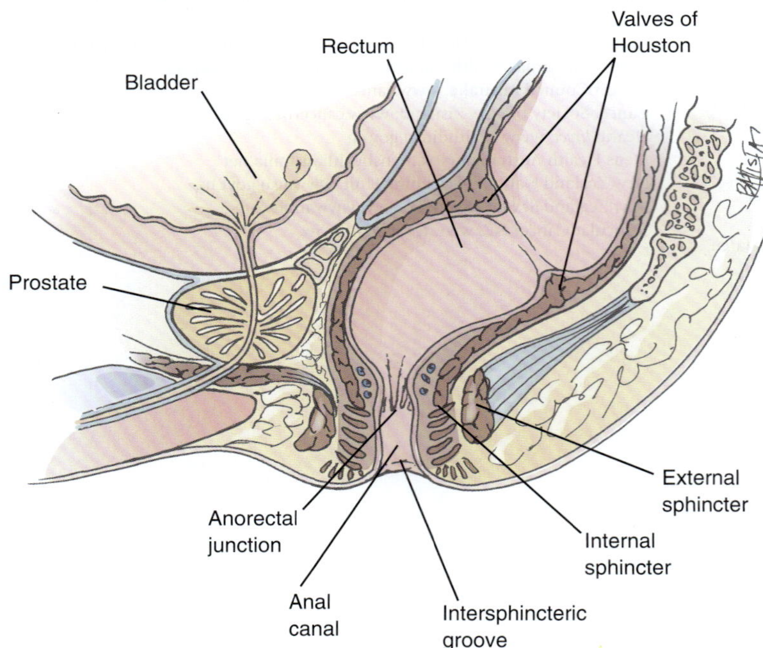

FIGURE 27-1 Anal and rectal structures.

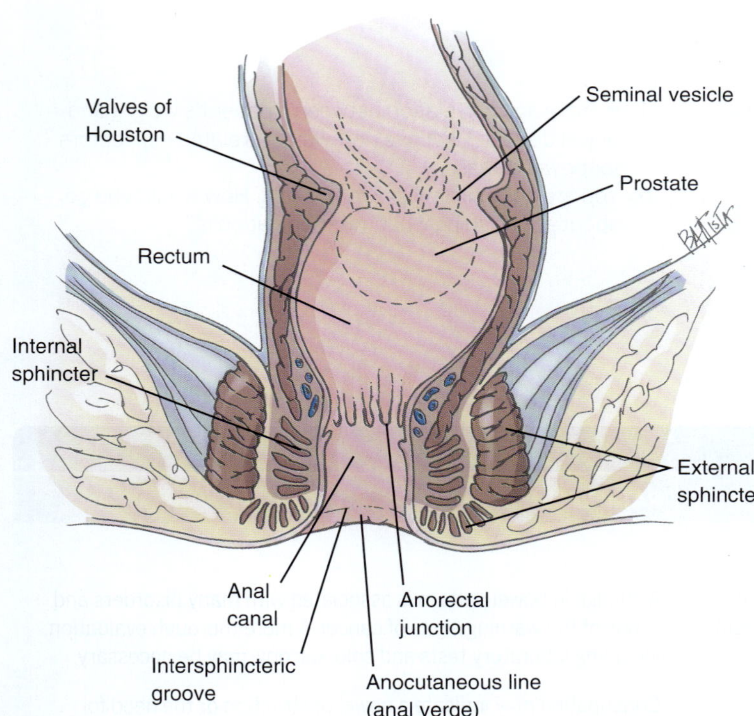

FIGURE 27-2 Prostate gland and nearby structures.

sigmoid colon to the anorectal junction. It enlarges above the anorectal junction and proceeds in a posterior direction towards the hollow of the sacrum and coccyx, forming the rectal ampulla. The anal canal and rectum are at approximately right angles to each other. The inside of the rectum contains three inward foldings called the valves of Houston. The function of these valves is unclear. The lowest valve may be felt, usually on the patient's left side.

The peritoneum lines the upper two-thirds of the anterior rectum and dips down enough so that it may be palpated where it forms the rectovesical pouch in men and the rectouterine pouch in women.

PROSTATE

The prostate gland is approximately 2.5 to 4 cm in diameter; it surrounds the neck of the bladder and the urethra and lies between these structures and the rectum in male patients. It consists of two lobes separated by a shallow groove called the median sulcus. It secretes a thin, milky substance that promotes sperm motility and neutralises female acidic vaginal secretions. This chestnut- or heart-shaped organ can be palpated through the anterior wall of the rectum.

OLDER ADULT CONSIDERATIONS

The prostate gland increases in size in most men over the age of 50. Benign prostatic hyperplasia is a commonly encountered condition, especially in men 65 years or older.

Located on either side of, and above, the prostate gland are the seminal vesicles (Fig. 27-2). These are rabbit-ear–shaped structures that produce the ejaculate that nourishes and protects sperm. They are not normally palpable. Cowper or bulbourethral glands are mucus-producing, pea-sized organs located posterior to the prostate gland. These glands surround and empty into the urethra. They are not normally palpable, either.

Health assessment

COLLECTING SUBJECTIVE DATA: THE NURSING HEALTH HISTORY

The data gathered during subjective assessment provide clues to the patient's overall health and whether the patient is at risk of diseases and disorders of the anus, rectum or prostate. The subjective assessment is a good time to teach the patient about risk factors related to diseases, such as colorectal or prostate cancer, and about ways to decrease those risk factors.

Collecting data about the anus, rectum and prostate can be embarrassing for both the examiner and the patient. Some questions are very personal. Therefore, it is important to ease the patient's anxiety as much as possible. Ask the questions in a straightforward manner, and let the patient voice any concerns throughout the assessment. In some cultural groups, only nurses of the same gender will be considered acceptable assessors of intimate body areas.

CASE STUDY

When questioned, Mr Kowalsky reports that he has observed small amounts of bright-red blood on his stools for the last 2 days and for about the last week his bowel movements have been quite painful—'like passing ground glass'. He states that he has had hard bowel movements for many years. He drinks 10 to 12 cups of coffee per day. For the most part his meals include traditional eggs and bacon for breakfast and meat and potatoes for dinner. He doesn't really like vegetables or fruit. He doesn't eat excessively and has maintained his weight 'within the chart norms' for more than 20 years. For years he has used Proctosedyl (Rectinol) ointment for his 'piles' with relief—until recently.

CRITICAL THINKING

1. What factor in Mr Kowalsky's history is suggestive of a disease of the bowel?
2. What questions would you, as the clinic nurse, ask Mr Kowalsky that would provide additional information pertinent to the assessment of his condition?
3. What risk factors for bowel disease does your assessment of Mr Kowalsky's history yield?
4. Is there any correlation between a patient's weight and bowel disease? List five non-weight–related risk factors for bowel disease.
5. You are unfamiliar with Proctosedyl. How would you go about establishing what this medication is?

History of present health concern

QUESTION	RATIONALE
Bowel patterns	
What is your usual bowel pattern? Have you noticed any recent change in the pattern? Any pain while passing a bowel movement?	A change in bowel pattern is associated with many disorders and is one of the warning signs of cancer. A more thorough evaluation, including laboratory tests and colonoscopy, may be necessary.
Do you experience constipation?	Constipation may indicate a bowel obstruction or the need for dietary counselling.
Do you experience diarrhoea? Is the diarrhoea associated with any nausea or vomiting?	Diarrhoea may signal impaction or infection, or indicate the need for dietary counselling.

COLDSPA

Example for rectal pain

Use the COLDSPA mnemonic as a guideline to collect needed information for each symptom the patient shares. In addition, the following questions help elicit important information.

Mnemonic	Question	Patient response example
Character	Describe the sign or symptom (feeling, appearance, sound or smell).	'My rectal area hurts right when I have a bowel movement and right after the bowel movement it really hurts.'
Onset	When did it begin?	'About 2 weeks ago, but I thought it would go away.'
Location	Where is it? Does it radiate? Does it occur anywhere else?	'I feel like I have a knot around my rectal area and I am worried about what it is.'
Duration	How long does it last? Does it recur?	'Sometimes it gets better. I had this 9 months ago, but it went away. This time, after taking a long car trip and sitting for long periods, it came back and is not getting any better.'
Severity	How bad is it? or How much does it bother you?	'Right now it really hurts badly. I would rate it a 9 on a scale of 1 to 10. The rectal knot is also getting bigger.'
Pattern	What makes it better or worse?	'A warm bath makes it feel better for a while. Straining if I am constipated makes it worse.'
Associated factors/How it Affects the patient	What other symptoms occur with it? How does it affect you?	'I am scared I may have cancer because of the knot down there.'

Past health history

QUESTION	RATIONALE
Do you have trouble controlling your bowels?	Faecal incontinence occurs with neurological disorders, some gastrointestinal infections and particular dietary habits.
Faecal stool	
What is the colour of your stool? Hard or soft? Have you noticed any blood on or in your stool? If so, how much?	Black stools may indicate gastrointestinal bleeding or the use of iron supplements or antacids. Red blood in the stool is found with haemorrhoids, polyps, cancer or colitis. Clay-coloured stools result from a lack of bile pigment.
Have you noticed any mucus in your stool?	Mucus in the stool may indicate steatorrhoea (excessive fat in the stool).
Itching and pain	
Do you experience any itching or pain in the rectal area?	Sexually transmitted infections, haemorrhoids, helminths or anal trauma may cause itching or pain (see Promote health—Haemorrhoids).
Have you ever had anal or rectal trauma or surgery? Were you born with any congenital deformities of the anus or rectum? Have you had prostate surgery? Have you had haemorrhoids or surgery for haemorrhoids?	Past conditions influence the findings of physical assessment. Congenital deformities, such as imperforate anus, are often surgically repaired when the patient is very young.
When was the last time you had a faecal stool test to detect blood, commonly known as FOBT (faecal occult blood test)?	The Royal Australian College of General Practitioners (RACGP) recommends an FOBT every 2 years from the age of 50 because of a known 16% reduction in colorectal cancer mortality (RACGP, 2018). Within Australia, the National Bowel Cancer Screening Program offers free FOBT for all people every 2 years between the ages of 50 and 74, and similarly in New Zealand every 2 years for those between the ages of 60 and 74 (Cancer Council, 2019; Time to Screen NZ, 2019)

Continued on following page

PROMOTE HEALTH — HAEMORRHOIDS

OVERVIEW

Haemorrhoids are formed when excessive pressure affects the veins in the pelvis and rectal areas. The tissues surrounding the inside of the anus fill with blood to help control bowel movements. With excessive pressure, the blood in the veins within these tissues causes veins to swell and stretch the surrounding tissue. There are many causes including straining when rushing to complete a bowel movement or with constipation or diarrhoea; being overweight; the last 6 months of pregnancy and delivery; prolonged standing or sitting; liver or heart disease if blood is pooled in the abdomen or pelvis; and, rarely, tumours in the pelvic area. Haemorrhoids can occur at any age but usually occur after 30 years of age, with approximately 50% of people over 50 having had some haemorrhoid problems during their lives.

Risk factors

- Poor bowel habits (rushing bowel movements with straining; not heeding the feeling of need for a bowel movement)
- Pregnancy (after 6 months and during labour)
- Inadequate fluid intake
- Inadequate fibre intake
- Prolonged standing or sitting
- Inadequate exercise
- Spending long periods of time on the toilet.

Teach risk reduction tips

- Avoid constipation.
- Avoid straining with bowel movements; avoid holding breath when passing bowel movement.
- Go to the bathroom as soon as urge occurs; leave as soon as bowel movement completed.
- Eat a diet with moderate fibre intake; whole grains, raw vegetables, raw and dried fruits, legumes (beans, lentils).
- Avoid a diet that has little or no fibre (ice cream, soft drinks, cheese, white bread, red meat).
- Drink 6 to 8 glasses of water daily. Avoid caffeine and alcohol.
- Evaluate foods that might worsen symptoms, such as nuts, spicy foods, coffee and alcohol.
- Avoid foods that may cause diarrhoea (intense diarrhoea resulting from food poisoning can cause haemorrhoids).
- Consult primary health care provider for safety of taking stool softeners with bran or psyllium.
- Avoid taking laxatives unless directed by a clinician (can cause diarrhoea or irritate haemorrhoids).
- Undertake exercise for at least 30 minutes per day.
- Avoid lifting heavy objects often and do not hold breath with lifting.
- Keep a food diary to determine what exacerbates or relieves the condition.

Past health history (continued)

QUESTION	RATIONALE
Have you ever had colonoscopy?	Colonoscopy is recommended every 5 years from the age of 50 based on the risk assessment made by a medical practitioner.
When was the last time you had a digital rectal examination (DRE)?	A DRE may reveal rectal masses, prostate enlargement or prostate nodules. Studies have shown that there is no evidence to support a DRE as a screening tool for bowel cancer, rather its use guides the determination of further investigations based on findings (Bowel Cancer Australia, 2019).
Have you ever had blood taken for a prostate screening, which measures the level of prostate-specific antigen (PSA) in your blood? When was the test and what was the result?	PSA is a biological marker for prostate cancer. The Prostate Cancer Foundation of Australia (2019) recommends males between the ages of 50 and 69 be offered a PSA every 2 years and in addition discuss with their medical practitioner the benefits and limitations of PSA testing.

Family history

QUESTION	RATIONALE
Is there a history of polyps, colon or rectal cancer, or prostate cancer in your family?	Colorectal and prostate cancer have a tendency to affect members of the same family (see Promote health—Prostate cancer and Promote health—Colorectal cancer below).

PROMOTE HEALTH **PROSTATE CANCER**

OVERVIEW

Prostate cancer is the most commonly diagnosed cancer in men. More men die of prostate cancer than women die of breast cancer each year, making prostate cancer the third leading cause of cancer death in men in Australia and New Zealand (Cancer Australia, 2019). One in five males will be diagnosed with prostate cancer and around 95% will survive for 5 years after diagnosis, although more than 3,100 males in Australia and 600 in New Zealand die each year as a result of prostate cancer (Cancer Australia, 2019; Prostate Cancer Foundation NZ, 2019). Prostate cancer is slow-growing and can be readily treated if found early. There is no sure way to prevent prostate cancer, but diet and lifestyle behaviours are thought to help with prevention.

Risk factors

- Age: increasing age is the most important and best-documented risk factor
- Family history: the genetic basis has not been fully determined; 5% to 10% of prostate cancers may be linked to genetic predisposition
- Ethnicity: Aboriginal and Torres Strait Islander peoples are less likely to be diagnosed with prostate cancer than non-Aboriginal and Torres Strait Islander Australians (Australian Institute of Health and Welfare [AIHW], 2019). New Zealand Māori males also have a much lower registration of prostate cancer, but a mortality rate almost twice that of non-Māori males (New Zealand Ministry of Health [NZMOH], 2018a).
- Dietary fat (especially high intake of red meat and high-fat dairy products)
- Dairy and calcium intake (some studies suggest this)
- Exposure to cadmium, dioxin or toxic combustion products (studies are limited)
- Frequent sexually transmitted infections (conclusive evidence is lacking)
- A multi-year large-scale research trial exploring whether selenium or vitamin E increases or reduces the risk of prostate cancer found that selenium did not prevent prostate cancer (Nicastro & Dunn, 2013). Furthermore, the same study found that vitamin E supplementation was associated with an increased risk of prostate cancer.

Teach risk reduction tips

- Avoid high-fat foods.
- Eat a diet rich in fruits and vegetables, high in fibre and high in omega-3 fatty acids.
- Maintain a healthy weight (avoid obesity).
- Get moderate exercise daily.
- Soy products and other legumes have phyto-oestrogens that may have a positive effect.
- Regular consumption of both green tea and cooked tomatoes (rich in lycopenes) may contribute to risk reduction.
- Drink no more than two alcoholic drinks per day.
- Have regular consultations with your health professional regarding prostate health.

COLLECTING OBJECTIVE DATA: PHYSICAL EXAMINATION

A physical examination of the anus and rectum should be performed on all adult men and women. It should be performed regardless of whether the patient complains of symptoms because some conditions, such as cancerous tumours, may be asymptomatic (Display 27-1). Detecting problems with the anus, rectum or prostate is the primary objective of this examination. Early detection of a problem is one way to promote early treatment and a more positive outcome. The examiner may also use this time to integrate teaching about ways to reduce risk factors for diseases and disorders of the anus, rectum and prostate.

PROMOTE HEALTH **COLORECTAL CANCER**

OVERVIEW

Colorectal cancer is the third most commonly diagnosed cancer in both males and females in Australia and New Zealand. It is also the second leading cause of cancer deaths in both countries (AIHW, 2019; NZMOH, 2018b).

Risk factors

- Any age, but 90% occur over age 50
- Personal history of rectal or colon polyps or cancer
- Inflammatory bowel diseases
- Genetics: family history of cancer or familial colorectal cancer syndromes
- Diet mostly from animal sources (high in fat and animal protein; low in fruits, vegetables and fibre)
- Physical inactivity
- Obesity
- Moderate to heavy alcohol consumption
- Smoking
- Diabetes mellitus

Teach risk reduction tips

- For people at average risk: Beginning at age 50, have a faecal occult blood test (FOBT) every 2 years and a sigmoidoscopic examination every 5 years, or a colonoscopic examination every 10 years, or a double contrast barium enema every 5 to 10 years.
- For people with a personal history of polyps or with first-degree relatives who are cancer patients: Have a colonoscopy at age 40 and every 5 to 10 years thereafter.
- Eat a diet high in fibre, fruit and vegetables, and low in fat and animal protein.
- Limit alcohol consumption.
- Get regular exercise for at least 30 minutes most days.
- Be aware of colorectal cancer symptoms, and if they develop, check with your doctor. Symptoms include:
    - A change in bowel habits, such as diarrhoea, constipation or narrowing of the stool (pencil thin) that lasts for more than a few days; the feeling you need to have a bowel movement that is not relieved by doing so
    - Rectal bleeding or blood in the stool
    - Cramping or steady abdominal pain
    - Decreased appetite
    - Weakness and fatigue
    - Jaundice.

DISPLAY 27-1 SCREENING GUIDELINES FOR THE EARLY DETECTION OF COLORECTAL CANCER

From the age of 50, men and women should follow one of the following examination schedules:

- For those with a low risk score, faecal occult blood testing every 2 years
- For those with a moderate risk score, colonoscopy every 5 years.

People at moderate to high risk for colorectal cancer need to talk with their doctor about a more rigorous testing schedule.

Royal Australian College of General Practitioners (2019 reprint).

Preparing the patient

The hands-on physical examination of the anus, rectum and prostate can cause most patients anxiety and embarrassment. It is important to proceed slowly, encourage relaxation and explain all steps of the examination as you proceed. Use gentle movements with your finger and make sure you use adequate lubrication. Listen to and watch the patient for signs of discomfort or tensing muscles. If the examination is being performed as part of a comprehensive physical examination, it is best to perform the examination of the anus, rectum and prostate at the end of the genitalia examination. It is also important to ask the patient to empty their bladder and bowels prior to physical assessment.

Positioning the patient is important for this examination, and several different positions can be assumed (Fig. 27-3). It is most logical for the female patient to stay in the lithotomy position after the vaginal examination for the anus and rectum examination. Some examiners find it easiest to perform the male anus, rectum and prostate examination while the patient stands and bends over the examining table with his hips flexed. Whichever position the examiner decides would be best for the particular patient and examination, it is important to determine if the patient is as comfortable as possible in that position.

The most frequently used position is the left lateral position. This position allows adequate inspection and palpation of the anus, rectum and prostate (in men) and is usually more comfortable for the patient. The patient's torso and legs should be draped during the examination, which helps to lessen the feeling of vulnerability. To help the patient into this position, ask them to lie on the left side, with the buttocks as close to the edge of the examining table as possible, and to bend the right knee. No matter which position is chosen, remember that you will only be able to examine up to a certain point in the rectum using your finger. If an examination of the upper rectum and sigmoid colon is necessary, a colonoscopy should be performed.

Equipment

- Gloves
- Water-soluble lubricant

Physical assessment

During examination of the patient, remember these key points:

- Understand the structures and functions of the anorectal region.
- Prepare the patient thoroughly for the physical examination to put the patient at the greatest ease.
- Perform the examination professionally and preserve the patient's modesty.
- Remember to wear gloves.

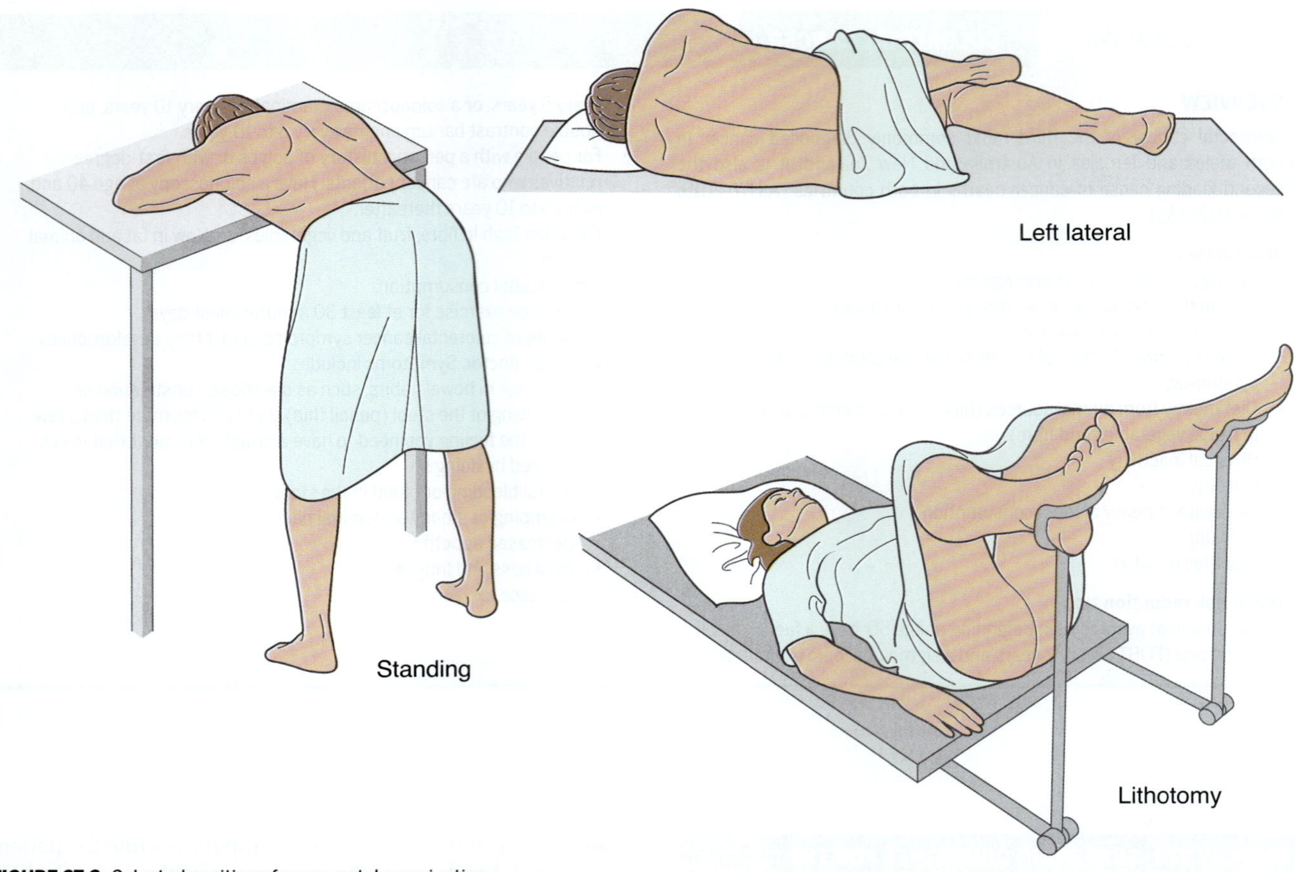

FIGURE 27-3 Selected positions for anorectal examination.

PHYSICAL ASSESSMENT

ASSESSMENT PROCEDURE	NORMAL FINDINGS	ABNORMAL FINDINGS
Anus and rectum		
INSPECTION		
Inspect the perianal area. Spread the patient's buttocks and inspect the anal opening and surrounding area (Fig. 27-4) for the following: • Lumps • Ulcers • Lesions • Rashes • Redness • Fissures • Thickening of the epithelium.	The anal opening should appear hairless, moist and tightly closed. The skin around the anal opening is more coarse and more darkly pigmented. The surrounding perianal area should be free of redness, lumps, ulcers, lesions and rashes.	Lesions may indicate sexually transmitted infections, cancer or haemorrhoids. A thrombosed external haemorrhoid appears swollen. It is itchy, painful and bleeds when the patient passes faecal stool. A previously thrombosed haemorrhoid appears as a skin tag that protrudes from the anus. A painful mass that is hardened and reddened suggests a perianal abscess.

PHYSICAL ASSESSMENT (continued)

ASSESSMENT PROCEDURE	NORMAL FINDINGS	ABNORMAL FINDINGS
Anus and rectum (continued)		
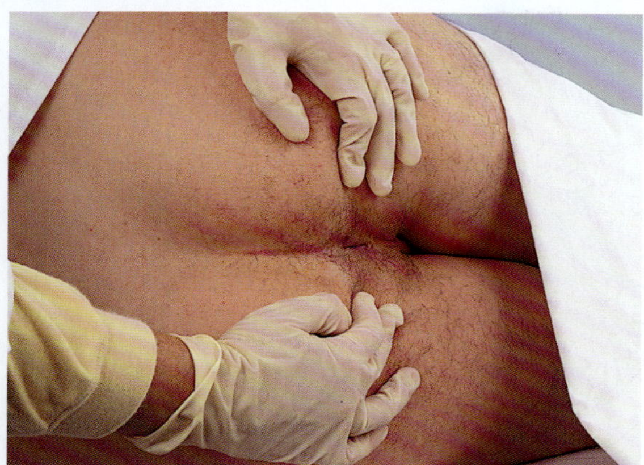 **FIGURE 27-4** Inspecting the perianal area. (© B. Proud.)		A swollen skin tag on the anal margin may indicate a fissure in the anal canal. Redness and excoriation may be from scratching an area infected by fungi or helminths. A small opening in the skin that surrounds the anal opening may be an anorectal fistula (see Abnormal findings 27-1). Thickening of the epithelium suggests repeated trauma from anal intercourse.
Ask the patient to perform the Valsalva manoeuvre by straining or bearing down. Inspect the anal opening for any bulges or lesions.	No bulging or lesions appear.	Bulges of red mucous membrane may indicate a rectal prolapse. Haemorrhoids or an anal fissure may also be seen (see Abnormal findings 27-1). **CLINICAL TIP** **Document any abnormalities by noting position in relation to a face of a clock.**
Inspect the sacrococcygeal area. Inspect this area for any signs of swelling, redness, dimpling or hair.	Area is normally smooth and free of redness and hair.	A reddened, swollen or dimpled area covered by a small tuft of hair located midline on the lower sacrum suggests a pilonidal cyst (see Abnormal findings 27-1).
PALPATION		
Palpate the anus. Inform the patient that you are going to perform the internal examination at this point. Explain that it may feel like his or her bowels are going to move but that this will not happen. Lubricate your gloved index finger; ask the patient to bear down. As the patient bears down, place the pad of your index finger on the anal opening and apply slight pressure; this will cause relaxation of the sphincter. **CLINICAL TIP** **Never use your fingertip—this causes the sphincter to tighten and, if forced into the rectum, may cause pain.**	Patient's sphincter relaxes, permitting entry.	Sphincter tightens, making further examination unrealistic. **CLINICAL TIP** **The use of a chaperone is a requirement in most Australian and New Zealand health settings to protect the interests of both the patient and the attending clinician both throughout and following an intimate assessment.**
When you feel the sphincter relax, insert your finger gently with the pad facing down (Figs 27-5 and 27-6).	Examination finger enters anus.	Examination finger cannot enter the anus. **CLINICAL TIP** **If severe pain prevents your entrance to the anus, do not force the examination.**

Continued on following page

PHYSICAL ASSESSMENT (continued)

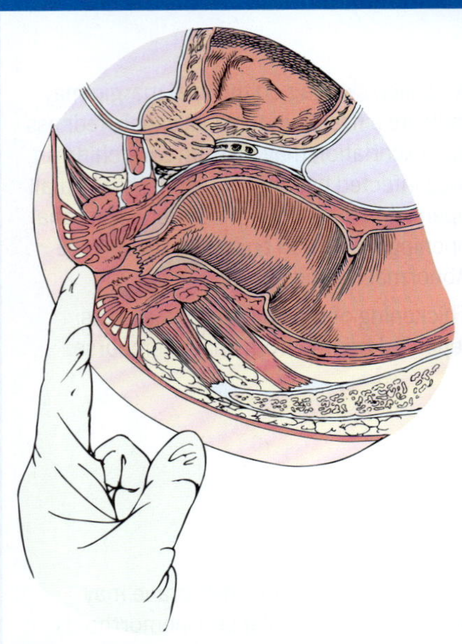

FIGURE 27-5 Relaxing the anal sphincter.

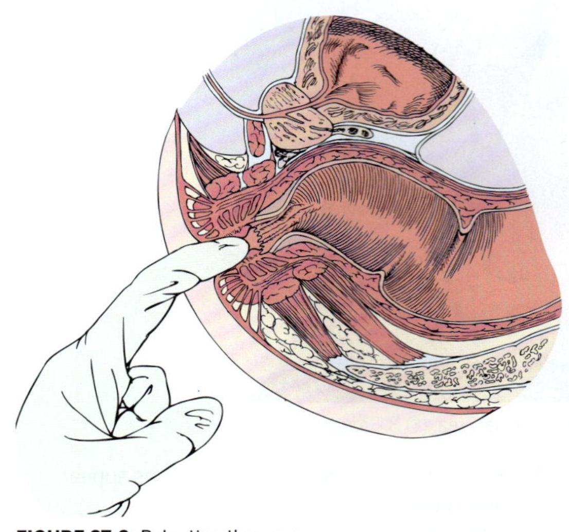

FIGURE 27-6 Palpating the anus.

ASSESSMENT PROCEDURE	NORMAL FINDINGS	ABNORMAL FINDINGS
If the sphincter does not relax and the patient reports severe pain, spread the gluteal folds with your hands in close approximation to the anus and attempt to visualise a lesion that may be causing the pain. If tension is maintained on the gluteal folds for 60 seconds, the anus will dilate normally.		
Ask the patient to tighten the external sphincter; note the tone.	The patient can normally close the sphincter around the gloved finger.	Poor sphincter tone may be the result of a spinal cord injury, previous surgery, trauma or a prolapsed rectum. Tightened sphincter tone may indicate anxiety, scarring or inflammation.
Rotate finger to examine the muscular anal ring. Palpate for tenderness, nodules and hardness.	The anus is normally smooth, non-tender and free of nodules and hardness.	Tenderness may indicate haemorrhoids, fistula or fissure. Nodules may indicate polyps or cancer. Hardness may indicate scarring or cancer.
Palpate the rectum. Insert your finger further into the rectum as far as possible (Fig. 27-7). Next, turn your hand clockwise then anticlockwise. This allows palpation of as much rectal surface as possible. Note tenderness, irregularities, nodules and hardness.	The rectal mucosa is normally soft, smooth, non-tender and free of nodules.	Hardness and irregularities may be from scarring or cancer. Nodules may indicate polyps or cancer (see Abnormal findings 27-1).
Palpate the peritoneal cavity. This area may be palpated in men above the prostate gland in the area of the seminal vesicles on the anterior surface of the rectum. In women, this area may be palpated on the anterior rectal surface in the area of the rectouterine pouch (behind the cervix and the uterus). Note tenderness or nodules.	This area is normally smooth and non-tender.	A peritoneal protrusion into the rectum, called a *rectal shelf* (see Abnormal findings 27-1) may indicate a cancerous lesion or peritoneal metastasis. Tenderness may indicate peritoneal inflammation.

PHYSICAL ASSESSMENT (continued)

ASSESSMENT PROCEDURE	NORMAL FINDINGS	ABNORMAL FINDINGS
Prostate gland		
PALPATION		
In male patients, palpate the prostate. The prostate can be palpated on the anterior surface of the rectum by turning the hand fully anticlockwise so the pad of your index finger faces towards the patient's umbilicus (Fig. 27-8). Tell the patient that he may feel an urge to urinate but that he will not. Move the pad of your index finger over the prostate gland, trying to feel the sulcus between the lateral lobes. Note the size, shape and consistency of the prostate, and identify any nodules or tenderness. **CLINICAL TIP** **You may need to move your body away from the patient to achieve the proper angle for examination.**	The prostate is normally non-tender and rubbery. It has two lateral lobes that are divided by a median sulcus. The lobes are normally smooth, 2.5 cm long and heart-shaped. Identify any tenderness with examination or nodules palpable.	A swollen, tender prostate may indicate acute prostatitis. An enlarged smooth, firm, slightly elastic prostate that may not have a median sulcus suggests benign prostatic hypertrophy. A hard area on the prostate or hard, fixed, irregular nodules on the prostate suggest cancer (see Abnormal findings 27-2). *Note:* Palpating prostate prior to drawing a prostate specific antigen (PSA) will raise the PSA level.

FIGURE 27-7 Palpating the rectal wall.

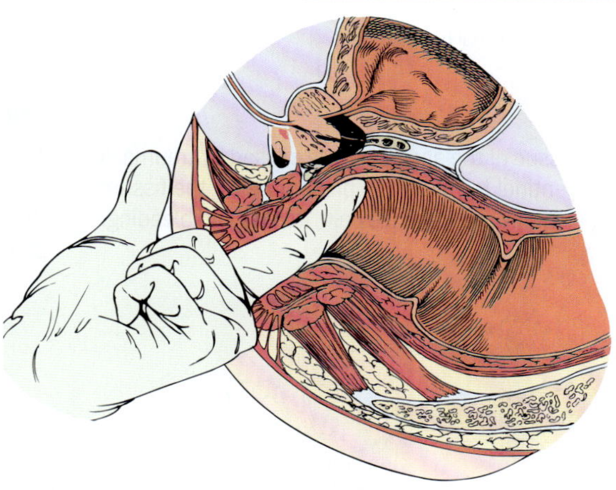

FIGURE 27-8 Palpating the prostate gland.

ASSESSMENT PROCEDURE	NORMAL FINDINGS	ABNORMAL FINDINGS
CHECK STOOL		
Inspect the stool. Withdraw your gloved finger. Inspect any faecal matter on your glove. Assess the colour, and test the faeces for occult blood. Provide the patient with a towel to wipe the anorectal area.	Stool is normally semi-solid, brown and free of blood.	Black stool may indicate upper gastrointestinal bleeding; grey or tan stool results from the lack of bile pigment; and yellow stool suggests steatorrhoea (increased fat content). Blood detected in the stool may indicate cancer of the rectum or colon. An endoscopic examination of the colon should be performed.

ABNORMAL FINDINGS 27-1 Abnormalities of the anus and rectum

EXTERNAL HAEMORRHOID

Haemorrhoids are usually painless papules caused by varicose veins. They can be internal or external (above or below the anorectal junction). This external haemorrhoid has become thrombosed—it contains clotted blood, is very painful and swollen, and itches and bleeds with bowel movements.

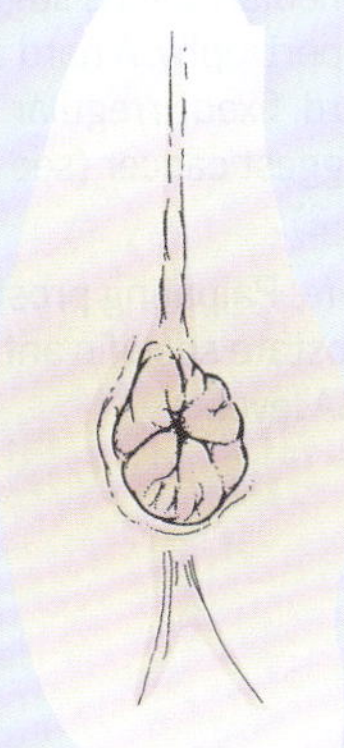

External haemorrhoid.

PERIANAL ABSCESS

Perianal abscess is a cavity of pus, caused by infection in the skin around the anal opening. It causes throbbing pain and is red, swollen, hard and tender.

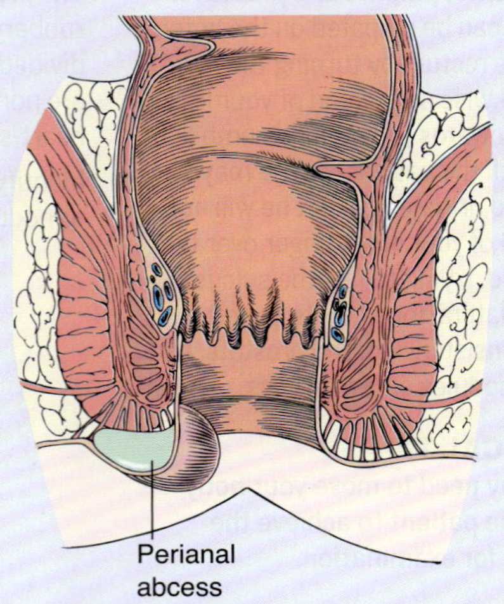

Perianal abscess.

ANAL FISSURE

These splits in the tissue of the anal canal are caused by trauma. A swollen skin tag ('sentinel tag') is often present below the fissure on the anal margin. They cause intense pain, itching and bleeding.

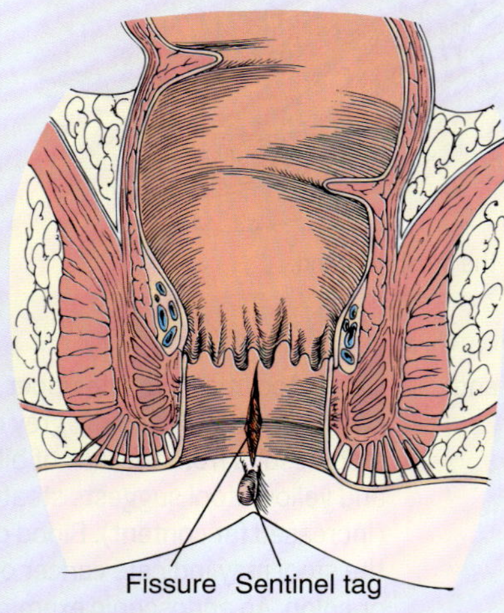

Anal fissure.

ANORECTAL FISTULA

This is evidenced by a small, round opening in the skin that surrounds the anal opening. It suggests an inflammatory tract from the anus or rectum out to the skin. A previous abscess may have preceded the fistula.

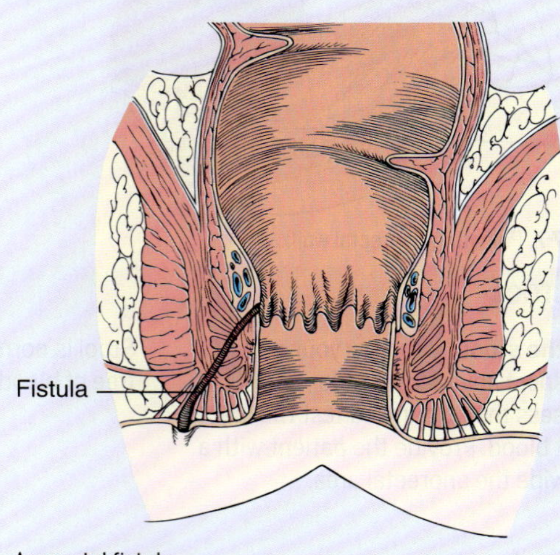

Anorectal fistula.

ABNORMAL FINDINGS 27-1 Abnormalities of the anus and rectum (continued)

RECTAL PROLAPSE

This occurs when the mucosa of the rectum protrudes out through the anal opening. It may involve only the mucosa or the mucosa and the rectal wall. It appears as a red, doughnut-like mass with radiating folds.

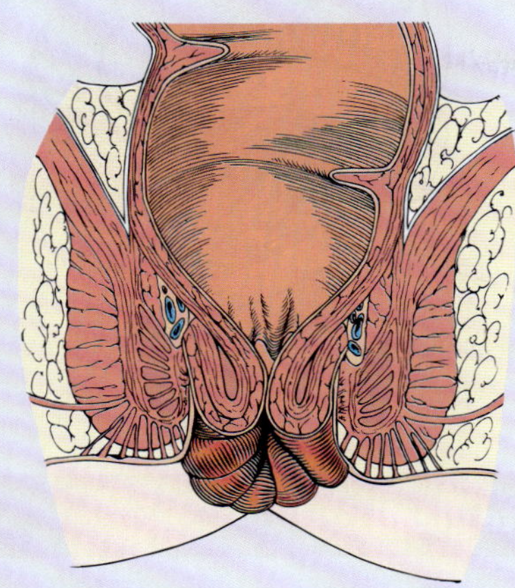

Rectal prolapse.

PILONIDAL CYST

This congenital disorder is characterised by a small dimple or cyst or sinus that contains hair. It is located midline in the sacro-coccygeal area and has a palpable sinus tract.

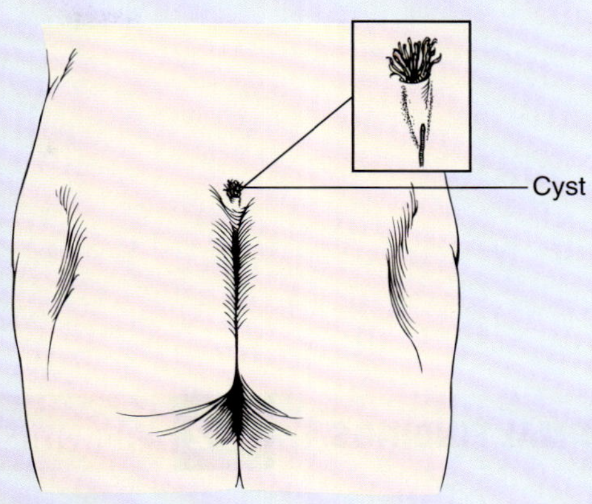

Pilonidal cyst.

RECTAL POLYPS

These soft structures are rather common and occur in varying size and number. There are two types: pedunculated (on a stalk) and sessile (on the mucosal surface).

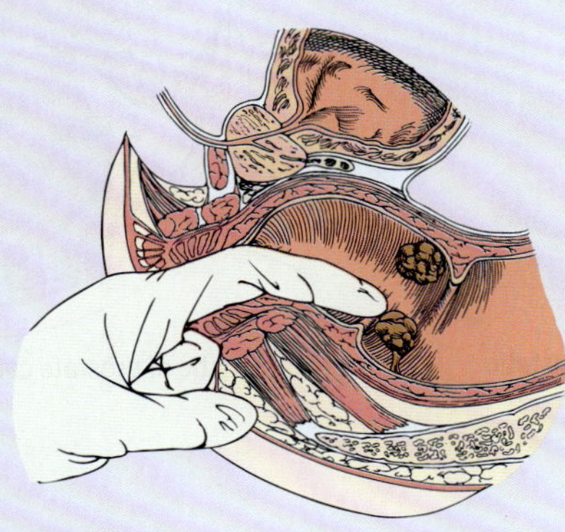

Rectal polyps.

RECTAL CANCER

A rectal carcinoma is usually asymptomatic until it is quite advanced. Thus, routine rectal palpation is essential. A cancer of the rectum may feel like a firm nodule, an ulcerated nodule with rolled edges, or, as it grows, a large, irregularly shaped, fixed, hard nodule.

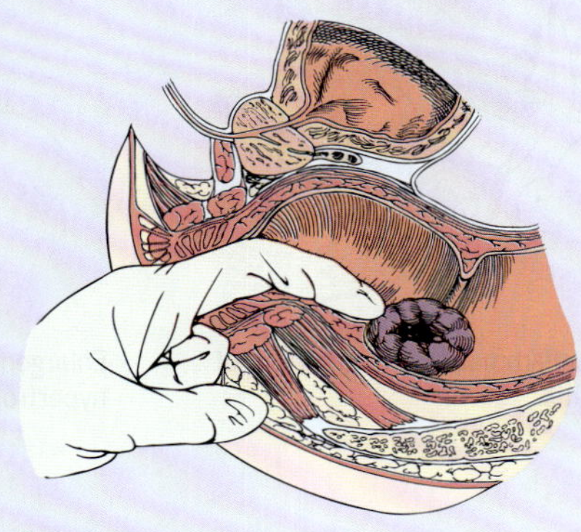

Rectal cancer.

Continued on following page

ABNORMAL FINDINGS 27-1 Abnormalities of the anus and rectum (continued)

RECTAL SHELF

If cancer metastasises to the peritoneal cavity, it may be felt as a nodular, hard, shelflike structure that protrudes onto the anterior surface of the rectum in the area of the seminal vesicles in men and in the area of the rectouterine pouch in women.

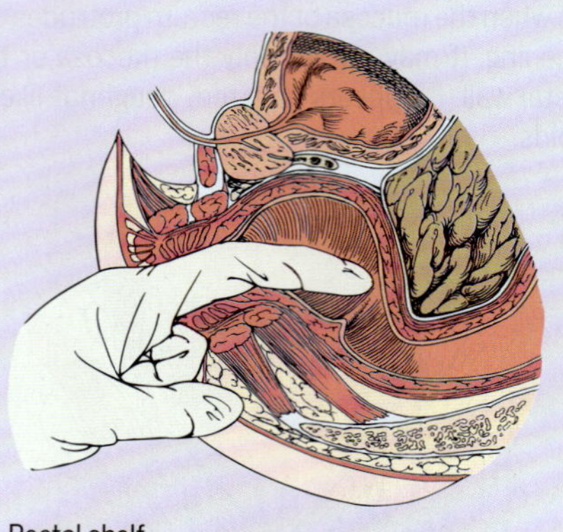

Rectal shelf.

ABNORMAL FINDINGS 27-2 Abnormalities of the prostate gland

ACUTE PROSTATITIS

The prostate is swollen, tender, firm and warm to the touch. Prostatitis is caused by a bacterial infection.

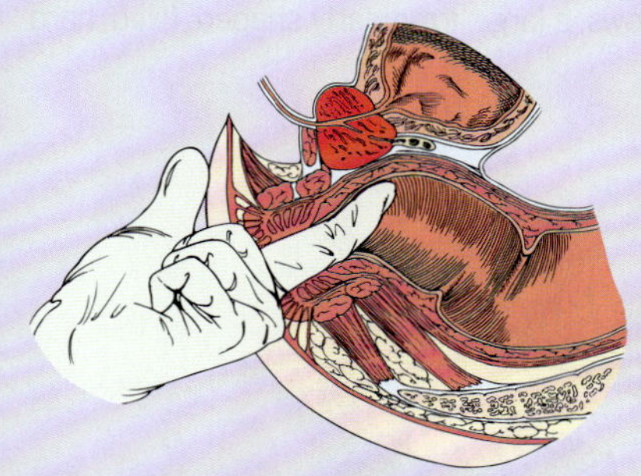

Swelling and inflammation characteristic of acute prostatitis.

BENIGN PROSTATIC HYPERTROPHY

The prostate is enlarged, smooth, firm and slightly elastic. The median sulcus may not be palpable. It is common in men older than age 50 years.

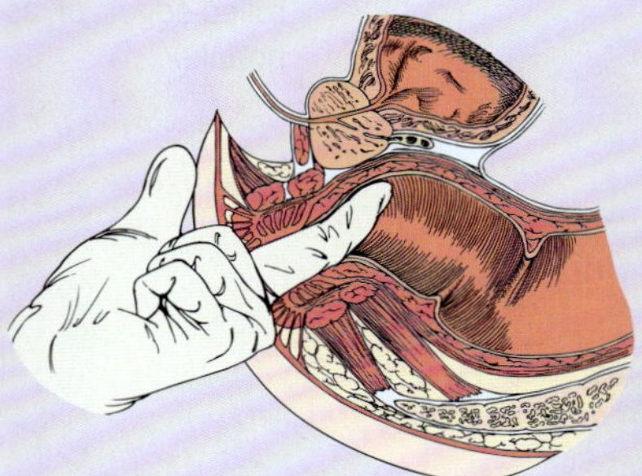

Enlargement characteristic of benign prostatic hypertrophy.

CANCER OF THE PROSTATE

A hard area on the prostate or hard, fixed, irregular nodules on the prostate suggest cancer. The median sulcus may not be palpable.

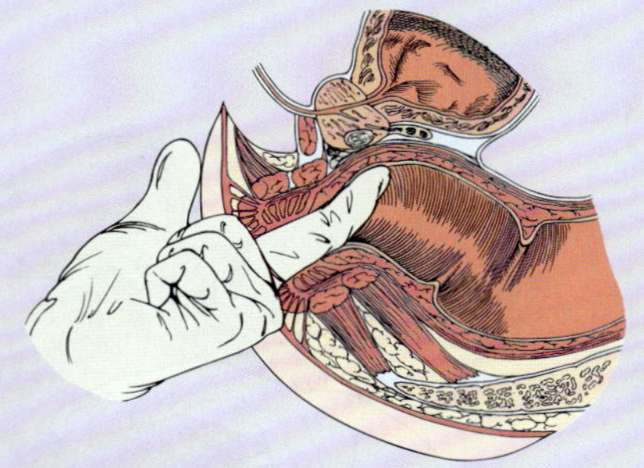

Mass characteristic of prostate cancer.

VALIDATING AND DOCUMENTING FINDINGS

Validate the anus, rectum and prostate assessment data you have collected. This is necessary to verify that the data are reliable and accurate. Document the assessment data following the health care facility or agency policy.

After you have collected the assessment data, you will need to analyse the data, using diagnostic reasoning skills. Refer to the discussion of the diagnostic reasoning process in Chapter 5.

Sample of subjective data

A 52-year-old male patient reports no recent change in bowel patterns, no constipation, diarrhoea or blood in his stools. He has no trouble controlling his bowels and denies pain and itching in the anal area. He has no history of anal or rectal surgery or trauma and no congenital deformities. He states that his last digital rectal examination, test for occult blood and prostate-specific antigen screening were 1 year ago. No significant findings were reported. He says he had a colonoscopy 2 years ago and the results were normal. He has no knowledge of polyps or cancer (colon, rectal or prostate) in his family. The patient explains that he seldom uses laxatives and has never used an enema. He denies engaging in anal sexual intercourse. He does not know exactly how much water and fibre he consumes but guesses a moderate to high amount.

Sample of objective data

The patient's anal opening is hairless, moist and closed tightly. The perianal area is free of redness, lumps, ulcers, lesions and rashes. No bulging or lesions appear when the patient performs the Valsalva manoeuvre. The sacrococcygeal area is smooth, free of redness and hair. The patient can close the external sphincter around gloved finger. Anus is smooth, non-tender and free of nodules and hardness. Rectal mucosa is soft, smooth, non-tender and free of nodules. Peritoneal cavity area is smooth and non-tender. Prostate gland palpated as two smooth, non-tender, rubbery lobes approximately 2.5 cm long. The median sulcus is palpated between the two lobes. The patient can close the external sphincter on command or voluntarily.

CASE STUDY

When the anorectal areas are inspected, several bluish, rounded swellings are present external to the anal sphincter and a small fissure is noted in the lining of the anus. A small amount of light-red blood is visible near the anal fissure.

CRITICAL THINKING

6. Following these findings, are there any other questions you would ask Mr Kowalsky that may provide additional information pertinent to the assessment of his condition?

Analysis of data

DIAGNOSTIC REASONING: POSSIBLE CONCLUSIONS

After collecting subjective and objective information pertaining to the anus, rectum and prostate, identify abnormal findings and patient strengths. Then cluster the data to reveal significant patterns or abnormalities; these data may be used to make clinical judgements about the status of the patient's anal, rectal and prostatic health.

Potential patient risks

- Risk of ineffective health maintenance (related to lack of knowledge of need for recommended colorectal and prostate examinations)
- Risk of impaired skin integrity in rectal area (related to chronic irritation secondary to diarrhoea)

Potential patient problems

- Acute rectal pain
- Diarrhoea (related to chronic inflammatory bowel disease)
- Ineffective sexuality patterns (related to feelings of loss of femininity or masculinity and sexual attractiveness secondary to chronic diarrhoea or pain)
- Situational low self-esteem (related to loss of control over bowel elimination)

Selected collaborative problems

After grouping the data, certain collaborative problems may become apparent. Remember that collaborative problems cannot be prevented by nursing interventions. However, the nurse can detect and monitor these physiological complications of medical conditions. In addition, the nurse can use doctor- and nurse-prescribed interventions to minimise the complications of these problems. The nurse may also have to refer the patient in such situations for further treatment of the problem. The following is a list of collaborative problems that may be identified when assessing the anus, rectum and prostate.

- Prostatic hypertrophy
- Fistula
- Fissure
- Haemorrhoids
- Rectal bleeding
- Rectal abscess.

Medical problems

After grouping the data, the patient's signs and symptoms—for example, rectal prolapse, benign prostatic hypertrophy—may clearly require medical diagnosis and treatment. Referral to a primary care provider is necessary.

CRITICAL THINKING

7. What risks and actual diagnoses would you arrive at following assessment of Mr Kowalsky?

ONLINE RESOURCES

An extensive range of additional resources to enhance teaching and learning and to facilitate understanding may be found online at the text's accompanying website, located on thePoint at http://thepoint.lww.com. These include Watch and Learn videos, Concepts in Action animations, journal articles, case studies, discussion topics and quizzes.

Subscribers may also access Lippincott Procedures, an extensive online point-of-care procedure guide that provides reliable step-by-step instructions for more than 1700 procedures, including 450 evidence-based Australian procedures, and skills in a variety of speciality settings, together with a wealth of supporting information.

CASE STUDY

The case study demonstrates how to analyse anus, rectum and prostate assessment data for a specific patient. The exercises included in the ancillary product on thePoint that complements this text offer further opportunities to enhance your skills.

George Kowalsky, 42 years old, is seeking advice from his local community health clinic because he has been 'bleeding from his rectum' and has pain and pressure in the rectal area. Mr Kowalsky is the head accountant and tax consultant for a high-profile company. He is currently preparing for the annual audit and reports to the nurse that he is 'very uptight'.

When questioned, Mr Kowalsky reports that he has observed small amounts of bright-red blood on his stools for the last 2 days and for about the last week his bowel movements have been quite painful—'like passing ground glass'. He states that he has had hard bowel movements for many years. He drinks 10 to 12 cups of coffee per day. For the most part his meals include traditional eggs and bacon for breakfast and meat and potatoes for dinner. He doesn't really like vegetables or fruit. He doesn't eat excessively and has maintained his weight 'within the chart norms' for more than 20 years. For years he has used Proctosedyl (Rectinol) ointment for his 'piles' with relief—until recently.

When the anorectal areas are inspected, several bluish, rounded swellings are present external to the anal sphincter and a small fissure is noted in the lining of the anus. A small amount of light-red blood is visible near the anal fissure.

The following concept map illustrates the diagnostic reasoning process.

Applying COLDSPA

Applying COLDSPA for patient symptoms: 'rectal bleeding'.

Mnemonic	Question	Data provided	Missing data
Character	Describe the sign or symptom (feeling, appearance, sound or smell).	Patient reports bleeding from rectum; has seen small amounts of bright-red blood with bowel movements.	
Onset	When did it begin?	Two days ago	
Location	Where is it? Does it radiate? Does it occur anywhere else?	Patient reports painful bowel movements.	
Duration	How long does it last? Does it recur?	Has occurred for the last 2 days.	
Severity	How bad is it? or How much does it bother you?	Bowel movements have been painful, 'like passing ground glass', for the last week.	
Pattern	What makes it better or worse?	Patient has used Preparation H in the past, but has not tried it recently.	
Associated factors/How it Affects the patient	What other symptoms occur with it? How does it affect you?	Patient reports 'pain and pressure in the rectal area' and states 'I am very uptight.' Eats a high-fat meat and potato diet; does not like fruits and vegetables.	

1) Identify abnormal findings and patient strengths

Subjective data

- 'Bleeding from his rectum'
- Pain and pressure in the rectal area
- Observed small amounts of bright-red blood on his stool for the last 2 days
- Bowel movements have been quite painful, 'like passing ground glass,' for about the last week
- Hard bowel movements for many years
- 'Very uptight'—preparing for annual audit
- Drinks 10 to 12 cups of coffee daily
- Traditional eggs and bacon for breakfast and meat and potatoes for dinner
- Has maintained his weight 'within the chart norms' for over 20 years
- Used Rectinol for relief for many years until recently

Objective data

- Bluish, rounded swellings noted external to the anal sphincter
- Small fissure in the anal lining
- Small amount of light-red blood visible near the anal fissure

2) Identify cue clusters

- Pain and pressure in the rectal area
- Observed small amounts of bright-red blood on his stool for the last 2 days
- Bowel movements have been quite painful, 'like passing ground glass', for about the last week
- Hard bowel movements for many years
- 'Very uptight'—preparing for annual audit
- Used Rectinol for many years with relief, until lately
- Bluish, rounded swellings noted external to the anal sphincter
- Small fissure in the lining of the anus
- Small amount of light red blood visible near the anal fissure

- Hard bowel movements for many years
- 'Very uptight'—preparing for annual audit
- Drinks 10 to 12 cups of coffee daily
- Traditional eggs and bacon for breakfast and meat and potatoes for dinner

3) Draw inferences

His history, the type of bleeding (bright, light red and on the stool), and physical findings are suggestive of haemorrhoids, which the patient has self-treated with OTC medication for some time. His bleeding and increased pain could be from a recent fissure or his tension, which may cause the sphincter to tighten and possibly cut off circulation to the external varices. **Mr Kowalsky needs to be referred to his own doctor for further work-up regarding the bleeding and increased pain.** Collaborative problems should also be identified.

Apparently, Mr Kowalsky has been living with and self-treating his bowel problem and has only sought assistance when he noted bleeding. His occupational stress and dietary habits tend to promote continuation of this problem. He does not indicate a desire to change his habits at this time.

4) List possible diagnoses

Constipation related to psychosomatic tension, improper diet and inadequate water intake to promote bowel health

Ineffective health maintenance related to insufficient knowledge of stress management and other health-promoting behaviours

Ineffective health maintenance related to lack of motivation to change lifestyle and not seeking treatment for chronic problem

5) Check for defining characteristics

Major: Hard, dry stool, painful defecation
Minor: Rectal pressure

Major: Demonstrates unhealthy practices and lifestyle
Minor: None

Major: Demonstrates unhealthy practices and lifestyle
Minor: None

6) Confirm or rule out diagnoses

Confirm because it meets the major and minor defining characteristics

Either or both may be confirmed because they meet the major defining characteristics. However, additional data must be collected to determine the correct cause of the disorder so proper nursing orders can be implemented.

7) Document conclusions

Diagnoses that are appropriate for this patient include:

- Constipation related to psychosomatic tension, and improper diet and inadequate water intake to promote bowel health
- Ineffective health maintenance related to insufficient knowledge of stress management and other health-promoting behaviours
- Ineffective health maintenance related to lack of motivation to change lifestyle and not seeking treatment for chronic problem

Potential collaborative problems include:

- Haemorrhage
- Variceal thrombosis
- Variceal strangulation

Mr Kowalsky should be referred to a doctor for evaluation and treatment of rectal bleeding and pain.

References

Australian Institute of Health and Welfare. (2019). Cancer in Australia 2019. Viewed July 2019 at www.aihw.gov.au/reports/cancer/cancer-in-australia-2019/data.

Bowel Cancer Australia. (2019). Tests and investigations used in the diagnosis of bowel cancer. Viewed July 2019 at www.bowelcanceraustralia.org/tests-investigations/advantages-disadvantages.

Cancer Australia. (2019). All cancers in Australia. Viewed July 2019 at https://canceraustralia.gov.au/affected-cancer/what-cancer/cancer-australia-statistics.

Cancer Council. (2019). Understanding your FOBT. Viewed July 2019 at www.cancer.org.au/about-cancer/early-detection/early-detection-factsheets/understanding-your-fobt.html.

New Zealand Ministry of Health (NZMOH). (2018a). Selected cancers 2015, 2016, 2017. Viewed July 2019 at www.health.govt.nz/publication/selected-cancers-2015-2016-2017.

New Zealand Ministry of Health (NZMOH). (2018b). New cancer registrations 2016. Viewed July 2019 at https://www.health.govt.nz/publication/new-cancer-registrations-2016.

Nicastro, H. L. & Dunn, B. K. (2013). Selenium and prostate cancer prevention: Insights from the Selenium and Vitamin E cancer prevention trial (SELECT). *Nutrients, 5*(4), 1122–1148.

Royal Australian College of General Practitioners (RACGP). (2018). Guidelines for preventive activities in general practice—The red book, 9.2 Colorectal cancer Viewed July 2019 at www.racgp.org.au/clinical-resources/clinical-guidelines/key-racgp-guidelines/view-all-racgp-guidelines/red-book/early-detection-of-cancers/colorectal-cancer.

Time to Screen NZ. (2019). Bowel screening, Viewed July 2019 at www.timetoscreen.nz/bowel-screening/.

Selected readings

Avellino, G., Theva, D. & Oates, R. D. (2017). Common urologic diseases in older men and their treatment: How they impact fertility. *Fertility and Sterility, 107*(2), 305–311.

Bell, N., Connor, G. S., et al. (2014). Recommendations on screening for prostate cancer with the prostate-specific antigen test. *Canadian Medical Association Journal, 186*(16), 1225–1234.

Bowel Cancer Australia. (2019). Piles (haemorrhoids). Available at www.bowelcanceraustralia.org.

Brenner, H., Chang-Claude, J., et al. (2014). Reduced risk of colorectal cancer up to 10 years after screening, surveillance, or diagnostic colonoscopy. *Gastroenterology, 146*(3), 709–717.

Lew, J. B., St John, D., et al. (2018). Evaluation of the benefits, harms and cost-effectiveness of potential alternatives to iFOBT testing for colorectal cancer screening in Australia. *International Journal of Cancer, 143*(2), 269–282.

Jideh, B. & Bourke, M. J. (2018). Colorectal cancer screening reduces incidence, mortality and morbidity. *The Medical Journal of Australia, 208*(11), 483–484.

Mayo Clinic. (2019). Haemorrhoids. Available at www.mayoclinic.org.

National Cancer Institute (NCI). (2019). Prostate cancer—Patient version. Available at www.cancer.gov.

Porkorny, C. S. (2017). Digital rectal examination: Indications and technique. *The Medical Journal of Australia, 207*(4), 147–148.

Prostate Cancer Foundation NZ. (2019). Prostate cancer. Viewed July 2019 at https://prostate.org.nz/prostate-cancer/.

Prostate Cancer Foundation of Australia. (2019). Clinical practice guidelines on PSA testing. Viewed July 2019 at www.prostate.org.au/awareness/for-healthcare-professionals/clinical-practice-guidelines-on-psa-testing/.

Prostate Cancer Foundation of Australia. (2019). PSA testing and early management of test-detected prostate cancer. Available at www.prostate.org.au/awareness/for-healthcare-professionals/clinical-practice-guidelines-on-psa-testing/.

Ranasinghe, W. K. B., Kim, S. P., et al. (2014). Population based analysis of prostate-specific antigen (PSA) screening in younger men (<55 years) in Australia. *BJU International, 113*(1), 77–83.

Royal Australian College of General Practitioners. (2019). *Guidelines for preventive activities in general practice—9.1 Prostate Cancer (the red book)*. Melbourne: Author.

Weight, C. J., Narayan, V. M., et al. (2017). The effects of population-based prostate-specific antigen screening beginning at age 40. *Urology, 110*, 127–133.

Online resources

Andrology Australia (Monash University Centre of Excellence for Male Health): www.andrologyaustralia.org

Australian Government Department of Health, cancer screening: www.cancerscreening.gov.au

Australian Institute of Health and Welfare, cancer rates: www.aihw.gov.au/reports/cancer/cancer-in-australia-2019/data

Bowel Cancer Australia: www.bowelcanceraustralia.org

BowelScreen Aotearoa™ service: www.bowelscreenaotearoa.org

BowelScreen Australia® program: www.bowelscreenaustralia.org

Cancer Australia: www.canceraustralia.gov.au

Cancer Council Australia: www.cancer.org.au

Cancer Society of New Zealand: www.cancernz.org.nz

New Zealand Ministry of Health: www.health.govt.nz

New Zealand National Screening Unit: www.nsu.govt.nz

Prostate Cancer Foundation of Australia: www.prostate.org.au

Prostate Cancer Foundation NZ: www.prostate.org.nz

Royal Australian College of General Practitioners, preventive guidelines (the red book): www.racgp.org.au/your-practice/guidelines/redbook

Urological Society of Australia New Zealand: www.usanz.org.au

CHAPTER 28

Musculoskeletal system

Australian and New Zealand perspective

Musculoskeletal disorders (MSDs) are defined as conditions of the bones, muscles and their attachments. Musculoskeletal disorders include joint disease such as osteoarthritis and rheumatoid arthritis, back and neck pain, osteoarthritis and fragility fractures, soft-tissue rheumatism, injuries due to sports and recreation and the workplace, and trauma commonly related to road traffic accidents. Musculoskeletal disorders such as low back pain, arthritis and other diseases of the joints are among the leading causes of disability worldwide (World Health Organization [WHO], 2019). The WHO's latest Global Burden Disease study indicates that MSDs, particularly lower back pain, are an emerging global health issue.

Musculoskeletal disorders affect people of all ages and ethnic backgrounds, causing pain, physical disability and the loss of personal and economic independence. Persons affected by MSDs are also likely to have depression or anxiety problems related to their condition. MSDs are the most common chronic condition in Australia, affecting almost one-third of the population. From 2017 to 2018, one in six Australians (16% or 4,000,000 people) had back problems, and back problems accounted for 4.1% of Australia's overall disease burden (Australian Institute of Health and Welfare [AIHW], 2019). In New Zealand, MSDs affect one in four adults and represent the second largest category of conditions, resulting in claims for sickness benefit. In 2010, 15.2% of New Zealanders aged 15 years and over were living with at least one type of arthritis (Bevan et al., 2012).

The nurse has a vital role in educating patients about the principles of safety and accident prevention. The morbidity associated with musculoskeletal injuries can be greatly reduced if people are aware of ways of avoiding environmental hazards in the home and the workplace, utilise appropriate safety equipment in sports and recreational activities, and abide by traffic safety rules. Falls are the leading cause of injury-related hospitalisation in persons aged 65 years and over and account for 4% of all hospital admissions in this age group (AIHW, 2013). In response to this, various prevention strategies have been developed in Australia and New Zealand. These include educating older people to wear shoes with functional and stable soles and heels, avoiding wet or slippery surfaces, carefully placing loose carpet mats so as not to trip over them, and removing obstacles from high-traffic areas in the home environment (Tricco et al., 2017).

Sports-related injuries such as sprains, strains and fractures make up almost 90% of all musculoskeletal injuries in patients between the ages of 5 and 24 years. The most common sprain and strain is an ankle strain, followed by muscle strain and back strain. The most common fractures are radial and metacarpal. In New Zealand, a high participation rate in rugby union makes it one of the costliest sports for injuries costing New Zealand over $70 million in claims per year (Accident Compensation Corporation [ACC], 2019).

The ACC (Te Kaporeihana Āwhina Hunga Whara) is a New Zealand Crown entity responsible for administering its *Injury Prevention, Rehabilitation, and Compensation Act 2001*. The Act provides support to all New Zealand citizens, residents and temporary visitors who have suffered an injury. The ACC's scheme is administered on a no-fault basis, so that anyone, regardless of the way in which they incurred an injury, is eligible for coverage under the scheme. For more information on the ACC, go to www.acc.co.nz.

CASE STUDY

Jacob Winter is a 16-year-old schoolboy who has presented to the emergency department (ED) after having a fall from his skateboard. His mother Debbie transported him to the ED after his friends carried him home. Jacob is complaining of pain in his left ankle, especially at the joint.

Before beginning the assessment of Jacob, it is important to have an understanding of the anatomy and physiology of the musculoskeletal system.

Structure and function

BONES

Bones provide structure, give protection, serve as levers, store calcium and produce blood cells. Two-hundred and six (206) bones make up the axial skeleton (head and trunk) and the appendicular skeleton (extremities, shoulders and hips; Fig. 28-1).

Composed of osseous tissue, bones can be divided into two types: compact bone, which is hard and dense and makes up the shaft and outer layers; and spongy bone, which contains numerous spaces and makes up the ends and centres of the bones. Bone tissue is formed by active cells called osteoblasts and broken down by cells referred to as osteoclasts. Bones contain red marrow that produces blood cells and yellow marrow composed mostly of fat.

The periosteum covers the bones and contains osteoblasts and blood vessels that promote nourishment and formation of new bone tissues. Bone shapes vary and include short bones (e.g. carpals), long bones (e.g. humerus, femur), flat bones (e.g. sternum, ribs) and bones with an irregular shape (e.g. vertebrae).

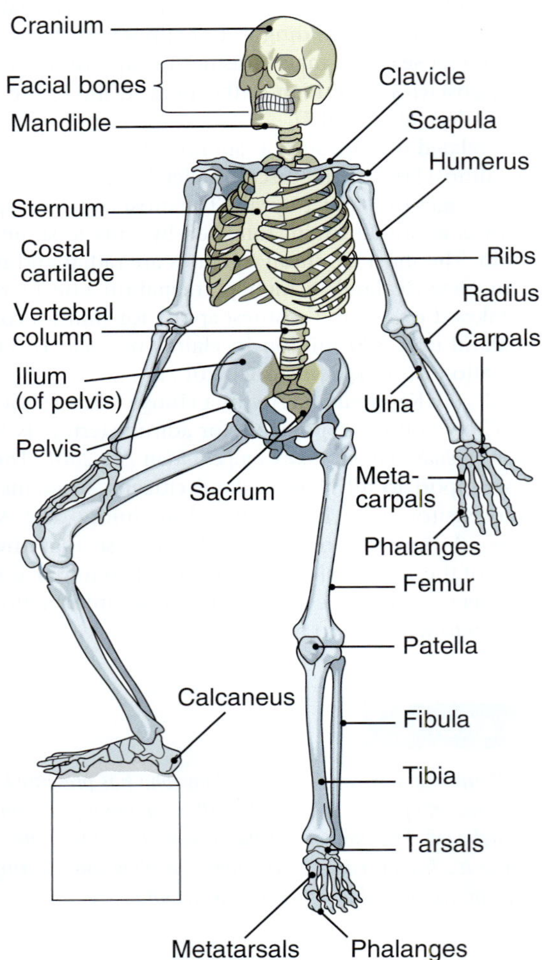

FIGURE 28-1 Major bones of the skeleton. The axial skeleton is shown in yellow; the appendicular, in blue. (Cohen, B. J. & Hull, K. L. [2015]. *Memmler's structure and function of the human body* [11th ed.]. Philadelphia: Lippincott Williams & Wilkins.)

SKELETAL MUSCLES

The body consists of three types of muscles: skeletal, smooth and cardiac. The musculoskeletal system is made up of 650 skeletal (voluntary) muscles, which are under conscious control (Fig. 28-2). Made up of long muscle fibres (fasciculi) that are arranged together in bundles and joined by connective tissue, skeletal muscles attach to bones by way of strong, fibrous cords called tendons. Skeletal muscles assist with posture, produce body heat and allow the body to move. Skeletal muscle movements (some of which are illustrated in Display 28-1) include:

Abduction: Moving away from midline of the body
Adduction: Moving towards the midline of the body
Circumduction: Circular motion
Inversion: Moving inwards
Eversion: Moving outwards
Extension: Straightening the extremity at the joint and increasing the angle of the joint
    Hyperextension: Joint bends greater than 180-degree angle
Flexion: Bending the extremity at the joint and decreasing the angle of the joint
    Dorsiflexion: Toes draw upwards to ankle
    Plantar flexion: Toes point away from ankle
Pronation: Turning or facing downwards
Supination: Turning or facing upwards
Protraction: Moving forwards
Retraction: Moving backwards
Rotation: Turning of a bone on its own long axis
    Internal rotation: Turning of a bone towards the centre of the body
    External rotation: Turning of a bone away from the centre of the body

JOINTS

The joint (or articulation) is the place where two or more bones meet. Joints provide a variety of *ranges of motion* (ROM) for the body parts and may be classified as fibrous, cartilaginous or synovial.

Fibrous joints (e.g. sutures between skull bones) are joined by fibrous connective tissue and are immovable. Cartilaginous joints (e.g. joints between vertebrae) are joined by cartilage. Synovial joints (e.g. shoulders, wrists, hips, knees and ankles; Fig. 28-3) contain a space between the bones that is filled with synovial fluid, a lubricant that promotes a sliding movement of the ends of the bones. Bones in synovial joints are joined by ligaments, which are strong, dense bands of fibrous connective tissue. Synovial joints are enclosed by a fibrous capsule made of connective tissue and connected to the periosteum of the bone. Articular cartilage smoothes and protects the bones that articulate with each other.

Some synovial joints contain bursae, which are small sacs filled with synovial fluid that serve to cushion the joint. Display 28-2 reviews the appearance, characteristics and motion of major joints.

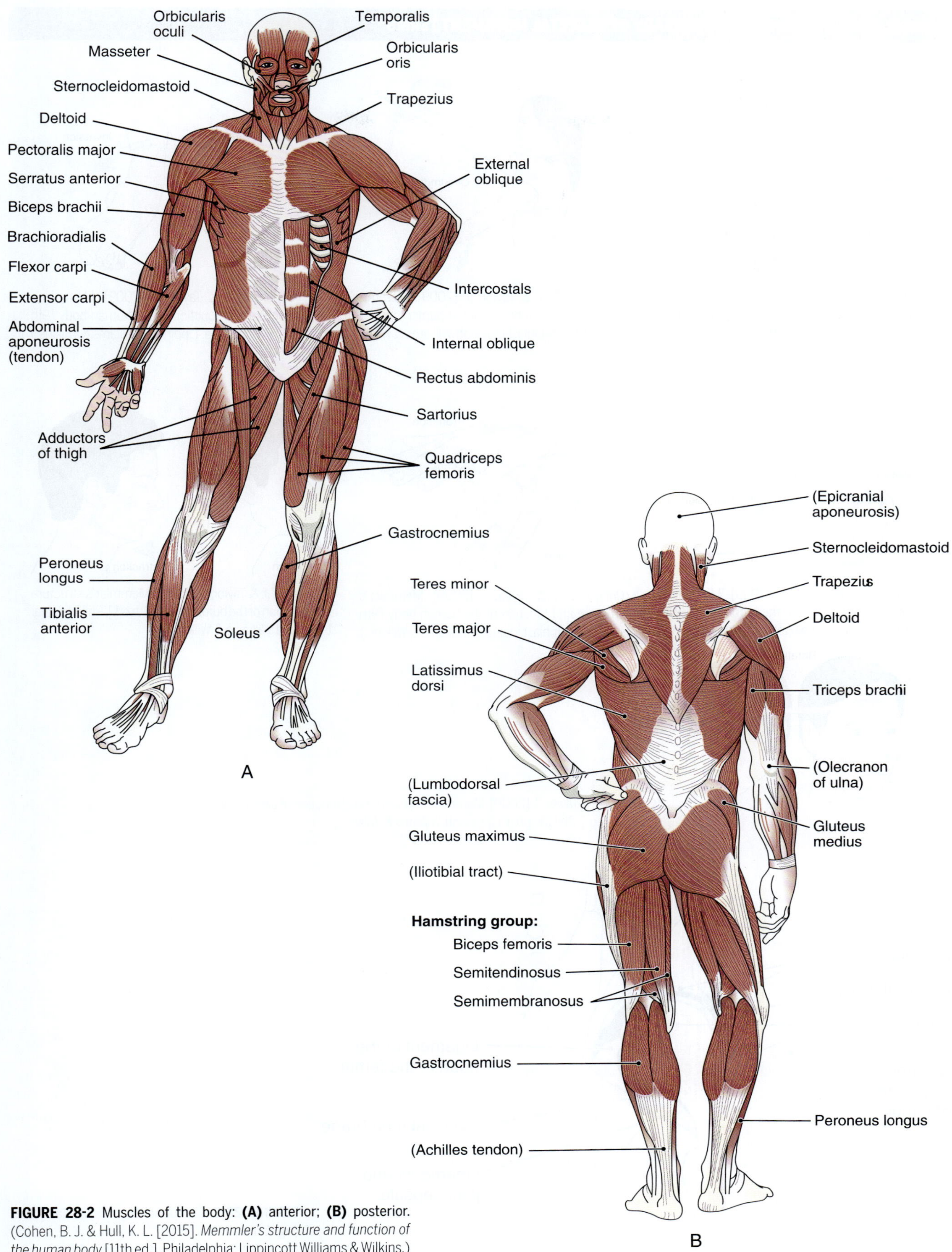

FIGURE 28-2 Muscles of the body: **(A)** anterior; **(B)** posterior. (Cohen, B. J. & Hull, K. L. [2015]. *Memmler's structure and function of the human body* [11th ed.]. Philadelphia: Lippincott Williams & Wilkins.)

DISPLAY 28-1 ILLUSTRATED GLOSSARY OF SKELETAL MOVEMENT TERMS

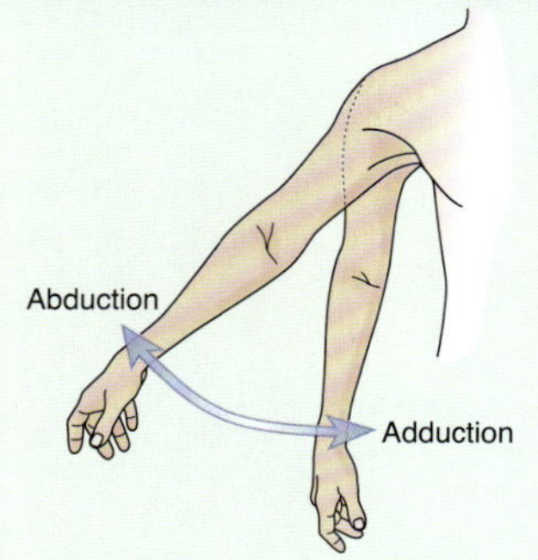

(Cohen, B. J. & Taylor, J. [2009]. Memmler's structure and function of the human body [9th ed.]. Philadelphia: Lippincott Williams & Wilkins.)

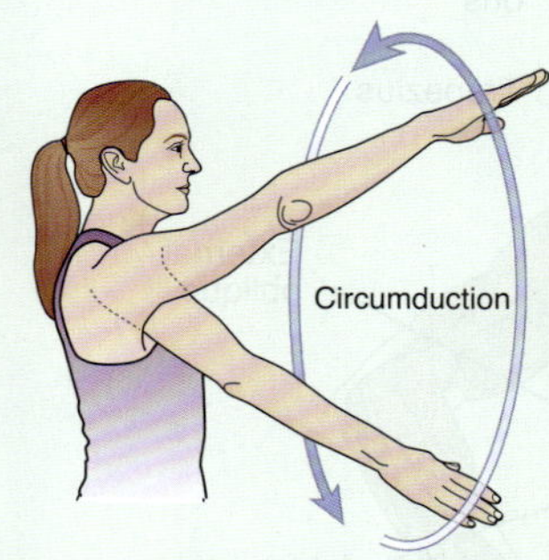

(Cohen, B. J. & Taylor, J. [2009]. Memmler's structure and function of the human body [9th ed.]. Philadelphia: Lippincott Williams & Wilkins.)

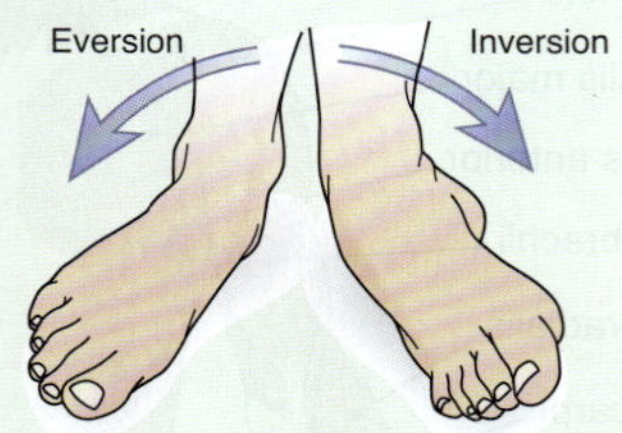

(Cohen, B. J. & Taylor, J. [2009]. Memmler's structure and function of the human body [9th ed.]. Philadelphia: Lippincott Williams & Wilkins.)

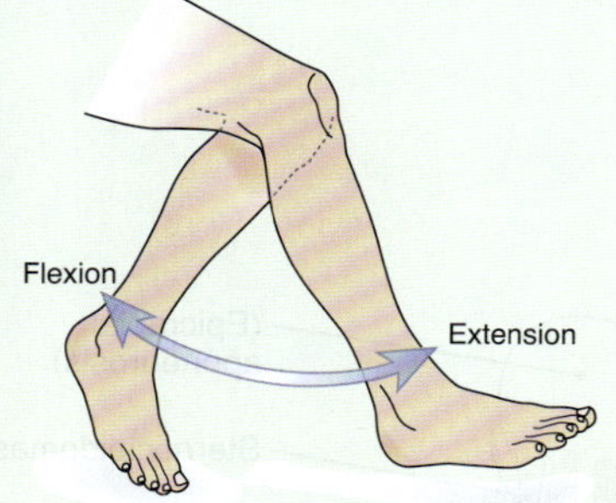

(Cohen, B. J. & Taylor, J. [2009]. Memmler's structure and function of the human body [9th ed.]. Philadelphia: Lippincott Williams & Wilkins.)

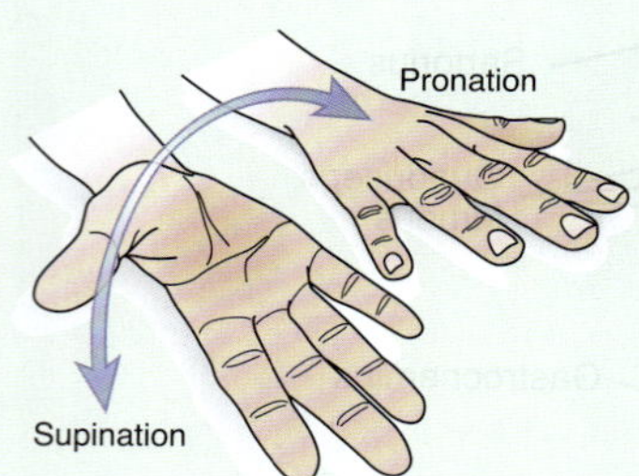

(Cohen, B. J. & Taylor, J. [2009]. Memmler's structure and function of the human body [9th ed.]. Philadelphia: Lippincott Williams & Wilkins.)

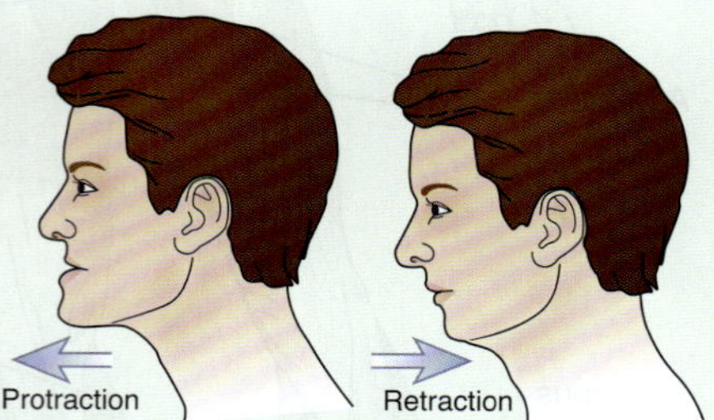

(Cohen, B. J. & Taylor, J. [2009]. Memmler's structure and function of the human body [9th ed.]. Philadelphia: Lippincott Williams & Wilkins.)

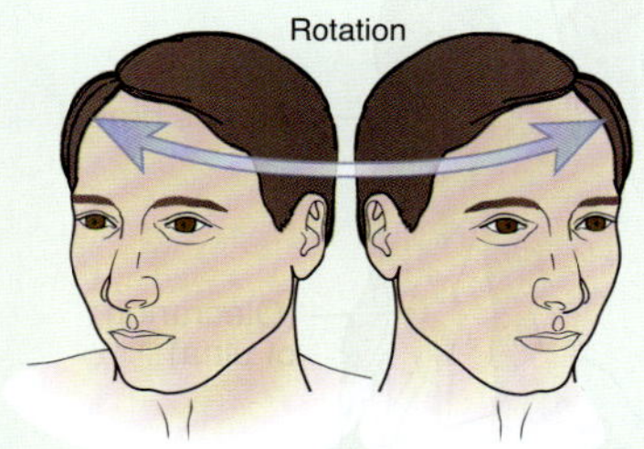

(Cohen, B. J. & Taylor, J. [2009]. Memmler's structure and function of the human body [9th ed.]. Philadelphia: Lippincott Williams & Wilkins.)

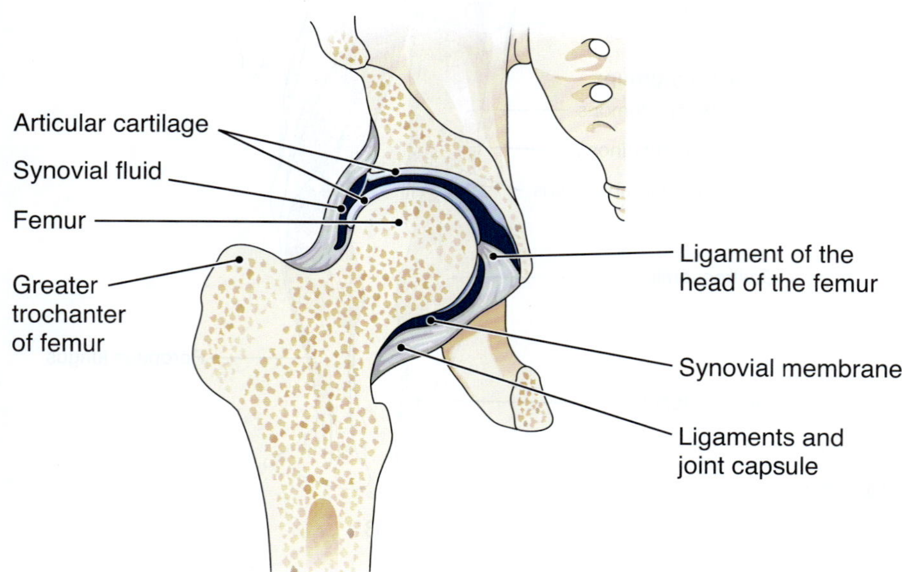

FIGURE 28-3 **Components of synovial joints (right hip joint).** (Cohen, B. J. & Hull, K. L. [2015]. *Memmler's structure and function of the human body* [11th ed.]. Philadelphia: Lippincott Williams & Wilkins.)

DISPLAY 28-2 UNDERSTANDING MAJOR JOINTS

Temporomandibular

Articulation between the temporal bone and mandible. Motion:

- Opens and closes mouth
- Projects and retracts jaw
- Moves jaw from side to side.

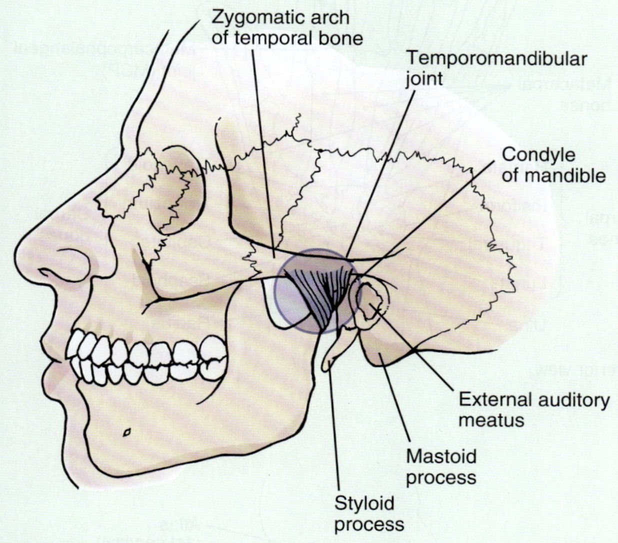

Sternoclavicular

Junction between the manubrium of the sternum and the clavicle; has no obvious movements.

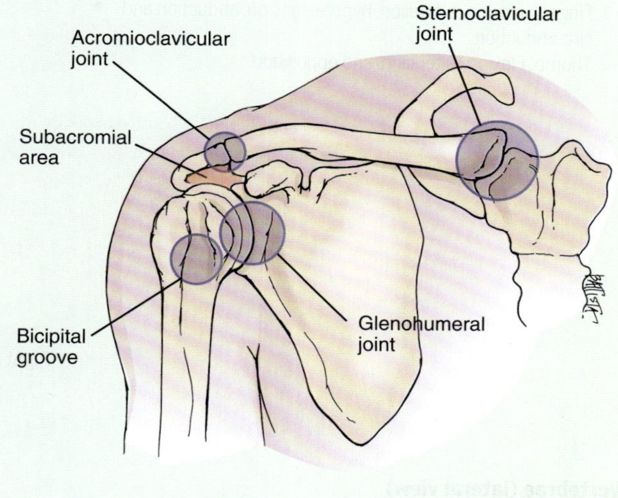

Shoulder

Articulation of the head of the humerus in the glenoid cavity of the scapula. The acromioclavicular joint includes the clavicle and acromion process of the scapula. It contains the subacromial and subscapular bursae. Motion:

- Flexion and extension
- Abduction and adduction
- Circumduction
- Rotation (internal and external).

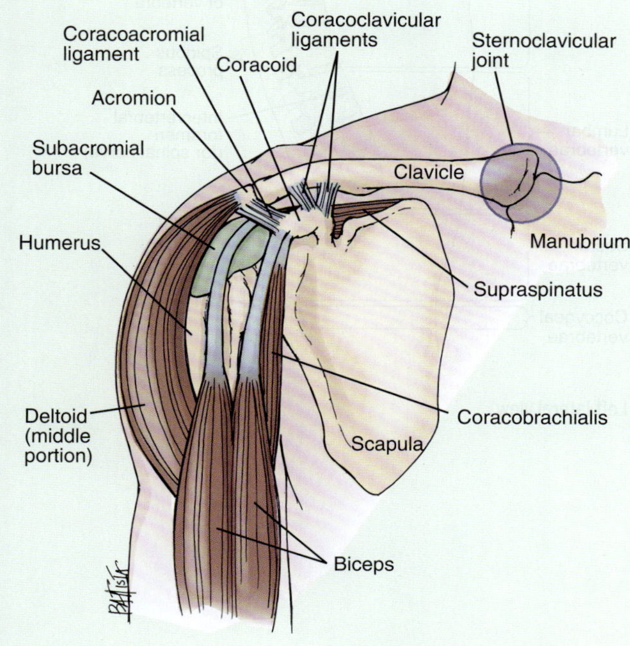

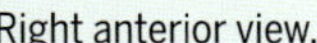

Right anterior view.

Elbow

Articulation between the ulna and radius of the lower arm and the humerus of the upper arm; contains a synovial membrane and several bursae. Motion:

- Flexion and extension of the forearm
- Supination and pronation of the forearm.

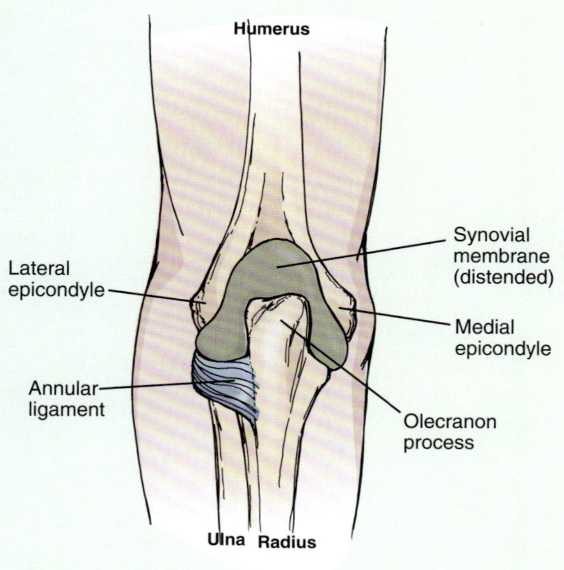

Left posterior view.

Continued on following page

DISPLAY 28-2 UNDERSTANDING MAJOR JOINTS (continued)

Wrist, fingers, thumb

Articulation between the distal radius, ulnar bone, carpals and metacarpals. Contains ligaments and is lined with a synovial membrane. Motion:

- Wrists: Flexion, extension, hyperextension, adduction, radial and ulnar deviation
- Fingers: Flexion, extension, hyperextension, abduction and circumduction
- Thumb: Flexion, extension, and opposition.

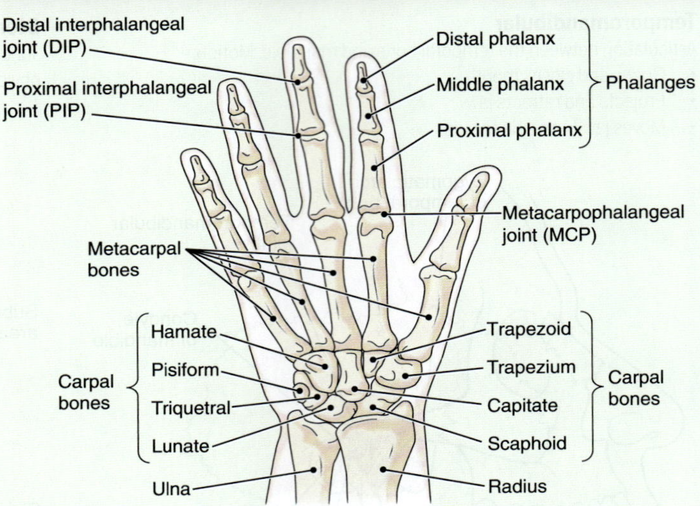

Right anterior view.

Vertebrae (lateral view)

Thirty-three (33) bones: 7 concave cervical (C), 12 convex thoracic (T), 5 concave lumbar (L), 5 sacral (S) and 3 to 4 coccygeal, connected in a vertical column. Bones are cushioned by elastic fibrocartilaginous plates (intervertebral discs) that provide flexibility and posture to the spine. Paravertebral muscles are positioned on both sides of vertebrae. Motion:

- Flexion
- Hyperextension
- Lateral bending
- Rotation.

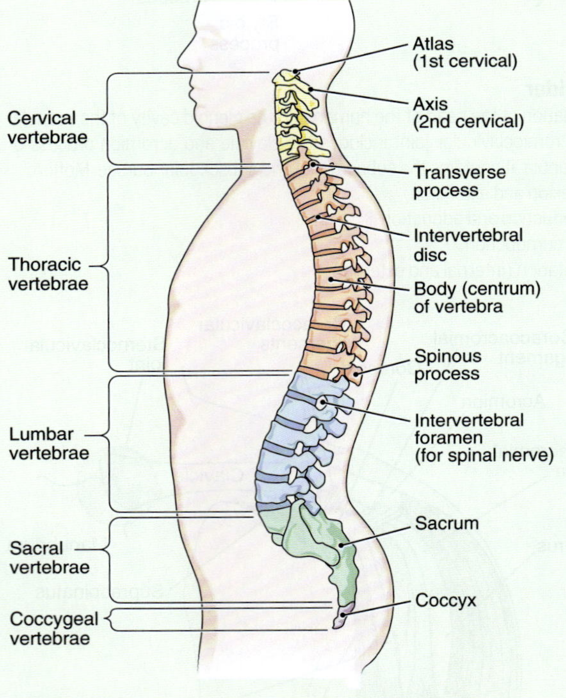

Left lateral view.

DISPLAY 28-2 UNDERSTANDING MAJOR JOINTS (continued)

Hip

Articulation between the head of the femur and the acetabulum. Contains a fibrous capsule. Motion:

- Flexion with knee flexed and with knee extended
- Extension and hyperextension
- Circumduction
- Rotation (internal and external)
- Abduction
- Adduction.

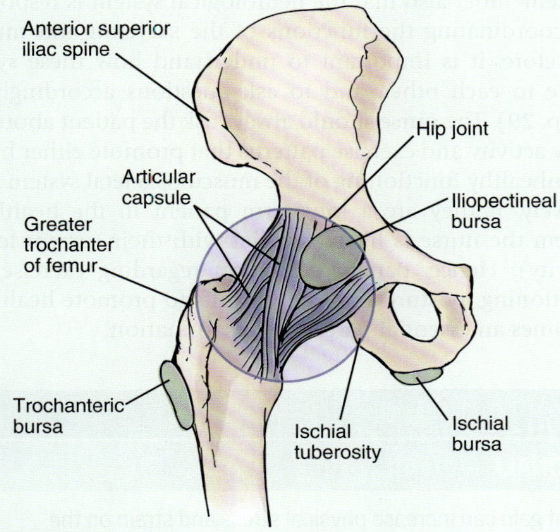

Right anterior view.

Knee

Articulation of the femur, tibia and patella; contains fibrocartilaginous discs (medial and lateral menisci) and many bursae. Motion:

- Flexion
- Extension.

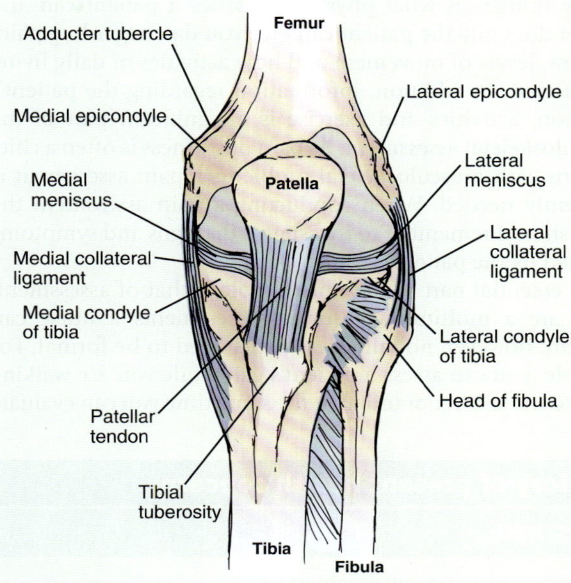

Left anterior view.

Ankle and foot

Articulation between the talus (large posterior foot tarsal), tibia and fibula. The talus also articulates with the navicular bones. The heel (calcaneus bone) is connected to the tibia and fibula by ligaments. Motion:

- Ankle: Plantar flexion and dorsiflexion
- Foot: Inversion and eversion
- Toes: Flexion, extension, abduction, adduction.

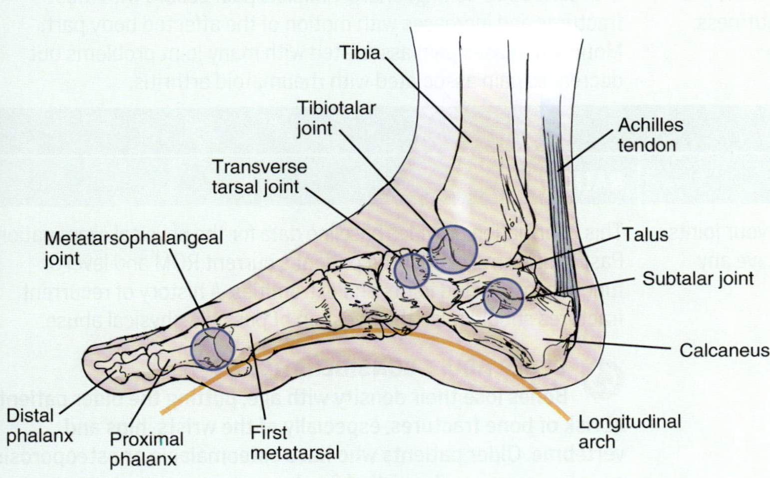

Right lateral view.

(Images from Cohen, B. J. & Hull, K. L. [2015]. *Memmler's structure and function of the human body* [11th ed.]. Philadelphia: Lippincott Williams & Wilkins.)

Health assessment

COLLECTING SUBJECTIVE DATA: THE NURSING HEALTH HISTORY

Assessment of the musculoskeletal system helps to evaluate the patient's level of functioning with activities of daily living. This system affects the entire body, from head to toe, and greatly influences what physical activities a patient can and cannot do. Only the patient can give you data regarding pain, stiffness, levels of movement and how activities of daily living are affected. In addition, information regarding the patient's nutrition, activities and exercise is a significant part of the musculoskeletal assessment. As pain or stiffness is often a chief concern with musculoskeletal problems a pain assessment is frequently needed. When conducting a pain assessment the nurse should remember to investigate the signs and symptoms reported by the patient.

An essential part of the nursing role is that of assessment. There are a multitude of formal assessments a nurse can perform; however, not all assessments need to be formal. For example, you can assess a patient's gait while you are walking them to the shower or toilet. At the same time you can evaluate if the patient is experiencing any pain, discomfort or shortness of breath associated with mobilisation.

As a nurse you should remember that assessing your patient is a continual process that should take place during any and all interactions you have with your patient during your shift. The information provided in the following pages can be utilised as a general guide to assist you in the assessment of the musculoskeletal system. Some of these assessments you may undertake using a formal process, whereas others you might note as you see the patient completing their activities of daily living.

Remember also that the neurological system is responsible for coordinating the functions of the skeleton and muscles. Therefore, it is important to understand how these systems relate to each other, and to ask questions accordingly (see Chap. 29). The nurse should always ask the patient about their daily activity and exercise patterns that promote either healthy or unhealthy functioning of the musculoskeletal system (alternatively, if they are a long-term patient in the health care system the nurse is likely familiar with their current level of activity). Hence, patient education regarding exercise, diet, positioning, posture and safety habits to promote health also becomes an essential part of this examination.

History of present health concern

QUESTION	RATIONALE
Have you had any recent weight gain?	Weight gain can increase physical stress and strain on the musculoskeletal system.
Describe any difficulty that you have chewing. Is it associated with tenderness or pain?	Patients with temporomandibular joint dysfunction may have difficulty chewing and may describe their jaws as 'getting locked or stuck'. Jaw tenderness, pain or a clicking sound may also be present with range of motion (ROM).
Describe any joint, muscle or bone pain you have. Where is the pain? What does the pain feel like (stab, ache)? When did the pain start? When does it occur? How long does it last? Any stiffness, swelling, limitation of movement?	Bone pain is often dull, deep and throbbing. Joint or muscle pain is described as aching. Sharp, knifelike pain occurs with most fractures and increases with motion of the affected body part. Motion increases pain associated with many joint problems but decreases pain associated with rheumatoid arthritis.

Past health history

QUESTION	RATIONALE
Describe any past problems or injuries you have had to your joints, muscles or bones. What treatment was given? Do you have any after-effects from the injury or problem?	This information provides baseline data for the physical examination. Past injuries may affect the patient's current ROM and level of function in affected joints and extremities. A history of recurrent fractures should raise the question of possible physical abuse. **OLDER ADULT CONSIDERATIONS** **Bones lose their density with age, putting the older patient at risk of bone fractures, especially of the wrists, hips and vertebrae. Older patients who have osteomalacia or osteoporosis are at an even greater risk of fractures.**
When were your last tetanus and polio immunisations?	Joint stiffening and other musculoskeletal symptoms may be a transient effect of the tetanus or polio vaccines. **OLDER ADULT CONSIDERATIONS** **Joint-stiffening conditions may be misdiagnosed as arthritis, especially in the older adult.**

COLDSPA

Example for pain in heels

Use the COLDSPA mnemonic as a guideline to collect needed information for each symptom the patient shares. In addition, the following questions help elicit important information.

Mnemonic	Question	Patient response example
Character	Describe the sign or symptom (feeling, appearance, sound, smell or taste, if applicable).	'I have sharp pains in my right foot, especially on the side and bottom of my heel.'
Onset	When did it begin?	'I first noticed the pain about 3 months ago. It has become worse over the past 2 weeks.'
Location	Where is it? Does it radiate? Does it occur anywhere else?	'The pain is mostly in my right heel and sometimes goes into the arch of my foot.'
Duration	How long does it last? Does it recur?	'I usually notice it in the morning when I first get up. It gets a little better during the day and then I notice it in the evening again.'
Severity	How bad is it? or How much does it bother you?	'It's bad enough that I can't take my daily walks. It's okay when I'm sitting but makes me hobble to the bathroom in the morning and hurts when I try to walk long distances.'
Pattern	What makes it better or worse?	'Naproxen helped some. I've tried taping the bottom of my foot, which helps a little. I've bought shoe inserts but can't tell that they help.'
Associated factors/How it **A**ffects the patient	What other symptoms occur with it? How does it affect you?	'I went through menopause a year ago and gained weight. I think those extra 8 kg have affected my foot. I'm discouraged because I can't walk. When I can't walk, I gain weight and then my foot gets worse.'

Past health history (continued)

QUESTION	RATIONALE
Have you ever been diagnosed with diabetes mellitus, sickle cell anaemia, systemic lupus erythematosus (SLE) or osteoporosis?	Having diabetes mellitus, sickle cell anaemia or SLE places the patient at risk of developing musculoskeletal problems such as osteoporosis and osteomyelitis. Patients who are immobile or have a reduced intake of calcium and vitamin D are especially prone to development of osteoporosis. **OLDER ADULT CONSIDERATIONS** **Osteoporosis is more common as a person ages because that is a time when bone resorption increases, calcium absorption decreases and production of osteoblasts decreases as well.**
For middle-aged women: Have you started menopause? Are you receiving oestrogen replacement therapy?	Women who begin menarche late or begin menopause early are at greater risk of developing osteoporosis because of decreased oestrogen levels, which tend to decrease the density of bone mass.

Family history

QUESTION	RATIONALE
Do you have a family history of rheumatoid arthritis, gout or osteoporosis?	These conditions tend to be familial and increase the patient's risk of developing these diseases.

Continued on following page

Family history (continued)

QUESTION	RATIONALE
What activities do you engage in to promote the health of your muscles and bones (e.g. exercise, diet, weight reduction)?	This question provides the examiner with knowledge of how much the patient understands and actively participates in trying to promote the health of the musculoskeletal system.
What medications are you taking?	Some medications can affect musculoskeletal function. Diuretics, for example, can alter electrolyte levels, leading to muscle weakness. Steroids can deplete bone mass, thereby contributing to osteoporosis. Adverse reactions to HMG-CoA reductase inhibitors (statins) can include myopathy, which can cause muscle aches or weakness.
Do you smoke tobacco? How much and how often?	Smoking increases the risk of osteoporosis (see Promote health—Osteoporosis).
Do you drink alcohol or caffeinated beverages? How much and how often?	Excessive consumption of alcohol or caffeine can increase the risk of osteoporosis.
Describe your typical 24-hour diet. Are you able to consume milk or milk-containing products? Do you take any calcium supplements?	Adequate protein in the diet promotes muscle tone and bone growth; vitamin C promotes healing of tissues and bones. A calcium deficiency increases the risk of osteoporosis. A diet high in purine (e.g. liver, sardines) can trigger gouty arthritis. **CULTURAL CONSIDERATIONS** **The ability to digest lactose varies between different races. The tendency to produce less lactase enzyme with age is more common in people of Asian, African, South American, Southern European and Australian Aboriginal heritage than in people of Northern European descent. There have been two studies in New Zealand, reported in the 1980s, which suggest that Māori and Pasifika have a higher prevalence of lactase deficiency than New Zealand Europeans (Pollard, 2008).**
Describe your activities during a typical day. How much time do you spend in the sunlight?	A sedentary lifestyle increases the risk of osteoporosis. Prolonged immobility leads to muscle atrophy. Exposure to 20 minutes of sunlight per day promotes the production of vitamin D in the body. Vitamin D deficiency can cause osteomalacia.
Describe any routine exercise that you do.	Regular exercise promotes flexibility, bone density, muscle tone and strength, and can help to slow the usual musculoskeletal changes (progressive loss of total bone mass and degeneration of skeletal muscle fibres) that occur with ageing. Improper body positioning in contact sports results in injury to the bones, joints or muscles.
Describe your occupation.	Certain job-related activities increase the risk of developing musculoskeletal problems. For example, incorrect body mechanics, heavy lifting or poor posture can contribute to back problems; consistent, repetitive wrist and hand movements can lead to the development of carpal tunnel syndrome.
Describe your posture at work and at leisure. What type of shoes do you usually wear? Do you use any special footwear (i.e. orthotics)?	Poor posture, prolonged forward bending (as in sitting) or backward leaning (as in working overhead), or long-term carrying of heavy objects on the shoulders can result in back problems. Contracture of the Achilles tendon can occur with prolonged use of high-heeled shoes.
Do you have difficulty performing normal activities of daily living (bathing, dressing, grooming, eating)? Do you use assistive devices (e.g. walker, cane, braces) to promote your mobility?	Impairment of the musculoskeletal system may affect the patient's ability to perform normal activities of daily living. Correct use of assistive devices can promote safety and independence. Some patients may feel embarrassed and not use their prescribed or needed assistive device.

Family history (continued)

QUESTION	RATIONALE
How have your musculoskeletal problems interfered with your ability to interact or socialise with others? Have they interfered with your usual sexual activity?	Musculoskeletal problems, especially chronic ones, can disable and cripple the patient, which may impair socialisation and prevent the patient from performing the same roles as in the past. Back problems, joint pain or muscle stiffness may interfere with sexual activities.
How did you view yourself before you had this musculoskeletal problem, and how do you view yourself now?	Body image disturbances and chronic low self-esteem may occur with a disabling or crippling problem.
Has your musculoskeletal problem added stress to your life? Describe.	Musculoskeletal problems often greatly affect activities of daily living and role performance, resulting in changed relationships and increased stress.

PROMOTE HEALTH **OSTEOPOROSIS**

OVERVIEW

Osteoporosis is a disease in which bones demineralise and become porous and fragile, making them susceptible to fractures. The International Osteoporosis Foundation (IOF, 2019) notes: 'The loss of bone occurs "silently" and progressively.' Because progress is silent, no symptoms are noted until the first fracture occurs, unless careful screening takes place in people over 50 with risk factors for osteoporosis.

Osteoporosis is internationally recognised as a serious health condition. In Australia and New Zealand, the burden of this disease is similar to other developed countries. According to the IOF (2019), around the world one in three women and one in five men aged 50 years and over are at risk of an osteoporotic fracture, with an osteoporotic fracture estimated to occur every 3 seconds. It is estimated that 1.2 million Australians have osteoporosis (AIHW, 2014). In New Zealand, a 2007 report estimated the number of fractures caused by osteoporosis at all sites in the skeleton to rise from 84,000 cases in 2007 to almost 116,000 by 2020. Based on costs in 2007 dollars, the direct costs for fracture care were expected to rise from almost $300 million in 2007 to $411 million by 2020. (Osteoporosis New Zealand, 2019).

To optimise bone health and diminish the risk of a person developing osteoporosis, a lifelong approach to building and maintaining a healthy skeleton is paramount. In 2011, Osteoporosis Australia began an undertaking to develop an evidence-informed national strategy to achieve its vision of healthy bones for all Australians. *Building healthy bones throughout life: An evidence-informed strategy to prevent osteoporosis in Australia* outlines a number of recommendations for health care professionals and can be sourced via www.mja.com.au.

The Royal Australian College of General Practitioners' 2017 guidelines also outline the current evidence-based recommendations for the prevention and treatment of osteoporosis in postmenopausal women and older men. These guidelines can be sourced via https://www.osteoporosis.org.au/clinical-guidelines.

Risk factors

- History of fractures
- Dowager hump
- Height reduction

Unmodifiable

- Age
- Female gender
- Family history
- Previous fracture
- Race and ethnicity
- Menopause and hysterectomy
- Long-term glucocorticoid therapy
- Rheumatoid arthritis
- Primary and secondary hypogonadism in men

Modifiable

- Alcohol (greater than 2 drinks a day)
- Smoking (past or current history)
- Low body mass index (<20 kg/m^2)
- Poor nutrition (low calcium intake and low protein intake)
- Vitamin D deficiency
- Eating disorders (lead to nutrition deficiencies)
- Insufficient exercise (especially sedentary lifestyle)

Risk factors are 'additive', meaning that the more risk factors you have, the greater your risk of developing osteoporosis.

Teach risk reduction tips

Teach parents of children and adolescents to help their children

- Ensure an adequate calcium intake that meets the relevant dietary recommendations in the country or region where they live.
- Avoid undernutrition and protein malnutrition.
- Maintain an adequate supply of vitamin D through sufficient exposure to the sun and through diet.
- Participate in regular physical activity.
- Avoid smoking.
- Be educated about the risk of high alcohol consumption.

Teach patients to prevent bone loss

- Ensure adequate calcium and vitamin D intake (recommendations range from country to country, varying between 800 and 1,300 mg/day, depending on age).
- Undertake regular, weight-bearing exercise.
- Avoid smoking or quit if smoking.
- Avoid heavy drinking.
- Middle-aged and older adults should follow these fundamental principles: Assess their risk of developing osteoporosis and, with medical advice, consider medications to help maintain an optimal bone mass and to decrease the risk of fracture.

CASE STUDIES

Jacob states that he was trying to do a jump over five steps and 'lost it'. He landed on a grassy area. He says that the pain happened straight away and is most severe over the outer aspect of his foot around the ankle area. He also says that his left hand and wrist are tender. He is unable to put any weight on his leg and walk because it is very painful. He tells you that he has full range of movement in his left wrist, but it is tender to touch. He says he is not injured anywhere else. He has nil complaints of neck pain or back pain and suffered no loss of consciousness in the accident.

CRITICAL THINKING

1. What questions would you ask about how Jacob injured himself?
2. Considering Jacob's age, what questions would you ask about his past medical history and lifestyle?

COLLECTING OBJECTIVE DATA: PHYSICAL EXAMINATION

Physical assessment of the musculoskeletal system provides data regarding the patient's posture, gait, bone structure, muscle strength and joint mobility, as well as the patient's ability to perform activities of daily living.

The physical assessment includes inspecting and palpating the joints, muscles and bones, testing range of motion (ROM), and assessing muscle strength. See Assessment tool 28-1 for guidelines to use when performing the musculoskeletal assessment.

Preparing the patient

Because this examination is lengthy, be sure the room is at a comfortable temperature and provide rest periods as necessary. Provide adequate draping to avoid unnecessary exposure of the patient yet adequate visualisation of the part being examined. Explain you will frequently ask the patient to change positions and to move various body parts against resistance and gravity. Clear, simple directions need to be given throughout the examination to help the patient understand how to move body parts to allow you to assess the musculoskeletal system, demonstrating to the patient how to move the various body parts and providing verbal directions to facilitate examination.

OLDER ADULT CONSIDERATIONS

Some positions required for this examination may be very uncomfortable for the older patient, who may have decreased flexibility. Be sensitive to the patient's needs and adapt your technique as necessary.

Equipment

- Tape measure
- Goniometer (optional)
- Skin marking pencil (optional)

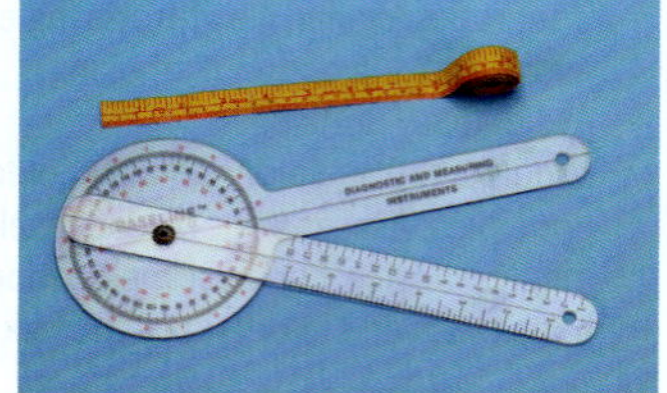

Physical assessment

- Observe gait and posture.
- Inspect joints, muscles and extremities for size, symmetry and colour.
- Palpate joints, muscles and extremities for tenderness, oedema, heat, nodules or crepitus.
- Test muscle strength and ROM of joints.
- Compare bilateral findings of joints and muscles.

CASE STUDY

Jacob is 165 cm tall and weighs 63 kg. Physical examination reveals bone tenderness over the posterior aspect of the tibia and lateral malleolus down to the fourth and fifth metatarsals. The area is swollen, deformed, warm and well perfused, and the skin is intact. Capillary refill is less than 2 seconds. There is no neurovascular injury, and a strong palpable pulse is noted in the dorsalis pedis and posterior tibial areas. Jacob has nil complaints of altered sensation or 'pins and needles' in the area. Jacob protects and guards his ankle and foot upon examination of the area.

CRITICAL THINKING

3. When assessing Jacob's ankle and wrist injury, there are a number of considerations—not all linked to Jacob's injury. What should be evaluated?
4. What should the initial management of the ankle and wrist injury involve to reduce further swelling?

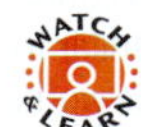

Assessing the musculoskeletal and neurological systems

CASE STUDY CONSIDERATIONS

In addition to using the COLDSPA mnemonic as a guide for the collection of information concerning Jacob's present condition, the following memory tip will aid your systematic assessment of Jacob's musculoskeletal injury.

Memory tip: Six Ps of assessing musculoskeletal injury:

Pain: Does the patient feel pain? If they do, assess its location, severity and quality.

Paraesthesia: Assess for loss of sensation by touching the injured area with the tip of an open safety pin. Abnormal sensation or loss of sensation indicates neurovascular involvement.

Paralysis: Can the patient move the affected area? If they are unable, they may have nerve or tendon damage.

Pallor: Paleness, discolouration and coolness on the injured side may indicate neurovascular compromise.

Pulse: Check all pulses distal to the injury site. If a pulse is decreased or absent, blood supply to the area is reduced.

Pressure: Monitor the calf for pressure measuring the circumference of the calf each time that you check the observations and also palpating to make sure that it is not becoming firmer which may indicate bleeding into one of the facial compartments of the muscle.

ASSESSMENT TOOL 28-1 Guidelines for Assessing Joints and Muscles

The following are guidelines for assessing joints and muscle strength.

Joints

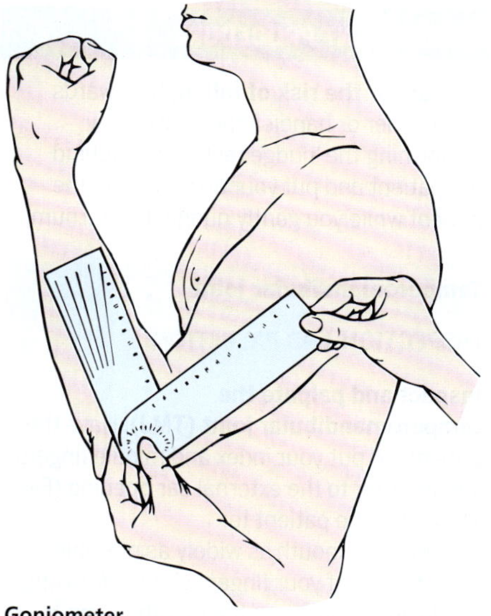
Goniometer

1. Inspect size, shape, colour and symmetry. Note any masses, deformities or muscle atrophy. Compare bilateral joint findings.
2. Palpate for oedema, heat, tenderness, pain, nodules or crepitus. Compare bilateral joint findings.
3. Test each joint's range of motion (ROM). Demonstrate how to move each joint through its normal ROM, then ask the patient actively to move the joint through the same motions. Compare bilateral joint findings.

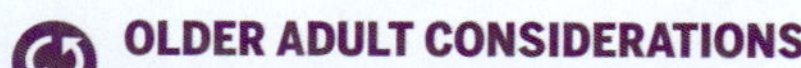

OLDER ADULT CONSIDERATIONS

Older patients usually have slower movements, reduced flexibility and decreased muscle strength because of age-related muscle fibre and joint degeneration, reduced elasticity of the tendons and joint capsule calcification.

If you identify a limitation in the ROM, measure ROM with a goniometer (a device that measures movement in degrees). To do so, move the arms of the goniometer to match the angle of the joint being assessed. Then describe the limited motion of the joint in degrees: for example, 'elbow flexes from 45 degrees to 90 degrees'.

Muscles

1. Test muscle strength by asking the patient to move each extremity through its full ROM against resistance. Do this by applying some resistance against the part being moved. Document muscle strength by using a standard scale (see Rating scale for muscle strength, below). If the patient cannot move the part against your resistance, ask the patient to move the part against gravity. If this is not possible, then attempt passively to move the part through its full ROM. If this is not possible, then inspect and feel for a palpable contraction of the muscle while the patient attempts to move it. Compare bilateral joint findings.

CLINICAL TIP

Do not force the part beyond its normal range. Stop passive motion if the patient expresses discomfort or pain. Be especially cautious with the older patient when testing ROM. When comparing bilateral strength, keep in mind that the patient's dominant side will tend to be the stronger side. As each person is different they strength and ROM should be checked against themselves (i.e. if you are checking one side, you should then check the other and determine if the strength and range are equivalent).

2. Rate muscle strength in accord with the strength table below.

Rating	Explanation	Strength classification
5	Active motion against full resistance	Normal
4	Active motion against some resistance	Slight weakness
3	Active motion against gravity	Average weakness
2	Passive ROM (gravity removed and assisted by examiner)	Poor ROM
1	Slight flicker of contraction	Severe weakness
0	No muscular contraction	Paralysis

PHYSICAL ASSESSMENT

ASSESSMENT PROCEDURE	NORMAL FINDINGS	ABNORMAL FINDINGS
Gait		
INSPECTION		
Observe gait. Observe the patient's gait as the patient enters and walks around the room. Note: • Base of support movements coordinated and rhythmic • Weight-bearing stability arms swing in opposition, stride length • Foot position appropriate • Stride and length and cadence of stride • Arm swing • Posture.	Evenly distributed weight. Patient able to stand on heels and toes. Toes point straight ahead. Equal on both sides. Posture erect, movements coordinated and rhythmic, arms swing in opposition, stride length appropriate.	Uneven weight-bearing is evident. Patient cannot stand on heels or toes. Toes point in or out. Patient limps, shuffles, propels forwards, or has wide-based gait. (See Chap. 29, Nervous system, for specific abnormal gait findings.)

Continued on following page

PHYSICAL ASSESSMENT (continued)

ASSESSMENT PROCEDURE	NORMAL FINDINGS	ABNORMAL FINDINGS
Assess for the risk of falling backwards in the older or handicapped patient by performing the 'nudge test'. Stand behind the patient and put your arms around the patient while you gently nudge the sternum.	Patient does not fall backwards. **OLDER ADULT CONSIDERATIONS** **Some older patients have an impaired sense of position in space, which may contribute to the risks of falling.**	Falling backwards easily is seen with cervical spondylosis and Parkinson disease.
Temporomandibular joint		
INSPECTION AND PALPATION		
Inspect and palpate the temporomandibular joint (TMJ). Have the patient sit; put your index and middle fingers just anterior to the external ear opening (Fig. 28-4). Ask the patient to: • Open the mouth as widely as possible. (The tips of your fingers should drop into the joint spaces as the mouth opens.) • Move the jaw from side to side. • Protrude (push out) and retract (pull in) jaw.	Jaw moves laterally 1 to 2 cm. Snapping and clicking may be felt and heard in the normal patient. Mouth opens 3 to 5 cm (distance between upper and lower teeth). Jaw protrudes and retracts easily. The patient's mouth opens and closes smoothly.	Decreased range of motion (ROM), swelling, tenderness, or crepitus may be seen in arthritis. Decreased muscle strength with muscle and joint disease. ROM and a clicking, popping or grating sound may be noted with TMJ dysfunction.
Test ROM. Ask the patient to open the mouth and move the jaw laterally against resistance. Next, as the patient clenches the teeth, feel for the contraction of the temporal and masseter muscles to test the integrity of cranial nerve V (trigeminal nerve).	Jaw has full ROM against resistance. Contraction palpated with no pain or spasms.	Lack of full contraction with cranial nerve V lesion. Pain or spasms occur with myofacial pain syndrome.
Sternoclavicular joint		
INSPECTION AND PALPATION		
With patient sitting, inspect the sternoclavicular joint for location in midline, colour, swelling and masses. Then palpate for tenderness or pain.	There is no visible bony overgrowth, swelling or redness; joint is non-tender.	Swollen, red or enlarged joint or tender, painful joint is seen with inflammation of the joint.
Cervical, thoracic and lumbar spine		
INSPECTION AND PALPATION		
Observe the cervical, thoracic and lumbar curves from the side then from behind. Have the patient standing erect with the gown positioned to allow an adequate view of the spine (Fig. 28-5). Observe for symmetry, noting differences in height of the shoulders, the iliac crests and the buttock creases.	Cervical and lumbar spines are concave; thoracic spine is convex. Spine is straight (when observed from behind).	A flattened lumbar curvature may be seen with a herniated lumbar disc or ankylosing spondylitis. Lateral curvature of the thoracic spine with an increase in the convexity on the curved side is seen in scoliosis. An exaggerated lumbar curve (lordosis) is often seen in pregnancy or obesity (see Abnormal findings 28-1). Unequal heights of the hips suggest unequal leg lengths. **OLDER ADULT CONSIDERATIONS** **An exaggerated thoracic curve (kyphosis) is common with ageing.**

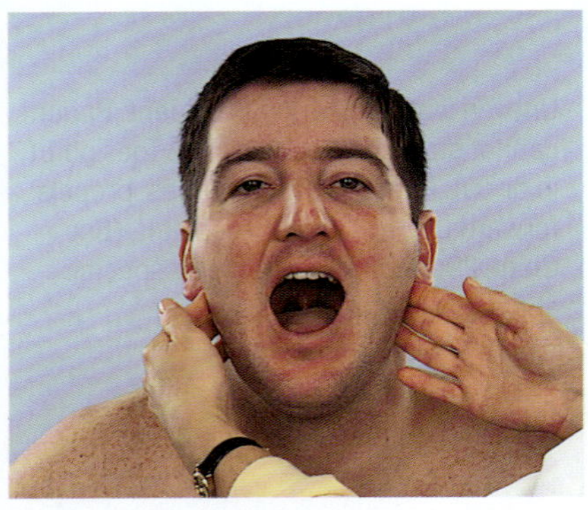
FIGURE 28-4 Palpating the temporomandibular joint. (© B. Proud.)

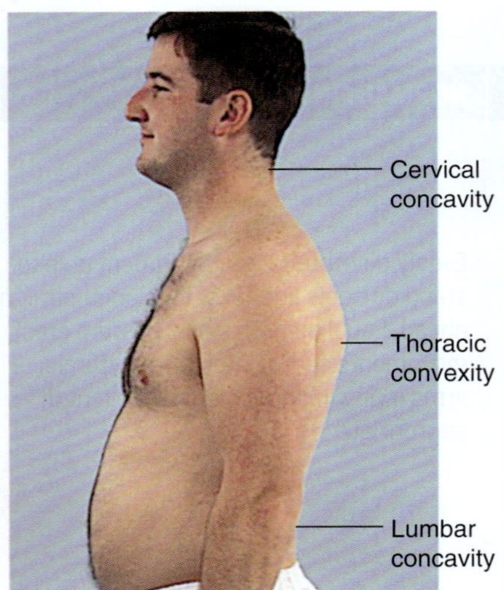

FIGURE 28-5 Normal curve of the spine (© B. Proud.)

PHYSICAL ASSESSMENT (continued)

ASSESSMENT PROCEDURE	NORMAL FINDINGS	ABNORMAL FINDINGS
Palpate the spinous processes and the paravertebral muscles on both sides of the spine for tenderness or pain.	Non-tender spinous processes; well-developed, firm and smooth, non-tender paravertebral muscles. No muscle spasm.	Compression fractures and lumbosacral muscle strain can cause pain and tenderness of the spinal processes and the paravertebral muscles.
Test ROM of the cervical spine. Test ROM of the cervical spine by asking the patient to touch the chin to the chest (flexion) and to look up at the ceiling (hyperextension) (Fig. 28-6).	Flexion of the cervical spine is 45 degrees. Extension of the cervical spine is 45 degrees.	Cervical strain is the most common cause of neck pain. It is characterised by impaired ROM and neck pain from abnormalities of the soft tissue (muscles, ligaments and nerves) due to straining or injuring the neck. Causes of strains can include sleeping in the wrong position, carrying a heavy suitcase or being in a car crash. Cervical disc degenerative disease and spinal cord tumours are associated with impaired ROM and pain that radiates to the back, shoulder or arms. Neck pain with a loss of sensation in the legs may occur with cervical spinal cord compression. **CLINICAL TIP** **Impaired ROM and neck pain associated with fever, chills and headache could be indicative of a serious infection such as meningitis.**
Next test lateral bending. Ask the patient to touch each ear to the shoulder on that side (Fig. 28-7).	Normally the patient can bend 40 degrees to the left side and 40 degrees to the right side.	
Evaluate rotation. Ask the patient to turn head to right and left (Fig. 28-8).	About 70 degrees of rotation is normal.	
Ask the patient to repeat the cervical ROM movements against resistance.	Patient has full ROM against resistance.	Decreased ROM against resistance is seen with joint or muscle disease.

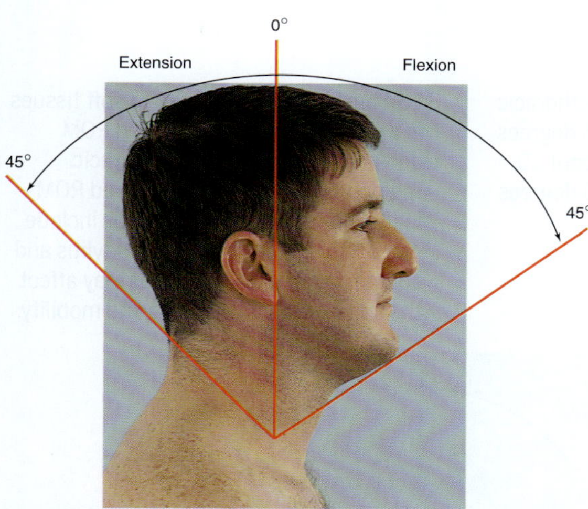

FIGURE 28-6 Normal range of motion of cervical spine: hyperextension–flexion. (© B. Proud.)

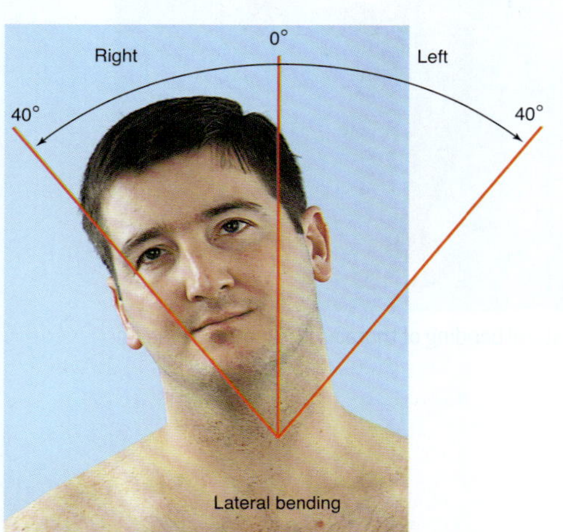

FIGURE 28-7 Normal range of motion of cervical spine: lateral bending. (© B. Proud.)

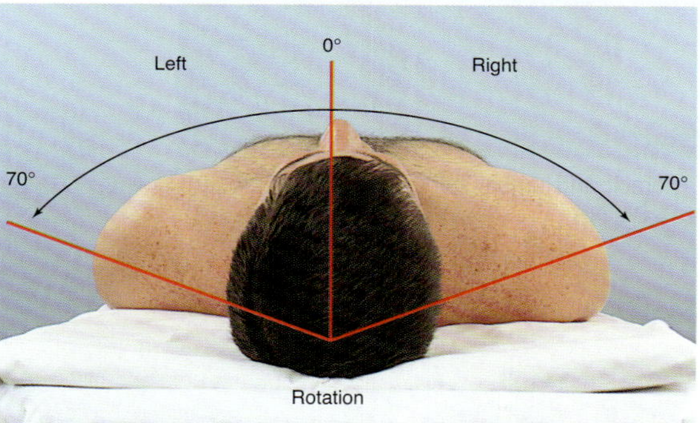

FIGURE 28-8 Normal range of motion of cervical spine: rotation. (© B. Proud.)

Continued on following page

PHYSICAL ASSESSMENT (continued)

ASSESSMENT PROCEDURE	NORMAL FINDINGS	ABNORMAL FINDINGS
Cervical, thoracic and lumbar spine (continued)		
Test ROM of the thoracic and lumbar spine. Ask the patient to bend forwards and touch the toes (flexion) (Fig. 28-9). Observe for symmetry of the shoulders, scapula and hips. **OLDER ADULT CONSIDERATIONS** **Similarly, ask older patients to bend forwards but do not insist that they touch their toes unless they are comfortable with this movement.**	Flexion of 75 degrees to 90 degrees, smooth movement, lumbar concavity flattens out and the spinal processes are in alignment.	Lateral curvature disappears in functional scoliosis; unilateral exaggerated thoracic convexity increases in structural scoliosis. Spinal processes are out of alignment.
Sit down behind the patient, stabilise the patient's pelvis with your hands and ask the patient to bend sideways (lateral bending), bend backwards towards you (hyperextension), and twist the shoulders one way then the other (rotation).	Lateral bending capacity of the thoracic and lumbar should be about 35 degrees (Fig. 28-10); hyperextension about 30 degrees; and rotation about 30 degrees (Fig. 28-11).	Low back strain from injury to soft tissues is a common cause of impaired ROM and pain in the lumbar and thoracic regions. Other causes of impaired ROM in the lumbar and thoracic areas include osteoarthritis, ankylosing spondylitis and congenital abnormalities that may affect the spinal vertebral spacing and mobility.

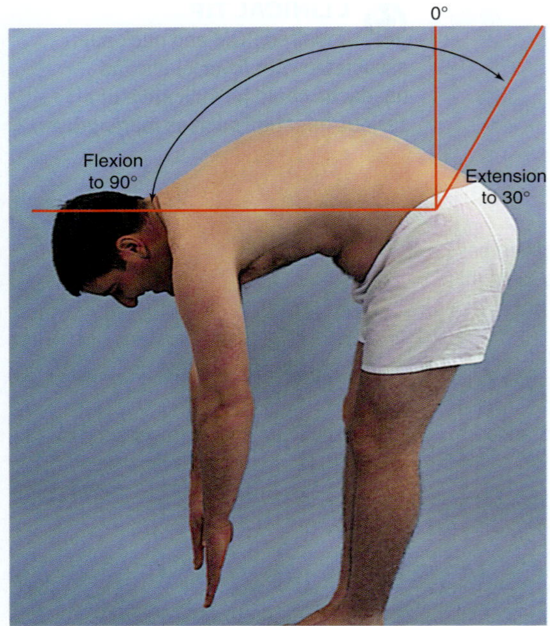

FIGURE 28-9 Thoracic and lumbar spine: flexion. (© B. Proud.)

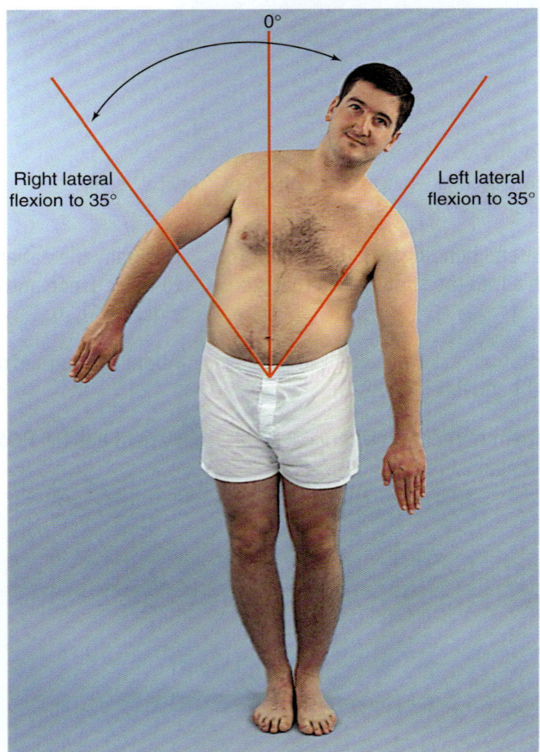

FIGURE 28-10 Lateral bending of thoracic and lumbar spine. (© B. Proud.)

PHYSICAL ASSESSMENT (continued)

ASSESSMENT PROCEDURE	NORMAL FINDINGS	ABNORMAL FINDINGS
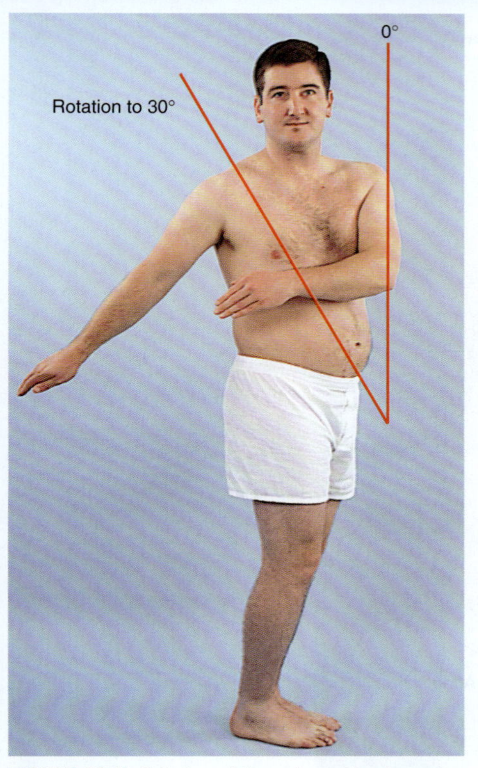 **FIGURE 28-11** Rotation of thoracic and lumber spines. (© B. Proud.)	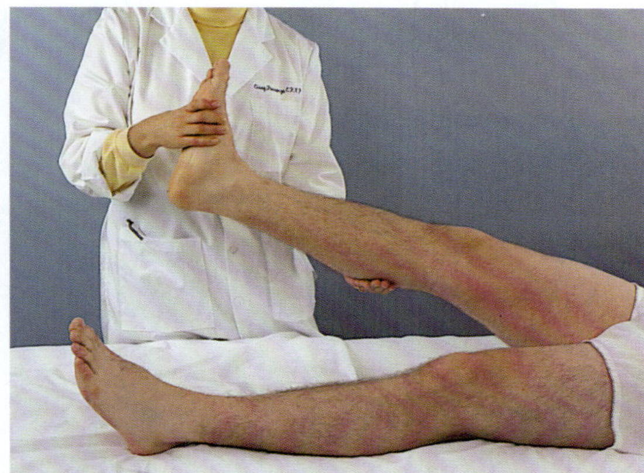 **FIGURE 28-12** Performing the Lasègue test. (© B. Proud.)	
Test for back and leg pain. If the patient has low back pain that radiates down the back, perform the Lasègue test (straight leg raising) to check a herniated nucleus pulposus. Ask the patient to lie flat and raise each relaxed leg independently to the point of pain. At the point of pain, dorsiflex the patient's foot (Fig. 28-12). Note the degree of elevation when pain occurs, the distribution and character of the pain, and the results from dorsiflexion of the foot.	Pain not reproduced. Patient is able to raise leg to 90-degree angle. Mild pain of the hamstring is a common finding and does not indicate sciatic pain.	Pain is reproduced. Pain that shoots and radiates down one or both legs (sciatica) below the knees may be due to a herniated intervertebral disc. Continuous, aching pain at night not relieved by rest may be from metastases. Lower back pain with tenderness and limited ROM is common in osteoporosis.
Shoulders and arms		
INSPECTION AND PALPATION		
Inspect and palpate shoulders and arms. With the patient standing or sitting, inspect anteriorly and posteriorly symmetry, colour, swelling and masses. Palpate for tenderness, swelling or heat. Anteriorly palpate the clavicle, acromioclavicular joint, subacromial area and biceps. Posteriorly palpate the glenohumeral joint, coracoid area, trapezius muscle and scapular area.	Shoulders are symmetrically round, no redness, swelling, deformity or heat. Muscles are fully developed. Clavicles and scapulae are even and symmetrical. The patient reports no tenderness.	Flat, hollow or less rounded shoulders are seen with dislocation. Muscle atrophy is seen with nerve or muscle damage or lack of use. Tenderness, swelling and heat may be noted with shoulder strains, sprains, arthritis, bursitis and degenerative joint disease.
Test ROM. Explain to the patient that you will be assessing range of motion (consisting of flexion, extension, adduction, abduction and motion against resistance).	Extent of forward flexion should be 180 degrees; hyperextension, 50 degrees; adduction, 50 degrees; and abduction 180 degrees.	Painful and limited abduction accompanied by muscle weakness and atrophy are seen with a rotator cuff tear. Patient has sharp catches of pain when

Continued on following page

PHYSICAL ASSESSMENT (continued)

ASSESSMENT PROCEDURE	NORMAL FINDINGS	ABNORMAL FINDINGS
Shoulders and arms (continued)		
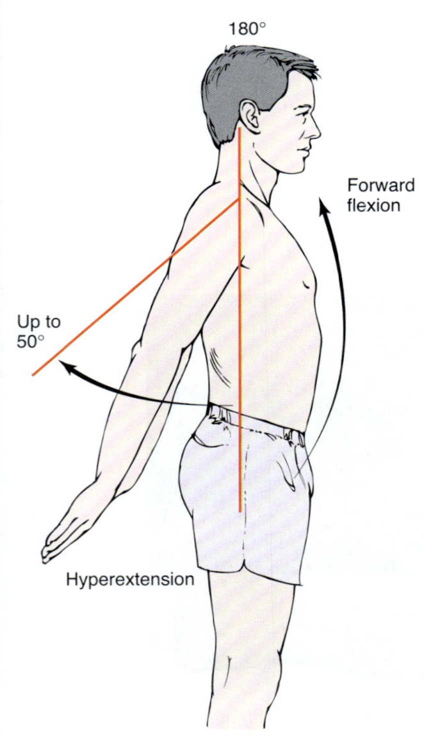 FIGURE 28-13 Normal range of motion of the shoulder: flexion–extension.	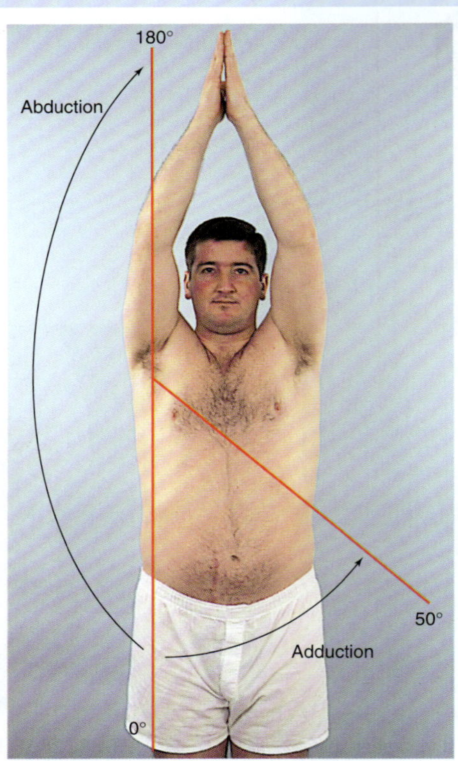 FIGURE 28-14 Normal range of motion of the shoulder: adduction–abduction. (© B. Proud.)	
Ask the patient to stand with both arms straight down at sides. Next ask the patient to move the arms forwards (flexion), then backwards with elbows straight (Fig. 28-13). Then have the patient bring both hands together overhead, elbows straight, followed by moving both hands in front of the body past the midline with elbows straight (this tests adduction and abduction) (Fig. 28-14).		bringing hands overhead when he or she has rotator cuff tendinitis. Chronic pain and severe limitation of all shoulder motions are seen with calcified tendinitis.
In a continuous motion, have the patient bring the hands together behind the head with elbows flexed (this tests external rotation) (Fig. 28-15A) and behind the back (internal rotation) (Fig. 28-15B). Repeat these two manoeuvres against resistance.	Extent of external and internal rotation should be about 90 degrees, respectively. The patient can flex, extend, adduct, abduct, rotate and shrug shoulders against resistance.	Inability to shrug shoulders against resistance is seen with a lesion of cranial nerve XI (spinal accessory). Decreased muscle strength is seen with muscle or joint disease.
Elbows		
INSPECTION AND PALPATION		
Inspect for size, shape, deformities, redness or swelling. Inspect elbows in both flexed and extended positions.	Elbows are symmetrical without deformities, redness or swelling.	Redness, heat and swelling may be seen with bursitis of the olecranon process due to trauma or arthritis.

PHYSICAL ASSESSMENT (continued)

ASSESSMENT PROCEDURE	NORMAL FINDINGS	ABNORMAL FINDINGS

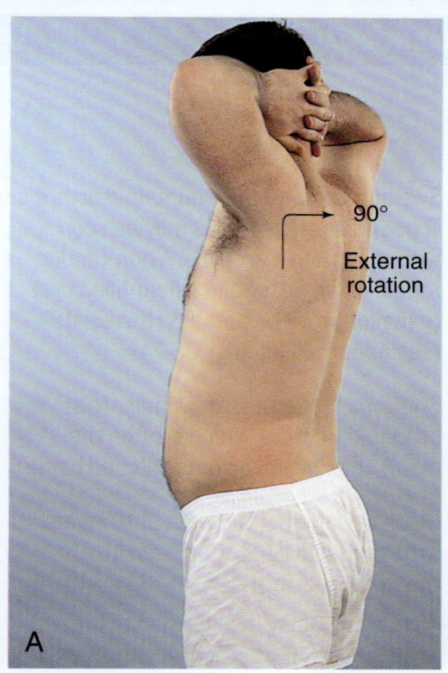

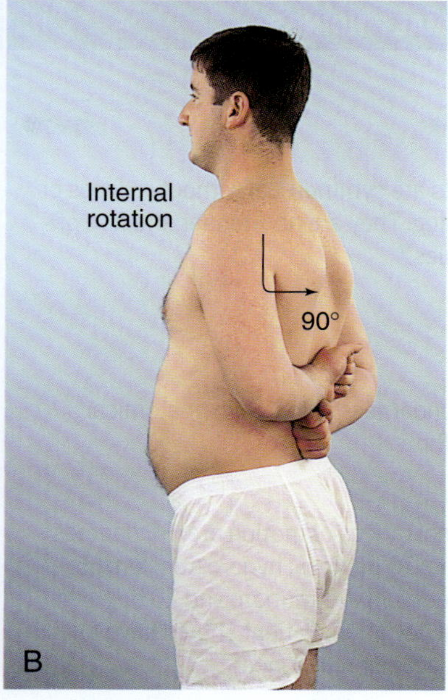

FIGURE 28-15 Normal range of motion of the shoulder: **(A)** external rotation; **(B)** internal rotation. (© B. Proud.)

ASSESSMENT PROCEDURE	NORMAL FINDINGS	ABNORMAL FINDINGS
With the elbow relaxed and flexed about 70 degrees, use your thumb and middle fingers to palpate the olecranon process and epicondyles.	Non-tender; without nodules.	Firm, non-tender, subcutaneous nodules may be palpated in rheumatoid arthritis or rheumatic fever. Tenderness or pain over the epicondyles may be palpated in epicondylitis (tennis elbow) due to repetitive movements of the forearm or wrists.
Test ROM. Ask the patient to perform the following movements to test ROM, flexion, extension, pronation and supination: Flex the elbow and bring the hand to the forehead (Fig. 28-16A). Straighten the elbow. Hold arm out, turn the palm down, then turn the palm up (Fig. 28-16B). Finally, have the patient repeat the movements against your resistance.	Normal ranges of motion are: 160 degrees of flexion; 180 degrees of extension; 90 degrees of pronation; and 90 degrees of supination. Some patients may lack 5 degrees to 10 degrees or have hyperextension. The patient should have full ROM against resistance.	Decreased ROM against resistance is seen with joint or muscle disease or injury.

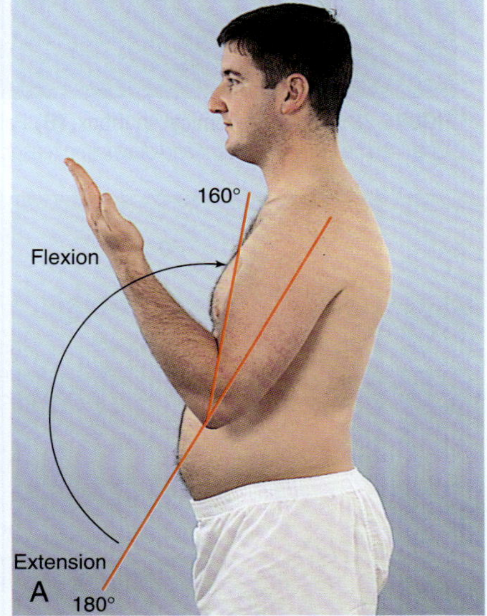

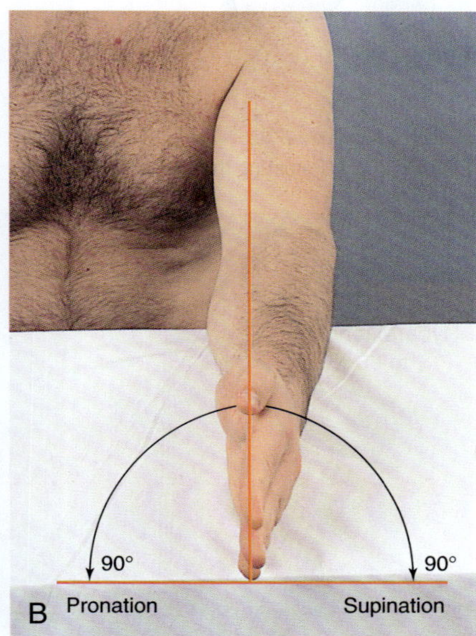

FIGURE 28-16 Normal range of motion of the elbow: **(A)** flexion–extension; **(B)** pronation–supination. (© B. Proud.)

Continued on following page

PHYSICAL ASSESSMENT (continued)

ASSESSMENT PROCEDURE	NORMAL FINDINGS	ABNORMAL FINDINGS
Wrists		
INSPECTION AND PALPATION		
Inspect wrist size, shape, symmetry, colour and swelling. Then palpate for tenderness and nodules (Fig. 28-17).	Wrists are symmetrical without redness or swelling. They are non-tender and free of nodules.	Swelling is seen with rheumatoid arthritis. Tenderness and nodules may be seen with rheumatoid arthritis. A non-tender, round, enlarged, swollen, fluid-filled cyst (ganglion) may be noted on the wrists (see Abnormal findings 28-2).
Palpate the anatomical snuffbox (the hollow area on the back of the wrist at the base of the fully extended thumb) (Fig. 28-18).	No tenderness palpated in anatomical snuffbox.	Snuffbox tenderness may indicate a scaphoid fracture, which is often the result of falling on an outstretched hand.
Test ROM. Ask the patient to bend wrist down and back (flexion and extension) (Fig. 28-19A). Next have the patient hold the wrist straight and move the hand outwards and inwards (deviation) (Fig. 28-19B). Repeat these manoeuvres against resistance.	Normal ranges of motion are: 90 degrees, flexion; 70 degrees, hyperextension; 55 degrees, ulnar deviation; and 20 degrees, radial deviation. Patient should have full ROM against resistance.	Ulnar deviation of the wrist and fingers with limited ROM is often seen in rheumatoid arthritis. Increased pain with extension of the wrist against resistance is seen in epicondylitis of the lateral side of the elbow. Increased pain with flexion of the wrist against resistance is seen in epicondylitis of the medial side of the elbow. Decreased muscle strength is noted with muscle and joint disease.

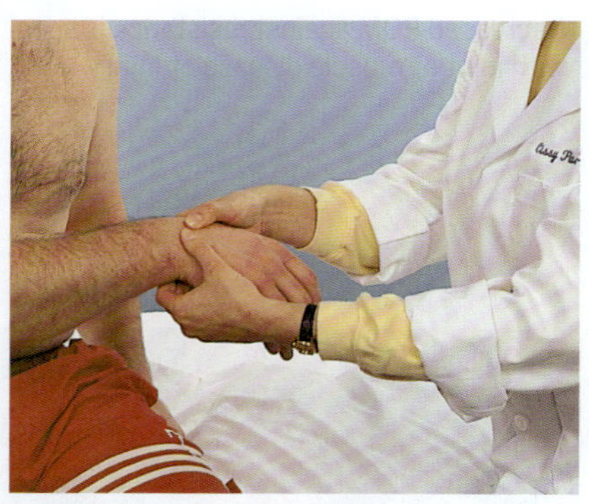

FIGURE 28-17 Palpating the wrists. (© B. Proud.)

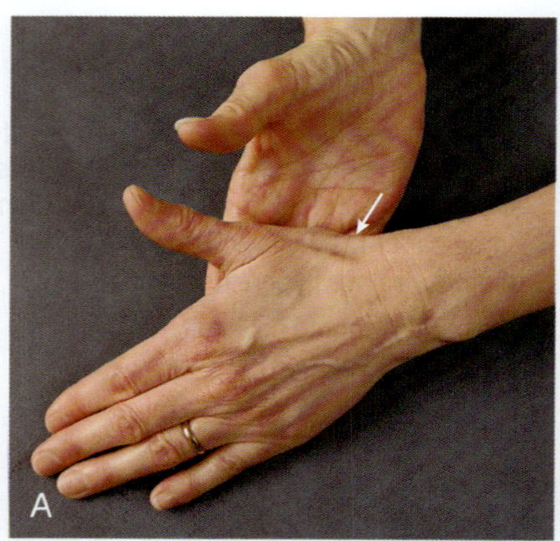

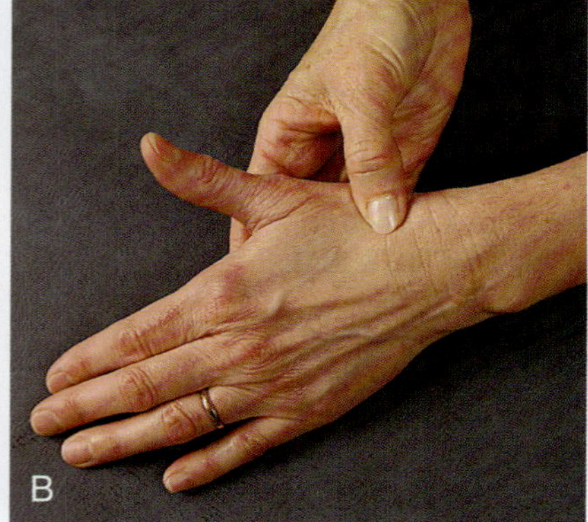

FIGURE 28-18 **(A)** Anatomical snuffbox. **(B)** Palpating the anatomical snuffbox. (Rhoads, J. [2006]. *Advanced health assessment and diagnostic reasoning.* Philadelphia: Lippincott Williams & Wilkins.)

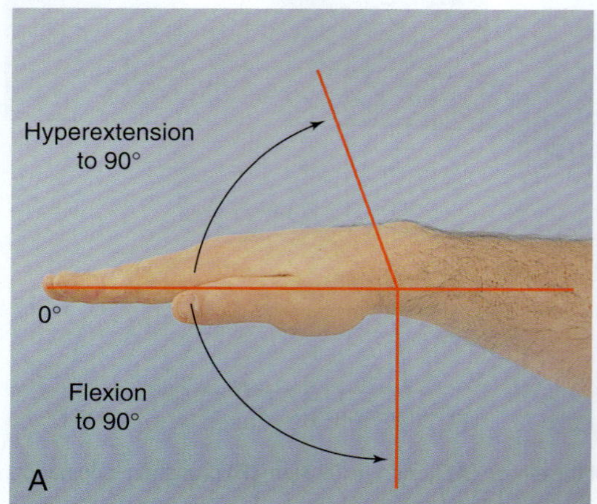

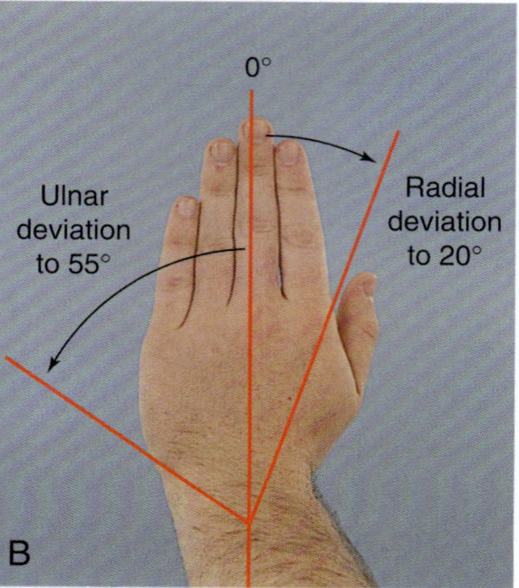

FIGURE 28-19 Range of motion of the wrists: **(A)** flexion–hyperextension; **(B)** radial–ulnar deviation. (© B. Proud.)

PHYSICAL ASSESSMENT (continued)

ASSESSMENT PROCEDURE	NORMAL FINDINGS	ABNORMAL FINDINGS
Test for carpal tunnel syndrome. Perform the Phalen test. Ask the patient to place the backs of both hands against each other while flexing the wrists 90 degrees downwards (Fig. 28-20A). Have the patient hold this position for 60 seconds. Optionally test for the Tinel sign. With your finger, percuss lightly over the median nerve (located on the inner aspect of the wrist) (Fig. 28-20B).	No tingling, numbness or pain result from the Phalen test or from the Tinel test.	After either test, patient may report tingling, numbness and pain with carpal tunnel syndrome. Median nerve entrapped in the carpal tunnel results in pain, numbness and impaired function of the hand and fingers (Fig. 28-21).

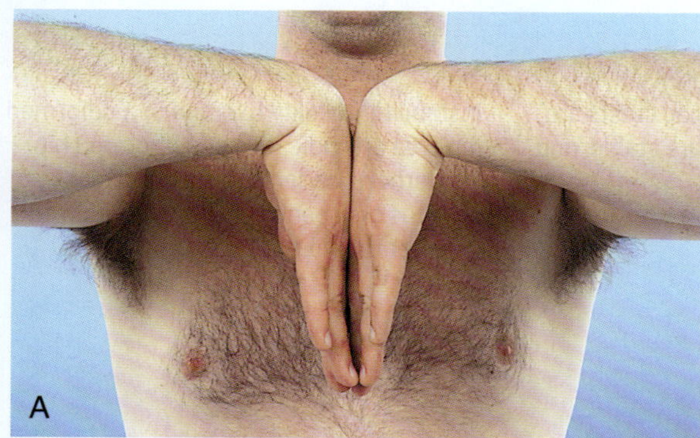

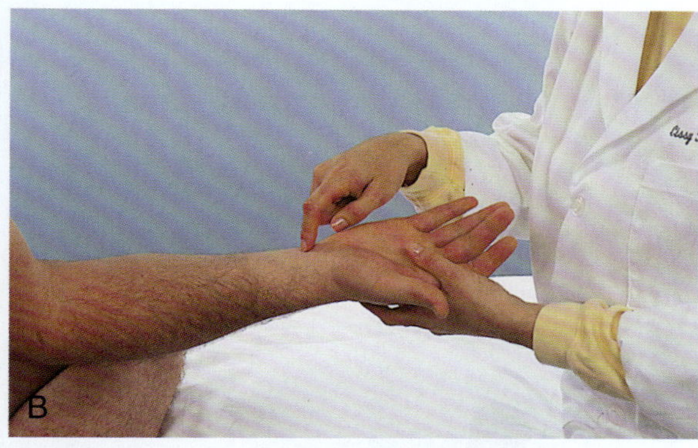

FIGURE 28-20 Tests for carpal tunnel syndrome: **(A)** Phalen test; **(B)** Tinel test. (© B. Proud.)

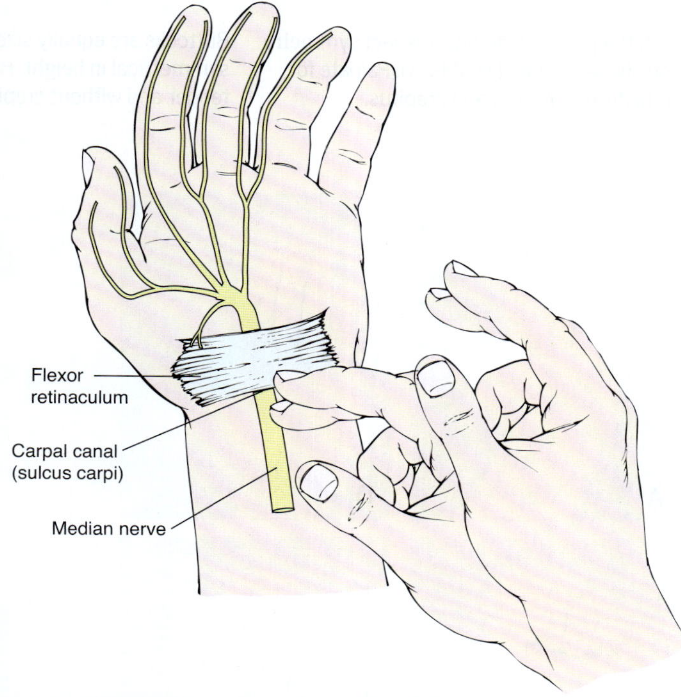

FIGURE 28-21 Median nerve entrapped in the carpal tunnel results in pain, numbness and impaired function of the hand and fingers.

Hands and fingers

INSPECTION AND PALPATION

Inspect size, shape, symmetry, swelling and colour. Palpate the fingers from the distal end proximally, noting tenderness, swelling, bony prominences, nodules or crepitus of each interphalangeal joint. Assess the metacarpophalangeal joints by squeezing the hand from each side between your thumb and fingers. Palpate each metacarpal of the hand, noting tenderness and swelling.	Hands and fingers are symmetrical, non-tender and without nodules. Fingers lie in straight line. No swelling or deformities. Rounded protuberance noted next to the thumb over the thenar prominence. Smaller protuberance seen adjacent to the small finger.	Swollen, stiff, tender finger joints are seen in acute rheumatoid arthritis. Boutonnière deformity and swan-neck deformity are seen in long-term rheumatoid arthritis (see Abnormal findings 28-2). Atrophy of the thenar prominence may be evident in carpal tunnel syndrome. In osteoarthritis, hard, painless nodules may be seen over the distal interphalangeal joints (Heberden nodes) and over the proximal interphalangeal joints (Bouchard nodes) (see Abnormal findings 28-2).

Continued on following page

PHYSICAL ASSESSMENT (continued)

ASSESSMENT PROCEDURE	NORMAL FINDINGS	ABNORMAL FINDINGS
Hands and fingers (continued)		
Test ROM (Fig. 28-22). Ask the patient to (*A*) spread the fingers apart (abduction), (*B*) make a fist (adduction), (*C*) bend the fingers down (flexion) and then up (hyperextension), (*D*) move the thumb away from other fingers and then (*E*) touch the thumb to the base of the small finger. Repeat these manoeuvres against resistance.	Normal ranges are 20 degrees of abduction, full adduction of fingers (touching), 90 degrees of flexion and 30 degrees of hyperextension. The thumb should easily move away from other fingers and 50 degrees of thumb flexion is normal. The patient normally has full ROM against resistance.	Inability to extend the ring and little fingers is seen in Dupuytren contracture. Painful extension of a finger may be seen in tenosynovitis (infection of the flexor tendon sheathes; see Abnormal findings 28-2). Decreased muscle strength against resistance is associated with muscle and joint disease.
Hips		
INSPECTION AND PALPATION		
With the patient standing, inspect symmetry and shape of hips (Fig. 28-23). Palpate for stability, tenderness and crepitus.	Buttocks are equally sized; iliac crests are symmetrical in height. Hips are stable, non-tender and without crepitus.	Instability, inability to stand or a deformed hip area are indicative of a fractured hip. Tenderness, oedema, decreased ROM and crepitus are seen in hip inflammation and degenerative joint disease.

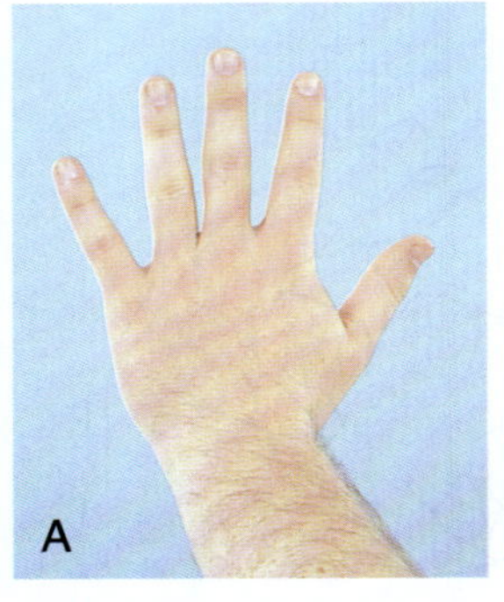

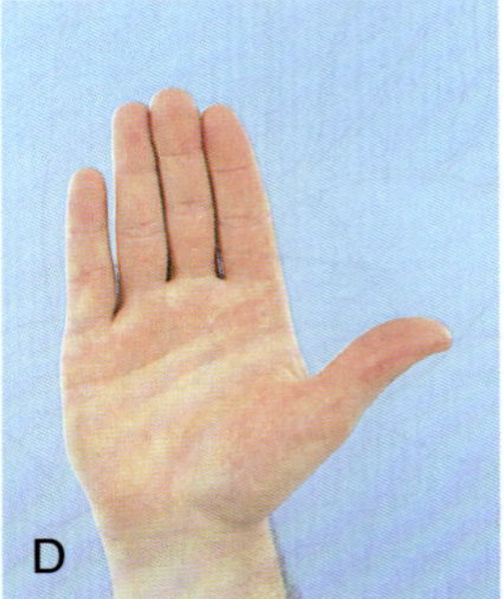

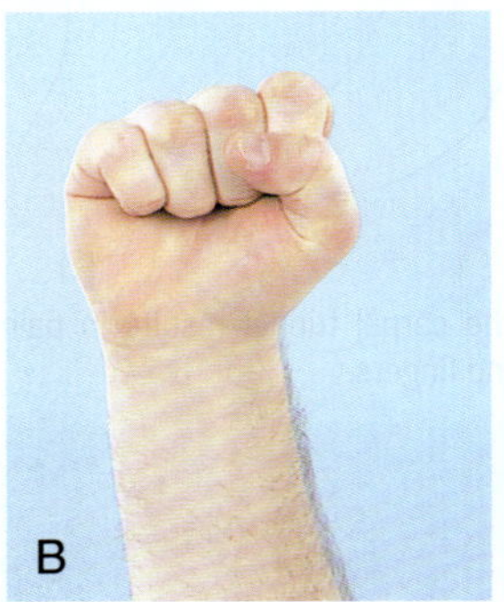

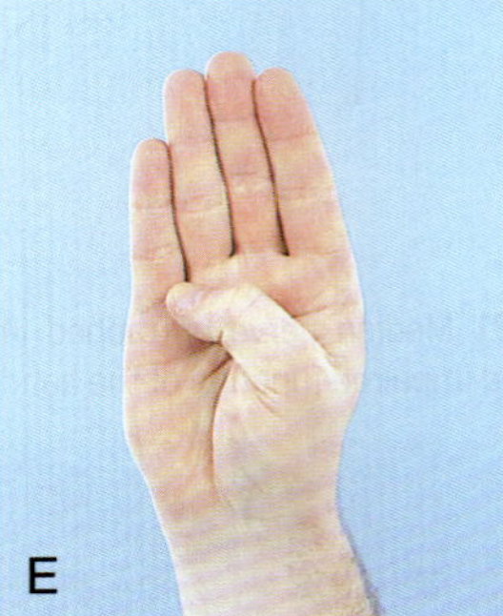

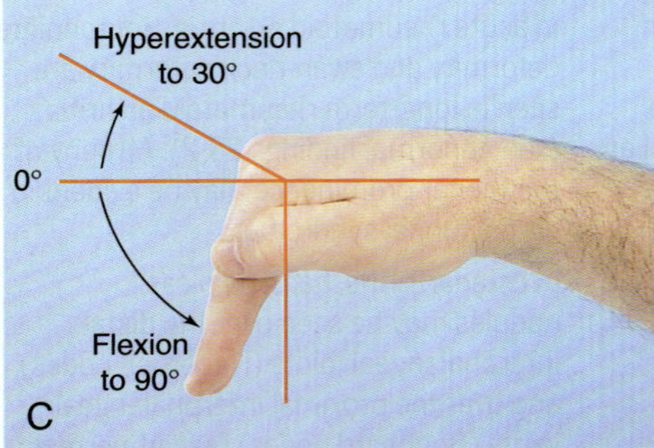

FIGURE 28-22 Normal range of motion of the fingers: **(A)** abduction, **(B)** adduction, **(C)** flexion–hyperextension, **(D)** thumb away from fingers, **(E)** thumb touching base of small finger. (© B. Proud.)

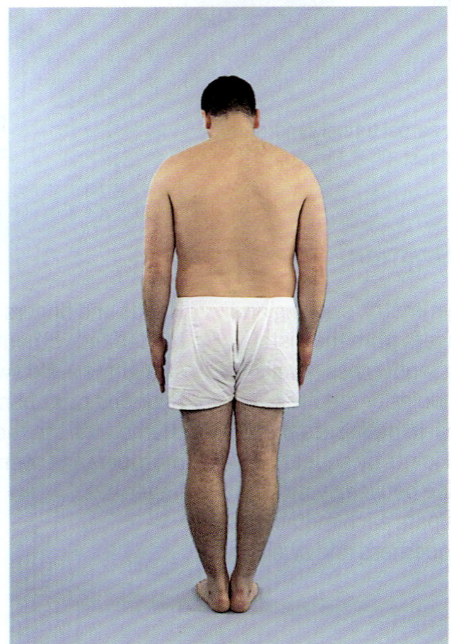

FIGURE 28-23 Inspecting the hips and buttocks. (© B. Proud.)

PHYSICAL ASSESSMENT (continued)

ASSESSMENT PROCEDURE	NORMAL FINDINGS	ABNORMAL FINDINGS
Test ROM (Fig. 28-24). With the patient supine, ask the patient to: • Raise extended leg (*A*). • Flex knee up to chest while keeping other leg extended (*B*). • Move extended leg (*C*) away from midline of body as far as possible and then towards midline of body as far as possible (abduction and adduction). • Bend knee and turn leg (*D*) inwards (rotation) and then outwards (rotation). • Ask the patient to lie prone (*E*) and lift extended leg off table. Alternatively, ask the patient to stand and swing extended leg backwards. Repeat these manoeuvres against resistance.	Normal ROM: 90 degrees of hip flexion with knee straight and 120 degrees of hip flexion with the knee bent and the other leg remaining straight. Normal ROM: • 45 degrees to 50 degrees of abduction; 20 degrees to 30 degrees of adduction. • 40-degree internal hip rotation, 45-degree external hip rotation. • 15-degree hip hyperextension. • Full ROM against resistance. **SAFETY TIP** **If the patient has had a total hip replacement, do not test ROM. Some movements (particularly adduction of the leg with the prosthesis will place stress on the joint and increase the risk of dislocating the hip.**	Inability to abduct hip is a common sign of hip disease. Pain and a decrease in internal hip rotation may be a sign of osteoarthritis or femoral neck stress fracture. Pain on palpation of the greater trochanter and pain as the patient moves from standing to lying down may indicate bursitis of the hip. Decreased muscle strength against resistance is seen in muscle and joint disease.

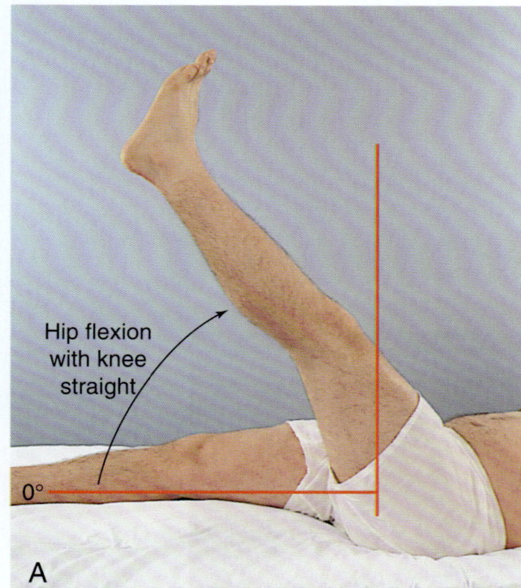

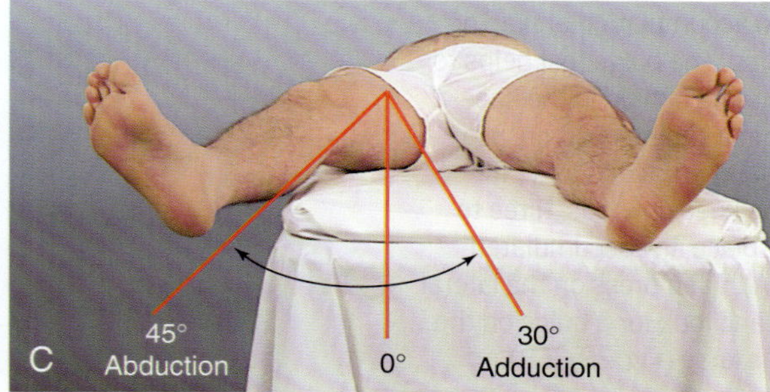

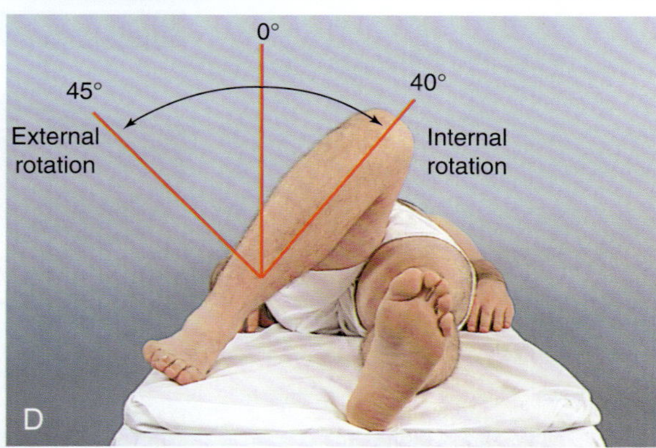

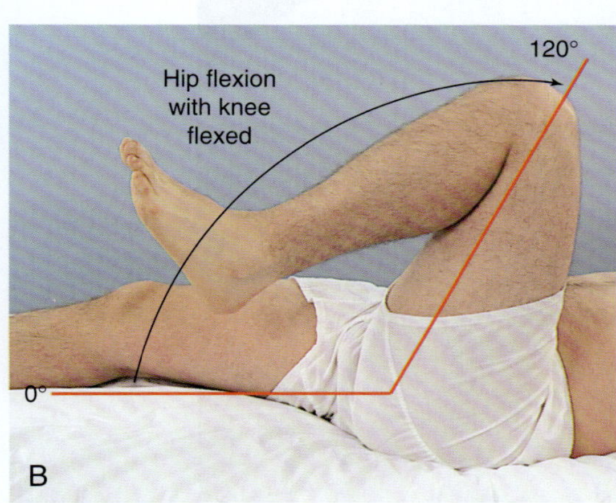

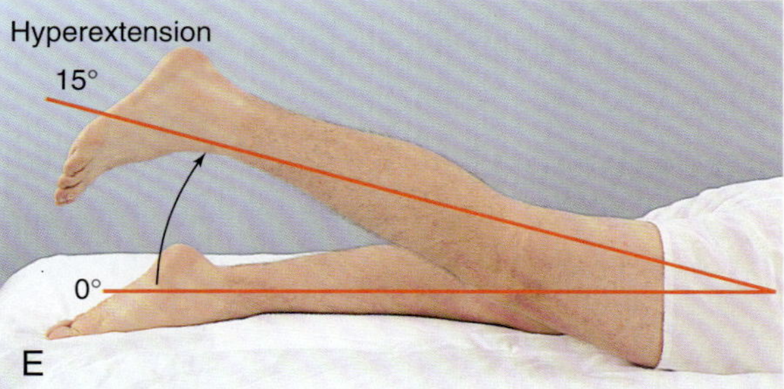

FIGURE 28-24 Normal range of motion of the hips: **(A)** hip flexion with extended knee straight; **(B)** hip flexion with knee bent; **(C)** abduction–adduction; **(D)** internal and external rotation; **(E)** hyperextension. (© B. Proud.)

Continued on following page

PHYSICAL ASSESSMENT (continued)

ASSESSMENT PROCEDURE	NORMAL FINDINGS	ABNORMAL FINDINGS
Knees		
INSPECTION AND PALPATION		
With the patient supine then sitting with knees dangling, inspect for size, shape, symmetry, swelling, deformities and alignment. Observe for quadriceps muscle atrophy.	Knees symmetrical, hollows present on both sides of the patella, no swelling or deformities. Lower leg in alignment with upper leg.	Knees turn in with knock knees (genu valgum) and turn out with bowed legs (genu varum). Swelling above or next to the patella may indicate fluid in the knee joint or thickening of the synovial membrane.
Palpate for tenderness, warmth, consistency and nodules. Begin palpation 10 cm above the patella, using your fingers and thumb to move downwards towards the knee (Fig. 28-25).	**OLDER ADULT CONSIDERATIONS** **Some older patients may have a bowlegged appearance because of decreased muscle control.** Non-tender and cool. Muscles firm. No nodules.	Tenderness and warmth with a boggy consistency may be symptoms of synovitis. Asymmetrical muscular development in the quadriceps may indicate atrophy.
Tests for swelling. If you notice swelling, perform the bulge test to determine if the swelling is due to accumulation of fluid or soft-tissue swelling. The bulge test helps to detect small amounts of fluid in the knee. With the patient in a supine position, use the ball of your hand firmly to stroke the medial side of the knee upwards, three to four times, to displace any accumulated fluid (Fig. 28-26A). Then press on the lateral side of the knee and look for a bulge on the medial side of the knee (Fig. 28-26B).	No bulge of fluid appears on medial side of knee.	Bulge of fluid appears on medial side of knee with a small amount of joint effusion.

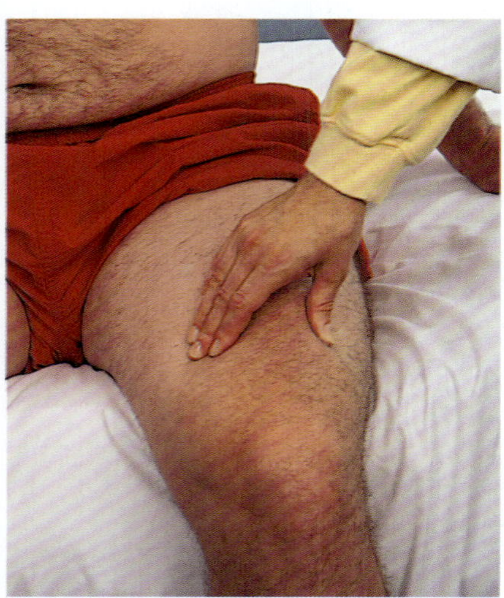

FIGURE 28-25 Palpating the knee area. (© B. Proud.)

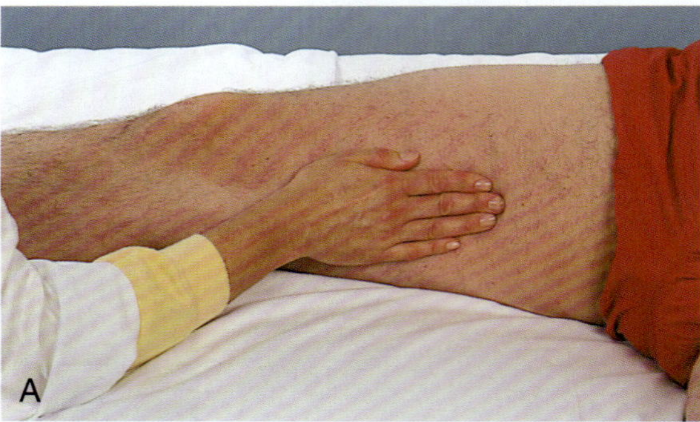

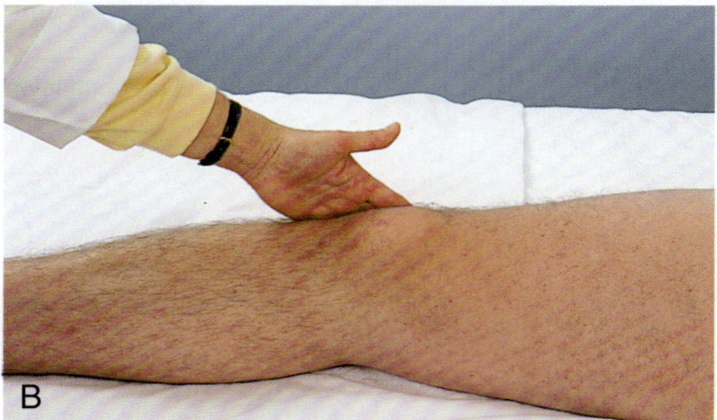

FIGURE 28-26 Performing the 'bulge' knee test: **(A)** stroking the knee; **(B)** observing the medial side for bulging. (© B. Proud.)

PHYSICAL ASSESSMENT (continued)

ASSESSMENT PROCEDURE	NORMAL FINDINGS	ABNORMAL FINDINGS
Perform the ballottement test. It helps to detect large amounts of fluid in the knee. With the patient in a supine position, firmly press your non-dominant thumb and index finger on each side of the patella. This displaces fluid in the suprapatellar bursa located between the femur and patella. Then with your dominant fingers, push the patella down on the femur (Fig. 28-27). Feel for a fluid wave or a click.	No movement of patella noted. Patella rests firmly over femur.	Fluid wave or click palpated with large amounts of joint effusion. A positive ballottement test may be present with meniscal tears.

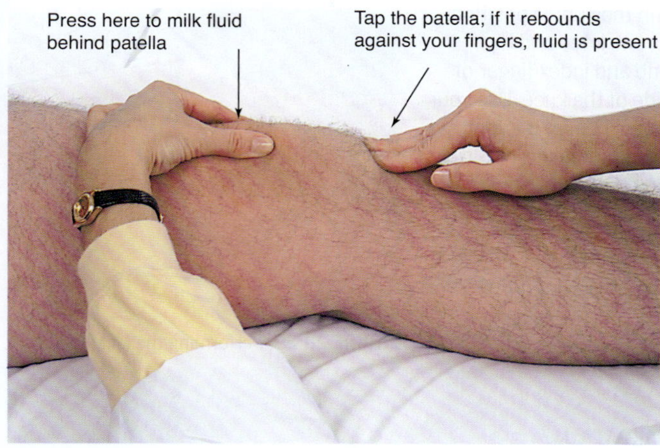

FIGURE 28-27 Performing the 'ballottement' knee test. (© B. Proud.)

ASSESSMENT PROCEDURE	NORMAL FINDINGS	ABNORMAL FINDINGS
Palpate the tibiofemoral space. As you compress the patella, slide it distally against the underlying femur. Note crepitus or pain.	There is no pain on examination. Crepitus may be present.	A patellofemoral disorder may be suspected if both crepitus and pain are present on examination.
Test ROM (Fig. 28-28). Ask the patient to: • Bend each knee up (flexion) towards the buttocks or back. • Straighten knee (extension and hyperextension). • Walk normally. Repeat these manoeuvres against resistance.	Normal ranges: 120 degrees to 130 degrees of flexion; 0 degrees of extension to 15 degrees of hyperextension. Patient should have full ROM against resistance.	Osteoarthritis is characterised by a decreased ROM with synovial thickening and crepitation. Flexion contractures of the knee are characterised by an inability to extend knee fully. Decreased muscle strength against resistance is seen in muscle and joint disease.

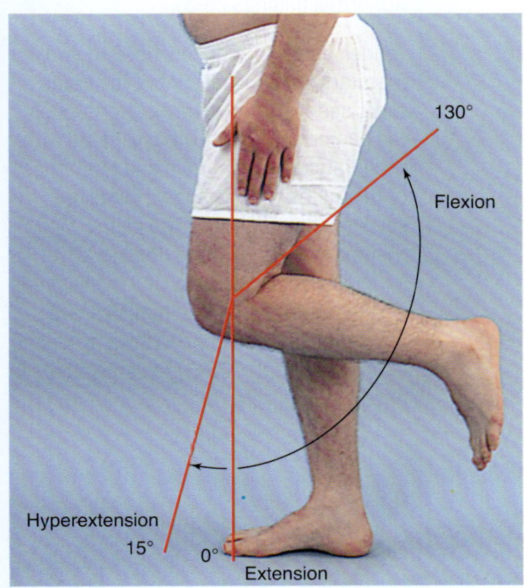

FIGURE 28-28 Normal range of motion of the knee. (© B. Proud.)

Continued on following page

PHYSICAL ASSESSMENT (continued)

ASSESSMENT PROCEDURE	NORMAL FINDINGS	ABNORMAL FINDINGS
Knees (continued)		
Test for pain and injury. If the patient complains of a 'giving in' or 'locking' of the knee, perform the McMurray test (Fig. 28-29). With the patient in the supine position, ask the patient to flex one knee and hip. Then place your thumb and index finger of one hand on either side of the knee. Use your other hand to hold up the heel of the foot. Rotate the lower leg and foot laterally. Slowly extend the knee, noting pain or clicking. Repeat, rotating lower leg and foot medially. Again note pain or clicking.	No pain or clicking noted. 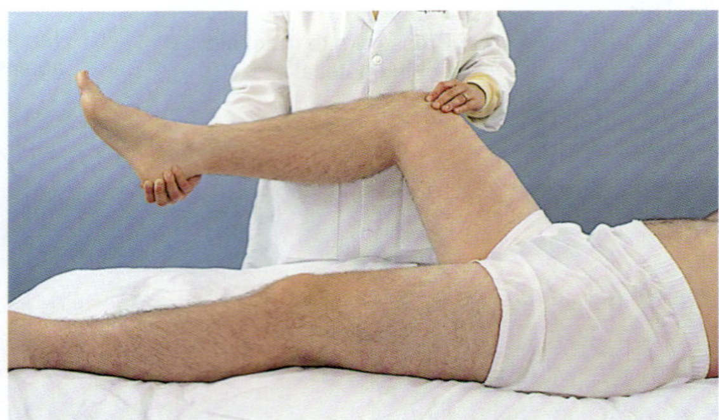 **FIGURE 28-29** Performing the McMurray test. (© B. Proud.)	Pain or clicking is indicative of a torn meniscus of the knee.
Ankles and feet		
INSPECTION AND PALPATION		
With the patient sitting, standing and walking, inspect position, alignment, shape and skin.	Toes usually point forwards and lie flat; however, they may point in (pes varus) or point out (pes valgus). Toes and feet are in alignment with the lower leg. Smooth, rounded medial malleolar prominences with prominent heels and metatarsophalangeal joints. Skin is smooth and free of corns and calluses. Longitudinal arch; most of weight-bearing is on foot midline.	A laterally deviated great toe with possible overlapping of the second toe and possible formation of an enlarged, painful, inflamed bursa (bunion) on the medial side is seen with hallux valgus. Common abnormalities include feet with no arches (pes planus or 'flat feet'), feet with high arches (pes cavus); painful thickening of the skin over bony prominences and at pressure points (corns); non-painful thickened skin that occurs at pressure points (calluses); and painful warts (verruca vulgaris) that often occur under a callus (plantar warts; see Abnormal findings 28-3).
Palpate ankles and feet for tenderness, heat, swelling or nodules (Fig. 28-30). Palpate the toes from the distal end proximally, noting tenderness, swelling, bony prominences, nodules or crepitus of each interphalangeal joint. Assess the metatarsophalangeal joints by squeezing the foot from each side with your thumb and fingers. Palpate each metatarsal, noting swelling or tenderness. Palpate the plantar area (bottom) of the foot noting pain or swelling. 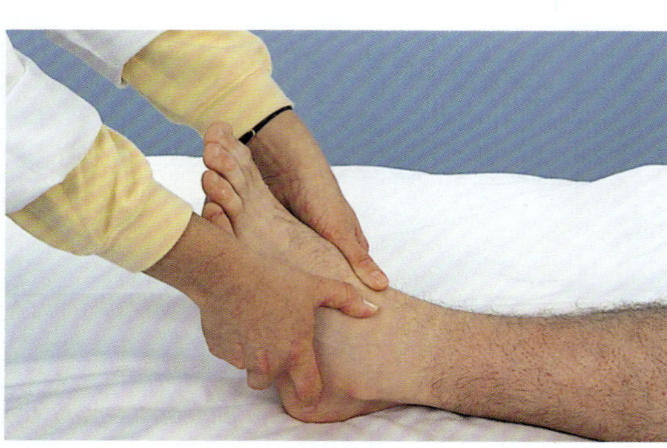 **FIGURE 28-30** Palpating the ankles and feet. (© B. Proud.)	No pain, heat, swelling or nodules are noted.	Tender, painful, reddened, hot and swollen metatarsophalangeal joint of the great toe is seen in gouty arthritis. Nodules of the posterior ankle may be palpated with rheumatoid arthritis. Pain and tenderness of the metatarsophalangeal joints are seen in inflammation of the joints, rheumatoid arthritis and degenerative joint disease. Tenderness of the calcaneus of the bottom of the foot may indicate plantar fasciitis. Use the Ottawa ankle and foot rules (Display 28-3) to determine need for X-ray referral.

PHYSICAL ASSESSMENT (continued)

ASSESSMENT PROCEDURE	NORMAL FINDINGS	ABNORMAL FINDINGS
Test ROM (Fig. 28-31). Ask the patient to: • Point toes upwards (dorsiflexion) and then downwards (plantar flexion) (A). • Turn soles outwards (eversion) and then inwards (inversion) (B). • Rotate foot outwards (abduction) and then inwards (adduction) (C). • Turn toes under foot (flexion) and then upwards (extension). • Repeat these manoeuvres against resistance.	Normal ranges: • 20-degree dorsiflexion of ankle and foot; 45-degree plantar flexion of ankle and foot. • 20 degrees of eversion; 30 degrees of inversion. • 10 degrees of abduction; 20 degrees of adduction. • 40 degrees of flexion; 40 degrees of extension. • Patient has full ROM against resistance.	Decreased strength against resistance is seen in muscle and joint disease. Hyperextension of the metatarsophalangeal joint and flexion of the proximal interphalangeal joint is apparent in hammer toe (see Abnormal findings 28-3). Decreased strength against resistance is common in muscle and joint disease.

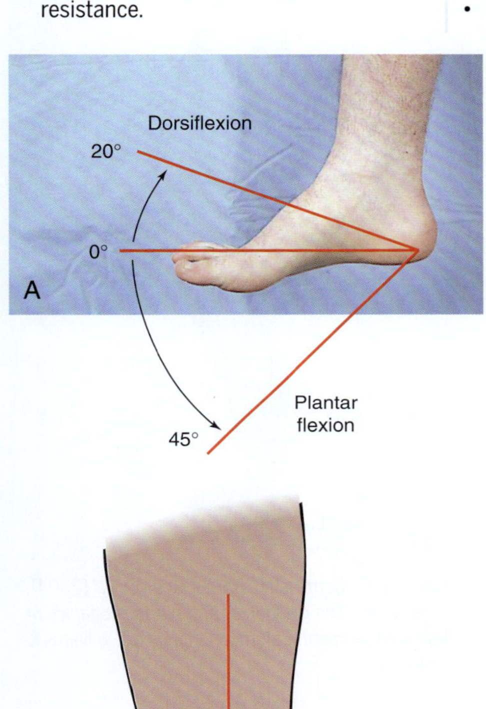

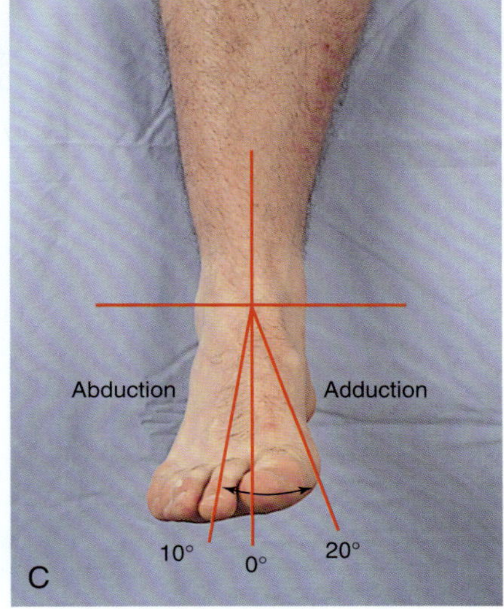

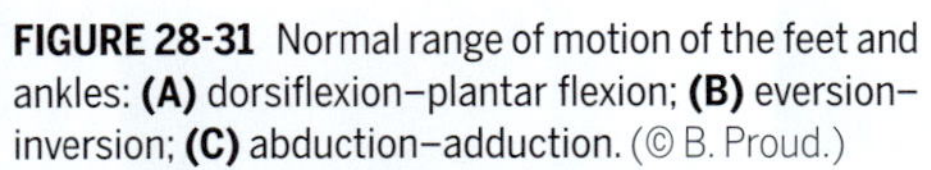
FIGURE 28-31 Normal range of motion of the feet and ankles: **(A)** dorsiflexion–plantar flexion; **(B)** eversion–inversion; **(C)** abduction–adduction. (© B. Proud.)

DISPLAY 28-3 OTTAWA ANKLE AND FOOT RULES

Ankle X-ray indicators

Malleolar area pain; and bone tenderness at the tips of 6 cm edges of the lateral malleolus or medial malleolus; or the inability to bear weight immediately or during examination indicate the need for an ankle X-ray.

Foot X-ray indicators

Pain in the midfoot area and bone tenderness at the base of the fifth metatarsal or the navicular bone area, or the inability to bear weight immediately or during examination indicate the need for a foot X-ray.

Adapted from Steill, I. G., Greenberg, G. H., McKnight, R. D., Nair, R. C., Mc Dowell, I. & Worthington, J. R. (1992). A study to develop clinical decision rules for the use of radiography in acute ankle injuries. *Annals of Emergency Medicine, 21*(4), 384–390.

ABNORMAL FINDINGS 28-1 Abnormal Spinal Curvatures

FLATTENING OF THE LUMBAR CURVE

Flattening of the lumbar curvature may be seen with a herniated lumbar disc or ankylosing spondylitis.

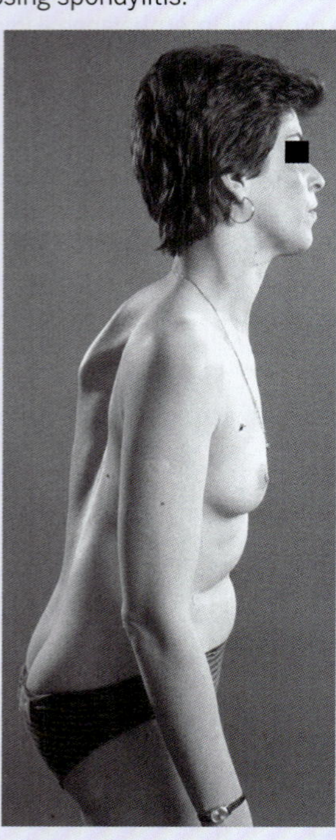

(Used with permission from Frymoyer, J. W., Wiesel, S. W. et al. [2004]. *The adult and pediatric spine.* Philadelphia: Lippincott Williams & Wilkins.)

KYPHOSIS

A rounded thoracic convexity (kyphosis) is commonly seen in older adults.

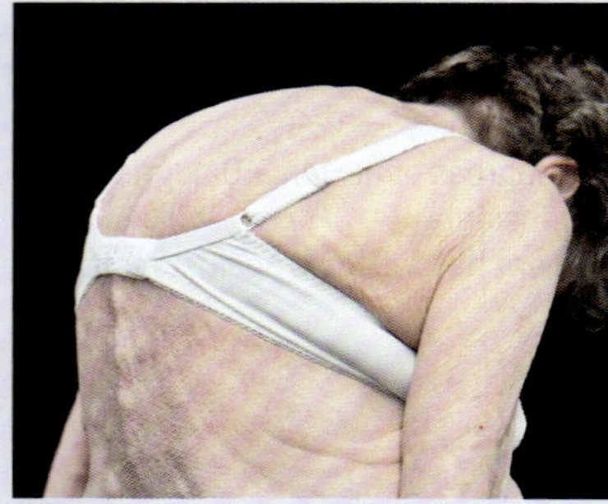

(Dr. P. Marazzi/Science Photo Library.)

LUMBAR LORDOSIS

An exaggerated lumbar curve (lumbar lordosis) is often seen in pregnancy or obesity.

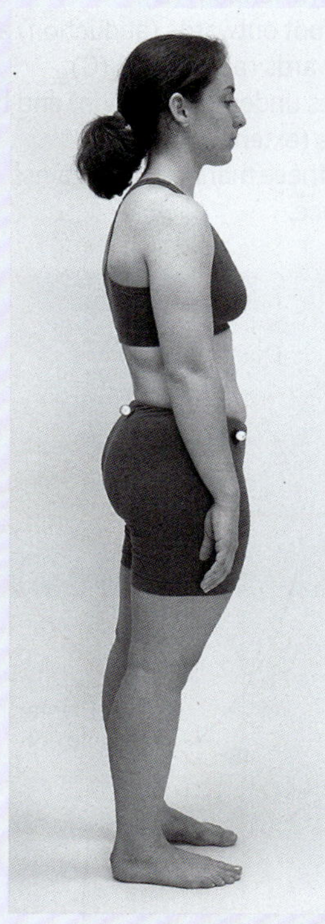

(Used with permission from Oatis, C. A. [2004]. *Kinesiology: The mechanics and pathomechanics of human movement.* Baltimore: Lippincott, Williams & Wilkins.)

SCOLIOSIS

Lateral curvature of the spine with an increase in convexity on the side that is curved is seen in scoliosis.

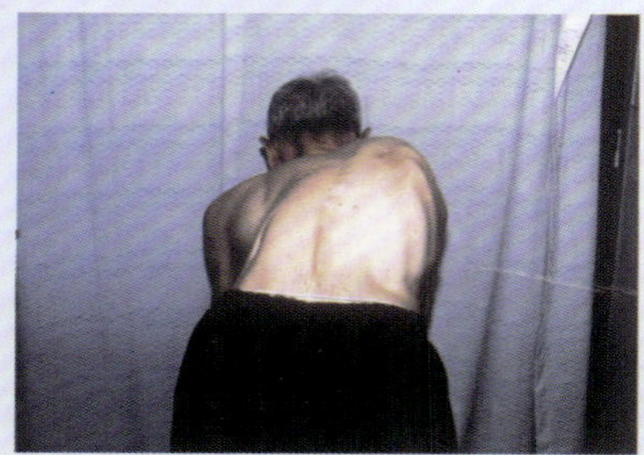

(Used with permission from Berg, D. & Worzala, K. [2006]. *Atlas of adult physical diagnosis.* Philadelphia: Lippincott Williams & Wilkins.)

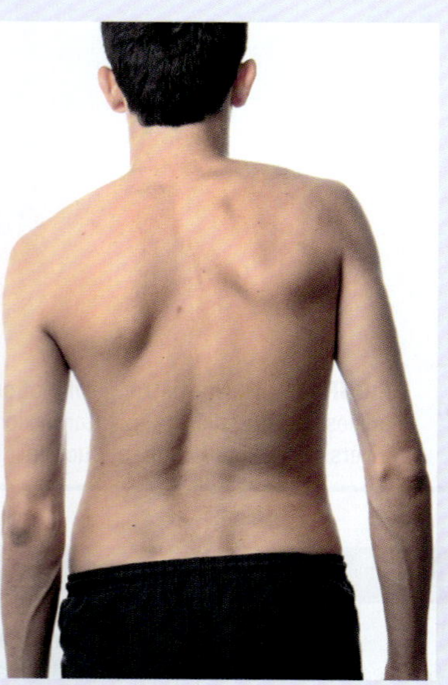

(Shutterstock.com/Kleber Cordeiro.)

ABNORMAL FINDINGS 28-2 Abnormalities Affecting the Wrists, Hands and Fingers

The following abnormalities are commonly associated with the upper extremities. Early detection is important because early intervention may help to preserve dexterity and daily function.

ACUTE RHEUMATOID ARTHRITIS

Tender, painful, swollen, stiff joints are seen in acute rheumatoid arthritis.

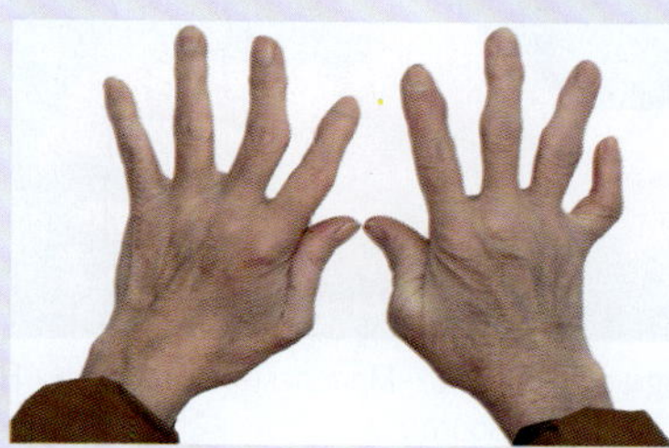

(Shutterstock.com/Gabdrakipova Dilyara.)

CHRONIC RHEUMATOID ARTHRITIS

Chronic swelling and thickening of the metacarpophalangeal and proximal interphalangeal joints, limited range of motion and finger deviation towards the ulnar side are seen in chronic rheumatoid arthritis.

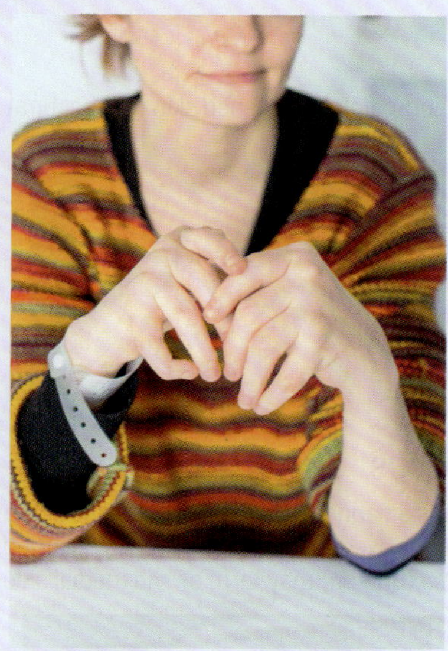

(Alamy Stock Photo/Phanie.)

THENAR ATROPHY

Atrophy of the thenar prominence due to pressure on the median nerve is seen in carpal tunnel syndrome.

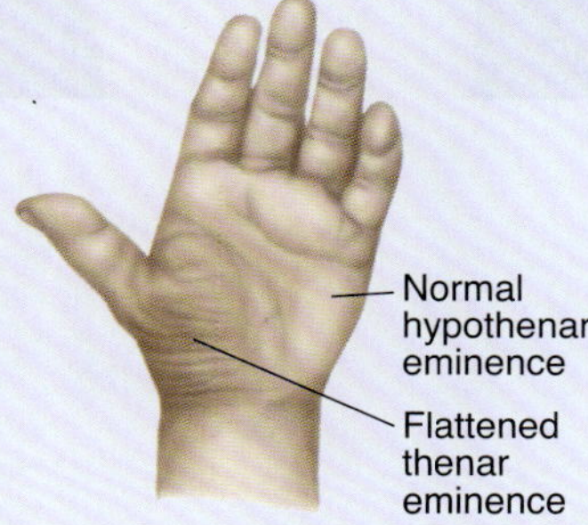

(Used with permission from Bickley, L.S. & Szilagyi, P. [2003]. *Bates' guide to physical examination and history taking* [8th ed.]. Philadelphia: Lippincott Williams & Wilkins.)

BOUTONNIÈRE AND SWAN-NECK DEFORMITIES

Flexion of the proximal interphalangeal joint and hyperextension of the distal interphalangeal joint (Boutonnière deformity) and hyperextension of the proximal interphalangeal joint with flexion of the distal interphalangeal joint (swan-neck deformity) are also common in chronic rheumatoid arthritis.

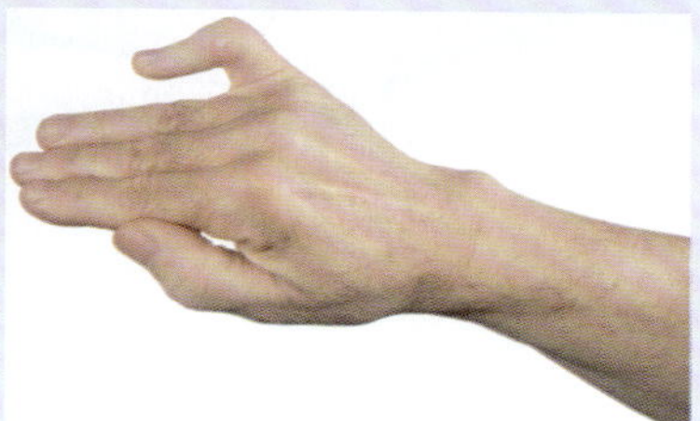

Boutonnière deformity. (Dreamstime.com/Fotokev)

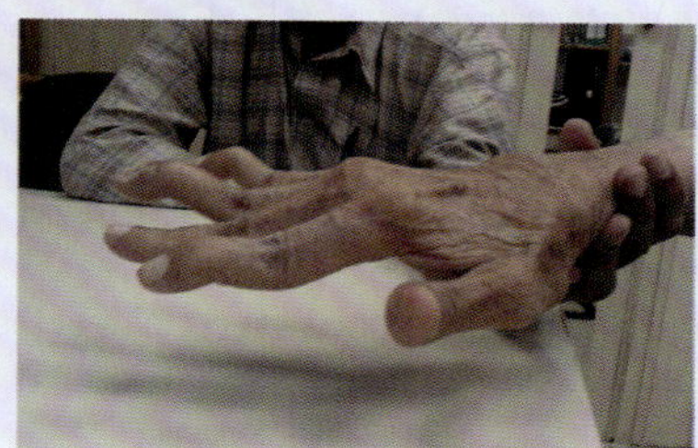

Swan-neck deformity. (Wikimedia Commons/Phoenix119 CC BY SA 3.0 Unported license, https://commons.wikimedia.org/wiki/File:Swan_neck_deformity_in_a_65_year_old_Rheumatoid_Arthritis_patient-_2014-05-27_01-49.jpg, accessed 1 May 2020.)

OSTEOARTHRITIS

Hard, painless nodules over the distal interphalangeal joints (Heberden nodes) and over the proximal interphalangeal joints (Bouchard nodes) are seen in osteoarthritis.

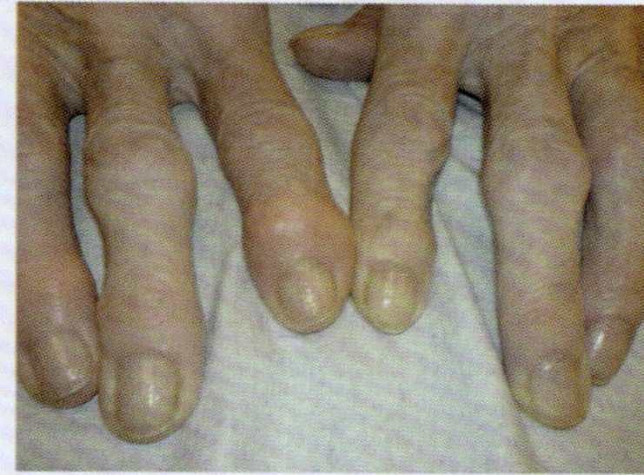

Heberden nodes. (Wikimedia Commons/Drahreg01 CC BY SA 3.0 Unported license, https://commons.wikimedia.org/wiki/File:Heberden-Arthrose.JPG, accessed 1 May 2020.)

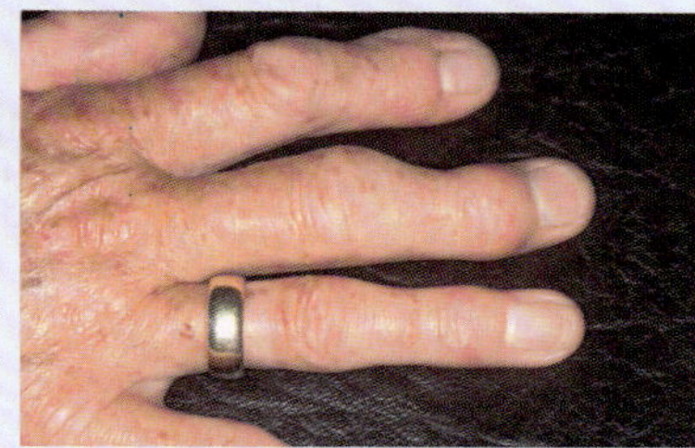

Bouchard nodes. (Hercules Robinson / Alamy Stock Photo.)

Continued on following page

ABNORMAL FINDINGS 28-2 Abnormalities Affecting the Wrists, Hands and Fingers (continued)

GANGLION

Non-tender, round, enlarged, swollen, fluid-filled cyst (ganglion) is commonly seen at the dorsum of the wrist.

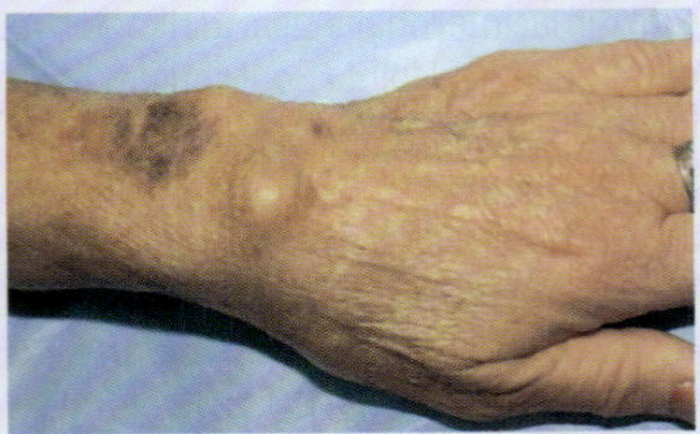

TENOSYNOVITIS

Painful extension of a finger may be seen in acute tenosynovitis (infection of the flexor tendon sheathes).

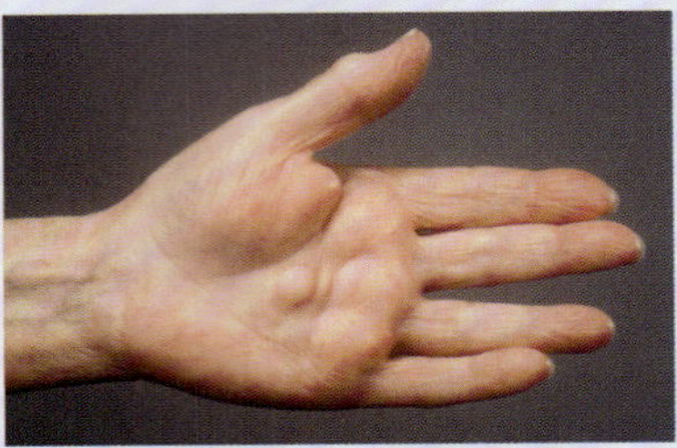

(Clinical Photography, Central Manchester University Hosptials NHS Foundation Trust/Science Soure.)

ABNORMAL FINDINGS 28-3 Abnormalities of the Feet and Toes

The following abnormalities affect the feet and toes, typically causing discomfort and impeding mobility. Early detection and treatment can help to restore or maximise function.

ACUTE GOUTY ARTHRITIS

In gouty arthritis, the metatarsophalangeal joint of the great toe is tender, painful, reddened, hot and swollen.

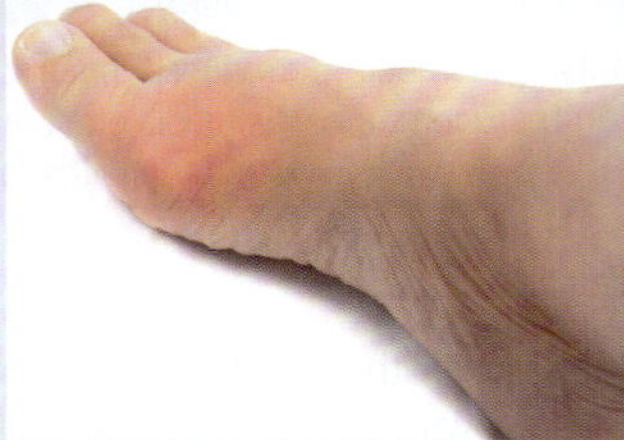

(Shutterstock.com/ThamKC.)

FLAT FEET

A flat foot (pes planus) has no arch and may cause pain and swelling of the foot surface.

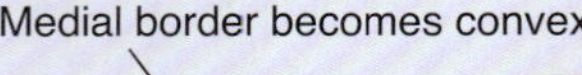

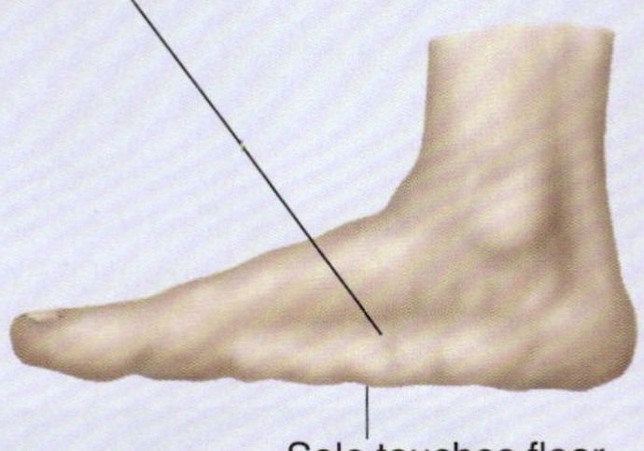

(Used with permission from Bickley, L. S. & Szilagyi, P. [2003]. *Bates' guide to physical examination and history taking* [8th ed.]. Philadelphia: Lippincott Williams & Wilkins.)

CALLUS

Calluses are non-painful, thickened skin that occur at pressure points.

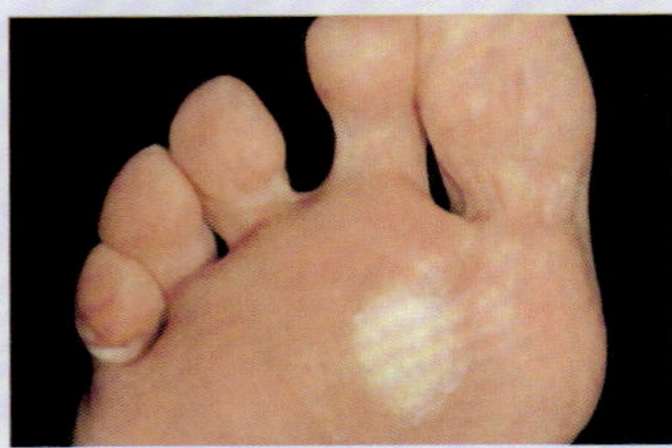

HALLUX VALGUS

Hallux valgus is an abnormality in which the great toe is deviated laterally and may overlap the second toe. An enlarged, painful, inflamed bursa (bunion) may form on the medial side.

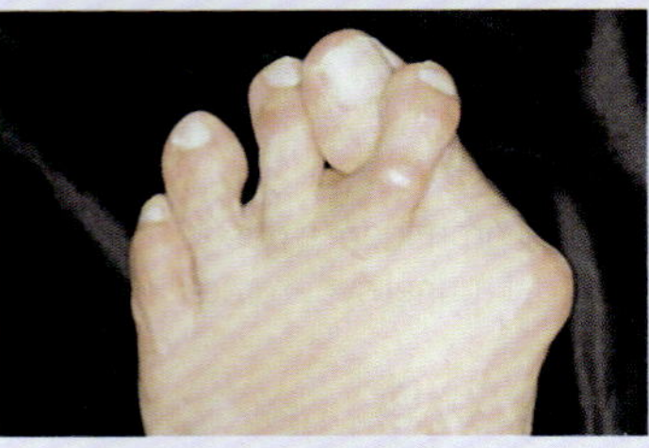

ABNORMAL FINDINGS 28-3 Abnormalities of the Feet and Toes (continued)

CORN

Corns are painful thickenings of the skin that occur over bony prominences and at pressure points.

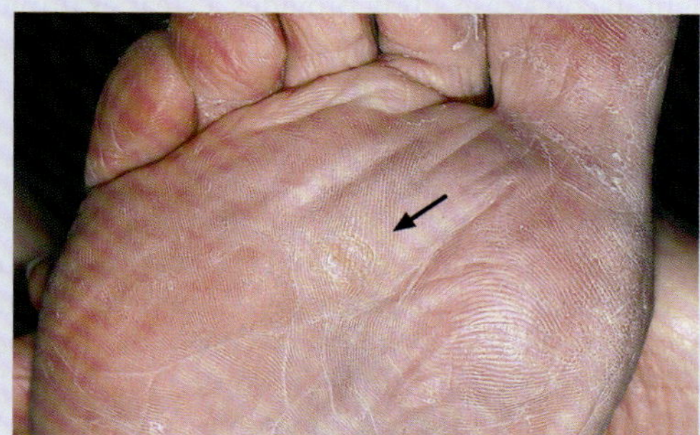

(Used with permission from Goodheart, H. P. [2003]. *Goodheart's photoguide to common skin disorders* [2nd ed.]. Philadelphia: Lippincott Williams & Wilkins.)

HAMMER TOE

Hyperextension at the metatarsophalangeal joint with flexion at the proximal interphalangeal joint (hammer toe) commonly occurs with the second toe.

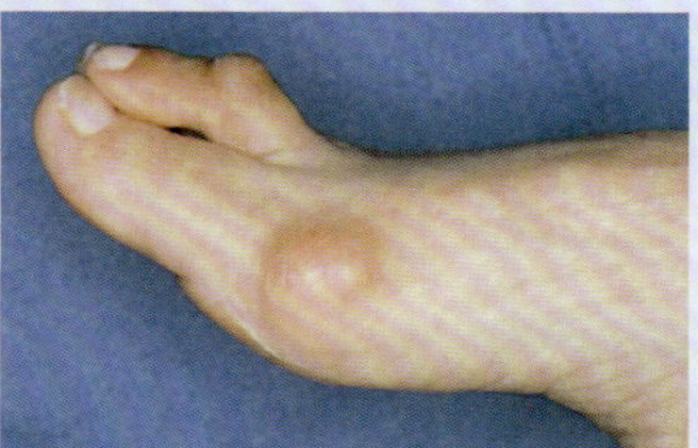

PLANTAR WART

Plantar warts are painful warts (verruca vulgaris) that often occur under a callus, appearing as tiny dark spots.

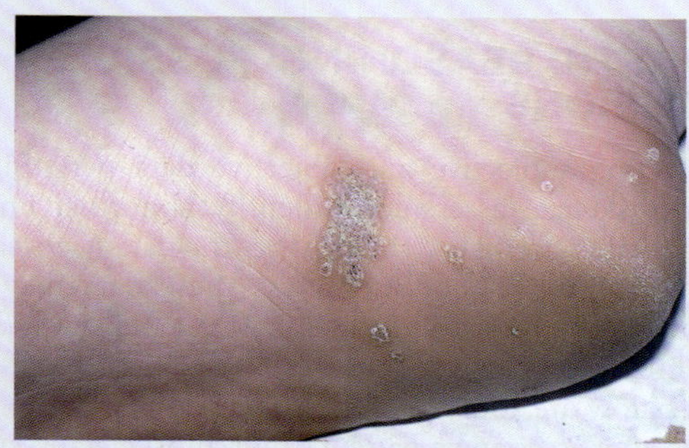

(Used with permission from Goodheart, H. P. [2003]. *Goodheart's photoguide to common skin disorders* [2nd ed.]. Philadelphia: Lippincott Williams & Wilkins.)

VALIDATING AND DOCUMENTING FINDINGS

Validate the musculoskeletal assessment data you have collected. This is necessary to verify that the data collected are reliable and accurate. Document the assessment data following the health care facility or agency policy.

Sample of subjective data

Sixteen-year-old schoolboy complaining of pain in his left ankle, especially at the joint. He states that he was trying to do a jump over five steps and 'lost it'. He states that the pain happened straight away and is most severe over the outer aspect of his left foot around the ankle area. He also states that his left hand and wrist are tender. He says he is unable to put any weight on his left leg and walk because it is very painful. He states that he has full range of movement in his left wrist, but it is tender to touch. He has nil complaints of neck pain or back pain and suffered no loss of consciousness in the accident.

There is no past history of problems with joints or muscles. The patient states that he broke his right arm when 5 years old after falling out of a tree, and had a cast for 6 weeks. He has had no problems with that arm since that time. All of his immunisations are up to date and he takes no regular medications. He recalls that his grandmother suffered from rheumatoid arthritis, while his other family members enjoy good health. The patient states that he drinks two caffeinated soft drinks per day, has a good appetite and consumes food from all food groups; he drinks milk daily. He reports no recent weight gain or loss.

Sample of objective data

The patient is 165 cm tall and weighs 63 kg. Physical examination reveals bone tenderness over the posterior aspect of the tibia and lateral malleolus down to the fourth and fifth metatarsals. The area is swollen, deformed, warm and well perfused, and the skin is intact. Capillary refill is less than 2 seconds. There is no neurovascular injury, and a strong palpable pulse is noted in the dorsalis pedis and posterior tibial areas. The patient protects and guards his ankle and foot upon examination of the area.

After you have collected the assessment data, you will need to analyse the data, using diagnostic reasoning skills. Refer to the discussion of the diagnostic reasoning process in Chapter 5.

Analysis of data

DIAGNOSTIC REASONING: POSSIBLE CONCLUSIONS

After collecting subjective and objective data pertaining to the musculoskeletal assessment, identify abnormal findings and the patient's strengths. Then cluster the data to reveal any significant patterns or abnormalities. These data may then be used to make clinical judgements about the status of the patient's musculoskeletal system.

Listed below are some possible conclusions that the nurse may make after assessing a patient's musculoskeletal system.

Potential patient risks

- Risk of trauma (related to repetitive movements of wrists or elbows with recreation or occupation)
- Risk of pathological fractures (related to osteoporosis)
- Risk of injury to joints, muscles or bones (related to environmental hazards)

Potential patient problems

- Potential for peripheral neurovascular dysfunction (related to vascular insufficiency and nerve compression secondary to peripheral oedema)
- Potential for acute pain (related to oedema, movement of bone fragments and muscular spasm)
- Potential for impaired physical mobility (related to limitations imposed by underlying condition and treatment modalities)
- Potential for ineffective coping (related to enforced immobility and altered lifestyle pattern)
- Potential for activity intolerance (related to muscle weakness or joint pain)
- Constipation (related to decreased gastric motility and muscle tone secondary to immobility)
- Impaired skin integrity (related to prolonged pressure on the skin secondary to immobility)
- Impaired social interaction (related to depression or immobility)
- Disturbed body image (related to skeletal deformities)

Selected collaborative problems

After grouping the data, certain collaborative problems may become apparent. Remember that collaborative problems cannot be prevented by nursing interventions alone. However, these physiological complications of medical conditions can be detected and monitored by the nurse. In addition, the nurse can use doctor- and nurse-prescribed interventions to minimise the complications of these problems. The nurse may also have to refer the patient in such situations for further treatment of the problem.

The following is a list of collaborative problems that may be identified when obtaining a general impression:

- Muscular spasm and pain
- Joint dislocation
- Compartmental syndrome
- Muscle atrophy
- Deep vein thrombosis.

Medical problems

Frequently musculoskeletal problems, despite nursing assessment and management, will require medical diagnosis and treatment. Jacob's case study provides a clear example of this.

CASE STUDY

It is apparent that Jacob's signs and symptoms clearly require further medical treatment. Jacob is examined by a doctor in the emergency department and sent for further radiological evaluation of his injured ankle and wrist. After the X-ray, Jacob is admitted to hospital and referred to an orthopaedic surgeon.

Jacob is admitted to the orthopaedic ward and is awaiting an open reduction and fixation of a malleolar fracture of his left ankle. Jacob's ankle has been stabilised in a backslab cast. The orthopaedic surgeon has ordered hourly circulation observations and the elevation of Jacob's leg on two pillows.

While awaiting surgery, Jacob continually complains of severe pain, despite receiving intravenous pain relief. Jacob describes the pain as burning in nature. He also complains of decreased sensation to touch in his toes and states that the area feels very cold.

CRITICAL THINKING

5. There are a number of complications associated with lower leg fractures. What complication do you think Jacob could be suffering from?
6. What further assessments could you undertake of Jacob's leg?
7. What would your nursing interventions be to address the issues highlighted?
8. Should you further elevate the leg and apply cold packs to help reduce Jacob's pain? Why or why not?

ONLINE RESOURCES

An extensive range of additional resources to enhance teaching and learning and to facilitate understanding may be found online at the text's accompanying website, located on thePoint at http://thepoint.lww.com. These include Watch and Learn videos, Concepts in Action animations, journal articles, case studies, discussion topics and quizzes.

Subscribers may also access Lippincott Procedures, an extensive online point-of-care procedure guide that provides reliable step-by-step instructions for more than 1700 procedures, including 450 evidence-based Australian procedures, and skills in a variety of speciality settings, together with a wealth of supporting information.

CASE STUDY

The case study demonstrates how to analyse musculoskeletal assessment data for a specific patient. The exercises included in the ancillary product on thePoint that complements this text offer further opportunities to enhance your skills.

Jacob Winter is a 16-year-old schoolboy who has presented to the emergency department (ED) after having a fall from his skateboard. His mother Debbie transported him to the ED after his friends carried him home. Jacob is complaining of pain in his left ankle, especially at the joint. Jacob states that he was trying to do a jump over five steps and 'lost it'. He landed on a grassy area. He says that the pain happened straight away and is most severe over the outer aspect of his foot around the ankle area. He also says that his left hand and wrist are tender. He is unable to put any weight on his leg and walk because it is very painful. He tells you that he has full range of movement in his left wrist, but it is tender to touch. He says he is not injured anywhere else. He has nil complaints of neck pain or back pain and suffered no loss of consciousness in the accident.

Jacob is 165 cm tall and weighs 63 kg. Physical examination reveals bone tenderness over the posterior aspect of the tibia and lateral malleolus down to the fourth and fifth metatarsals. The area is swollen, deformed, warm, well perfused and the skin is intact. Capillary refill is less than 2 seconds. There is no neurovascular injury with a strong palpable pulse noted in the dorsalis pedis and posterior tibial areas. Jacob has nil complaints of altered sensation or 'pins and needles' in the area. Jacob protects and guards his ankle and foot upon examination of the area.

It is apparent that Jacob's signs and symptoms clearly require further medical treatment. Jacob is reviewed by a doctor in the emergency department and sent for further radiological evaluation of his injured ankle and wrist. After the X-ray, Jacob is admitted to hospital and referred to an orthopaedic surgeon.

Jacob is admitted to the orthopaedic ward and is awaiting an open reduction and fixation of a malleolar fracture of his left ankle. Jacob's ankle has been stabilised in a backslab cast. The orthopaedic surgeon has ordered hourly circulation observations and the elevation of Jacob's leg on two pillows.

While awaiting surgery, Jacob continually complains of severe pain, despite receiving intravenous pain relief. Jacob describes the pain as burning in nature. He also complains of decreased sensation to touch in his toes and states that the area feels very cold.

The following concept map illustrates the diagnostic reasoning process.

Applying COLDSPA

Applying COLDSPA for patient with symptoms of 'ankle pain' upon presentation to the emergency department.

Mnemonic	Question	Data provided	Missing data
Character	Describe the sign or symptom.	'I have pain in my ankle, especially at the joint.'	Describe the type of pain you are having. Is it sharp, dull or throbbing?
Onset	How did you injure your ankle?	'I took a tumble on my skateboard. I was trying to do a jump over some steps.'	Did you hear any noises when you fell on your ankle? What position was your ankle and foot in when you fell? How far did you fall? What did you land on?
Location	Where is the pain?	'It is mostly on the outer aspect on my foot and over my ankle.'	Did you injure anywhere else when you fell? Were you knocked out?
Duration	When did you first notice the pain in your ankle?	'The pain happened straight away after I fell.'	Were you able to walk after the accident?
Severity	How bad is the pain? How much does it bother you?	'Oh, it really hurts.'	Rate the pain on a scale of 1 to 10, with 10 being the worst pain and 1 being no pain.
Pattern	Does anything make it worse?	'I can't walk on my ankle due to the pain.'	Have you done any first aid treatment on your ankle?
Associated factors/How it Affects the patient	Do you have any pins and needles or altered sensation in your ankle?	'No, it feels normal.' 'Just really painful!'	Did you hit your head or have any loss of consciousness associated with the fall?

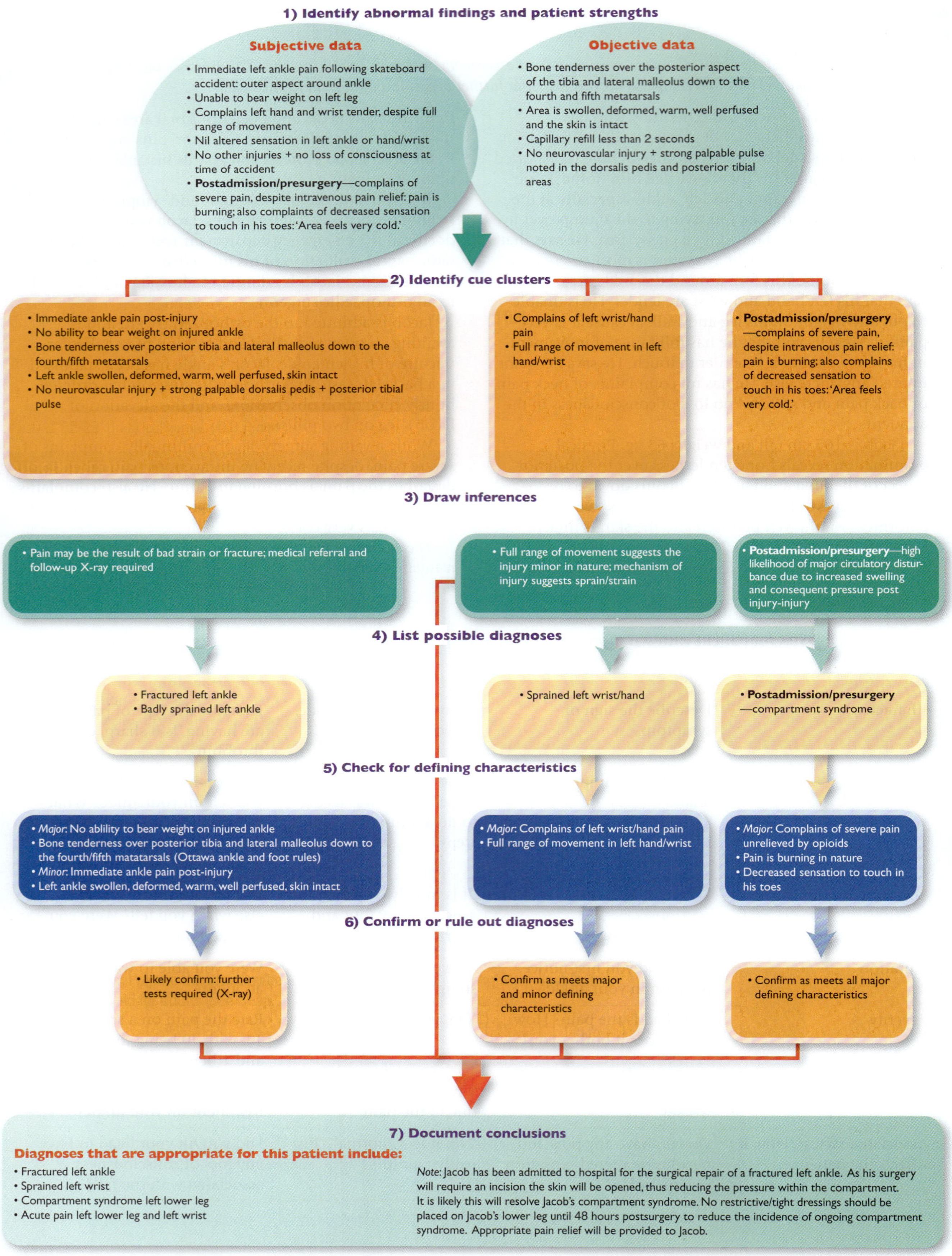

1) Identify abnormal findings and patient strengths

Subjective data

- Immediate left ankle pain following skateboard accident: outer aspect around ankle
- Unable to bear weight on left leg
- Complains left hand and wrist tender, despite full range of movement
- Nil altered sensation in left ankle or hand/wrist
- No other injuries + no loss of consciousness at time of accident
- **Postadmission/presurgery**—complains of severe pain, despite intravenous pain relief: pain is burning; also complaints of decreased sensation to touch in his toes: 'Area feels very cold.'

Objective data

- Bone tenderness over the posterior aspect of the tibia and lateral malleolus down to the fourth and fifth metatarsals
- Area is swollen, deformed, warm, well perfused and the skin is intact
- Capillary refill less than 2 seconds
- No neurovascular injury + strong palpable pulse noted in the dorsalis pedis and posterior tibial areas

2) Identify cue clusters

- Immediate ankle pain post-injury
- No ability to bear weight on injured ankle
- Bone tenderness over posterior tibia and lateral malleolus down to the fourth/fifth metatarsals
- Left ankle swollen, deformed, warm, well perfused, skin intact
- No neurovascular injury + strong palpable dorsalis pedis + posterior tibial pulse

- Complains of left wrist/hand pain
- Full range of movement in left hand/wrist

- **Postadmission/presurgery**—complains of severe pain, despite intravenous pain relief: pain is burning; also complains of decreased sensation to touch in his toes: 'Area feels very cold.'

3) Draw inferences

- Pain may be the result of bad strain or fracture; medical referral and follow-up X-ray required

- Full range of movement suggests the injury minor in nature; mechanism of injury suggests sprain/strain

- **Postadmission/presurgery**—high likelihood of major circulatory disturbance due to increased swelling and consequent pressure post injury-injury

4) List possible diagnoses

- Fractured left ankle
- Badly sprained left ankle

- Sprained left wrist/hand

- **Postadmission/presurgery**—compartment syndrome

5) Check for defining characteristics

- *Major:* No ability to bear weight on injured ankle
- Bone tenderness over posterior tibia and lateral malleolus down to the fourth/fifth matatarsals (Ottawa ankle and foot rules)
- *Minor:* Immediate ankle pain post-injury
- Left ankle swollen, deformed, warm, well perfused, skin intact

- *Major:* Complains of left wrist/hand pain
- Full range of movement in left hand/wrist

- *Major:* Complains of severe pain unrelieved by opioids
- Pain is burning in nature
- Decreased sensation to touch in his toes

6) Confirm or rule out diagnoses

- Likely confirm: further tests required (X-ray)

- Confirm as meets major and minor defining characteristics

- Confirm as meets all major defining characteristics

7) Document conclusions

Diagnoses that are appropriate for this patient include:

- Fractured left ankle
- Sprained left wrist
- Compartment syndrome left lower leg
- Acute pain left lower leg and left wrist

Note: Jacob has been admitted to hospital for the surgical repair of a fractured left ankle. As his surgery will require an incision the skin will be opened, thus reducing the pressure within the compartment. It is likely this will resolve Jacob's compartment syndrome. No restrictive/tight dressings should be placed on Jacob's lower leg until 48 hours postsurgery to reduce the incidence of ongoing compartment syndrome. Appropriate pain relief will be provided to Jacob.

References

Accident Compensation Corporation (ACC). (2019). Statistics on our claims. Viewed October 2019 at https://www.acc.co.nz/about-us/statistics/.

Australian Institute of Health and Welfare (AIHW). (2013). Hospitalisations due to falls by older people, Australia: 2009–10 Injury research and statistics. Series no. 70. Cat. no. INJCAT 146. Canberra: Author.

Australian Institute of Health and Welfare (AIHW). (2014). Estimating the prevalence of osteoporosis in Australia. Viewed October 2019 at https://www.aihw.gov.au/reports/chronic-musculoskeletal-conditions/estimating-the-prevalence-of-osteoporosis-in-austr/contents/summary.

Australian Institute of Health and Welfare. (2019). Back problems. Viewed October 2019 at https://www.aihw.gov.au/reports/chronic-musculoskeletal-conditions/back-problems/contents/what-are-back-problems.

Bevan, S., Gunning, N. & Thomas, R. (2012). Fit for work: Musculoskeletal disorders and the New Zealand labour market. Brussels: Fit for Work Coalition. Available at www.fitforworkeurope.eu.

Cohen, B. J. & Hull, K. L. (2015). *Memmler's structure and function of the human body* (11th ed.). Philadelphia: Lippincott Williams & Wilkins.

International Osteoporosis Foundation (IOF). (2019). What is osteoporosis? Viewed October 2019 at https://www.iofbonehealth.org/what-is-osteoporosis.

Osteoporosis New Zealand. (2019). *Fractures caused by osteoporosis*. Wellington: Author. Viewed October 2019 at https://osteoporosis.org.nz/osteoporosis-fractures/fractires-caused-by-osteoporosis/.

Pollard, T. M. (2008). *Western diseases: An evolutionary perspective*. New York: Cambridge University Press.

Royal Australian College of General Practitioners. (2017). Clinical guideline for the prevention and treatment of osteoporosis in postmenopausal women and older men. Viewed October 2019 at https://www.osteoporosis.org.au/clinical-guidelines.

Steill, I. G., Greenberg, G. H., McKnight, R. D., et al. (1992). A study to develop clinical decision rules for the use of radiography in acute ankle injuries. *Annals of Emergency Medicine, 21*(4), 384–390.

Tricco, A. C., Thomas, S. M., Veroniki, A. A., et al. (2017). Comparisons of interventions for preventing falls in older adults: A systematic review and meta-analysis. *JAMA, 318*(17), 1687–1699.

World Health Organisation (WHO). (2019). *Musculoskeletal conditions*. Geneva: Author. Viewed October 2019 at https://www.who.int/news-room/fact-sheets/detail/musculoskeletal-conditions.

Selected readings

Haley, C. (Ed). (2015). *Pillitteri's child and family health nursing in Australia and New Zealand* (2nd ed.). Sydney: Lippincott Williams & Wilkins.

Hawker, G. A. (2017). The assessment of musculoskeletal pain. *Clinical and Experimental Rheumatology, 35*(107), S8–S12.

Hunter, S. & Miller, C. (2015). *Miller's nursing for wellness in older adults* (2nd Australian & New Zealand ed.). Sydney: Lippincott Williams & Wilkins.

Murray, C., et al. (2012). Disability-adjusted life years (DALYs) for 291 diseases and injuries in 21 regions, 1990–2010: A systematic analysis for the Global Burden of Disease Study 2010. *The Lancet, 380*(9859), 2197–2223.

Royal College of Physicians' Clinical Effectiveness and Evaluation Unit. (2011). *Falling standards, broken promises: Report of the national audit of falls and bone health in older people 2010*. Sydney: Author.

Willis, L. (Ed). (2017). *Anatomy & physiology made incredibly easy* (5th ed.). Sydney: Lippincott Williams & Wilkins.

Online resources

Accident Compensation Corporation (ACC): www.acc.co.nz
Arthritis Australia: www.arthritisaustralia.com.au
Arthritis New Zealand: www.arthritis.org.nz
Australia and New Zealand Falls Prevention Society: www.anzfallsprevention.org
Australian & New Zealand Orthopaedic Nurses Association: www.anzona.net
Australian Institute of Health and Welfare: www.aihw.gov.au
Independent Living Centre Australia: ilcaustralia.org.au
Independent Living Service New Zealand: www.ilsnz.org
International Osteoporosis Foundation (IOF): www.iofbonehealth.org
Osteoporosis Australia: www.osteoporosis.org.au
Osteoporosis New Zealand: https://osteoporosis.org.nz/
Rheumatoid Arthritis: www.rheumatoidarthritis.com.au

CHAPTER 29

Nervous system

CASE STUDY

Thomas Walker is 65 years old and has just been admitted to the neurosurgical ward. He is lean and athletic in stature and looks much younger than his age. He has an abrasion on the left side of his face, a result of a fall while jogging. Witnesses at the scene stated that he seemed to 'stumble and fall' and that he was unconscious for 2 to 3 minutes. His wife arrived with him and stated that he is normally very fit and well, although over the past 3 to 4 weeks he has been complaining of headaches and intermittent numbness and tingling in his right arm. Mr Walker has refused to see a doctor, saying he is only experiencing stress from his job as an air traffic controller.

Structure and function

The complex neurological system is responsible for coordinating and regulating all body functions. It consists of two structural components: the central nervous system (CNS) and the peripheral nervous system.

THE CENTRAL NERVOUS SYSTEM

The CNS encompasses the brain and the spinal cord and is covered by the meninges. The meninges consist of three layers of connective tissue that protect and nourish the CNS. The subarachnoid space surrounds the brain and spinal cord and is filled with cerebrospinal fluid, which is formed in the ventricles. This fluid-filled space cushions the brain and spinal cord, nourishes the CNS and removes waste materials. Electrical activity of the CNS is governed by neurons located throughout the sensory and motor neural pathways. The CNS contains upper motor neurons that influence activity of the lower motor neurons. Upper motor neurons are located entirely within the CNS. Lower motor neurons are also found within the CNS but are located mostly in the peripheral nervous system.

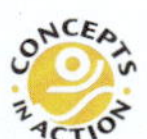

Neurological: Nerve synapse
Neurological: Simple cell
Neurological: Action potential
Neurological: Saltatory conduction

Brain

Located in the cranial cavity, the brain has four major divisions: the cerebrum, the diencephalon, the brainstem and the cerebellum (Fig. 29-1A).

Cerebrum

The cerebrum consists of two hemispheres, the thalamus, the hypothalamus and the basal ganglia. The right and left hemispheres are incompletely separated by the great longitudinal fissure and joined at the lower portion of the fissure by the corpus callosum. The outside surface of the hemispheres has a wrinkled appearance due to convolutions and creases (gyri and sulci), which increase the surface area of the brain. The outer portion of the cerebrum (cerebral cortex) is made up of grey matter approximately 2 to 5 mm in depth and contains billions of neurons, giving it a grey appearance.

White matter makes up the innermost layer and is composed of nerve fibres and neuroglia that form tracts connecting various parts of the brain with one another (transverse and association pathways) and the cortex to lower portions of the brain and spinal cord (projection fibres). The cerebral hemispheres are divided into pairs of frontal, parietal, temporal and occipital lobes (Fig. 29-1B).

Table 29-1 describes the specific functions of each lobe. Damage to a lobe results in impairment of the specific function directed by that lobe.

Diencephalon

The diencephalon lies beneath the cerebral hemispheres and consists of the thalamus and the hypothalamus. Most sensory impulses travel through the grey matter of the thalamus, which is responsible for screening and directing the impulses to specific areas in the cerebral cortex. The hypothalamus controls the autonomic nervous system (which is a part of the peripheral nervous system) and is responsible for regulating body functions including water balance, appetite, temperature, blood pressure, pulse, respiratory rate, sleep cycles, pain perception and emotional status.

Brainstem

The brainstem consists of the midbrain, the pons and the medulla oblongata (Fig 29-1A). The midbrain connects the pons and the cerebellum with the cerebral hemispheres; it contains sensory and motor pathways and serves as the centre

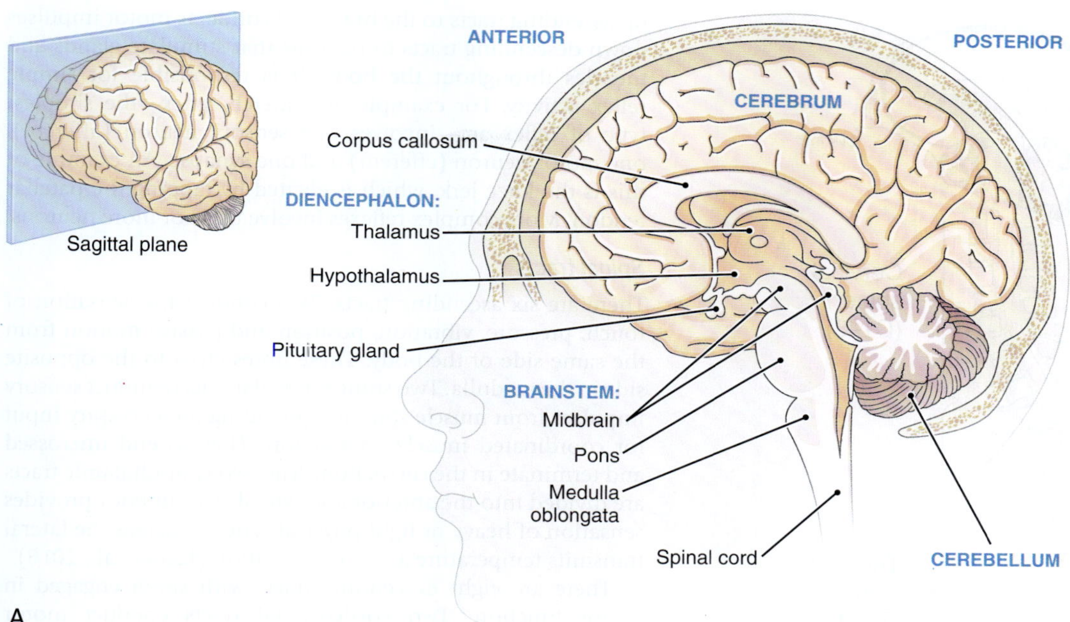

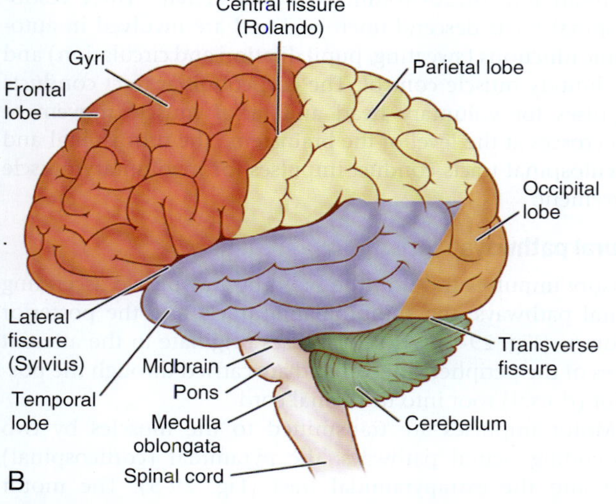

FIGURE 29-1 (A) Structures of the brain (sagittal section). **(B)** View of the external surface of the brain, showing the lobes, cerebellum and brainstem (Farrell & Dempsey, 2014).

Table 29-1 Lobes of the cerebral hemispheres and their function

Lobe	Function
Frontal	Directs voluntary, skeletal actions (left side of lobe controls right side of body and right side of lobe controls left side of body). Also influences communication (talking and writing), emotions, intellect, reasoning ability, judgement and behaviour. Contains the Broca area, which is responsible for speech.
Parietal	Interprets tactile sensations, including touch, pain, temperature, shapes and two-point discrimination.
Occipital	Influences the ability to read with understanding and is the primary visual receptor centre.
Temporal	Receives and interprets impulses from the ear. Contains the Wernicke area, which is responsible for interpreting auditory stimuli.

for auditory and visual reflexes. Cranial nerves III and IV originate in the midbrain. The pons is situated in front of the cerebellum between the midbrain and the medulla and is a bridge between the two halves of the cerebellum, the medulla and the cerebrum. Cranial nerves V to VIII connect to the brain in the pons. The pons contains motor and sensory pathways. Portions of the pons also control the heart, respiration and blood pressure.

The medulla oblongata contains motor fibres from the brain to the spinal cord, and sensory fibres from the spinal cord to the brain. Most of these fibres cross at this level. Cranial nerves IX to XII connect to the brain in the medulla.

Cerebellum

The cerebellum, located behind the brainstem and under the cerebrum, also has two hemispheres. Although the cerebellum does not initiate movement, its primary functions include coordination and smoothing of voluntary movements, maintenance of equilibrium and maintenance of muscle tone.

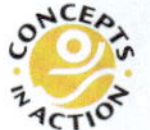

Neurological: Equilibrium potential

Spinal cord

The spinal cord (Fig. 29-2) is located in the vertebral canal and extends from the medulla oblongata to the first lumbar vertebra. (Note that the spinal cord is not as long as the vertebral canal.) The inner part of the cord has an H-shaped appearance and is made up of two pairs of columns (dorsal and ventral) consisting of grey matter. The outer surface of the spinal cord is made up of white matter and surrounds the internal grey matter (Fig. 29-3). The spinal cord conducts sensory impulses

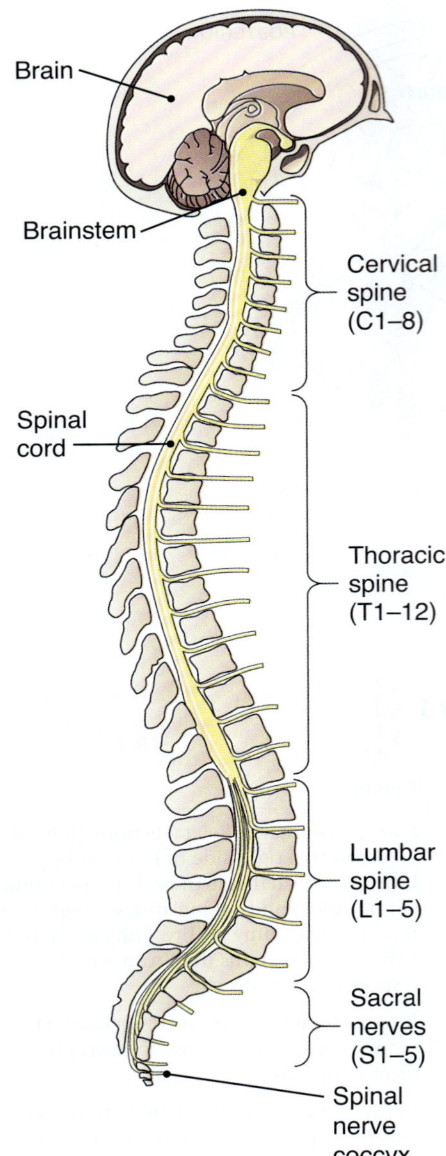

FIGURE 29-2 Spinal cord.

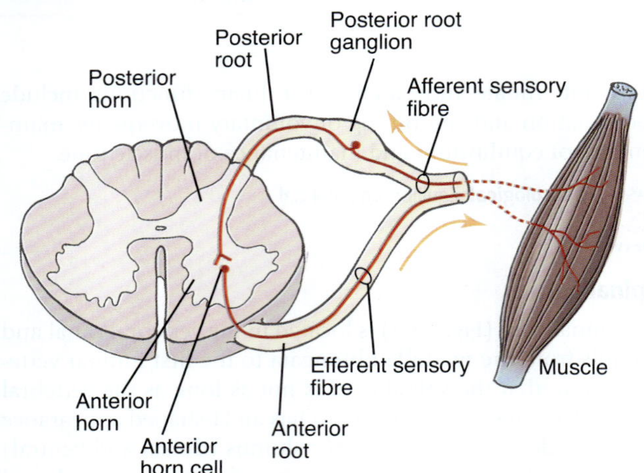

FIGURE 29-3 Cross-section of the spinal cord. (Cohen, B.J. and Taylor, J. (2009). Memmler's Structure and Function of the Human Body, 9th edition, LWW.)

up ascending tracts to the brain and conducts motor impulses down descending tracts to neurons that stimulate glands and muscles throughout the body. It is responsible for simple reflex activity. For example, the stretch reflex—the simplest type of reflex arc—involves one sensory neuron (afferent), one motor neuron (efferent) and one synapse. An example of this is the knee jerk, which is elicited by tapping the patellar tendon. More complex reflexes involve three or more neurons.

Spinal tracts

There are six ascending tracts. Two conduct the sensation of touch, pressure, vibration, position and passive motion from the same side of the body. These fibres cross to the opposite side in the medulla. Two spinocerebellar tracts conduct sensory impulses from muscle spindles, providing the necessary input for coordinated muscle contraction. They ascend uncrossed and terminate in the cerebellum. The two spinothalamic tracts are divided into the anterior and lateral. The anterior provides sensation of heavy or light physical touch, whereas the lateral transmits temperature and pain sensation (Estes et al., 2016).

There are eight descending tracts with seven engaged in motor function. Two corticospinal tracts conduct motor impulses to the anterior horn cells from the opposite side of the brain and control voluntary muscle activity. Three vestibulospinal tracts descend uncrossed and are involved in autonomic functions (sweating, pupil dilation and circulation) and involuntary muscle control. The corticobulbar tract conducts impulses for voluntary head and facial muscle movement and crosses at the level of the brainstem. The rubrospinal and reticulospinal tracts conduct impulses for involuntary muscle movement.

Neural pathways

Sensory impulses travel to the brain by way of two ascending neural pathways: the spinothalamic tracts and the posterior columns (Fig. 29-4). These impulses originate in the afferent fibres of the peripheral nerves and are carried through the posterior (dorsal) root into the spinal cord.

Motor impulses are transmitted to the muscles by two descending neural pathways: the pyramidal (corticospinal) tract and the extrapyramidal tract (Fig. 29-5). The motor neurons of the pyramidal tract originate in the motor cortex and travel down to the medulla where they cross over to the opposite side, then travel down the spinal cord where they synapse with a lower motor neuron in the anterior horn of the spinal cord. These impulses are carried to muscles and produce voluntary movements that involve skill and purpose. The extrapyramidal tract motor neurons consist of those motor neurons that originate in the motor cortex, basal ganglia, brainstem and spinal cord outside the pyramidal tract. They travel from the frontal lobe to the pons, where they cross over to the opposite side and travel down the spinal cord, where they connect with lower motor neurons that conduct impulses to the muscles. These neurons conduct impulses related to maintenance of muscle tone and body control.

The voluntary motor system consists of upper motor neurons and lower motor neurons. Upper motor neurons originate in the cerebral cortex, the cerebellum and the brainstem and modulate the activity of the lower motor neurons. Upper motor neuron fibres make up the descending motor pathways and are located entirely within the CNS. Lower motor neurons are located either in the anterior horn of the spinal cord grey

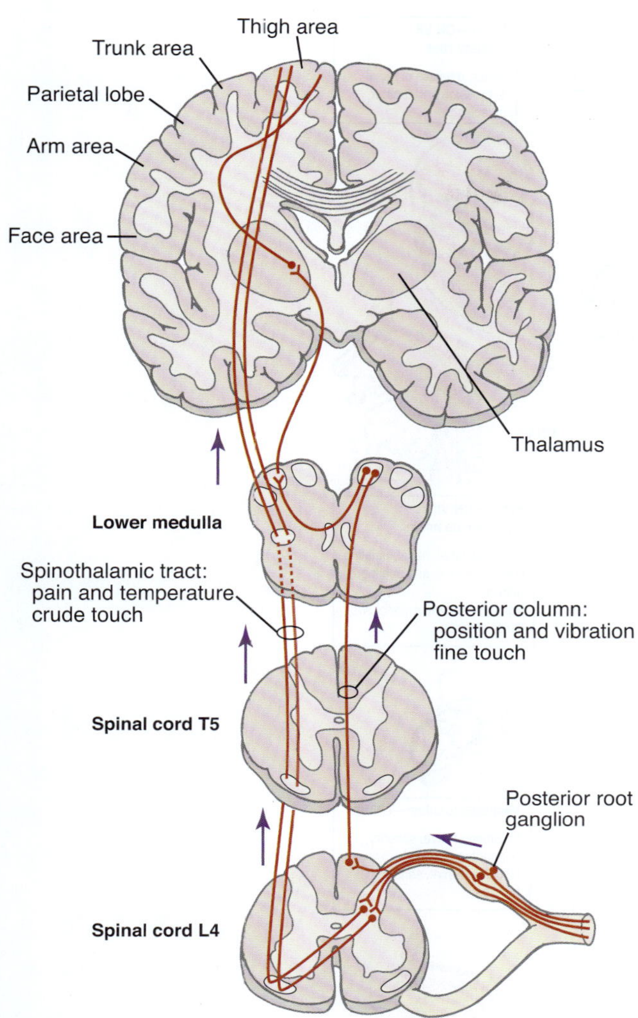

FIGURE 29-4 Sensory (ascending) neural pathways.

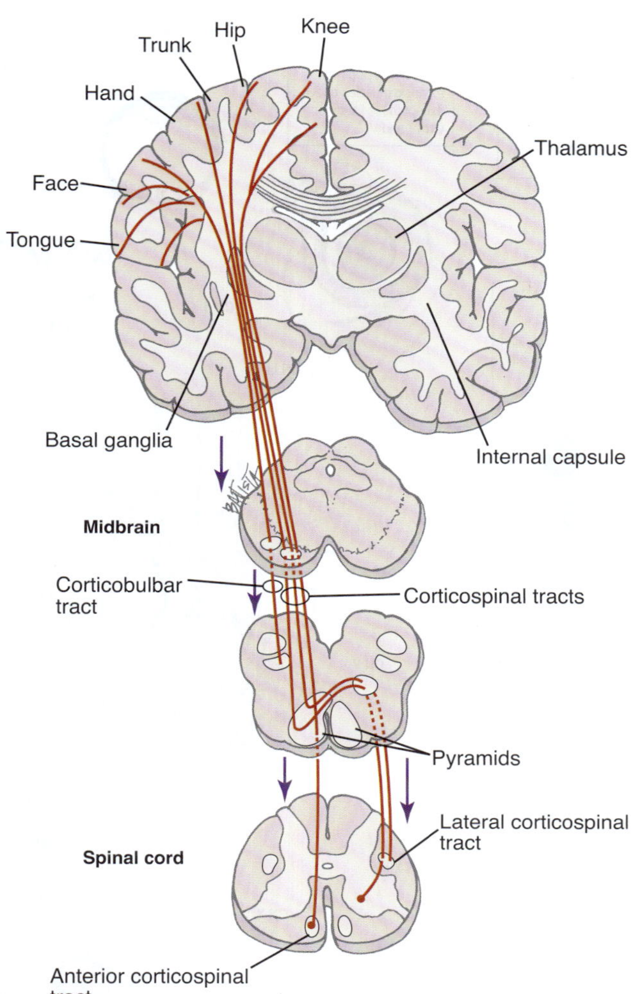

FIGURE 29-5 Motor (descending) neural pathways.

matter or within cranial nerve nuclei in the brainstem. Axons of both extend through peripheral nerves and terminate in skeletal muscle. Lower motor neurons are located in both the CNS and the peripheral nervous system, receive the impulse in the posterior part of the cord and run to the myoneural junction located in the peripheral muscle.

THE PERIPHERAL NERVOUS SYSTEM

Carrying information to and from the CNS, the peripheral nervous system consists of 12 pairs of cranial nerves and 31 pairs of spinal nerves. These nerves are categorised as two types of fibres: somatic and autonomic. Somatic fibres carry CNS impulses to voluntary skeletal muscles, whereas autonomic fibres carry CNS impulses to smooth, involuntary muscles (in the heart and glands). The somatic nervous system mediates conscious, or voluntary, activities, whereas the autonomic nervous system mediates unconscious, or involuntary, activities, such as heart rate, pupillary dilation and constriction, and blood pressure.

Cranial nerves

Twelve pairs of cranial nerves evolve from the brain or brainstem and transmit motor or sensory messages. Figures 29-6

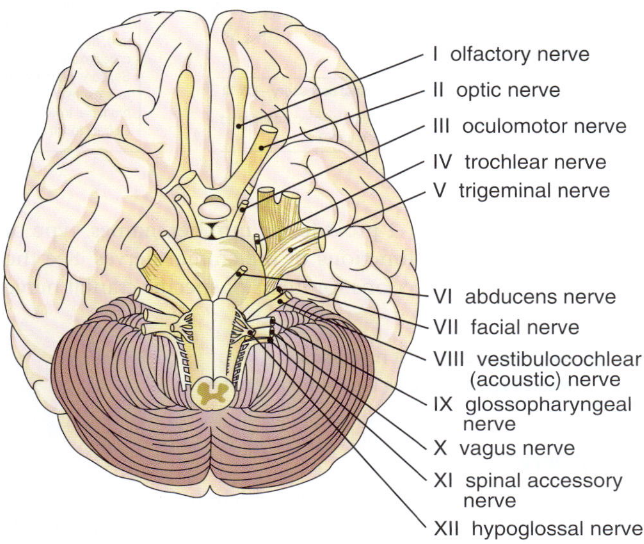

FIGURE 29-6 Cranial nerves, inferior view. (Cohen, B.J. & Taylor, J. [2009]. *Memmler's Structure and Function of the Human Body* [9th ed.]. LWW.)

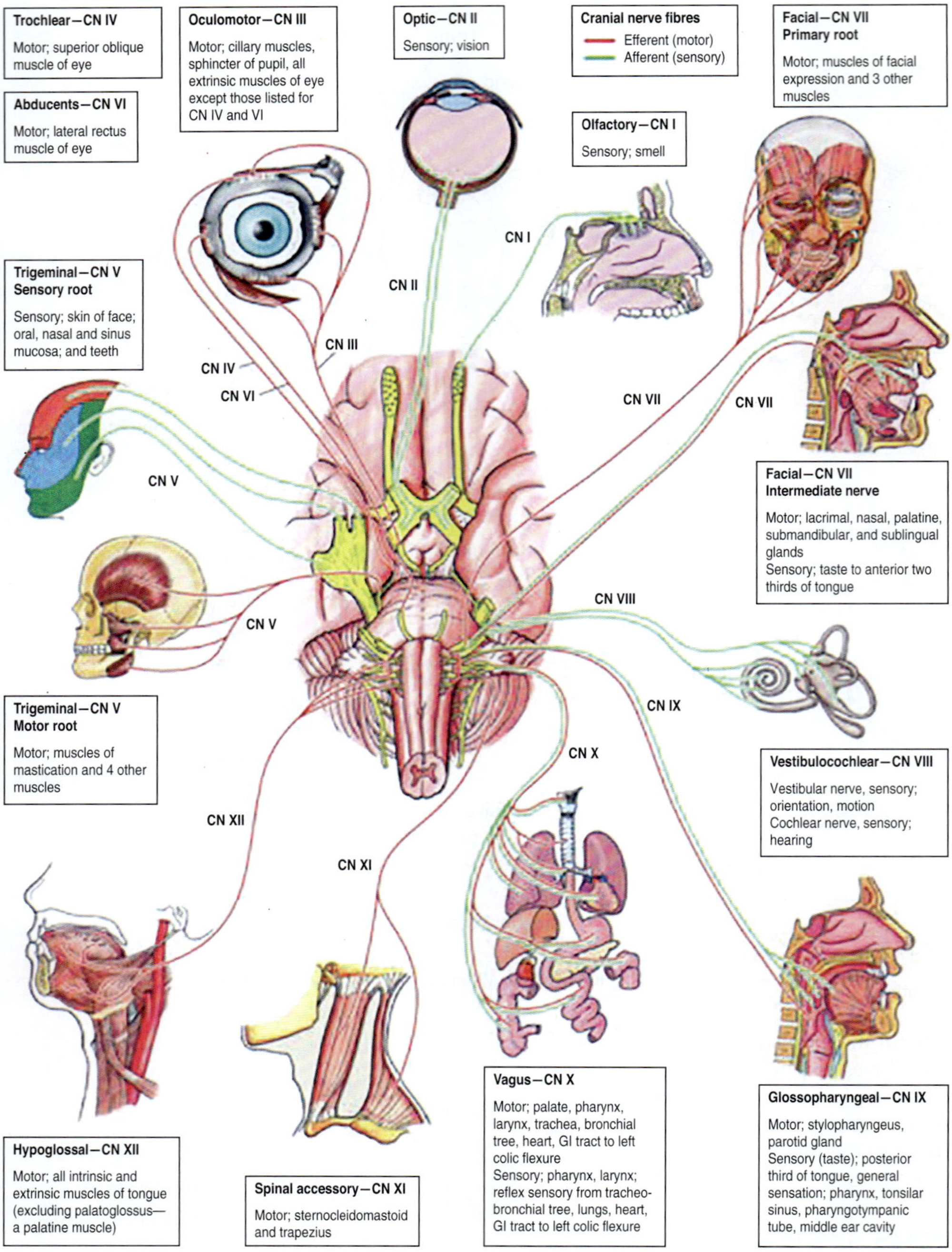

Trochlear—CN IV
Motor; superior oblique muscle of eye

Abducents—CN VI
Motor; lateral rectus muscle of eye

Oculomotor—CN III
Motor; cillary muscles, sphincter of pupil, all extrinsic muscles of eye except those listed for CN IV and VI

Optic—CN II
Sensory; vision

Cranial nerve fibres
Efferent (motor)
Afferent (sensory)

Olfactory—CN I
Sensory; smell

Facial—CN VII Primary root
Motor; muscles of facial expression and 3 other muscles

Trigeminal—CN V Sensory root
Sensory; skin of face; oral, nasal and sinus mucosa; and teeth

CN I
CN II
CN III
CN IV
CN VI
CN V
CN VII
CN VII

Facial—CN VII Intermediate nerve
Motor; lacrimal, nasal, palatine, submandibular, and sublingual glands
Sensory; taste to anterior two thirds of tongue

CN VIII
CN V
CN IX
CN X
CN XII
CN XI

Trigeminal—CN V Motor root
Motor; muscles of mastication and 4 other muscles

Vestibulocochlear—CN VIII
Vestibular nerve, sensory; orientation, motion
Cochlear nerve, sensory; hearing

Hypoglossal—CN XII
Motor; all intrinsic and extrinsic muscles of tongue (excluding palatoglossus—a palatine muscle)

Spinal accessory—CN XI
Motor; sternocleidomastoid and trapezius

Vagus—CN X
Motor; palate, pharynx, larynx, trachea, bronchial tree, heart, GI tract to left colic flexure
Sensory; pharynx, larynx; reflex sensory from tracheobronchial tree, lungs, heart, GI tract to left colic flexure

Glossopharyngeal—CN IX
Motor; stylopharyngeus, parotid gland
Sensory (taste); posterior third of tongue, general sensation; pharynx, tonsilar sinus, pharyngotympanic tube, middle ear cavity

FIGURE 29-7 Cranial nerves, overview (from Rubin, P. & Hansen, J. T. [2012]. *TNM Staging atlas with oncoanatomy*. Philadelphia: Lippincott Williams & Wilkins.)

and 29-7 and Table 29-2 provide the number, names, type of impulse and primary functions of the cranial nerves. See the Physical assessment sections for items of specific cranial nerve testing.

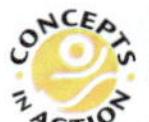

Neurological: Basilar membrane
Neurological: Flipping the membrane potential

Spinal nerves

There are 31 pairs of spinal nerves, which are named after the vertebrae below each one's exit point along the spinal cord: 8 cervical nerves, 12 thoracic nerves, 5 lumbar nerves, 5 sacral nerves and 1 coccygeal nerve (see Fig. 29-2). Each nerve is attached to the spinal cord by two nerve roots. The sensory (afferent) fibre enters through the dorsal (posterior) roots of the cord, whereas the motor (efferent) fibre exits through the ventral (anterior) roots of the cord. The sensory root of each spinal nerve innervates an area of the skin called a dermatome (Fig. 29-8).

CLINICAL TIP

If you look after a patient who has an epidural during surgery, you may be required to check the patient's dermatome levels. You can do this using an ice block, to ascertain at which spinal nerve the epidural anaesthetic is effective. Local anaesthetics work by blocking nerve impulses on sensory, motor and autonomic nerve fibres. Fibres with the smallest diameters

Table 29-2 Cranial nerves: Type and function

Cranial nerve (name)	Type of impulse	Function
I (olfactory)	Sensory	Carries smell impulses from nasal mucous membrane to brain
II (optic)	Sensory	Carries visual impulses from eye to brain
III (oculomotor)	Motor	Contracts eye muscles to control eye movements (interior lateral, medial and superior), constricts pupils and elevates eyelids
IV (trochlear)	Motor	Contracts one eye muscle to control inferomedial eye movement
V (trigeminal)	Sensory	Carries sensory impulses of pain, touch and temperature from the face to the brain
	Motor	Influences clenching and lateral jaw movements (biting, chewing)
VI (abducens)	Motor	Controls lateral eye movements
VII (facial)	Sensory	Contains sensory fibres for taste on anterior two-thirds of tongue and stimulates secretions from salivary glands (submaxillary and sublingual) and tears from lacrimal glands
	Motor	Supplies the facial muscles and affects facial expressions (smiling, frowning, closing eyes)
VIII (acoustic, vestibulocochlear)	Sensory	Contains sensory fibres for hearing and balance
IX (glossopharyngeal)	Sensory	Contains sensory fibres for taste on posterior third of tongue and sensory fibres of the pharynx that result in the 'gag reflex' when stimulated
	Motor	Provides secretory fibres to the parotid salivary glands; promotes swallowing movements
X (vagus)	Sensory	Carries sensations from the throat, larynx, heart, lungs, bronchi, gastrointestinal tract and abdominal viscera
	Motor	Promotes swallowing, talking and production of digestive juices
XI (spinal accessory)	Motor	Innervates neck muscles (sternocleidomastoid and trapezius) that promote movement of the shoulders and head rotation. Also promotes some movement of the larynx
XII (hypoglossal)	Motor	Innervates tongue muscles that promote the movement of food and talking

are most sensitive to the effects of local anaesthetics: autonomic fibres will be blocked first, then sensory fibres, then motor fibres. The sensory fibres respond to pain, temperature, touch and pressure. Because pain and temperature nerve fibres are similarly affected by local anaesthetics, changes in temperature perception indicate the area where the epidural is working. The area of sensory block can be assessed using cold sensation (i.e. ice) to establish which dermatome levels are covered. Both left and right sides need to be assessed and recorded, as per your hospital's protocol.

THE AUTONOMIC NERVOUS SYSTEM

Some peripheral nerves have a special function associated with automatic activities; they are referred to as the autonomic nervous system. Autonomic nervous system impulses are carried by both cranial and spinal nerves. These impulses are carried from the CNS to the involuntary smooth muscles that make up the walls of the heart and glands. The autonomic nervous system, which maintains the internal homeostasis of the body, incorporates the sympathetic and parasympathetic nervous systems. The sympathetic nervous system ('fight-or-flight' system) is activated during stress and elicits responses such as decreased gastric secretions, bronchiole dilation, increased pulse rate and pupil dilatation. These sympathetic fibres arise from the thoracolumbar level (T1 to L2) of the spinal cord. The parasympathetic nervous system functions to restore and maintain normal body functions, for example, by decreasing heart rate. The parasympathetic fibres arise from the craniosacral regions (S1 to S4 and cranial nerves III, VI, IX and X).

CLINICAL TIP

As you learn pharmacological therapeutics, you will notice that many drug actions are directed at the autonomic nervous system. For example, beta-blockers block some of the sympathetic nervous system, slowing the heart rate and lowering the blood pressure; and atropine blocks the parasympathetic nervous system, increasing the heart rate.

Health assessment

COLLECTING SUBJECTIVE DATA: THE NURSING HEALTH HISTORY

Problems with other body systems may affect the CNS, and CNS disorders can affect all other body systems. Regardless of the source of the neurological problem, the patient's lifestyle and level of functioning are often affected. Because of their subjective nature, CNS problems related to activities of daily

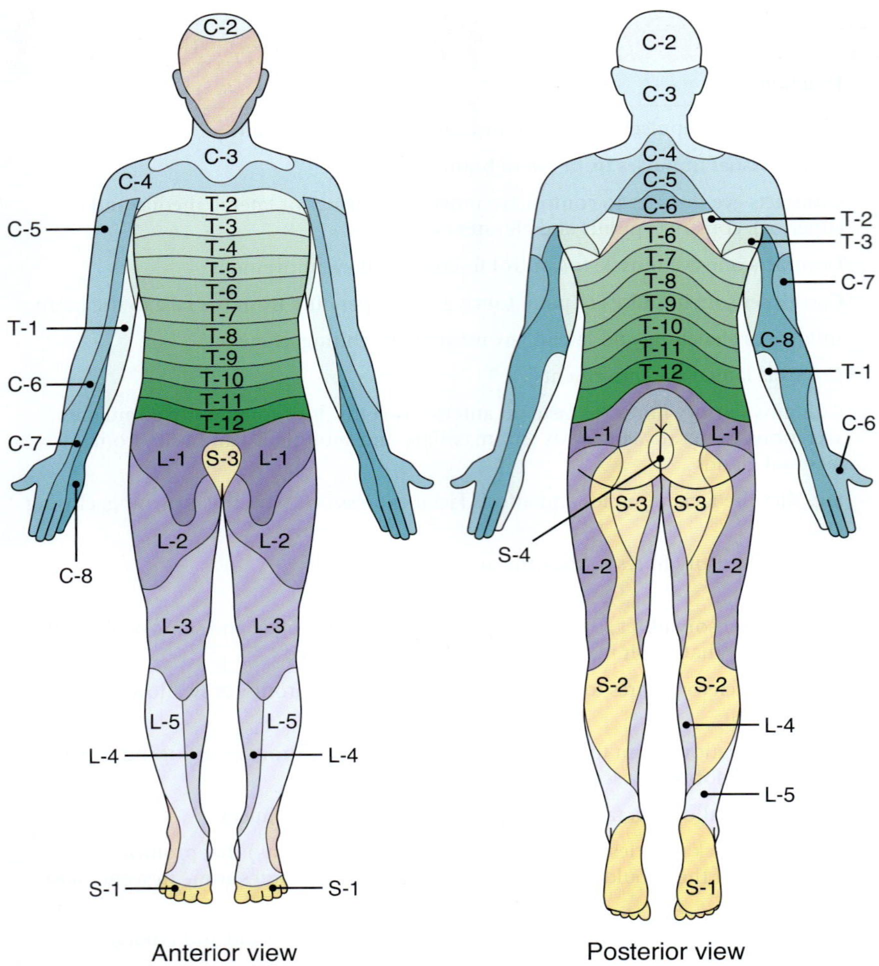

FIGURE 29-8 Anterior and posterior dermatomes (areas of skin innervated by spinal nerves). (Cohen, B.J. & Taylor, J. [2009]. *Memmler's Structure and Function of the Human Body* [9th ed.]. LWW.)

living are typically detected through a comprehensive nursing history. For example, problems of concentration, sensation or dizziness may occasionally be identified, but only through precise questioning during the patient interview.

Patients who are experiencing symptoms associated with the CNS (such as headaches or memory loss) may be very fearful that they have a serious condition such as a metastatic brain tumour or a difficult-to-treat disease such as Alzheimer disease. Fear of losing control and independence, along with threatened self-esteem or role performance, is common. Symptoms are often reversible and may be due to medication side effects, electrolyte disturbances or imbalances in other body systems such as renal or cardiac failure. You need to be sensitive to these fears and concerns because the patient may decline to share important information with you if these fears and concerns are not addressed.

Neurological assessments such as the ones described in this chapter should be integrated into your nursing practice as a matter of course. A thorough and routine neurological assessment can be vital to the discovery and subsequent effective management of patients in your care. This is not to say it should be a standard assessment. Rather, your assessment needs to be patient centred; that is, it should be individualised yet holistic in its implementation.

History of present health concerns

QUESTION	RATIONALE
Headaches	
Do you experience headaches? When do they occur and what do they feel like? (See related questions in Chap. 16.)	See Chapter 16 for a description of various types of headaches. Morning headaches that subside after rising may be an early sign of increased intracranial pressure such as with a brain tumour.

History of present health concerns (continued)

QUESTION	RATIONALE
Head injury	
Have you had a head injury? If so, what part of your head was involved? Did you lose consciousness at all? If so, for how long?	Head injuries can produce long-term neurological deficits and affect level of functioning.
Dizziness	
Do you experience dizziness or light-headedness or problems with balance or coordination? If so, how often? Does it occur with activity? Or have you experienced any falling? Do you have any clumsy movement?	Dizziness or light-headedness may be related to carotid artery disease, cerebellar abscess, Menière disease, medications such as angiotensin–converting enzyme inhibitors or inner ear infection. Imbalance and difficulty coordinating or controlling movements are seen in neurological diseases involving the cerebellum, basal ganglia, extrapyramidal tracts or the vestibular part of cranial nerve VIII (acoustic). Diminished cerebral blood flow and vestibular response may increase the risk of falls.
Seizures	
Do you experience seizures? How often? Can you tell me how long these seizures last? When was your last seizure? Were there any complications or injuries related to the seizure? Did you have any follow up with a neurologist or other health professional? What was the result? Did you have any further testing after your last seizure? What was your understanding of what was said and done as a result of your last seizure?	Seizures occur with epilepsy, metabolic disorders, head injuries, space occupying masses, some drugs and high fevers.
Describe what happens before you have the seizure and where on your body the seizure starts. Does anything seem to initiate a seizure? Do you lose control of your bladder during the seizure? How do you feel afterwards? Do you take medications for the seizures? Do you wear medical identification to alert others that you have seizures? Do you take safety precautions regarding driving or operating dangerous machinery?	In some cases, an aura (an auditory, visual or motor sensation) forewarns the patient that a seizure is about to occur. Where the seizure starts and what occurs before and after can aid in determining the type of seizure (e.g. generalised seizure, formerly known as grand mal and affecting both hemispheres of the brain; or absence seizure, also known as petit mal) and its treatment. Patients with generalised seizures often experience bladder incontinence during the seizure. Anti-epileptic medications (anticonvulsants) must be distributed at a therapeutic level in the blood to be effective. Wearing a medical identification tag, such as a MedicAlert bracelet, and the patient's knowledge of the medication regimen and the importance of safety measures provide information on the patient's willingness to be involved in and adhere to the treatment plan.
Muscle control	
Have you lost bowel or bladder control or do you retain urine?	Loss of bowel control or urinary retention and bladder distension are seen with spinal cord injury or tumours.
Do you have muscle weakness? If so, where?	Unilateral weakness or paralysis may result from cerebrovascular accident (CVA), compression of the spinal cord or nerve injury. Progressive weakness is a symptom of several nervous system diseases.

Continued on following page

History of present health concerns (continued)

QUESTION	RATIONALE
Do you experience any tremors? If so, where?	Tremors are typical in degenerative neurological disorders, such as Parkinson disease (3 to 6 per second while muscles are at rest), or in cerebellar disease and multiple sclerosis (variable rate, and especially with intentional movement). **OLDER ADULT CONSIDERATIONS** **Older adults may experience tremors with movement. Tremors may involve the hands, head (yes or no nodding) and the tongue, which may protrude back and forth. Such tremors are not associated with disease, but they may cause embarrassment or emotional distress.** **PAEDIATRIC CONSIDERATIONS** **The neurological system is not fully developed at birth and most actions in the newborn are primitive reflexes.**
Numbness and tingling	
Do you experience any numbness or tingling? When and where does this occur?	Loss of sensation or tingling may occur with damage to the brain, spinal cord or peripheral nerves.
Senses	
Have you noticed a decrease in your ability to smell or to taste?	A decrease in the ability to smell may be related to a dysfunction of cranial nerve I (olfactory) or a brain tumour. A decrease in the ability to taste may be related to dysfunction of cranial nerves VII (facial) or IX (glossopharyngeal). **OLDER ADULT CONSIDERATIONS** **Decreased taste and scent sensation occurs normally in older adults.**
Have you experienced any ringing in your ears or hearing loss?	Ringing in the ears (tinnitus) and decreased ability to hear may occur with dysfunction of cranial nerve VIII (acoustic). **OLDER ADULT CONSIDERATIONS** **There is a normal degenerative process in the older person's ability to hear.** **PAEDIATRIC CONSIDERATIONS** **Newborns can hear loud sounds at 90 decibels and react with the startle reflex. They respond to low-frequency sounds, such as a heartbeat or lullaby, by decreasing crying and motor movement.**
Have you noticed any change in your vision?	Changes in vision may occur with dysfunction of cranial nerve II (optic), increased intracranial pressure or brain tumours. Damage to cranial nerves III (oculomotor), IV (trochlear) or VI (abducens) may cause double or blurred vision. Transient blind spots may be an early sign of a stroke. **OLDER ADULT CONSIDERATIONS** **There is a normal degenerative process in the older person's ability to see.**

History of present health concerns (continued)

QUESTION	RATIONALE
Difficulty speaking	
Do you have difficulty understanding when people are talking to you? Do you have difficulty making others understand you? Do you have difficulty forming words or verbally interpreting your thoughts?	Injury to the cerebral cortex can impair the ability to use or understand verbal language. This is related to the Broca area (associated with understanding and producing spoken language) and Wernicke area (associated with processing words or language). These two areas work closely together to make sense out of the words we are hearing and to be able to respond using language. They are connected by a large bundle of nerve fibres called the arcuate fasciculus.
Difficulty swallowing	
Do you experience difficulty swallowing?	Difficulty swallowing may relate to CVA, Parkinson disease, myasthenia gravis, Guillain-Barré syndrome or dysfunction of cranial nerves IX (glossopharyngeal), X (vagus) or XII (hypoglossal).
Memory loss	
Do you experience any memory loss?	Recent memory (24-hour memory) is often impaired in amnestic disorders, Korsakoff syndrome, delirium and dementia. Remote memory (past dates and historical accounts) may be impaired in cerebral cortex disorders.

Continued on following page

COLDSPA

Example

Use the COLDSPA mnemonic as a guideline to collect needed information for each symptom the patient shares. In addition, the following questions help elicit important information.

Mnemonic	Question	Patient response example
Character	Describe the sign or symptom (feeling, appearance, sound, smell or taste, if applicable)	'Numbness and aching in my right hand.'
Onset	When did it begin?	'Since I started typing at my office 4 months ago.'
Location	Where is it? Does it radiate? Does it occur anywhere else?	'At the centre of my hand below the wrist.'
Duration	How long does it last? Does it recur?	'It lasts for several hours and recurs.'
Severity	How bad is it? or How much does it bother you?	'It hurts so much I cannot type for long and is beginning to affect my productivity at work.'
Pattern	What makes it better or worse?	'It gets worse after I type for 10 minutes or more. It goes away when I rest it and stop typing.'
Associated factors/How it Affects the patient	What other symptoms occur with it? How does it affect you?	'It also tingles at times.'

Past health history

QUESTION	RATIONALE
Have you ever had any type of head injury with or without loss of consciousness (e.g. sports injury, motor vehicle accident, fall)? If so, describe any physical or mental changes that have occurred as a result. What type of treatment did you receive?	Head injuries, even if minor, can produce long-term neurological deficits and affect level of functioning.
Have you ever had meningitis, encephalitis, injury to the spinal cord or a stroke? If so, describe any physical or mental changes that have occurred as a result. What type of treatment did you receive?	These disorders can affect the long-term physical and mental status of the patient.

Family history

QUESTION	RATIONALE
Do you have a family history of high blood pressure, stroke, Alzheimer disease, epilepsy, brain cancer or Huntington disease?	These disorders may be genetic.

Lifestyle and health practices

QUESTION	RATIONALE
Do you take any prescription or non-prescription medications? How much alcohol do you drink? Do you use recreational drugs such as marijuana, tranquilisers, barbiturates or cocaine?	Prescription and non-prescription drugs can cause various neurological symptoms such as tremors or dizziness, altered level of consciousness, decreased response times, and changes in mood and temperament.
Do you smoke?	Nicotine, which is found in cigarettes, constricts the blood vessels, which decreases blood flow to the brain. Cigarette smoking is a risk factor for CVA. See Promote health—Cerebrovascular accident (stroke).
Do you wear your seat belt when riding in vehicles? Do you wear protective headgear when riding a bicycle or playing sports?	Risk taking behaviours have a known increased risk of injury. Seat belts and protective headgear can prevent head injury.
Describe your usual daily diet.	Peripheral neuropathy can result from a deficiency in niacin, folic acid or vitamin B12, or progressive and non-controlled diabetes
Have you ever had prolonged exposure to lead, insecticides, pollutants or other chemicals?	Prolonged exposure to these substances can alter neurological status.
Do you frequently lift heavy objects or perform repetitive motions?	Intervertebral disc injuries may result when heavy objects are lifted improperly. Peripheral nerve injuries can occur from repetitive movements.
Can you perform your normal activities of daily living?	Neurological symptoms and disorders often negatively affect the ability to perform activities of daily living.
Has your neurological problem changed the way you view yourself? Describe.	Low self-esteem and body image problems may lead to depression and changes in role functions.
Has your neurological problem added much stress to your life? Describe.	Neurological problems can impair ability to fulfil role responsibilities, greatly increasing stress. Stress can increase existing neurological symptoms.

PROMOTE HEALTH — CEREBROVASCULAR ACCIDENT (STROKE)

OVERVIEW

Cerebrovascular accident (CVA), commonly called stroke, results when the blood supply to an area of the brain is disrupted. This blood supply disruption can be caused by thrombosis, embolism, infarction or haemorrhage. All four of these may result from underlying cerebrovascular disease.

The Stroke Foundation (2019a) describes the different types of strokes: ischaemic and haemorrhagic. Ischaemic strokes may be due to narrowing of the artery from clot formation (thrombotic stroke), or from a clot breaking off from another location in the brain or body, causing blockage as it lodges in the smaller brain artery (embolic stroke). Haemorrhagic strokes occurs when a vessel becomes weak (aneurysm) and ruptures. A mini-stroke that causes no damage but indicates stroke risk is called a transient ischaemic attack (TIA).

Stroke is Australia's second biggest killer following coronary heart disease and is a leading cause of disability (Australian Institute of Health and Welfare [AIHW], 2017), as many stroke survivors have disabilities and need significant daily support for the rest of their lives. Stroke is 1.5 times more likely to cause death in Aboriginal and Torres Strait Islander peoples than in the non-Aboriginal and Torres Strait Islander population (Stroke Foundation, 2019b). In 2017, more than 80,200 people were admitted to hospital within Australia with either primary or subsequent diagnosis of stroke (AIHW, 2017). It is estimated that in 2019 in excess of $54 billion will be spent on stroke-related costs within Australia (Queensland Brain Institute, 2019).

Each year approximately 9,000 New Zealanders are diagnosed with having a stroke (Ministry of Health, 2019), and on average one New Zealander has a stroke each hour, making stroke the leading cause of death in New Zealand (Stroke Foundation NZ, 2019a). Statistics in New Zealand indicate that one-quarter of all people who suffer a stroke are of working age; as a result, significant disabilities cause financial, social and health impact on the individual and families (Stroke Foundation NZ, 2019b). Māori are more likely to die at a younger age from stroke than non-Māori: Māori who die from stroke are on average 62 years old, in comparison with non-Māori who are 75 years old. Furthermore, stroke rates for Māori and Pasifika have increased by 19% and 66%, respectively, over the last decade; these groups also suffer disproportionately more severe strokes and poorer outcomes (Mahawish et al., 2018).

RISK FACTORS

Modifiable	Unmodifiable
Hypertension	Older adulthood: risk increases twofold each decade after age 55
Smoking	Male sex (slightly higher risk)
Chronic alcohol intake (more than two drinks per day)	History of stroke or transient TIA
Sleep apnoea	History of cardiovascular disease such as coronary artery disease, heart failure, rhythm abnormalities (especially atrial fibrillation), mitral valve prolapse
High serum levels of fibrinogen, beta-lipoproteins, cholesterol, haematocrit	High oestrogen levels
Diabetes mellitus	Postmenopausal woman
Drug abuse (especially cocaine and methamphetamines)	Sickle cell anaemia
High-dose oral contraceptives (especially with coexisting hypertension, smoking)	Family history of stroke
Overweight	
Sedentary lifestyle	
Newly industrialising environment	

TEACH RISK REDUCTION TIPS

- Monitor blood pressure regularly and take part in 30 minutes of moderate exercise on most days.
- Stop smoking, especially if taking oral contraceptives. (Quitting smoking reduces risk to non-smoker level in 5 years.)
- Limit intake of alcohol to less than three drinks per day.
- Schedule regular health care checkups.
- Adhere to a diet low in fat and cholesterol; follow cardiovascular disease risk factor modifications.
- Have regular blood tests to measure cholesterol and haematocrit levels.
- If diabetic, follow diabetes treatment plan.
- Monitor blood sugar regularly, if diabetic.
- Avoid use of drugs such as cocaine and methamphetamines.

The Stroke Foundation Australia's Stride-4-Stroke program was developed to raise community awareness of the risks associated with cardiovascular disease through the encouragement of activities such as their November event where participants raise both funds and recognition of the impact stroke has on the Australian community. The Australian government in collaboration with the Stroke Foundation and the Heart Foundation are currently drafting a national action plan for heart and stroke aimed at reducing the impact of disease for all Australians (Stroke Foundation, 2019c).

WARNING SIGNS OF STROKE

- Sudden numbness (face, arm, leg), especially if on only one side of body
- Sudden confusion, trouble speaking or understanding speech
- Sudden vision problems in one or both eyes
- Sudden trouble walking, dizziness, loss of balance or coordination
- Sudden severe headache with no known cause

The Stroke Foundation (2019d) has released a simple mnemonic, FAST, which aims to educate those within the community on the common and recognisable signs of stroke so they recognise a stroke more quickly and thus reduce the time to management.

Using the FAST test involves asking these simple questions:

Face: Check their face. Has their mouth drooped?
Arms: Can they lift both arms?
Speech: Is their speech slurred? Do they understand you?
Time: Is critical. If you see any of these signs call 000 straight away.

The signs of stroke may occur alone or in combination. They can last a few seconds or up to 24 hours and then disappear. As indicated in the FAST test, the importance of early identification, presentation, assessment, imaging and referral plays a significant role in achieving positive patient outcomes associated with stroke management. Interventions such as thrombolytic therapy are known to be time critical and have shown to have significant recovery outcomes (Nindra et al., 2019).

Do not wait for the symptoms to improve or worsen. Calling early for medical help can make the difference in avoiding a lifelong disability.

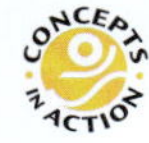

Neurological: Stroke

COLLECTING OBJECTIVE DATA: PHYSICAL EXAMINATION

A complete neurological examination consists of evaluating the following five areas:

- Mental status
- Cranial nerves
- Motor and cerebellar systems
- Sensory system
- Reflexes.

The examinations may be performed in an order that moves from a level of higher cerebral integration to a lower level of reflex activity. *Note:* A nervous system assessment is considered an advanced skill, and this knowledge is often gained after many years in specialist practice.

Mental status examinations provide information about cerebral cortex function. Cerebral abnormalities disturb the patient's intellectual ability, communication ability or emotional behaviours. A mental status examination is often performed at the beginning of the head-to-toe examination because it provides clues to the validity of the subjective information provided by the patient. For example, if the nurse finds that the patient's thought processes are distorted and his or her memory is impaired, another means of obtaining necessary subjective data must be identified (refer to Chap. 6).

The *cranial nerve evaluation* provides information regarding the transmission of motor and sensory messages, primarily to the head and neck. Many of the cranial nerves are evaluated during the head, neck, eye and ear examinations.

The *motor and cerebellar systems* are assessed to determine functioning of the pyramidal and extrapyramidal tracts. The cerebellar system is assessed to determine the patient's level of balance and coordination. The motor system examination is usually performed during the musculoskeletal examination.

Examining the *sensory system* provides information regarding the integrity of the spinothalamic tract, the posterior columns of the spinal cord and the parietal lobes of the brain, whereas testing reflexes provides clues to the integrity of deep and superficial *reflexes*. Deep reflexes depend on an intact sensory nerve, a functional synapse in the spinal cord, an intact motor nerve, a neuromuscular junction and competent muscles. Superficial reflexes depend on skin receptors rather than muscles.

If meningitis is suspected, you may try to elicit the Brudzinski sign (flexion of the neck produces movement of the ankle, knee and hip) and Kernig sign (when sitting or lying with the thigh flexed upon the abdomen, the leg cannot be completely extended), which are characteristic of meningeal irritation. Sometimes, a complete neurological examination is unnecessary. In such cases, the nurse performs 'neuro obs'—a brief screening of the patient's neurological observations. 'Neuro obs' include the following assessment points:

- Level of consciousness, using either the Glasgow Coma Scale (see Display 29-1), the AVPU (Alert, Voice, Pain, Unresponsive) mnemonic or the FOUR (Full Outline of UnResponsiveness) Score Coma Scale (FOUR Score; see Display 29-2)
- Pupillary response to light
- Movement and strength of arms and legs
- Sensation in the extremities
- Vital signs.

DISPLAY 29-1 ASSESSMENT FOR GLASGOW COMA SCALE

The Glasgow Coma Scale is a tool for assessing a patient's response to stimuli. Scores range from 3 (deep coma) to 15 (normal).*

Eye opening response	Spontaneous	4
	To voice	3
	To pain	2
	None	1
Best verbal response	Orientated	5
	Confused	4
	Inappropriate words	3
	Incomprehensible sounds	2
	None	1
Best motor response	Obeys command	6
	Localises pain	5
	Withdraws	4
	Flexion	3
	Extension	2
	None	1
Total		3 to 15

Source: Teasdale, G. & Jennett, B. (1974). Assessment of coma and impaired consciousness: A practical scale (later called the 'Glasgow Coma Scale'). Lancet, 2(7872), 81–84. © Sir Graham Teasdale via Copyright Clearance Center.

*See Chapter 6 for more information on interpreting the GCS score.

DISPLAY 29-2 FOUR SCORE COMA SCALE

Eye response

4 Eyelids open or opened, tracking or blinking to command
3 Eyelids open but not tracking
2 Eyelids closed but opens to loud voice
1 Eyelids closed but opens to pain
0 Eyelids remain closed with pain

Motor response

4 Thumbs up, fist or peace sign to command
3 Localising to pain
2 Flexion response to pain
1 Extensor posturing
0 No response to pain or generalised myoclonus status epilepticus

Brainstem reflexes

4 Pupil and corneal reflexes present
3 One pupil wide and fixed
2 Pupil *or* corneal reflexes absent
1 Pupil *and* corneal reflexes absent
0 Absent pupil, corneal and cough reflex

Respiration

4 Not intubated, regular breathing pattern
3 Not intubated, Cheyne–Stokes breathing pattern
2 Not intubated, irregular breathing pattern
1 Breathes above ventilator rate
0 Breaths at ventilator rate or apnoea

Source: Wijdicks, E. F. M., Bamlet, W. R., Maramattorn, B. V., Manno, E. M. & McClelland, R. L. (2005). Validation of a new coma scale: The FOUR Score. *Annals of Neurology, 58,* 585–593. (Copyright © 2005 American Neurological Association.)

Neurological observation can be performed for any patient at any time but is particularly useful when frequent assessments are needed during an acute phase of illness, to detect rapid changes in neurological status. 'Neuro obs' are also useful for the patient who has already had a complete neurological examination but needs to be rechecked for changes related to therapy or other potential deteriorations in neurological function.

The need for patients to be screened early in the stroke trajectory is well established in the nursing literature (Middleton et al., 2015). Furthermore, implementation of multidisciplinary evidence-based protocols initiated by nurses for the management of fever, hyperglycaemia and swallowing dysfunction has been found to deliver better patient outcomes after discharge from stroke units.

In Australia and elsewhere, the mnemonic FAST is used to identify the warning signs of a stroke (National Stroke Foundation Australia, 2019a) and involves asking these simple questions:

- Face: Check their face. Has their mouth drooped?
- Arm: Can they lift both arms?
- Speech: Is their speech slurred? Do they understand you?
- Time: Is critical. If any of the above signs are present, make an emergency call straight away.

Patients who are assessed to be at high risk of aspiration should be screened using an appropriate stroke assessment chart in collaboration with a speech pathologist. This ensures that reliable screening has occurred and will establish if it is safe for the patient to commence oral intake, or is at risk of aspiration and requires further assessment and management from the speech pathology team, or is in need of alternative (non-oral) routes of nutrition, hydration and medication administration.

If it has been established it is not safe for a patient to receive oral intake, the nurse should place the patient on a nil by mouth order while awaiting a formal speech pathology assessment; notify the medical team; seek alternative routes of medication administration; hydration and nutrition (for example IV or nasogastric tube); and, finally, instigate an oral care program as recommended by the local health service (Bray et al., 2017).

Preparing the patient

Prepare for the examination by ensuring that the patient's clothing allows accessibility; if not, you may ask the patient to put on an examination gown. Initially have the patient sit comfortably on the examination table or bed but explain that several different position changes are necessary throughout the course of the examination. Assure the patient that you will explain each position before starting that particular examination. Also advise your patient that the examination will take a considerable amount of time to perform and that you will provide rest periods as needed. Explain that actions the patient will be asked to perform, such as counting backwards or hopping on one foot, may seem unusual but that these activities are parts of a comprehensive evaluation.

CLINICAL TIP

Demonstrate what you want the patient to do especially during the cerebellar examination, when the patient will need to perform several different coordinated movements.

Equipment

General

- Examination gloves

Cranial nerve examination

- Cotton wool applicators
- Magazine, book or newspaper to read
- Ophthalmoscope
- Paper clip
- Penlight
- Snellen chart
- Sterile woven ball (or gauze ball)
- Substances to smell or taste such as soap, coffee, vanilla, salt, sugar, lemon and juice
- Tongue depressor
- Tuning fork

Motor and cerebellar examination

- Tape measure

Sensory examination

- Woven ball (or gauze ball)
- Objects to feel such as a coin and keys
- Paper clip
- Cups containing hot and cold water
- Tuning fork (low-pitched)

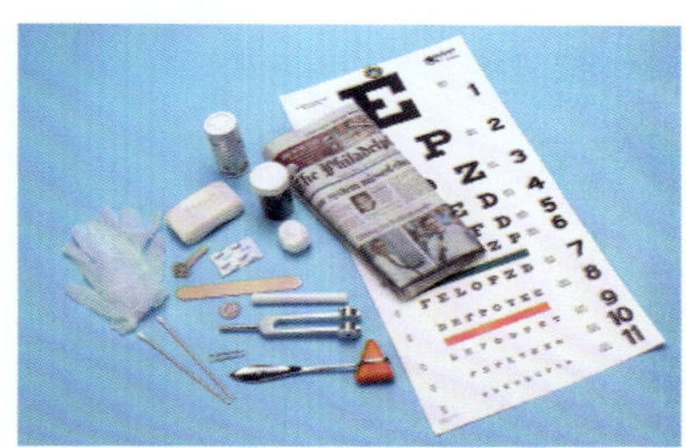

Reflex examination

- Cotton wool applicator
- Reflex (percussion) hammer

Physical assessment

Prior to the examination, review these key points:

- Understand what is meant by mental status and level of consciousness.
- Know how to correctly apply and interpret mental status examinations and the Glasgow Coma Scale.
- Identify the 12 cranial nerves and their sensory and motor functions.
- Thoroughly assess movement, balance, coordination, sensation and reflexes during physical examination.
- Know how to use a reflex hammer (Equipment spotlight 29-1).
- Coordinate patient education—particularly in regard to risks related to stroke—with the health interview and physical examination.

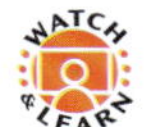

Assessing the musculoskeletal and neurological systems

EQUIPMENT SPOTLIGHT 29-1 HOW TO USE THE REFLEX HAMMER

The reflex (or percussion) hammer is used to elicit deep tendon reflexes. Proceed as follows to elicit a deep tendon reflex:

1. Encourage the patient to relax because tenseness can inhibit a normal response.
2. Position the patient properly.
3. Hold the handle of the reflex hammer between your thumb and index finger so it swings freely.
4. Palpate the tendon that you will need to strike to elicit the reflex.
5. Using a rapid wrist movement, briskly strike the tendon. Observe the response. Avoid a slow or weak movement for striking.
6. Compare the response of one side with the other.
7. To prevent pain, use the pointed end to strike a small area, and the wider, blunt (flat) end to strike a wider area or a more tender area.

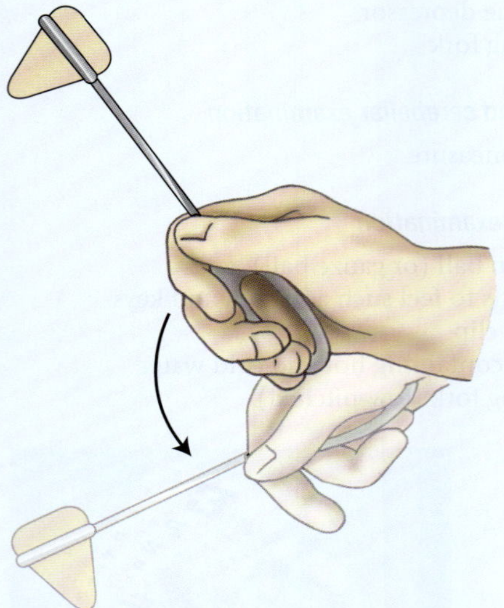

8. Use a reinforcement technique, which causes other muscles to contract and thus increases reflex activity, to assist in eliciting a response if no response can be elicited.
9. For arm reflexes, ask the patient to clench his or her jaw or to squeeze one thigh with the opposite hand, then immediately strike the tendon. For leg reflexes, ask the patient to lock the fingers of both hands and pull them against each other, then immediately strike the tendon.
10. Rate and document reflexes using the following scale and figure.
    - Grade 4+ Hyperactive, very brisk, rhythmic oscillations (clonus); abnormal and indicative of disorder
    - Grade 3+ More brisk or active than normal, but not indicative of a disorder
    - Grade 2+ Normal, usual response
    - Grade 1+ Decreased, less active than normal
    - Grade 0 No response

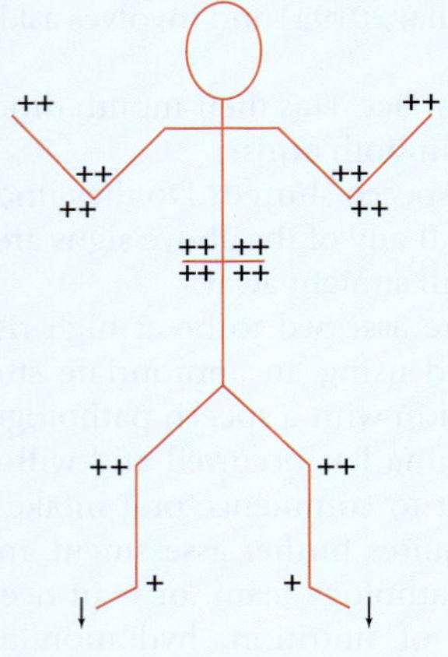

CASE STUDY

On physical assessment, Mr Walker's observations are as follows: blood pressure 155/92 mmHg, pulse 48 beats/minute and respiratory rate 12 breaths/minute, with deep slow breaths. He has a Glasgow Coma Scale score of 13 and is moving all his limbs, but he is not obeying verbal commands. He localises to painful stimuli and is mumbling incoherently. His left pupil is 2 mm and brisk, and his right pupil is 4 mm and sluggish to light. His eyes are open.

CRITICAL THINKING

1. Given Mr Walker's presenting history, would his observations be of concern? Why or why not?
2. What is the significance of a dilated pupil? Suggest three possible causes of a dilated pupil, providing a rationale for each.
3. Suggest possible causes of Mr Walker's altered level of consciousness. (Consider organic and non-organic causes.)
4. If a patient's thought processes are distorted and his or her memory is impaired, another means of obtaining the necessary subjective data must be identified. Suggest other ways these data could be found.

PHYSICAL ASSESSMENT

ASSESSMENT PROCEDURE	NORMAL FINDINGS	ABNORMAL FINDINGS
Cranial nerves (CN)		
Test CN I (olfactory). For all assessments of the cranial nerves, have the patient sit in a comfortable position at your eye level. Ask the patient to clear the nose to remove any mucus then to close the eyes, occlude one nostril and identify a scented object that you are holding such as soap, coffee or vanilla (Fig. 29-9). Repeat this procedure for the other nostril.	Patient correctly identifies scent presented to each nostril.  **OLDER ADULT CONSIDERATIONS** **Some older patients' sense of smell may be decreased.**	Inability to smell (neurogenic anosmia) or identify the correct scent may indicate olfactory tract lesion or tumour or lesion of the frontal lobe. Loss of smell may also be congenital or due to other causes such as nasal disease, smoking and use of cocaine.
Test CN II (optic). Use a Snellen chart to assess vision in each eye (see Chap. 17 for additional information).	Patient has 20/20 (6/6, dependent on Snellen chart) vision OD (right eye) and OS (left eye).	Abnormal findings include difficulty reading Snellen chart, missing letters and squinting.
Ask the patient to read a newspaper or magazine paragraph to assess near vision.	Patient reads print at 35 cm without difficulty.	Patient reads print by holding closer than 35 cm or holds print further away as in presbyopia, which occurs with ageing.
Assess visual fields of each eye by confrontation. 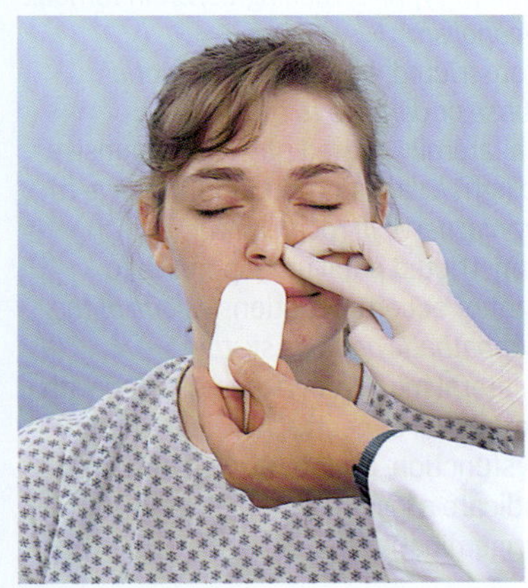 **FIGURE 29-9** Testing cranial nerve I. (© B. Proud.)	Full visual fields (see Chap. 17).	Loss of visual fields may be seen in retinal damage or detachment, with lesions of the optic nerve, or with lesions of the parietal cortex (see Chap. 17).
Use an ophthalmoscope to view the retina and optic disc of each eye.	Round red reflex is present, optic disc is 1.5 mm, round or slightly oval, well-defined margins, creamy pink with paler physiological cup. Retina is pink (see Chap. 17).	Papilloedema (swelling of the optic nerve) results in blurred optic disc margins and dilated, pulsating veins. Papilloedema occurs with increased intracranial pressure from intracranial haemorrhage or a brain tumour. Optic atrophy occurs with brain tumours (see Chap. 17).

Continued on following page

PHYSICAL ASSESSMENT (continued)

ASSESSMENT PROCEDURE	NORMAL FINDINGS	ABNORMAL FINDINGS
Assess CN III (oculomotor), IV (trochlear) and VI (abducens). Inspect margins of the eyelids of each eye.	Eyelid covers about 2 mm of the iris.	Ptosis (drooping of the eyelid) is seen with weak eye muscles such as in myasthenia gravis.
Assess extraocular movements. If nystagmus is noted, determine the direction of the fast and slow phases of movement (see Chap. 17).	Eyes move in a smooth, coordinated motion in all directions (the six cardinal fields).	Some abnormal eye movements and possible causes follow (causes are in italics): • Nystagmus: rhythmic oscillation of the eyes), *cerebellar disorders* • Limited eye movement through the six cardinal fields of gaze, *increased intracranial pressure* • Paralytic strabismus, *paralysis of the oculomotor, trochlear or abducens* nerves (see Chap. 17).
Assess pupillary response to light (direct and indirect) and accommodation in both eyes (see Chap. 17).	Bilateral illuminated pupils constrict simultaneously. Pupil opposite the one illuminated constricts simultaneously.	Some abnormalities and their implications follow (implications in italics): • Dilated pupil (6 to 7 mm), *oculomotor nerve paralysis* • Argyll Robertson pupils, *central nervous system syphilis, meningitis, brain tumour, alcoholism* • Constricted, fixed pupils, *narcotics abuse or damage to the pons* • Unilaterally dilated pupil unresponsive to light or accommodation, *damage to cranial nerve III (oculomotor)* • Constricted pupil unresponsive to light or accommodation, *lesions of the sympathetic nervous system* • Bilateral muscle weakness is seen with peripheral or central nervous system dysfunction. Unilateral weakness may indicate a lesion of cranial nerve V (trigeminal).
Assess CN V (trigeminal). Test motor function. Ask the patient to clench the teeth while you palpate the temporal and masseter muscles for contraction (Fig. 29-10). **CLINICAL TIP** **This test may be difficult to perform and evaluate in the patient without teeth.**	Temporal and masseter muscles contract bilaterally.	

PHYSICAL ASSESSMENT (continued)

ASSESSMENT PROCEDURE	NORMAL FINDINGS	ABNORMAL FINDINGS
Cranial nerves (CN) (continued)		

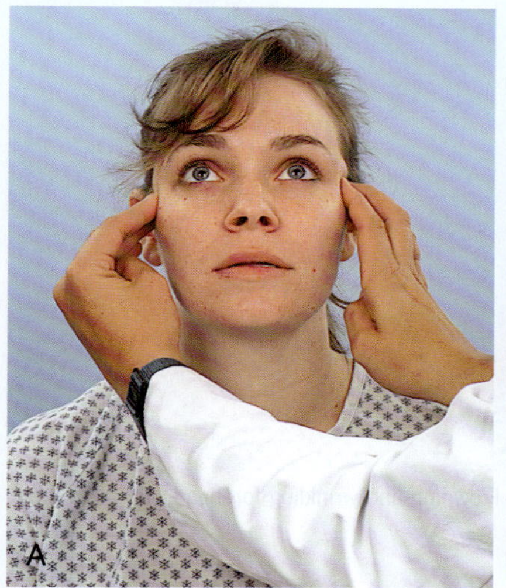

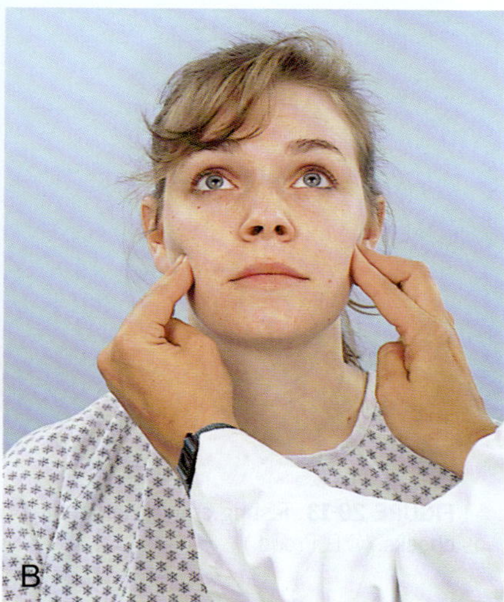

FIGURE 29-10 Testing motor function of cranial nerve V: **(A)** Palpating temporal muscles; **(B)** palpating masseter muscles. (© B. Proud.)

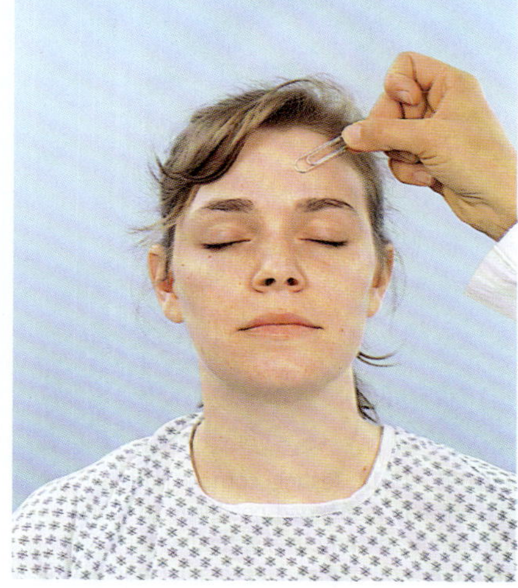

FIGURE 29-11 Testing sensory function of cranial nerve V: Dull stimulus using a paper clip. (© B. Proud.)

ASSESSMENT PROCEDURE	NORMAL FINDINGS	ABNORMAL FINDINGS
Test sensory function. Tell the patient: 'I am going to touch your forehead, cheeks and chin with the sharp or dull side of this safety pin or paper clip [a paper clip is less hazardous]. Please close your eyes and tell me if you feel a sharp or dull sensation. Also tell me where you feel it' (Fig. 29-11). Vary the sharp and dull stimulus in the facial areas and compare sides. Repeat test for light touch with a wisp of cottonwool. **SAFETY TIP** **To avoid transmitting infection, use a new object with each patient. Avoid 'stabbing' the patient with the object's sharp side.**	The patient correctly identifies sharp and dull stimuli and light touch to the forehead, cheeks and chin.	Inability to feel and correctly identify facial stimuli occurs with lesions of the trigeminal nerve or lesions in the spinothalamic tract or posterior columns.
Test corneal reflex. Ask the patient to look away and up while you lightly touch the cornea with a fine wisp of cottonwool (Fig. 29-12). Repeat on the other side.	Eyelids blink bilaterally. **CLINICAL TIP** **This reflex may be absent or reduced in patients who wear contact lenses.**	An absent corneal reflex may be noted with lesions of the trigeminal nerve or lesions of the motor part of cranial nerve VII (facial).
Test CN VII (facial). Test motor function. Ask the patient to: • Smile • Frown and wrinkle forehead (Fig. 29-13A) • Show teeth • Puff out cheeks (Fig. 29-13B) • Purse lips • Raise eyebrows • Close eyes tightly against resistance.	Patient smiles, frowns, wrinkles forehead, shows teeth, puffs out cheeks, purses lips, raises eyebrows and closes eyes against resistance. Movements are symmetrical.	Inability to close eyes, wrinkle forehead or raise forehead along with paralysis of the lower part of the face on the affected side is seen with Bell palsy (a peripheral injury to cranial nerve VII [facial]). Paralysis of the lower part of the face on the opposite side affected may be seen with a central lesion that affects the upper motor neurons such as from cerebrovascular accident.

Continued on following page

PHYSICAL ASSESSMENT (continued)

ASSESSMENT PROCEDURE	NORMAL FINDINGS	ABNORMAL FINDINGS
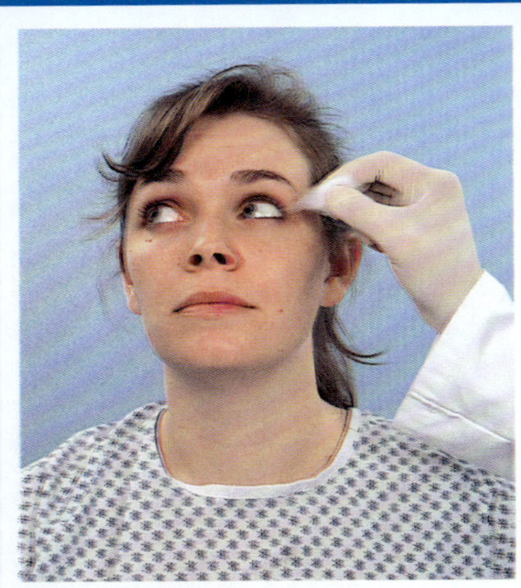 **FIGURE 29-12** Testing corneal reflex. If the patient has responded positively to touch on the forehead and cheeks, testing the corneal reflex is not required as cranial nerve V is intact. (© B. Proud.)	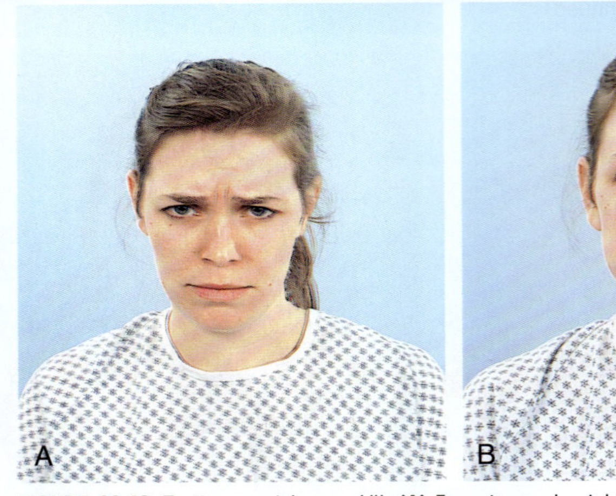 **FIGURE 29-13** Testing cranial nerve VII: **(A)** Frowning and wrinkling forehead; **(B)** puffing out cheeks. (© B. Proud.)	
Sensory function is not routinely tested. If it is, however, touch the anterior two-thirds of the tongue with a moistened applicator dipped in salt, sugar or lemon juice, and ask the patient to identify the flavour. If the patient is unsuccessful, repeat the test using one of the other solutions. If needed, repeat the test using the remaining solution. **CLINICAL TIP** **Make sure the patient leaves the tongue protruded to identify the flavour. Otherwise the substance may move to the posterior third of the tongue (vagus nerve innervation). The posterior portion is tested similarly to evaluate functioning of cranial nerves IX and X. The patient should rinse the mouth with water between each taste test.**	Patient identifies correct flavour. **OLDER ADULT CONSIDERATIONS** **In some older patients, the sense of taste may be decreased.**	Inability to identify correct flavour on anterior two-thirds of the tongue suggests impairment of cranial nerve VII (facial).
Test CN VIII (acoustic/ vestibulocochlear). Test the patient's hearing ability in each ear and perform the Weber test and the Rinne test to assess the cochlear (auditory) component of cranial nerve VIII (see Chap. 18 for detailed procedures). *Note:* The vestibular component, responsible for equilibrium, is not routinely tested. In comatose patients, the test is used to determine integrity of the vestibular system. (See a neurology textbook for detailed testing procedures.)	Patient hears whispered words from 30 to 60 cm. *Weber test:* Vibration heard equally well in both ears. *Rinne test:* AC > BC (air conduction is twice as long as bone conduction).	Vibratory sound lateralises to good ear in sensorineural loss. Air conduction is longer than bone conduction but not twice as long in sensorineural loss (see Chap. 18).

PHYSICAL ASSESSMENT (continued)

ASSESSMENT PROCEDURE	NORMAL FINDINGS	ABNORMAL FINDINGS
Cranial nerves (CN) (continued)		
Test CN IX (glossopharyngeal) and X (vagus). Test motor function. Ask the patient to open the mouth wide and say 'ah' while you use a tongue depressor on the patient's tongue (Fig. 29-14).	Uvula and soft palate rise bilaterally and symmetrically on phonation.	Soft palate does not rise with bilateral lesions of cranial nerve X (vagus). Unilateral rising of the soft palate and deviation of the uvula to the normal side are seen with a unilateral lesion of cranial nerve X (vagus).
Test the gag reflex by touching the posterior pharynx with the tongue depressor. Warn the patient that you are going to do this and that the test may feel a little uncomfortable.	Gag reflex intact. Some normal patients may have a reduced or absent gag reflex.	An absent gag reflex may be seen with lesions of cranial nerve IX (glossopharyngeal) or X (vagus).
Check the patient's ability to swallow by giving the patient a drink of water. Also note the patient's voice quality.	Patient swallows without difficulty. No hoarseness noted.	Dysphagia or hoarseness may indicate a lesion of cranial nerve IX (glossopharyngeal) or X (vagus) or other neurological disorder.
Test CN XI (spinal accessory). Ask the patient to shrug the shoulders against resistance to assess the trapezius muscle (Fig. 29-15).	There is symmetrical, strong contraction of the trapezius muscles.	Asymmetrical muscle contraction or drooping of the shoulder may be seen with paralysis or muscle weakness due to neck injury or torticollis.
Ask the patient to turn the head against resistance, first to the right then to the left, to assess the sternocleidomastoid muscle (Fig. 29-16).	There is strong contraction of sternocleidomastoid muscle on side opposite the turned face.	Atrophy with fasciculations may be seen with peripheral nerve disease.
Test CN XII (hypoglossal). To assess strength and mobility of the tongue, ask the patient to protrude the tongue, move it to each side against the resistance of a tongue depressor, then put it back in the mouth.	Tongue movement is symmetrical and smooth and bilateral strength is apparent.	Fasciculations and atrophy of the tongue may be seen with peripheral nerve disease. Deviation to the affected side is seen with a unilateral lesion.

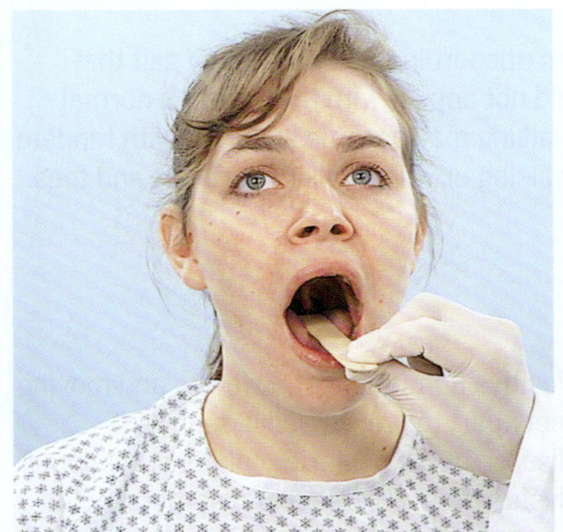

FIGURE 29-14 Testing cranial nerves IX and X: Checking uvula rise and gag reflex. (© B. Proud.)

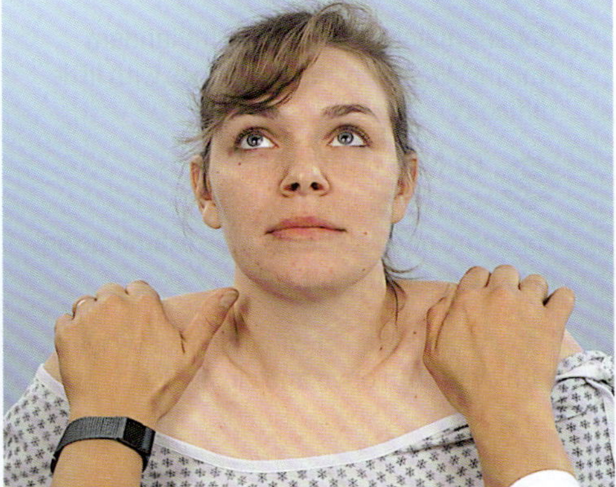

FIGURE 29-15 Testing cranial nerve XI: Assessing strength of trapezius muscle. (© B. Proud.)

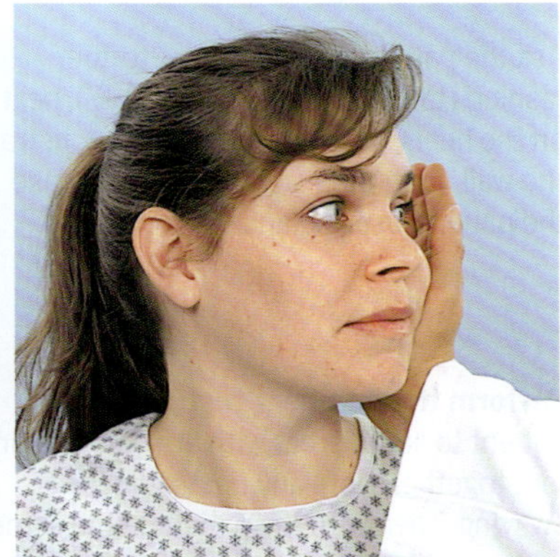

FIGURE 29-16 Testing cranial nerve XI: assessing strength of sternocleidomastoid muscle. (© B. Proud.)

ASSESSMENT PROCEDURE	NORMAL FINDINGS	ABNORMAL FINDINGS
Motor and cerebellar systems		
Assess condition and movement of muscles. Assess the size and symmetry of all muscle groups (see Chap. 28 for detailed procedures).	Muscles are fully developed and symmetrical in size (bilateral sides may vary 1 cm from each other). **OLDER ADULT CONSIDERATIONS** **Some older patients may have reduced muscle mass from degeneration of muscle fibres.**	Muscle atrophy may be seen in diseases of the lower motor neurons or muscle disorders (see Chap. 28).

Continued on following page

PHYSICAL ASSESSMENT (continued)

ASSESSMENT PROCEDURE	NORMAL FINDINGS	ABNORMAL FINDINGS
Assess the strength and tone of all muscle groups (see Chap.28).	Relaxed muscles contract voluntarily and show mild, smooth resistance to passive movement. All muscle groups equally strong against resistance, without flaccidity, spasticity or rigidity.	Soft, limp, flaccid muscles are seen with lower motor neuron involvement. Spastic muscle tone is noted with involvement of the corticospinal motor tract. Rigid muscles that resist passive movement are seen with abnormalities of the extrapyramidal tract.
Note any unusual involuntary movements such as fasciculations, tics or tremors.	No fasciculations, tics or tremors are noted. **OLDER ADULT CONSIDERATIONS** **Some older patients may normally have hand or head tremors or dyskinesia (repetitive movements of the lips, jaw or tongue).**	Abnormal findings include: • Tic (twitch of the face, head or shoulder) from stress or neurological disorder • Unusual, bizarre face, tongue, jaw or lip movements from chronic psychosis or long-term use of psychotropic drugs • Tremors (rhythmic, oscillating movements) from Parkinson disease, cerebellar disease, multiple sclerosis (with movement), hyperthyroidism or anxiety • Slow, twisting movements in the extremities and face from cerebral palsy • Brief, rapid, irregular, jerky movements (at rest) from Huntington chorea.
Evaluate balance. To assess gait, ask the patient to walk naturally across the room. Note posture, freedom of movement, symmetry, rhythm and balance. **CLINICAL TIP** **It is best to assess gait when the patient is not aware that you are directly observing their gait.**	Gait is steady; opposite arm swings. **OLDER ADULT CONSIDERATIONS** **Some older patients may have a slow and uncertain gait. The base may become wider and shorter and the hips and knees may be flexed for a bent-forward appearance.**	Gait and balance can be affected by disorders of the motor, sensory, vestibular and cerebellar systems. Therefore, a thorough examination of all systems is necessary when an uneven or unsteady gait is noted (see Abnormal findings 29-1 for more information about abnormal gaits).
Ask the patient to walk in heel-to-toe fashion (tandem walking; Fig. 29-17), next on the heels, then on the toes. Demonstrate the walk first, then stand close by in case the patient loses balance.	Patient maintains balance with tandem walking. Walks on heels and toes with little difficulty. **OLDER ADULT CONSIDERATIONS** **For some older patients, this examination may be very difficult.**	An uncoordinated or unsteady gait that did not appear with the patient's normal walking may become apparent with tandem walking or when walking on heels and toes.
Perform the Romberg test. Ask the patient to stand erect with arms at side and feet together. Note any unsteadiness or swaying. Then with the patient in the same body position, ask the patient to close the eyes for 20 seconds. Again note any imbalance or swaying. **SAFETY TIP** **Stand near the patient to prevent a fall should they lose balance.**	Patient stands erect with minimal swaying with eyes both open and closed.	Positive Romberg test: Swaying and moving feet apart to prevent fall is seen with disease of the posterior columns, vestibular dysfunction or cerebellar disorders.
Now ask the patient to stand on one foot and to bend the knee of the leg he or she is standing on (Fig. 29-18). Then ask the patient to hop on that foot. Repeat on the other foot.	Patient bends knee while standing on one foot; hops on each foot without losing balance.	Inability to stand or hop on one foot is seen with muscle weakness or disease of the cerebellum.

PHYSICAL ASSESSMENT (continued)

ASSESSMENT PROCEDURE	NORMAL FINDINGS	ABNORMAL FINDINGS

Motor and cerebellar systems (continued)

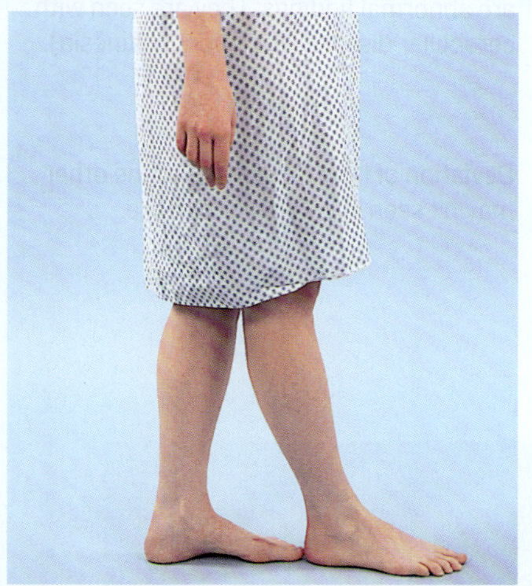

FIGURE 29-17 Testing balance: Tandem walking. (© B. Proud.)

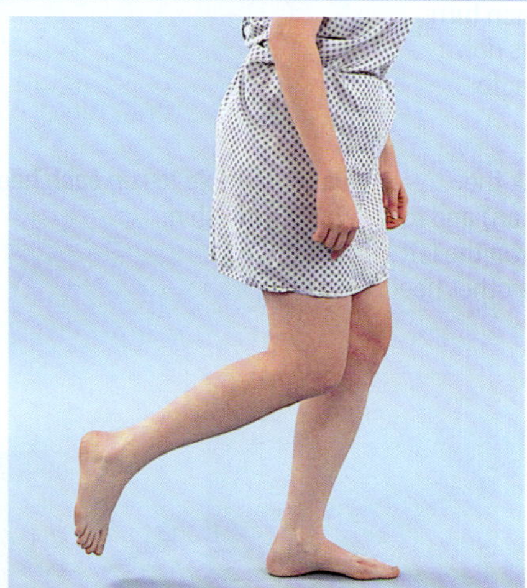

FIGURE 29-18 Tandem balance: Standing and hopping on one foot. (© B. Proud.)

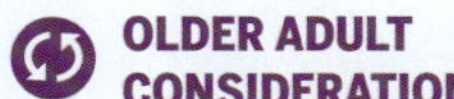

OLDER ADULT CONSIDERATIONS

This test is often impossible for the older adult to perform because of decreased flexibility and strength. Moreover, it is not usual to perform this test with the older adult because it puts the patient at risk.

Assess coordination. Demonstrate the finger-to-nose test to assess accuracy of movements then ask the patient to extend and hold arms out to the side with eyes open. Next say 'Touch the tip of your nose first with your right index finger, then with your left index finger. Repeat this three times' (Fig. 29-19). Next ask the patient to repeat these movements with eyes closed.

Normal findings: Patient touches finger to nose with smooth, accurate movements with little hesitation.

CLINICAL TIP
When assessing coordination of movements, bear in mind that normally the patient's dominant side may be more coordinated than the non-dominant side.

Abnormal findings: Loss of positional sense and inability to touch tip of nose are seen with cerebellar disease.

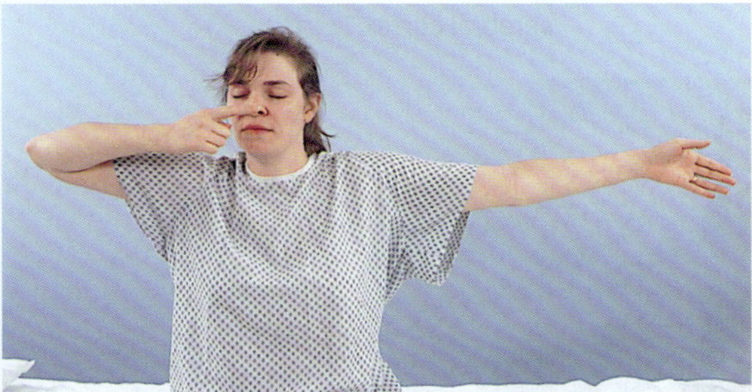

FIGURE 29-19 Testing coordination: Finger-to-nose test. (© B. Proud.)

Next assess rapid alternating movements. Have the patient sit down. First ask the patient to touch each finger to the thumb and to increase the speed as the patient progresses. Repeat with the other side.

Normal findings: Patient touches each finger to thumb rapidly.

OLDER ADULT CONSIDERATIONS
For some older patients, rapid alternating movements are difficult because of decreased reaction time and flexibility.

Abnormal findings: Inability to perform rapid alternating movements may be seen with cerebellar disease, upper motor neuron weakness or extrapyramidal disease.

Continued on following page

PHYSICAL ASSESSMENT (continued)

ASSESSMENT PROCEDURE	NORMAL FINDINGS	ABNORMAL FINDINGS
Next ask the patient to put the palms of both hands down on both legs, then turn the palms up, then turn the palms down again (Fig. 29-20). Ask the patient to increase the speed.	Patient rapidly turns palms up and down.	Uncoordinated movements or tremors are abnormal findings. They are seen with cerebellar disease (dysdiadochokinesia).
Perform the heel-to-shin test. Ask the patient to lie down (supine position) and to slide the heel of the right foot down the left shin (Fig. 29-21). Repeat with the other heel and shin.	Patient is able to run each heel smoothly down each shin.	Deviation of heel to one side or the other may be seen in cerebellar disease.

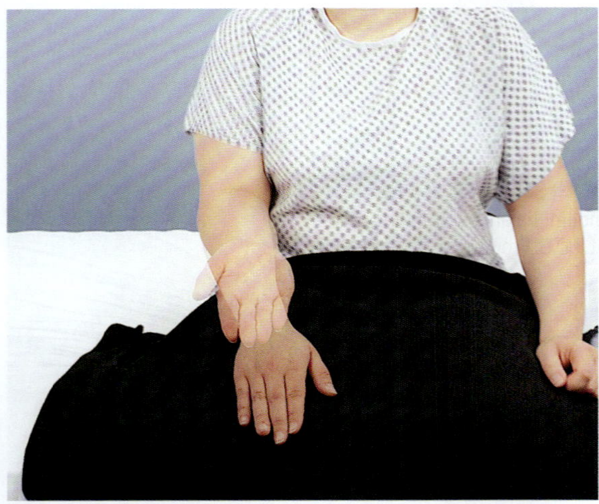

FIGURE 29-20 Testing rapid alternating movements: Palms. (© B. Proud.)

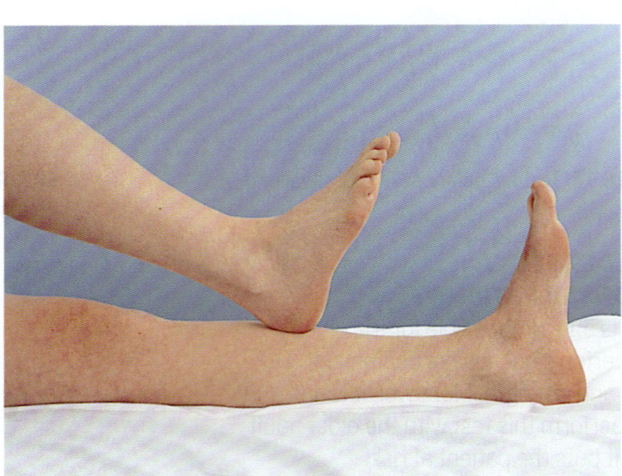

FIGURE 29-21 Performing heel-to-shin test. (© B. Proud.)

Sensory system

ASSESSMENT PROCEDURE	NORMAL FINDINGS	ABNORMAL FINDINGS
Assess light touch, pain and temperature sensations. For each test, ask the patient to close both eyes and tell you what they feel and where they feel it. Scatter stimuli over the distal and proximal parts of all extremities and the trunk to cover most of the dermatomes. It is not necessary to cover the entire body surface unless you identify abnormal symptoms such as pain, numbness or tingling. To test light touch sensation, use a wisp of a woven or gauze ball to touch the patient (Fig. 29-22).	Patient correctly identifies light touch. 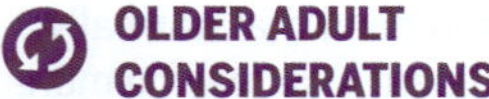 **OLDER ADULT CONSIDERATIONS** **In some older patients, light touch and pain sensations may be decreased.** 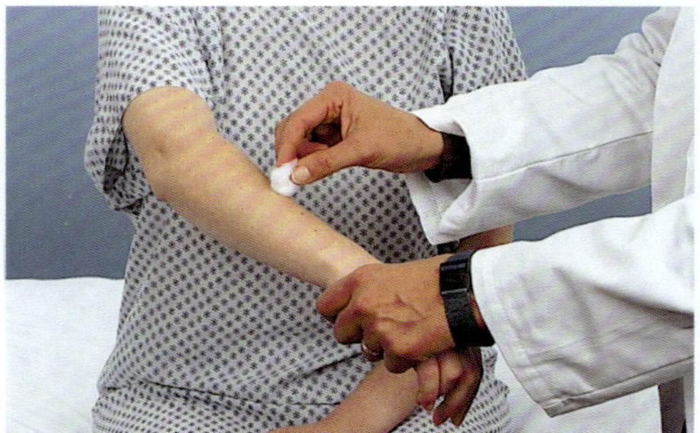 **FIGURE 29-22** Testing light touch sensation. (© B. Proud.)	Many disorders can alter a person's ability correctly to perceive sensations. These include peripheral neuropathies (due to diabetes mellitus, folic acid deficiencies or alcoholism) and lesions of the ascending spinal cord, brainstem, cranial nerves and cerebral cortex.

PHYSICAL ASSESSMENT (continued)

ASSESSMENT PROCEDURE	NORMAL FINDINGS	ABNORMAL FINDINGS
Sensory system (continued)		
To test pain sensation, use the blunt (Fig. 29-23A) and sharp ends (Fig. 29-23B) of a safety pin or paper clip. To test temperature sensation, use test tubes filled with hot and cold water. **CLINICAL TIP** **Test temperature sensation only if abnormalities are found in the patient's ability to perceive light touch and pain sensations. Temperature and pain sensations travel in the lateral spinothalamic tract, so temperature need not be tested if pain sensation is intact.**	Patient correctly differentiates between dull and sharp sensations and hot and cold temperatures over various body parts.	Patient reports: • Anaesthesia (absence of touch sensation) • Hypaesthesia (decreased sensitivity to touch) • Hyperaesthesia (increased sensitivity to touch) • Analgesia (absence of pain sensation) • Hypalgesia (decreased sensitivity to pain) • Hyperalgesia (increased sensitivity to pain).
Test vibratory sensation. Strike a low-pitched tuning fork on the heel of your hand and hold the base on a bony surface of the fingers or big toe (Fig. 29-24). Ask the patient to indicate what he or she feels. Repeat on the other side. **CLINICAL TIP** **If vibratory sensation is intact distally, then it is intact proximally.**	Patient correctly identifies sensation (although, unless clear markers of vibration perception are included, this is not relevant).	Inability to sense vibrations may be seen in posterior column disease or peripheral neuropathy (e.g. as seen with diabetes or chronic alcohol abuse).
Test sensitivity to position. Ask the patient to close both eyes. Then move the patient's toes or a finger up or down (Fig. 29-25). Ask the patient to tell you the direction it is moved. Repeat on the other side. **CLINICAL TIP** **If position sense is intact distally, then it is intact proximally.**	Patient correctly identifies directions of movements.  **OLDER ADULT CONSIDERATIONS** **In some older patients, the sense of position of great toe may be reduced.**	Inability to identify the directions of the movements may be seen in posterior column disease or peripheral neuropathy (e.g. as seen with diabetes or chronic alcohol abuse).

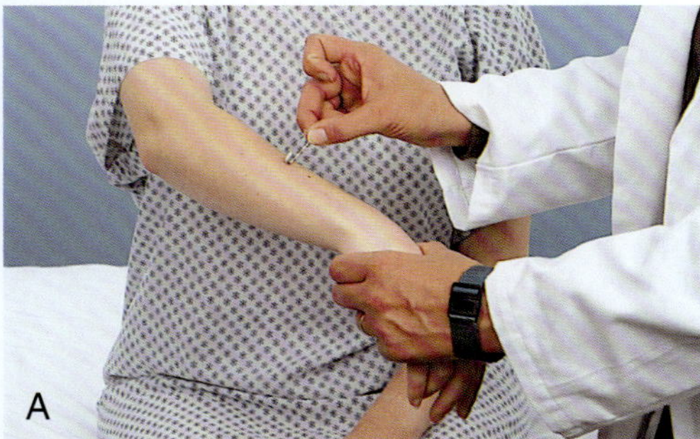

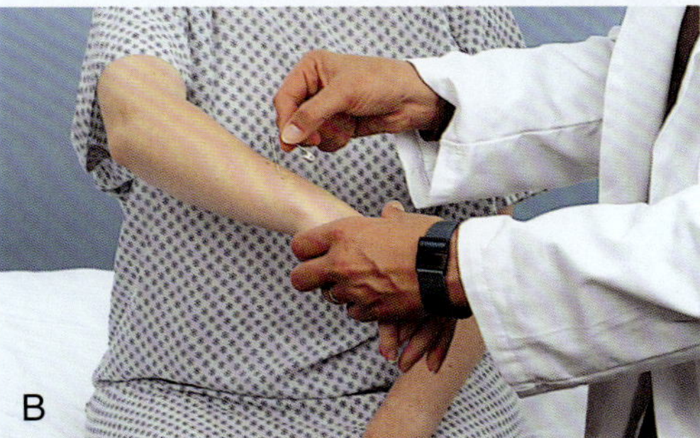

FIGURE 29-23 Testing pain sensation: **(A)** Dull stimulus and **(B)** sharp stimulus. (© B. Proud.)

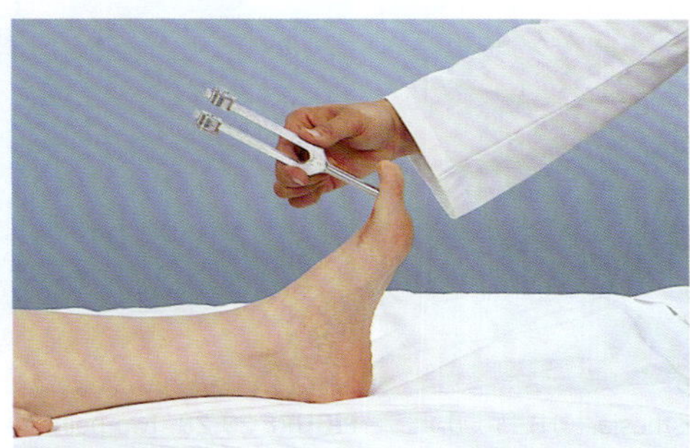

FIGURE 29-24 Testing vibratory sensation. (© B. Proud.)

Continued on following page

PHYSICAL ASSESSMENT (continued)

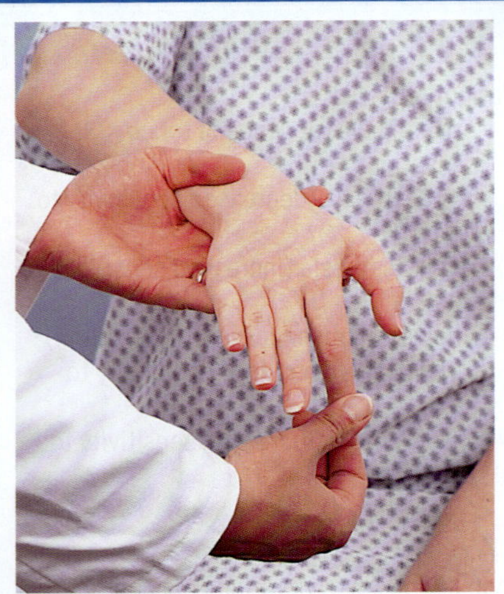

FIGURE 29-25 Testing position sense. (© B. Proud.)

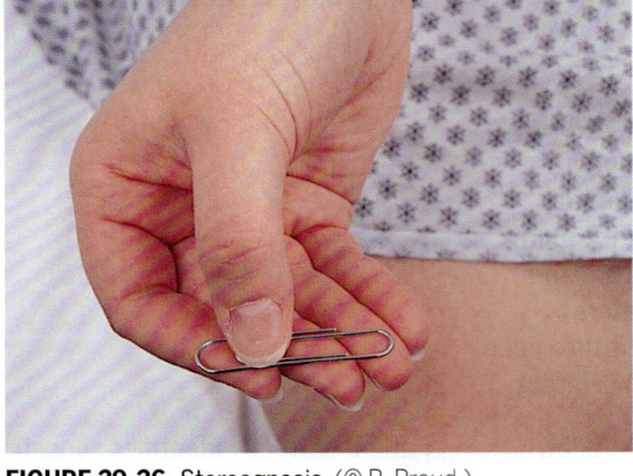

FIGURE 29-26 Stereognosis. (© B. Proud.)

ASSESSMENT PROCEDURE	NORMAL FINDINGS	ABNORMAL FINDINGS
Assess tactile discrimination (fine touch). Remember that the patient should have his or her eyes closed. To test stereognosis, place a familiar object such as a coin, paperclip or key in the patient's hand and ask the patient to identify it (Fig. 29-26). Repeat with another object in the other hand.	Patient correctly identifies object.	Inability to correctly identify objects (astereognosis), area touched or number written in hand, to discriminate between two points or to identify areas simultaneously touched may be seen in lesions of the sensory cortex.
To test point localisation, briefly touch the patient and ask the patient to identify the points touched.	Patient correctly identifies area touched.	Same as above.
To test graphaesthesia, use a blunt instrument to write a number, such as 2, 3 or 5, on the palm of the patient's hand (Fig. 29-27). Ask the patient to identify the number. Repeat with another number on the other hand.	Patient correctly identifies number written.	Same as above.

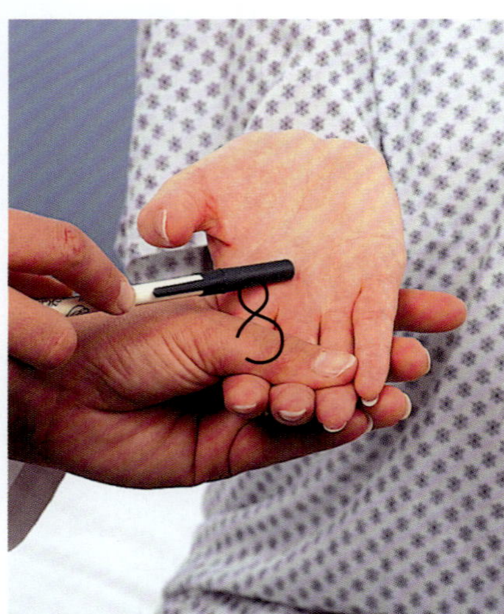

FIGURE 29-27 Graphaesthesia. (© B. Proud.)

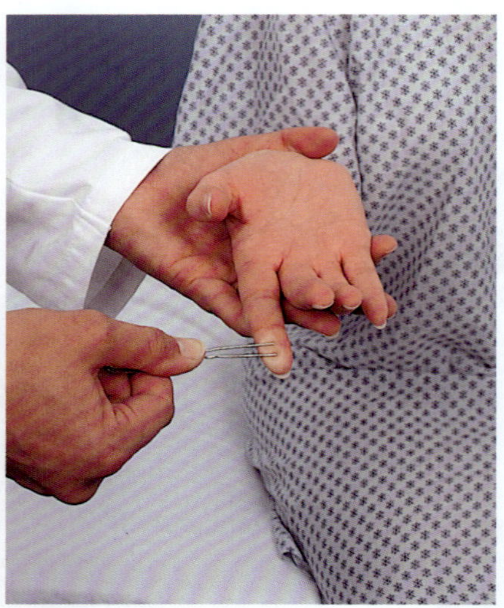

FIGURE 29-28 Two-point discrimination. (© B. Proud.)

PHYSICAL ASSESSMENT (continued)

ASSESSMENT PROCEDURE	NORMAL FINDINGS	ABNORMAL FINDINGS
Sensory system (continued)		
To test two-point discrimination, ask the patient to identify the number of points felt when touched with the ends of two applicators at the same time (Fig. 29-28). Touch the patient on the fingertips, forearm, dorsal hands, back and thighs. Note the distance between the applicators.	Identifies two points on: • Fingertips at 2 to 5 mm apart • Forearm at 40 mm apart • Dorsal hands at 20 to 30 mm apart • Back at 40 mm apart • Thighs at 70 mm apart.	Same as above.
To test extinction, simultaneously touch the patient in the same area on both sides of the body at the same point. Ask the patient to identify the area touched.	Correctly identifies points touched.	Same as above.
Reflexes		
Test deep tendon reflexes. Position patient in a comfortable sitting position. Use the reflex hammer to elicit reflexes (see Equipment spotlight 29-1).  **CLINICAL TIP** **If deep tendon reflexes are diminished or absent, two reinforcement techniques may be used to enhance their response:** • When testing the arm reflexes, have the patient clench their teeth. • When testing the leg reflexes, have the patient interlock their hands. 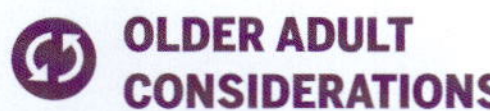 **OLDER ADULT CONSIDERATIONS** **Reinforcement techniques may also help the older patient who has difficulty relaxing.**	**OLDER ADULT CONSIDERATIONS:** **Older adults usually have deep tendon reflexes intact, although a decrease in reaction time may slow the response (Estes et al., 2016).** Normal reflex scores range from 1+ (present but decreased) to 2+ (normal) to 3+ (increased or brisk but not pathological).	**OLDER ADULT CONSIDERATIONS:** **Deep tendon reflexes are often reduced and of note the Achilles tendon reflex may be absent (Maher, 2016).** Markedly hyperactive (hyper-reflexia) deep tendon reflexes (rated 4+) may be seen with lesions of the upper motor neurons and when the higher cortical levels are impaired.  **OLDER ADULT CONSIDERATIONS** **Some older patients may have decreased deep tendon reflexes because of a numeric decrease in nerve axons and increased demyelination of nerve axons. Impulse transmission may also decrease along with a delay in reaction time.**
Test biceps reflex. Ask the patient to partially bend the arm at elbow with palm up. Place your thumb over the biceps tendon and strike your thumb with the reflex hammer (Fig. 29-29). Repeat on the other side. (This evaluates the function of spinal levels C5 and C6.)	Elbow flexes and contraction of the biceps muscle is seen or felt. Ranges from 1+ to 3+.	No response or an exaggerated response is abnormal.

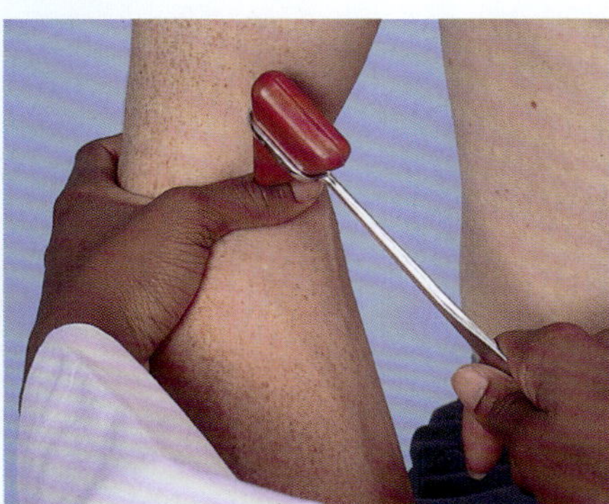
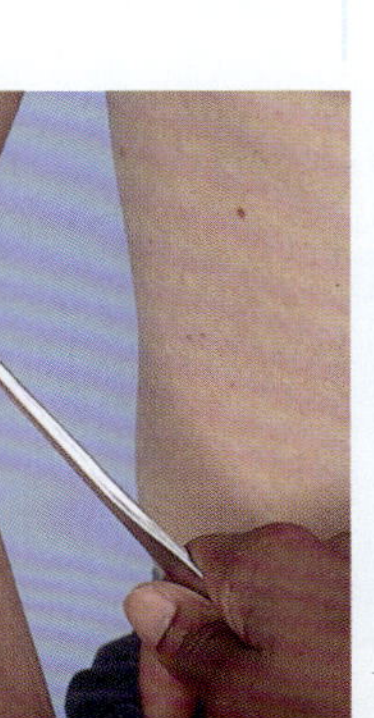

FIGURE 29-29 Eliciting biceps reflex. (© B. Proud.)

Continued on following page

PHYSICAL ASSESSMENT (continued)

ASSESSMENT PROCEDURE	NORMAL FINDINGS	ABNORMAL FINDINGS
Assess brachioradialis reflex. Ask the patient to flex the elbow with the palm down and hand resting on the abdomen or lap. Tap the tendon at the radius about 5 cm above the wrist (Fig. 29-30). Repeat on the other side. (This evaluates the function of spinal levels C5 and C6.)	Forearm flexes and supinates. Ranges from 1+ to 3+.	No response or an exaggerated response is abnormal.
Test triceps reflex. Ask the patient to hang their arm freely ('limp like it is hanging from a clothesline to dry') while you support it with your non-dominant hand. With the elbow flexed, tap the tendon above the olecranon process (Fig. 29-31). Repeat on the other side. (This evaluates the function of spinal levels C6, C7 and C8.)	Elbow extends, triceps contracts. Ranges from 1+ to 3+.	No response or an exaggerated response is abnormal.

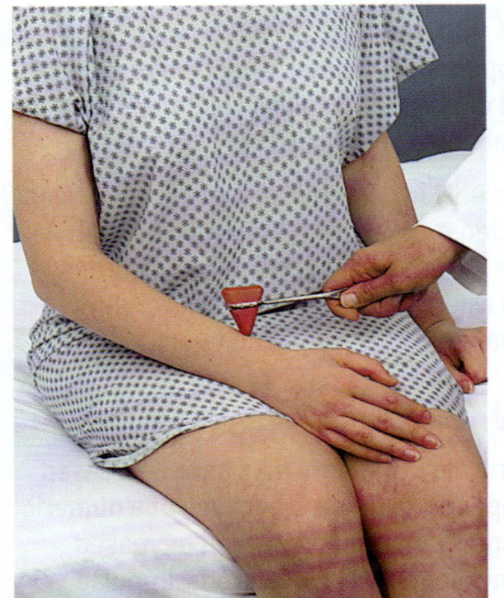

FIGURE 29-30 Eliciting brachioradialis reflex. (© B. Proud.)

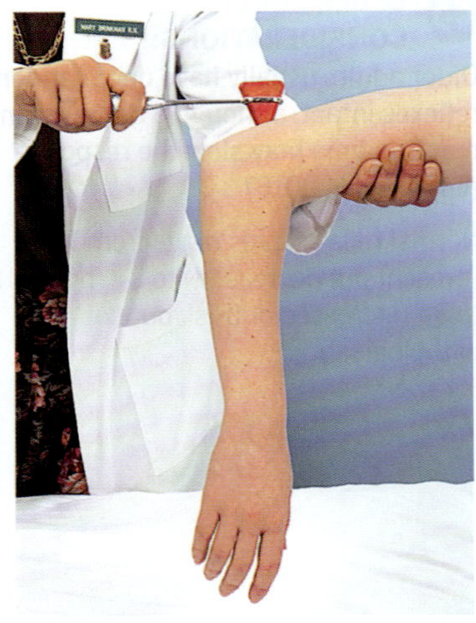

FIGURE 29-31 Eliciting triceps reflex. (© B. Proud.)

ASSESSMENT PROCEDURE	NORMAL FINDINGS	ABNORMAL FINDINGS
Assess patellar reflex. Ask the patient to let both legs hang freely off the side of the examination table. Tap the patellar tendon, which is located just below the patella (Fig. 29-32A). Repeat on the other side. See Figure 29-32B for the patient who cannot sit up. (This evaluates the function of spinal levels L2, L3 and L4.)	Knee extends, quadriceps muscle contracts. Ranges from 1+ to 3+.	No response or an exaggerated response is abnormal.

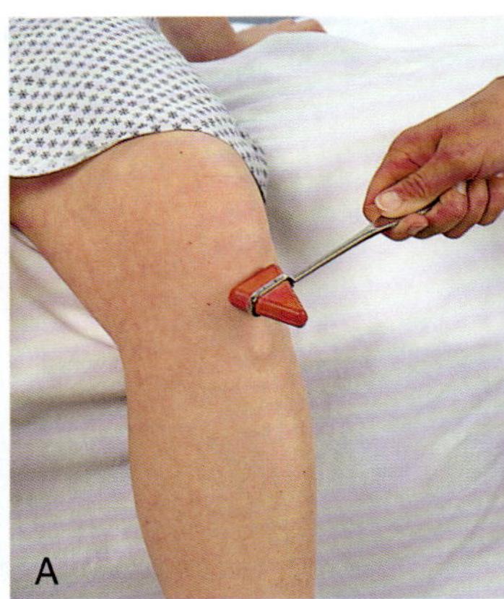

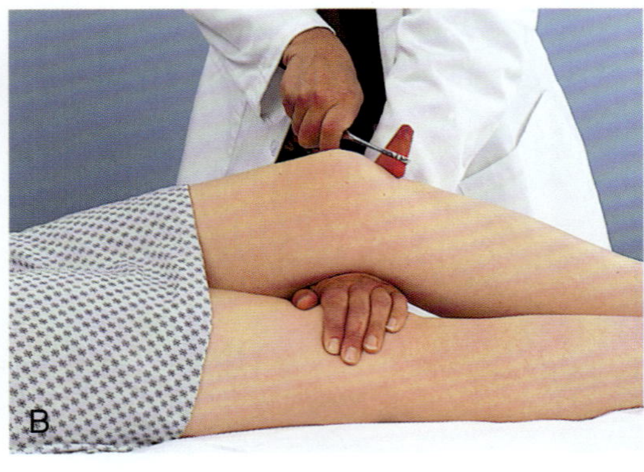

FIGURE 29-32 Eliciting **(A)** patellar reflex and **(B)** patellar reflex (supine position). (© B. Proud.)

PHYSICAL ASSESSMENT (continued)

ASSESSMENT PROCEDURE	NORMAL FINDINGS	ABNORMAL FINDINGS
Reflexes (continued)		
Achilles reflex. With the patient's leg still hanging freely, dorsiflex the foot. Tap the Achilles tendon with the reflex hammer (Fig. 29-33A). Repeat on the other side. See Figure 29-33B for assessing the reflex in the patient who cannot sit up. (This evaluates the function of spinal levels S1 and S2.)	Normal response is plantar flexion of the foot. Ranges from 1+ to 3+. **OLDER ADULT CONSIDERATIONS** **In some older patients, the Achilles reflex may be absent or difficult to elicit.**	No response or an exaggerated response is abnormal.

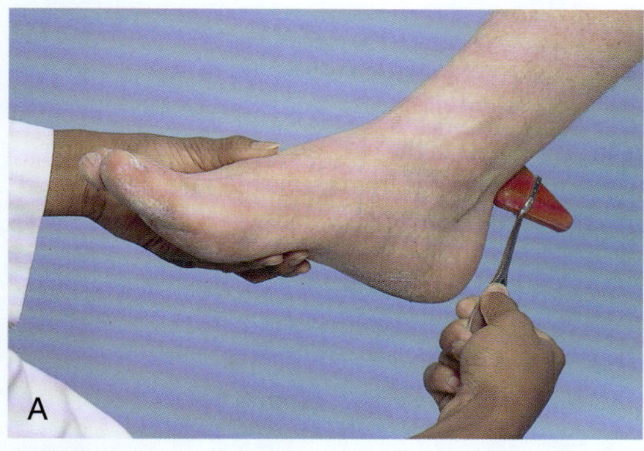

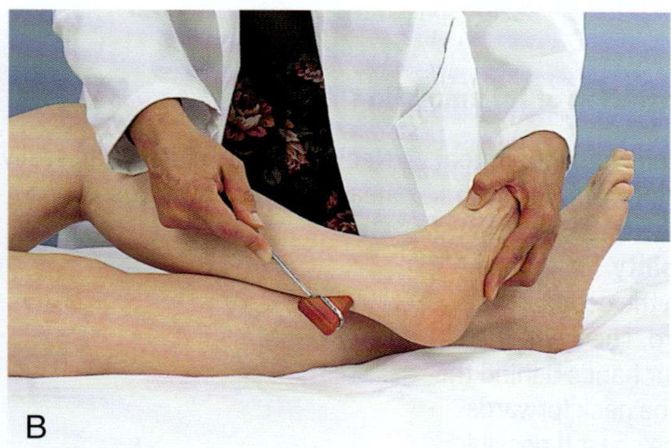

FIGURE 29-33 Eliciting **(A)** Achilles reflex and **(B)** Achilles reflex (supine position). (© B. Proud.)

ASSESSMENT PROCEDURE	NORMAL FINDINGS	ABNORMAL FINDINGS
Test ankle clonus when the other reflexes tested have been hyperactive. Place one hand under the knee to support the leg then briskly dorsiflex the foot towards the patient's head (Fig. 29-34). Repeat on the other side.	No rapid contractions or oscillations (clonus) of the ankle are elicited.	Repeated rapid contractions or oscillations of the ankle and calf muscle are seen with lesions of the upper motor neurons.
TEST SUPERFICIAL REFLEXES. **Assess plantar reflex.** **CLINICAL TIP** **Use the handle end of the reflex hammer to elicit superficial reflexes, whose receptors are in the skin rather than the muscles.** With the end of the reflex hammer, stroke the lateral aspect of the sole from the heel to the ball of the foot, curving medially across the ball (Fig. 29-35A). Repeat on the other side. (This evaluates the function of spinal levels L4, L5, S1 and S2.)	Flexion of the toes occurs (plantar response; Fig. 29-35B). 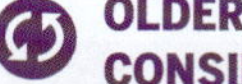 **OLDER ADULT CONSIDERATIONS** **In some older patients, flexion of the toes may be difficult to elicit and may be absent.**	Except in infancy, extension (dorsiflexion) of the big toe and fanning of all toes (positive Babinski response) are seen with lesions of upper motor neurons. Unconscious states resulting from drug and alcohol intoxication, brain injury or subsequent to an epileptic seizure may also cause it.

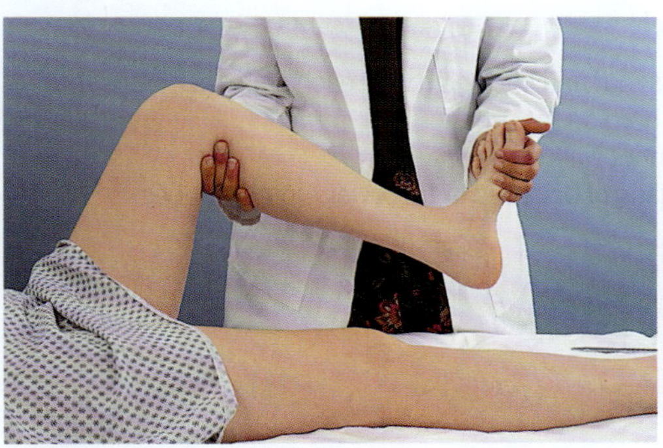

FIGURE 29-34 Testing for ankle clonus. (© B. Proud.)

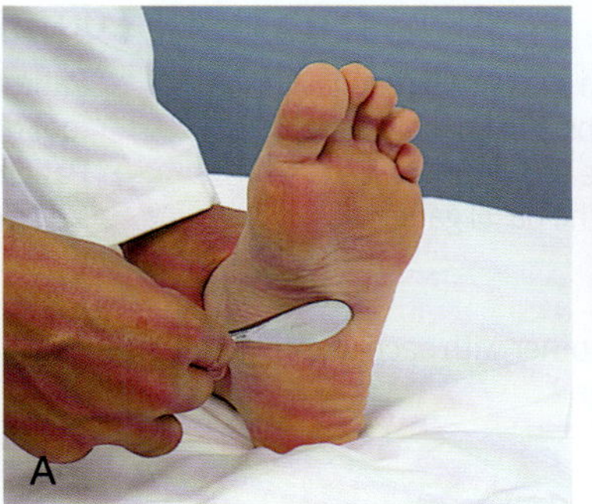

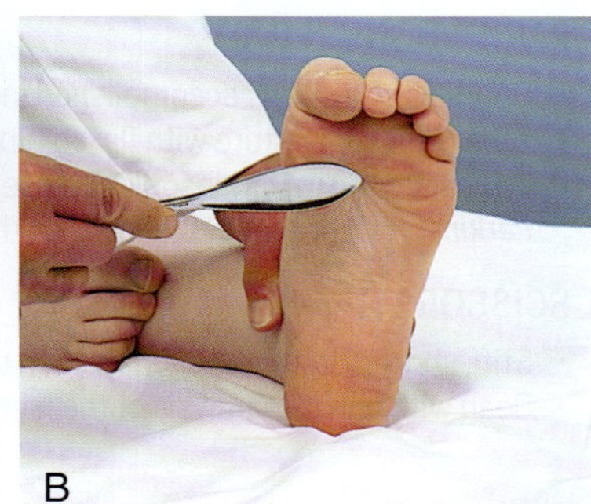

FIGURE 29-35 Eliciting **(A)** plantar reflex and **(B)** normal plantar response. (© B. Proud.)

Continued on following page

PHYSICAL ASSESSMENT (continued)

ASSESSMENT PROCEDURE	NORMAL FINDINGS	ABNORMAL FINDINGS
Test abdominal reflex. Lightly stroke the abdomen on each side, above and below the umbilicus. (This evaluates the function of spinal levels T8, T9 and T10 with the upper abdominal reflex and spinal levels T10, T11, and T12 with the lower abdominal reflex.)	Abdominal muscles contract; umbilicus deviates towards the side being stimulated.	Superficial reflexes may be absent with lower or upper motor neuron lesions. *Caution:* The abdominal reflex may be concealed because of obesity or muscular stretching from pregnancies. This is not an abnormality.
Test cremasteric reflex in male patients. Lightly stroke the inner aspect of the upper thigh. (This evaluates the function of spinal levels T12, L1 and L2.)	Scrotum elevates on stimulated side.	Absence of reflex may indicate motor neuron disorder.
Tests for meningeal irritation or inflammation		
If you suspect the patient has meningeal irritation or inflammation from infection or subarachnoid haemorrhage, assess the patient's neck mobility. First make sure there is no injury to the cervical vertebrae or cervical cord. Then with the patient supine, place your hands behind the patient's head and flex the neck forwards until the chin touches the chest if possible.	Neck is supple; patient can easily bend head and neck forwards.	Pain in the neck and resistance to flexion can arise from meningeal inflammation, arthritis or neck injury.
Test for Brudzinski sign. As you flex the neck, watch the hips and knees in reaction to your manoeuvre.	Hips and knees remain relaxed and motionless.	Pain and flexion of the hips and knees are positive Brudzinski signs and suggest meningeal inflammation.
Test for Kernig sign. Flex the patient's leg at both the hip and the knee, then straighten the knee.	No pain is felt. Discomfort behind the knee during full extension occurs in many normal people.	Pain and increased resistance to extending the knee are a positive Kernig sign. When Kernig sign is bilateral, the examiner suspects meningeal irritation.

ABNORMAL FINDINGS 29-1 Abnormal gaits

Everyone normally walks a little bit differently from everyone else, but sometimes a person's gait is distinctively abnormal, suggesting that the person has a neurological problem. Some common abnormal gaits and their causes follow.

CEREBELLAR ATAXIA

- Wide-based, staggering, unsteady gait
- Romberg test results are positive (patient cannot stand with feet together)
- Seen with cerebellar diseases or alcohol or drug intoxication

PARKINSONIAN GAIT

- Shuffling gait, turns accomplished in a very stiff manner
- Stooped-over posture with flexed hips and knees
- Typically seen in Parkinson's disease and *drug-induced Parkinsonian* because of effects on the basal ganglia

SCISSORS GAIT

- Stiff, short gait; thighs overlap each other with each step
- Seen with partial paralysis of the legs

SPASTIC HEMIPARESIS

- Flexed arm held close to body while patient drags toe of leg or circles it stiffly outwards and forwards
- Seen with lesions of the upper motor neurons in the cortical spinal tract, such as occurs in stroke

FOOTDROP

- Patient lifts foot and knee high with each step, then slaps the foot down hard on the ground
- Patient cannot walk on heels
- Characteristic of diseases of the lower motor neurons

ABNORMAL FINDINGS 29-1 Abnormal gaits (continued)

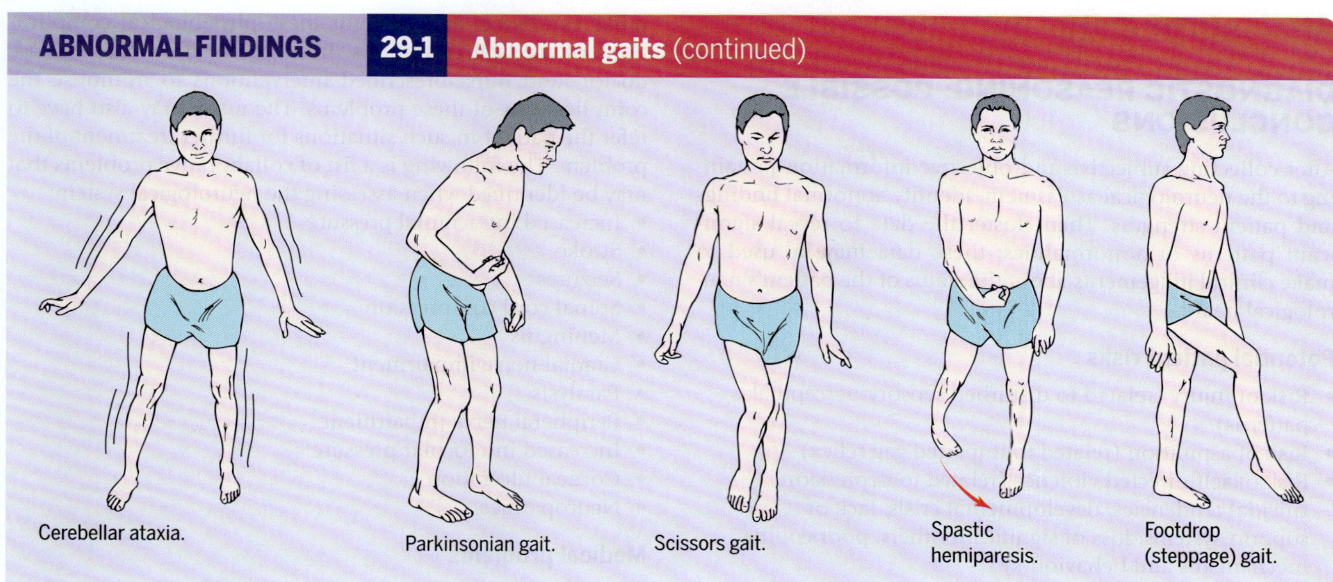

VALIDATING AND DOCUMENTING FINDINGS

Validate the neurological assessment data you have collected. This is necessary to verify that the data are reliable and accurate. Document the data following the health care facility or hospital policy.

After you have collected your assessment data, you will need to analyse the data using diagnostic reasoning skills. Refer to the discussion of the diagnostic reasoning process in Chapter 5.

CLINICAL TIP

When documenting your assessment findings, it is better to describe the patient's response than to label the behaviour.

Sample of subjective data

No history of head injury, spinal cord injury, seizures, meningitis. No dizziness, tinnitus, severe or chronic headache. No difficulty swallowing or communicating. No memory loss.

Sample of objective data

Mental status: Alert, oriented to person, place, day and time. Good eye contact. Positive about daily activities and the future. Short-term and long-term memory intact. Able to follow directions, compare unlike objects and explain simple proverbs.

Cranial nerves:

I: Identifies correct scents.

II: Vision 20/20 [or 6/6] OS, 20/20 [or 6/6] OD [dependent on Snellen chart used], full visual fields intact, red reflex present, optic disc round with well-defined borders. Retinal background pink. No haemorrhages or arteriovenous nicking noted.

III, IV and VI: No ptosis, full extraocular movements, pupils equally round, react to light and accommodation (PERRLA). [Or: Pupils equal and react to light (PEARL).]

V: Temporal and masseter muscles contract bilaterally. Able to identify light, sharp and dull touch to forehead, cheek and chin. Corneal reflex present.

VII: Able to smile, frown, wrinkle forehead, show teeth, puff out cheeks, purse lips, raise eyebrows and close eyes against resistance.

VIII: Whispered words heard bilaterally. Vibration heard equally well in both ears; air conduction greater than bone conduction .

IX and X: Uvula and soft palate rise symmetrically on phonation. Gag reflex present. Swallows without difficulty.

XI: Equal shoulder shrug against resistance; turns head in both directions against resistance.

XII: Protrudes tongue in midline with no tremors. Able to push tongue blade to right and left without difficulty.

Motor and cerebellar systems: No atrophy, tremors or weakness; full range of motion of all extremities. No fasciculations, tics or tremors. Gait and tandem walk normal and steady. Negative Romberg test. Performs repetitive alternating movements, finger-to-nose at smooth, good pace. Runs each heel down each shin with no deviation.

Sensory system: Identifies light touch, dull and sharp sensations to trunk and extremities. Vibratory sensation, stereognosis, graphaesthesia, two-point discrimination intact.

Reflexes: Reflexes 2 bilaterally, except Achilles 1. No ankle clonus noted. Abdominal reflex present. No Babinski sign present.

CRITICAL THINKING

5. The list of possible causes for abnormal findings on a nervous system examination is very extensive. List five of the most common causes of abnormal findings seen in hospital presentations. (Again, consider organic and non-organic causes.)
6. Describe the most common symptoms of each one.
7. How are pupil size, reactions and limb power recorded at your place of work?

Analysis of data

DIAGNOSTIC REASONING: POSSIBLE CONCLUSIONS

After collecting subjective and objective information pertaining to the neurological assessment, identify abnormal findings and patient strengths. Then cluster the data to reveal significant patterns or abnormalities; these data may be used to make clinical judgements about the status of the patient's neurological health.

Potential patient risks

- Risk of injury (related to disturbed sensory-perceptual patterns)
- Risk of aspiration (related to impaired gag reflex)
- Risk of self-directed violence (related to depression, suicidal tendencies, developmental crisis, lack of support systems, loss of significant others, poor coping mechanisms and behaviours)

Potential patient problems

- Disturbed thought processes (related to abuse of alcohol or drugs, psychotic disorder or organic brain dysfunction)
- Impaired verbal communication (related to aphasia, psychological impairment or organic brain disorder)
- Acute or chronic confusion (related to dementia, head injury, stroke, or alcohol or drug abuse)
- Impaired memory (related to dementia, stroke, head injury, or alcohol or drug abuse)
- Sexual dysfunction
- Impaired environmental interpretation syndrome (related to dementia, depression or alcoholism)
- Self-care deficit (bathing, hygiene, toileting or feeding) (related to paralysis, weakness or confusion)
- Reflex urinary incontinence (related to spinal cord or brain damage)
- Unilateral neglect (related to poor vision on one side, trauma or neurological disorder)

Selected collaborative problems

After grouping the data, certain collaborative problems may become apparent. Remember that collaborative problems cannot be prevented by nursing interventions. However, the nurse can detect and monitor these physiological complications of medical conditions. In addition, the nurse can use doctor- and nurse-prescribed interventions to minimise the complications of these problems. The nurse may also have to refer the patient in such situations for further treatment of the problem. The following is a list of collaborative problems that may be identified when assessing the neurological system:

- Increased intracranial pressure
- Stroke
- Seizures
- Spinal cord compression
- Meningitis
- Cranial nerve impairment
- Paralysis
- Peripheral nerve impairment
- Increased intraocular pressure
- Corneal ulceration
- Neuropathies.

Medical problems

After grouping the data, the patient's signs and symptoms may clearly require medical diagnosis and treatment. Referral to a primary care provider is necessary.

ONLINE RESOURCES

An extensive range of additional resources to enhance teaching and learning and to facilitate understanding may be found online at the text's accompanying website, located on thePoint at http://thepoint.lww.com. These include Watch and Learn videos, Concepts in Action animations, journal articles, case studies, discussion topics and quizzes.

Subscribers may also access Lippincott Procedures, an extensive online point-of-care procedure guide that provides reliable step-by-step instructions for more than 1700 procedures, including 450 evidence-based Australian procedures, and skills in a variety of speciality settings, together with a wealth of supporting information.

CASE STUDY

The case study demonstrates how to analyse neurological assessment data for a specific patient. The exercises included in the ancillary product on thePoint that complements this text offer further opportunities to enhance your skills.

Thomas Walker is 65 years old and has just been admitted to the neurosurgical ward. He is lean and athletic in stature and looks much younger than his age. He has an abrasion on the left side of his face, a result of a fall while jogging. Witnesses at the scene stated that he seemed to 'stumble and fall' and that he was unconscious for 2 to 3 minutes. His wife arrived with him and stated that he is normally very fit and well, although over the past 3 to 4 weeks he has been complaining of headaches and intermittent numbness and tingling in his right arm. He has refused to see a doctor, saying he is only experiencing stress from his job as an air traffic controller.

On physical assessment, Mr Walker's observations are as follows: blood pressure of 155/92 mmHg, pulse rate of 48 beats/minute and respiratory rate of 12 breaths/minute, with deep, slow breaths. He has a Glasgow Coma Scale score of 13 and is moving all his limbs, but he is not obeying verbal commands. He localises to painful stimuli and is mumbling incoherently. His left pupil is 2 mm and brisk, and his right pupil is 4 mm and sluggish to light. His eyes are open.

The following concept map illustrates the diagnostic reasoning process.

Applying COLDSPA

Applying COLDSPA for patient symptoms: 'loss of consciousness with corresponding decreased Glasgow Coma Scale, dilated pupil, altered vital signs'.

Mnemonic	Question	Data provided	Missing data
Character	Describe the sign or symptom (feeling, appearance, sound, smell or taste, if applicable.)	Wife reports patient has had some headaches over the last few weeks and intermittent numbness and tingling to right arm	Does anything precipitate the headaches? Have you had a recent head injury?
Onset	When did it begin?	3 to 4 weeks ago	
Location	Where is it? Does it radiate? Does it occur anywhere else?	Head and left arm	Does the pain radiate anywhere else? Does anything precipitate the pain? Do the headache and tingling come on at the same time?
Duration	How long does it last? Does it recur?		How long do the headache and tingling last? How often do they occur?
Severity	How bad is it? Or How much does it bother you?		Does the pain make you miss work, or stop what you are doing?
Pattern	What makes it better or worse?	The stress of work exacerbates the symptoms	Does resting make it better?
Associated factors/How it Affects the patient	What other symptoms occur with it? How does it affect you?	The patient is mumbling incoherently; thus, his wife will be asked to supply information	

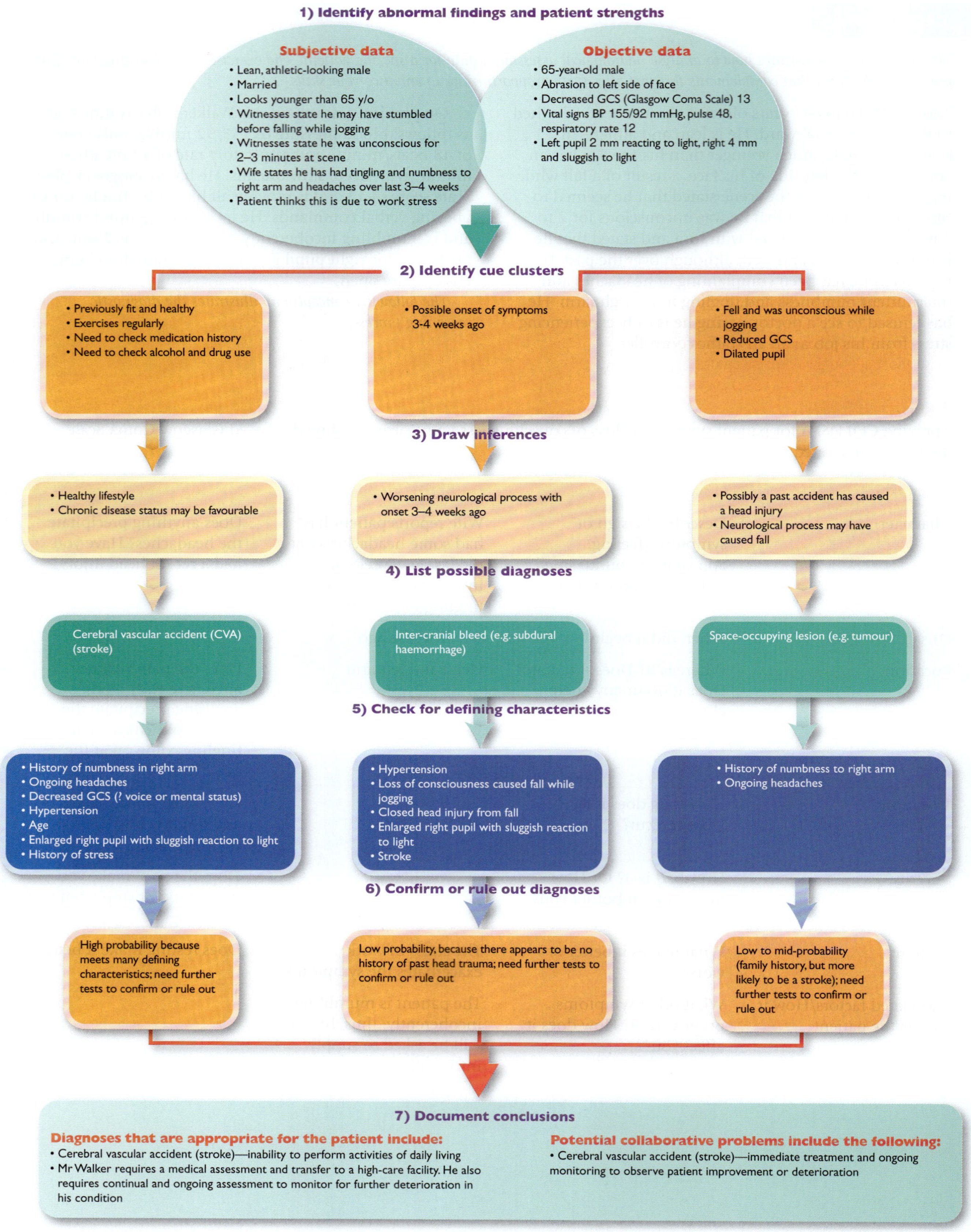

1) Identify abnormal findings and patient strengths

Subjective data
- Lean, athletic-looking male
- Married
- Looks younger than 65 y/o
- Witnesses state he may have stumbled before falling while jogging
- Witnesses state he was unconscious for 2–3 minutes at scene
- Wife states he has had tingling and numbness to right arm and headaches over last 3–4 weeks
- Patient thinks this is due to work stress

Objective data
- 65-year-old male
- Abrasion to left side of face
- Decreased GCS (Glasgow Coma Scale) 13
- Vital signs BP 155/92 mmHg, pulse 48, respiratory rate 12
- Left pupil 2 mm reacting to light, right 4 mm and sluggish to light

2) Identify cue clusters

- Previously fit and healthy
- Exercises regularly
- Need to check medication history
- Need to check alcohol and drug use

- Possible onset of symptoms 3-4 weeks ago

- Fell and was unconscious while jogging
- Reduced GCS
- Dilated pupil

3) Draw inferences

- Healthy lifestyle
- Chronic disease status may be favourable

- Worsening neurological process with onset 3–4 weeks ago

- Possibly a past accident has caused a head injury
- Neurological process may have caused fall

4) List possible diagnoses

Cerebral vascular accident (CVA) (stroke)

Inter-cranial bleed (e.g. subdural haemorrhage)

Space-occupying lesion (e.g. tumour)

5) Check for defining characteristics

- History of numbness in right arm
- Ongoing headaches
- Decreased GCS (? voice or mental status)
- Hypertension
- Age
- Enlarged right pupil with sluggish reaction to light
- History of stress

- Hypertension
- Loss of consciousness caused fall while jogging
- Closed head injury from fall
- Enlarged right pupil with sluggish reaction to light
- Stroke

- History of numbness to right arm
- Ongoing headaches

6) Confirm or rule out diagnoses

High probability because meets many defining characteristics; need further tests to confirm or rule out

Low probability, because there appears to be no history of past head trauma; need further tests to confirm or rule out

Low to mid-probability (family history, but more likely to be a stroke); need further tests to confirm or rule out

7) Document conclusions

Diagnoses that are appropriate for the patient include:
- Cerebral vascular accident (stroke)—inability to perform activities of daily living
- Mr Walker requires a medical assessment and transfer to a high-care facility. He also requires continual and ongoing assessment to monitor for further deterioration in his condition

Potential collaborative problems include the following:
- Cerebral vascular accident (stroke)—immediate treatment and ongoing monitoring to observe patient improvement or deterioration

References

Australian Institute of Health and Welfare (AIHW). (2017). Source data tables: Risk factors to health. Available at https://www.aihw.gov.au/reports-data/health-conditions-disability-deaths/heart-stroke-vascular-diseases/data#page1.

Bray, B. D., Smith, C. J., Cloud, G. C., et al. (2017). The association between delays in screening for and assessing dysphagia after acute stroke, and the risk of stroke-associated pneumonia. *Journal of Neurology, Neurosurgery, and Psychiatry, 88*(1), 25–30.

Estes, M. E., Calleja, P., Theobald, K., et al. (2016). *Health assessment and physical examination* (2nd ed.). South Melbourne: Cengage Learning.

Farrell, M. & Dempsey, J. (2014). *Smeltzer and Bare's textbook of medical surgical nursing*. North Ryde, New South Wales: Lippincott Williams & Wilkins.

Mahawish, K., Barber, P. A., McRae, A., et al. (2018). Why the new 'living' Australian stroke guidelines matter to New Zealand. *The New Zealand Medical Journal, 131*(1487), 7763.

Maher, A. B. (2016). Neurological assessment. *International Journal of Orthopeadic and Trauma Nursing (2016)*, 44–53.

Middleton, S., Grimley, R. & Alexandrov, A. W. (2015). Triage, treatment and transfer: Evidence-based clinical practice recommendations and models of nursing care for the first 72 hours of admission to hospital for acute stroke. *Stroke—A Journal of Cerebral Circulation, 46*(2), e18–e25.

Ministry of Health (2019). Stroke. Available at https://www.health.govt.nz/your-health/conditions-and-treatments/diseases-and-illnesses/stroke.

Nindra, U., Wonson, T. M. & Fuller, K. (2019). Delayed CT imaging leading to delays in acute stroke management in regional Australia. *Journal of Neurology, Neurosurgery, and Psychiatry, 90*(E7).

Queensland Brain Institute. (2019) Stroke facts. Available at https://qbi.uq.edu.au/brain/brain-diseases/stroke/stroke-facts.

Reith, F., Brande, R., Synnot, A., et al. (2016). The reliability of the Glasgow Coma Scale: A systematic review. *Intensive Care Medicine, 42*(1), 3–15.

Stroke Foundation Australia (2019a) Types of strokes. Available online at https://strokefoundation.org.au/About-Stroke/Types-of-stroke.

Stroke Foundation Australia (2019b) Aboriginal and Torres Strait Islander project. Available at https://strokefoundation.org.au/About-Stroke/Facts-and-figures-about-stroke/Aboriginal-and-Torres-Strait-Islander-project.

Stroke Foundation Australia (2019c) National action plan for heart and stroke. Available at https://strokefoundation.org.au/What-we-do/National-Action-Plan-for-Heart-and-Stroke.

Stroke Foundation Australia (2019d) Stroke symptoms, FAST. Available at https://strokefoundation.org.au/About-Stroke/Stroke-symptoms.

Stroke Foundation of New Zealand. (2019a). What is stroke; what you need to know. Available at https://www.stroke.org.nz/what-strokeStroke.

Stroke Foundation of New Zealand. (2019b). Fact sheet—Signs of stroke. Available at https://www.stroke.org.nz/sites/default/files/inline-files/What%20is%20a%20Stroke.pdf.

Wijdicks, E. F. M., Bamlet, W. R., Maramattorn, B. V., et al. (2005). Validation of a new Coma Scale: The FOUR Score. *Annals of Neurology, 58*, 585–593. Viewed January 2014 at www.coma.ulg.ac.be/images/four_e.pdf.

Selected readings

Green, S. M., Haukoos, J. S. & Schringer, D. L. (2017). How to measure the Glasgow Coma Scale. *Annals of Emergency Medicine, 70*(2), 158–160.

Kim, J., Andrew, N. E., Thrift, A. G., et al. (2017). The potential health and economic impact of improving stroke care standards for Australia. *International Journal of Stroke: Official Journal of the International Stroke Society, 12*(8), 875–885.

Samaniego, E. A. & Hasan, D. (2019). *Acute stroke management in the era of thrombectomy*. Cham: Springer.

Tomoyuki, T. (2018). Post-stroke depression: Risk assessment. *Journal of the Neurological Sciences, 387*, 228.

CHAPTER 30

Pulling it all together

Using a head-to-toe assessment framework

Although most nursing health assessment textbooks culminate in a chapter that presents a step-by-step approach to a comprehensive health assessment in an attempt to pull all content together, this is rarely applied in the acute care setting. Given this, it is far more important for you to learn the key elements of a systematic, brief head-to-toe assessment and expand this with specialised or focused assessment skills relevant to the presenting problem of each patient and his or her context of care.

It has been emphasised throughout this text that you must use your judgement in each clinical situation to determine which data are important to collect. Each of the preceding chapters provides an excellent resource for conducting a focused body system assessment based on the patient's presenting problem. However, for practical reasons, these system assessments are usually integrated into a head-to-toe approach when performing a comprehensive patient assessment.

When using a head-to-toe approach, some body systems may be assessed in combination with others. For example, when performing an eye assessment you will also be performing part of the neurological examination for cranial nerves II, III, IV and VI, which affect vision and eye movements. When you assess the legs, you will also be assessing parts of the skin (colour and condition of the skin on the legs), peripheral vascular system (pulses, colour, oedema, lesions of the legs), and neurological and musculoskeletal systems (movement, strength and tone of the legs). There is no one correct way to integrate the entire health history and physical examination. However, it is important to develop a routine in order to avoid omitting an important step and therefore missing significant data from your assessment.

Pulling all these skills together takes time and practice. The more you practise, the faster you will perform the assessment. Do not get discouraged; no one becomes an expert without practice. Develop a routine that is comfortable for you and your patients. Each patient's physical and mental status will determine how much of the total examination you may perform at any one time. For example, if a patient is experiencing severe pain, an extensive assessment may need to wait until the patient is more comfortable. If a patient is confused or suffers any cognitive impairment, you will need to proceed in a manner that does not agitate the patient. You will also need to gather data from the next of kin or accompanying adult; relatives and friends may also be of benefit.

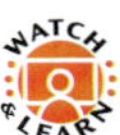

There are numerous videos illustrating the head-to-toe physical assessment. The full list appears at the end of this chapter.

APPROACH TO PHYSICAL ASSESSMENT IN THE ACUTE CARE SETTING

The following is a brief head-to-toe physical assessment guide that may be used to establish a patient's physical status. This type of assessment is frequently used by nurses at the beginning of a hospital shift when nurses have multiple patients for whom they will provide nursing care or when receiving a new admission. Often, a total physical examination is completed by the doctor or nurse practitioner when the patient is admitted to the hospital. Therefore, this shorter format is more practical for ongoing patient assessment.

The Registered Nurse (RN) will frequently use a brief head-to-toe assessment

- to evaluate their patients' health status at the beginning of a shift
- when indicated by a change in a patient's condition
- to gather baseline data as part of an initial nursing assessment or admission
- to evaluate the physiological outcomes of care.

CLINICAL TIP

Expert RNs know that one of the best times to undertake health assessment is during nursing care, as the patient is usually unaware that the assessment is being undertaken and this can often provide more accurate data. Additionally, it takes less time, as the assessment is incorporated into patient care rather than being carried out separately. However, more important, by incorporating assessment into patient care the RN is constantly monitoring patients and thus will be aware of any deterioration or improvement when it occurs. Consider what important nursing assessments can be made in the following situations: giving a patient a shower or sponge bath; assisting a patient to mobilise on the ward; taking a bedpan to a patient; answering a patient's questions about the medications he or she is taking.

There are many variations in the manner in which a head-to-toe assessment may be performed. As an RN who is continually assessing the patients in your care, you need to develop a routine so that you do not forget any important parts. The focus and depth in each instance will change, depending on the context of care (e.g. medical–surgical, critical care, emergency, palliative, community).

Table 30-1 presents an abbreviated assessment guide appropriate for the acute care setting. As one example of working

Table 30-1 Abbreviated head-to-toe physical assessment

Assessment procedure	Normal findings	Abnormal findings
General survey		
Assess level of consciousness (LOC).	Awake, alert and oriented to person, place and time.	If altered LOC, consider the Glasgow Coma Scale.
Assess speech.	Speech clear. Makes and maintains conversation appropriately.	
Assess comfort level.	Denies complaints of pain or discomfort.	If the patient reports or complains of pain: rate the pain using the 0 to 10 pain scale, intervene to provide comfort measures and evaluate the effectiveness of such interventions.
Assess skin colour, temperature, moisture, turgor, pressure areas.	Skin intact, pink, warm and dry.	Pressure area Pale, pallor → anaemia Erythema → infection Warmth → infection Increased tenting → dehydration
Eyes		
Assess pupils.	Pupils equal, round, react to light and accommodation.	Pupils unequal or non-reactive to light.
Chest		
Assess breath sounds.	Lungs: clear to auscultation anterior and posterior, bilaterally. Respiratory rate = 18 per minute, no reports of dyspnoea.	Note any wheezes or crackles and identify their location (anterior or posterior, upper or lower lobes, right or left).
Assess heart sounds. Note if rhythm is irregular.	Heart: S_1 and S_2 present, regular rate (82) and rhythm. No S_3 or S_4 appreciated. No murmur, rub or gallop.	If heart sounds are irregular, note whether they are regularly irregular or irregularly irregular. Note any murmurs, rub or gallop.
Abdomen		
Assess contour and firmness.	Non-distended, soft and non-tender.	Distended and firm, visible palpations.
Assess bowel sounds.	Active bowel sounds noted in all four quadrants (+ABS × 4Q).	Absence of bowel sounds in one or more quadrants. One must listen for 5 minutes to document absent bowel sounds. Normal bowel sounds = 5 to 35 per minute.
Extremities		
Assess mobility of extremities, strength of extremities, and peripheral pulses.	Able to actively move all extremities. Equal strength, 5/5. Radial, dorsalis pedis and posterior tibia pulses 2+. No peripheral oedema.	Unable to actively or passively move one or more extremities.
Other		
Note any wounds or lesions.	Describe: size, shape, location, colour, characteristics of any drainage, type of dressing.	
Note any drains: Foley catheter, Hemovac, nasogastric tube.	Describe insertion site; colour, consistency and odour of any drainage.	
Note any venous access devices.	Describe the location, appearance, type and size of device, type of intravenous fluids and rate of infusion, and infusion devices.	
Note any other therapies: external ice and heat devices, continuous passive motion devices, transcutaneous electrical nerve stimulation unit, etc.	Describe the presence of correct functioning of any of these devices.	

from head to toe, comparing side to side, it is a guide for students to use as they develop their own confidence and competence with the head-to-toe assessment. As you systematically proceed through body regions:

- Inspect any wounds and dressings for signs of bleeding, drainage, infection or dehiscence.
- Inspect the placement, patency, securing and consistency of drainage for any drains or catheters, such as postoperative drains, indwelling catheters or nasogastric tubes.
- Inspect and palpate IV insertion sites for signs of infiltration, phlebitis or infection. Ensure the device is secure. (Also be aware of the date on which these devices were inserted, as many hospitals have a policy to remove them after 48 hours.)
- Assess the patient's fluid balance, noting intake and output and whether the patient is in an overall positive or negative balance (over the past 24 hours, as well as over the past 4 or 5 days).
- Collect and document data from any specific monitoring device (e.g. bedside electrocardiogram monitoring).
- Remove and inspect skin under anti-thromboembolic stockings.

CLINICAL TIP

Remember that you should continually assess each patient at each contact or during nursing care, so the initial brief head-to-toe or shift assessment becomes more comprehensive with each interaction.

Pulling it all together: Case study challenge

Apply your health assessment skills to the following nursing case studies and critical thinking questions. Refer back to the relevant chapters of this text as you work through each case study.

CASE STUDY 1

Charlotte Davies is a 3-year-old girl being admitted to your paediatric medical ward with atopic dermatitis. She has an itchy, red rash covering most of her body. It appears to be worst in her flexures, but also around her eyes, cheeks and neck, and on her feet. She was brought in by her mother, who reports that Charlotte's skin is usually very dry, with itchy red patches, but has become much worse over the past 2 days. She describes Charlotte as scratching her skin 'constantly', day and night, often until it bleeds.

You assess Charlotte, who is sitting on her mother's lap. Her unaffected skin is pale, and she cries irritably as you approach. When you observe the rash, you note marked erythema, with widespread excoriations and weeping, and lichenification in her flexures. You also note patches of thick, yellow crusting in places. Her vital signs are temperature 38.9 °C, heart rate 152, respiratory rate 28 per minute, blood pressure 90/60 mmHg and SpO_2 99% on room air.

Charlotte's mother hands you a bag full of creams and ointments. She appears tired and frustrated, and tells you she has tried all of them to improve Charlotte's skin but nothing is helping. She has trouble finding time to apply the creams regularly, since she works full-time and has to get Charlotte and her 2-year-old brother Oliver to day care by 8 a.m. each day. When she does try to put the creams on, Charlotte is uncooperative, screaming and running around the house. She is separated from Charlotte's father, and receives little support from family and friends.

Charlotte appears small for her age, with height 88 cm and weight 11.52 kg. Her mother thinks Charlotte is allergic to dairy, eggs and wheat, and has put Charlotte on an 'allergy diet' she found on the Internet, which excludes a wide range of foods. She has never had formal allergy testing.

Charlotte has blood cultures collected and skin swabs taken from the most severely affected areas. You administer IV antibiotics as prescribed and organise oral analgesia and cool compresses for pain relief. You prepare Charlotte for an emollient bath and arrange the prescribed corticosteroid ointments, emollients and dressings that you will need to apply after the bath. Charlotte's mother appears stressed and anxious, saying that she gets confused about which creams to apply where, and she forgets what they are all for. She is also worried about bathing Charlotte, who does not cope well and often kicks and screams at bath time.

CRITICAL THINKING

Refer to Case Study 1.

1. Apply a nursing assessment framework to organise the data into relevant categories. Justify why you chose this framework.
2. Identify the significant or abnormal assessment data. Explain how and why these data are abnormal given the patient's presenting problem.
3. Construct a concept map that demonstrates all the significant assessment data and the relationships or links among these data.
4. What additional data would you want to validate?
5. Outline the key psychosocial aspects of the case that might require intervention or referral by the RN.

CASE STUDY 2

Accompanied by his mother, Mandu Hovane, age 16, arrived at your emergency department complaining of difficulty breathing, coughing and wheezing, which started about 2 hours ago. He appears anxious and short of breath and can talk only in phrases. You help him to a bed and attach him to pulse oximetry. His vital signs are temperature 37 °C, heart rate

120, respiratory rate 28 per minute, blood pressure 140/74 mmHg and SpO_2 90% on room air.

Mandu says his symptoms began shortly after he went to a friend's house. His mother tells you that Mandu's friend recently acquired a cat and that Mandu has a history of asthma and environmental allergies (including pets) since age 4. He has no known drug allergies or other past medical history. Mandu's mother says her son takes a daily antihistamine, loratadine (Claratyne), and has a salbutamol (Ventolin) inhaler that he uses once every few months. He has misplaced his Ventolin inhaler, so he did not use it today.

Mandu tells you he has not been taught how to use a peak flow meter. He denies a history of smoking, alcohol or drug use and says he has no fever or pain. His cough is non-productive. He is alert and oriented. His respirations are regular but rapid and laboured, and he is using accessory muscles of respiration. He also has 'tracheal tug' and intercostal recession. He does not appear cyanotic. When you auscultate his lungs, you hear an expiratory wheeze throughout all lung fields.

You show Mandu how to use a peak flow meter to measure the peak expiratory flow rate (PEFR), which helps determine the severity of airway obstruction. His PEFR value is 60% of the predicted value for his age, height and sex. You notify the emergency department doctor and administer supplemental oxygen to relieve hypoxaemia, aiming to maintain SpO_2 at >94%. You quickly begin administration of the prescribed inhaled short-acting beta-2 agonist (Ventolin) via a nebuliser to relieve airflow obstruction. You monitor Mandu's vital signs, lung sounds, pulse oximetry and PEFR to determine his response to treatment. You also administer the prescribed oral corticosteroid to help decrease airway inflammation.

CRITICAL THINKING

Refer to Case Study 2.

1. Apply a nursing assessment framework to organise the data into relevant categories. Justify why you chose this framework.
2. Identify the significant or abnormal assessment data. Explain how and why these data are abnormal given the patient's presenting problem.
3. Construct a concept map that demonstrates all the significant assessment data and the relationships or links among these data.
4. What additional data would you want to validate?
5. What data would indicate that the nursing interventions have been effective? That is, what evaluation criteria would be appropriate for this patient?
6. An expiratory wheeze was identified on auscultation. What is a wheeze and how does it differ from crackles or rhonchi?
7. Briefly discuss what patient teaching topics are indicated by the assessment data.

CASE STUDY 3

You are caring for Piripi Sullivan, a 65-year-old man who has been admitted to your unit for investigation of chest pain that has occurred several times over the past few weeks. Mr Sullivan describes his chest pain as 'a heavy pressure, like someone sitting on my chest'. He states that it first occurred while he was mowing the grass. He later felt the same heavy sensation while raking leaves. The pain was located in the substernal area and resolved after about 5 minutes of rest. While carrying some boxes today, however, he experienced chest pain that was more severe and was not relieved by resting. He says he attributed the chest pain to indigestion after eating, and has tried Mylanta (an antacid) with no relief.

Mr Sullivan has a past history of hypertension controlled with medication that was diagnosed 7 years ago. His family history is significant for coronary artery disease (his father had a myocardial infarction at age 50). He smokes half to one pack of cigarettes per day and has 1 or 2 glasses of red wine per night.

His wife looks pale and anxious. She complains, 'I don't know what to do with him. I work so hard to keep him healthy, but he goes out eating fast food. I'm so tired of dealing with him when he won't help himself.' Mr Sullivan grins and says, 'I just got to have my junk food! That low-fat, low-salt diet my doctor put me on is impossible.'

Mr Sullivan appears to be in no acute distress. He is alert and cooperative. His vital signs are temperature 37.4°C, heart rate 94, respiratory rate 22 per minute, blood pressure 154/90, SpO_2 99% on 3L/min O_2 via nasal prongs. His skin is pink, warm and dry, with capillary refill <2 seconds in all extremities. He has a patent intravenous cannula in his left hand. His neck veins are flat at 45degrees and no carotid bruits are noted. His apical pulse rate is also 94 and regular; heart sounds: S_1 and S_2, without murmur or added sounds. His lungs are clear to auscultation. His abdomen is centrally obese, without tenderness or masses. Bowel sounds are active in all quadrants. Full and equal strength is noted in all extremities. Pedal pulses are strong. He has no ankle oedema.

Mr Sullivan has serial electrocardiograms and bloods are taken for full blood count, urea and electrolytes, cardiac markers, serum lipids and coagulation profile.

CRITICAL THINKING

Refer to Case Study 3.

1. Apply a nursing assessment framework to organise the data into relevant categories. Justify why you chose this framework.
2. Identify the significant or abnormal assessment data. Explain how and why these data are abnormal given the patient's presenting problem.
3. Construct a concept map that demonstrates all the significant assessment data and the relationships or links among these data.

4. What other assessment data not given in the case study would you want to collect or validate? How would you assess these data—that is, what questions would you ask or what physical assessment techniques would you use?
5. The case documents 'Heart sounds: S_1 and S_2, without murmur or added sounds.' What is a cardiac murmur? What extra heart sounds does the RN listen for and what do these sounds represent?

CASE STUDY 4

Chien Tran is an alert and oriented 81-year-old who has been admitted to the hospital after a fall with complaints of dizziness and syncope. His blood pressure on admission is 110/70 mmHg. At the aged-care nursing facility where he lives, he had been ambulating with a walker independently; however, since a recent episode of syncope, he has complained of weakness and needs another person to assist him while walking as a precaution against falls.

Nursing staff at the facility found Mr Tran lying on the floor on his right hip. He explains, 'I had to go to the bathroom. I know I should have called for help, but the nurses are so busy. I figured I could go myself. Only two more steps and I could have reached my walker. I just slipped, that's all.' He reports pain in his right hip that is a 7 on a 0 to 10 numerical pain rating scale (with 10 being the worst). He describes the pain as a 'dull ache' that is worse with movement of his right leg.

An X-ray of his right hip is negative for a fracture. You complete a set of orthostatic vital signs: lying blood pressure 120/84 mmHg, heart rate 73 per minute; sitting blood pressure 114/70 mmHg, heart rate 83; standing blood pressure 96/60 mmHg and heart rate 92 per minute. His other vital signs are temperature 36.8 °C, respiratory rate 16 per minute and SpO_2 99% on room air. You note no injuries on inspection and palpation of his head and neck. His pupils are equal, round and react briskly to light. His chest is clear to auscultation, and his heart sounds are irregularly irregular. He has full range of motion in the upper extremities and his handgrip strength is bilaterally equal. His abdomen is soft and non-tender. There is no physical deformity of the right hip and no other injuries are apparent, but a moderate amount of ecchymosis is visible over his right hip that extends around to his lower back and right upper buttock. He demonstrates normal movement and sensation in both feet. He has requested the urinal once for 200 mL of clear yellow urine. An electrocardiogram confirms his known history of atrial fibrillation.

Mr Tran's plan of care includes assessment of his orthostatic vital signs every shift and fall precautions. You explain to Mr Tran how to use the call light, and he remains on bed rest with the side rails up. He confides to you that he is worried about the consequences of this fall for his mobility and independence.

CRITICAL THINKING

Refer to Case Study 4.

1. Apply a nursing assessment framework to organise the data into relevant categories. Justify why you chose this framework.
2. Identify the significant or abnormal assessment data. Explain how and why these data are abnormal given the patient's presenting problem.
3. Construct a concept map that demonstrates all the significant assessment data and the relationships or links among these data.
4. What other assessment data not given in the case study would you want to collect or validate? How would you assess these data—that is, what questions would you ask or what physical assessment techniques would you use?
5. Discuss some of the falls risk assessment tools commonly used in clinical practice. Identify the predisposing risk factors relevant to Mr Tran using one of these tools.

CASE STUDY 5

Rachael Oosterman, a 22-year-old nursing student, was recently treated for acute tonsillitis caused by infection by group A streptococcus. She presents to the emergency department 10 days later appearing acutely ill. She states that her throat is so sore ('like swallowing razor blades') that she even has difficulty swallowing liquids.

Rachael explains that she thought she was getting better after taking about half of her prescribed antibiotics, so she discontinued the medication. However, over the last 2 days she has had a worsening fever with chills, swollen glands and general fatigue. She admits that she has been studying 'day and night' for end-of-semester exams and has 'only one more exam to go'. 'This is the third time I've had this problem this year', she says. 'I didn't even bother coming in the first two times. I just stayed in bed between classes and treated myself.'

Upon examination, you note her face and neck are flushed, with dark circles underlying her eyes. Her vital signs are temperature 39.2 °C tympanic, heart rate 104 per minute, respiratory rate 22 per minute, blood pressure 100/60 mmHg and SpO_2 99% on room air. Her skin is warm with sluggish skin turgor. You also note she has dry oral mucous membranes. She has an acutely swollen and reddened area of the soft palate in her mouth, half occluding the orifice from the mouth into the pharynx. Yellow exudate is present on the tonsillar areas. She has enlarged and very tender cervical lymph nodes, particularly on the right. The chest and abdominal examinations are unremarkable. She reports decreased urine output and that 'it's a lot darker in colour than normal'.

Rachel is worried about missing her final examination for nursing health assessment, as it is her favourite subject. She has been unable to study since this last episode of illness began. She lives in shared on-campus accommodation with two other students, who suggest she 'drinks some straight whiskey to kill the bugs in her throat'.

A full blood count reveals a WBC of 17.0×10^9/L. A diagnosis of peritonsillar abscess is made and a needle aspiration of the abscess is performed.

CRITICAL THINKING

Refer to Case Study 5.

1. Apply a nursing assessment framework to organise the data into relevant categories. Justify why you chose this framework.
2. Identify the significant or abnormal assessment data. Explain how and why these data are abnormal given the patient's presenting problem.
3. Construct a concept map that demonstrates all the significant assessment data and the relationships or links among these data.
4. What other assessment data not given in the case study would you want to collect or validate? How would you assess these data—that is, what questions would you ask or what physical assessment techniques would you use?
5. Consider the nursing history data and identify some of the key topics for health education that could be provided by the RN.

CASE STUDY 6

Aziza Sohal is a 28-year-old social worker and part-time master's student. On returning home from class one evening, she developed a fever with chills. She alternated between chills and sweats all night. Staying home from work, she remained in bed most of the next day. Her fever continued, and she developed a cough and dull aching chest pain. When her cough became productive of rust-coloured sputum the following day, she sought treatment.

Aziza denies any previous history of respiratory diseases 'other than the usual colds, flu, and such'. She also denies any history of smoking. She says her symptoms began abruptly with the onset of the chills. She describes her chest pain as a 'dull ache' that was initially substernal but now is localised in her lower lateral right chest. The pain increases with deep breathing, coughing and moving. Her cough is increasing in frequency and severity, and her sputum appears rusty brown.

Aziza reports anorexia and nausea associated with coughing, and decreased urine output, which she attributes to drinking less fluid since her illness began. She usually has excellent exercise tolerance but has been too weak and fatigued to do anything but rest in bed.

Her vital signs are temperature 38.7 °C, blood pressure 116/74 mmHg, heart rate 104 per minute and regular, respiratory rate 26 per minute and SpO_2 92% on room air. Her skin is warm and flushed, with no evidence of cyanosis. Capillary refill is <3 seconds. Her respirations are shallow and unlaboured; and chest expansion L > R. Auscultation reveals diminished lung sounds in bases bilaterally, with coarse crackles noted in the right lower lobe not cleared by coughing. You discuss your assessment findings with the doctor and she orders a full blood count with WBC differential, sputum culture and chest X-ray.

CRITICAL THINKING

Refer to Case Study 6.

1. Apply a nursing assessment framework to organise the data into relevant categories. Justify why you chose this framework.
2. Identify the significant or abnormal assessment data. Explain how and why these data are abnormal given the patient's presenting problem.
3. Construct a concept map that demonstrates all the significant assessment data and the relationships or links among these data.
4. What other assessment data not given in the case study would you want to collect or validate? How would you assess these data—that is, what questions would you ask or what physical assessment techniques would you use?
5. Discuss what findings would be likely on the WBC, sputum culture and chest X-ray given a medical diagnosis of acute bacterial pneumonia.

CASE STUDY 7

Frank Logan is a 64-year-old retired truck driver who is admitted to your cardiac unit with a medical diagnosis of congestive heart failure. Six months ago he had a large anterior wall myocardial infarction and subsequently underwent a coronary artery bypass graft. This evening he presents with acute shortness of breath. He tells you, 'I woke up suddenly from my sleep feeling like I was suffocating. I just can't catch my breath.'

He states that up to a week ago he could walk up to one block before feeling slightly short of breath; now he becomes short of breath after walking a few metres. He sleeps with three pillows in order to get to sleep without breathlessness. Moreover, his sleep is disturbed because he awakens several times a night to urinate.

Mr Logan is accompanied by his wife and daughter. They mention that he has started smoking again and eating fatty takeaway foods, despite his promise to give these up after his heart surgery.

His current medications include aspirin (Cartia), metoprolol (Betaloc), lisinopril (Zestril) and atorvastatin (Lipitor), and Mr Logan assures you that he takes them regularly. He has no known drug allergies.

He is sitting upright and appears very anxious and restless. His respiratory rate is 30 per minute and laboured with accessory muscle use. His SpO_2 is 89% on room air.

He has pale, cool and clammy skin. Capillary refill is 3 seconds. His other vital signs are temperature 36.5 °C, blood pressure 100/72 mmHg sitting and apical pulse rate 110 per minute and regular. His neck veins are visibly distended at 45 degrees. You hear an S_3 heart sound with the bell of the stethoscope over the apex, and note bibasilar crackles to the mid-zones posteriorly. You also palpate pitting oedema over the sacrum. His abdomen is rounded, soft and non-tender. You see in the medical admission progress notes that his liver span was 10 cm at the midclavicular line by percussion. The lower extremities have pitting oedema to the mid-tibia. The bedside electrocardiogram shows sinus tachycardia.

CRITICAL THINKING

Refer to Case Study 7.

1. Apply a nursing assessment framework to organise the data into relevant categories. Justify why you chose this framework.
2. Identify the significant or abnormal assessment data. Explain how and why these data are abnormal given the patient's presenting problem.
3. Construct a concept map that demonstrates all the significant assessment data and the relationships or links among these data.
4. What other assessment data not given in the case study would you want to collect or validate? How would you assess these data—that is, what questions would you ask or what physical assessment techniques would you use?
5. Mr Logan is placed on fluid restriction, needs to be weighed daily and have all intake and output (I&O) strictly recorded on a fluid balance chart. Discuss how and why this patient should be weighed daily. Also discuss and demonstrate how to record accurately the patient's I&O on a fluid balance chart.

Selected reading

Douglas, C., Windsor, C. & Lewis, P. A. (2015). Too much knowledge for a nurse? Use of physical assessment by final-semester nursing students. *Nursing and Health Sciences, 17*(4), 492–499.

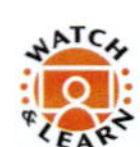

Beginning the physical assessment
Assessing the head
Assessing the eyes
Assessing the ears
Assessing the nose and sinuses
Assessing the mouth and throat
Assessing the neck
Assessing the arms, hands and fingers
Assessing the posterior and lateral thorax
Assessing the anterior thorax
Assessing the heart
Assessing the abdomen
Assessing the legs, feet and toes
Assessing the musculoskeletal and neurological systems
Physical assessment: Conclusion
Thorax and lungs: Introduction
Thorax and lungs: Health history taking
Thorax and lungs: Anatomy review: Thorax
Thorax and lungs: Anatomy review: Lungs
Thorax and lungs: Surveying the chest and respiration
Thorax and lungs: Examining the posterior thorax and lungs
Thorax and lungs: Normal and adventitious breath sounds
Thorax and lungs: Auscultation of the posterior thorax
Thorax and lungs: Examining the anterior thorax and lungs
Thorax and lungs: Auscultation of the anterior chest
Thorax and lungs: Summary
Cardiovascular neck vessels and heart: Introduction
Cardiovascular neck vessels and heart: Health history taking
Cardiovascular neck vessels and heart: Anatomy review: Vascular structures of the neck
Cardiovascular neck vessels and heart: Estimating jugular venous pressure (JVP)
Cardiovascular neck vessels and heart: Assessing the carotid pulse
Cardiovascular neck vessels and heart: Anatomy review: Heart
Cardiovascular neck vessels and heart: Inspection and palpation of the heart
Cardiovascular neck vessels and heart: Auscultation of heart sounds
Cardiovascular neck vessels and heart: Heart sounds
Cardiovascular neck vessels and heart: Attributes and grading of murmurs
Cardiovascular neck vessels and heart: Auscultation of murmurs
Cardiovascular neck vessels and heart: Summary
Performing a physical examination: Introduction
Performing a physical examination: The head
Performing a physical examination: The eyes
Performing a physical examination: The ears
Performing a physical examination: The nose and sinuses
Performing a physical examination: The mouth and throat
Performing a physical examination: The neck
Performing a physical examination: The arms, hands and fingers
Performing a physical examination: The posterior and lateral thorax
Performing a physical examination: The anterior thorax
Performing a physical examination: The heart
Performing a physical examination: The abdomen
Performing a physical examination: The legs, feet and toes
Performing a physical examination: The musculoskeletal and neurological systems
Performing a physical examination: Conclusion

UNIT 4 NURSING ASSESSMENT OF SPECIAL GROUPS

CHAPTER 31

Assessing childbearing women

CASE STUDY

Sarah Lees is a 25-year-old woman and is married to Sam. She is currently pregnant for the first time and has presented to the emergency department because she was involved in a minor motor vehicle accident.

MODELS OF MATERNITY CARE

It is important to understand that pregnancy is a physiological process and normal life event. The primary maternity care provider should seek to establish a two-way partnership with the woman, where each party shares their expertise in order to individualise and optimise the care provided to the woman and her family throughout pregnancy, childbirth and the postnatal period (Pairman et al., 2019; Sandall et al., 2013; Tracy et al., 2013). In Australia and New Zealand, maternity care is provided through different models of care, as described below.

Australian models

The Australian models of maternity care are:

- *Midwifery-led model,* in which maternity care is provided by midwives through a team midwifery model or a case load model. The midwife is the primary care provider throughout the antenatal, intrapartum and postnatal period.
- *Eligible midwife model,* in which a midwife is endorsed with access to the Medicare Benefits Schedule and Pharmaceutical Benefits Scheme and is self-employed to provide private midwifery care covering antenatal services, birth in a hospital or birth centre, and postnatal services up to 6 weeks.
- *Obstetric model,* in which an obstetrician is the primary care provider. This care may be provided through the public or private health care system.
- *Public hospital model,* in which care is provided in a public hospital. Women will receive care from a range of different midwives or medical staff throughout pregnancy, birth and the early postnatal period.
- *Shared care model,* in which general practitioners (GPs) provide the majority of antenatal and postnatal care for women but work in collaboration with midwives and medical staff who provide care at designated intervals throughout the pregnancy, during labour and birth and, sometimes, the early postnatal period (Department of Health, 2019; South Australian Department of Health, 2017; Willis & Reynolds, 2016).

New Zealand models

The New Zealand models of maternity care are:

- *Self-employed midwife model,* in which care is provided by a midwife as the lead maternity carer (LMC) for antenatal, intrapartum and postpartum care.
- *Employed midwife model,* in which care is provided by the midwife as the LMC, or as a small midwifery team, through the maternity hospital.
- *Shared care model,* where care is provided by the GP as the LMC, but care is often shared with a self-employed midwife or hospital midwife.
- *Obstetric model,* in which care is provided by private obstetrician or hospital specialist as the LMC.

There are times, however, when the care of a pregnant woman may require collaboration between a range of health professionals. It is therefore important for the nurse who may be involved in such complex episodes of care to understand the physiological adaptations in pregnancy.

This chapter focuses on providing that understanding in order to equip the nurse to provide appropriate care. In doing so, it is important for the nurse to remember that while they are working with a pregnant woman and her unborn baby, neither the mother nor her baby exists independently of the woman's psychosocial needs and expectations and these should also be considered in the assessment and provision of care (Department of Health, 2019). If the episode of care has not come through a referral from the woman's primary maternity care provider, such as presentation to an emergency department, the primary maternity provider should always be notified.

PHYSIOLOGICAL CHANGES DURING PREGNANCY

The body experiences physiological and anatomical changes during pregnancy. Most of these changes are influenced by the hormones of pregnancy, primarily *oestrogen* and *progesterone*. Normal physiological and anatomical changes during pregnancy are discussed in this chapter.

SKIN, HAIR AND NAILS

During pregnancy, integumentary system changes occur primarily because of hormonal influences. Many of these skin, hair and nail changes fade or completely resolve after the end of the gestational period. As the pregnancy progresses, the breasts and abdomen enlarge and *striae gravidarum*, or stretch marks—pinkish-red streaks with slight depressions in the skin—may begin to appear over the abdomen, breasts, thighs and buttocks. These marks usually fade to a white or silvery colour, but they typically never completely resolve after the pregnancy.

Hyperpigmentation also results from hormonal influences (e.g. oestrogen, progesterone and melanocyte-stimulating hormone). It is most noted on the abdomen (linea nigra, a dark line extending from the umbilicus to the mons pubis) and face (chloasma, a darkening of the skin on the face, known as the facial 'mask of pregnancy'; some women who take oral contraceptives may also have chloasma because of the hormones in the medication).

Other skin changes during pregnancy include darkening of the areolae and nipples, axillae, umbilicus and perineum. Scars and moles may also darken from the influence of melanocyte-stimulating hormone. Vascular changes, such as spider naevi (tiny red angiomas occurring on the face, neck, chest, arms and legs), may occur because of elevated oestrogen levels. Palmar erythema (a pinkish colour on the palms of the hands) may also be noted. Pruritic urticarial papules and plaques of pregnancy is a skin disorder sometimes seen during the third trimester of pregnancy, characterised by erythematous papules, plaques and urticarial lesions. The rash begins on the abdomen and may soon spread to the thighs, buttocks and arms. The intense itching and rash usually resolve within weeks of birth.

Acne vulgaris is an unpredictable response during pregnancy. Acne may worsen or improve. It consists of erythema, pustules, comedones or cysts that appear on the face, back, neck or chest. The activity of the eccrine sweat glands and the excretion rate of sebum onto the skin increase in normal pregnancy, whereas the activity of the apocrine sweat glands appears to decrease. The changes that occur in the endocrine system help to maintain optimal maternal and fetal health. Oestrogen is primarily responsible for the changes that occur to the pituitary, thyroid, parathyroid and adrenal glands. The increased production of the hormones, especially triiodothyronine (T3) and thyroxine (T4), increases the basal metabolic rate, cardiac output, vasodilation, heart rate and heat intolerance. The basal metabolic rate increases up to 30% in a term pregnancy.

Growth of hair and nails also tends to increase during pregnancy. Some women note excessive oiliness or dryness of the scalp and a softening and thinning of the nails by the sixth week of gestation. Pregnancy hormones increase the growing phases of the hair follicle and decrease the resting phase of the hair follicle. During the postpartum period, hormone withdrawal increases the resting phase of the hair follicle and transient hair loss may be noticed, commonly peaking at 3 to 4 months postpartum. This loss is normally resolved within 9 months to 1 year after birth.

Hirsutism of the face, abdomen and back may also be experienced during the second and third trimesters of pregnancy. Hormonal changes (androgens) cause this hair growth, which may reduce after birth.

EARS AND HEARING

Pregnant women may report a decrease in hearing, a sense of fullness in the ears or earaches because of the increased vascularity of the tympanic membrane and blockage of the eustachian tubes.

MOUTH, THROAT, NOSE AND SINUS

Some women may note changes in their gums during pregnancy. Gingival bleeding when brushing the teeth and hypertrophy are common. Occasionally, epulis, which are small, irritating nodules of the gums, develop. These nodules usually resolve on their own; however, occasionally the lesion may need to be surgically excised if the nodule bleeds excessively.

Vocal changes may be noted due to the oedema of the larynx. Nasal 'stuffiness' and epistaxis are also common during pregnancy because of the oestrogen-induced oedema and vascular congestion of the nasal mucosa and sinuses.

THORAX AND LUNGS

As the pregnancy progresses, progesterone influences the relaxation of the ligaments and joints. This relaxation allows the rib cage to flare, thus increasing the anteroposterior and transverse diameters. This accommodation is necessary as the pregnancy progresses and the enlarging uterus pushes up on the diaphragm. The woman's respiratory pattern changes from abdominal to costal. Shortness of breath is a common complaint during the last trimester. The woman may be more aware of her breathing pattern and of deep respirations and more frequent sighing. Oxygen requirements increase during pregnancy because of the additional cellular growth of the body and the fetus. Pulmonary requirements also increase, with the tidal volume increasing by 30% to 40%. All of these changes are normal and are to be expected during the last trimester.

BREASTS

Soon after conception, the surge of oestrogen and progesterone begins, causing notable changes in the mammary glands (Fig. 31-1). Breast changes noted by many women include:

- Tingling sensations and tenderness
- Enlargement of breast and nipple
- Hyperpigmentation of areola and nipple
- Enlargement of Montgomery tubercles
- Prominence of superficial veins

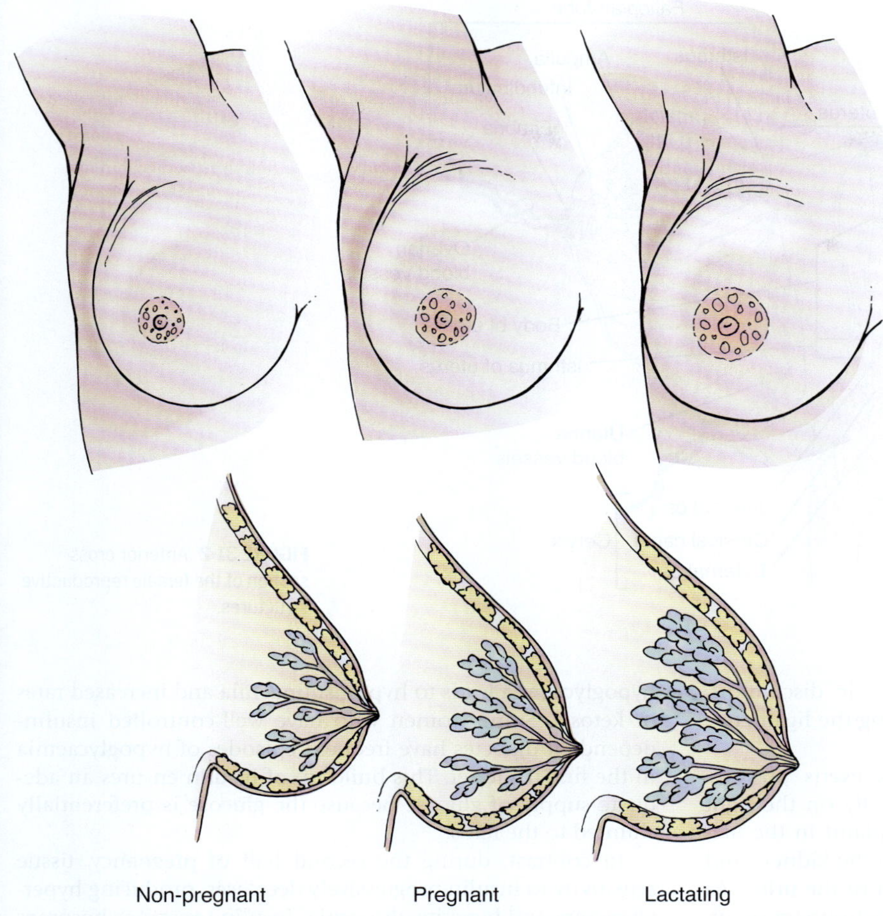

FIGURE 31-1 Breast changes during pregnancy.

- Development of striae
- Expression of colostrum in the second and third trimester.

HEART

Significant cardiovascular changes occur during pregnancy. One of the most dynamic changes is the increase in cardiac output and maternal blood volume by approximately 40% to 50%. Because the heart is required to pump much harder, it actually increases in size. Its position is rotated up and to the left approximately 1 cm to 1.5 cm. The heart rate may increase by 10 to 15 beats/minute and systolic murmurs may be heard.

PERIPHERAL VASCULAR SYSTEM

With the dynamic increase in maternal blood volume, a physiological anaemia (pseudoanaemia) commonly develops. This anaemia results primarily from the disproportionate increase in blood volume compared with the increased red blood cell (RBC) production. By 30 to 34 weeks, gestation plasma volume increases by 40% to 50%, whereas RBC volume increase is between 18% and 30%.

As the plasma blood volume increases, the blood vessels must accommodate for this volume, so progesterone acts on the vessels to make them relax and dilate. Subsequently, women often complain of dizziness and light-headedness, beginning with the second trimester and peaking at approximately 32 to 34 weeks. As the pregnancy progresses, the arterial blood pressure stabilises and symptoms begin to resolve. Prepregnant values return in the third trimester.

Other changes that occur during pregnancy include dependent oedema and varicosities. Two-thirds of all pregnant women will experience swelling of the lower extremities in the third trimester, usually noted late in the day after standing for long periods. Fluid retention is caused by the increased hormones of pregnancy, increased hydrophilicity of the intracellular connective tissue and the increased venous pressure in the lower extremities. As the expanding uterus applies pressure on the femoral venous area, femoral venous pressure increases. This uterine pressure restricts the venous blood flow return, causing stagnation of the blood in the lower extremities and resulting in dependent oedema. Varicose veins in the lower extremities, vulva and rectum are also common during pregnancy. Pregnant women are also more prone to development of thrombophlebitis because of the hypercoagulable state of pregnancy.

ABDOMEN

During pregnancy, the abdominal muscles stretch as the uterus enlarges. These muscles, known as the rectus abdominis muscles, may stretch to the point that permanent separation occurs. This condition is known as diastasis recti abdominis. Four paired ligaments (broad ligaments, uterosacral ligaments, cardinal ligaments, round ligaments) support the uterus and keep it in position in the pelvic cavity (Fig. 31-2). As the uterus

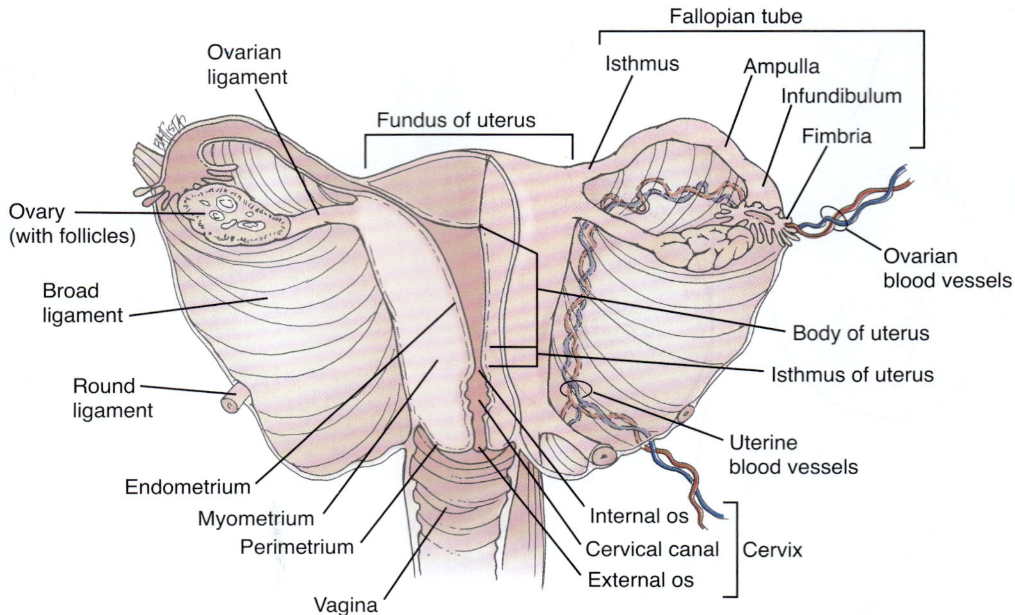

FIGURE 31-2 Anterior cross-section of the female reproductive structures.

enlarges, the woman may report lower pelvic discomfort, which quite commonly results from stretching the ligaments, especially the round ligaments.

In the abdomen, the expanding uterus exerts pressure on the bladder, kidneys and ureters (especially on the right side). Urinary frequency is a common complaint in the first and third trimesters. The applied pressure on the kidneys and ureters causes decreased flow and stagnation of the urine. As a result, physiological hydronephrosis and hydroureter occur. During the second trimester, bladder pressure subsides and urinary frequency is relieved by the uterus enlarging and being lifted out of the pelvic area. Nevertheless, throughout pregnancy women are at increased risk of urinary tract infections.

The enlarging uterus also applies pressure and displaces the small intestine. This pressure, along with the secretion of progesterone, decreases gastric motility. Gastric tone is decreased and the smooth muscles relax, decreasing emptying time of the stomach. Constipation results from these physiological events. Heartburn, which may also result, may be related to the decreased gastrointestinal motility and displacement of the stomach, causing the reflux of stomach acid into the oesophagus. Progesterone secretion relaxes the smooth muscles of the gallbladder; as a result, gallstone formation may occur because of the prolonged emptying time of the gallbladder.

Other gastrointestinal symptoms include ptyalism and pica. Ptyalism, or excessive salivation, may occur in the first trimester. Pica, a craving for or ingestion of non-nutritional substances such as dirt or clay, is rare but observed across all socio-economic classes and cultures. Pica can be a major concern if the craving interferes with proper nutrition during pregnancy.

Carbohydrate metabolism is also altered during pregnancy. Glucose use increases, leading to decreased maternal glucose levels. The rise in serum levels of oestrogen, progesterone and other hormones stimulates beta-cell hypertrophy and hyperplasial; additionally, insulin secretion increases. Glycogen is stored, and gluconeogenesis is reduced. In addition, the woman's body tissues develop an increased sensitivity to insulin, thus decreasing her need. As a result, maternal hypoglycaemia leads to hypoinsulinaemia and increased rates of ketosis. Some women who have well-controlled insulin-dependent diabetes have frequent episodes of hypoglycaemia in the first trimester. This build-up of insulin ensures an adequate supply of glucose because the glucose is preferentially shunted to the fetus.

In contrast, during the second half of pregnancy, tissue sensitivity to insulin progressively decreases, producing hyperglycaemia and hyperinsulinaemia. Insulin resistance becomes maximal in the latter half of the pregnancy.

REPRODUCTIVE ORGANS

Before conception, the uterus is a small, pear-shaped organ that weighs approximately 44 g. Its cavity can hold approximately 10 mL of fluid. Pregnancy changes this organ, giving it the capacity of weighing approximately 1,000 g and potentially holding approximately 5 L of amniotic fluid. This dynamic change is mainly due to the hypertrophy of pre-existing myometrial cells and the hyperplasia of new cells. Once conception occurs, the uterus prepares itself for the pregnancy: ovulation ceases, the uterine endometrium thickens, and the number and size of uterine blood vessels increase. Oestrogen is primarily responsible for these early changes.

With fetal growth, the uterus continues to expand throughout the pregnancy. At approximately 10 to 12 weeks' gestation, the uterus should be palpated at the top of the symphysis pubis. At 16 weeks' gestation, the top of the uterus, known as the fundus, should reach halfway between the symphysis pubis and the umbilicus. At 20 weeks' gestation, the fundus should be at the level of the umbilicus. For the rest of the pregnancy, the uterus grows approximately 1 cm per week, so the fundal height should equal the number of weeks pregnant (e.g. at 25 weeks' gestation, the fundal height should measure 25 cm). This formula is known as the McDonald rule and can be calculated by taking the fundal height in centimetres and multiplying it by 1.143. With a full-term pregnancy, the fundus should reach the xiphoid process. The fundal height measurement may drop in the last few weeks of the pregnancy if the fetal head is engaged and descended in the maternal pelvis. This occurrence is known as 'lightening'.

At near-term gestation, the uterine wall begins thinning out to approximately 5 mm or less. In the absence of obesity, fetal parts are usually easily palpated on the external abdomen in a term pregnancy. Braxton Hicks contractions (painless, irregular contractions of the uterus) may also occur sporadically in the third trimester. These contractions are normal as long as no cervical change is noted.

Normal changes in the cervix, vagina and vulva also occur during pregnancy. Cervical softening (Goodell sign), bluish discolouration (Chadwick sign) and hypertrophy of the glands in the cervical canal all occur. With these glands secreting more mucus, there is an increase in vaginal discharge, which is acidic. The mucus collects in the cervix to form the mucus plug. This plug acts to seal the endocervical canal and prevent bacteria from ascending into the uterus, thus preventing infection. The vaginal smooth muscle and connective tissue soften and expand to prepare for the passage of the fetus through the birth canal.

ANUS AND RECTUM

Constipation is a common problem during pregnancy. Progesterone decreases intestinal motility, allowing more time for nutrients to be absorbed for the woman and fetus. This also increases the absorption time for water into the circulation, taking fluid from the large intestine and contributing to hardening of the stool and decreased frequency of bowel movements. It should be noted that iron supplementation can also contribute to constipation for those women who take additional iron. As a result, haemorrhoids (varicose veins in the rectum) may develop because of the pressure on the venous structures from straining during bowel movement. Vascular congestion of the pelvis also contributes to haemorrhoid development.

MUSCULOSKELETAL SYSTEM

Anatomical changes of the musculoskeletal system during pregnancy result from fetal growth, hormonal influences and maternal weight gain. As the pregnancy progresses, uterine growth pulls the pelvis forward, which causes the spine to curve forward also, thus creating a gradual *lordosis* (Fig. 31-3). The enlarging breasts influence the shoulders to droop forward, and the pregnant woman may find herself pulling her shoulders back and straightening her head and neck to accommodate for this extra weight. Progesterone and *relaxin* (non-steroidal hormone) influence the pelvic joints and ligaments to relax; subsequently, the symphysis pubis, sacroiliac and sacrococcygeal joints all become more flexible during pregnancy. This flexibility allows the pelvic outlet diameter to increase slightly, which reduces the risk of trauma during childbirth. After the postpartum period, the pelvic diameter will generally remain larger than the size before childbirth.

The relaxin hormone contributes to changing the woman's gait during pregnancy, often observed as a side-to-side movement when walking with short steps and a swinging of the body. Gait changes are also attributed to weight gain of the uterus, fetus and breasts. At approximately 24 weeks' gestation the woman's centre of gravity and stance shift, often causing the woman to lean back slightly to balance herself. Backaches are also common during pregnancy. Along with these changes, the woman may even see an increase in shoe size, especially with regard to width.

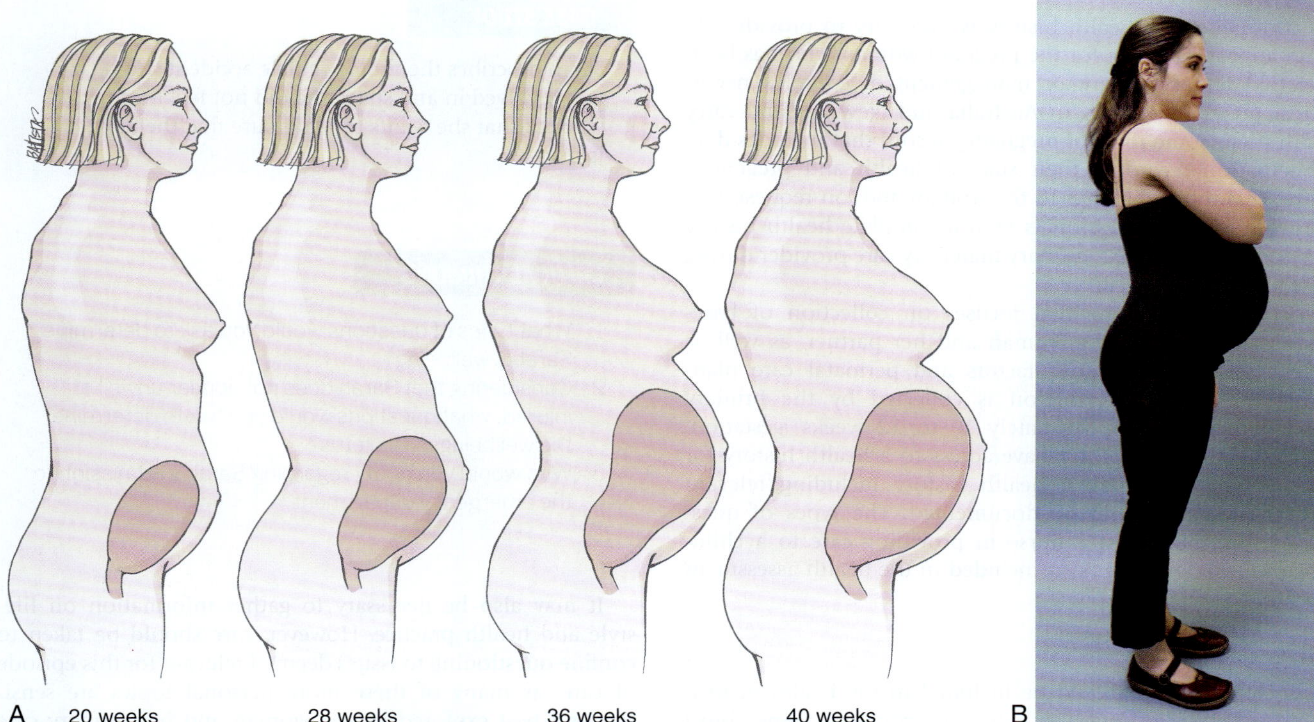

FIGURE 31-3 (A) Postural changes during pregnancy; **(B)** lordosis in pregnant patient. (**B,** © B. Proud.)

NEUROLOGICAL SYSTEM

Neurological changes that occur during pregnancy can be discomforting to the woman. Common issues include:

- *Pain or tingling sensations in the thigh:* Pressure on the lateral femoral cutaneous nerve causes these sensations.
- *Carpal tunnel syndrome*: Pressure on the median nerve below the carpal ligament of the wrist causes a tingling sensation in the hand. Because fluid retention occurs during pregnancy, swollen tissues compress the median nerve in the wrist and produce the tingling sensations. Pain can be reproduced by performing the Tinel sign and the Phalen test (see Chap. 28). Up and down movement of the wrist aggravates this condition.
- *Leg cramps:* Inadequate calcium or magnesuim intake, dehydration, fatigue or decreased circulation may cause leg cramps.
- *Dizziness and light-headedness:* In early pregnancy, the woman may experience dizziness because of the slight decrease in blood pressure resulting from vasodilation and decreased vascular resistance. In later pregnancy, a woman in the supine position may experience dizziness caused by the heavy uterus compressing the vena cava and aorta. This compression reduces cardiac return, cardiac output, blood pressure and the subsequent effect known as *supine hypotensive syndrome. Therefore, when examining pregnant women, a wedge or towel should be placed under the right hip to achieve a left-lateral tilt.*

Health assessment

COLLECTING SUBJECTIVE DATA: THE NURSING HEALTH HISTORY

A comprehensive health history is necessary to provide safe and appropriate care for the pregnant woman who has been referred for assessment or management of complex needs. Most pregnant women in Australia and New Zealand carry with them some form of pregnancy record that includes documentation regarding their state of health and pregnancy care. This record belongs to the woman and, on request, will provide health professionals with a complete health history as documented by the primary maternity care provider during the first antenatal visit.

The first antenatal visit focuses on collection of baseline data regarding the woman and her partner, as well as identification of any risk factors and perinatal care planning. Generally, information is collected by the primary care provider at approximately 10 to 12 weeks' gestation. If the examiner does not have access to a health history for the pregnant woman, a health history including relevant maternal data should be documented. The types of questions that may assist a nurse in providing care to a childbearing woman have been included in the health assessment tables.

Biographical data

Biographical data should be included in the health history. This information may include the woman's name, birth date, address and phone number. Obtaining the woman's educational level, occupation and employment status helps the staff to tailor their approach to the client's level of health literacy. The health history should also include the woman's primary support person, together with their phone number and other contact details in case of emergency. Any cultural or spiritual requirements need to be noted and observed in order to provide holistic and culturally safe care that honours human dignity.

The woman's *estimated due date* (EDD) should be noted and is an important factor in considering care for her. The EDD will enable the nurse to determine the gestation of this pregnancy. The EDD will be documented in the woman's pregnancy record but can be calculated based on the Naegele rule or a pregnancy calculator. The Naegele rule uses the formula of adding 9 months and 7 days to the first day of the woman's last menstrual period. A variation of this formula can be followed if the woman's normal menstrual cycle is shorter or longer than 28 days. Previous pregnancies and perinatal outcomes should be noted, as well as previous surgical or medical history. Most women will have had mental health and wellbeing screening completed by their primary care provider and referrals offered as appropriate (Department of Health, 2019; Gray & Smith, 2018; Hanley, 2009; Pairman et al., 2019; South Australian Department of Health, 2015).

It is also important to gather data regarding the reason for the health care visit. Documenting the description of the women's experience is important. Consideration must also be given to the holistic wellbeing of the mother and fetus. Questions regarding the woman's perception of her wellbeing are vital. In addition, questions regarding fetal wellbeing are important and help to inform clinical approach (Johnson & Taylor, 2019; Radestad & Lindgren, 2012).

CASE STUDY

Sarah describes the motor vehicle accident she was involved in and states she did not feel hurt in any way but that she wants to make sure that the baby is okay.

CRITICAL THINKING

1. What types of questions would you ask to determine Sarah's wellbeing?
2. Considering that Sarah does not appear unwell or injured, what questions would you ask to determine the wellbeing of the fetus?
3. Who would you notify regarding Sarah's admission to the emergency department?

It may also be necessary to gather information on lifestyle and health practice. However, care should be taken to confine questioning to issues deemed relevant for this episode of care, as many of these more personal topics are sensitive and best explored by the woman and her primary care provider.

COLDSPA

Example

Use the COLDSPA mnemonic as a guideline to collect needed information for each symptom the pregnant woman shares. In addition, the following questions help elicit important information.

Mnemonic	Question	Client response example
Character	Describe the sign or symptom (feeling, appearance, sound, smell or taste, if applicable).	'Nausea; occasional small amounts of vomiting with some dry heaves.'
Onset	When did it begin?	'One week ago.'
Location	Where is it? Does it radiate? Does it occur anywhere else?	Not applicable
Duration	How long does it last? Does it recur?	'Usually all morning and seems to subside by lunch time.'
Severity	How much does it bother you?	'I can't eat breakfast in the morning.'
Pattern	Is there anything that makes it better or worse?	'Some odours like meat cooking make me more nauseated.'
Associated factors/How it **A**ffects the patient	What other symptoms occur with it? How does it affect you?	'Some vomiting and belching and dry heaves. It is hard for me to concentrate at work.'

Past maternal history, including health history

QUESTION	RATIONALE

Can you list the number of times you have been pregnant, beginning with your first pregnancy?	Determine the women's gravida and parity status:
	• Gravida (G): total number of pregnancies
	• Parity (P): number of pregnancies that have birthed at 20 weeks' gestation or greater or where the fetus weighed over 400 g:
	  • Term gestation: birth of baby >37 weeks
	  • Preterm gestation: birth of baby after 20 weeks and before the beginning of 37 weeks' gestation
	  • Miscarriage or abortion: termination of pregnancy prior to the 20th week of pregnancy (elective or spontaneous).
	Example: G2 P1
	This represents a woman who has been pregnant twice and has birthed once. This woman may currently be pregnant or, if not currently pregnant, this would indicate a miscarriage.

Describe your previous pregnancies including birth date, birth weight, sex, gestational age, type of birth (if operative, discuss reasons). Did you experience any complications during these pregnancies (e.g. high blood pressure, diabetes, bleeding, depression)? Did you have twins or other multiple gestation? Discuss any previous abortion (spontaneous or elective) including procedures required and gestational age of fetus.	History of previous pregnancies helps identify women at risk of complications during current pregnancy. Knowledge may be relevant to this episode of care.
Describe any neonatal complications within the first 2 weeks of life. Describe any perinatal or neonatal losses, including when the loss occurred and the reason for the loss if known.	Previous neonatal complications may be hereditary and may recur in future births. Knowledge may be relevant to this episode of care with regard to fetal wellbeing.
Do you have a history of any major medical problems (e.g. heart trouble, rheumatic fever, hypertension, lung problems, asthma, diabetes, tuberculosis, trouble with nerves and/or depression, kidney disease, cancer, convulsions, epilepsy, abnormality of female organs, thyroid problems).	Identification of any medical problem is important during pregnancy because the body undergoes many physiological changes; certain medical conditions may put the woman and fetus at risk of complications. This history may be relevant to this episode of care.

Continued on following page

Past maternal history, including health history (continued)

QUESTION	RATIONALE
Do you have a history of sexually transmitted infections (STIs) such as *Chlamydia*, gonorrhoea, herpes, genital warts or syphilis? If so, please describe when it occurred and the treatment. Does your partner have a history of STIs? If so, when was he treated?	Early detection and treatment of STIs may prevent intrauterine complications from long-term exposure to infections. This also allows the nurse (and other health professionals) to plan and provide safe and appropriate care.
When was your last cervical screening test and what were the results?	Human papillomavirus can lead to the development of genial warts, abnormal cervical cells or even cervical cancer. Early detection can prompt follow-up monitoring, further testing or treatment of malignant and premalignant cells of the cervix. It is important to note that any treatment for cervical cancer will increase the woman's risk of an incompetent cervix during pregnancy (Royal Australian and New Zealand College of Obstetricians and Gynaecologists [ANZCOG], 2017).
Do you have a history of any vaginal infections such as bacterial vaginosis, yeast infections or others? If so, when did the last infection occur and what was the treatment?	Vaginal infections require timely treatment to reduce the risk of adverse perinatal outcome (e.g. premature labour).
Do you have a history of medication, food or other allergies? If so, list the allergies and describe the reactions.	Identification of medication allergies is necessary to prevent complications.
Have you ever been hospitalised or had surgery? If so, discuss the reason for hospitalisation or surgery, the date, and if the problem is resolved today.	Previous hospitalisations or surgeries must be noted to assess for potential medical complications during pregnancy and may be relevant to this episode of care.
Family history	
Has anyone in your family (grandparents, parents, siblings, children) suffered from any medical conditions (e.g. heart trouble, lung problems, diabetes, asthma, cancer)?	Cardiovascular disease or heart defects may be inherited. Pulmonary or endocrine disorders may be familial. There is a genetic component associated with certain types of cancer.
Has anyone in your family been born with any birth defects, inherited diseases, blood disorders, intellectual disability or any other problems?	There is a genetic risk factor for Down syndrome, spina bifida, brain defects, anencephaly, heart defects, muscular dystrophy, cystic fibrosis, haemophilia, thalassaemia and other inherited diseases. Genetic testing may be offered during preconception counselling, and all women should be offered screening for chromosomal abnormalities and neural tube defects during antenatal care.
Current pregnancy	
Do you know your estimated due date (EDD)? Can you tell me how many weeks pregnant you are?	Many women keep excellent records of their pregnancy and will be able to provide this information.
When was the first day of your last menstrual period? Do you have regular periods when not pregnant? Do you know the normal length of your menstrual cycle (i.e. 28 days)?	If the woman does not know her EDD, menstrual history can help to determine this and, subsequently, gestation. Calculate EDD based on the Naegele rule and note gestational age.
Have you experienced any complications during this pregnancy (i.e. diabetes, high blood pressure, bleeding)? If so, please describe these complications.	It is important to identify any current complications in this pregnancy as this information may influence this episode of care.
Are you expecting just one baby? If not, are you pregnant with twins or more?	It is important to ascertain whether this is a single or multiple gestation in order to assess fetal wellbeing; additionally, perinatal risks associated with multiple gestation should be considered.
Do you know your blood type and Rh factor?	Rh-negative mothers should receive Rho immune globulin at 28 weeks, 34 weeks or with any sensitising event (e.g. abdominal injury, episode of vaginal bleeding).

Past maternal history, including health history (continued)

QUESTION	RATIONALE
Are you currently taking any medications (either prescription or non-prescription), or have you taken any since you have become pregnant? If so, list the medications, the amount taken, the date you started taking it and the reason for taking it.	Some medications are teratogenic (i.e. cause birth defects) for the fetus during pregnancy, so medications should be managed by the woman's primary care provider; however, it is helpful to note medications the pregnant woman is taking and that may be relevant to this episode of care.
Are your immunisations up to date? Have you received the influenza and whooping cough immunisations this year?	Assessment for rubella and hepatitis B is performed at the first antenatal visit. Vaccination of pregnant women against influenza is supported by evidence and may be offered to women at any stage of their pregnancy but preferably prior to the influenza season; pertussis is also recommended and can be given during the third trimester (Rowe et al., 2019).
Do you have vaginal bleeding, leakage of fluid or vaginal discharge at the moment?	Vaginal bleeding, leakage or discharge may indicate pregnancy complications, membrane rupture or vaginal infection (e.g. bacterial vaginosis, trichomoniasis, STI). If the woman suspects vaginal loss of any sort, she should be given a sanitary pad to wear which can then be reviewed during the physical examination and obstetric assessment.
Have you recently experienced any stinging or burning sensation when urinating?	Pregnant women may have asymptomatic bacteriuria. Urinary tract infections (UTIs) need to be diagnosed and treated with antibiotics. Untreated UTIs predispose the woman to complications such as preterm labour. A routine urinalysis should be performed, and a midstream urine sample collected (Pairman et al., 2019).
Have you experienced any pain recently, or are you experiencing pain? Where was or is this pain? Was or is this pain continual or intermittent? Was or is this pain sharp or more of a dull, periodlike pain?	Pain may indicate a pregnancy complication, depending on the type of pain, where it is experienced and at what stage during the gestation the woman is experiencing the pain. Women may experience pain in their back or pelvic joints because of pregnancy hormones that relax the ligaments. It is common for women in the late last trimester to experience Braxton Hicks contractions, but these are generally painless or mildly uncomfortable. Contractions are experienced as intermittent pain, sometimes extending to the back or upper thighs, and can suggest premature labour if they occur prior to 37 weeks' gestation. Headaches, epigastric discomfort or continual abdominal pain may indicate a pregnancy complication and requires immediate obstetric assessment.
Are there any other concerns you have that we have not discussed yet? What is most important to you right now and how can we help?	This questioning provides the woman with an opportunity to discuss any other concerns she may have, including personal or sensitive issues. For example, there is an increase in the risk of women experiencing domestic violence when pregnant than at other times (Eustace et al., 2016). Universal screening by the primary care provider is recommended. It also allows the woman to share any cultural, spiritual, social or pragmatic needs.

Lifestyle and health practices

QUESTION	RATIONALE
Are you currently drinking alcohol? If yes, can you describe how much and how often?	Drinking while pregnant increases the risk of miscarriage, premature labour, low birth weight and stillbirth. Heavy drinking can cause fetal alcohol spectrum disorder (Bailey & Sokol, 2011).

Continued on following page

Lifestyle and health practices (continued)

QUESTION	RATIONALE
Do you smoke cigarettes? If so, how many do you smoke per day?	Maternal cigarette smoking correlates with an increased incidence of premature rupture of membranes, preterm birth, placental abruption, bleeding during pregnancy and perinatal mortality (Pairman et al., 2019). Smoking is also associated with low birth weight, attention deficit hyperactivity disorder, and behavioural and learning disorders in school (Wehby et al., 2011). Women who quit or reduce smoking during pregnancy will benefit not only the health of themselves but also that of the fetus. These women may also have a lower relapse rate of smoking again compared with women who are not pregnant (American College of Obstetricians and Gynecologists [ACOG], 2017).
Do you take partake in any recreational drugs?	Drug use in pregnancy has been linked with miscarriage, pre-eclampsia, intrauterine growth restriction, low birth weight, premature labour, placental abruption, stillbirth and neonatal abstinence syndrome (Forray, 2016).
What is a normal daily intake of food for you? Are you on any special diet? Do you have any diet intolerances or restrictions? If so, what are they?	Maternal nutrition has a direct relationship to maternal–fetal wellbeing.
As you probably know, there are some foods that need to be cooked well or avoided in pregnancy. Have you eaten any unpasteurised milk products, deli meats, raw fish or prepackaged salads recently?	Changes in hormone levels and immune system function during pregnancy can make women more vulnerable to infections such aslisteriosis. Maternal infection can cause fetal infection and mortality may approach 50%; listeria can also cause neonatal sepsis or meningitis (Madjunkov et al., 2017).
Do you currently take any vitamin supplements? If so, what are they?	All women of childbearing age are recommended to consume 500 µg of folic acid daily to help prevent neural tube defects in the fetus, and women who are pregnant or breastfeeding are advised to also take an iodine supplement of 150 µg/day (Department of Health, 2019). The woman's balanced diet should provide an appropriate supply of the other vitamins required for pregnancy. Nutritional intake should be from protein-rich foods, wholegrain breads and cereals, dairy products, and fruits and vegetables. Routine multivitamin supplementation for women is based solely on individual assessment; where this is required, often iron, vitamin B12 and vitamin D require consideration.
Activity and exercise	
Do you exercise daily? If so, what do you do and for how long?	Daily exercise is highly recommended as long as it is tolerated well by the pregnant woman. Women who are physically active tend to have shorter, less difficult labours compared with women who are not fit (Hinman et al., 2015). However, new forms of exercise or an increase in effort in exercise may not be advisable; rather, women are encouraged to maintain their prepregnancy activities or consider the introduction of gentle, low-impact movement such as walking.
Toxic exposure	
Have you or your partner ever worked around chemicals or radiation? If so, please explain. Are you exposed to an excessive amount of smoke daily?	Assessment of toxic exposure can identify potential teratogens to the fetus. This helps to identify environmental exposures/risks for the woman.
Role and relationships	
Can you tell me about your schooling? What is the highest level of education you have completed?	These questions identify psychosocial issues for the woman. Assess social support systems for the family.

Lifestyle and health practices (continued)

QUESTION	RATIONALE
How are you feeling about this pregnancy? Do you have a primary support person we can call for you? What type of support systems do you have at home?	Identification of the woman's primary social support is necessary. Permission to contact this person may be sought. If the women does not identify a primary support person, assessment of social structures may be indicated.
Who is your primary maternity care provider for this pregnancy?	The primary maternity care provider should be contacted and advised of the woman's presentation to the health service.

COLLECTING OBJECTIVE DATA: PHYSICAL EXAMINATION

There is debate as to the degree of physical examination that is required during the first antenatal visit. Pairman et al. (2019, p. 450) provide discussion regarding this process, concluding, 'There is no consensus as to the detail, make-up and content of 'routine' initial physical examination of a well pregnant woman.' Pairman et al. (2019, p. 450) suggest that 'it is important to distinguish between something that is offered routinely, and that which is offered in response to risk markers'. For example, if a woman has a history of unsafe sexual practice, a vaginal swab for sexually transmitted infections (STIs) may be appropriate. Accordingly, the examiner should only undertake relevant and necessary physical examinations in response to the reasons for these episodes of care.

Based on the information gathered during the first antenatal visit and the appropriate physical examination undertaken, the midwife and woman would have discussed the relevance and need for particular screening and diagnostic tests (Pairman et al., 2019). Antenatal blood tests generally include a complete blood picture, blood group, Rh status and antibody screen, rubella titre, Trepinostika screening assay for syphilis, and hepatitis B surface antigen. Universal screening for human immunodeficiency virus and hepatitis C is recommended. There are some tests that may be offered to specific groups, including screening for haemoglobinopathies (sickle cell disease or thalassaemia), varicella, haemoglobin electrophoresis, and ferritin and vitamin D deficiency.

In addition, the woman may be offered specific screening options, for example, first trimester screening—nuchal translucency between 11 + 0 and 13 + 6 weeks and biochemistry between 10 + 0 and 13 + 6 weeks—to detect risk for Trisomy 18 and 21. Second trimester screening includes biochemistry between 14 + 0 and 20 + 6 weeks for the detection of neural tube defects as well as Trisomy 18 and 21. The morphology ultrasound generally occurs at 18 to 20 weeks. It also screens for fetal growth and development as well as amniotic fluid and placental position. An earlier dated ultrasound may be appropriate if a pregnancy date is unknown or uncertain (South Australian Department of Health, 2015). All records of tests and investigations are documented in the woman's pregnancy record, providing important background data for the nurse providing care and avoiding unnecessary repetition of investigations (Department of Health, 2019; Johnson & Taylor, 2019).

Preparing the woman for assessment

Pregnancy is a time when women may feel more vulnerable or be susceptible to anxiety, so it is important that, after meeting the woman, the nurse should explain the sequence of events for this episode of care. The nurse should provide a warm and comfortable environment for any physical assessment. It is not expected that the nurse would conduct an examination of the pregnant abdomen, referred to as an *abdominal palpation*, because this requires specialised skills; however, locating and listening to the fetal heart rate (FHR) and measuring the size of the uterus maybe appropriate if the primary maternity care provider or an appropriately trained health professional are unavailable. The nurse should note any fetal movements. An ultrasound can be conducted to determine the wellbeing of the fetus if necessary. It is important to document the woman's vital signs, understanding that the woman's vital signs may reflect fetal wellbeing; for example, tachycardia in the mother may also result in tachycardia in the fetus. An elevated or significantly low blood pressure in pregnancy can signal possible complications that may affect both woman and fetus. Any examination of the woman that requires her to be in a supine position should be conducted with the woman tilted to her left side. This may be achieved by placing a wedge under the mattress or a pillow or rolled towel under her right side.

It is important to note any changes to normal experiences that the woman may have experienced such as pain or vaginal loss; this should be considered carefully and her primary maternity provider contacted immediately. The nurse should not conduct a pelvic examination. Pelvic examination of the woman should only be conducted in discussion with her primary maternity care provider and should be undertaken by an appropriately trained health professional if deemed necessary. It is important that, prior to any pelvic examination, the position of the placenta is identified (Department of Health, 2019; Johnson & Taylor, 2019; Pairman et al., 2019).

Physical assessment

Remember these key points during examination:

- Obtain an accurate and complete antenatal history.
- Understand and recognise cardiovascular changes of pregnancy.
- Recognise common skin changes.
- Identify common discomforts of pregnancy and explain what causes them.
- Note any variations from normal physiological changes.
- Note any vaginal loss or pain.
- If required, correctly measure growth of uterus during pregnancy and locate the FHR.
- Note fetal movements.

PHYSICAL ASSESSMENT

ASSESSMENT PROCEDURE	NORMAL FINDINGS	ABNORMAL FINDINGS
General survey: Vital signs, height and weight		
Measure blood pressure (BP). Take the blood pressure on the right arm where possible.	BP range: systolic 90 to 139 mmHg and diastolic 60 to 89 mmHg. BP decreases during the second trimester because of the relaxation effect on the blood vessels. By 32 to 34 weeks, the woman's BP should be back to normal.	Elevated BP at 9 to 11 weeks may be indicative of chronic hypertension hydatidiform mole pregnancy or thyroid storm. After 20 weeks, increased BP (>140/90 mmHg) may be associated with pregnancy-induced hypertension. Decreased blood pressure may indicate supine hypotensive syndrome.
Measure pulse rate.	60 to 90 beats/minute; may increase 10 to 15 beats/minute higher than prepregnant levels	Irregularities in heart rhythm, chest pain, dyspnoea and oedema may indicate cardiac disease.
Take the woman's temperature.	35.8°C to 37.3°C	During pregnancy, hormones and an increased metabolic rate may result in a temperature rise of 0.5 (Johnson & Taylor, 2019). An elevated temperature above 38.0°C may indicate infection.
Measure weight on admission.	Appropriate gestational weight gain is determined by prepregnancy body mass index; however, if a woman is in a healthy weight range prior to conception, then ideally she will gain between 1 and 1.5 kg in the first 3 months and then 1.5 to 2 kg each month thereafter (Gilmore & Redman, 2015).	A sudden weight gain of 2 kg a week may be associated with pregnancy-induced hypertension and fluid retention. Weight gain of less than 1 kg a month after 20 weeks may indicate insufficient nourishment.
Observe behaviour.	*First trimester:* Fatigue. *Second trimester:* Introspective, energetic. *Third trimester:* Restless, preparing for baby.	Denial of pregnancy, withdrawal, depression or psychosis may be seen in the woman with psychological problems.
Systems examinations		
Body systems should be examined only as relevant to this episode of care according to nursing assessment requirements. The data outlined in this table provide some of the changes you may expect to see if you need to perform any of the following systems examinations. *Note:* If the woman is in the third trimester, a pillow or rolled towel should be placed under her right side or a wedge placed under the mattress to ensure she is not lying flat on her back for any of the examinations.		
Skin, hair and nails		
Inspect the skin. Note hyperpigmented areas associated with pregnancy.	Linea nigra, striae, gravidarum, chloasma and spider nevi may be present.	Pale skin suggests anaemia. Yellow discolouration suggests jaundice.
Observe skin for vascular markings associated with pregnancy.	Angiomas and palmar erythema are common.	
Inspect the hair and nails.	Hair and nails tend to increase in growth; softening and thinning are common.	
Head and neck		
INSPECTION AND PALPATION		
Inspect and palpate the neck. Assess the anterior and posterior cervical chain lymph nodes. Also palpate the thyroid gland.	Smooth, non-tender, small cervical nodes may be palpable. Slight enlargement of the thyroid may be noted during pregnancy.	Hard, tender, fixed or prominent nodes may indicate infection or cancer. Marked enlargement of the thyroid gland indicates thyroid disease. Benign and malignant nodules as well as tenderness are noted in thyroiditis.

PHYSICAL ASSESSMENT (continued)

ASSESSMENT PROCEDURE	NORMAL FINDINGS	ABNORMAL FINDINGS
Eyes		
INSPECTION		
Inspect the eyes. Examine cornea, lens, iris and pupil. Use an ophthalmoscope to examine the fundus of the eye.	Pupils are equal and round, reactive to light and accommodate.	Narrowing of the arterioles or arteriovenous nicking may indicate hypertension.
Ears		
INSPECTION		
Inspect the ears.	Tympanic membrane clear: landmarks visible.	Tympanic membrane red and bulging with pus indicates infection.
Mouth, throat and nose		
INSPECTION		
Inspect the mouth. Pay particular attention to the teeth and the gingival tissues, which may normally appear swollen and slightly reddened.	Hypertrophy of gingival tissue is common. Bleeding may occur due to brushing teeth or dental examinations.	Epulis nodules may be present.
Inspect the throat.	Throat pink, no redness or exudate.	Throat red, exudate present, tonsillary hypertrophy indicates infection.
Inspect the nose.	Nasal mucosal swelling and redness may result from increased oestrogen production. Epistaxis is a common variation because of the increased vascular supply to the nares during pregnancy.	Abnormal findings are the same as those in non-pregnant women.
Thorax and lungs		
Inspect, palpate, percuss and auscultate the chest.	Normal findings include increased anteroposterior diameter, thoracic breathing, slight hyperventilation; shortness of breath in late pregnancy. Lung sounds are clear to auscultation bilaterally.	Dyspnoea, rales, rhonchi, wheezes, rubs, absence of breath sounds and unequal breath sounds are signs of respiratory distress. Women with a history of asthma have increased risk of perinatal morbidity or mortality, pregnancy-induced hypertension, preterm labour and low birth weight (Gilbert, 2011).
Breasts		
INSPECTION AND PALPATION		
Inspect and palpate the breasts and nipples for symmetry and colour (Fig. 31-4).	Venous congestion is noted with prominence of veins. Montgomery tubercles are prominent. Breast size is increased and nodular. Breasts are more sensitive to touch. Colostrum is excreted, especially in the third trimester. Hyperpigmentation of nipples and areolae is evident (Fig. 31-5).	Bloody discharge of the nipple and retraction of the skin could indicate breast cancer.
Heart		
AUSCULTATION		
Auscultate the heart.	Normal sinus rhythm.	Irregular rhythm.
	Soft systolic murmurs are audible during pregnancy secondary to the increased blood volume.	Progressive dyspnoea, palpitations and markedly decreased activity tolerance indicate cardiovascular disease.

Continued on following page

PHYSICAL ASSESSMENT (continued)

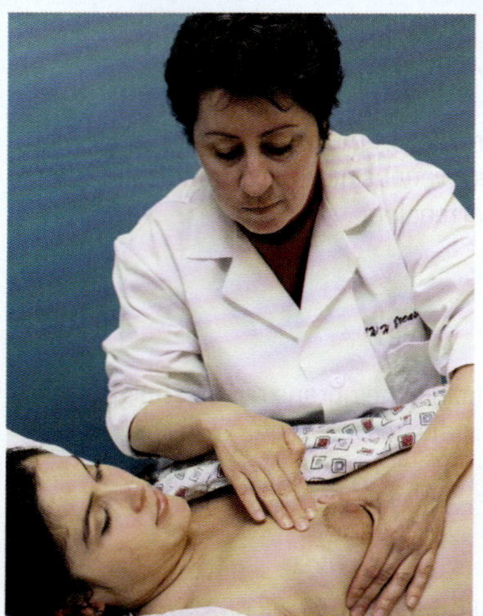

FIGURE 31-4 Palpating the breasts. (© B. Proud.)

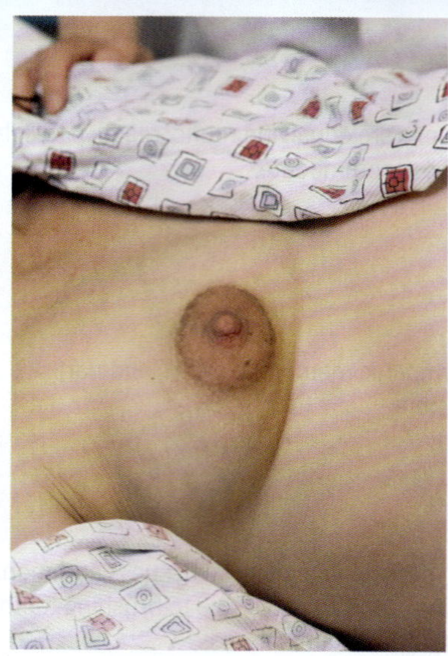

FIGURE 31-5 Hyperpigmentation of the nipples and areolae. (© B. Proud.)

ASSESSMENT PROCEDURE	NORMAL FINDINGS	ABNORMAL FINDINGS
Peripheral vascular		
INSPECTION AND PERCUSSION		
Inspect the face and extremities. Note colour and oedema.	During the third trimester, dependent oedema is normal. Varicose veins may also appear.	Abnormal findings include calf pain, positive Homans sign, generalised oedema (or facial oedema) and diminished pedal pulses. These findings may indicate thrombophlebitis. Facial oedema may indicate pregnancy-induced hypertension, especially in the presence of elevated blood pressure and proteinuria.
Percuss deep tendon reflexes.	Normal reflexes 1 to 2+. Clonus is absent.	Reflexes 3 to 4+ and positive clonus require evaluation for pregnancy-induced hypertension.
Abdomen—Performed only by a pracititoner with specialist skills		
INSPECTION		
Inspect the abdomen. For this part of the examination, ask the woman to recline with a pillow under her head and her knees flexed. Note striae, scars and the shape and size of the abdomen.	Striae and linea nigra are normal. The size of the abdomen may indicate gestational age. The shape of the uterus may suggest fetal presentation and position in later pregnancy.	Scars indicate previous surgery; be careful to note cesarean section scars and location. A transverse lie may be suspected by abdominal palpation, noting enlargement of the width of the uterus.
PALPATION		
Palpate the abdomen. If the abdomen is soft, note organs and any masses.	The uterus is palpable from 10 to 12 weeks' gestation.	Abnormal masses palpable in the abdomen may indicate uterine fibroids or hepatosplenomegaly.
Palpate for fetal movement after 24 weeks.	Fetal movement should be felt by the woman from approximately 18 to 20 weeks.	If fetal movement is not felt, the expected date of delivery may be wrong, or intrauterine fetal demise may have occurred.

PHYSICAL ASSESSMENT (continued)

ASSESSMENT PROCEDURE	NORMAL FINDINGS	ABNORMAL FINDINGS
Palpate for uterine contractions. Contractions are felt as the uterine muscles begin to contract and the abdomen becomes firm. Generally this is felt by placing the palms of your hands on the fundus of the uterus, located in the upper portion of the abdomen, depending on gestation. Once the uterine muscles relax and the contraction ceases, the abdomen becomes soft to palpate. Note the intensity of contractions. Notice the difference between the uterus at rest and during a contraction.	The uterus contracts and feels firm to the examiner and then relaxes (note normal labour is considered after 37 weeks' gestation).	Regular contractions before 37 weeks' gestation may suggest premature labour. If you determine contractions and the woman is less than 37 weeks you should avoid palpating the abdomen more than necessary. Additionally, if the uterus appears continually rigid you should seek emergency obstetric assistance immediately.
Time the length of the contraction from the beginning to the end. Also note the frequency of the contractions, timing from the beginning of one contraction until the beginning of the next (Fig. 31-6).	Contractions may last 30 to 60 seconds and occur every 2 to 10 minutes, depending on the stage of labour.	Contractions lasting too long or occurring too frequently can cause fetal distress.
FUNDAL HEIGHT		
Measure fundal height. Do this by placing one hand on each side of the abdomen and walking your hands up the sides of the uterus until you feel the uterus curve; your hands should meet. Take a tape measure and place the zero point on the symphysis pubis and measure to the top of the fundus (Fig. 31-7).	Uterine size should approximately equal the number of weeks of gestation (e.g. the uterus at 28 weeks' gestation should measure approximately 28 cm) (Fig. 31-8). Measurements may vary by about 2 cm, and examiners' techniques may vary, but measurements should be approximately the same.	Measurements below or beyond 4 cm of gestational age need to be further evaluated. Measurements greater than expected may indicate a multiple gestation, polyhydramnios (excess of amniotic fluid), fetal anomalies or macrosomia (great increase in size similar to obesity). Measurements smaller than expected may indicate intrauterine growth restriction.

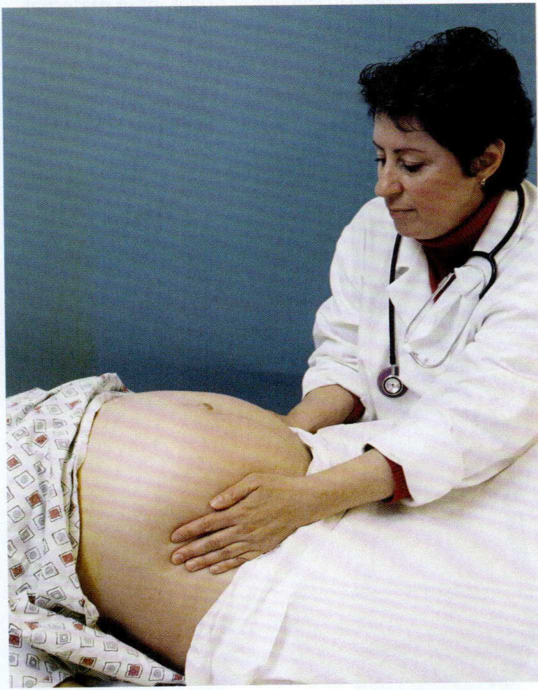

FIGURE 31-6 Palpating for uterine contractions. (© B. Proud.)

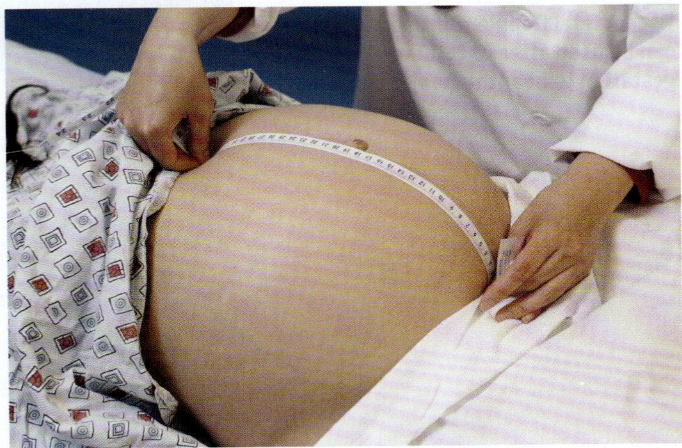

FIGURE 31-7 Measuring the fundal height. (© B. Proud.)

Continued on following page

PHYSICAL ASSESSMENT (continued)

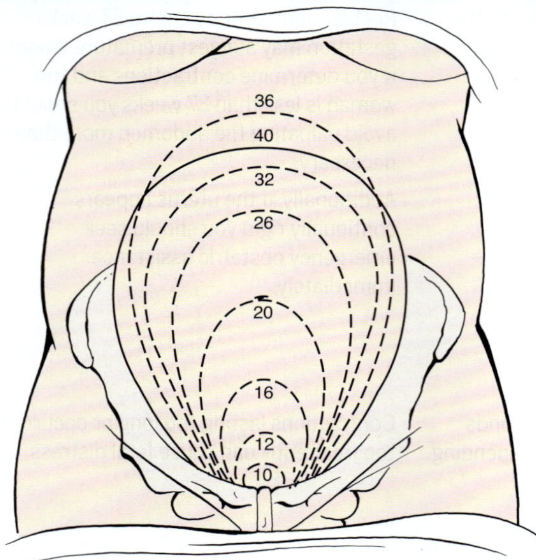

FIGURE 31-8 Approximate height of fundus at various weeks of gestation. (© B. Proud.)

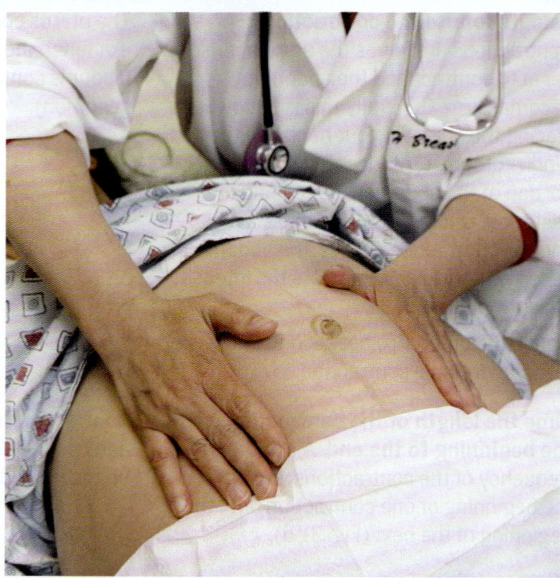
FIGURE 31-9 Palpating fetal back to locate fetal heart sounds. (© B. Proud.)

ASSESSMENT PROCEDURE	NORMAL FINDINGS	ABNORMAL FINDINGS
FETAL HEART		
Determine the location, rate and rhythm of the fetal heart. In order to auscultate the fetal heart rate, it is helpful to locate the fetal back. This can be achieved by placing your hands on the lateral sides of the abdomen (see Fig. 31-9).	On one side of the abdomen you will feel round nodules; these are the fists and feet of the fetus. Kicking and movement are expected to be felt. The woman will confirm this with you. This should be noted as 'fetal movements felt by woman'. The other side of the abdomen feels smooth; this is the fetal back.	Inability to auscultate fetal heart tones with a fetal Doppler at 12 weeks may indicate a retroverted uterus, uncertain dates, fetal demise or false pregnancy. Fetal heart rate decelerations could indicate poor placental perfusion. In breech presentations, fetal heart rate is heard in the upper quadrant of maternal abdomen.
The fetal heart will be heard through the fetal shoulder, depending on the position of the fetus. Display 31-1 provides possible locations, depending on position of the fetus to guide you.	Fetal heart rate ranges from 110 to 160 beats/minute. During the third trimester, the fetal heart rate should accelerate with fetal movement (Fig. 31-10).	An inability to hear the fetal heart or a fetal heart rate that is not within normal limits requires immediate obstetric assessment.

CLINICAL TIP

A fetal Doppler ultrasound device can be used after 10 to 12 weeks' gestation to hear the fetal heartbeat.

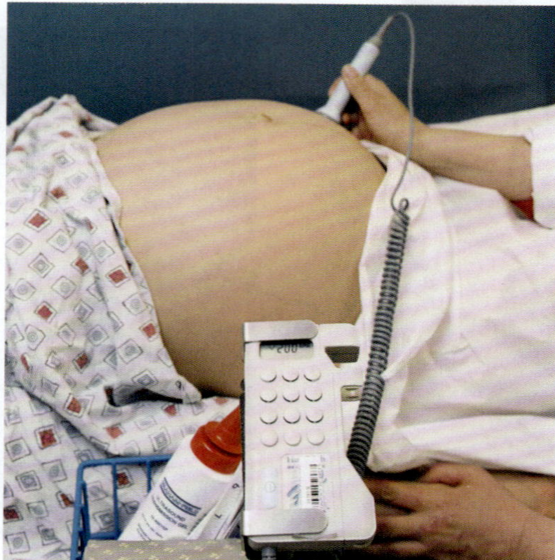
FIGURE 31-10 Auscultating the fetal heart rate with a Doppler ultrasound device. (© B. Proud.)

DISPLAY 31-1 WHERE TO AUSCULTATE FETAL HEART RATE

The illustrations below represent the best locations for auscultating the fetal heart rate: Left occiput anterior (LOA), right occiput anterior (ROA), left occiput posterior (LOP), right occiput posterior (ROP), left sacrum anterior (LSA) and right sacrum posterior (RSP).

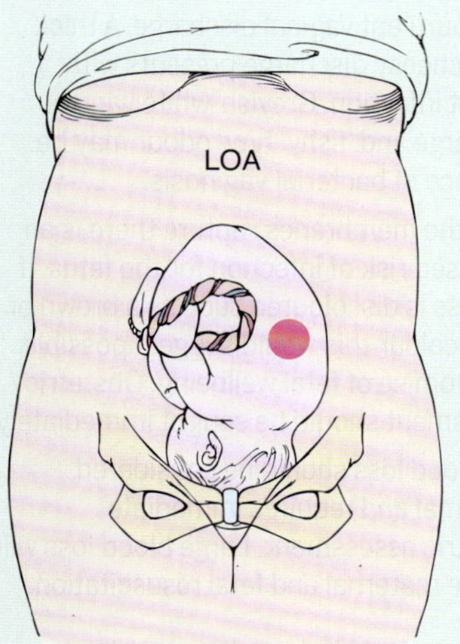

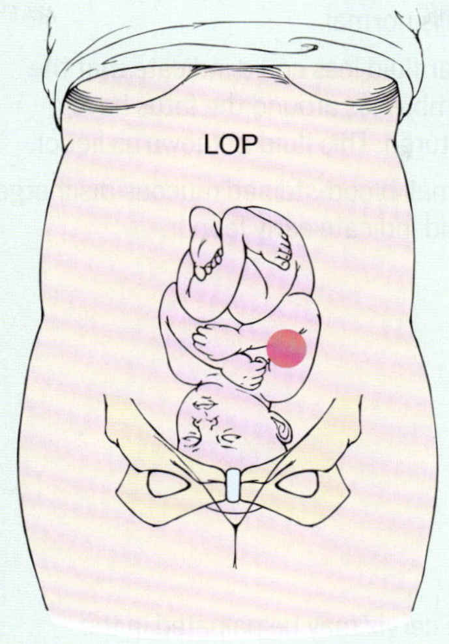

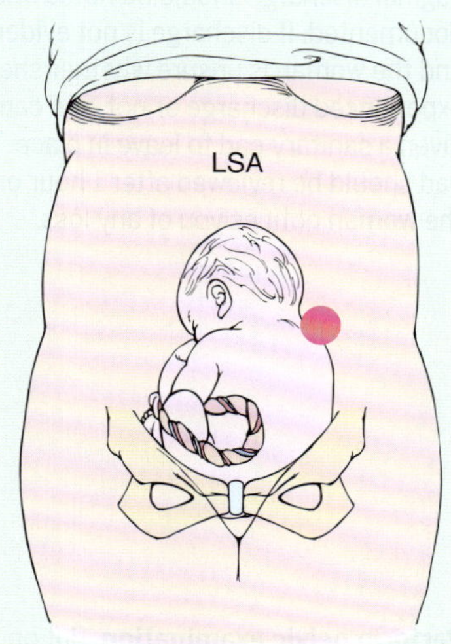

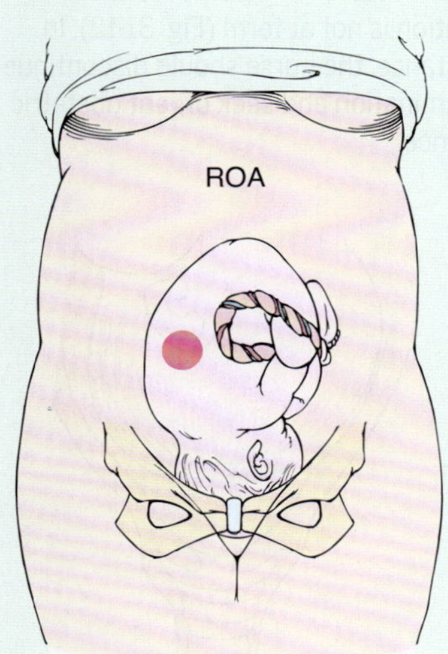

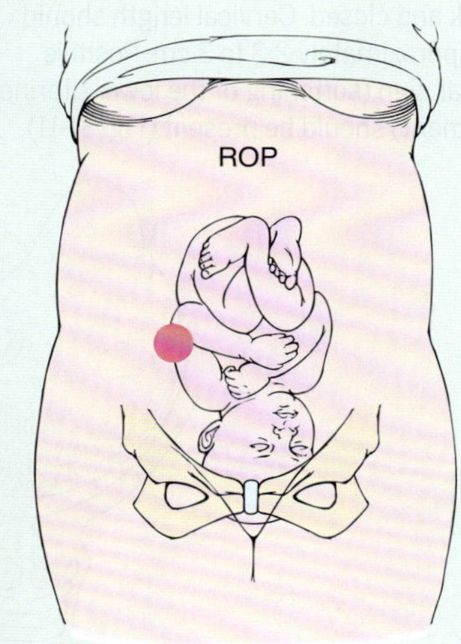

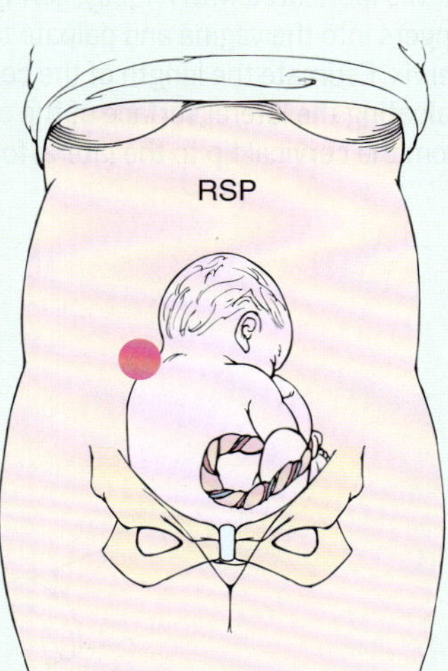

PHYSICAL ASSESSMENT (continued)

ASSESSMENT PROCEDURE	NORMAL FINDINGS	ABNORMAL FINDINGS
Genitalia—performed only by a pracititoner with specialist skills		
EXTERNAL GENITALIA		
Inspect the external genitalia. Note hair distribution, colour of skin, varicosities and scars.	Normal findings include enlarged labia and clitoris, parous relaxation of the introitus, and scars from an episiotomy or perineal lacerations (in multiparous women).	Labial varicosities, which can be painful.
Palpate the Bartholin and Skene glands.	There should be no discomfort or discharge with examination.	Discomfort and discharge noted with palpation may indicate infection.
Inspect vaginal opening for cystocele or rectocele.	No cystocele or rectocele.	Cystocele or rectocele may be more pronounced because of the muscle relaxation of pregnancy.

Continued on following page

PHYSICAL ASSESSMENT (continued)

ASSESSMENT PROCEDURE	NORMAL FINDINGS	ABNORMAL FINDINGS
Vaginal discharge should be noted and documented. If discharge is not evident and the woman is unsure whether she has experienced discharge or not, she can be given a sanitary pad to leave in place. The pad should be reviewed after 1 hour or if the woman notifies you of any loss.	Whitish vaginal discharge may be evident and is normal. Clear fluid loss could indicate that the membranes around the fetus have ruptured. This fluid is known as liquor. A small blood-stained mucous discharge could indicate early labour.	Gonorrhoea infection may present with thick purulent vaginal discharge. A thick white cheesy discharge presents with a yeast infection. Greyish-white vaginal discharge and 'fishy' type odour may be evidence of bacterial vaginosis. Once the membranes rupture there is an increased risk of infection for the fetus. If this loss is discoloured such as a brown or green colour this would suggest possible compromise of fetal wellbeing. Obstetric assessment should be sought immediately. Any blood loss should be considered abnormal and requires immediate obstetric assessment. Large blood loss will require maternal and fetal resuscitation.
Perform pelvic examination. Put on gloves lubricated with KY jelly, gently insert fingers into the vagina and palpate the cervix. Estimate the length of the cervix by palpating the lateral surface of the cervix from the cervical tip to the lateral fornix.	The cervix may be palpated in the posterior vaginal vault. It should be long, thick and closed. Cervical length should be approximately 2.3 to 3 cm. Positive Hegar sign (softening of the lower uterine segment) should be present (Fig. 31-11).	An effaced opened cervix may indicate preterm labour or an incompetent cervix if gestation is not at term (Fig. 31-12). In this instance, the nurse should discontinue the examination and seek urgent obstetric assistance.

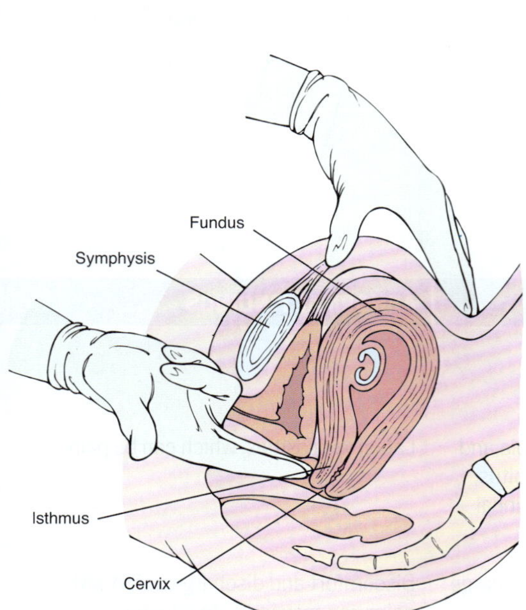

FIGURE 31-11 Positive Hegar sign.

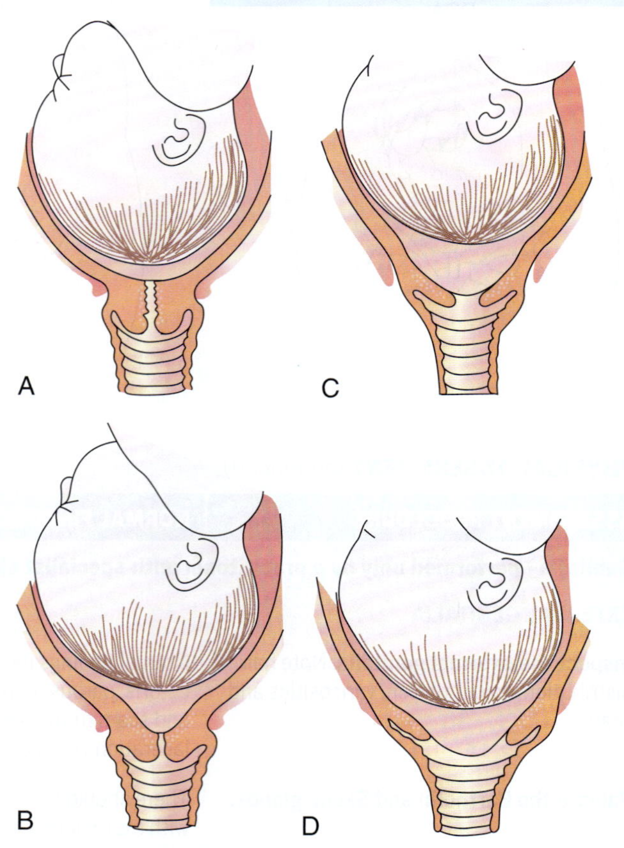

FIGURE 31-12 Effacement and dilation. **(A)** Before labour, 0% effacement. **(B)** Early effacement, 30%. **(C)** Complete effacement, 100%. **(D)** Complete effacement and dilation. (Haley, C. [2012]. *Pillitteri's child and family health nursing in Australia and New Zealand.* Sydney: Lippincott Williams & Wilkins.)

PHYSICAL ASSESSMENT (continued)

ASSESSMENT PROCEDURE	NORMAL FINDINGS	ABNORMAL FINDINGS
Feel for uterus. While leaving the fingers in the vagina, place the other hand on the abdomen and gently press down towards the internal hand until you feel the uterus between the two hands.	The uterus should feel about the size of an orange at 10 weeks (palpable at the suprapubic bone) and about the size of a grapefruit at 12 weeks.	If uterine size is not consistent with dates, consider the possibility of incorrect dates, uterine fibroids or multiple gestation.
Palpate the left and right adnexa.	No masses should be palpable. Discomfort with examination is due to stretching of the round ligaments throughout the pregnancy.	Adnexal masses may indicate ectopic pregnancy (Fig. 31-13).
Anus and rectum		
Inspect the anus and rectum. Note colour, varicosities, lesions, tears or discharge.	Mucosa should be pink and intact. No varicosities, lesions, tears or discharge present. Haemorrhoids or varicose veins may be present. Haemorrhoids usually get bigger and more uncomfortable during pregnancy. Bleeding and infection may occur.	Masses may indicate cancer.

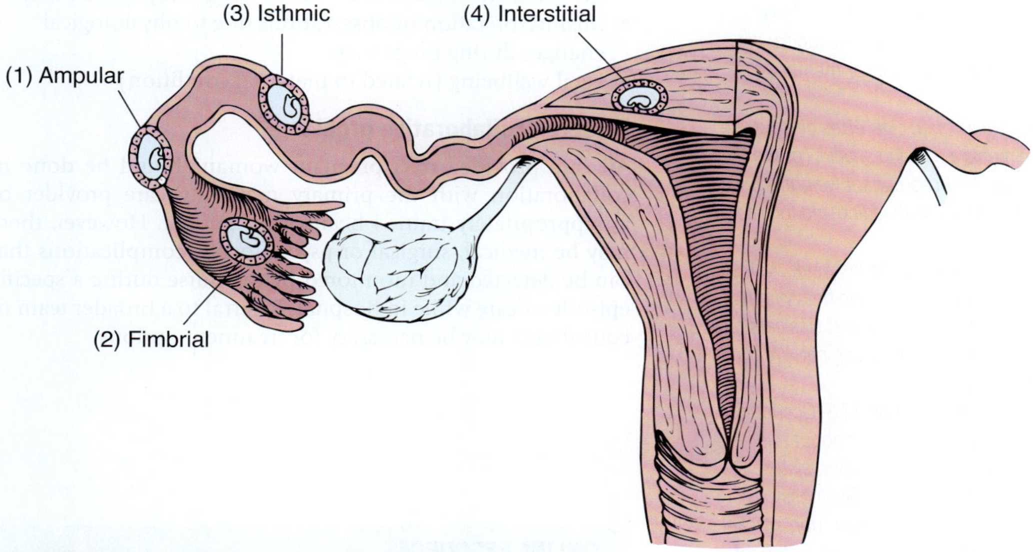

(3) Isthmic
(4) Interstitial
(1) Ampular
(2) Fimbrial

FIGURE 31-13 Sites of ectopic pregnancy.

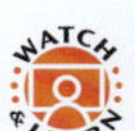

Developmental tasks of pregnancy: 1st trimester: Accepting the pregnancy

Developmental tasks of pregnancy: 2nd trimester: Accepting the baby

Developmental tasks of pregnancy: 3rd trimester: Preparing for parenthood

VALIDATING AND DOCUMENTING FINDINGS

Validate the assessment data that you have collected with the childbearing woman. This is necessary to verify that the data are reliable and accurate. Document the health history and examination data following the health care facility or agency policy. This would include completing the pregnancy record appropriate for the district in which you work. Any concerns voiced by the woman should be noted and considered.

Sample of subjective data

The woman is 28 weeks pregnant and has been well during her pregnancy with occasional nausea. She lives with her partner of 4 years. Non-smoker, and no alcohol since she found out she was pregnant. No vaginal loss or bleeding at present. No pain. States she can feel the baby moving since the accident.

Past history: Gravida 1 Parity 0 LMP 2/20/05. Normal period: 28-day cycle. No reported history of vaginal infections or STIs; partner also negative for STIs. Blood type: A positive. Medical history: unremarkable. Allergies: no known drug allergies. Surgeries: none. Hospitalisations: none. Gynaecological: no problems. Cervical screening: up to date and normal. Breasts: unremarkable. Current medications: pregnancy multivitamin one daily. Ethnicity: Causcasian.

Family history: No history of early deaths, diabetes, tuberculosis, asthma, cancer, birth defects, blood abnormalities or mental disorders.

Lifestyle and health practices: No alcohol, cigarettes or drug use since LMP. Diet consists of three meals a day and snacks (primarily meats, vegetables, fruits, bread, water). Prepregnant weight is 58 kg. Current vitamins: pregnancy multivitamin (with iodine and folic acid) once daily.

Activity and exercise: Exercises three to five times week. Walks 30 minutes; occasional weightlifting with aerobics. No heavy lifting or heavy labour. Reports no exposure to toxic substances. Has cats but does not change litter. Washes hands well after petting cat. Wears gloves if working outdoors in dirt or plants.

Role and relationships: Highest level education: M.S. Occupation: Registered Nurse. Lives with husband, who is excited about this planned pregnancy. Additional support: parents, in-laws, sister and friends. Partner: highest level education B.S. in Business Administration; current occupation: business manager; non-smoker; drinks alcohol occasionally on weekends with friends; no history of recreational drug use.

Sample of objective data

Blood pressure 120/80 mmHg; pulse 95 beats/minute; temperature 36.6°C; height 170 cm; weight 65 kg. Behaviour: anxious. Skin: some hyperpigmentation. Hair/nails: soft, smooth, clean. Thorax/lungs: clear to auscultate bilaterally. Heart: normal sinus rhythm without murmur. Abdomen: soft, non-tender; fundal height measured 28 cm above symphysis pubis. Fetal heart tones: audible with fetal Doppler, rate 158 beats/minute. Peripheral vascular: face/extremities: no oedema; pink, well perfused; pulses equal bilaterally.

Analysis of data

Diagnostic reasoning: Possible conclusions

After collecting subjective and objective data pertaining to the assessment of the pregnant woman during an episode of care, you will need to identify abnormalities and cluster the data to reveal any significant patterns or abnormalities. This information will then be used in collaboration with the primary maternity provider to make clinical judgements about the status of the woman during the specific episode of care.

Potential client risks

- Maternal stress (related to anxiety regarding assessment)
- Misinterpretation of observations due to physiological changes during pregnancy
- Fetal wellbeing (related to maternal condition)

Selected collaborative problems

All care provided to a pregnant woman should be done in collaboration with the primary maternity care provider or an appropriately trained health professional. However, there may be medical, surgical or psychological complications that can be detected and monitored by the nurse during a specific episode of care while in hospital. Referral to a broader team of consultants may be necessary for treatment options.

ONLINE RESOURCES

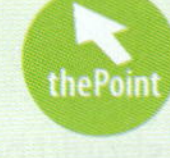

An extensive range of additional resources to enhance teaching and learning and to facilitate understanding may be found online at the text's accompanying website, located on thePoint at http://thepoint.lww.com. These include Watch and Learn videos, Concepts in Action animations, journal articles, case studies, discussion topics and quizzes.

Subscribers may also access Lippincott Procedures, an extensive online point-of-care procedure guide that provides reliable step-by-step instructions for more than 1700 procedures, including 450 evidence-based Australian procedures, and skills in a variety of speciality settings, together with a wealth of supporting information.

CASE STUDY

Another case study below demonstrates how to analyse pregnancy assessment data for a specific client. The exercises included in the ancillary product on thePoint that complements this text offer further opportunities to enhance your skills.

Mrs Hani Yusuf is a 29-year-old woman, gravida 3, parity 2, who presents to the clinic today for her initial antenatal examination. She states that her last menstrual period was on 15 September, approximately 16 weeks ago. Because she was unable to get transportation to the clinic, she did not come in for antenatal care earlier in this pregnancy. 'I do know how important early antenatal care is, but I just couldn't get here. And I feel good—no problems so far.'

Mrs Yusuf lives with her husband and two sons in a two-bedroom granny flat on land owned by her in-laws. She states that her in-laws are very supportive and help out during tough times by not charging rent. Her husband works full-time at a fast-food restaurant chain but is looking for a job that pays more money. It is often hard for them to meet their financial responsibilities; however, they believe it is important for her to stay home with the children, so she does not contribute financially. She reports that, in general, she encourages healthy practices for herself and family, but because her husband gets a discount on food from his work, they don't eat as well as she knows they should. 'But I am eating less so I don't gain so much weight this time.' Mrs Yusuf's past medical history is unremarkable; her two pregnancies were term gestations that she birthed vaginally. However, during the last pregnancy, she was diagnosed with pregnancy-induced hypertension and gestational diabetes, and labour was induced at 38 weeks' gestation. She states that she gained 28 kg with that pregnancy and that her son weighed 4.2 kg.

Your physical assessment of Mrs Yusuf reveals a blood pressure of 100/60 mmHg (right arm, sitting); a pulse rate of 86 beats/minute, regular and strong; respirations of 18 breaths/minute, regular and moderately shallow; and a temperature of 36.7 °C. Her apical beat is also 86 beats/minute and strong; heart sounds: S_1 and S_2 with no murmurs or clicks. Mrs Yusuf's skin is warm and dry, slightly pale with light-pink nail beds, pale palpebral conjunctiva and oral mucous membranes. Her abdomen is moderately rounded with striae; fundal height is 20 cm; fetal heart rate is 158 beats/minute per Doppler, right lower quadrant. Mrs Yusuf's current weight is 63 kg, 1 kg less than her stated usual weight, and height is 175 cm. Results of laboratory tests show haemoglobin at 10.2 g/dL, haematocrit at 29.9% and red blood cell count at $3.20 \times 10^{-6}/mm^3$. The remainder of the blood values is within normal limits. Urinalysis results are negative for protein and glucose.

The following concept map illustrates the diagnostic reasoning process.

Applying COLDSPA

Applying COLDSPA for symptoms: '29-year-old woman G3 P2; LMP 16 weeks ago'.

Mnemonic	Question	Data provided	Missing data
Character	Describe the sign or symptom (feeling, appearance, sound, smell or taste, if applicable).	Woman says she feels good but has no transportation to get to clinic for antenatal care during the last 16 weeks.	How did you get to the clinic today?
Onset	When did it begin?	During the woman's last pregnancy, she gained 28 kg and her son weighed 4.2 kg at birth. She tries to eat healthy, but says her husband brings home free 'fast-food' often.	
Location	Where is it? Does it radiate? Does it occur anywhere else?		
Duration	How long does it last? Does it recur?		What is your typical fluid and food intake at this time? Are you taking any antenatal vitamins? What proteins do you typically eat?
Severity	How bad is it? or How much does it bother you?	Woman is 175 cm and weighs 63 kg; 1 kilogram less than normal stated weight. Oral mucous membranes and conjunctiva are pale.	
Pattern	What makes it better or worse?	During her last pregnancy, the woman was diagnosed with pregnancy-induced hypertension and gestational diabetes. Labour was induced at 38 weeks.	
Associated factors/How it Affects the client	What other symptoms occur with it? How does it affect you?	The woman has financial concerns; her husband works at a fast-food chain and is looking for a betterpaying job.	What antenatal resources does the woman qualify for and which ones has the woman used in the past?

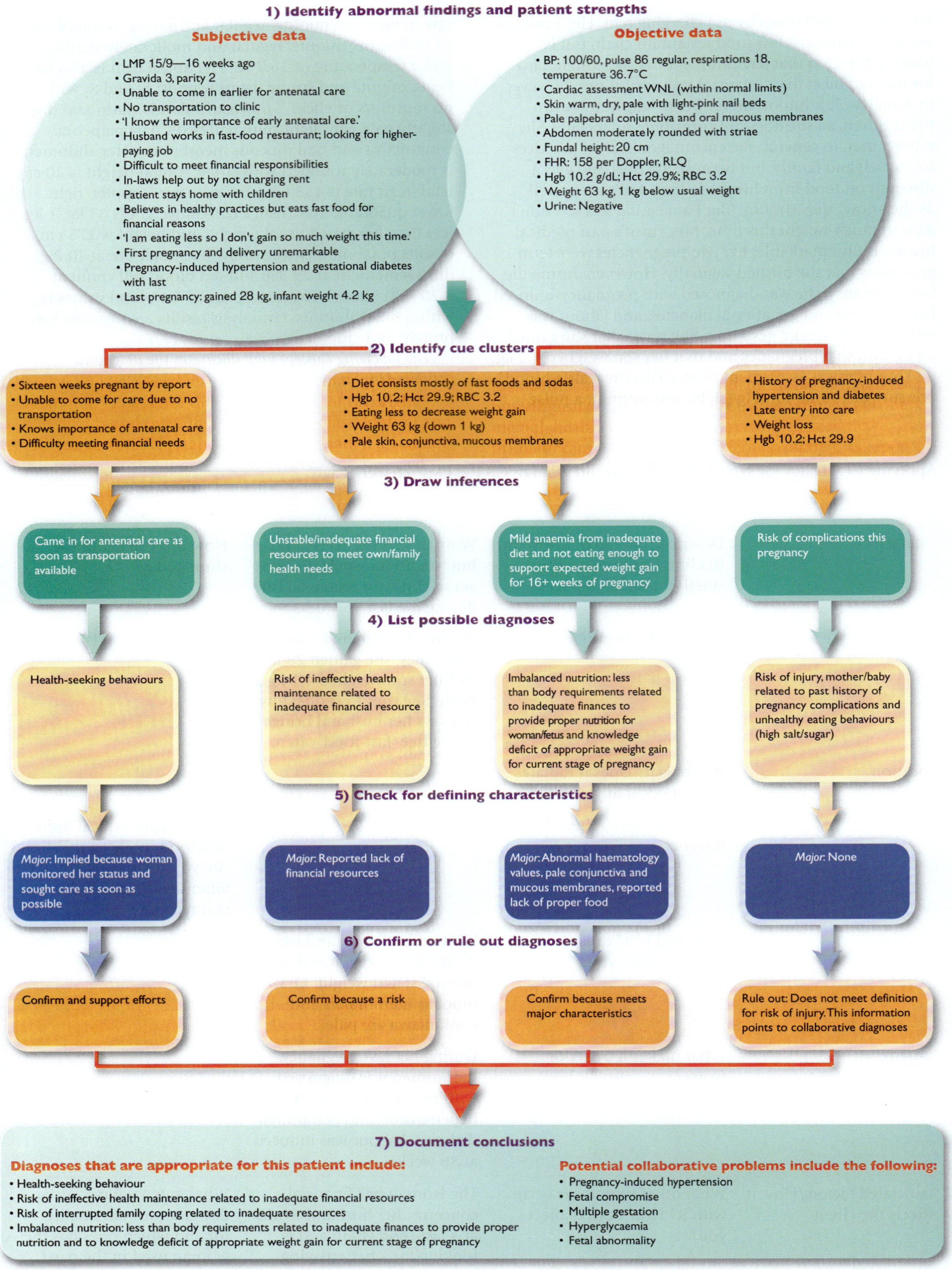

1) Identify abnormal findings and patient strengths

Subjective data

- LMP 15/9—16 weeks ago
- Gravida 3, parity 2
- Unable to come in earlier for antenatal care
- No transportation to clinic
- 'I know the importance of early antenatal care.'
- Husband works in fast-food restaurant; looking for higher-paying job
- Difficult to meet financial responsibilities
- In-laws help out by not charging rent
- Patient stays home with children
- Believes in healthy practices but eats fast food for financial reasons
- 'I am eating less so I don't gain so much weight this time.'
- First pregnancy and delivery unremarkable
- Pregnancy-induced hypertension and gestational diabetes with last
- Last pregnancy: gained 28 kg, infant weight 4.2 kg

Objective data

- BP: 100/60, pulse 86 regular, respirations 18, temperature 36.7°C
- Cardiac assessment WNL (within normal limits)
- Skin warm, dry, pale with light-pink nail beds
- Pale palpebral conjunctiva and oral mucous membranes
- Abdomen moderately rounded with striae
- Fundal height: 20 cm
- FHR: 158 per Doppler, RLQ
- Hgb 10.2 g/dL; Hct 29.9%; RBC 3.2
- Weight 63 kg, 1 kg below usual weight
- Urine: Negative

2) Identify cue clusters

- Sixteen weeks pregnant by report
- Unable to come for care due to no transportation
- Knows importance of antenatal care
- Difficulty meeting financial needs

- Diet consists mostly of fast foods and sodas
- Hgb 10.2; Hct 29.9; RBC 3.2
- Eating less to decrease weight gain
- Weight 63 kg (down 1 kg)
- Pale skin, conjunctiva, mucous membranes

- History of pregnancy-induced hypertension and diabetes
- Late entry into care
- Weight loss
- Hgb 10.2; Hct 29.9

3) Draw inferences

Came in for antenatal care as soon as transportation available

Unstable/inadequate financial resources to meet own/family health needs

Mild anaemia from inadequate diet and not eating enough to support expected weight gain for 16+ weeks of pregnancy

Risk of complications this pregnancy

4) List possible diagnoses

Health-seeking behaviours

Risk of ineffective health maintenance related to inadequate financial resource

Imbalanced nutrition: less than body requirements related to inadequate finances to provide proper nutrition for woman/fetus and knowledge deficit of appropriate weight gain for current stage of pregnancy

Risk of injury, mother/baby related to past history of pregnancy complications and unhealthy eating behaviours (high salt/sugar)

5) Check for defining characteristics

Major: Implied because woman monitored her status and sought care as soon as possible

Major: Reported lack of financial resources

Major: Abnormal haematology values, pale conjunctiva and mucous membranes, reported lack of proper food

Major: None

6) Confirm or rule out diagnoses

Confirm and support efforts

Confirm because a risk

Confirm because meets major characteristics

Rule out: Does not meet definition for risk of injury. This information points to collaborative diagnoses

7) Document conclusions

Diagnoses that are appropriate for this patient include:

- Health-seeking behaviour
- Risk of ineffective health maintenance related to inadequate financial resources
- Risk of interrupted family coping related to inadequate resources
- Imbalanced nutrition: less than body requirements related to inadequate finances to provide proper nutrition and to knowledge deficit of appropriate weight gain for current stage of pregnancy

Potential collaborative problems include the following:

- Pregnancy-induced hypertension
- Fetal compromise
- Multiple gestation
- Hyperglycaemia
- Fetal abnormality

References

American College of Obstetricians and Gynecologists (ACOG). (2017). Smoking cessation during pregnancy. Available at www.acog.org.

Bailey, B. & Sokol, R. (2011). Antenatal alcohol exposure and miscarriage, stillbirth, preterm delivery and sudden infant death syndrome. *Alcohol Research & Health, 34*(1), 86–91.

Department of Health. (2019). *Clinical practice guidelines: Pregnancy care*. Canberra: Australian Government Department of Health.

Eustace, J., Baird, K., Saito, A., et al. (2016). 'Midwives' experiences of routine enquiry for intimate partner violence in pregnancy. *Women and Birth: Journal of the Australian College of Midwives, 29*(6), 503–510.

Forray, A. (2016). Substance use during pregnancy. *F1000Research, 5*, F1000 Faculty Rev-887. doi:10.12688/f1000research.7645.1.

Gilbert, E. (2011). *Manual of high risk pregnancy and delivery* (5th ed.). Phoenix, AZ: Mosby/Elsevier.

Gilmore, L. & Redman, L. (2015). Weight gain in pregnancy and application of the 2009 IOM guidelines: Toward a uniform approach. *Obesity, 23*(3), 507–511.

Gray, J. & Smith, R. (2018). *Midwifery essentials* (2nd ed.). Sydney: Churchill Livingstone.

Haley, C. (2012). *Pillitteri's child and family health nursing in Australia and New Zealand* (1st ed.). Sydney: Lippincott Williams & Wilkins.

Hanley, J. (2009). *Perinatal mental health*. West Sussex: Wiley Blackwell.

Hinman, S., Smith, K., Quillen, D., et al. (2015). Exercise in pregnancy: A clinical review. *Sports Health, 7*(6), 527–531.

Johnson, R. & Taylor, W. (2019). *Skills for midwifery practice* (ANZ ed.). Edinburgh: Churchill Livingstone.

Madjunkov, M., Chaudhry, S. & Ito, S. (2017). Listeriosis during pregnancy. *Archives of Gynaecology and Obstetrics, 296*(2), 143–152.

Pairman, S., Tracy, S., Dahlen, H., et al. (Eds). (2019). *Midwifery preparation for practice* (4th ed.). Sydney: Elsevier.

Radestad, I. & Lindgren, H. (2012). Women's perceptions of fetal movements in full-term pregnancy. *Sexual & Reproductive Healthcare, 3*(3), 113–116.

Rowe, S., Perrett, K., Morey, R., et al. (2019). Influenza and pertussis vaccination of women during pregnancy in Victoria, 2015-2017. *The Medical Journal of Australia, 210*(10), 454–462.

Royal Australian and New Zealand College of Obstetricians and Gynaecologists (RANZCOG). 2017. Cervical cancer screening in Australia. Available at https://ranzcog.edu.au/RANZCOG_SITE/media/RANZCOG-MEDIA/Women%27s%20Health/Statement%20and%20guidelines/Clinical-Obstetrics/Cervical-cancer-screening-in-Australia-(C-Gyn-19)-Review-July-2017.pdf?ext=.pdf.

Sandall, J., Soltani, H., Gates, S., et al. (2013). Midwife-led continuity models versus other models of care for childbearing women. *The Cochrane Database of Systematic Reviews*, (8), Art. no.: CD004667.

South Australian Department of Health. (2015). Normal pregnancy, labour and puerperium management clinical guideline. South Australian perinatal practice guidelines. Available at https://www.sahealth.sa.gov.au/wps/wcm/connect/26cf8d004ee52a4fa536add150ce4f37/Normal+Pregnancy%2C+Labour+and+Puerperium_Sept2015.pdf?MOD=AJPERES&CACHEID=ROOTWORKSPACE-26cf8d004ee52a4fa536add150ce4f37-mN5MAUV.

South Australian Department of Health. (2017). South Australian GP obstetric shared care protocols 2017. South Australian perinatal practice guidelines. Available at https://www.sahealth.sa.gov.au/wps/wcm/connect/950d1700491685ff975eff9006c065a9/SA+GPOSC+Protocols_CD_v3_0.pdf?MOD=AJPERES&CACHEID=ROOTWORKSPACE-950d1700491685ff975eff9006c065a9-mMHHSYx.

Tracy, S., Hartz, D., Tracy, M., et al. (2013). Caseload midwifery care versus standard maternity care for women of any risk: M@NGO, a randomised controlled trial. *The Lancet, 382*(9906), 1723–1732.

Wehby, G., Prater, K., McCarthy, A., et al. (2011). The impact of maternal smoking during pregnancy on early child neurodevelopment. *Journal of Human Capital, 5*(2), 207–254.

Willis, E. & Reynolds, L. (Eds). (2016). *Understanding the Australian health care system* (3rd ed.). Melbourne: Elsevier.

Selected readings

Australian Nursing & Midwifery Council (ANMC). (2018a). Code of ethics midwives. Viewed September 2019 at www.nursingmidwiferyboard.gov.au.

Australian Nursing & Midwifery Council (ANMC). (2018b). *Midwife standards for practice*. Dickson, ACT: Author. Available at www.nursingmidwiferyboard.gov.au.

Australian Nursing and Midwifery Council (ANMC). (2018c). Code of conduct for midwives. Viewed September 2019 at www.nursingmidwiferyboard.gov.au.

Cunningham, E., Levano, K., Bloom, S., et al. (2018). *William's obstetrics* (25th ed.). New York: McGraw-Hill.

Daemers, D., Limbeek, E., Wijnen, H., et al. (2017). Factors influencing the clinical decision-making of midwives: A qualitative study. *BMC Pregnancy and Childbirth, 17*(345), doi:10.1186/s12884-017-1511-5.

Feghali, M., Venkataramanan, R. & Caritis, S. (2015). Pharmacokinetics of drugs in pregnancy. *Seminars in Perinatology, 39*(7), 512–519.

Naughton, F., Hopewell, S., Sinclair, L., et al. (2018). Barriers and facilitators to smoking cessation in pregnancy and in the postpartum period: The health care professionals' perspective. *British Journal of Health Psychology, 23*(3), 741–757.

Reitan, T. (2017). Substance abuse during pregnancy: A 5-year follow-up of mothers and children. *Drugs: Education, Prevention and Policy, 26*(3), 219–228.

Stables, D. & Rankin, J. (2017). *Physiology in childbearing with anatomy and related biosciences* (4th ed.). London: Elsevier.

Online resources

Australian College of Midwives Incorporated: www.midwives.org.au
Australian Department of Health and Ageing: www.health.gov.au
Australian Indigenous Health*InfoNet*: www.healthinfonet.ecu.edu.au
Cancer Council Australia: www.cancer.org.au
Cancer Society of New Zealand: www.cancernz.org.nz
Centre for Culture, Ethnicity and Health: www.ceh.org.au
Congress of Aboriginal and Torres Strait Islander Nurses and Midwives (CATSINaM): http://catsin.org.au
Midwifery Council of New Zealand/Te Tatau o te Whare Kahu (Wellington): www.midwiferycouncil.health.nz
New Zealand College of Midwives Incorporated (Christchurch): www.midwife.org.nz
New Zealand Ministry of Health: www.health.govt.nz
Nursing and Midwifery Board of Australia (NMBA): www.nursingmidwiferyboard.gov.au
Royal Australian and New Zealand College of Obstetricians and Gynaecologists, guidelines: www.ranzcog.edu.au

CHAPTER **32**

Assessing newborns and infants

> **CASE STUDY**
>
> *Two-month-old Lee Simpson is admitted to the ward with bronchiolitis. It is her first presentation after being unwell for 3 days with a runny nose and fever. Today she has been wheezy and had decreased feeding. She has been admitted for monitoring, oxygen therapy and small frequent feeds. As the nurse caring for Lee, you begin to attend to her admission, where a full physical assessment needs to be completed. While you are doing the assessment, Lee's mother Bianca tells you she is anxious and isn't sure how to care for Lee when she is so unwell.*

> **CRITICAL THINKING**
>
> Note that when assessing an infant, you are really assessing the mother and infant as a pair.
> 1. What do you know about assessing an infant?
> 2. What type of questions would you ask to establish Lee's wellbeing?
> 3. What type of questions would you ask to determine how Bianca is coping with parenthood?

Structure and function

A *newborn,* or neonate, is the term used to describe a child from birth to 28 days old. It can also refer to a premature infant by corrected age (premature baby's chronological age minus the number of weeks born early) (Harel-Gadassi et al., 2018). An *infant* refers to a child between the ages of 28 days and 1 year. In Australia, the immediate care of a newborn is attended to by a midwife or a neonatal nurse.

SKIN, HAIR AND NAILS

At birth, the newborn's skin is smooth and thin. In a term baby (born from the 38th to the 42nd week gestation), the skin should be soft and may have mild peripheral peeling. The skin is pink with acrocyanosis and has varying amounts of vernix, which is normal and is absorbed (Kain & Mannix, 2018).

In a preterm baby, the skin may appear reddish because of visible blood circulation through the newborn's thin layer of subcutaneous fat. This thin layer of fat, combined with the skin's inability to contract and shiver, results in ineffective temperature regulation. The skin may appear mottled on the trunk, arms or legs. The dermis and epidermis are thin and loosely bound together, increasing the skin's susceptibility to infection and irritation and creating a poor barrier, which results in fluid loss.

After birth, the newborn's sebaceous glands are active because of high levels of maternal androgen. Milia, white spots found on the face and chest, develop when these glands become plugged. Eccrine glands function at birth, creating palmar sweating, which is helpful when assessing pain. Apocrine glands stay small and non-functional until puberty.

The fine, downy hairs called lanugo, which appear on the newborn's body, shoulders or back at birth, develop in the fetus at 3 months' gestation and disappear within the first 2 weeks of life. Scalp hair–follicle growth phases occur concurrently at birth but are disrupted during early infancy. This may result in overgrowth or alopecia (hair loss).

Nails are usually present at birth. Missing or short nails usually signify prematurity, and long nails usually signify postmaturity. Nails are usually pink, convex and smooth throughout childhood and adolescence.

The baby may also have areas of pigmentation or birthmarks, such as hyperpigmented macules, superficial nevi, erythema toxicum and milia. Although these areas commonly disappear without treatment, they may need review by a paediatrician, and parents will need education for ongoing care (Pairman et al., 2019).

HEAD AND NECK

Head growth predominates during the fetal period. At birth, the circumference of the head is larger (by 2 cm) than that of the chest. The cranial bones are soft and separated by the coronal, lambdoid and sagittal sutures, which intersect at the anterior and posterior fontanelle (Fig. 32-1). Ossification begins in infancy and continues into adulthood.

The newborn's skull is typically asymmetrical (plagiocephaly) because of moulding that occurs as the newborn passes through the birth canal. The skull moulds easily during birth, allowing for overlapping of the cranial bones.

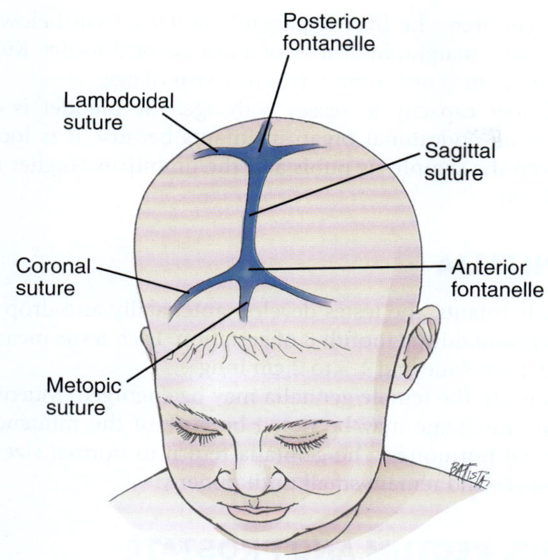

FIGURE 32-1 The infant head.

The posterior fontanelle usually measures 1 to 2 cm at birth and usually closes by 6 weeks. The anterior fontanelle usually measures 1 to 4 cm at birth and closes between 12 and 18 months (Marshall & Raynor, 2014).

CLINICAL TIP
A full anterior fontanelle may be palpable when the newborn cries.

Visible pulsations may also appear, representing the peripheral pulse. The sutures and fontanelles allow the skull to expand to accommodate brain growth. Brain growth is reflected by head circumference (occipital–frontal circumference), which may be smaller on the first day compared with day 2 or 3. An oedematous area over the presenting part of the scalp at birth is a caput succedaneum that extends over the suture lines and resolves within 36 hours. A cephalhaematoma is a soft mass of blood in the subperiosteal space on the surface of the skull bone. This mass does not cross suture lines, appears 12 hours after the birth and may take weeks to resolve (Marshall & Raynor, 2014). The head circumference increases six times as much during the first year as it does during the second. Half of postnatal brain growth is achieved within the first year of life.

The neck is usually short during infancy (lengthening at about age 3 or 4 years). Lymphoid tissue is well developed at birth and reaches adult size by age 6 years.

EYES

Eyes should be observed for position, with the space between one eye and the nose and the other eye equal at one-third each. Hypotelorism may be a characteristic of fetal alcohol syndrome. Eye structure and function are not fully developed at birth (Kain & Mannix, 2018). The iris shows little pigment and the pupils are small. The macula, which is absent at birth, develops at 4 months and is mature by 8 months. Pupillary reflex is poor at birth and improves at age 5 months. The sclera is clear. Small subconjunctival haemorrhages are normal after birth. Peripheral vision is developed, but central vision is not. The newborn is farsighted and has a visual acuity of 20/200. At 4 months, an infant can fixate on a singular object with both eyes simultaneously (binocularity). Tearing and voluntary control over eye muscles begin at 2 to 3 months; by 4 months, infants establish binocular vision and focus on a single image with both eyes simultaneously. These functions are better developed by 9 months. Newborns cannot distinguish between colours; this ability develops by 8 months.

EARS

The ear pinna should be positioned above a line extended from the inner to outer canthus of the eye. Low set ears should act as an alert for congenital anomalies. Skin tags may be present most commonly in front of the earlobe and are usually benign (Pairman et al., 2019). The inner ear develops during the first trimester of gestation. Therefore, maternal problems during this time, such as rubella, may impair hearing. Newborns can hear loud sounds at 90 decibels and react with the startle reflex. They respond to low-frequency sounds, such as a heartbeat or lullaby, by decreasing crying and motor movement. They react to high-frequency sounds with an alerting reaction. In infants, the external auditory canal curves upwards and is short and straight. Therefore, the pinna must be pulled down and back to perform an otoscopic examination. The eustachian tube is wider, shorter and more horizontal, increasing the possibility of infection rising from the pharynx.

FACE, MOUTH, THROAT, NOSE AND SINUS

The facial features should be symmetrical. Asymmetry may be due to facial palsy following forceps application (Kain & Mannix, 2018). Saliva is minimal at birth, but drooling is evident by 3 months because of the increased secretion of saliva. Drooling persists for a few months until the infant learns to swallow the saliva. Drooling does not signify tooth eruption. The development of both temporary (deciduous) and permanent teeth begins in utero. Deciduous tooth eruption takes place between the ages of 6 and 24 months.

The tonsils and adenoids are small in relation to body size and hard to see at birth. The pharynx is best seen when the newborn is crying.

Newborns are obligatory nose breathers and, therefore, have significant distress when their nasal passages are obstructed. The maxillary and ethmoid sinuses are present at birth, but they are small and cannot be examined until they develop.

THORAX AND LUNGS

At term gestation, the fetal lungs should be developed and the alveoli should be collapsed. Gas exchange is performed by the placenta. Immediately after birth, the lungs aerate; blood flows through them more vigorously, causing greater expansion and relaxation of the pulmonary arteries. The decrease in pulmonary pressure closes the foramen ovale, increasing oxygen tension and closing the ductus arteriosus. The lungs continue to develop after birth, and new alveoli form until about 8 years of age.

BREASTS

Ventral epidermal ridges (milk lines), which run from the axilla to the medial thigh, are present during gestation. True breasts develop along the thoracic ridge; the other breasts along the milk line atrophy. Occasionally, a supernumerary nipple persists along the ridge track. At birth, lactiferous ducts are present in the nipple, but there are no alveoli. Although the newborn's breasts may be temporarily enlarged from the effects of maternal oestrogen, they are usually flat and remain so until puberty.

HEART

Because oxygenation takes place in the placenta in fetal circulation, the lungs are bypassed and arterial blood is returned to the right side of the heart. Blood is shunted through the foramen ovale and ductus arteriosus into the left side of the heart and out the aorta. At birth, lung aeration causes circulatory changes. The foramen ovale closes within the first hour because of the newly created low pressure in the right side of the heart, and the ductus arteriosus closes about 10 to 15 hours after birth.

During auscultation of the heart in the infant, systolic murmurs may be audible due to the transition from intrauterine to extrauterine life. This murmur generally resolves within 24 to 48 hours after birth. The pulse rate at birth is usually between 120 and 160 beats/minute. The rate decreases as the child ages, declining to approximately 120 at 6 months and 110 from 6 months to 1 year old. The heart should be auscultated at approximately the fourth intercostal margin to the left of the midclavicular line. The heart lays more horizontal in the chest and may seem enlarged with percussion. Heart sounds are also more audible in the newborn secondary to the thin subcutaneous layer of skin on the newborn.

PERIPHERAL VASCULAR SYSTEM

The skin should appear pink and well perfused. The hands and feet may appear blue at times (acrocyanosis), which is normal, especially when the newborn is cold. With warming the extremities, skin colour should return to pink normal colour. If the infant does not respond to this technique, consider a congenital heart defect in the newborn.

Pulses should be felt in the extremities, with assessment of the radial, brachial and femoral pulses bilaterally. Weakness or absence of femoral pulses may indicate coarctation of the aorta. Bounding pulses can be seen with patent ductus arteriosus.

ABDOMEN

The umbilical cord is prominent in the newborn and contains two arteries and one vein. The umbilicus consists of two parts: the amniotic portion and the cutaneous portion. The amniotic portion is covered with a gel-like substance and dries up and falls off within 2 weeks of life. The cutaneous portion is covered with skin and draws back to become flush with the abdominal wall.

The abdomen of infants is cylindrical. Peristaltic waves may be visible and may be indicative of a disease or disorder. Bowel sounds can be audible on auscultation within 1 hour of birth after feeding and crying (Marshall & Raynor, 2014).

The liver of the newborn is palpable at 0.5 to 2.5 cm below the right costal margin, thereby occupying proportionately more space than at any other time after birth. In infants and small children, the liver is palpable at 1 to 2 cm below the right costal margin, indicative of a disease or disorder. Kidney development is not complete until 1 year of age.

Bladder capacity increases with age; the bladder is considered an abdominal organ in infants because it is located between the symphysis pubis and the umbilicus (higher than in adults).

GENITALIA

In male infants, the testes develop antenatally and drop into the scrotum during month 8 of gestation. Each testis measures about 1 cm wide and 1.5 to 2 cm long.

At birth, the female genitalia may be engorged. Mucoid or bloody discharge may be noted because of the influence of maternal hormones. The genitalia return to normal size in a few weeks and remain small until puberty.

ANUS, RECTUM AND PROSTATE

Meconium is passed during the first 24 hours of life, signifying anal patency. Stools are passed by reflex, and anal sphincter control is not reached until age 1.5 to 2 years, after the nerves supplying the area have become fully myelinated. Meconium not passed within 24 hours of birth could signify a problem. In boys, the prostate gland is underdeveloped and not palpable.

MUSCULOSKELETAL SYSTEM

At birth the newborn should have full range of motion of all extremities. Many newborns have feet that may appear deformed because of the intrauterine position of the extremities. The examiner should turn the feet to the normal position with ease.

The hips should also be checked for dislocation and ease of movement by the assessing doctor performing the Ortolani and Barlow tests.

The vertebral column of the newborn differs in contour from that of the normal adult. The spine has a single C-shaped curve at birth. By 3 to 4 months, the anterior curve in the cervical region develops from the infant raising its head when prone.

NEUROLOGICAL SYSTEM

The neurological system is not fully developed at birth. Motor control is maintained by the spinal cord and medulla, and most actions in the newborn are primitive reflexes. As myelinisation develops and the number of brain neurons grows rapidly, from the 30th week of gestation through to the first year of life, voluntary control and advanced cerebral functions appear and the more primitive reflexes diminish or disappear. The nervous system grows rapidly during fetal and early postnatal life, reaching 25% of adult capacity at birth, 50% by age 1 year, 80% by age 3 and 90% by age 7.

Newborns have rudimentary sensation; any stimulus must be strong to cause a reaction, and the response is not localised. A strong stimulus causes a vigorous response of crying with whole-body movements. As myelinisation develops, stimulus localisation becomes possible and the child responds in a more localised manner. Motor control develops in a head-to-neck to trunk-to-extremities sequence.

Health assessment

COLLECTING SUBJECTIVE DATA: THE NURSING HEALTH HISTORY

Interviewing parents

The initial assessment of the newborn occurs immediately after birth. Therefore, parent interviewing is not performed. However, the nurse needs to get a complete maternal history of the mother before and during pregnancy. Labour and birth record information is also imperative for the initial newborn assessment. This information is usually obtained from the maternal hospital chart. For assessment following initial birth assessment, the nurse or midwife interviews the parents.

Subjective assessment of the infant encompasses interviewing and compiling a complete nursing history from the parents or the primary carer. The nurse should:

- Use a friendly, non-judgemental approach when interviewing the family; use active listening skills; and provide empathy as appropriate.
- Portray proficiency and competence when talking with the parents.
- Explain the purpose of the interview and clarify any misunderstandings during this time.
- Explain the importance of obtaining accurate information about the infant to ensure that the correct diagnosis and treatment are provided for the infant.
- Realise that common behaviours of the family may not be portrayed at this setting.
- Appreciate that the unfamiliar setting and concern for the infant, especially if the infant is ill, may cause the parents to be very nervous and anxious during the interview. Provide a safe, relaxed environment to help the parents to be calm and be able to answer questions accurately.
- Understand that cultural variations may exist with the family.
- Be aware of barriers to effective communication between the nurse or midwife and the parents. These include time constraints, frequent interruptions, lack of privacy and language differences as well as provider callousness and cultural insensitivity. Make every effort to prevent these barriers.
- Provide enough time for the interview; keeping interruptions to a minimum, maintaining patient privacy and using interpreters when language barriers exist will help with obtaining accurate information regarding the newborn's history.

CASE STUDY

Bianca summarises the type of care provided to Lee before she became unwell. She states that Lee responds well to her voice and is generally content, drinks her bottle well, and sleeps through the night. You notice Bianca is attentive to the baby during the interview. When undressing Lee to obtain her weight, you notice she has slight intercostal recession and tracheal tug. You also notice her nose is blocked.

CRITICAL THINKING

4. What do these symptoms indicate to you?
5. How can you help Lee to become more comfortable?
6. What other observations should you consider?

Biographical data

QUESTION	RATIONALE
What is the child's name? Nickname? What are the parents' or carers' names?	Knowing personal information about the child and carers helps to establish rapport with the child and family.
Who is the child's primary health care provider, and when was the child's last well-child care appointment?	This determines the child's access to health care. It tells the nurse where to find the patient's previous medical information or record.
Where does the child live? (Address)	In addition, assess the family's living conditions.
Do the parents and child live in the same residence? Are the child's parents married, single, divorced, other? Who else lives in this residence? What are the parents' ages?	This indicates the availability of potential carers and support people for the patient. It also helps to define familial relationships.
What is the child's age? What is the child's date of birth?	This provides a reference for assessing developmental level.
Is the child adopted, foster, naturally conceived?	Certain health problems run in families. It is helpful to know the child's genetic relationship with the parents.
What is the child's ethic origin? Religion?	This information helps the nurse to examine special needs and beliefs that may affect the patient or family's health care.
What is occupation of child's parents?	What the parents do for a living provides insight into the economic status of the family.

History of present health concern/current health status

Elicit the reason for seeking care and ask questions about the child's current health status. During the first year of life, many visits to the health care provider will be well visits (checkups).

QUESTION	RATIONALE
Describe the child's general state of health. Does the child have a chronic illness?	Obtaining baseline information about the patient helps to identify important areas of assessment.
Does the child have any allergies? If so, what is the specific allergen? How does the child react to it?	This identifies allergens and helps the nurse plan to prevent exposure.
What prescriptions, over-the-counter medications, devices, treatments and home or natural remedies is the child taking? Please provide the name of the drug, dosage, frequency and reason it is administered.	It is always important to know what medications a patient is taking, especially if he or she is young.

COLDSPA

Example for difficulty with breastfeeding

If there is a health concern, use the COLDSPA mnemonic as a guideline to collect needed information for each symptom the patient shares.

Mnemonic	Question	Patient response example
Character	Describe the sign or symptom (feeling, appearance, sound, smell or taste, if applicable).	Difficulty with breastfeeding
Onset	When did it begin?	'On day 2 post birth.'
Location	Where is it? Does it radiate? Does it occur anywhere else?	'There is a lump on the outside of my right breast and I have a bleeding nipple.'
Duration	How long does it last? Does it recur?	'It is very painful from the start of my feed. Has been painful each time I have tried with the last two feeds.'
Severity	How bad is it? or How much does it bother you?	'It is painful even to attach my baby.'
Pattern	What makes it better or worse?	'I've tried many positions and still feeling pain.'
Associated factors/How it Affects the patient	What other symptoms occur with it? How does it affect you?	'I am really worried because this is the best way to bond with my baby and I want him to have the immunity from my milk. I'm very stressed about being unable to breastfeed.'

Past health history

QUESTION	RATIONALE
Ask about the pregnancy: Was the pregnancy planned? How did you feel when you found out you were pregnant? When did you first receive antenatal care? How was your general health during pregnancy? Did you have any problems with your pregnancy?	The carer's answer may provide insight into her feelings about the child. Antenatal information helps to identify potential health problems for the child.
Did you have any accidents during this pregnancy? Did you take any medications during pregnancy?	Certain medications should not be taken during pregnancy and may be harmful to the child.

Past health history (continued)

QUESTION	RATIONALE
Did you use any tobacco, alcohol or drugs during this pregnancy?	Smoking, alcohol and drug use may cause complications or anomalies with the fetus.
Ask about the birth of the child: Where was the child born? What type of delivery did you have? Were there any problems during the delivery? Did you have any vaginal infections at time of delivery? What was the child's Apgar score? What were the child's weight, length and head circumference? Did the child have any problems after birth (e.g. feeding, jaundice)?	Delivery details and complications are pertinent for assessing fetal injury and potential risk for infection.
Ask about past illnesses or injuries: Has the child ever been hospitalised? Has the child ever had any major illnesses?	Previous illnesses and hospitalisations may affect the present examination.
What immunisations has the child received thus far? Has your child had any reactions to immunisations?	This helps identify risk for infection and potential reactions to immunisations.

Family history

QUESTION	RATIONALE
Please list any chronic health conditions in the family.	Certain conditions tend to run in families and increase the patient's risk for such conditions.
Please list the age and cause of death for blood relatives.	This helps to identify risk factors.
Does the child have family members with communicable diseases?	This also helps to identify risk factors.

Review of systems

QUESTION	RATIONALE
Skin, hair, nails	
Has your child had any changes in hair texture?	Changes may indicate an underlying problem.
Does your child exhibit scaling on her scalp?	Cradle cap is a common problem.
Has your child been exposed to any contagious disease such as measles, chickenpox, lice, ringworm and scabies?	This helps to identify risks for health problems.
Has your child ever had any rashes or sores? Does your child have nappy rash?	Nappy rash is a common finding in infants.
Has your child had any excessive bruising or burns?	This helps to assess for child abuse. Excessive bruising or burns suggest abuse.
Does your child have any birthmarks?	Birthmarks are normal findings.
Head and neck	
Has your child ever had a head injury?	Head injuries may cause neurological problems.
Did the fontanelles close on schedule? Does the child have head control? If so, at what age did this occur?	These questions assess normal growth and development.

Continued on following page

Review of systems (continued)

QUESTION	RATIONALE
Eyes and vision	
Does your infant have any unusual eye movements? Does your infant/child excessively cross eyes?	This helps to determine eye and vision development.
Does your infant blink when necessary?	Absent blinking is abnormal.
Is your infant able to focus on moving objects?	By 1 month, the infant should be able to follow a moving object or light.
Has your infant ever had cloudiness in the eyeball?	Cloudiness of the eyeball may indicate the presence of cataracts.
Ears and hearing	
Does your child appear to be paying attention when you speak? (Infants should respond to the human voice.) Does the child respond to loud noise?	Infants who do not respond to the human voice or loud noises may have a hearing loss.
Has your child had frequent ear infections? Tubes in ears?	Frequent otitis media is a risk factor for hearing loss.
Does anyone in the child's home smoke?	Smoking increases the risk of otitis media.
Mouth, throat, nose and sinuses	
Does your child have any teeth?	No teeth by age 1 is a variation of normal.
Does your child attend day care?	Attending day care increases risk of upper respiratory infections (through exposure to other children).
Thorax and lungs	
Has your child ever had cough, wheezing, shortness of breath or nocturnal dyspnoea; if so, when does it occur? Has your child had frequent or severe colds?	Positive answers to any of these questions may indicate upper respiratory disorders.
Heart and neck vessels	
Does your infant become fatigued or short of breath during feedings?	Infants who fatigue easily with feedings may have congenital heart defect or disorder.
Peripheral vascular system	
Does your child ever experience bluing of the extremities? Do your child's hands and/or feet get unusually cold?	These questions assess vascular supply and perfusion.
Abdomen	
Are you breast- or bottle feeding? What foods does the infant eat?	Feeding patterns help the nurse to assess nutrition and gastrointestinal function.
Has your child ever had any excessive vomiting? Abdominal pain? Please describe.	Excessive vomiting may indicate neurological disorder.
Genitalia	
How often does your child urinate? How many wet nappies do you change per day?	The carer's answer helps the nurse to assess the genitourinary system.
Is the child prone to frequent nappy rash?	Nappy rash (irritant contact dermatitis) is common in infants.

Review of systems (continued)

QUESTION	RATIONALE
Anus and rectum	
How often does your child have a bowel movement? What does it look like?	These questions help to assess gastrointestinal function.
Is there any history of bleeding, constipation, diarrhoea or haemorrhoids?	
Musculoskeletal system	
Has your child ever had limited range of motion, joint pain, stiffness, paralysis?	These questions assess musculoskeletal development.
Has your child ever had any fractures? Have you noticed any bone deformities?	Frequent fractures may indicate child abuse.
Neurological system	
Has your child ever had a seizure?	Seizures indicate a neurological or other systemic disorder.
Has your child ever experienced any problems with motor coordination?	If the child is not meeting developmental landmarks, he or she may have a developmental delay or a developmental disorder.

Growth and development

Growth and development of the newborn or infant may be assessed using the Parent's Evaluation of Developmental Status (see Assessment 32-1). This questionnaire is completed by the parent and is scored with the nurse to detect concerning development and behaviour. Children from birth to eight years can be assessed with this method.

Motor development

Gross motor

Newborns can turn their heads from side to side when prone unless they are lying on a soft surface. This inability to turn their head while lying on a soft surface makes suffocation a real concern. Hence, newborns should be placed only on their backs.

By 3 to 4 months, there is almost no head lag and the infant may push up to a prone position. Infants roll from front to back at 5 months and sit unsupported by 6 to 7 months. They pull to standing by 9 months, cruise by 10 months and walk when hand-held by 12 months. Figure 32-2 displays gross motor development of the infant.

Fine motor

The grasp reflex is present at birth and strengthens at 1 month. This reflex fades at 3 months, at which time an infant can actively hold a rattle. Five-month-old infants can grasp voluntarily and 7-month-old infants can transfer hand-to-hand. The pincer grasp develops by 9 months (Fig. 32-3), and 12-month-old infants will attempt to build a two-block tower.

Sensory perception (vision, hearing and other senses)

Visual

The newborn's visual impressions are unfocused and the ability to distinguish between colours is not developed until the newborn is approximately 8 months of age. Therefore, stimuli should be bright, simple, moving and, preferably, black and white (e.g. a mobile that consists of black and white circles and cubes).

Auditory

Newborns can distinguish sounds and turn towards voices and other noises. They may be very familiar with their mother's voice, and other sounds gradually gain significance when associated with pleasure.

Olfactory

Smell is fully developed at birth, and at age 2 weeks an infant can differentiate the smell of his or her mother's milk and parents' body odours.

Tactile

Touch is well developed at birth, especially the lips and tongue. Touch should be used frequently because infants enjoy rocking, warmth and cuddling. Infants normally attend to the human voice; therefore, ask parents as to whether their child appears to be paying attention when they speak.

Cognitive and language development (Piaget)

The sensorimotor stage, from birth to around 18 months, involves the development of intellect and knowledge of the environment gained through the senses. During this stage, development progresses from reflexive activity to purposeful acts. At the completion of this stage, the infant achieves a sense of object permanence (retains a mental image of an absent object; sees self as separate from others). An emerging sense of body image parallels sensorimotor development.

Crying is the first means of communication, and parents can usually differentiate cries. Cooing begins by 1 to 2 months, laughing and babbling by 3 to 4 months and consonant sounds by 3 to 4 months. The infant begins to imitate sounds by 6 months. Combined syllables ('mama') are vocalised by 8 months and the infant understands 'no-no' by 9 months. 'Mama' and 'dada' are said with meaning by 10 months, and the infant says a total of 2 to 4 words with meaning by 12 months.

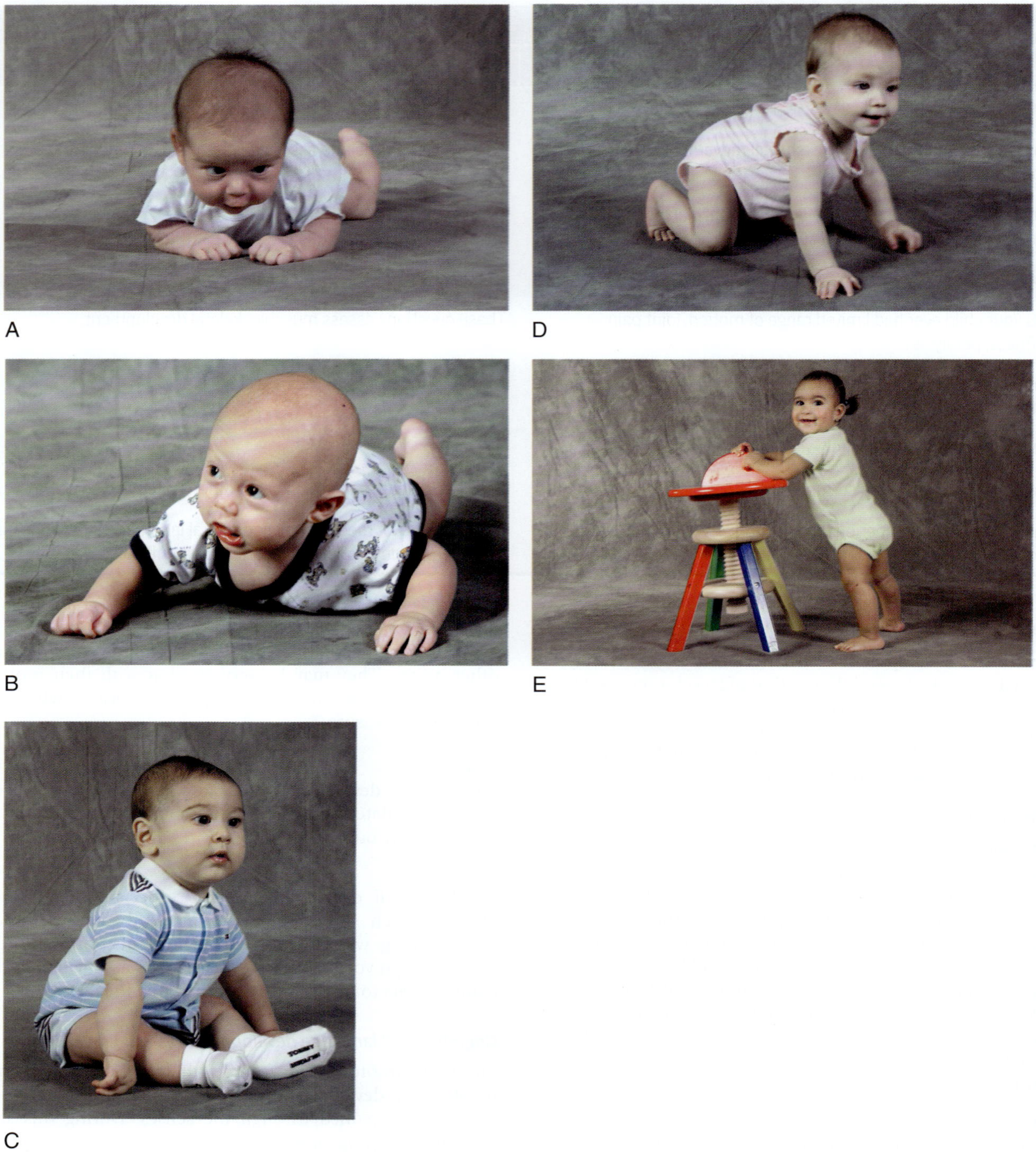

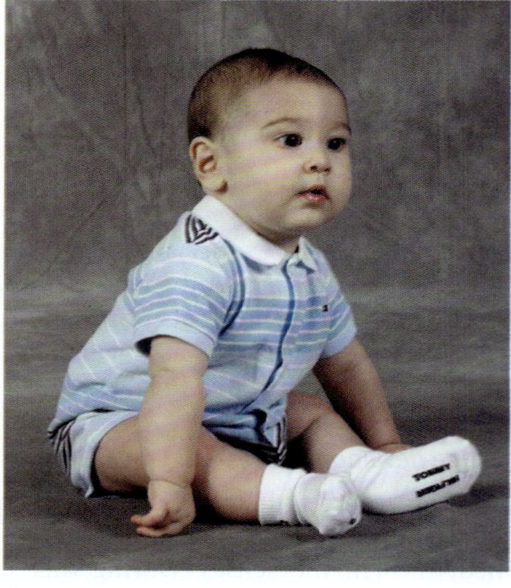

A D B E C

FIGURE 32-2 Growth and development of the infant. **(A)** At 4 weeks, this infant turns his head when lying in a prone position. **(B)** At 12 weeks, this infant pushes up from a prone position. **(C)** At 21 weeks, this infant sits up but tilts forwards for balance. **(D)** At 30 weeks, this infant is crawling around and on the go. **(E)** At 43 weeks, this infant is getting ready to walk. (Klossner, N. J. & Hatfield, N. [2006]. *Introductory maternity and pediatric nursing.* Philadelphia: Lippincott Williams & Wilkins.)

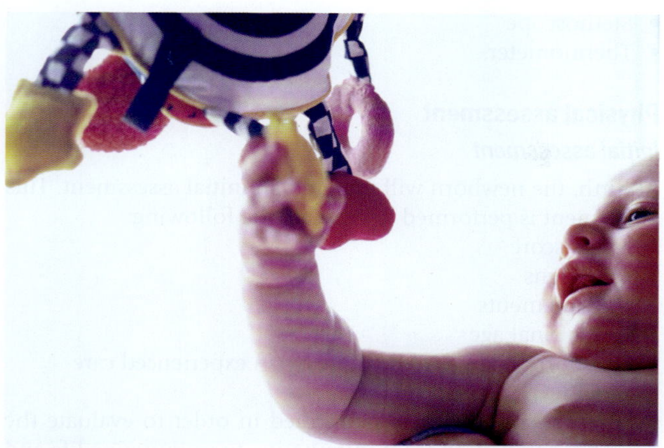

FIGURE 32-3 Development of the pincer grasp. (Used with permission from Kyle, T. & Carman, S. (2012). *Essentials of pediatric nursing* [2nd ed.]. Philadelphia: Lippincott Williams & Wilkins, p. 77.)

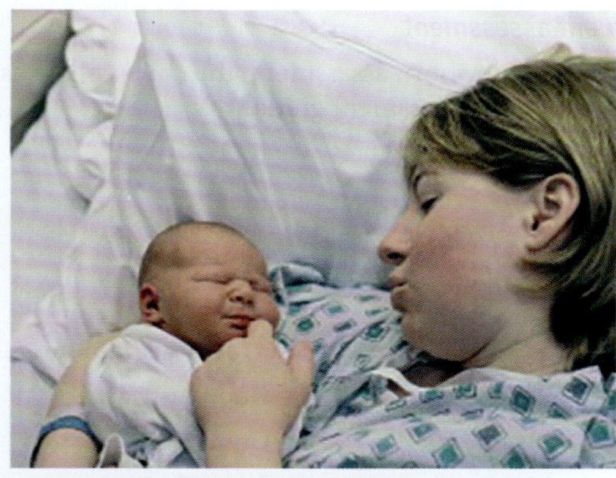

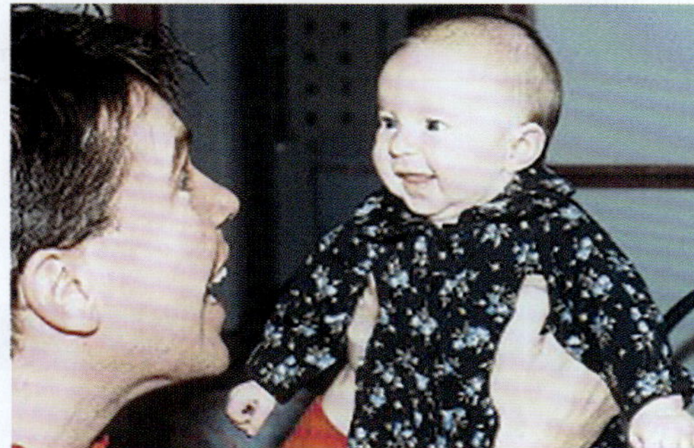

FIGURE 32-4 The infant–carer relationship fosters trust.

Moral development (Kohlberg)

Although the Kohlberg theory of moral development begins with toddlerhood, infants cannot be overlooked. Child moral development begins with the value and belief system of the parents and the infant's own development of trust. Parental discipline patterns may start with the young infant in the form of interventions for crying behaviours. Stern discipline and withholding love and affection may affect infant moral development. Love and affection are the building blocks of an infant's developing sense of trust (Fig. 32-4).

Psychosocial development (Erikson)

The crisis faced by an infant (birth to 1 year) is termed trust versus mistrust. In this stage, the infant's significant other is the 'caretaking' person. Developing a sense of trust in carers and the environment is a central focus for an infant. This sense of trust forms the foundation for all future psychosocial tasks.

The quality of the carer–child relationship is a crucial factor in the infant's development of trust. An infant who receives attentive care learns that life is predictable and that his or her needs will be met promptly; this fosters trust. In contrast, an infant experiencing consistently delayed needs gratification develops a sense of uncertainty, leading to mistrust of carers and the environment. An infant commonly seeks comfort from a security blanket or other objects such as a favourite stuffed animal.

Psychosexual development (Freud)

In the *oral stage* of development, from birth to 18 months, the erogenous zone is the mouth, and sexual activity takes the form of sucking, swallowing, chewing and biting. In this stage, the infant meets the world by crying, tasting, eating and early vocalisation; biting, to gain a sense of having a hold on and having greater control of the environment; and grasping and touching to explore texture variations in the environment.

Lifestyle and health practices

Normal nutritional requirements

Breast milk is the most desirable complete food for the first 6 months of a child's life as milk contains the most appropriate nutritional components for developing infants; it also has anti-infective properties and may lower the incidence of many conditions and diseases. However, commercially prepared, iron-fortified formula may be used if necessary. Formula intake varies per infant. Most infants take 420 kJ/kg of body weight per day. This amount of formula should be offered to the infant every 3 to 4 hours, approximately four to six times a day. Cow's milk is not recommended for the first 12 months. Solids are not recommended before the age of 6 months because of the presence of the protrusion or sucking reflexes and the immaturity of the gastrointestinal tract and the immune system. Infant rice cereal is usually the initial solid food given because it is easy to digest, contains iron and rarely triggers allergy. Additional foods usually include other cereals followed by fruits and vegetables and finally meats. Finger foods are introduced at 8 or 9 months. Weaning from breast or bottle to cup should be gradual. The desire to imitate at 8 to 9 months increases the success of weaning. Check for current infant nutrition guidelines via the National Health and Medical Research Council (2013) and the New Zealand Ministry of Health (2013).

SAFETY TIP

Honey should be discouraged during the first year of life because it may cause infant botulism.

Normal sleep requirements and patterns

Sleep patterns vary among infants. During the first month, most infants sleep when not eating. By 3 to 4 months, most infants sleep 9 to 11 hours at night. By 12 months, most infants take morning and afternoon naps. Bedtime rituals should begin in infancy to prepare the infant for sleep and prevent future sleep problems.

SAFETY TIP

Because of the possibility of sudden unexplained death of an infant (Australian Breastfeeding Association, 2013; NZMOH, 2013), it is suggested that young infants sleep in the supine or side-lying position.

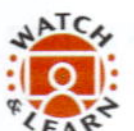

Developmental considerations in caring for children: Infants

COLLECTING OBJECTIVE DATA: PHYSICAL EXAMINATION

Preparing the neonate

Make sure the carer understands the examination process. Describe what will be performed and how it will be performed. Explain that the neonatal examination is a physical examination that occurs soon after birth and prior to discharge from the care provider. Encourage the carer to ask questions during the examination. For most of the examination, the infant should be unclothed.

Equipment

- Measuring tape
- Ophthalmoscope—this is frequently used in the advanced eye assessment (see Equipment spotlight 17-1)
- Otoscope—this is frequently used in the advanced ear assessment (see Equipment spotlight 18-1)
- Scales
- Stethoscope
- Thermometer.

Physical assessment

Initial assessment

At birth, the newborn will undergo an initial assessment. This assessment is performed to evaluate the following:

- Apgar score
- Vital signs
- Measurements
- Gestational age
- Newborn reflexes (to be done by an experienced care provider).

These assessments are performed in order to evaluate the newborn's transition from intrauterine to extrauterine life and to detect any health concerns that may require prompt intervention. The assessment is performed immediately after birth, while the infant is supine and under a radiant warmer.

Subsequent assessment

After the initial newborn assessment, the child will be assessed using the physical assessment guide.

Table 32-1 Apgar scoring

	Score 0	Score 1	Score 2
Heart rate	Absent	<100 beats/minute	>100 beats/minute
Respiratory rate	Absent	Slow, irregular	Good lusty cry
Reflex irritability	No response	Grimace, some motion	Cry, cough
Muscle tone	Flaccid, limp	Flexion of extremities	Active flexion
Colour	Cyanotic, pale	Pink body, acrocyanosis	Pink body, pink extremities

INITIAL NEWBORN ASSESSMENT

ASSESSMENT PROCEDURE	NORMAL FINDINGS	ABNORMAL FINDINGS
Apgar score		
Assign Apgar scores at 1 and at 5 minutes after delivery. The Apgar score is an assessment of a newborn's ability to adapt to extrauterine life. Perform the following:	The score is 8 to 10. See Table 32-1 for Apgar scoring.	A score of less than 8 may indicate poor transition from intrauterine to extrauterine life.
Auscultate apical pulse.	The pulse is less than 100 beats/minute.	Pulse is greater the 100 beats/minute, indicating bradycardia. Absent heartbeat indicates fetal demise.
Inspect chest and abdomen for respiratory effort.	The newborn is crying.	The newborn has absent, slow or irregular respirations.
Inspect muscle tone by extending legs and arms. Observe degree of flexion and resistance in extremities.	The extremities are flexed, and you note active movement.	Delayed neurological function may be seen in grimace, no response.
Inspect body and extremities for skin colour.	The full body should be pink (acrocyanosis).	The newborn is cyanotic, pale.

INITIAL NEWBORN ASSESSMENT (continued)

ASSESSMENT PROCEDURE	NORMAL FINDINGS	ABNORMAL FINDINGS
Vital signs		
Monitor axillary temperature (Fig. 32-5).	Temperature is 36.5°C to 37.2°C.	A temperature of less than 36.5°C indicates hypothermia, which may suggest sepsis. A temperature of greater than 37.2°C indicates hyperthermia. (Consider infection or improper monitoring of temperature probe.)
Inspect and auscultate lung sounds.	Breathing is easy and non-laboured. The lungs are clear bilaterally.	Abnormal findings include laboured breathing, nasal flaring, rhonchi, rales, retractions or grunting.
Monitor respiratory rate.	Rate is 30 to 60 breaths/minute.	A rate less than 30 or greater than 60 breaths/minute is seen with respiratory distress.
Auscultate apical pulse.	Pulse is regular and within a range of 100 to 140 beats/minute while at rest. The rate may rise to 180 beats/minute when crying or fall to 100 beats/minute when sleeping.	Pulse is irregular or the rate is above 180 beats/minute while crying; below 100 beats/minute while sleeping may indicate cardiac abnormalities.
Measurements		
Weigh the newborn using a newborn scale (Fig. 32-6). The child should be unclothed.	The newborn weighs between 2,500 and 4,000 g.	Weight is less than 2,500 g or greater than 4,000 g.
Measure length (Fig. 32-7).	The newborn is 44 to 55 cm.	Length is less than 44 or greater than 55 cm.
Measure head circumference (Fig. 32-8). (See instructions below, in 'Subsequent physical assessment'.)	Circumference is 33 to 35.5 cm.	Circumference less than 33 cm may indicate microcephaly, improper brain growth, premature closing of the sutures, intrauterine infection or chromosomal defect. Greater than 35.5 cm may indicate bulging fontanelles, 'split sutures' or swollen scalp veins or hydrocephaly.
Measure chest circumference. Place tape measure at nipple line and wrap around newborn.	Circumference is 30 to 33 cm (1 to 2 cm less than head).	Circumference is less than 29 cm or greater than 34 cm.

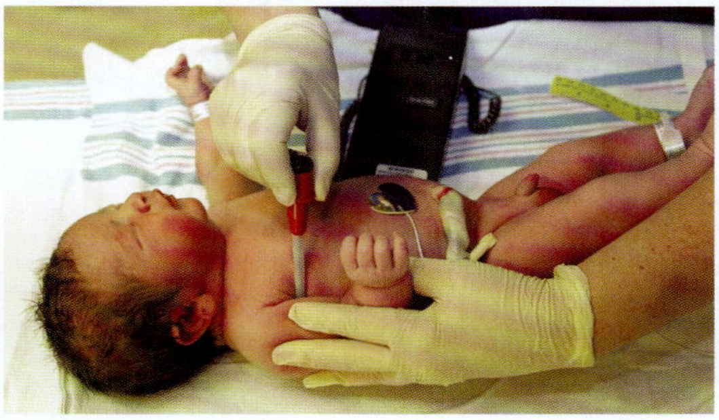

FIGURE 32-5 Measuring the newborn's axillary temperature. (Klossner, N. J. & Hatfield, N. [2006]. *Introductory maternity and pediatric nursing*. Philadelphia: Lippincott Williams & Wilkins.)

Continued on following page

INITIAL NEWBORN ASSESSMENT (continued)

ASSESSMENT PROCEDURE	NORMAL FINDINGS	ABNORMAL FINDINGS

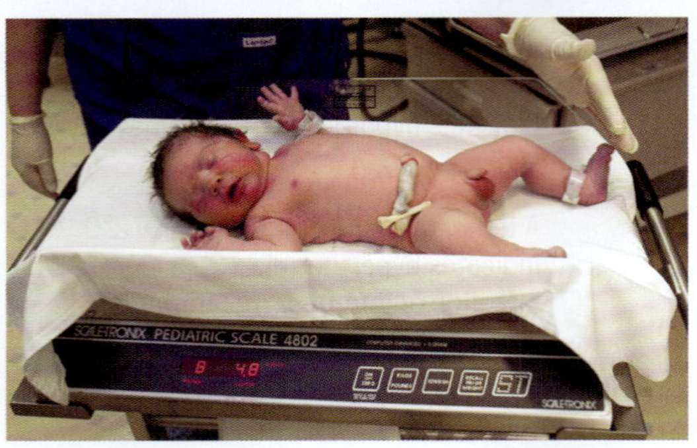

FIGURE 32-6 Weighing the newborn. (Klossner, N. J. & Hatfield, N. [2006]. *Introductory maternity and pediatric nursing*. Philadelphia: Lippincott Williams & Wilkins.)

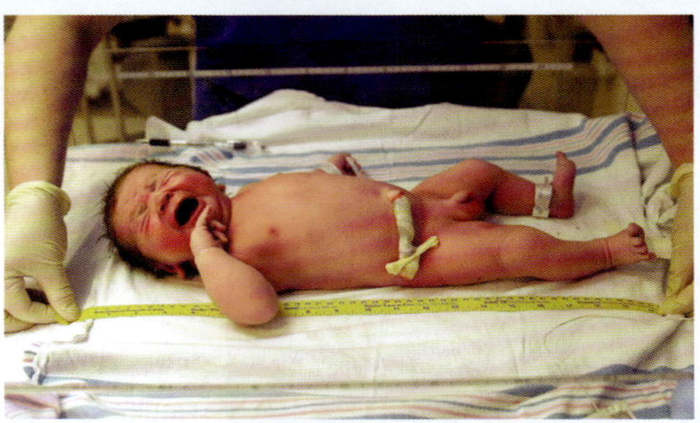

FIGURE 32-7 Measuring the length of the newborn. (Klossner, N. J. & Hatfield, N. [2006]. *Introductory maternity and pediatric nursing*. Philadelphia: Lippincott Williams & Wilkins.)

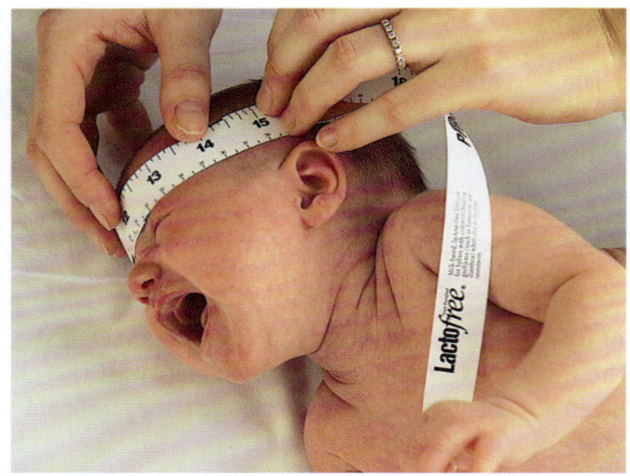

FIGURE 32-8 Measuring head circumference. (© B. Proud.)

Gestational age

Assess gestational age within 4 hours after birth to identify any potential age-related problems that may occur within the next few hours. This examination requires assessing the newborn's neuromuscular and physical maturity. Use the Ballard Scale to rate (Figure 32-11).

ASSESSMENT PROCEDURE	NORMAL FINDINGS	ABNORMAL FINDINGS
To assess neuromuscular maturity (with the newborn in supine position):		
Inspect posture (with the newborn undisturbed).	Arms and legs are flexed.	In premature children, the newborn's arms and legs may be limp and extend away from the body.
Assess for square window sign. Bend wrist towards ventral forearm until resistance is met. Measure angle.	Angle is 0 to 30 degrees (Fig. 32-9).	Premature newborns may have a square window measurement of more than 30 degrees and very premature newborns may have an angle of 90 degrees (www.atitesting.com/ati_next_gen/skillsmodules/content/maternal-newborn/equipment/gestational_age.html).

INITIAL NEWBORN ASSESSMENT (continued)

ASSESSMENT PROCEDURE	NORMAL FINDINGS	ABNORMAL FINDINGS
Gestational age (continued)		

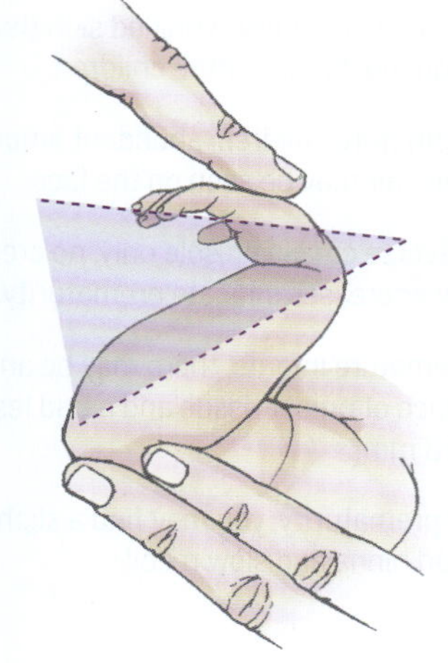

FIGURE 32-9 Square window sign: **(A)** term infant; **(B)** preterm infant.

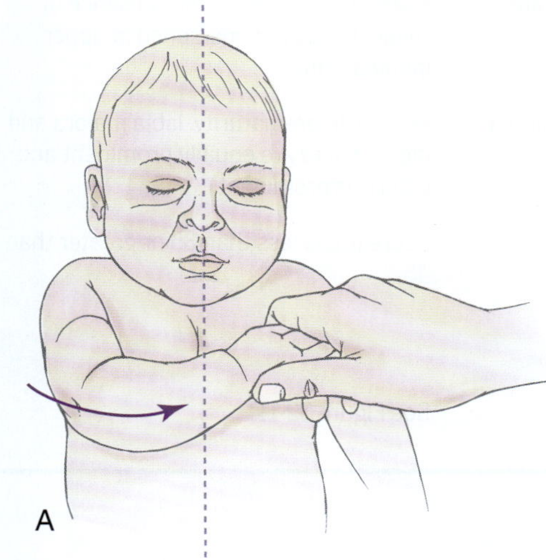

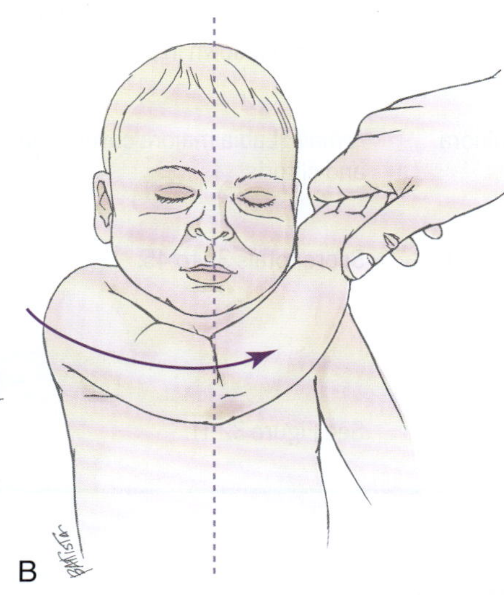

FIGURE 32-10 Scarf sign: **(A)** term infant; **(B)** preterm infant.

ASSESSMENT PROCEDURE	NORMAL FINDINGS	ABNORMAL FINDINGS
Test arm recoil. Bilaterally flex elbows up.	Elbow angle is less than 90 degrees and the arm rapidly recoils to a flexed state.	In premature children, elbow angle may be greater than 110 degrees, and delayed recoil may be seen.
Assess popliteal angle. Flex thigh on top of the abdomen; push behind the ankle and extend the lower leg up towards the head until resistance is met. Measure the angle behind the knee.	The angle should be less than 100 degrees.	Premature children may have a popliteal angle of greater than 100 degrees.
Assess for Scarf sign. Lift the arm across the chest towards the opposite shoulder until resistance is met; note location of elbow in relation to midline of chest.	Elbow position is less than midline of chest (Fig. 32-10).	In premature children, elbow position is at midline of chest or greater (towards opposite shoulder) (Fig. 32-10).
Perform heel-to-ear test. Keeping buttocks flat on the bed, pull leg towards ear on same side of the body; inspect popliteal angle and proximity of heel to ear.	Popliteal angle is less than 90 degrees; heel is distal from ear.	In premature infants, popliteal angle may be greater than 90 degrees, and the heel may be proximal to ear.

Continued on following page

INITIAL NEWBORN ASSESSMENT (continued)

ASSESSMENT PROCEDURE	NORMAL FINDINGS	ABNORMAL FINDINGS
To assess for physical maturity:		
Inspect skin.	Inspection reveals parchment, few or no vessels on the abdomen, and crackling, especially in the ankle area.	Inspection reveals translucent, visible veins; rash; leathery, wrinkled skin that is seen in most postmature children.
Inspect for lanugo.	Normally there is thinning and balding on the back, shoulders and knees.	In premature children, abundant amounts of fine hair may be seen on the face.
Inspect the plantar surface of the feet for creases.	There are creases on the anterior two-thirds or entire sole.	Transverse crease on sole only, no creases or fewer creases indicate prematurity.
Inspect and palpate breast bud tissue with middle finger and forefinger; measure bud in millimetres.	The areola is raised and full.	In premature infants, there may be an absence of breast tissue and a bud less than 3 mm.
Observe ear cartilage in upper pinna for curving. Fold pinna down towards side of the head and release; note recoil of the ear.	Normally you find a well-curved pinna, well-formed cartilage and instant recoil.	With prematurity, you may find a slightly curved pinna and slow recoil.
Inspect the genitals.		
Male: Assess scrotum for rugae and palpate position of testes.	*Male:* There are deep rugae; testes are positioned down in scrotal sac.	*Male*: There is decreased presence of rugae; testes are positioned in upper inguinal canal.
Female: Inspect labia majora, labia minora and clitoris.	*Female:* Labia majora cover labia minora and clitoris.	*Female:* In prematurity, labia majora and labia minora are equally prominent and clitoris is prominent.
Determine score rating: Use Figure 32-11. Mark the boxes that most closely represent each observation.	Score totals 35 to 45.	Score totals less than 35 or greater than 45.
Newborn reflexes		
Assess newborn reflexes. See Figure 32-11 for techniques.	See Figure 32-11.	See Figure 32-11.

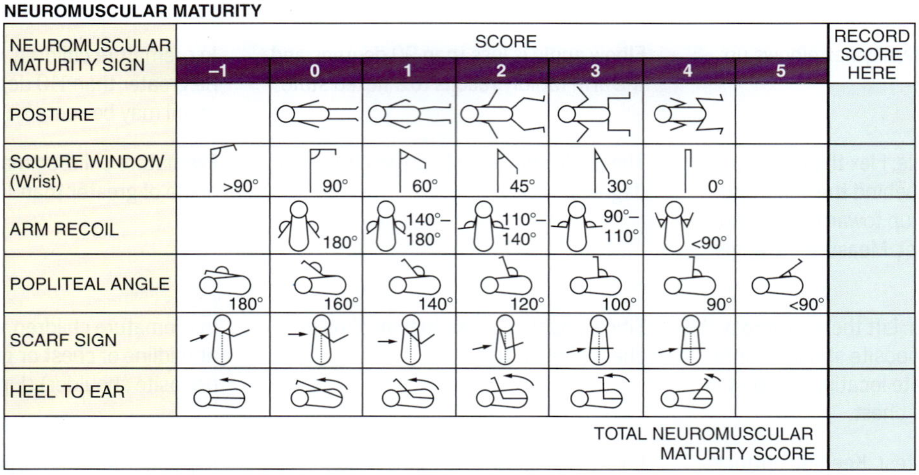

NEUROMUSCULAR MATURITY

NEUROMUSCULAR MATURITY SIGN	SCORE −1	0	1	2	3	4	5	RECORD SCORE HERE
POSTURE								
SQUARE WINDOW (Wrist)	>90°	90°	60°	45°	30°	0°		
ARM RECOIL		180°	140°–180°	110°–140°	90°–110°	<90°		
POPLITEAL ANGLE	180°	160°	140°	120°	100°	90°	<90°	
SCARF SIGN								
HEEL TO EAR								
							TOTAL NEUROMUSCULAR MATURITY SCORE	

FIGURE 32-11 New Ballard scale. Used to rate neuromuscular and physical maturity of gestational age.

PHYSICAL MATURITY

PHYSICAL MATURITY SIGN	SCORE −1	0	1	2	3	4	5	RECORD SCORE HERE
SKIN	sticky, friable, transparent	gelatinous, red, translucent	smooth, pink, visible veins	superficial peeling and/or rash, few veins	cracking pale areas, rare veins	parchment, deep cracking, no vessels	leathery, cracked, wrinkled	
LANUGO	none	sparse	abundant	thinning	bald areas	mostly bald		
PLANTAR SURFACE	heel-toe 40–50 mm: −1 <40 mm: −2	>50 mm no crease	faint red marks	anterior transverse crease only	creases ant. 2/3	creases over entire sole		
BREAST	impercep-tible	barely perceptible	flat areola no bud	stippled areola 1–2 mm bud	raised areola 3–4 mm bud	full areola 5–10 mm bud		
EYE-EAR	lids fused loosely: −1 tightly: −2	lids open pinna flat stays folded	sl. curved pinna; soft; slow recoil	well-curved pinna; soft but ready recoil	formed and firm instant recoil	thick cartilage, ear stiff		
GENITALS (Male)	scrotum flat, smooth	scrotum empty, faint rugae	testes in upper canal, rare rugae	testes descending, few rugae	testes down, good rugae	testes pendulous, deep rugae		
GENITALS (Female)	clitoris prominent and labia flat	prominent clitoris and small labia minora	prominent clitoris and enlarging minora	majora and minora equally prominent	majora large, minora small	majora cover clitoris and minora		
							TOTAL PHYSICAL MATURITY SCORE	

SCORE
Neuromuscular ____
Physical ____
Total ____

MATURITY RATING

Score	Weeks
−10	20
−5	22
0	24
5	26
10	28
15	30
20	32
25	34
30	36
35	38
40	40
45	42
50	44

GESTATIONAL AGE (weeks)
By dates ________
By ultrasound ________
By exam ________

FIGURE 32-11 (continued)

DISPLAY 32-1 NEWBORN REFLEXES: DIFFERENTIATING NORMAL AND ABNORMAL FINDINGS

The reflexes illustrated and described below are the most commonly tested newborn reflexes. These reflexes are present in all normal newborns, and most disappear within a few months after birth. Therefore, absence of a reflex at birth or persistence of a reflex past a certain age may indicate a problem with central nervous system (CNS) function.

Rooting reflex

To elicit the rooting reflex, touch the newborn's upper or lower lip or cheek with a gloved finger or sterile nipple. The newborn will move the head towards the stimulated area and open the mouth.

Disappearance of reflex

The rooting reflex disappears by 3 to 4 months.

Abnormal findings

Absence of a rooting indicates serious CNS disease.

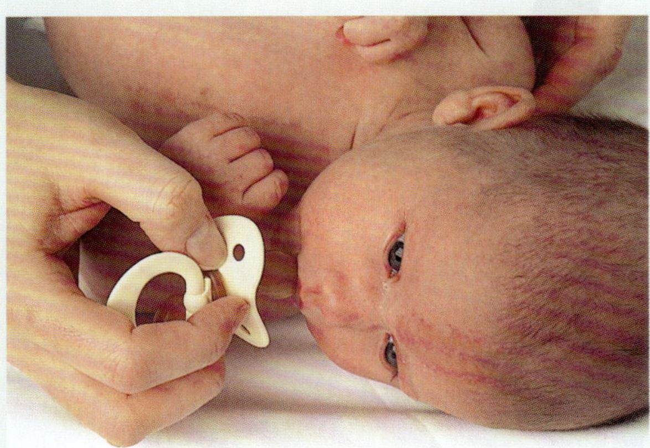

(© B. Proud.)

Sucking reflex

Place a gloved finger or nipple in the newborn's mouth and note the strength of the sucking response. (A diminished response is normal in a recently fed newborn.)

Disappearance of reflex

This reflex disappears at 10 to 12 months.

Abnormal findings

A weak or absent sucking reflex may indicate a neurological disorder, prematurity or CNS depression caused by maternal drug use or medication during pregnancy.

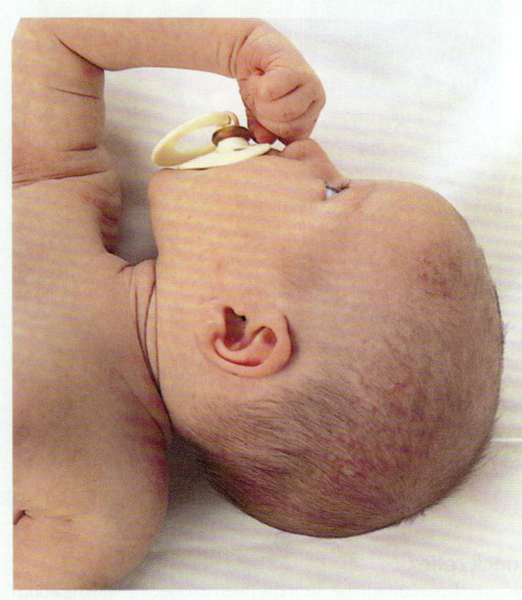

(© B. Proud.)

Continued on following page

DISPLAY 32-1 NEWBORN REFLEXES: DIFFERENTIATING NORMAL AND ABNORMAL FINDINGS (continued)

Palmar grasp reflex

Press your fingers against the palmar surface of the newborn's hand from the ulnar side. The grasp should be strong—you may even be able to pull the newborn to a sitting position.

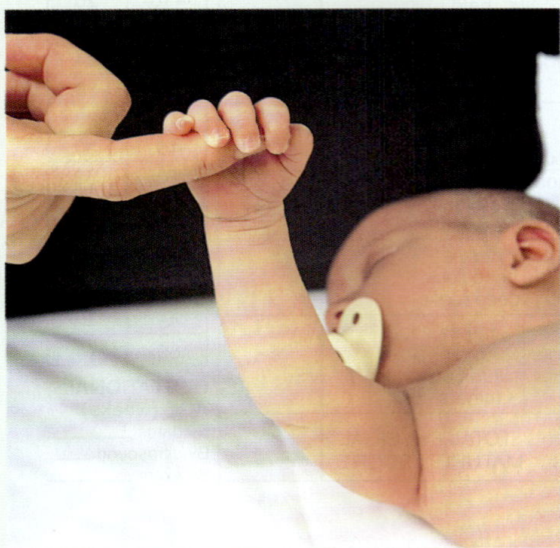

(© B. Proud.)

Disappearance of reflex

This reflex disappears at 3 to 4 months.

Abnormal findings

A diminished response usually indicates prematurity; no response suggests neurological deficit; asymmetrical grasp suggests fracture of the humerus or peripheral nerve damage. If this reflex persists past 4 months, cerebral dysfunction may be present.

Plantar grasp reflex

Touch the ball of the newborn's foot. The toes should curl downwards tightly.

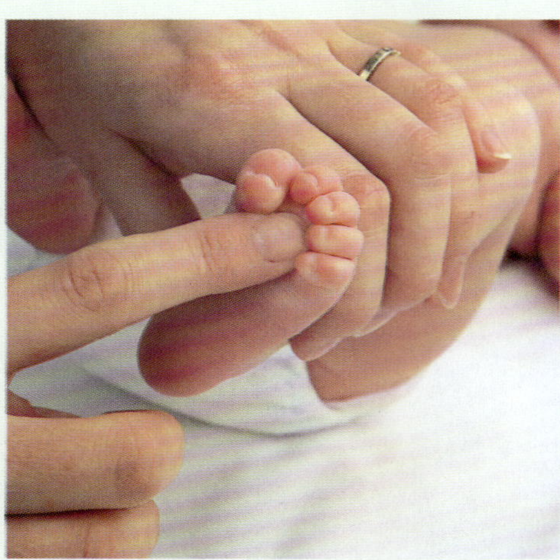

(© B. Proud.)

Disappearance of reflex

This reflex disappears at 8 to 10 months.

Abnormal findings

A diminished response usually indicates prematurity; no response suggests neurological deficit.

Tonic neck reflex

The newborn should be supine. Turn the head to one side with newborn's jaw at the shoulder. The tonic neck reflex is present when the arm and leg on the side to which the head is turned extend and the opposite arm and leg flex. This reflex usually does not appear until age 2 months.

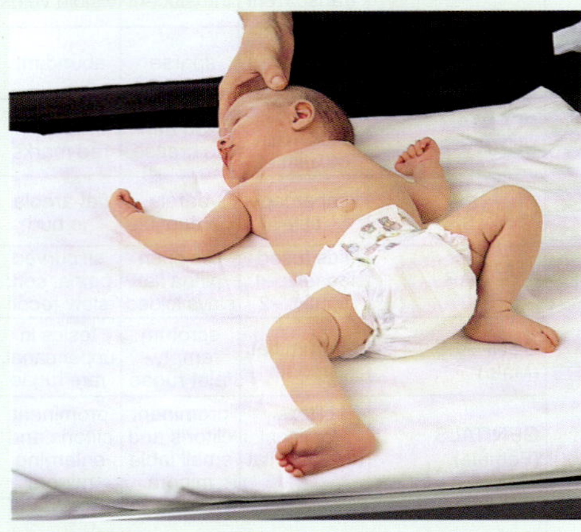

(© B. Proud.)

Disappearance of reflex

This reflex disappears by 4 to 6 months. The reflex may not occur every time that the examiner tries to elicit it, in which case, repeat stimulus of turning head to one side to re-elicit the response.

Abnormal findings

If this reflex persists until later in infancy, brain damage is usually present.

Moro (or startle) reflex

The Moro reflex is a response to sudden stimulation or an abrupt change in position. This reflex can be elicited by using either one of the following two methods:

1. Hold the infant with the head supported and rapidly lower the whole body a few inches.
2. Place the infant in the supine position on a flat, soft surface. Hit the surface with your hand or startle the infant in some way.

The reflex is manifested by the infant slightly flexing and abducting the legs, laterally extending and abducting the arms, forming a 'C' with thumb and forefinger and fanning the other fingers. This is immediately followed by anterior flexion and adduction of the arms. All movements should be symmetrical.

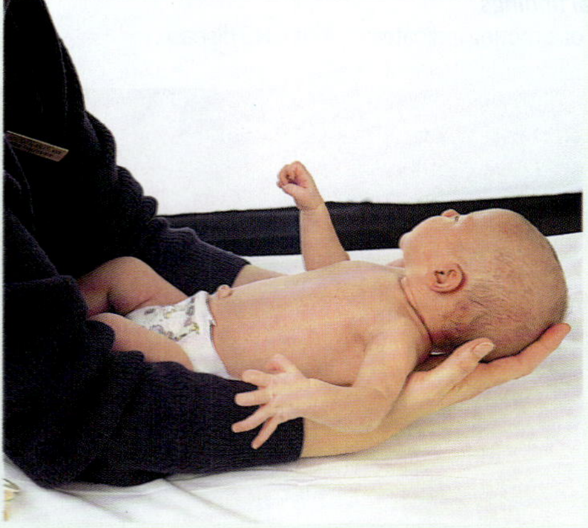

(© B. Proud.)

Disappearance of reflex

This reflex disappears by 3 months.

DISPLAY 32-1 NEWBORN REFLEXES: DIFFERENTIATING NORMAL AND ABNORMAL FINDINGS (continued)

Abnormal findings
An asymmetrical response suggests injury of the part that responds more slowly. Absence of a response suggests CNS injury. If the reflex was elicited at birth and disappears later, cerebral oedema or intracranial haemorrhage is suspected. Persistence of the response after 4 months suggests CNS injury.

Babinski reflex

Hold the newborn's foot and stroke up the lateral edge and across the ball. A positive Babinski reflex is fanning of the toes. Many normal newborns will not exhibit a positive Babinski reflex; instead, they will exhibit the normal adult response, which is flexion of the toes. Response should always be symmetrical bilaterally.

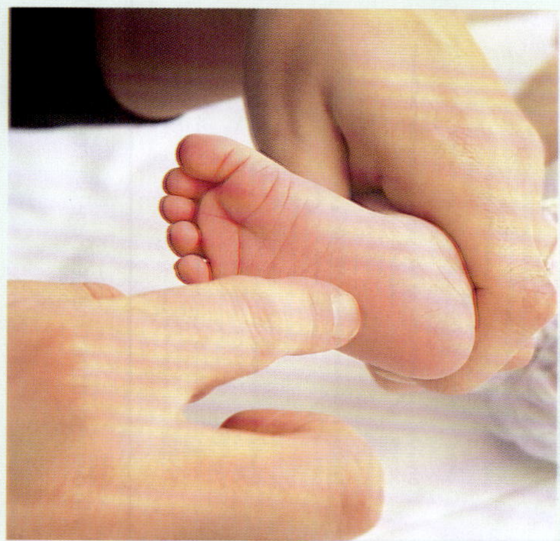

(© B. Proud.)

Disappearance of reflex
This reflex disappears within 2 years.

Abnormal findings
A positive response after 2 years suggests pyramidal tract disease.

Stepping reflex

Hold the newborn upright from behind, provide support under the arms and let the newborn's feet touch a surface. The reflex response is manifested by the newborn stepping with one foot and then the other in a walking motion.

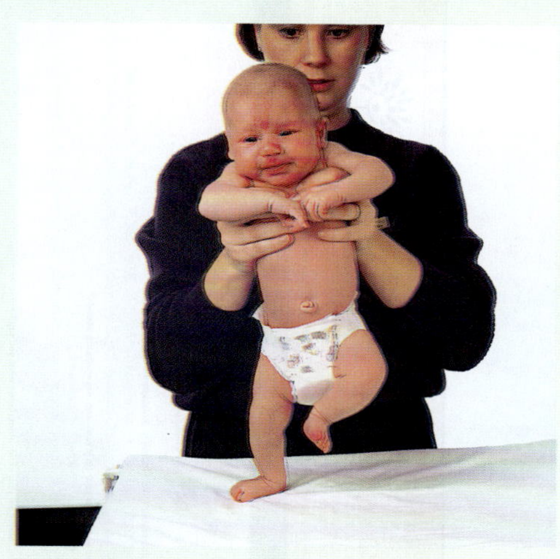

(© B. Proud.)

Disappearance of reflex
This reflex usually disappears within 2 months.

Abnormal findings
An asymmetrical response may indicate injury of the leg, CNS damage or peripheral nerve injury.

SUBSEQUENT PHYSICAL ASSESSMENT

ASSESSMENT PROCEDURE	NORMAL FINDINGS	ABNORMAL FINDINGS
General appearance and behaviour		
Observe general appearance. Observe hygiene. Note interaction with parents and yourself (and siblings if present). Note also facial expressions and posture.	Child appears stated age, is clean and has no unusual body odour, and clothing is in good condition and appropriate for climate. Child is alert, active, responds appropriately to stress of the situation. Child is appropriately interactive for age, seeks comfort from parent; appears happy. Newborn's arms and legs are in flexed position.	Note any facial expressions that indicate acute illness or respiratory distress. Flaccidity or rigidity in newborn may be from neurological damage, sepsis or pain. Poor hygiene and clothes may indicate neglect or poverty. Child does not appear stated age (mental retardation, abuse, neglect).
Developmental assessment		
Screen for cognitive, language, social, and gross and fine motor developmental delays in the beginning of the physical assessment in infants. Assessment tool 32-1 presents the PEDS and directions for its use.	Child meets normal parameters for age. See information contained in subjective data section.	Child lags in earlier stages.

Continued on page 668

ASSESSMENT TOOL 32-1 Using the Parents' Evaluation of Developmental Status

The following is an example of the Parents' Evaluation of Developmental Status (PEDS) a method for identifying children with concerning development and behaviour from birth to seven years and 11 months. It must be used with the PEDS Brief administration and scoring guide.

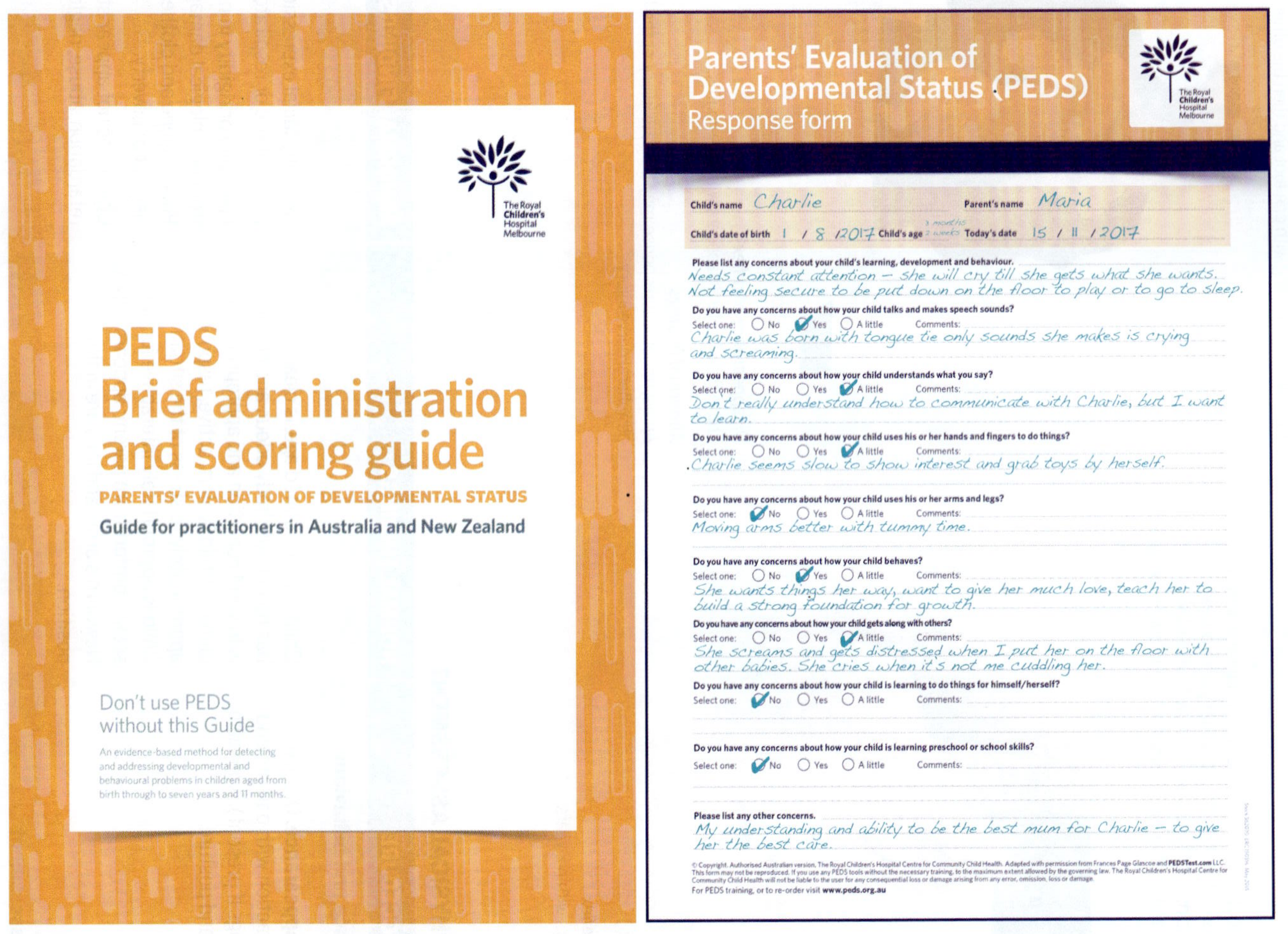

PEDS
Brief administration and scoring guide
PARENTS' EVALUATION OF DEVELOPMENTAL STATUS
Guide for practitioners in Australia and New Zealand

The Royal Children's Hospital Melbourne

Don't use PEDS without this Guide

An evidence-based method for detecting and addressing developmental and behavioural problems in children aged from birth through to seven years and 11 months.

Parents' Evaluation of Developmental Status (PEDS)
Response form

The Royal Children's Hospital Melbourne

Child's name: Charlie   Parent's name: Maria
Child's date of birth: 1 / 8 / 2017   Child's age: 3 months 2 weeks   Today's date: 15 / 11 / 2017

Please list any concerns about your child's learning, development and behaviour.
Needs constant attention – she will cry till she gets what she wants. Not feeling secure to be put down on the floor to play or to go to sleep.

Do you have any concerns about how your child talks and makes speech sounds?
Select one: ○ No ✔ Yes ○ A little
Comments: Charlie was born with tongue tie only sounds she makes is crying and screaming.

Do you have any concerns about how your child understands what you say?
Select one: ○ No ○ Yes ✔ A little
Comments: Don't really understand how to communicate with Charlie, but I want to learn.

Do you have any concerns about how your child uses his or her hands and fingers to do things?
Select one: ○ No ○ Yes ✔ A little
Comments: Charlie seems slow to show interest and grab toys by herself.

Do you have any concerns about how your child uses his or her arms and legs?
Select one: ✔ No ○ Yes ○ A little
Comments: Moving arms better with tummy time.

Do you have any concerns about how your child behaves?
Select one: ○ No ✔ Yes ○ A little
Comments: She wants things her way, want to give her much love, teach her to build a strong foundation for growth.

Do you have any concerns about how your child gets along with others?
Select one: ○ No ○ Yes ✔ A little
Comments: She screams and gets distressed when I put her on the floor with other babies. She cries when it's not me cuddling her.

Do you have any concerns about how your child is learning to do things for himself/herself?
Select one: ✔ No ○ Yes ○ A little
Comments:

Do you have any concerns about how your child is learning preschool or school skills?
Select one: ✔ No ○ Yes ○ A little
Comments:

Please list any other concerns.
My understanding and ability to be the best mum for Charlie – to give her the best care.

For PEDS training, or to re-order visit www.peds.org.au

ASSESSMENT TOOL 32-1 Using the Parents' Evaluation of Developmental Status (continued)

Parents' Evaluation of Developmental Status (PEDS) Score form

The Royal Children's Hospital Melbourne

Child's name *Mohammed* Child's date of birth *26 / 5 / 2013*

You must refer to the PEDS Brief Administration and Scoring Guide in order to correctly administer, score and interpret PEDS.

Child's age in months	0–3	4–5	6–11	12–14	15–17	18–23	24–35	36–47	48–53	54–71	72–83	84–96
Today's date						*28 Nov 2014*						
Global/cognitive	○	○	○	○	○	○	○	○	○	○	○	○
Expressive language and articulation	○	○	○	○	○	○	○	○	○	○	○	○
Receptive language	☐	☐	☐	☐	☐	✓	○	*Mohammed doesn't listen*				○
Fine motor	☐	☐	☐	☐	☐	☐	☐	☐	☐	○	○	○
Gross motor	☐	☐	☐	☐	☐	✓	☐	*Took ages to walk*				○
Behavior	☐	☐	☐	☐	☐	✓	☐	*Can be naughty. Runs away when I call him.*				
Social-emotional	○	○	○	○	○	☐	☐	☐	☐	☐	☐	☐
Self-help	☐	☐	☐	☐	☐	☐	☐	☐	☐	☐	☐	☐
School	☐	☐	☐	☐	☐	☐	☐	☐	☐	○	○	○
Other	○	○	○	○	○	✓	○	*Lots of ear infections*				○

Count the number of small circles with checkmarks and place the total in the large circle below.

Child's age in months	0–3	4–5	6–11	12–14	15–17	18–23	24–35	36–47	48–53	54–71	72–83	84–96
	○	○	○	○	○	*2*	○	○	○	○	○	○

If the number shown in the large circle is 2 or more, follow **Path A** on the PEDS Interpretation Form. If the number shown is exactly 1, follow **Path B**. Then count the number of small boxes and place the total in the large box below.

Child's age in months	0–3	4–5	6–11	12–14	15–17	18–23	24–35	36–47	48–53	54–71	72–83	84–96
	☐	☐	☐	☐	☐	*2*	☐	☐	☐	☐	☐	☐

If the number shown in the large box is 1 or more, also follow **Path C**. If the number 0 is shown, consider **Path D** if relevant. Otherwise, follow **Path E**.

For PEDS training, or to re-order visit **www.peds.org.au**

Parents' Evaluation of Developmental Status (PEDS) Interpretation form

The Royal Children's Hospital Melbourne

Child's name *Eleanor* Child's date of birth *21 / 1 / 2016*

Path A Two or more predictive concerns? → Yes → Two or more concerns about self-help, social, school or receptive language skills?
- Yes → Refer for audiological and speech-language testing. Use professional judgement to decide if referrals are also needed for social work, occupational/physiotherapy, mental health services etc.
- No → Refer for intellectual and educational assessments. Use professional judgement to decide if speech-language, audiological, or other evaluations are also needed.

Path B One predictive concern? → Yes → Health concerns only?
- Yes → Screen for health/sensory problems; consider second-stage developmental screen.
- No → Administer second-stage developmental screen.
- If screen is passed, counsel in areas of concern and watch vigilantly.
- If screen is failed, refer for testing in areas of difficulty.

Path C Non-predictive concerns? → Yes → Counsel in areas of difficulty and follow up in several weeks. → If unsuccessful, screen for emotional/behavioral problems and refer as indicated. Otherwise refer for parent training, behavioral intervention etc. If concerns still exist at age 4 ½ and older, refer for mental health services.

Path D Parental difficulties communicating? → Yes → Foreign language a barrier?
- Yes → Use foreign language versions; send PEDS home in preparation for a second visit; seek an interpreter; or refer for screening elsewhere.
- No → Use a second screen that directly elicits children's skills or refer for screening elsewhere.

Path E No concerns? → Yes → Elicit concerns at next checkpoint. → No → Use PEDS between checkpoints (eg sick or return visit).

Specific decisions

0–3 months		24–35 months	
4–5 months	*Path C – see notes*	36–47 months	
6–11 months		48–53 months	
12–14 months		54–71 months	
15–17 months		72–83 months	
18–23 months		84–96 months	

For PEDS training, or to re-order visit **www.peds.org.au**

SUBSEQUENT PHYSICAL ASSESSMENT (continued)

ASSESSMENT PROCEDURE	NORMAL FINDINGS	ABNORMAL FINDINGS
Vital signs		
Assess temperature. Use rectal, axillary, skin or tympanic route when assessing the temperature of an infant. The rectal temperature is most accurate. To take a rectal temperature in a newborn, lay the child supine and lift lower legs up into the air, bending the legs at the hips. Insert lubricated rectal thermometer no more than 2 cm into rectum. Temperature registers in 3 to 5 minutes on a rectal thermometer. Axillary and/or tympanic temperature may also be used. For axillary temperature, place the thermometer under axilla, holding arm close to chest for approximately 3 to 5 minutes. For tympanic temperature, use digital tympanic thermometer as directed in manufacturer's instructions.	Temperature is 37.5°C (because of excess heat production).	Temperature may be altered by exercise, stress, crying, environment, diurnal variation (highest between 4 and 6 p.m.). Both hyperthermic and hypothermic conditions are noted in children.
Note apical pulse rate. Count the pulse for a full minute (Fig. 32-12).	Awake and resting rates vary with the age of the child. For a newborn to 1-month-old child it should be 120 to 160 beats/minute. Rate decreases gradually with age. At 6 months to 1 year, rate is approximately 110 beats/minute.	Pulse may be altered by medications, activity and pain as well as pathological conditions. Bradycardia (<100 beats/minute) in an infant is usually an ominous finding.
Assess respiratory rate. Measure respiratory rate and character in infants by observing abdominal movements.	Newborns: Rate is 30 to 60 breaths/minute. Breathing is unlaboured; lung sounds clear. Newborns are obligatory nose breathers.	Respiratory rate and character may be altered by medications, positioning, fever or activity as well as pathological conditions.
Evaluate blood pressure. Newborn blood pressure: A Doppler stethoscope should be used or an electronic Dinamap (device for indirect non-invasive mean arterial pressure) machine may be used to record blood pressure readings in the newborn. **CLINICAL TIP** **The child should not be crying as this can elevate blood pressure.**	Specific to age and size.	**CLINICAL TIP** **If the blood pressure reading is too high for age, the cuff may be too small; it should cover two-thirds of the child's upper arm. If the blood pressure reading is too low for age, the cuff may be too large. Chapter 7 explains how to take a blood pressure reading.**

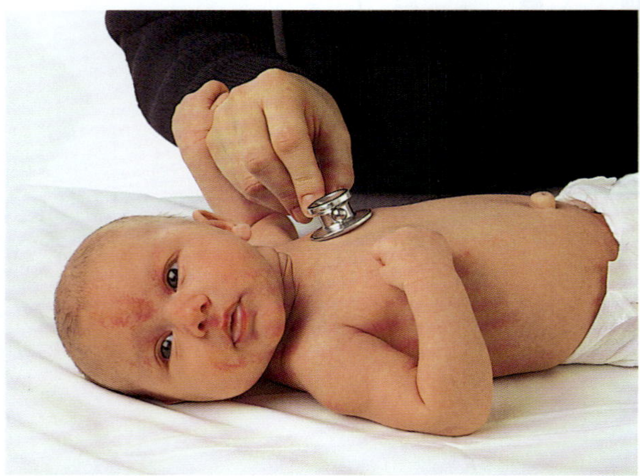

FIGURE 32-12 Auscultating apical pulse rate in the infant. (© B. Proud.)

SUBSEQUENT PHYSICAL ASSESSMENT (continued)

ASSESSMENT PROCEDURE	NORMAL FINDINGS	ABNORMAL FINDINGS
Measurements		
Measure height. Determine height by measuring the recumbent length. Fully extend the body, holding the head in midline and gently grasping the knees and pushing them downwards until the legs are fully extended and touching the table (Fig. 32-13). If using a measuring board, place the head at the top of the board and the heels firmly at the bottom. Without a board, use paper under the child and mark the paper at the top of the head and bottom of the heels. Then measure the distance between the two points. Plot height measurement on an age- and gender-appropriate growth chart.	See Appendix A for growth charts. **CULTURAL CONSIDERATIONS** **Asian and Aboriginal and Torres Strait Islander newborns are smaller than Caucasian newborns. Asian children are smaller at all ages.**	Significant deviation from normal in the growth charts would be considered abnormal.
Measure weight. Measure weight on an appropriately-sized beam scale with non-detectable weights. Weigh an infant lying or sitting on a scale that measures to the nearest 10 g (Fig. 32-14). Weigh an infant naked. Plot weight measurement on age- and gender-appropriate growth chart.	See the growth charts in Appendix A for normal findings.	Deviation from the wide range of normal weights is abnormal. See Appendix A and compare differences.
Determine head circumference. Measure head circumference (HC) or occipital frontal circumference (OFC) at every physical examination for infants and toddlers younger than 2 years and older children when conditions warrant. Plot the measurement on standardised growth charts specific for gender from birth to 36 months.	HC (OFC) measurement should fall between the 5th and 95th percentiles and should be comparable to the child's height and weight percentiles.	HC (OFC) not within the normal percentiles may indicate pathology. Those greater than 95% may indicate macrocephaly. Those under the fifth percentile may indicate microcephaly.

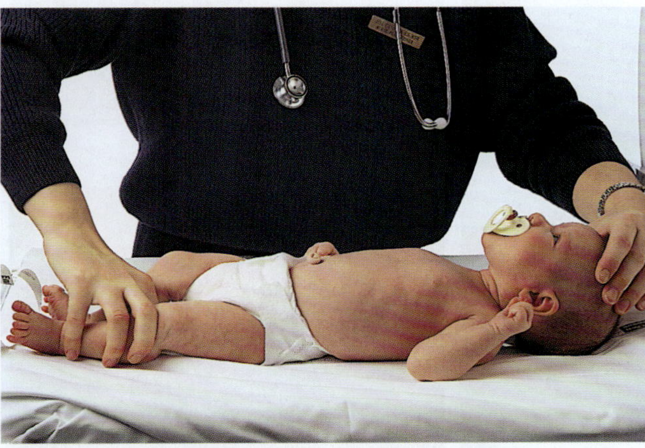

FIGURE 32-13 Positioning for measuring an infant's height. (© B. Proud.)

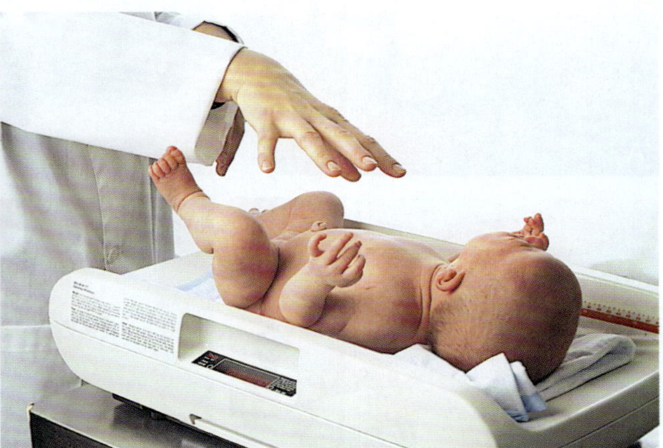

FIGURE 32-14 Weighing an infant. (© B. Proud.)

Continued on following page

SUBSEQUENT PHYSICAL ASSESSMENT (continued)

ASSESSMENT PROCEDURE	NORMAL FINDINGS	ABNORMAL FINDINGS
Skin, hair and nails		
Assess for skin colour, odour and lesions.	Skin colour ranges from pale white with pink, yellow, brown or olive tones to dark brown or black. No strong odour should be evident, and the skin should be lesion-free. Skin should be soft, warm, slightly moist with good turgor and without oedema or lesions. Common newborn skin variations include: • Physiological jaundice • Birthmarks • Milia (Fig. 32-15) • Erythema toxicum (Fig. 32-15) • Telangiectatic naevi (stork bites). (Fig. 32-15). Another common variation is harlequin sign (one side of the body turns red; the other side is pale). There is a distinct colour line separation at midline. The cause is unknown. **CULTURAL CONSIDERATIONS** **Dark-skinned newborns have lighter skin colour than their parents. Their colour darkens with age. Bluish pigmented areas called Mongolian spots (Fig. 32-15) may be noted on the sacral areas of Asian and Aboriginal and Torres Strait Islander infants.**	Yellow skin may indicate jaundice or passage of meconium in utero secondary to fetal distress. Jaundice within 24 hours after birth is pathological and may indicate haemolytic disease of the newborn. Blue skin suggests cyanosis; pallor suggests anaemia; and redness suggests fever or irritation.

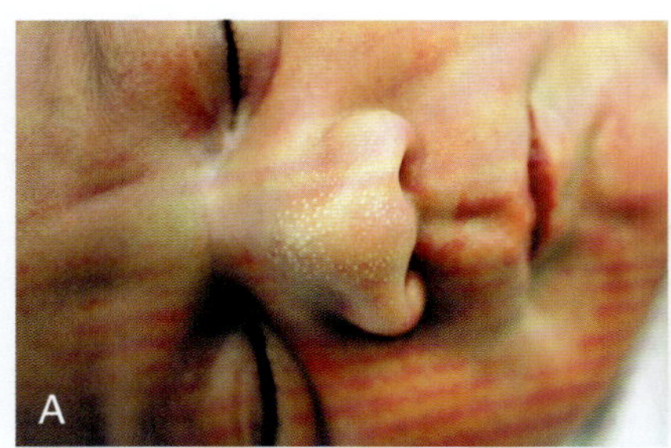

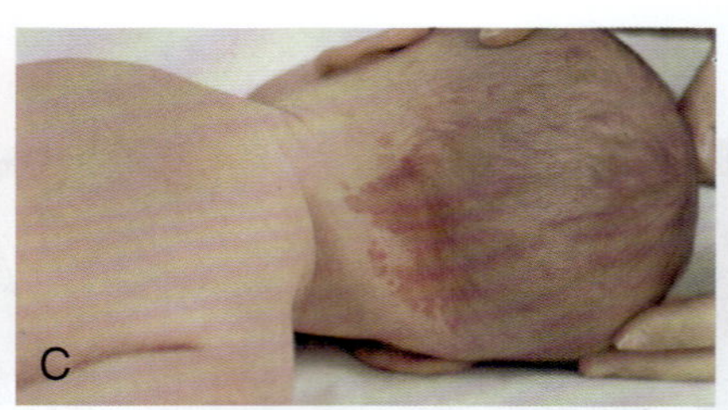

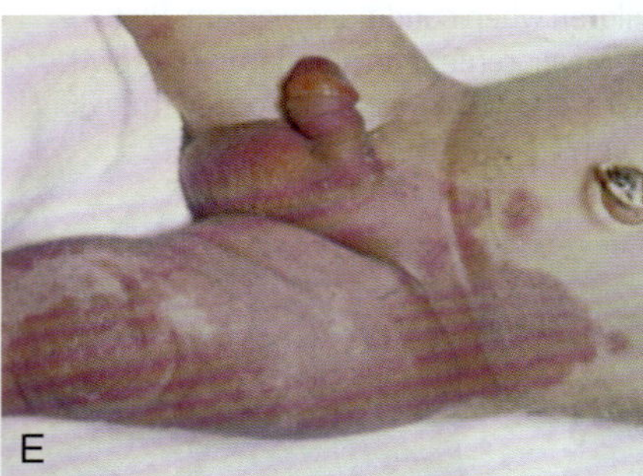

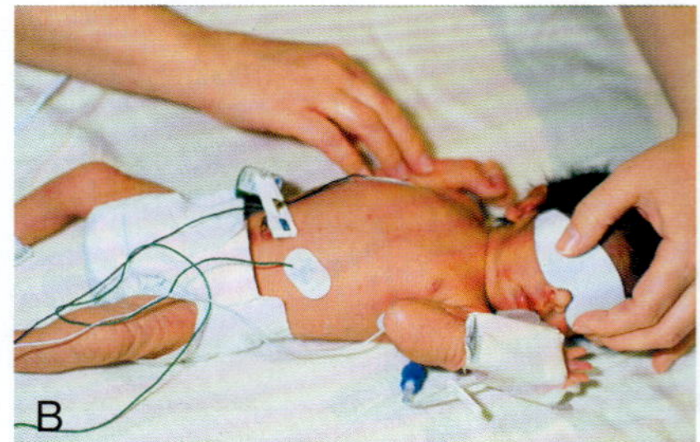

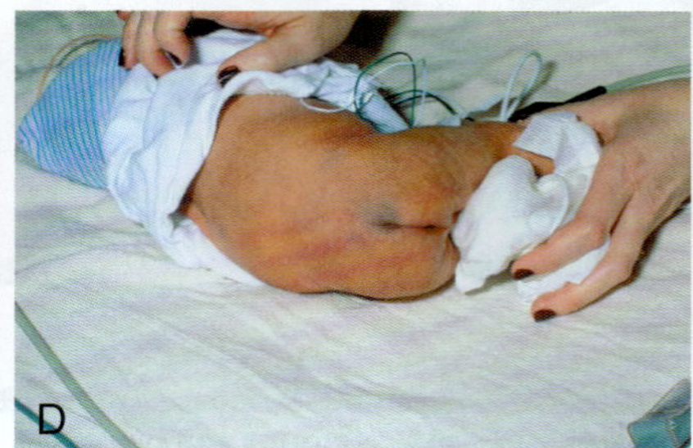

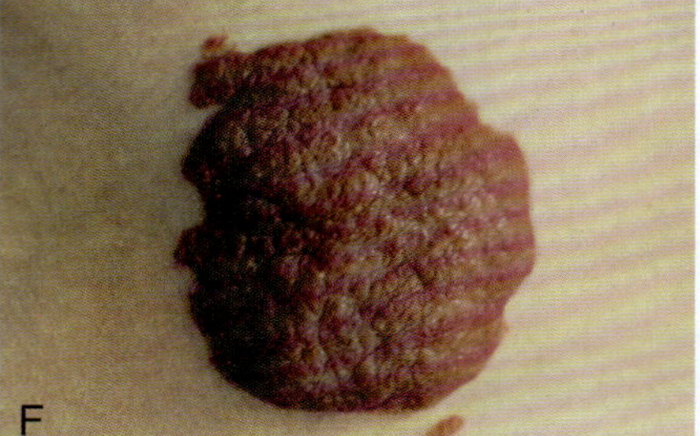

FIGURE 32-15 Common skin variations found in newborns: **(A)** milia; **(B)** erythema toxicum; **(C)** telangiectatic naevi; **(D)** Mongolian spot; **(E)** port-wine stain (naevus flammeus); **(F)** strawberry haemangioma. (Klossner, N. J. & Hatfield, N. [2006]. *Introductory maternity and pediatric nursing*. Philadelphia: Lippincott Williams & Wilkins.)

SUBSEQUENT PHYSICAL ASSESSMENT (continued)

ASSESSMENT PROCEDURE	NORMAL FINDINGS	ABNORMAL FINDINGS
Skin, hair and nails (continued)		
Palpate for texture, temperature, moisture, turgor and oedema.	Skin is warm and slightly moist. Vernix caseosa (cheesy, white substance that is found on the skin, especially in skin folds) is a common finding; it eventually absorbs into the skin.	Ecchymoses in various stages or in unusual locations or circular burn areas suggest child abuse, although bruising or burning may also be from cultural practices such as *cupping* or *coining.* Petechiae, lesions or rashes may indicate serious disorders.
Inspect and palpate hair. Observe for distribution, characteristics and presence of any unusual hair on body.	Hair is normally lustrous, silky, strong and elastic. Fine, downy hair covers the body. Children of African descent usually have hair that is curlier and coarser than white children.	Dirty, matted hair may indicate neglect. Tufts of hair over spine may indicate spina bifida occulta.
Inspect and palpate nails. Note colour, texture, shape and condition of nails.	Nails extend to end of fingers or beyond and are well-formed. **CULTURAL CONSIDERATIONS** **Dark-skinned children have deeper nail pigment.**	Blue nailbeds indicate cyanosis. Yellow nailbeds indicate jaundice. Blue-black nailbeds suggest a nailbed haemorrhage.
Head, neck and cervical lymph nodes		
Inspect and palpate the head. Note shape and symmetry. In newborns, inspect and palpate the condition of fontanelles and sutures (Fig. 32-16).	Head is normocephalic and symmetrical. In newborns, the head may be oddly shaped from moulding (overriding of the sutures) during vaginal birth. The diamond-shaped anterior fontanelle measures about 4 to 5 cm at its widest part; it usually closes by 12 to 18 months. The triangular posterior fontanelle measures about 0.5 to 1 cm at its widest part and should close at age 2 months.	A very large head is found with hydrocephalus. An oddly shaped head is found with premature closure of sutures (possibly genetic). One-sided flattening of the head suggests prolonged positioning on one side. A third fontanelle between the anterior and posterior fontanelle is seen with Down syndrome. Premature closure of sutures (craniosynostosis) may result in caput succedaneum (oedema from trauma), which crosses the suture line, and cephalohaematoma (bleeding into the periosteal space), which does not extend across the suture line (Fig. 32-17). Craniotabes may result from osteoporosis of the outer skull bone. Palpating too firmly with the thumb or forefinger over the temporoparietal area will leave an indentation of the bone. Bulging fontanelle indicates increased cranial pressure. Microcephaly is seen with infants who have been exposed to congenital infections.

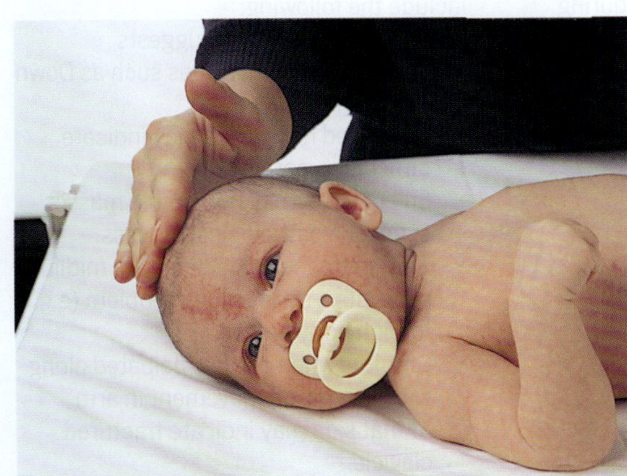

FIGURE 32-16 Palpating the anterior fontanelle. (© B. Proud.)

Continued on following page

SUBSEQUENT PHYSICAL ASSESSMENT (continued)

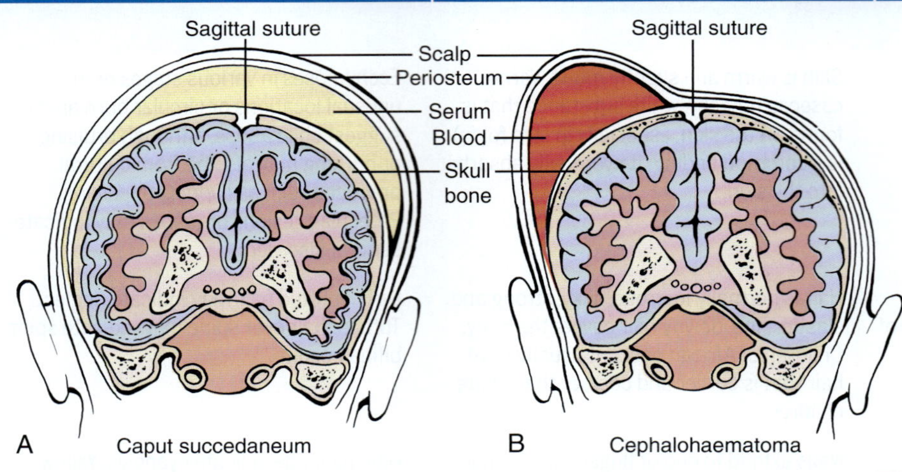

FIGURE 32-17 Premature suture closure may result in **(A)** caput succedaneum and **(B)** cephalohaematoma.

ASSESSMENT PROCEDURE	NORMAL FINDINGS	ABNORMAL FINDINGS
Test head control, head posture, range of motion.	Full range of motion—up, down and sideways—is normal. **Infant should have head control at 4 months.**	Hyperextension is seen with opisthotonos or significant meningeal irritation. Limited range of motion may indicate torticollis (wryneck).
Inspect and palpate the face. Note appearance, symmetry and movement. Palpate the parotid glands for swelling.	Face is normally proportionate and symmetrical. Movements are equal bilaterally. Parotid glands are normal size.	Unusual proportions (short palpebral fissures, thin lips, and wide and flat philtrum, which is the groove above the upper lip) may be hereditary or may indicate specific syndromes such as Down syndrome and fetal alcohol syndrome. Unequal movement may indicate facial nerve paralysis. Abnormal facial expressions may indicate chromosomal anomaly.
Inspect and palpate the neck. Palpate the thyroid gland and the trachea. Also inspect and palpate the cervical lymph nodes for swelling, mobility, temperature and tenderness. **CLINICAL TIP** **The thyroid is very difficult to palpate in an infant because of the short, thick neck.**	The neck is usually short with skin folds between the head and shoulder during infancy. The isthmus is the only portion of the thyroid that should be palpable. The trachea is midline. Lymph nodes are usually non-palpable in infants. Clavicles are symmetrical and intact.	Implications of some abnormal findings include the following: • Short, webbed neck suggests anomalies or syndromes such as Down syndrome. • Distended neck veins may indicate difficulty breathing. • Enlarged thyroid or palpable masses suggest a pathological process. • Shift in tracheal position from midline suggests a serious lung problem (e.g. foreign body or tumour). • Crepitus when clavicle palpated along with decreased movement in arm of that side may indicate fractured clavicle.

SUBSEQUENT PHYSICAL ASSESSMENT (continued)

ASSESSMENT PROCEDURE	NORMAL FINDINGS	ABNORMAL FINDINGS
Eyes		
Inspect the external eye. Note the position, slant and epicanthal folds of the external eye.	Inner canthus distance approximately 2.5 cm, horizontal slant, no epicanthal folds. Outer canthus aligns with tips of the pinnas. **CULTURAL CONSIDERATIONS** **Epicanthal folds (excess of skin extending from roof of nose that partially or completely covers the inner canthus) are normal findings in Asian children, whose eyes also slant upwards.**	Wide-set position (hypertelorism), upward slant and thick epicanthal folds suggest Down syndrome. 'Sun-setting' appearance (upper lid covers part of the iris) suggests hydrocephalus.
Observe eyelid placement, swelling, discharge and lesions.	Eyelids have transient oedema, absence of tears.	Eyelid inflammation may result from infection. Swelling, erythema or purulent discharge may indicate infection or blocked tear ducts. Purulent discharge seen with sexually transmitted infections (gonorrhoea, *Chlamydia*).
Inspect the sclera and conjunctiva for colour, discharge, lesions, redness and lacerations.	Sclera and conjunctiva are clear and free of discharge, lesions, redness or lacerations. Small subconjunctival haemorrhages may be seen in newborns.	Yellow sclera suggests jaundice; blue sclera may indicate osteogenesis imperfecta ('brittle bone disease').
Observe the iris and the pupils.	Typically the iris is blue in light-skinned infants and brown in dark-skinned infants; permanent colour develops within 9 months. Brushfield spots (white flecks on the periphery of the iris) may be normal in some infants. Pupils are equal, round and reactive to light and accommodation.	Brushfield spots may indicate Down syndrome. Sluggish pupils indicate a neurological problem. Miosis (constriction) indicates iritis or narcotic use or abuse. Mydriasis (pupillary dilation) indicates emotional factors (fear), trauma or certain drug use.
Finally, inspect the eyebrows and eyelashes.	Eyebrows should be symmetrical in shape and movement. They should not meet midline. Eyelashes should be evenly distributed and curled outwards.	Sparseness of eyebrows or lashes could indicate skin disease.
Perform visual acuity tests. Assess visual acuity by observing infant's inability to gaze at object.	Visual acuity is difficult to test in infants; it is usually tested by observing the infant's ability to fix on and follow objects. Normal visual acuity is as follows: Birth: 20/100 to 20/400 1 year: 20/200 By 4 weeks of age, child should be able to fixate on objects. By 6 to 8 weeks, eyes should follow a moving object. By 3 months, the child is able to follow and reach for an object.	Children with a one-line difference between eyes should be referred. Abnormal findings include congenital defects such as cataracts.
Perform extraocular muscle tests. Hirschberg test: Shine light directly at the cornea while the child looks straight ahead.	In the Hirschberg test, the light reflects symmetrically in the centre of both pupils. Light causes pupils to vasoconstrict bilaterally and blink reflex occurs. Blink reflex also occurs as an object is brought towards the eyes.	Unequal alignment of light on the pupils in the Hirschberg test signals strabismus.

Continued on following page

SUBSEQUENT PHYSICAL ASSESSMENT (continued)

ASSESSMENT PROCEDURE	NORMAL FINDINGS	ABNORMAL FINDINGS
Perform ophthalmoscopic examination. The procedure is the same as for adults. Distraction is preferred over the use of restraint, which is likely to result in crying and closed eyes. Careful ophthalmoscopic examination of newborns is difficult without the use of mydriatic medications.	Red reflex is present. This reflex rules out most serious defects of the cornea, aqueous chamber, lens and vitreous humour. When visualised, the optic disc appears similar to an adult's. A newborn's optic discs are pale; peripheral vessels are not well developed.	Absence of the red reflex indicates cataracts. Papilloedema is unusual in children of this age owing to the ability of the fontanelles and sutures to open during increased intracranial pressure. Disc blurring and haemorrhages should be reported immediately.
Ears		
Inspect external ears. Note placement, discharge or lesions of the ears.	Top of pinna should cross the eye-occiput line and be within a 10-degree angle of a perpendicular line drawn from the eye-occiput line to the lobe. No unusual structure or markings should appear on the pinna.	Low-set ears with an alignment greater than a 10-degree angle (Fig. 32-18) suggest retardation or congenital syndromes. Abnormal shape may suggest renal disease process, which may be hereditary. Preauricular skin tags or sinuses suggest other anomalies of ears or the renal system.
Inspect internal ear. The internal ear examination requires using an otoscope. The nurse should always hold the otoscope in a manner that allows for rapid removal if the child moves. Have the carer hold and restrain the child. Because an infant's external canal is short and straight, pull the pinna down and back (Fig. 32-19).	No excessive cerumen, discharge, lesions, excoriations or foreign body in external canal. Amniotic fluid or vernix may be present in canal of ear of newborn. Tympanic membrane is pearly grey to light pink with normal landmarks. Tympanic membranes redden bilaterally when child is crying or febrile.	Presence of foreign bodies or cerumen impaction. Purulent discharge may indicate otitis externa or presence of foreign body. Purulent, serous discharge suggests otitis media. Bloody discharge suggests trauma, and clear discharge may indicate cerebrospinal fluid leak. Perforated tympanic membrane may also be noted.

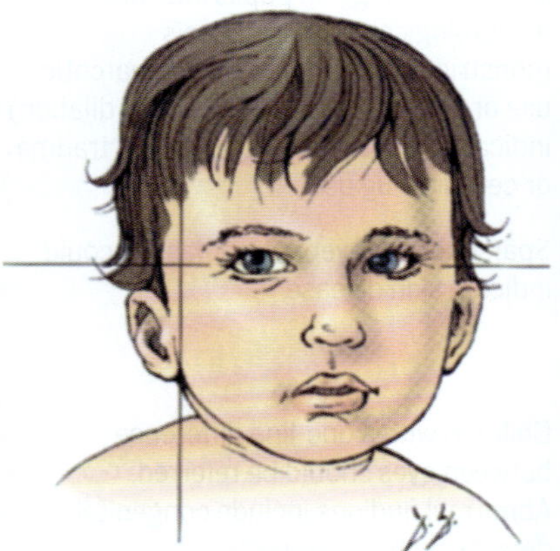

FIGURE 32-18 Low-set ears with an alignment greater than a 10-degree angle suggest retardation or congenital syndromes.

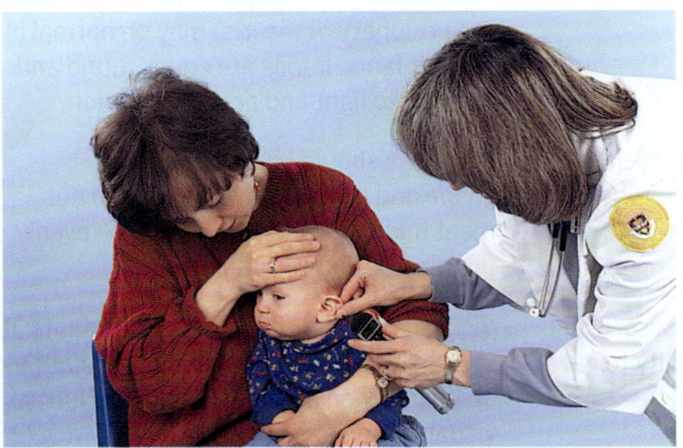

FIGURE 32-19 To examine the ears of an infant, restrain the child and pull the pinna down and back. (© B. Proud.)

ASSESSMENT PROCEDURE	NORMAL FINDINGS	ABNORMAL FINDINGS
Hearing acuity. In the infant, test hearing acuity by noting the reaction to noise. Stand approximately 30 cm from the infant and create a loud noise (e.g. clap hands, shake or squeeze a noisy toy). Routine newborn hearing screening is performed in most newborn nurseries 24 to 48 hours after birth or prior to discharge.	A newborn will exhibit the startle (Moro) reflex and blink eyes (acoustic blink reflex) in response to noise. Older infant will turn head.	No reactions to noise may indicate a hearing deficit. Audiometry results outside normal range suggest hearing deficit.

SUBSEQUENT PHYSICAL ASSESSMENT (continued)

ASSESSMENT PROCEDURE	NORMAL FINDINGS	ABNORMAL FINDINGS
Mouth, throat, nose and sinuses		
INSPECTION		
Inspect mouth and throat. Note the condition of the lips, palates, tongue and buccal mucosa.	Epstein pearls—small yellow-white retention cysts on the hard palate and gums—are common in newborns and usually disappear in the first weeks of life. In infants, a sucking tubercle (pad) from the friction of sucking may be evident in the middle of the upper lip.	Cleft lip or palate are congenital abnormalities.
Observe the condition of the gums. When teeth appear, count teeth and note location.	Gums appear pink and moist. Teeth may begin erupting at 4 to 6 months. Teeth develop in sequential order. By 10 months, most infants have two upper and two lower central incisors.	Abnormal findings include lesion and oedema.
Note the condition of the throat and tonsils. Also observe the insertion and ending point of the frenulum.	Tonsils are not visible in newborns. As the infant gets older, it is possible but still difficult to see the tonsils.	Extension of the frenulum to the tip of the tongue may interfere with extension of the tongue, which causes speech difficulties.
Inspect nose and sinuses. To inspect the nose and sinuses, avoid using the nasal speculum in infants and young children. Instead push up the tip of the nose and shine the light into each nostril. Observe the structure and patency of the nares, discharge, tenderness and any colour or swelling of the turbinates. **CLINICAL TIP** **Infants are obligatory nose breathers. Consequently obstructed nasal passages may precipitate serious health conditions, making it very important to assess the patency of the nares in the newborn. If, after suctioning fluid and mucus from the nares, you suspect obstruction, insert a small-lumen catheter into each nostril to assess patency.**	Nose is midline in face, septum is straight and nares are patent. No discharge or tenderness is present. Turbinates are pink and free of oedema. Milia are small, white papules found on the nose, forehead and chin. They develop from retention of sebum in sebaceous pores. They usually resolve spontaneously within a few weeks.	Choanal atresia is blockage of the posterior nares in the newborn. If the blockage is bilateral, the newborn is at risk of acute respiratory distress. Immediate referral is necessary. Deviated septum may be congenital or caused by injury. Foul discharge from one nostril may indicate a foreign body.
Thorax		
INSPECTION		
Inspect the shape of the thorax.	Infant's thorax is smooth, rounded and symmetrical.	Abnormal shapes of the thorax include pectus excavatum and pectus carinatum.
Observe respiratory effort, keeping in mind newborns and young infants are obligatory nose breathers.	Respirations should be unlaboured and regular in all ages except for immediate newborn period when respirations are irregular (see 'Vital signs' section, previous). Some newborns, especially the premature, have periodic irregular breathing, sometimes with apnoea (episodes when breathing stops) lasting a few seconds. This is a normal finding if bradycardia does not accompany irregular breathing.	Retractions (suprasternal, sternal, substernal, intercostal) and grunting suggest increased inspiratory effort, which may be due to airway obstruction. Periods of apnoea that last longer than 20 seconds and are accompanied by bradycardia may be a sign of a cardiovascular or central nervous system (CNS) disease. Nasal flaring, tachypnoea, see-saw movement of chest indicate respiratory distress.

Continued on following page

SUBSEQUENT PHYSICAL ASSESSMENT (continued)

ASSESSMENT PROCEDURE	NORMAL FINDINGS	ABNORMAL FINDINGS
PERCUSSION AND AUSCULTATION		
Percuss the chest. During percussion of the lungs, note tone elicited.	Hyper-resonance is the normal tone elicited in infants because of thinness of the chest wall.	A dull tone may indicate a mass, fluid or consolidation.
Auscultate for breath sounds and adventitious sounds. If a newborn's lung sounds seem noisy, auscultate the upper nostrils.	Breath sounds may seem louder and harsher in young children because of their thin chest walls. No adventitious sounds should be heard, although transmitted upper airway sounds may be heard on auscultation of the thorax.	Diminished breath sounds suggest respiratory disorders such as pneumonia or atelectasis. Stridor (inspiratory wheeze) is a high-pitched, piercing sound that indicates a narrowing of the upper tracheobronchial tree. Expiratory wheezes indicate narrowing in the lower tracheobronchial tree. Rhonchi and rales (crackles) may indicate a number of respiratory diseases such as pneumonia, bronchitis and bronchiolitis.
Breasts		
INSPECTION AND PALPATION		
Inspect and palpate breasts. Note shape, symmetry, colour, tenderness, discharge, lesions and masses.	Newborns may have enlarged and engorged breasts with a white liquid discharge because of the influence of maternal hormones (Fig. 32-20). This condition resolves spontaneously within days.	A palpable mass of the breast is abnormal. The newborn or infant may have extra nipples noted on the chest or abdomen called supernumerary nipples.
Heart		
INSPECTION AND PALPATION		
Inspect and palpate the praecordium. Note lifts, heaves and apical impulse (Fig. 32-21).	The apical pulse is at the fourth intercostal space until the age of 7 years, when it drops to the fifth. It is to the left of the midclavicular line until age 4.	A systolic heave may indicate right ventricular enlargement. Apical impulse that is not in proper location for age may indicate cardiomyopathy, pneumothorax or diaphragmatic hernia.

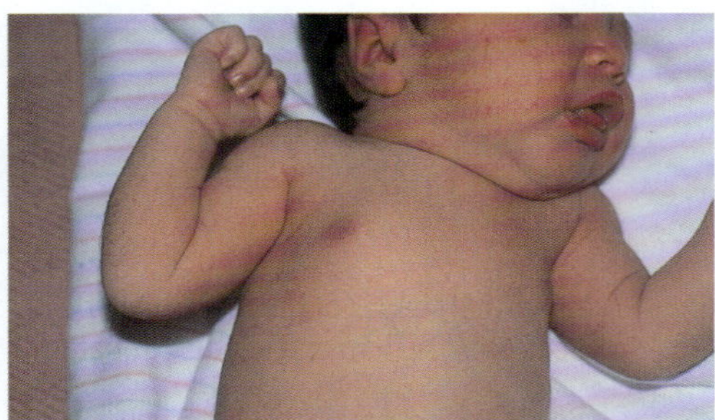

FIGURE 32-20 The enlarged breasts of this newborn are normal and result from the influence of maternal hormones. (Evans, R.J., Brown, Y.M., & Evans, M.K. [2014]. *Canadian Maternity, Newborn and Women's Health Nursing: Comprehensive Care Across the Lifespan* [2nd ed.]. Philadelphia: Wolters Kluwer.)

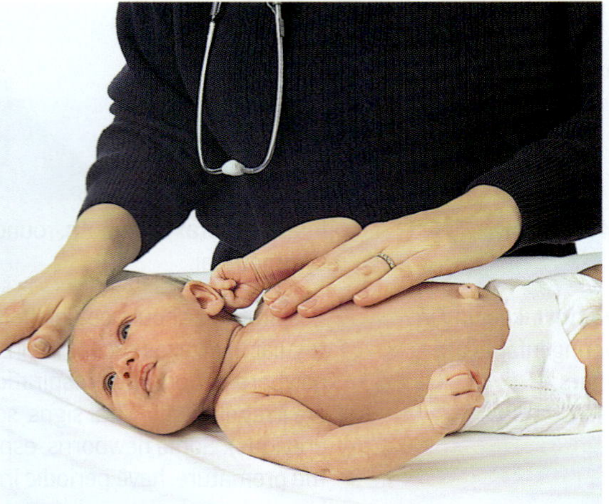

FIGURE 32-21 Palpate the infant's chest for lifts and heaves. (© B. Proud.)

SUBSEQUENT PHYSICAL ASSESSMENT (continued)

ASSESSMENT PROCEDURE	NORMAL FINDINGS	ABNORMAL FINDINGS
AUSCULTATION		
Auscultate heart sounds. Listen to the heart. Note rate and rhythm of apical impulse, S_1, S_2, extra heart sounds and murmurs. Keep in mind that sinus arrhythmia is normal in infants. Heart sounds are louder, higher pitched and of shorter duration in infants. A split S_2 at the apex occurs normally in some infants and S_3 is a normal heart sound in some children. A venous hum also may be normally heard in children.	Normal heart rates are cited in the 'Vital signs' section. Innocent murmurs, which are common throughout childhood, are classified as systolic, of short duration, show no transmission to other areas, grade III or less, loudest in pulmonic area (base of heart), low-pitched, musical or groaning, varying in intensity in relation to position, respiration, activity, fever and anaemia. No other associated signs of heart disease should be found.	Murmurs that do not fit the criteria for innocent murmurs may indicate a disease or disorder. Extra heart sounds and variations in pulse rate and rhythm also suggest pathological processes.
Abdomen		
INSPECTION		
Inspect the shape of the abdomen.	In infants, the abdomen is prominent in the supine position.	A scaphoid (boat-shaped; i.e. sunken with prominent rib cage) abdomen may result from malnutrition or dehydration. Distended abdomen may indicate pyloric stenosis.
Inspect umbilicus. Note colour, discharge, evident herniation of the umbilicus.	Umbilicus is pink, no discharge, odour, redness or herniation. Cord should demonstrate three vessels (two arteries and one vein). Remnant of cord should appear dried 24 to 48 hours after birth.	Inflammation, discharge and redness of umbilicus suggest infection. Diastasis recti (separation of the abdominal muscles) is seen as midline protrusion from the xiphoid to the umbilicus or pubis symphysis. This condition is secondary to immature musculature of abdominal muscles and usually has little significance. As the muscles strengthen, the separation resolves on its own. A bulge at the umbilicus suggests an umbilical hernia (Fig. 32-22), which may be seen in newborns; it usually disappears by age 1 year. Abnormal insertion of cord, discoloured cord or two-vessel cord could indicate genetic abnormalities; however, these are also seen in newborns without abnormalities.

Continued on following page

SUBSEQUENT PHYSICAL ASSESSMENT (continued)

ASSESSMENT PROCEDURE	NORMAL FINDINGS	ABNORMAL FINDINGS
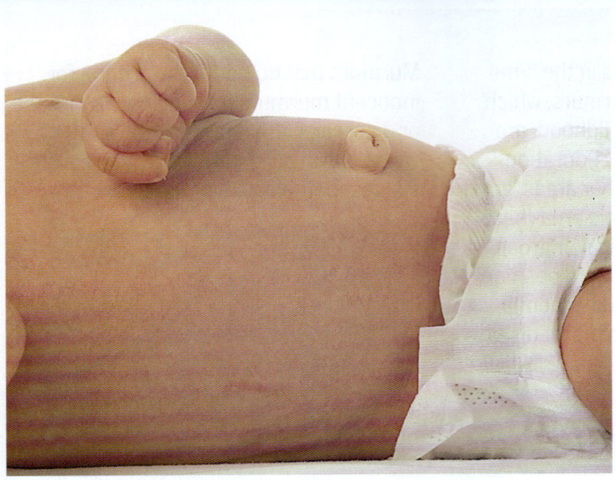 **FIGURE 32-22** Umbilical hernia. (© B. Proud.)		
AUSCULTATION		
Auscultate bowel sounds. Follow auscultation guidelines for adult patients provided in Chapter 24.	Normal bowel sounds occur every 10 to 30 seconds. They sound like clicks, gurgles or growls.	Marked peristaltic waves almost always indicate a pathological process such as pyloric stenosis.
PALPATION		
Palpate for masses and tenderness. Palpate abdomen for softness or hardness.	Abdomen is soft to palpation and without masses or tenderness.	A rigid abdomen is almost always an emergent problem. Masses or tenderness warrants further investigation. Hirschsprung disease could also be considered, especially with suprapubic mass palpable.
Palpate liver. Palpate the liver the same as you would for adults (see Chap. 24).	Liver is usually palpable 1 to 2 cm below the right costal margin in young children. The liver is hard to palpate in the newborn.	An enlarged liver with a firm edge that is palpated more than 2 cm below the right costal margin usually indicates a pathological process.
Palpate spleen. Palpate the spleen the same as you would for adults (see Chap. 24).	Spleen tip may be palpable during inspiration. The spleen is difficult to palpate in the newborn.	Enlarged spleen is usually indicative of a pathological process.
Palpate kidneys. Palpate the kidneys the same as you would for adults (see Chap. 24).	The tip of the right kidney may be palpable during inspiration.	Enlarged kidneys are usually indicative of a pathological process.
Palpate bladder. Palpate the bladder the same as you would for adults (see Chap. 24).	The bladder may be slightly palpable in infants and small children.	An enlarged bladder is usually due to urinary retention but may be due to a mass.

SUBSEQUENT PHYSICAL ASSESSMENT (continued)

ASSESSMENT PROCEDURE	NORMAL FINDINGS	ABNORMAL FINDINGS
Male genitalia		
INSPECTION AND PALPATION		
Inspect penis and urinary meatus. Inspect the genitalia, observing size for age and any lesions.	Penis is normal size for age, and no lesions are seen. Nappy rash, however, is a common finding in infants (Fig. 32-23). The foreskin is retractable in uncircumcised child. Urinary meatus is at tip of glans penis and has no discharge or redness. Penis may appear small in large for gestational-age boys because of overlapping skin folds. For circumcised boys, the site is dry with minimal swelling and drainage.	An unretractable foreskin in a child older than 3 months suggests phimosis. Paraphimosis is indicated when the foreskin is tightened around the glans penis in a retracted position. Hypospadias, urinary meatus on ventral surface of glans, and epispadias, urinary meatus on dorsal surface of glans, are congenital disorders (see Chap. 26).
Inspect and palpate scrotum and testes. To rule out cryptorchidism, it is important to palpate for testes in the scrotum in infants. **CLINICAL TIP** **When palpating the testicles in the infant, you must keep the cremasteric reflex in mind. This reflex pulls the testicles up into the inguinal canal and abdomen and is elicited in response to touch, cold or emotional factors.**	Scrotum is free of lesions. Testes are palpable in scrotum, with the left testicle usually lower than the right. Testes are equal in size, smooth, mobile and free of masses. If a testicle is missing from the scrotal sac but the scrotal sac appears well developed, suspect physiological cryptorchidism. The testis has originally descended into the scrotum but has moved back up into the inguinal canal because of the cremasteric reflex and the small size of the testis. You should be able to milk the testis down into the scrotum from the inguinal canal. This normal condition subsides at puberty.	Absent testicles and atrophic scrotum suggest true cryptorchidism (undescended testicles). This suggests that the testicles never descended. This condition occurs more frequently in preterm than term infants because testes descend at 8 months of gestation. It can lead to testicular atrophy and infertility, and increases the risk for testicular cancer. Hydrocoeles are common in infants. They are fluid-filled masses that can be transilluminated (see Chap. 26, Abnormal findings 26-2). They usually resolve spontaneously. A scrotal hernia is usually caused by an indirect inguinal hernia that has descended into the scrotum. It can usually be pushed back into the inguinal canal. This mass will not transilluminate.

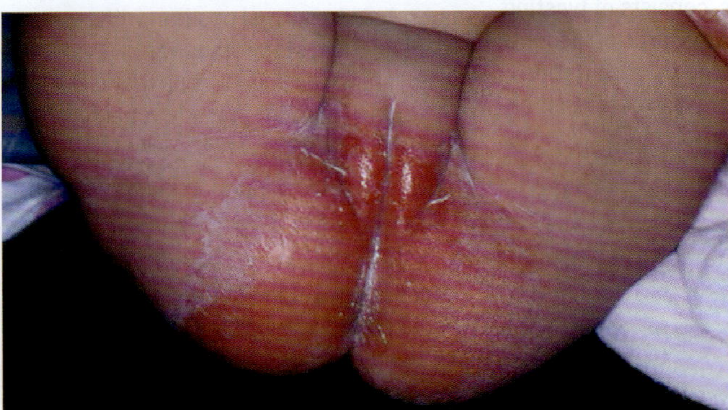

FIGURE 32-23 Nappy rash, a common finding in infants.

ASSESSMENT PROCEDURE	NORMAL FINDINGS	ABNORMAL FINDINGS
Inspect and palpate inguinal area for hernias. Observe for any bulge in the inguinal area. Using your little finger, palpate up the inguinal canal to the external inguinal ring if a hernia is suspected.	No inguinal hernias are present.	A bulge in the inguinal area or palpation of a mass in the inguinal canal suggests an inguinal hernia. Indirect inguinal hernias occur most frequently in children (see Chap. 26).

Continued on following page

SUBSEQUENT PHYSICAL ASSESSMENT (continued)

ASSESSMENT PROCEDURE	NORMAL FINDINGS	ABNORMAL FINDINGS
Female genitalia		
INSPECTION		
Inspect external genitalia. Note labia majora, labia minora, vaginal orifice, urinary meatus and clitoris.	Labia majora and minora are pink and moist. Newborn's genitalia may appear prominent because of influence of maternal hormones. Bruises and swelling may be caused by breech vaginal delivery.	Enlarged clitoris in newborn combined with fusion of the posterior labia majora suggests ambiguous genitalia.
Anus and rectum		
INSPECTION		
Inspect the anus. Spread the buttocks with gloved hands; note patency of anal opening, presence of any lesions and fissures, and condition and colour of perianal skin.	The anal opening should be visible and moist. Perianal skin should be smooth and free of lesions. Perianal skin tags may be noted. Meconium passed within 24 to 48 hours after birth.	Imperforate anus (no anal opening) should be referred. Pustules may indicate secondary infection of nappy rash. No passage of stool could indicate no patency of anus or cystic fibrosis.
PALPATION		
Palpate rectum. This internal examination is not routinely performed in infants.		
Musculoskeletal		
INSPECTION		
Assess arms, hands, feet and legs. Note symmetry, shape, movement and positioning of the feet and legs. Perform neurovascular assessment. **CLINICAL TIP** **If the patient is a newborn, keep in mind that the feet may retain their intrauterine position and appear deformed (positioned outwards or inwards from normal right angle to the leg). This is normal if the foot easily returns to its normal position with manipulation (either scratch along the lateral edge of the affected foot or gently push the forefoot into its normal position).**	Feet and legs are symmetrical in size, shape and movement. Extremities should be warm and mobile with adequate capillary refill. All pulses (radial, brachial, femoral, popliteal, pedal) should be strong and equal bilaterally. There may be an inwards (pointing towards centre of the body) positioning of the forefoot with the heel in normal straight position; it resolves spontaneously. Tibial torsion, also common in infants and toddlers, consists of twisting of the tibia inwards or outwards on its long axis and is usually caused by intrauterine positioning; this typically corrects itself by the time the child is 2 years old.	Short, broad extremities, hyperextensible joints and palmar simian crease may indicate Down syndrome. Polydactyly (extra digits) and syndactyly (webbing) are sometimes found in children with mental retardation. Absent femoral pulses may indicate coarctation of the aorta. Neurovascular deficit in children is usually secondary to trauma (e.g. fracture). Fixed-position (true) deformities do not return to normal position with manipulation. Metatarsus varus is inversion (a turning inwards that elevates the medial margin) and adduction of the forefoot. Talipes varus is adduction of the forefoot and inversion of the entire foot. Talipes equinovarus (clubfoot) is indicated if foot is fixed in the following position: adduction of forefoot, inversion of entire foot and equinus (pointing downwards) position of entire foot.
Assess for congenital hip dysplasia. Assessing for hip dysplasia is an important aspect of the physical examination for infants. The assessment should be performed at each visit until the child is about 1 year old. (Several tests are described below.)		

SUBSEQUENT PHYSICAL ASSESSMENT (continued)

ASSESSMENT PROCEDURE	NORMAL FINDINGS	ABNORMAL FINDINGS
Musculoskeletal (continued)		
Begin by assessing the symmetry of the gluteal folds. Also assess hip abduction using the manoeuvres below.	Equal gluteal folds and full hip abduction are normal findings.	Unequal gluteal folds and limited hip abduction are signs of congenital hip dysplasia.
Perform the Ortolani manoeuvre to test for congenital hip dysplasia (Fig. 32-24). With the infant supine, flex infant's knees while holding your thumbs on midthigh and your fingers over the greater trochanters; abduct the legs, moving the knees outwards and down towards the table.	Negative Ortolani sign is normal.	Positive Ortolani sign: A click heard along with feeling the head of the femur slip in or out of the hip.
Perform the Barlow manoeuvre (Fig. 32-25). With the infant supine, flex the infant's knees while holding your thumbs on midthigh and your fingers over the greater trochanters; adduct legs until thumbs touch.	Negative Barlow sign is normal.	Positive Barlow sign: A feeling of the head of the femur slipping out of the hip socket (acetabulum).
Assess spinal alignment. Observe spine and posture.	In newborns, the spine is flexible, with convex dorsal and sacral curves. In infants younger than 3 months, the spine is rounded (Fig. 32-26). The newborn's spine is flexed.	In newborns, flaccid or rigid posture is considered abnormal. In older infants and children, abnormal posture suggests neuromuscular disorders such as cerebral palsy.

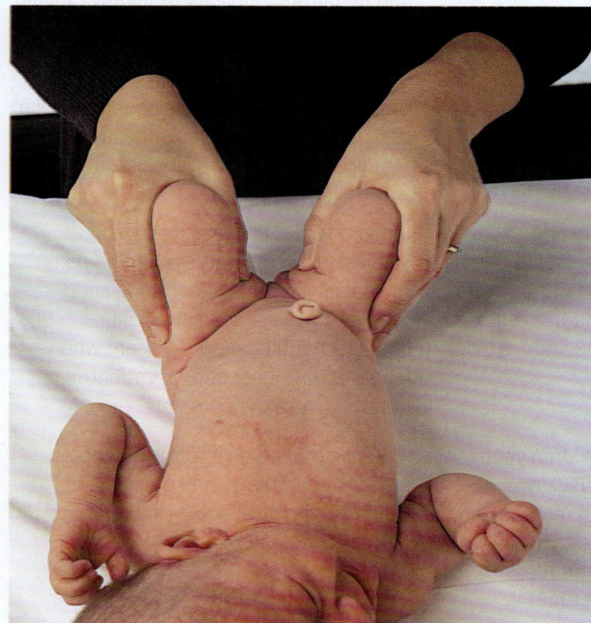

FIGURE 32-24 Performing the Ortolani manoeuvre.

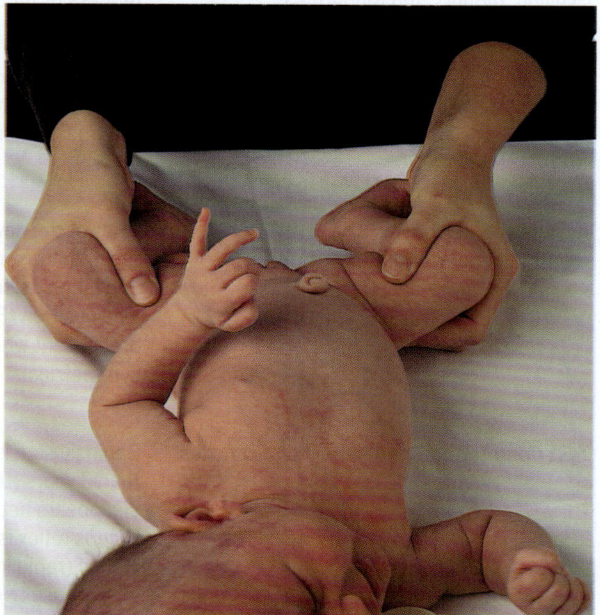

FIGURE 32-25 Performing the Barlow manoeuvre.

Continued on following page

SUBSEQUENT PHYSICAL ASSESSMENT (continued)

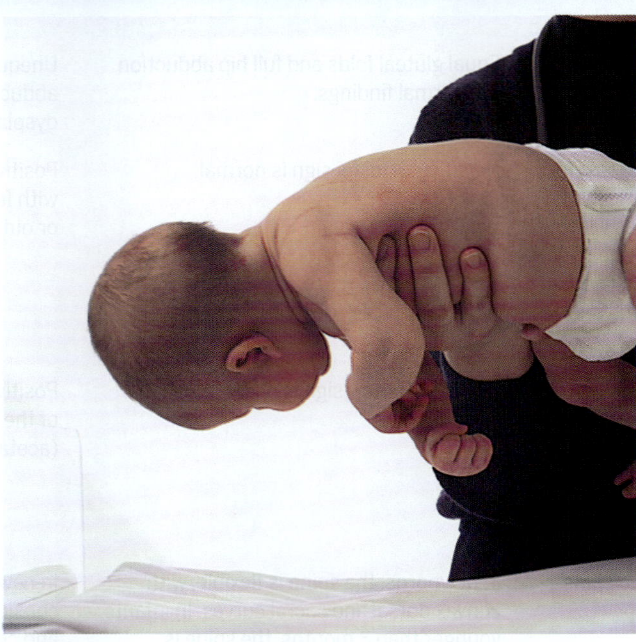

FIGURE 32-26 The spine is rounded in infants under 3 months old. (© B. Proud.)

ASSESSMENT PROCEDURE	NORMAL FINDINGS	ABNORMAL FINDINGS
Assess joints. Note range of motion, swelling, redness and tenderness.	Full range of motion and no swelling, redness or tenderness.	Limited range of motion, swelling, redness and tenderness indicate problems ranging from mild injuries to serious disorders.
Assess muscles. Note size and strength. (For example, can the infant bear weight on his or her legs?)	Muscle size and strength should be adequate for the particular age and should be equal bilaterally.	Inadequate muscle size and strength for the particular age indicate neuromuscular disorders such as muscular dystrophy.
NEUROLOGICAL SYSTEM		
Assess the newborn's cry, responsiveness and adaptation.	Cries of the newborn are lusty and strong; the infant responds appropriately to stimuli and quiets to soothing when held in the *en face* position (Fig. 32-27). Infantile reflexes are present when appropriate and are symmetrical.	Inappropriate response to stimuli suggests CNS disorders or problems. An inability to quiet to soothing and gaze aversion are seen in 'cocaine babies'. Infantile reflexes present when inappropriate, absent or asymmetrical may indicate a CNS problem.
Test deep tendon and superficial reflexes.	Babinski sign is normal in children younger than 2 years (this response usually disappears between 2 and 24 months), and triceps reflex is absent until age 6. Ankle clonus (rapid, rhythmic plantar flexion) in response to eliciting ankle reflex is common in newborns.	Absence or marked intensity of these reflexes, asymmetry and presence of Babinski sign after age 2 years may demonstrate pathology.
Test motor function. See the Parents' Evaluation of Developmental Status (PEDS) examination (see Assessment tool 32-1).	Gross and fine motor skills should be appropriate for the child's developmental age. Head control should be acquired by age 4 months. Hand preference is developed during the preschool years.	Gross and fine motor skills that are inappropriate for developmental age and lack of head control by age 6 months may indicate cerebral palsy. Hand preference that is not developed during preschool years may indicate paresis on opposite side.

SUBSEQUENT PHYSICAL ASSESSMENT (continued)

ASSESSMENT PROCEDURE	NORMAL FINDINGS	ABNORMAL FINDINGS
Musculoskeletal (continued)		

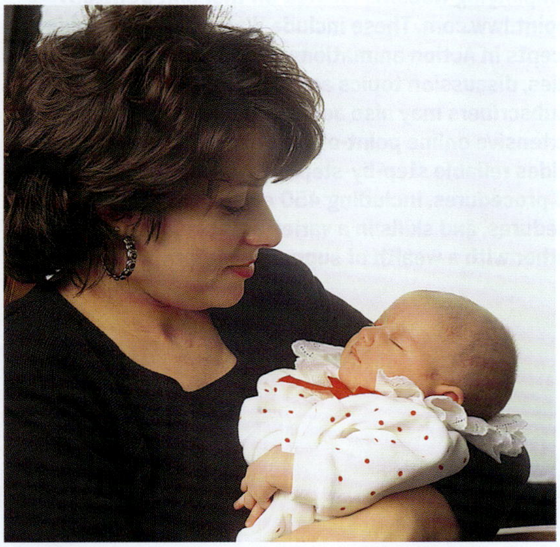

FIGURE 32-27 The newborn quiets to soothing when held *en face.*

VALIDATING AND DOCUMENTING FINDINGS

Validate the assessment data you have collected. This is necessary to verify that the data are reliable and accurate. Document the assessment data following the health care facility or agency policy.

After you have collected your assessment data, you will need to analyse the data using diagnostic reasoning skills. Refer to the discussion of the diagnostic reasoning process in Chapter 5.

Sample of subjective data

JM is a 4-month-old male in for well-child visit. Primary carer is mother. Father works in sales. Mother remains at home with child. She reports the child is healthy and happy. Child pushes himself up when in prone position. Responds to mother's voice. Sleeps through the night. Child breastfeeds. Mother reports no problems with feeding. Stools normal and regular. Immunisations are up to date.

Sample of objective data

Child is 4 months old, weighs 8.10 kg and is 63 cm long. Temperature is 37.5°C. Pulse, normal and regular. Head circumference 42 cm. Skin, soft and warm; no lesions present. Head symmetrical. Child holds head erect and midline. Mouth free of lesions. Nose free of obstruction. Eye placement normal. Infant follows object with eyes. Red reflex present. Ears aligned and symmetrical. Internal ears free of discharge or lesions. Respirations even and unlaboured. Breath sounds clear bilaterally. S_1 *and* S_2 *auscultated and normal. No herniation of umbilicus. Bowel sounds normal. Genitalia appropriate size for age; no lesions. Testes palpable, equal in size, smooth and mobile. Anus free of lesions and haemorrhoids. Negative Ortolani sign and Barlow manoeuvre. Full range of motion in joints.*

Analysis of data

DIAGNOSTIC REASONING: POSSIBLE CONCLUSIONS

After collecting subjective and objective data, identify abnormal findings and patient strengths. Then cluster the data to reveal any significant patterns or abnormalities. These data may be used to make clinical judgements about the health status of the neonate or infant.

Potential patient risks

- Risk of impaired parent–infant attachment
- Risk of delayed development
- Risk of disproportionate growth
- Risk of disorganised infant behaviour

Potential patient problems

- Ineffective breastfeeding (related to poor infant sucking reflex)
- Delayed growth and development (related to inadequate caretaking)
- Disorganised infant behaviour (related to malnutrition)
- Ineffective infant feeding pattern

Selected collaborative problems

After grouping the data, it may become apparent that certain collaborative problems emerge. Remember that collaborative problems cannot be prevented with nursing interventions alone. However, these physiological complications of medical conditions can be detected and monitored by the nurse. In addition, the nurse can use doctor- and nurse-prescribed interventions to minimise the complications of these problems. The nurse may also have to refer the patient in such situations for further treatment of the problem. The following is a list of collaborative problems seen more frequently in the newborn or infant. However, other collaborative problems seen in the adult are also seen in paediatric patients.

- Severe malnutrition or dehydration
- Delayed growth
- Failure to thrive
- Respiratory distress
- Permanently deformed femoral head
- Hydrocephalus or shunt infections.

Medical problems

If, after grouping the data, it becomes apparent that the patient has signs and symptoms that may require medical diagnosis and treatment, referral to a primary care provider is necessary.

ONLINE RESOURCES

An extensive range of additional resources to enhance teaching and learning and to facilitate understanding may be found online at the text's accompanying website, located on thePoint at http://thepoint.lww.com. These include Watch and Learn videos, Concepts in Action animations, journal articles, case studies, discussion topics and quizzes.

Subscribers may also access Lippincott Procedures, an extensive online point-of-care procedure guide that provides reliable step-by-step instructions for more than 1700 procedures, including 450 evidence-based Australian procedures, and skills in a variety of speciality settings, together with a wealth of supporting information.

CASE STUDY

The case study demonstrates how to analyse assessment data for newborns and infants. The exercises included in the ancillary product on thePoint that complements this text offer further opportunities to enhance your skills.

Two-month-old Lee Simpson is admitted to the ward with bronchiolitis. It is her first presentation after being unwell for 3 days with a runny nose and fever. Today she has been wheezy and had decreased feeding. She has been admitted for monitoring, oxygen therapy and small frequent feeds. As the nurse caring for Lee, you begin to attend to her admission, where a full physical assessment needs to be completed. While you are doing the assessment, Lee's mother Bianca tells you she is anxious and isn't sure how to care for her when she is so unwell.

Bianca summarises the type of care provided to Lee before she became unwell. She states that Lee responds well to her voice and is generally content, drinks her bottle well and sleeps through the night. You notice Bianca is attentive to the baby during the interview. When undressing Lee to obtain her weight, you notice she has slight intercostal recession and tracheal tug. You also notice her nose is blocked.

The following concept map illustrates the diagnostic reasoning process.

Applying COLDSPA

Applying COLDSPA for a 2-month-old infant with bronchiolitis. Mother reports that she is anxious and isn't sure how to care for her daughter when she is so unwell. Note that when assessing an infant, you are really assessing the mother and infant as a pair.

Mnemonic	Question	Data provided	Missing data
Character	Describe the sign or symptom (feeling, appearance, sound, smell or taste, if applicable).	Mother is anxious about not knowing how to care for her child who is unwell with bronchiolitis	
Onset	When did it begin?	Three days ago following a runny nose and fever. The child is now fussy and seems uncomfortable	
Location	Where is it? Does it radiate? Does it occur anywhere else?	She has intercostal recession, tracheal tug and a blocked nose	What is her respiration rate? Is her chest wheezy? Has she been coughing? Has she been coughing up phlegm?
Duration	How long does it last? Does it recur?		Has she had this before? When did you notice the symptoms starting? Has anyone else in the family been unwell?
Severity	How bad is it? or How much does it bother you?		Is the child settled? How does mother respond to settling the child? Is the child able to feed with the oxygen? How much nasal discharge? What colour is it?
Pattern	What makes it better or worse?		Has the mother been using anything to help clear the blocked nose? What helps the baby to settle?
Associated factors/How it **A**ffects the patient	What other symptoms occur with it? How does it affect you?	Mother is attentive to child and reports that the child responds to her voice, is generally content, and eats and sleeps well	How does the mother respond to education regarding babies with bronchiolitis and the associated care?

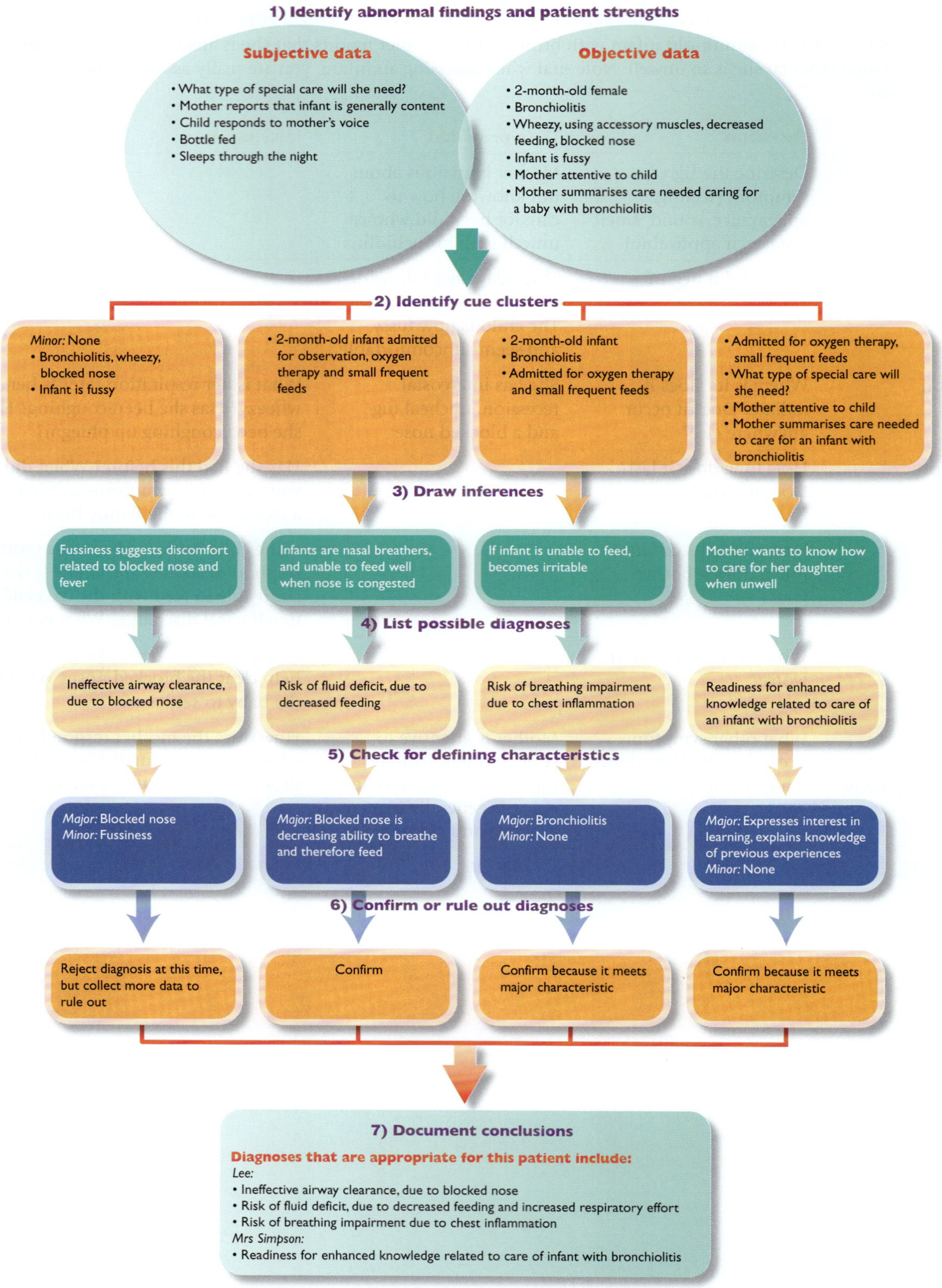

1) Identify abnormal findings and patient strengths

Subjective data

- What type of special care will she need?
- Mother reports that infant is generally content
- Child responds to mother's voice
- Bottle fed
- Sleeps through the night

Objective data

- 2-month-old female
- Bronchiolitis
- Wheezy, using accessory muscles, decreased feeding, blocked nose
- Infant is fussy
- Mother attentive to child
- Mother summarises care needed caring for a baby with bronchiolitis

2) Identify cue clusters

Minor: None
- Bronchiolitis, wheezy, blocked nose
- Infant is fussy

- 2-month-old infant admitted for observation, oxygen therapy and small frequent feeds

- 2-month-old infant
- Bronchiolitis
- Admitted for oxygen therapy and small frequent feeds

- Admitted for oxygen therapy, small frequent feeds
- What type of special care will she need?
- Mother attentive to child
- Mother summarises care needed to care for an infant with bronchiolitis

3) Draw inferences

Fussiness suggests discomfort related to blocked nose and fever

Infants are nasal breathers, and unable to feed well when nose is congested

If infant is unable to feed, becomes irritable

Mother wants to know how to care for her daughter when unwell

4) List possible diagnoses

Ineffective airway clearance, due to blocked nose

Risk of fluid deficit, due to decreased feeding

Risk of breathing impairment due to chest inflammation

Readiness for enhanced knowledge related to care of an infant with bronchiolitis

5) Check for defining characteristics

Major: Blocked nose
Minor: Fussiness

Major: Blocked nose is decreasing ability to breathe and therefore feed

Major: Bronchiolitis
Minor: None

Major: Expresses interest in learning, explains knowledge of previous experiences
Minor: None

6) Confirm or rule out diagnoses

Reject diagnosis at this time, but collect more data to rule out

Confirm

Confirm because it meets major characteristic

Confirm because it meets major characteristic

7) Document conclusions

Diagnoses that are appropriate for this patient include:

Lee:
- Ineffective airway clearance, due to blocked nose
- Risk of fluid deficit, due to decreased feeding and increased respiratory effort
- Risk of breathing impairment due to chest inflammation

Mrs Simpson:
- Readiness for enhanced knowledge related to care of infant with bronchiolitis

References

Apgar, V. (1953). A proposal for a new method of evaluation of the newborn infant. *Current Researches in Anesthesia and Analgesia*, Viewed January 2014 at http://profiles.nlm.nih.gov/ps/access/CPBBKG.pdf.

Australian Breastfeeding Association. (2013). Breastfeeding, co-sleeping and sudden unexpected deaths in infancy [SUDI]. Available via www.breastfeeding.asn.au.

Erikson, E. H. (1963). *Childhood and society* (2nd ed.). New York: Norton.

Freud, S. (1923/1974). *The ego and the id*. London: Hogarth.

Harel-Gadassi, A., Friedlander, E., Yaari, M., et al. (2018). Developmental assessment of preterm infants: Chronological or corrected age? *Research in Developmental Disabilities, 80*, 35–43.

Kain, V. & Mannix, T. (2018). *Neonatal nursing*. Chatswood, Australia: Elsevier.

Kohlberg, L. (1969). Stage and sequence: The cognitive developmental approach to socialization. In D. Gaslin (Ed). *Handbook of socialization: Theory and research* (pp. 347–380). Chicago: Rand McNally.

Kohlberg, L. (1976). Moral stages and moralization: The cognitive-developmental approach. In T. Lickona (Ed). *Moral development and behaviour*. New York: Holt, Rinehart & Winston.

Kohlberg, L. (1984). *The psychology of moral development: The nature and validity of moral stages* (Vol. 2). New York: Harper & Row.

Marshall, J. & Raynor, M. (2014). *Myles textbook for midwives*. London, England: Elsevier.

New Zealand Ministry of Health (NZMOH). (2013). Babies and toddlers [includes breastfeeding and SUDI]. Available via www.health.govt.nz.

Pairman, S., Tracy, S., Dahlen, H., et al. (2019). *Midwifery: Preparation for practice*. Chatswood, Australia: Elsevier.

Piaget, J. (1932). *The moral judgement of the child*. New York: Harcourt Brace Jovanovich.

Piaget, J. (1952). *The origins of intelligence in children*. New York: International Universities Press.

Piaget, J. & Inhelder, B. (1969). *The psychology of the child*. New York: Basic Books.

Selected readings

Association of Women's Health, Obstetric and Neonatal Nurses (AWHONN). (2011). Newborn screening. Position statement. *Journal of Obstetric, Gynaecologic, and Neonatal Nursing, 40*(1), 136–137. Available January 2014 via www.awhonn.org.

Dempsey, J., Hillege, S. & Hill, R. (2014). *Fundamentals of nursing: A person-centred approach to care* (2nd ed.). Sydney: Lippincott Williams & Wilkins.

Gyland, E. A. (2012). Infant pain assessment: A quality improvement project in a level III neonatal intensive care unit in Northeast Florida. *Newborn and Infant Nursing Reviews, 12*(1), 44–50.

Haley, C. (2012). *Pillitteri's child and family health nursing in Australia and New Zealand* (1st ed.). Sydney: Lippincott Williams & Wilkins.

Royal Children's Hospital Melbourne. (2014). *Paediatric handbook* (8th ed.). Melbourne: Wiley Blackwell.

Online resources

Australasian Newborn Hearing Screening Committee: www.newbornhearingscreening.com.au

Australian Breastfeeding Association: www.breastfeeding.asn.au

Australian Institute of Family Studies: www.aifs.gov.au

Child, Youth & Family, New Zealand: www.cyf.govt.nz

Kiwi Families: www.kiwifamilies.co.nz

National Health and Medical Research Council, infant feeding guidelines: www.nhmrc.gov.au/guidelines/publications/n56

New Zealand Breastfeeding Authority: www.babyfriendly.org.nz

New Zealand Ministry of Health: www.health.govt.nz

Nutrition Australia: www.nutritionaustralia.org

Pregnancy Birth & Baby (Australian Government support portal): www.pregnancybirthbaby.org.au

Royal Children's Hospital Melbourne, clinical guidelines: https://www.rch.org.au/clinicalguide/

Vision Australia: www.visionaustralia.org

CHAPTER 33

Assessing children and adolescents

CASE STUDY

Mrs Carter brings her 2-year-old child Michael to the paediatric emergency department because he has been 'irritable and feverish since last night'. Further history reveals Michael has also had a runny nose and cough for 2 days, and his appetite and fluid intake have decreased since his fever started. His mother tells you that she is concerned as this has never happened before. Michael is otherwise healthy. You are the assessing nurse.

CRITICAL THINKING

1. What do you understand about the physical, mental, social and emotional development of a 2-year-old child?
2. How would you approach the assessment?
3. How would you communicate with and support both Michael and his mother?

Structure and function

SKIN, HAIR AND NAILS

During early childhood, the skin develops a tighter bond with the dermis, making it more resistant to infection, irritation and fluid loss. Skin colour appears pink and evenly distributed and may include normal variations such as freckles. The texture is smooth because the skin has not had years of exposure to the environment and because the hair is less coarse than in adulthood. The sebaceous glands and eccrine glands are minimally active, with the eccrine glands producing little sweat.

During the toddler years, scalp hair grows coarser, thicker and darker and usually loses its curliness. Fine hair becomes visible on the distal portions of the upper and lower extremities.

As the child ages, skin structure and function remain stable until puberty, when *adrenarche* (adrenocortical maturation) signals the onset of increased sebum production from the sebaceous glands, a process that continues until late adolescence. Sebum is involved in the development of acne. The apocrine glands also respond more to emotional stimulation and heat, with the end result being body odour.

HEAD AND NECK

During infancy, body growth predominates and the head grows proportionately to body size, reaching 90% of its full adult size by age 6 years. Facial bone growth is variable, especially for the nasal and jaw bones. During the toddler years, the nasal bridge is low and the mandible and maxilla are small, making the face seem small compared with the whole skull. During the school-age years, the face grows proportionately faster than the rest of the cranium, and secondary teeth appear too large for the face. In adolescence, the nose and thyroid cartilage enlarge in boys. Lymph tissue is well developed at birth and continues to grow rapidly until age 10 or 11 years, exceeding adult size before puberty, after which the tissue atrophies and stabilises to adult dimensions by the end of adolescence.

EYES

During childhood, the eyes are less spherical than adult eyes. Visual acuity reaches the adult level of 6/6 (20/20) by age 3 to 5 years, although many young children will not perform well in visual acuity testing at this age.

EARS

As the child grows, the inner ear matures. In older children, the Eustachian tube lengthens, but it may become occluded from growth of lymphatic tissue, specifically the adenoids. The canal shortens and straightens as the child ages, and the pinna can be pulled up and back, as in the adult.

MOUTH, NOSE, THROAT AND SINUSES

Children have 20 deciduous teeth, which are lost between the ages of 6 and 12 years. Permanent teeth begin forming in the jaw by age 6 months and begin to replace temporary teeth at age 6 years, usually starting with the central incisors. Permanent teeth appear earlier in Aboriginal and Torres Strait Islander children than in Caucasians, and in girls before boys.

Nasal cartilage grows during adolescence with the secondary sex characteristics. Growth starts at age 12 or 13 years and reaches full size by 16 years in girls and 18 years in boys. The maxillary and ethmoid sinuses are present at birth, but they are small and cannot be examined until they develop, when the child is much older. The frontal sinuses develop around age 7 to 8 years, and the sphenoid sinuses develop after puberty.

The tonsils and adenoids rapidly grow, reaching maximum development by age 10 to 12 years. At this point, they may be about twice their adult size. However, as with other lymphoid tissue, they atrophy to stable adult dimensions by the end of adolescence.

THORAX AND LUNGS

The lungs continue to develop after birth and new alveoli form until about age 8 years. Thus, in a child with pulmonary damage or disease at birth, pulmonary tissue may regenerate and the lungs can eventually attain normal respiratory function. The child will have 300 million alveoli by adolescence.

The chest wall is thin with very little musculature. The ribs are soft and pliable with the xiphoid process movable. The airways of children are also smaller and narrower than in adults; therefore, children are at risk of airway obstruction from oedema and infections in the lungs. A child's respiratory rate is much faster than an adult's rate: children younger than 7 years old tend to be abdominal breathers. In children between 8 and 10 years old, respiratory rates are lower and breathing becomes thoracic, like the adult's.

BREASTS

In girls, breast growth is stimulated by oestrogen at the onset of puberty. Between the ages of 8 and 13 years, *thelarche* may occur and breasts continue to develop in stages (Table 33-1). Breasts enlarge primarily as a result of fat deposits. However, the duct system also grows and branches, and masses of small cells develop at the duct endings. These masses are potential alveoli. Tenderness and asymmetrical development are common, and anticipatory guidance and reassurance are needed. Gynaecomastia, the enlargement of breast tissue in boys, may be noted in some male adolescents. This is related to pubertal changes and is usually temporary. However, use of marijuana and anabolic steroids are two of several external causes of gynaecomastia.

HEART

In children, the heart is positioned more horizontally in the chest. The apical impulse is felt at the fourth intercostal space left of the midclavicular line in young children. By the time the child is 7 years old, the apical pulse reaches the fifth intercostal space and the midclavicular line. Heart sounds are louder, higher pitched and of shorter duration in children. Physiological splitting of the second sound, which widens with inspiration, may be heard in the second left intercostal space. A third heart sound (S_3) may be heard at the apex and is present in one-third of all children. Sinus arrhythmia is normal and reaches its greatest degree during adolescence. Some children may have physiological murmurs that do not indicate disease. The heart rate decreases as the child gets older, usually dropping to about 85 beats/minute by age 8 years. Athletic adolescents may have even lower heart rates.

Table 33-1 Tanner sexual maturity ratings: Female breast development

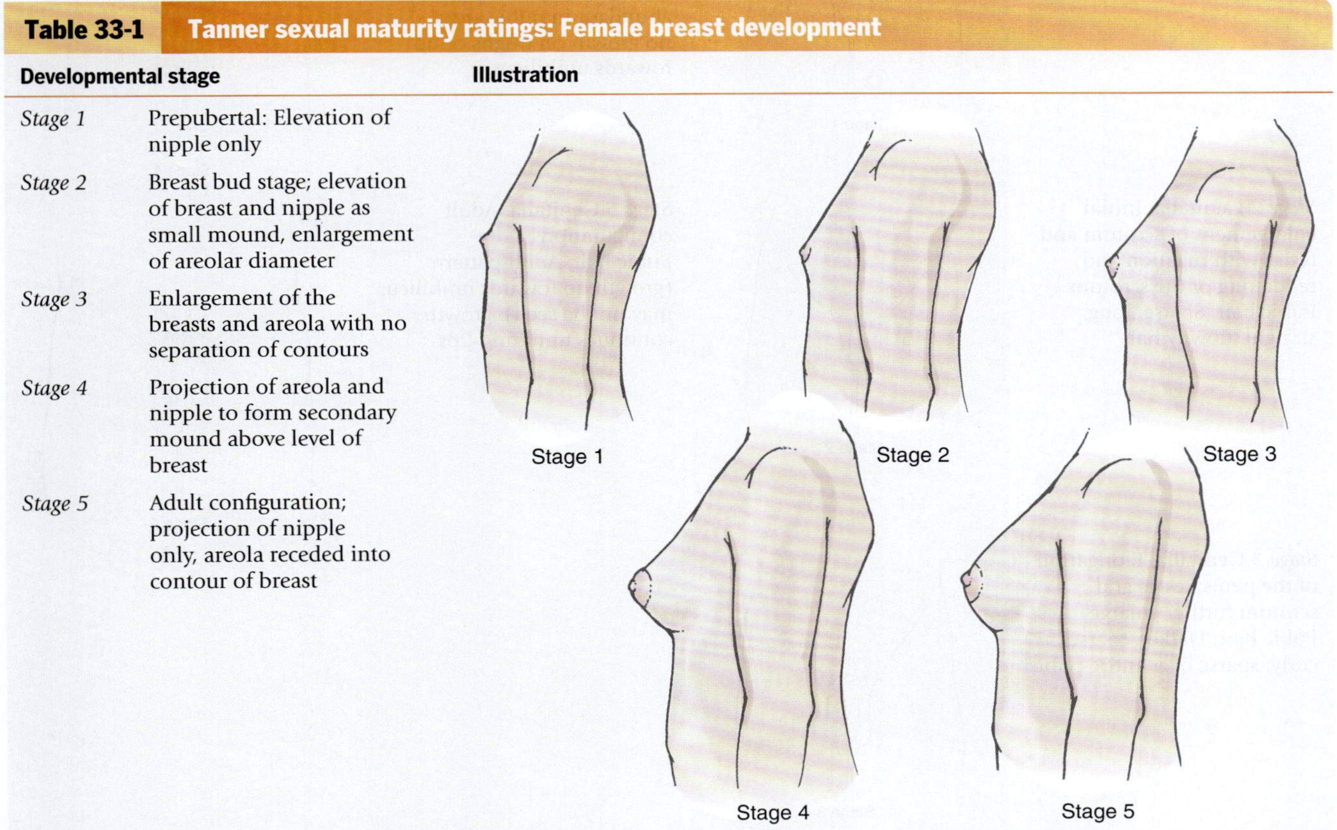

Developmental stage		Illustration
Stage 1	Prepubertal: Elevation of nipple only	
Stage 2	Breast bud stage; elevation of breast and nipple as small mound, enlargement of areolar diameter	
Stage 3	Enlargement of the breasts and areola with no separation of contours	
Stage 4	Projection of areola and nipple to form secondary mound above level of breast	
Stage 5	Adult configuration; projection of nipple only, areola receded into contour of breast	

Tanner, J. M. (1962). *Growth at adolesence* (2nd ed.). Oxford: Blackwell Scientific Publications.

ABDOMEN

The abdomen of small children is cylindrical, prominent in the standing position and flat when supine. The abdomen of toddlers appears prominent and gives the child what is popularly called a pot-belly appearance. The contours of the abdomen change to adult shapes during adolescence. Peristaltic waves may be visible in thin children; they may also be indicative of a disease or disorder.

The tip of the right kidney may be felt in young children, especially during inspiration.

In small children, the liver is palpable at 1 to 2 cm below the right costal margin. The spleen may be palpable below the left costal margin at 1 to 2 cm. Often in older children these structures are not palpable.

GENITALIA

Male genitalia generally develop over a 2- to 5-year period, beginning from preadolescence to adulthood. In the adolescent male, the enlargement of the testes is an early sign of puberty, occurring between the ages of 9.5 and 13.5 years. Pubic hair signifies the onset of puberty in boys. Pubic hair development and penile enlargement are concurrent with testicular growth (Table 33-2). Axillary hair development occurs late in puberty. It follows definitive penile and testicular enlargement in boys. Facial hair in boys also develops at this time. The onset of spontaneous nocturnal emission of seminal fluid is a sign of puberty similar to menarche in females. During puberty, the prostate gland grows rapidly to twice its prepubertal size under the influence of androgens.

In female adolescents, puberty is the time that oestrogen stimulates the development of the reproductive tract and secondary sex characteristics. The external genitalia increase in size and sensitivity, whereas the internal reproductive organs increase in weight and mass. Pubic hair begins growing early in puberty (2 to 6 months after thelarche [breast development]) and follows a distinct pattern (Table 33-3). Axillary hair development precedes *menarche* (first menstrual period) in girls. Menarche takes place in the latter half of puberty, after breast and pubic hair begin to develop. Menarche typically begins 2.5 years after the onset of puberty. The menstrual cycle is usually irregular during the first 2 years because of physiological anovulation.

Table 33-2 Tanner sexual maturity rating: Male genitalia and pubic hair

Developmental stage	Illustration	Developmental stage	Illustration
Stage 1 Genitalia: Prepubertal: No pubic hair; fine vellus hair	Stage 1	*Stage 4* Genitalia: Increase in size and width of penis and the development of the glans; scrotum darkens Pubic hair: Dark, curly and abundant in pubic area; no growth on thighs or up towards umbilicus	Stage 4
Stage 2 Genitalia: Initial enlargement of scrotum and testes with rugation and reddening of the scrotum Pubic hair: Sparse, long, straight, downy hair	Stage 2	*Stage 5* Genitalia: Adult configuration Pubic hair: Adult pattern (growth up towards umbilicus may not be seen); growth continues until mid-20s	Stage 5
Stage 3 Genitalia: Elongation of the penis; testes and scrotum further enlarge Pubic hair: Darker, coarser, curly; sparse over entire pubis	Stage 3		

Tanner, J. M. (1962). *Growth at adolescence* (2nd ed.). Oxford: Blackwell Scientific Publications.

Table 33-3 Tanner sexual maturity rating: Female pubic hair

Developmental stage	Illustration	Developmental stage	Illustration
Stage 1 Prepubertal: No pubic hair; fine vellus hair	Stage 1	*Stage 4* Dark, curly and abundant on mons pubis; no growth on medial thighs	Stage 4
Stage 2 Sparse, long, straight, downy hair	Stage 2	*Stage 5* Adult pattern of inverse triangle; growth on medial thighs	Stage 5
Stage 3 Darker, coarser, curly; sparse over mons pubis	Stage 3		

Tanner, J. M. (1962). *Growth at adolescence* (2nd ed.). Oxford: Blackwell Scientific Publications.

ANUS AND RECTUM

The anus and rectum appear and function like those in the adult. Anorectal malformations are a common congenital abnormality with an incidence of 1 in every 3,000 live births.

MUSCULOSKELETAL SYSTEM

The skeleton of small children is made chiefly of cartilage, accounting for the relative softness and malleability of the bones and the relative ease with which certain deformities can be corrected. Bone formation occurs by ossification, beginning during the gestational period and continuing throughout childhood. Bones grow rapidly during infancy. As children grow into adolescence, they will experience a skeletal growth spurt, usually seen in correlation with Tanner stage 2 for girls and Tanner stage 3 for boys. Skeletal growth continues throughout Tanner stage 5 for both sexes.

Bone growth occurs in two dimensions: diameter and length. Growth in diameter takes place predominantly in children and adolescents and slows as the person ages because of the predominance of bone breakdown over bone formation. Growth in length takes place at the epiphyseal plates, vascular areas of active cell division. Bones increase in circumference and length under the influence of hormones, primarily pituitary growth hormone and thyroid hormone.

Muscle growth is related to growth of the underlying bone. Individual fibres, ligaments and tendons grow throughout childhood. Bone and muscle development is influenced by use of the extremities. If extremities are not used, minimal growth of the muscle will occur. Walking and weight-bearing activities stimulate bone and muscle growth.

The anterior curve in the lumbar region of the vertebral column develops between ages 12 and 18 months, when the toddler starts to stand erect and walk.

Muscle growth contributes significantly to weight gain in the child. Individual fibres grow throughout childhood, and growth is considerable during the adolescent growth spurt, which usually peaks at 12 years in girls and 14 years in boys.

NEUROLOGICAL SYSTEM

Motor control develops in a head-to-neck to trunk-to-extremities sequence. Development takes place in an orderly progression, but each child develops at his or her own pace. The norms demonstrate wide variation among individuals as well as within a single individual under different circumstances. The developmental milestones of children are discussed below.

Health assessment

COLLECTING SUBJECTIVE DATA: THE NURSING HEALTH HISTORY

The complete paediatric nursing history is one of the most crucial components of child health care. Many of the materials and questions are unique to this population. The nursing history interview usually provides an opportunity to observe the carer– or parent–child interaction and to participate in early detection of health problems and prevention of future difficulties.

CASE STUDY

Michael's physical examination reveals he is a slightly irritable, 2-year-old boy, who is pulling at his ears, with a temperature of 38 °C and nasal congestion with clear discharge. When the medical officer examined him he was found to have bilateral red, bulging tympanic membranes; his pharynx was lightly red without exudate; his chest was clear; his abdomen was soft without hepatosplenomegaly, and there were no meningeal signs.

He is diagnosed with an upper respiratory tract infection (URTI) and a bilateral otitis media (BOM). The doctor orders amoxicillin 250 mg TDS for 10 days.

You are to provide Michael's mother with discharge education regarding the care and management of his URTI and BOM at home.

CRITICAL THINKING

4. What considerations do you need to make when communicating to parents and children?

Nurses must have the communication skills needed to elicit data about the child and family within a framework that incorporates biographical data, current health status, past history, family history, a review of each body system, knowledge of growth and development, and lifestyle and health practices information. It is important to keep in mind that data collected in one category may have relevance to another category. For example, data collected about the condition of the child's skin, hair and nails may indicate a problem in the area of nutrition.

Because infants and children are uniquely different from adults, a separate subjective assessment that focuses on questions suited for this population is vital. Nurses must ask age-appropriate questions, in a manner in which the child will understand. How you interview a 2-year-old will be markedly different from how you elicit information from a 15-year-old. It is for this reason that nurses must have a sound understanding of developmental theories and milestones. The subjective assessment of children encompasses interviewing and compiling a complete nursing history. Although general interviewing techniques used for adults can be used in the paediatric setting, in most cases someone other than the patient, usually the parent, gives the history. Having said that, the child's point of view, and interpretation of the situation, should never be discounted. Thus, the interview becomes the onset of a relational triad between the nurse, the child or adolescent, and the parents. Nurses establish a comfortable, yet professional, rapport that forms the foundation for an ongoing therapeutic relationship. Nurses accomplish this by developing communication and interviewing skills that incorporate the needs of both the parent and the child or adolescent, treating both as equal partners, in an age and developmentally appropriate way.

Interviewing

Interviewing parents

The parental interview entails more than just fact gathering. The tone of future contacts is established as parents begin to develop a trusting relationship with the nurse (Fig. 33-1). Parents expect health professionals to be sources of information and education, and they assess professional competence during the initial contact. Therefore, it is important that the nurse uses a friendly, non-judgemental approach while demonstrating proficiency as a practitioner. Rarely is the interview just data gathering; it is also a forum for rapport building, explaining and health teaching.

Introductory stage

As with all patients, the nurse–parent relationship begins with the introduction, when nurses explain their roles and

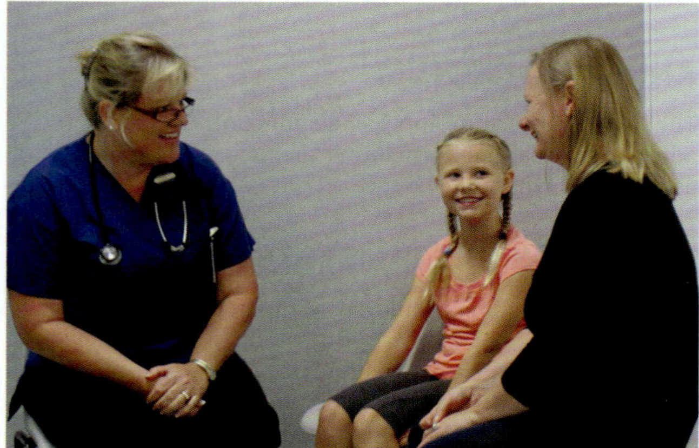

FIGURE 33-1 Developing a trusting relationship with the parent is an essential aspect of the interview process.

the purpose of the interview. Clarification and consistency are crucial from the start because parents may be anxious about the child's condition or uncomfortable about their roles, especially if the setting is a hospital. Anxiety may be overt or masked, even demonstrated by negative behaviours such as hostility.

CULTURAL CONSIDERATIONS
Cultural variations and past experiences may also affect parental reactions and responses.

Active listening facilitates the use of leads and better enables nurses to keep the interview focused on specific concerns. It also allows nurses to uncover clues that further the interview, to seek validation of perceptions and responses that may have alternate meanings, and to provide reassurance for both the expressed and hidden concerns that parents may be experiencing.

Encouraging talk

By encouraging parents to talk, you can identify information that affects all aspects of a child's life. Some parents take the lead without prompting (e.g. 'He's been pulling up his legs like he's in pain.'). Others offer vague concerns (e.g. '. . . she's just not acting right.') and need more direction. However, all have significant information about their child. You can further encourage verbalisation through communication techniques such as open-ended questioning ('How does Sarah behave when she isn't acting just right?') and focus directing ('When does Darryl have the pain?'). Communication skills allow nurses to elicit information in all patient groups, even in the most difficult situations.

The atmosphere should create an exchange of information rather than one directed solely by the nurse. Nurses use *problem solving, collaboration* and *anticipatory guidance.* For example, ask the parent, 'What do you see as the problem?' Once the problem is identified, lead the parent through the problem-solving process to arrive at a solution. Parents should also be asked what they found to be effective or ineffective in managing their child's problems. Anticipatory guidance promotes an exchange because parents can better participate in discussions of their child's future developmental trends.

Nurses should also take into account any experiences either the parent or the child might have had with health professionals in the past. The child may have a chronic illness and regularly attend the emergency department, or the parent may have felt unheard, judged or dismissed in a previous encounter. These experiences may have an impact on their willingness to be open and share information.

Be aware of the barriers to effective nurse–parent communication. These include time constraints, frequent interruptions, lack of privacy and language differences as well as provider callousness and cultural insensitivity. Make every effort possible to avoid these barriers. Allow adequate time and privacy for every interview and keep interruptions at a minimum.

CULTURAL CONSIDERATIONS
Interpreters can assist when language differences are present. Nurses should always display a warm, professional manner when interacting with patients and families, and they should be sensitive to cultural differences displayed in values, beliefs and customs.

Interviewing children and adolescents

As noted earlier, the child or adolescent and the parents are treated as equal partners in the healthcare triad. Include the child in the introductory stage of the interview and observe for signs of readiness to evaluate the level of participation. *Readiness evaluation* includes questioning the parents about how the child copes with stressful situations and what the child has been told about this particular health encounter.

Communication techniques

Direct communication—such as open-ended and closed-ended questions, age-appropriate humour, and dialogue strategies—is usually more beneficial when used with indirect communication techniques, including sentence completion, mutual storytelling, using drawings, play (the universal language of children) and 'magic'.

Play as communication

Nurses should talk to the child at eye level and actively engage children through play and verbalisation.

CULTURAL CONSIDERATIONS
Be aware of cultural variations for making direct eye contact (see, for example, Chap. 11).

Play is one of the most valuable communication techniques when working with children; it allows for the discovery of important clues to children's development and illness behaviours. Rushing creates anxiety; therefore, time should be taken to listen and allow children to feel comfortable. Privacy and confidentiality are important in paediatric nursing, especially when assessing the adolescent. Children or adolescents may be anxious, fearful or embarrassed. Their emotions should be respected.

The interview process and assessment procedures should be explained in clear and honest terms. Directions should be stated in a positive manner, and choices should be offered only when available and appropriate. Honest praise is used to reinforce positive behaviours; gratuitous praise is quickly recognised by children and may decrease the child's trust in the nurse.

Touch

Touch is a powerful communication tool. However, the child may find touch intrusive if the nurse has not yet begun to formulate a relationship with the child. Therefore, it is prudent to communicate with the child at a 'safe distance' until the relationship begins to form.

CULTURAL CONSIDERATIONS
Cultural taboos may also prohibit touch; prior approval is to be requested (see, for example, Chaps 11 and 12).

Developmental considerations

Nurses should also be familiar with developmentally oriented approaches to interviewing children. Display 33-1 presents specific developmentally oriented approaches that may be used in interviewing children and adolescents.

These approaches are important to know because barriers can exist when communicating with children. For example, some nurses overestimate the understanding abilities of young children and underestimate those of older children and adolescents. This creates frustration for all involved. Nurses need to be habitually aware of children's cognitive status when interacting with them. Another barrier develops when the child is excluded altogether. Children and adolescents can be eager participants and should be treated as such.

Finally, although many children are eager participants, others need encouragement, especially toddlers and preschoolers, who may react with crying and a lack of cooperation.

DISPLAY 33-1: AGE-SPECIFIC INTERVIEW TECHNIQUES

Each child responds differently during the assessment interview according to his or her developmental status, severity and perception of illness, experience with health care, the intrusiveness of procedures and the child's own uniqueness. The following are some guidelines for adapting interview techniques to the child's status.

Toddlers: Sensorimotor to preoperational stages

Trial and error experimentation and relentless exploration are typical in the early toddler stage; later, the toddler uses representational thought in intellectual development. Children age under 5 years are egocentric. A toddler's attention span ranges between 5 and 10 minutes.

- Encourage parental presence.
- Provide careful and simple explanations just before procedure.
- Use play as a communication technique.
- Tell the child it is okay to cry.
- Encourage expression through toys.
- Use simple terminology; the child's receptive language is more advanced than his or her expressive language.
- Allow the child to be close to their parent—be alert for separation anxiety.
- Acknowledge the child's favourite toy or a unique characteristic about the child.
- Use the child's toys for expression; use miniature equipment on toys.

Preschoolers: Preoperational stage

Preschoolers progress from making simple classifications and associating one event with a simultaneous one to classifying and quantifying and exhibiting intuitive thought processes. A preschooler's attention span ranges between 10 and 15 minutes. Preschoolers use magical thinking.

- Explain why things are as they are, simply.
- Validate the child's perceptions.
- Avoid threatening words.
- Use simple visual aids.
- Involve the child in teaching by doing something (handling equipment).
- Allow the child to ask questions.
- Use the child's toys for expression; use miniature equipment on toys.
- Avoid using words that have double meaning.
- Explain sensations that the child will experience.
- Answer 'why' questions with simple explanations.
- Be direct and concrete; do not use analogies, abstractions or words with more than one meaning; avoid slang (such as 'laugh your head off'—preschoolers interpret literally).
- Ask simple questions.
- Allow the child to manipulate equipment.
- Use the child's active imagination—use toys, puppets and play.

School-age children: Operational stage

Egocentric thinking progresses to objective thinking in school-age children who begin using inductive reasoning, logical operations and reversible concrete thought. A school-age child's attention span ranges between 30 and 45 minutes. Use books and other visual aids to advance the assessment interview.

- Remember to remain concrete (i.e. avoid abstractions).
- Use group discussion to educate children among their peers; also use games.
- Provide health teaching; perform demonstrations.
- Give more responsibility to the child.
- School-age children like explanations and need assistance in vocalising their needs.
- Allow children to engage in discussions.

Adolescents: Formal operations stage

Abstract thought develops, as does thinking beyond the present and forming theories about everything.

- Give adolescents control whenever possible.
- Use scientific explanations and make expectations clear.
- Explore expected parental level of involvement before initiating it.
- Involve adolescents in planning.
- Clearly explain how body will be affected.
- Anticipate feelings of anger and grief.
- Use peers with common situation to help with teaching.
- Encourage expression of ideas and feelings.
- Maintain confidentiality; facilitate trust.
- Give adolescents your undivided attention.
- Make expectations clear.
- Ask to speak to the adolescent alone.
- Encourage open and honest communication.
- Be non-judgemental; respect views, differences and feelings.
- Ask open-ended questions.

Nurses should avoid power struggles and instead rely on empathy, developmental strategies, parental assistance and a good sense of humour.

Adolescent concerns

Adolescents are neither children nor adults and, therefore, should be treated accordingly. Privacy is essential, as are respect and confidentiality. This group of patients rarely access routine health care, so any visit to a health care provider gives them an opportunity to assess and explore a broad range of issues. General health issues may or may not be discussed with the parent present. However, sensitive issues, such as sex, sexuality, drugs and alcohol, are best handled without parental presence. Trust and genuineness are important; nurses should not 'talk down' to adolescents or mimic their language style. The approach should be as a professional, not as a peer, parent or big sister or brother (Fig. 33-2). Use open-ended and specific questions to avoid 'yes/no' answers; use silence sparingly because it may be viewed as threatening to this age group. Be aware of your own non-verbal and facial expressions. Delicate issues should be approached with sensitivity

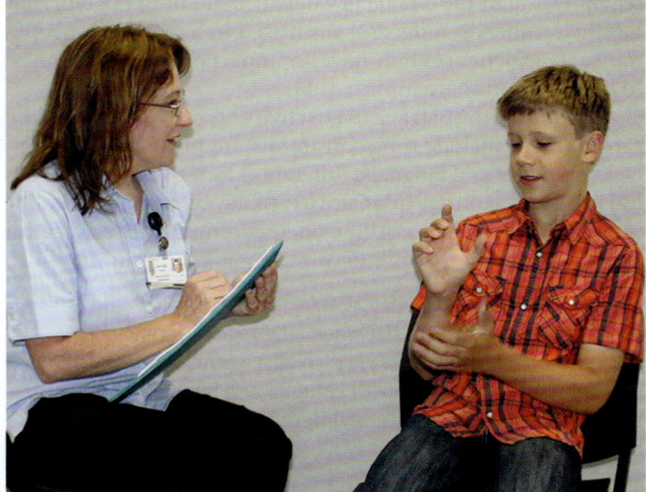

FIGURE 33-2 It is important to establish trust and genuineness when talking to adolescents.

and a non-judgemental, matter-of-fact manner to keep them from appearing to be focal points. Although it is important to gain trust and empathy, the nurse should be vigilant of professional boundaries. History taking provides an excellent opportunity for health teaching with adolescents, who are eager to learn about their ever-changing bodies. Questions should be encouraged and answered throughout the history.

Biographical data

Gathering biographical information is a good way to begin the health history. It consists of general, easy-to-answer information that puts the parent and child at ease. It can also provide the nurse with important clues that can benefit the rest of the subjective examination. For example, discovering that a 5-year-old child lives in the city with his 40-year-old professional parents and no brothers or sisters may give the nurse clues about his developmental level, activity, relationships and socio-economic status. However, the nurse must be careful not to make quick assumptions based on demographic or biographical data.

These types of questions are often asked on a form that the parent fills out before the assessment. However, the nurse should go over the form with the parent and child (if feasible) at the beginning of the assessment. Typical data are included in the Biographical data box.

CASE STUDY

During your discussion with Mrs Carter, she informs you she is concerned Michael may be jealous of his new baby sister because he has occasional tantrums when she holds the baby. She is also concerned about Michael's development because he has recently started to refuse using the potty, a newly acquired skill.

CRITICAL THINKING

5. Is this a normal stage of development for a 2-year-old?
6. What other information do you need to know?

Biographical data

QUESTION	RATIONALE
What is the child's name? Nickname? What are the parents' or carers' names?	Knowing personal information about the child and carers helps to establish rapport with the child and family.
Who is the child's primary health care provider, and when was the child's last well-child care appointment? (Table 33-4 provides guidelines for primary health care provider visits developed by the Bright Futures and American Academy of Pediatrics [2019]).	This determines the child's access to health care. It tells the nurse where to find the patient's previous medical information or record.
Where does the child live? (Address) Do the parents and child live in the same residence? Who else lives in this residence? Are the child's parents married, single, divorced, same-sex, or transgender and gender diverse? What are the parents' ages?	This provides insight into living conditions and family dynamics, which contribute to the child's health.
What is the child's age? What is the child's date of birth?	This provides a reference for assessing the child's developmental level.
Is the child adopted, foster, natural?	Certain health problems run in families. It is helpful to know the child's genetic relationship with the parents.
What is the child's ethic origin? Religion?	This information helps the nurse to examine special needs and beliefs that may affect the child or family's health care.
What do the child's parents do for a living?	This provides insight into the economic status of the family.

History of present health concern and current health status

As with adults, it is important to obtain information regarding the child's current status of health. Nurses should ask the parent, and child if possible, to describe the child's general state of health and compare it with how it was 1 and 5 years ago (if age appropriate). If the answer is 'good', ask what 'good' means to them. 'Good' could mean 'only one cold this year' for a generally healthy child or 'only two hospitalisations this year' for a child with a chronic illness such as cystic fibrosis.

Current health status includes information regarding chronic illnesses and allergies. Chronic illness, such as asthma, or disability, such as cerebral palsy, must be established early in the history to allow for better assessment and teaching strategies. Allergies are very common during childhood. Nurses need to ask what the specific allergen is and how the child reacts to it.

Finally nurses must ask for complete medication and treatment information. This includes prescription and over-the-counter medications, devices and treatments (e.g. hot and cold compresses, respiratory therapy, assistive devices, such as orthopaedic braces), and home or folk remedies. The child may be taking a combination of medications and folk remedies that are incompatible.

The purpose of asking about the child's current health status is to determine why the child was brought in for an examination. For some examinations, the child and parents may have no symptoms to report. In this case, the parent and child should be asked to describe the general state of the child's health and the reason for seeking medical attention.

Continued on following page

History of present health concern and current health status (continued)

If there is a perceived problem with the child's health or if the child or parent notices symptoms, the same focus questions that are asked for each body system for the adult patient are used for the child (e.g. location, intensity, duration). However, for the child, it is important to ask both the parent and the child (if possible) to get accurate information. Conflicting information may clue the nurse in to other areas that may need to be assessed. When asking the child about symptoms, the following techniques are usually helpful:

- Ask the child to point with one finger to where the pain or symptom is located.
- Use a pain scale developed for children, such as the Wong–Baker FACES Pain Rating Scale characters, ranging from a happy face signifying no pain to a tearful face signifying the worst pain; six photographs of children's faces ranging from 'no hurt' to 'hurts worst'; also comes with a scale from 0 to 10; or a numeric scale (straight line with numbers from 0 to 10 representing no pain to worst pain). Figure 33-3 illustrates the Wong–Baker FACES and numeric pain rating scales.

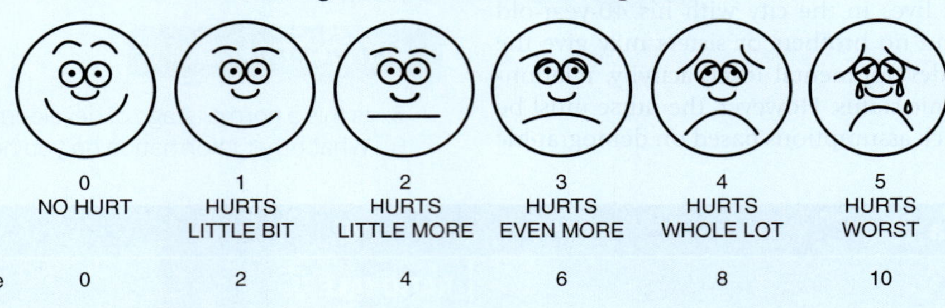

Explain to the person that each face is for a person who feels happy because he has no pain (hurt) or sad because he has some or a lot of pain. Face 0 is very happy because he doesn't hurt at all. Face 1 hurts just a little bit. Face 2 hurts a little more. Face 3 hurts even more. Face 4 hurts a whole lot. Face 5 hurts as much as you can imagine, although you don't have to be crying to feel this bad. Ask the person to choose the face that best describes how he is feeling.

Rating scale is recommended for persons age 3 years and older.

Brief word instructions: Point to each face using the words to describe the pain intensity. Ask the child to choose face that best describes own pain and record the appropriate number.

FIGURE 33-3 FACES and numeric pain rating scales. (From Hockenberry, M. & Wilson, D. [2013]. *Wong's essentials of pediatric nursing* [9th ed.]. St Louis: Mosby. Used with permission. Copyright Mosby.)

Explain to the person that each face is for a person who feels happy because he has no pain (hurt) or sad because he has some or a lot of pain. Face 0 is very happy because he doesn't hurt at all. Face 1 hurts just a little bit. Face 2 hurts a little more. Face 3 hurts even more. Face 4 hurts a whole lot. Face 5 hurts as much as you can imagine, although you don't have to be crying to feel this bad. Ask the person to choose the face that best describes how he is feeling.

Rating scale is recommended for persons age 3 years and older.

Brief word instructions: Point to each face using the words to describe the pain intensity. Ask the child to choose face that best describes own pain and record the appropriate number.

QUESTION	RATIONALE
Describe the child's general state of health.	Obtaining baseline information about the patient helps to identify important areas of assessment.
Does the child have a chronic illness?	Chronic illnesses may explain or affect assessment findings.
Does the child have any allergies? If so, what is the specific allergen? How does the child react to it?	This identifies allergens and helps the nurse plan to prevent exposure.

CLINICAL TIP

Some parents consider medication side effects to be allergic responses (e.g. diarrhoea that is common after antibiotic use) and need information to differentiate side effects from actual allergies.

QUESTION	RATIONALE
What prescriptions, over-the-counter medications, devices, treatments and home or folk remedies is the child taking? Note the name of the drug, dosage, frequency and reason it is administered.	It is always important to know what medications a patient is taking, especially young patients.

Past health history

Past history is important information to collect when assessing children. Certain problems and conditions can be associated with a difficult birth experience, whether the child was immunised, genetic conditions acquired from parents. Obviously, most of this information must come from the birth parent. If the child is a foster child or adopted, some of the information may be obtained from hospital records.

QUESTION	RATIONALE
Sample nursing history questions include:	
Was this pregnancy planned? How did you feel when you found out you were pregnant?	The carer's answer may provide insight into her feelings about the child.
When did you first receive antenatal care? How was your general health during pregnancy?	Antenatal information helps to identify potential health problems for the child.
Did you have any problems with your pregnancy?	It is important to identify problems during pregnancy to help identify potential complications for the child.
Did you have any accidents during this pregnancy?	Trauma or domestic violence that involved any type of physical trauma to the abdomen should be identified for possible complications for the child. Family violence is a major health issue in Australia, affecting 1 in 4 women, half of these will have children in their care. Medical and nursing staff are required by law to report suspected child abuse.
Did you take any medications during pregnancy?	Certain medications should not be taken during pregnancy and may be harmful to the child.
Did you use any tobacco, alcohol or drugs during this pregnancy?	Smoking, alcohol and drug use may cause complications or anomalies with the fetus.

COLDSPA

Example

Use the COLDSPA mnemonic as a guideline to collect needed information for each symptom the patient shares. In addition, the following questions help elicit important information.
Assessment of a 9-year-old child.

Mnemonic	Question	Patient response example
Character	Describe the sign or symptom (feeling, appearance, sound, smell or taste, if applicable).	'My ear hurts.'
Onset	When did it begin?	'Yesterday.'
Location	Where is it? Does it radiate? Does it occur anywhere else?	'Inside my right ear and down to my jaw.'
Duration	How long does it last? Does it recur?	'It hurts all the time.'
Severity	How bad is it? or How much does it bother you?	'Really bad.' Patient gives the pain a rating of 8 on a scale of 1–10.
Pattern	What makes it better or worse?	'Paracetamol and heat made it a little better.'
Associated factors/How it **A**ffects the patient	What other symptoms occur with it? How does it affect you?	'My head hurts and my nose is stuffy. I keep coughing. I can't sleep and I can't think in school either because I feel bad all over.'

Table 33-4 Recommendations for preventive paediatric health care

Each child and family is unique; therefore, these recommendations for preventive pediatric health care are designed for the care of children who are receiving competent parenting, have no manifestations of any important health problems, and are growing and developing in a satisfactory fashion. Developmental, psychosocial and chronic disease issues for children and adolescents may require frequent counseling and treatment visits separate from preventive care visits. Additional visits also may become necessary if circumstances suggest variations from normal.

These recommendations represent a consensus by the American Academy of Pediatrics (AAP) and Bright Futures. The AAP continues to emphasize the great importance of continuity of care in comprehensive health supervision and the need to avoid fragmentation of care.

Refer to the specific guidance by age as listed in the *Bright Futures guidelines* (Hagan, J. F., Shaw, J. S., Duncan, & P. M. [Eds]. [2017]. *Bright Futures: Guidelines for health supervision of infants, children, and* adolescent (4th ed.). Elk Grove Village, IL: American Academy of Pediatrics).

	Infancy								Early Childhood				
Age[1]	**Antenatal[2]**	**Newborn[3]**	**3-5 d[4]**	**By 1 mo**	**2 mo**	**4 mo**	**6 mo**	**9 mo**	**12 mo**	**15 mo**	**18 mo**	**24 mo**	**30 mo**
HISTORY Initial/interval	•	•	•	•	•	•	•	•	•	•	•	•	•
MEASUREMENTS													
Length/height and weight		•	•	•	•	•	•	•	•	•	•	•	•
Head circumference		•	•	•	•	•	•	•	•	•	•	•	
Weight for length		•	•	•	•	•	•	•	•	•	•		
Body mass index[5]												•	•
Blood pressure[6]		★	★	★	★	★	★	★	★	★	★	★	★
SENSORY SCREENING													
Vision[7]		★	★	★	★	★	★	★	★	★	★	★	★
Hearing		•[8]	•[9] →	→	→	★	★	★	★	★	★	★	★
DEVELOPMENTAL/BEHAVIORAL HEALTH													
Developmental screening[11]								•			•		•
Autism spectrum disorder screening[12]											•	•	
Developmental surveillance		•	•	•	•	•	•		•	•		•	
Psychosocial/behavioral assessment[13]		•	•	•	•	•	•	•	•	•	•	•	•
Tobacco, alcohol or drug use assessment[14]													
Depression screening[15]													
Maternal depression screening[16]				•	•	•	•						
PHYSICAL EXAMINATION[17]		•	•	•	•	•	•	•	•	•	•	•	•
PROCEDURES[18]													
Newborn blood		•[19]	•[20] →	→	→								
Newborn bilirubin[21]		•											
Critical congenital heart defect[22]		•											
Immunization[23]		•	•	•	•	•	•	•	•	•	•	•	•
Anemia[24]						★			•	★	★	★	★
Lead[25]							★	★	• or ★[26]		★	• or ★[26]	
Tuberculosis[27]				★			★		★			★	
Dyslipidemia[28]												★	
Sexually transmitted infections[29]													
HIV[30]													
Cervical dysplasia[31]													
ORAL HEALTH[32]							•[33]	•[33]	★		★	★	★
Fluoride varnish[34]							←	—	—	—	•	—	—
Fluoride supplementation[35]							★	★	★		★	★	★
ANTICIPATORY GUIDANCE	•	•	•	•	•	•	•	•	•	•	•	•	•

Adapted from United States Department of Health and Human Services, National Instututes of Health, National Heart, Lung, and Blood InstituteThe Fourth Report on the Diagnosis, Evaluation, and Treatment of High Blood Pressure in Children and Adolescents, Sept. 1996, Rev. May 2005, Tables 3 and 4, pp. 10-13. https://www.nhlbi.nih.gov/files/docs/resources/heart/hbp_ped.pdf.

[1] If a child comes under care for the first time at any point on the schedule, or if any items are not accomplished at the suggested age, the schedule should be brought up-to-date at the earliest possible time.

[2] A antenatal visit is recommended for parents who are at high risk, for first-time parents and for those who request a conference. The antenatal visit should include anticipatory guidance, pertinent medical history and a discussion of benefits of breastfeeding and planned method of feeding, per 'The antenatal visit' (http://pediatrics.aappublications.org/content/124/4/1227.full).

[3] Newborns should have an evaluation after birth, and breastfeeding should be encouraged (and instruction and support should be offered).

[4] Newborns should have an evaluation within 3 to 5 days of birth and within 48 to 72 hours after discharge from the hospital to include evaluation for feeding and jaundice. Breastfeeding newborns should receive formal breastfeeding evaluation, and their mothers should receive encouragement and instruction, as recommended in 'Breastfeeding and the use of human milk' (http://pediatrics.aappublications.org/content/129/3/e827.full). Newborns discharged less than 48 hours after delivery must be examined within 48 hours of discharge, per 'Hospital stay for healthy term newborns' (http://pediatrics.aappublications.org/content/125/2/405.full).

[5] Screen, per 'Expert Committee recommendations regarding the prevention, assessment, and treatment of child and adolescent overweight and obesity: Summary report' (http://pediatrics.aappublications.org/content/120/Supplement_4/S164.full).

[6] Screening should occur per 'Clinical Practice Guideline for Screening and Management of High Blood Pressure in Children and Adolescents' (http://pediatrics.aappublications.org/content/140/3/e20171904). Blood pressure measurement in infants and children with specific risk conditions should be performed at visits before age 3 years. [Revised December 2018].

[7] A visual acuity screen is recommended at ages 4 and 5 years, as well as in cooperative 3-year-olds. Instrument-based screening may be used to assess risk at ages 12 and 24 months, in addition to the well visits at 3 through 5 years of age. See 'Visual system assessment in infants, children, and young adults by pediatricians' (http://pediatrics.aappublications.org/content/137/1/e20153596) and 'Procedures for the evaluation of the visual system by pediatricians' (http://pediatrics.aappublications.org/content/137/1/e20153597).

[8] Confirm initial screen was completed, verify results and follow up, as appropriate. Newborns should be screened, per 'Year 2007 position statement: Principles and guidelines for early hearing detection and intervention programs' (http://pediatrics.aappublications.org/content/120/4/898.full).

[9] Verify results as soon as possible, and follow up, as appropriate.

[10] Screen with audiometry including 6,000- and 8,000-Hz–high frequencies once between 11 and 14 years, once between 15 and 17 years, and once between 18 and 21 years. See 'The sensitivity of adolescent hearing screens significantly improves by adding high frequencies' (http://www.jahonline.org/article/S1054-139X(16)00048-3/fulltext).

[11] See 'Identifying infants and young children with developmental disorders in the medical home: An algorithm for developmental surveillance and screening' (http://pediatrics.aappublications.org/content/118/1/405.full).

[12] Screening should occur per 'Identification and evaluation of children with autism spectrum disorders' (http://pediatrics.aappublications.org/content/120/5/1183.full).

[13] This assessment should be family centred and may include an assessment of child social–emotional health, caregiver depression and social determinants of health. See 'Promoting optimal development: Screening for behavioral and emotional problems' (http://pediatrics.aappublications.org/content/135/2/384) and 'Poverty and child health in the United States' (http://pediatrics.aappublications.org/content/137/4/e20160339).

[14] A recommended assessment tool is available at http://crafft.org.

[15] Recommended screening using the Patient Health Questionnaire (PHQ)-2 or other tools available in the GLAD-PC toolkit and at http://www.aap.org/en-us/advocacy-and-policy/aap-health-initiatives/Mental-Health/Documents/MH_ScreeningChart.pdf).

[16] Screening should occur per 'Incorporating recognition and management of perinatal and postpartum depression into pediatric practice' (http://pediatrics.aappublications.org/content/126/5/1032).

[17] At each visit, age-appropriate physical examination is essential, with infant totally unclothed and older children undressed and suitably draped. See 'Use of chaperones during the physical examination of the pediatric patient' (http://pediatrics.aappublications.org/content/127/5/991.full).

[18] These may be modified, depending on entry point into schedule and individual need.

Table 33-4 Recommendations for preventive paediatric health care—cont'd

		Middle Childhood						Adolescence										
3 y	4 y	5 y	6 y	7 y	8 y	9 y	10 y	11 y	12 y	13 y	14 y	15 y	16 y	17 y	18 y	19 y	20 y	21 y
•	•	•	•	•	•	•	•	•	•	•	•	•	•	•	•	•	•	•
•	•	•	•	•	•	•	•	•	•	•	•	•	•	•	•	•	•	•
•	•	•	•	•	•	•	•	•	•	•	•	•	•	•	•	•	•	•
•	•	•	•	•	•	•	•	•	•	•	•	•	•	•	•	•	•	•
•	•	•	•	★	•	★	•	★	•	★	★	•	★	★	★	★	★	★
★	•	•	•	★	•	★	•	←		•[10]	→	←	•	→	←		•	→
•	•	•	•	•	•	•	•	•	•	•	•	•	•	•	•	•	•	•
•	•	•	•	•	•	•	•	•	•	•	•	•	•	•	•	•	•	•
								★		★	★	★	★	★	★	★	★	★
									•	•	•	•	•	•	•	•	•	•
•	•	•	•	•	•	•	•	•	•	•	•	•	•	•	•	•	•	•
•	•	•	•	•	•	•	•	•	•	•	•	•	•	•	•	•	•	•
★	★	★	★	★	★	★	★	★	★	★	★	★	★	★	★	★	★	★
★	★	★	★															
★	★	★	★	★	★	★	★	★	★	★	★	★	★	★	★	★	★	★
	★		★		★	←	•	→	★	★	★	★	★	←			•	→
								★	★	★	★	★	★	★	★	★	★	★
								★	★	★	★	←		•	→	★	★	★
																		•
★	★	★	★															
→																		
★	★	★	★	★	★	★	★	★	★	★	★	★	★					
•	•	•	•	•	•	•	•	•	•	•	•	•	•	•	•	•	•	•

[19] Confirm initial screen was accomplished, verify results, and follow up, as appropriate. The Recommended Uniform Screening Panel (https://www.hrsa.gov/advisory-committees/heritable-disorders/rusp/index.html), as determined by The Secretary's Advisory Committee on Heritable Disorders in Newborns and Children, and state newborn screening laws/regulations (http://genes-r-us.uthscsa.edu/home) establish the criteria for and coverage of newborn screening procedures and programs.
[20] Verify results as soon as possible, and follow up, as appropriate.
[21] Confirm initial screening was accomplished, verify results, and follow up, as appropriate. See 'Hyperbilirubinemia in the newborn infant ≥35 weeks' gestation: An update with clarifications' (http://pediatrics.aappublications.org/content/124/4/1193).
[22] Screening for critical congenital heart disease using pulse oximetry should be performed in newborns, after 24 hours of age, before discharge from the hospital, per 'Endorsement of Health and Human Services recommendation for pulse oximetry screening for critical congenital heart disease' (http://pediatrics.aappublications.org/content/129/1/190.full).
[23] Schedules, per the AAP Committee on Infectious Diseases, are available at http://redbook.solutions.aap.org/SS/Immunization_Schedules.aspx. Every visit should be an opportunity to update and complete a child's immunizations.
[24] Perform risk assessment or screening, as appropriate, per recommendations in the current edition of the AAP *Pediatric Nutrition: Policy of the American Academy of Pediatrics* (Iron chapter). [Revised December 2018].
[25] For children at risk of lead exposure, see 'Prevention of Childhood Lead Toxicity' (http://pediatrics.aappublications.org/content/138/1/e20161493) and 'Low Level Lead Exposure Harms Children: A Renewed Call for Primary Prevention' (https://www.cdc.gov/nceh/lead/ACCLPP/Final_Document_030712.pdf). [Revised December 2018].
[26] Perform risk assessments or screenings as appropriate, based on universal screening requirements for patients with Medicaid or in high prevalence areas.
[27] Tuberculosis testing per recommendations of the AAP Committee on Infectious Diseases, published in the current edition of the AAP *Red book: Report of the Committee on Infectious Diseases*. Testing should be performed on recognition of high-risk factors.
[28] See 'Integrated guidelines for cardiovascular health and risk reduction in children and adolescents' (http://www.nhlbi.nih.gov/guidelines/cvd_ped/index.htm).
[29] Adolescents should be screened for sexually transmitted infections (STIs) per recommendations in the current edition of the AAP *Red book: Report of the Committee on Infectious Diseases*.
[30] Adolescents should be screened for HIV according to the USPSTF recommendations (http://www.uspreventiveservicestaskforce.org/uspstf/uspshivi.htm) once between the ages of 15 and 18, making every effort to preserve confidentiality of the adolescent. Those at increased risk of HIV infection, including those who are sexually active, participate in injection drug use, or are being tested for other STIs, should be tested for HIV and reassessed annually.
[31] See USPSTF recommendations (https://www.uspreventiveservicestaskforce.org/Page/Document/UpdateSummaryFinal/cervical-cancer-screening2). Indications for pelvic examinations prior to age 21 are noted in 'Gynecologic examination for adolescents in the pediatric office setting' (http://pediatrics.aappublications.org/content/126/3/583.full).
[32] Assess whether the child has a dental home. If no dental home is identified, perform a risk assessment (https://www.aap.org/en-us/advocacy-and-policy/aap-health-initiatives/Oral-Health/Pages/Oral-Health-Practice-Tools.aspx) and refer to a dental home. Recommend brushing with fluoride toothpaste in the proper dosage for age. See 'Maintaining and improving the oral health of young children' (http://pediatrics.aappublications.org/content/134/6/1224).
[33] Perform a risk assessment. See 'Maintaining and improving the oral health of young children' (http://pediatrics.aappublications.org/content/134/6/1224).
[34] See USPSTF recommendations (https://www.uspreventiveservicestaskforce.org/Page/Document/UpdateSummaryFinal/dental-caries-in-children-from-birth-through-age-5-years-screening). Once teeth are present, fluoride varnish may be applied to all children every 3–6 months in the primary care or dental office. Indications for fluoride use are noted in 'Fluoride use in caries prevention in the primary care setting' (http://pediatrics.aappublications.org/content/134/3/626).
[35] If primary water source is deficient in fluoride, consider oral fluoride supplementation. See 'Fluoride use in caries prevention in the primary care setting' (http://pediatrics. aappublications.org/content/134/3/626).

KEY: • = to be performed ★ = risk assessment to be performed with appropriate action to follow, if positivel ←•→ = range during which a service may be provided

Past health history (continued)

QUESTION	RATIONALE
Ask about delivery of the child: Where was the child born? What type of delivery did you have? Were there any problems during the delivery? Did you have any vaginal infections at time of delivery? What was the child's Apgar score? What were the child's weight, height and head circumference? Did the child have any problems after birth (e.g. feeding, jaundice)?	Delivery details and complications are pertinent for assessing fetal injury and potential risk for infection.
Ask about past illnesses or injuries: Has the child ever been hospitalised? Has the child ever had any major illnesses? Has the child ever experienced any major injuries?	Previous illnesses and hospitalisations may affect the present examination.
What immunisations has the child received thus far? Has your child had any reactions to immunisations?	These questions help to identify the risk of infection or potential reactions. The latest immunisation schedules (see Display 2-4) and catch-up guidelines are published by relevant state and federal agencies (e.g. Australian Technical Advisory Group on Immunisation [2018]).

Family history

The questions asked about family history for the child are basically the same types of questions that are asked of the adult patient (e.g. whether certain diseases or conditions run in the family, the age and cause of death for blood relatives, and family members with communicable diseases). This is an area of the subjective assessment in which the nurse focuses primarily on the parent for the necessary information. An exception might be if the child is older and knows a great deal about his or her family history. As with the past history information, if the child is adopted or is a foster child, family history information may not be known. An important reason for collecting these data is to implement preventive teaching at a young age.

QUESTION	RATIONALE
Do certain diseases or conditions run in the family?	Certain conditions tend to run in families and increase the patient's risk for such conditions.
Please list the ages and causes of death for blood relatives.	This helps to identify risk factors.
Does the child have family members with communicable diseases?	This also helps to identify risk factors.

Review of systems

It is essential that pertinent subjective data be collected for each body system. Many of the questions for each body system asked of the adult are asked of the parent or child.

The additional nursing history questions listed in the following sections for each system are of special concern in children.

QUESTION	RATIONALE
Skin, hair, nails	
Has your child had any changes in hair texture?	Changes may indicate an underlying problem.
Does your child complain of scalp itching?	Itching may indicate lice, seborrhoea, allergies or ringworm.
Have you noticed any changes in your child's nails? Colour? Cracking? Shape? Lines?	Changes may indicate an underlying problem.
Has your child been exposed to any contagious disease such as measles, chickenpox, lice, ringworm, scabies and the like?	These communicable diseases are common in childhood.

Review of systems (continued)

QUESTION	RATIONALE
Has your child ever had any rashes or sores? Acne?	Rashes may represent a number of diseases and disorders. Acne is a common problem for adolescents. They often have a hard time talking about it but they want treatment.
Has your child had any excessive bruising or burns?	This helps to assess for child abuse. Excessive bruising or burns suggest abuse.
Does your child use any cosmetics? Have tattoos? Have any pierced body parts?	This provides insight into personal habits.
Does your child have any birthmarks?	This helps to identify any lesions and lets the examiner know to assess areas for changes.
Head and neck	
Has your child ever had a head injury?	Head injuries may cause neurological problems.
Does your child experience headaches? How frequently?	Many neurological disorders cause headaches.
Has your child ever had swollen neck glands for any significant length of time?	This may indicate an underlying disorder.
Has your child ever experienced any neck stiffness?	Stiffness may indicate disorders such as meningitis.
Eyes	
Does your child excessively cross eyes?	Eye crossing may indicate visual or neurological problems.
Does your child frequently rub his or her eyes or blink repeatedly?	This could indicate visual problems.
Does your child strain or squint to see distant objects?	These suggest visual problems.
Has your child's vision been tested?	Children require regular vision screening.
Does your child wear glasses or contact lenses? Does he or she wear them when needed? Do the glasses help your child to see better?	This helps to gauge usage and if the prescription needs to be reassessed.
Ears	
Does your child appear to be paying attention when you speak?	Children should respond. A child who often appears to not be paying attention may have a hearing deficit or neurological disorder.
Does your child speak? At what age did he or she start talking?	It is important to assess developmental milestones.
Does your child or adolescent listen to loud music?	This is common behaviour among adolescents and usually does not indicate hearing deficit. However, it can lead to a hearing deficit. Preventive education may be needed.
Does your child use a hearing aid? If so, has it improved the child's ability to interact with and understand others.	This helps to evaluate the effectiveness of the hearing aid.
Has your child had frequent ear infections? Tubes in ears?	Frequent ear infections may contribute to hearing loss.
How frequently does your child have his or her hearing tested?	Screening for hearing deficits should be done regularly.
Mouth, throat, nose and sinuses	
Has your child ever had any difficulty swallowing or chewing?	Difficulty may indicate a mechanical or neurological disorder.
Has your child ever had strep throat, tonsillitis or any other mouth or throat infections? Does your child get frequent oral lesions?	Past infections may affect current condition.

Continued on following page

Review of systems (continued)

QUESTION	RATIONALE
When did your child's teeth erupt? When did the child lose his or her baby teeth? When did adult teeth erupt?	See Chapter 32 for a schedule for teeth eruption.
Does your child have any dental problems? Does he or she visit the dentist regularly? Does he or she wear any dental appliances?	Children should visit the dentist twice a year. If the child has frequent dental problems, provide education about dental care and preventive care.
Does your child experience nosebleeds?	Nosebleeds may occur with allergies, trauma, nose-picking or foreign bodies.
Does your child have any sinus problems?	Sinus pain may indicate allergies or infection.
Thorax and lungs	
Has your child ever had cough, wheezing, shortness or breath, or nocturnal dyspnoea; if so, when does it occur?	Many respiratory problems, such as asthma and bronchitis, are frequently seen in children. They may affect current health status.
Has your child received the influenza vaccine?	Annual influenza vaccination is recommended for children aged 6 months and above with certain medical risk factors and all Aboriginal and Torres Strait Islander people. In New Zealand the vaccine is recommended for children aged under 4 years who have been hospitalised with, or have a history of significant respiratory illness.
Does your child smoke? When did the child start smoking? How much does he or she smoke? **CLINICAL TIP** **Adolescents and older school-age children should be asked about smoking, including smokeless tobacco, in private.**	Smoking increases the risk for many diseases, including lung cancer. Provide appropriate patient teaching.
Is your child exposed to second-hand smoke?	Respiratory infections are more common in children exposed to second-hand smoke.
Breasts and lymphatics	
Has your daughter started developing breasts (thelarche)? If so, when did development start?	This helps to determine the child's sexual development stage.
Have you noticed any abnormal breast development in your son or young daughter?	Gynaecomastia is enlargement of breast tissue in males. It is a normal finding during puberty.
Heart and neck vessels	
Has your child ever experienced chest pain, heart murmurs, congenital heart disease or hypertension?	All of these symptoms indicate possible cardiac problems.
Has your child ever complained of fatigue? Does your child have difficulty keeping up with peers when running or exercising?	Fatigue may result from decreased cardiac output. Heart problems may impede the child's ability to perform physical activities.
Has your child ever fainted?	Children who faint should be screened for cardiac problems.
Has your child ever turned 'blue' during activity?	This may suggest cardiac arrhythmia.
Do you believe that your child is meeting the normal growth requirements for his or her age?	Children with congenital heart disease may grow and develop more slowly than other children.
Peripheral vascular system	
Does your child ever experience bluing of the extremities? Do your child's hands or feet get unusually cold?	Cyanosis or coldness in the extremities suggests vascular problems.
Has your child ever had problems with blood clots?	A history of blood clots increases the risk of recurrence.

Review of systems (continued)

QUESTION	RATIONALE
Abdomen	
Has your child ever had any excessive vomiting? Abdominal pain? Please describe.	Excessive vomiting may be associated with gastrointestinal problems. Abdominal pain may accompany many disorders or problems.
Does your child have any digestive problems (i.e. irritable bowel, constipation)?	Bowel problems should be explored further.
Has your child ever experienced any trauma to the abdomen?	Trauma may result in injuries or contribute to disorders.
Does your child have any hernias?	
Genitalia and sexuality	
How often does your child urinate? How many wet nappies do you change per day?	This helps to determine nutritional habits, e.g. is the child receiving enough fluids?
At what age was your child toilet (bladder) trained? Night?	This helps to determine whether and when child reaches developmental milestones.
Does your child ever wet his or her pants?	If there is a history of enuresis, obtain routine that family follows to deal with problem.
Is there any history of frequency, burning or pain during urination?	These genitourinary problems should be further explored.
Do you have any concerns about your child related to masturbation, asking or answering questions about sex, not respecting other's privacy or wanting too much privacy?	This helps to assess the child's sexual development.
Has anyone ever touched your child in a way that made him or her feel uncomfortable? (Make sure to ask the parent and the child this question.)	It is important to screen for sexual abuse.
Has your child started puberty, thelarche, menarche?	See Tables 33-1, 33-2 and 33-3 for Tanner stages of sexual development.
Has the child started having wet dreams (nocturnal emissions)?	Pubescent patients should be reassured that nocturnal emissions are normal.
Who is the source of sex or AIDS education? Questions to the adolescent about sexuality and reproductive issues should be asked privately. Gynaecologists recommend that the first visit to the gynaecologist be between the ages of 13 and 15 years for health screening, guidance and preventive services (American College of Obstetricians and Gynecologists, 2014).	This helps to determine the child's need for sexual education.
Do you know how to perform breast self-examination or testicular self-examination?	Self-examination is an important screening tool and should be taught.
Ask about menstruation: How old were you when you started menstruating (menarche)? When was your last menstrual period? What is your menstrual cycle schedule? Has it always been this way? What is your bleeding like? Light, moderate, heavy? Do you experience any cramps? Tell me about them. Do you experience any other physical or emotional discomfort associated with menstruation? Do you use tampons? How frequently do you change them?	This assesses the patient's development and gynaecological needs.

Continued on following page

Review of systems (continued)

QUESTION	RATIONALE
Assess sexual history: What was your age at first intercourse? Have you received information regarding the human papillomavirus vaccine (HPV) that can reduce the incidence of cervical cancer? Have you received the vaccine?	A careful sexual history should be taken for all sexually active patients. Adolescents aged 9 to 18 years are recommended to receive the 9vHPV vaccine. The recommended schedule for adolescents aged 9 to 14 years is two doses with a 6- to 12-month interval between doses. The recommended schedule for adolescents aged 15 to 18 years at the time of their first HPV vaccine is three doses, with an interval of 2 months between dose 1 and 2, and 4 months between dose 2 and 3. The vaccine prevents development of the nine types of HPV (6, 11, 16, 18, 31, 33, 45, 52 and 58). Types 16 and 18 are the two main causes of HPV-related cancers. The next five most common are 31, 33, 45, 52 and 58. Two non-cancer–causing HPV types are 6 and 11, which cause 90% of genital warts.
Have you ever had a Pap smear? Do you experience any discomfort or pain with intercourse? How many sexual partners do you have or have you had?	Cervical screening starts at age 25.
What type of contraception do you use and how do you use it? Do you use condoms? How do you use them? Have you ever had a sexually transmitted infection? Were you ever pregnant? What was the result of that pregnancy?	Contraceptive education (preventive education) should be provided.
Have you had or considered having a gynaecological examination?	This exam should be performed based on appropriate medical indications, circumstances of the presentation and willingness of child, parent or guardian. The rationale for the exam should be clearly explained; privacy and dignity should be maintained at all times. The use of a chaperone is highly recommended.
Anus and rectum	
How often does your child have a bowel movement? What does it look like?	This helps to assess the child's nutritional intake and gastrointestinal function.
At what age was your child toilet trained (bowel)?	This helps to determine whether and when the child reached developmental milestones.
Does your child ever soil his or her pants?	With a history of encopresis, obtain the routine that the family follows to deal with problem.
Is there any history of bleeding, constipation, diarrhoea, rectal itching or haemorrhoids?	Haemorrhoids are very unusual in children. They may indicate an intra-abdominal mass or child abuse (sodomy). *Note:* In Australia, state and territory governments are responsible for receiving reports from mandated reporters of suspected child neglect or physical, sexual or emotional abuse. In New Zealand, legislation does not require mandatory reporting of suspected child abuse, but District Health Boards have within their child protection policies the requirement to report concerns to the police.
Musculoskeletal system	
Has your child ever had limited range of motion, joint pain, stiffness, paralysis? Have you noticed any bone deformity?	A positive history of any of these requires further investigation.
Has your child ever had any fractures?	Frequent fractures may suggest a disorder of the musculoskeletal system or child abuse.
Has your child ever used any corrective devices (orthopaedic shoes, scoliosis brace)?	This should be noted as it may affect or explain findings during the physical examination.

Review of systems (continued)

QUESTION	RATIONALE
Describe your child's posture.	Children, especially females, should be screened for scoliosis.
Is your child involved in any sports? What type of protective gear does he or she use?	Provide appropriate patient teaching about safety and protective gear as needed.
Neurological system	
Does your child have any learning disabilities? Does your child have any attention problems at home or at school?	Learning disabilities may hinder a child's performance at school or indicate a neurological disorder.
Has your child ever experienced any problems with memory?	Memory problems may indicate neurological disorders.
Has your child ever had a seizure?	Seizures may indicate a neurological or cardiovascular disorder.
Has your child ever had a head injury?	Head trauma may cause intracranial bleeding or other injuries.
Has your child ever experienced any problems with motor coordination?	Uncoordinated movements or difficulty with coordination may indicate neurological disorders.

Growth and development

Nurses must possess baseline knowledge of the fundamental principles of growth and development as well as strategies for assessment and patient teaching. Several theories exist regarding the various stages and phases of development. It is suggested that nurses review the basic principles of the major theorists, such as Freud, Erikson and Piaget, to refresh their frames of reference. Information about these theorists is readily accessible in any basic or developmental psychology text. Developmental monitoring and assessment should comprise a number of tools, as it guides clinical judgement and can be universally applied. The Ages and Stages Questionnaire (ASQ) and the Parents' Evaluation of Developmental Status (PEDS) are two validated tools that are appropriate for general developmental monitoring. The ASQ can be used to identify developmental delay in children ages 3 months to 5 years. The PEDS can detect developmental and behavioural problems in children from birth to age 8 years. Both tools utilise parent report.

Growth patterns

Appendix A includes paediatric growth charts.

Toddlers

Height and weight increase in a steplike rather than a linear fashion, reflecting the growth spurts and lags characteristic of toddlerhood. The toddler's characteristic protruding abdomen results from underdeveloped abdominal muscles. Bow leggedness typically persists through toddlerhood because the leg muscles must bear the weight of the relatively large trunk. The height at age 2 years approximately equals one-half of the child's adult height. The child's birth weight quadruples by age 2.5 years. Head circumference (HC) equals chest circumference by 1 to 2 years. Total increase in HC in the second year of life is 2.5 cm, and the rate then increases slowly at 1.27 cm per year until age 5 years. Primary dentition (20 deciduous teeth) is completed by 2.5 years.

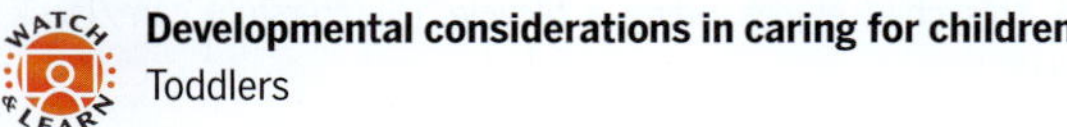

Preschoolers

Preschoolers are generally slender, graceful and agile. The average 4-year-old child is 101.25 cm tall and weighs 16.8 kg.

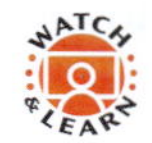
Developmental considerations in caring for children: Preschoolers

School-age children

During school age, girls often grow faster than boys and commonly surpass boys in height and weight. During pre-adolescence, extending from about ages 10 to 13, children commonly experience rapid and uneven growth compared with age mates. The average 6-year-old child is 112.5 cm tall and weighs 21 kg (whereas the average 12-year-old child is 147.5 cm tall and weighs 40 kg). Beginning around age 6, permanent teeth erupt and deciduous teeth are gradually lost. Caries, malocclusion and periodontal disease become evident.

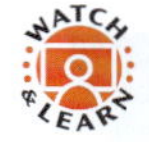
Developmental considerations in caring for children: School agers

Adolescents

From 20% to 25% of adult height is achieved in adolescence. Girls grow 5 cm to 20 cm until about age 16 or 17. Boys grow 10 cm to 30 cm until about age 18 or 20 years. From 30% to 50% of adult weight is achieved during adolescence (see Appendix A). Adolescence encompasses puberty—the period during which primary and secondary sex characteristics begin to develop and reach maturity. In girls, puberty begins between the ages of 8 and 14 years and is completed within 3 years. In boys, puberty begins between the ages of 9 and 16 years and is completed by age 18 or 19. During adolescence, hormonal influence causes important developmental changes.

Body mass reaches adult size, sebaceous glands become active and eccrine sweat glands become fully functional. Apocrine sweat glands develop, and hair grows in the axillae, areola of the breast, and genital and anal regions. Body hair assumes characteristic distribution patterns and texture changes (see Tables 33-1, 33-2 and 33-3). During puberty, girls experience growth in height, weight, breast development and pelvic girth with expansion of uterine tissue. Menarche typically occurs about 2.5 years after onset of puberty. Boys experience increases in height, weight, muscle mass, and penis and testicle size. Facial and body hair growth and voice deepening also occur. The onset of spontaneous nocturnal emissions of seminal fluid is an overt sign of puberty, analogous to menarche in girls. Sexual development is evaluated by noting the specific stages that take place in boys and girls.

Developmental considerations in caring for children: Adolescents

Motor development

Toddlers

Motor development should be evaluated at well-child visits. Using either the ASQ or PEDS tool can assist the nurse in noting the developmental milestones of the child at a particular age.

The major gross motor skill is locomotion. At 15 months, toddlers walk without help (Fig. 33-4). At 18 months, they walk upstairs with one hand held. At 24 months, toddlers walk up and down stairs one step at a time. At 30 months, they jump with both feet.

Fifteen-month-old toddlers can build a two-block tower and scribble spontaneously. At 18 months, they can build a three- to four-block tower. Toddlers at 24 months imitate a vertical stroke; at 30 months, they build an eight-block tower and copy a cross.

Sample questions for toddlerhood include:

- When did your child first walk?
- Can your child walk up and down steps?
- Can your child jump with both feet?
- Does your child spontaneously scribble?

Preschoolers

At 3 years old, children can ride a tricycle, go upstairs using alternate feet, stand on one foot for a few seconds and broad jump. Four-year-old children can skip, hop on one foot, catch a ball and go downstairs using alternate feet. At 5 years, children can skip on alternate feet, throw and catch a ball, jump rope, and balance on alternate feet with their eyes closed.

Three-year-old children can build a tower of up to 10 blocks, build three-block bridges, copy a circle and imitate a cross. At 4 years old, children can lace shoes, copy a square shape, trace a diamond shape and add three parts to a stick figure. A 5-year-old child can tie shoelaces, use scissors well, copy diamond and triangle shapes, add seven to nine parts to a stick figure, and print a few letters and numbers and her or his first name.

Sample questions for preschoolers include:

- Can your child run, hop and skip?
- Can your child lace shoes?
- Can your child write his or her first name?

School-age children

Skills acquired during the school years include cycling (Fig. 33-5), rollerskating, rollerblading and skateboarding (Fig. 33-6). Running and jumping improve progressively, and swimming is added to the child's repertoire.

Printing skills develop in the early school years; script skills in later years. School-age children also develop greater dexterity and competence for crafts, video games and computers.

Sample questions for school-age children include:

- Can your child ride a bicycle?
- Can your child write script?

Adolescents

Gross motor skills have reached adult levels, and fine motor skills continue to be refined.

Sample questions for the adolescent include:

- Does your son or daughter have a job, hobby or interest that involves hand skills? If so, how is his or her performance?
- Does your son or daughter participate in sports?

Sensory perception

Toddlers

Toddlers' visual acuity and depth perception improve, and they are able to recall visual images. Toddlers begin learning the ability to listen and comprehend. As every parent knows, listening is different from hearing. This ability includes attending

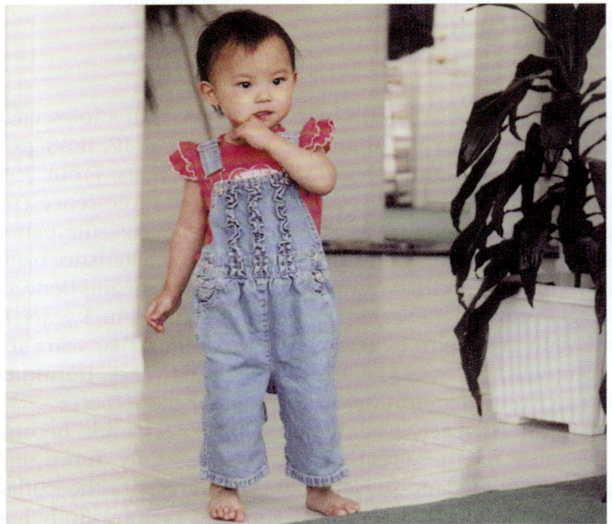

FIGURE 33-4 The toddler is proud of her ability to stand and walk without help. (Klossner, N. J. & Hatfield, N. [2006]. *Introductory maternity and pediatric nursing*. Philadelphia: Lippincott Williams & Wilkins.)

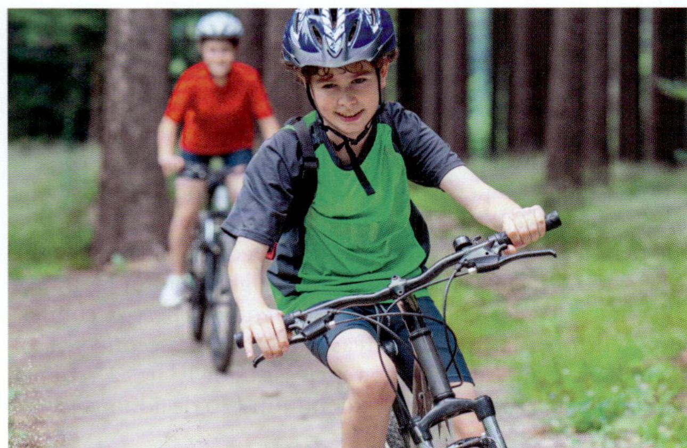

FIGURE 33-5 This child enjoys riding a bicycle. (Shutterstock.com/Jacek Chabraszewski)

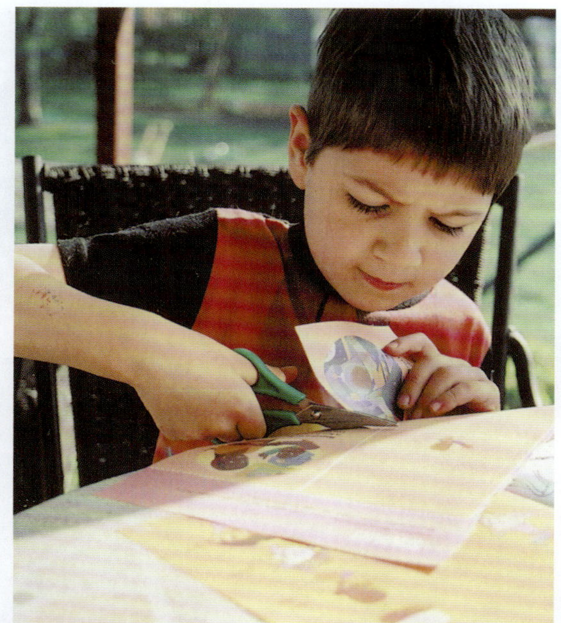

FIGURE 33-6 School-aged children become accomplished at a number of skills. (Weber, J.R., & Kelley, J.H. [2017] *Health Assessment in Nursing* [6th ed.]. © Wolters Kluwer Health.)

to what is heard, discriminating sound qualities, creating cognitive associations with previous learning, and remembering. The olfactory and gustatory senses are influenced by voluntary control and are associated with other sensory and motor areas. Therefore, toddlers refuse to eat anything that looks unpleasant to them. Children also begin to learn conditioned reactions to odours at this age.

Preschoolers

Colour and depth perception become fully developed. Preschoolers may be aware of visual difficulties. Hearing reaches its maximum level and listening further develops. Preschoolers usually enjoy vision and hearing testing.

School-age children

Visual capacity reaches adult level (6/6) by age 6 or 7 years. Hearing acuity is almost complete.

Adolescents

All senses have reached their mature capacity by adolescence.

Sample questions to assess for vision problems include:

- Does your child frequently rub his or her eyes?
- Does your child become irritable with close work?
- Does your child blink repeatedly?
- Does your child ever appear cross-eyed?
- Does your child strain to see distant objects or sit close to the TV?
- Does your child reverse letters or numbers?
- Does your child ever complain of headaches?

Sample questions to assess for hearing deficits include:

- Does your child respond to verbal commands? (Remember that we can only test hearing, not listening.)
- Does your child sit too close to the TV?
- Does your adolescent blast the stereo? (This may not indicate a hearing deficit, as it is typical behaviour; however, it can lead to hearing deficit.)
- How much screen time does your child have per day?
- Does your child have any speech difficulties?

Sample questions to assess sense of smell and taste include:

- Does your child ever complain of having difficulty with his or her sense of smell?
- Does your child experience difficulty with taste?

Cognitive and language and development

Toddlers

The sensorimotor phase (between ages 12 and 24 months) involves two substages in toddlerhood: tertiary circular reactions (age 12 to 18 months) involving trial-and-error experimentation, and relentless exploration and mental combinations (age 18 to 24 months) during which the toddler begins to devise new means for accomplishing tasks through mental calculations.

Toddlers go through a preconceptual substage of the preoperational phase typical of preschoolers. During this time, the child uses representational thought to recall the past, represent the present and anticipate the future. As toddlers get older, they begin to enter the preoperational phase. This phase is described in the following section on preschoolers.

At 15 months, toddlers use expressive jargon. At 2 years, they say 300 words and use 2- to 3-word phrases and pronouns. At 2.5 years, toddlers give their first and last names and use plurals.

Sample nursing history questions for toddlers include:

- Can your child name some body parts?
- Can your child state his or her first and last name?
- Does your child imitate adults?
- Does your child put two words together to form a sentence (e g. 'me go')?

Preschoolers

This stage of preoperational thought (age 2 to 7 years) consists of two phases. In the preconceptual phase, extending from age 2 to 4, the child forms concepts that are not as complete or logical as an adult's; makes simple classifications; associates one event with a simultaneous one (transductive reasoning); and exhibits egocentric thinking.

In the intuitive phase, extending from age 4 to 7, the child becomes capable of classifying, quantifying and relating objects but remains unaware of the principles behind these operations; exhibits intuitive thought processes (is aware that something is right but cannot say why); is unable to see the viewpoint of others; and uses many words appropriately but without a real knowledge of their meaning. Preschoolers exhibit 'magical thinking', believing that thoughts are all-powerful. They may feel guilty and responsible for bad thoughts, which, at times, may coincide with the occurrence of a wished event (e.g. wishing a sibling were dead and the sibling suddenly needs to be hospitalised).

Three-year-old children can say 900 words, use 3- to 4-word sentences and talk incessantly. Four-year-old children can say 1,500 words, tell exaggerated stories and sing simple songs. This is also the peak age for 'why' questions. Five-year-old children can say 2,100 words, and they know four or more colours, the names of the days of the week and the months.

Sample questions for preschoolers include:

- Does your child tell fantasy stories or have an imaginary friend?
- Does your child have an invisible friend?

- Can your child make simple classifications (e.g. dogs and cats)?
- Is your child 'chatty'? Does your child frequently ask 'why'?
- Can your child name at least four colours?

School-age children

A child aged 7 to 11 years is in the stage of concrete operations marked by inductive reasoning, logical operations and reversible concrete thought. Specific characteristics of this stage include movement from egocentric to objective thinking: seeing another's point of view; seeking validation and asking questions; focusing on immediate physical reality with inability to transcend the here and now; difficulty dealing with remote, future or hypothetical matters; development of various mental classifying and ordering activities; and development of the principle of conservation of volume, weight, mass and numbers. Typical activities of a child at this stage may include collecting and sorting objects (e.g. football cards, dolls, marbles); ordering items according to size, shape, weight and other criteria; and considering options and variables when problem solving.

Children develop formal adult articulation patterns by age 7 to 9. They learn that words can be arranged in terms of structure. The ability to read is one of the most significant skills learned during these years (Fig. 33-7).

Sample questions for school-age children include:

- Can your child see another's point of view?
- Does your child collect things (e.g. football cards, dolls)?
- Does your child try to solve problems?
- How well does your child do in school? (Also ask the school-age child and compare the answers.)
- How well does your child read?

Adolescents

In the development of formal operations, which commonly occurs from age 11 to 15 years, the adolescent develops abstract reasoning. This period consists of three substages:

- *Substage 1*: The adolescent sees relationships involving the inverse of the reciprocal.
- *Substage 2:* The adolescent develops the ability to order triads of propositions or relationships.
- *Substage 3:* The adolescent develops the capacity for true formal thought.

In *true formal thought,* the adolescent thinks beyond the present and forms theories about everything, delighting especially in considerations of 'that which is not'. However, adolescents in this age group do not have futuristic thoughts. They do not relate current events 'here and now' to long-term results (i.e. 2 years from now). An example of this includes teenagers who are sexually active and who may not consider the consequences of sexual activity (pregnancy and parenthood).

Sample nursing history questions for adolescents include:

- Do you consider your son or daughter to be a problem solver?
- How well does your son or daughter do in school? (Also ask the adolescent and compare the responses.)

Moral development (Kohlberg)

The moral development of children and adolescents outlined here is based on the work of Lawrence Kohlberg and his colleagues, from the mid- to late 1900s.

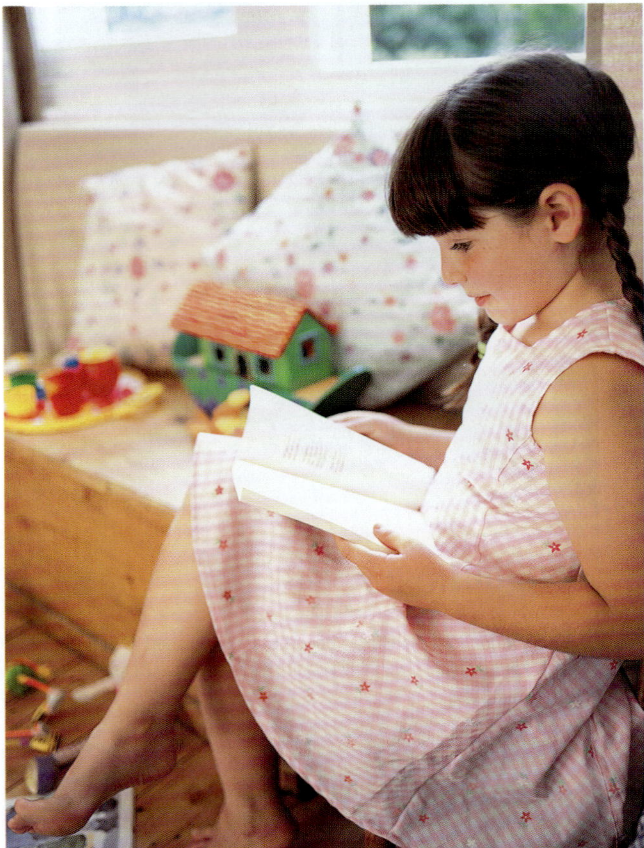

FIGURE 33-7 Reading is a milestone achievement for a school-aged child. (Weber, J.R., & Kelley, J.H. [2018]. *Health Assessment in Nursing* [6th ed.]. © Wolters Kluwer Health.)

Toddler

A toddler is typically at the first substage of the preconventional stage, which involves punishment and obedience orientation, in which he or she makes judgements on the basis of avoiding punishment or obtaining a reward. Discipline patterns affect a toddler's moral development. For example, physical punishment and withholding privileges tend to give the toddler a negative view of morals; withholding love and affection as punishment leads to feelings of guilt in the toddler. Appropriate disciplinary actions include providing simple explanations about why certain behaviours are unacceptable, praising appropriate behaviour and using distraction when the toddler is headed for danger.

Preschooler

A preschooler is in the preconventional stage of moral development, which extends to 10 years. In this phase, conscience emerges and the emphasis is on external control. The child's moral standards are those of others, and he or she observes them either to avoid punishment or to reap rewards.

School-age child

A child at the conventional level of the role conformity stage (generally age 10 to 13 years) has an increased desire to please others. The child observes and, to some extent, externalises the standards of others. The child wants to be considered 'good' by those people whose opinion matters to him or her.

Adolescent

Development of the postconventional level of morality occurs at about age 13, marked by the development of an individual conscience and a defined set of moral values. For the first time, the adolescent can acknowledge a conflict between two socially accepted standards and try to decide between them. Control of conduct is now internal, both in standards observed and in reasoning about right or wrong.

Sample nursing history questions for toddlerhood through to adolescence include:

- Does your child understand the difference between right and wrong?
- Do you discuss family values with your child?
- Do you have family rules? How are they implemented?
- How are disciplinary measures handled?
- Has your child ever had any problems with lying, cheating or stealing?
- Has your child ever required disciplinary action at school?
- Has your child ever violated the law?

CASE STUDY

Mrs Carter is very attentive to both the new baby and Michael throughout the interview, and she asks you for suggestions in how to help Michael cope with the new arrival. While doing so, she points out that her husband has been extra attentive to Michael since his sister was born.

CRITICAL THINKING

7. What suggestions could you provide to Michael's mother?

Psychosocial development (Erikson)

Toddler

E. H. Erikson (1963) termed the psychosocial crises facing a child between ages 1 and 3 years *autonomy versus shame and doubt*. The psychosocial theme is 'to hold on; to let go'. The toddler has developed a sense of trust and is ready to give up dependence to assert his or her budding sense of control, independence and autonomy (Fig. 33-8). The toddler begins to master the following:

- Individuation—differentiation of self from others
- Separation from parents
- Control over bodily functions
- Communication with words
- Acquisition of socially acceptable behaviour
- Egocentric interactions with others.

The toddler has learned that his or her parents are predictable and reliable. The toddler begins to learn that his or her own behaviour has a predictable, reliable effect on others. The toddler learns to wait longer for needs gratification. The toddler often uses 'no' even when he or she means 'yes'. This is done to assert independence (negativistic behaviour). A sense of shame and doubt can develop if the toddler is kept dependent in areas where he or she is capable of using newly

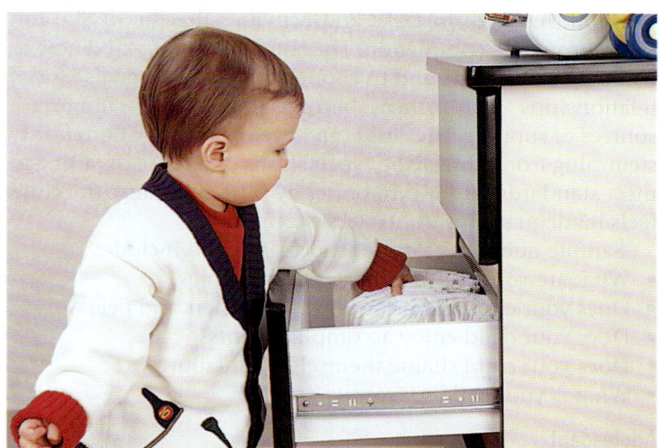

FIGURE 33-8 Toddlers love to assert their sense of control, independence and autonomy.

acquired skills or if made to feel inadequate when attempting new skills. A toddler often continues to seek a familiar security object, such as a blanket, during times of stress.

Sample questions for the toddler include:

- Does your child try to do things for himself or herself (e.g. feed, dress)?
- Does your child have temper tantrums? How are they handled?
- Does your child frequently use the word 'no'?
- At what age was your child completely toilet trained?
- Does your child actively explore the environment?

Preschooler

Between ages 3 and 6 years, a child faces a psychosocial crisis that Erikson termed *initiative versus guilt*. The child's significant other is the family. At this age, the child has normally mastered a sense of autonomy and moves on to master a sense of initiative. A preschooler is an energetic, enthusiastic and intrusive learner with an active imagination. Conscience (an inner voice that warns and threatens) begins to develop. The child explores the physical world with all his or her senses and powers.

Development of a sense of guilt occurs when the child is made to feel that his or her imagination and activities are unacceptable. Guilt, anxiety and fear result when the child's thoughts and activities clash with parental expectations. A preschooler begins to use simple reasoning and can tolerate longer periods of delayed gratification.

Sample questions for the preschooler include:

- Does your child have an active imagination?
- Does your child imitate adult activities?
- Does your child engage in fantasy play?
- Does your child frequently ask questions?
- Does your child enjoy new activities?

School-age child

Erikson termed the psychosocial crisis faced by a child age 6 to 12 years *industry versus inferiority*. During this period, the child's radius of significant others expands to include school and instructive adults. A school-age child normally has mastered the first three developmental tasks—trust, autonomy and initiative—and now focus on mastering industry. A child's sense of industry grows out of a desire for real achievement.

The child engages in tasks and activities that he or she can carry through to completion. The child learns rules and how to compete with others and to cooperate to achieve goals. Social relationships with others become increasingly important sources of support. The child can develop a sense of inferiority stemming from unrealistic expectations or a sense of failing to meet standards set for him or her by others. Because the child feels inadequate, his or her self-esteem sags.

Sample questions for the school-age child include:

- What are your child's interests and hobbies?
- Does your child interact well with teachers and peers?
- Does your child enjoy accomplishments?
- Does your child shame themselves for failures?
- What is your child's favourite activity?

Adolescent

Erikson termed the psychosocial crisis faced by adolescents (ages 13 to 18 years) *identity versus role diffusion.* For an adolescent, the radius of significant others is the peer group. To an adolescent, development of who he or she is and where he or she is going becomes a central focus. The adolescent continues to redefine his or her self-concept and the roles that he or she can play with certainty. As rapid physical changes occur, adolescents must reintegrate previous trust in their body, themselves and how they appear to others. The inability to develop a sense of who he or she is, and what he or she can become, results in role diffusion and inability to solve core conflicts.

Sample questions for adolescents include:

- Does your son or daughter have a peer group?
- Does your son or daughter have a best friend?
- Does your son or daughter exhibit rebellious behaviour at home?
- How does your son or daughter see themselves as fitting in with peers?
- What does your son or daughter want to do with their life?

Psychosexual development (Freud)

It is suggested that children of all ages be questioned about sexual abuse. This may be elicited by asking, 'Has anyone ever touched you where or when you did not want to be touched?'

The stages of a child's psychosexual development outlined here derive from the work of psychopathologist Sigmund Freud from the late 1800s and early 1900s.

Toddler

In Freud's *anal stage,* typically extending from age 8 months to 4 years, the erogenous zone is the anus and buttocks, and sexual activity centres on the expulsion and retention of body waste. In this stage, the child's focus shifts from the mouth to the anal area with emphasis on bowel control as he or she gains neuromuscular control over the anal sphincter. The toddler experiences both satisfaction and frustration as he or she gains control over withholding and expelling, containing and releasing. The conflict between 'holding on' and 'letting go' gradually resolves as bowel training progresses; resolution occurs once control is firmly established.

Toilet training is a major task of toddlerhood (Fig. 33-9). Readiness is not usual until age 18 to 24 months. Bowel training occurs before bladder; night bladder training usually does not occur until age 3 to 5 years. Masturbation can occur from body exploration. Toddlers learn words associated with anatomy and elimination and can distinguish between the sexes.

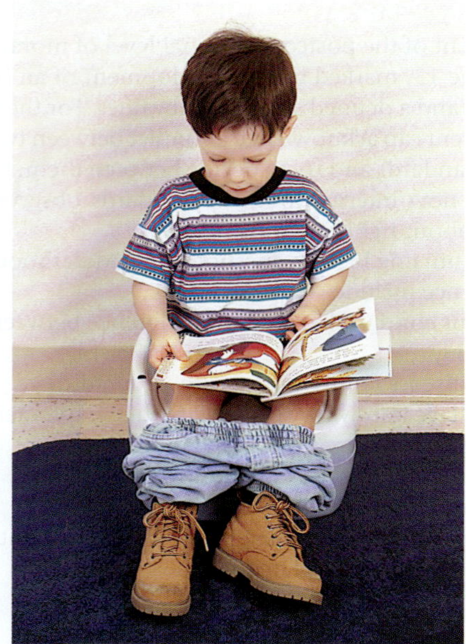

FIGURE 33-9 Toilet training is a major task of toddlerhood.

Sample questions for the toddler include:

- Does your child have any problems with toilet training?
- Does your child play with his or her genitals?

Preschooler

In the Freudian *phallic stage,* extending from about age 3 to 7 years, the child's pleasure centres on the genitalia and masturbation. Many preschoolers masturbate for physiological pleasure.

The *Oedipal stage* occurs, marked by jealousy and rivalry towards the same-sex parent and love of the opposite-sex parent. The Oedipal stage typically resolves in the late preschool period, with a strong identification with the same-sex parent.

Sexual identity is developed during this time. Modesty may become a concern, and the preschooler may have fears of castration. Because preschoolers are keen observers but poor interpreters, the child may recognise but not understand sexual activity. Before answering a child's questions about sex, parents should clarify what the child is really asking and what the child already thinks about the specific subject. Questions about sex should be answered simply and honestly, providing only the information that the child requests; additional details can come later.

Sample questions for the preschooler include:

- Does your child play with his or her genitals?
- Does your child know what sex he or she is?
- Has your child asked questions about sex, childbirth and the like?

School-age child

The *latency period,* extending from about 5 to 12 years, represents a stage of relative sexual indifference before puberty and adolescence. During this period, development of self-esteem is closely linked with a developing sense of industry in gaining a concept of one's value and worth. Preadolescence begins near the end of the school-age years, and discrepancies in growth and maturation between the sexes become apparent.

A school-age child has acquired much of his or her knowledge of, and many of his or her attitudes towards, sex at a very early age. During the school-age years, the child refines this knowledge and these attitudes. Questions about sex require honest answers based on the child's level of understanding.

Sample questions for the school-age child include:

- Does your child interact with same-sex peers?
- What has your child been told about puberty and sex?

Adolescent

In the *genital stage,* which extends from about age 12 to 20 years, an adolescent focuses on the genitals as an erogenous zone and engages in masturbation and sexual relations with others. During this period of renewed sexual drive, an adolescent experiences conflict between his or her own needs for sexual satisfaction and society's expectations for control of sexual expression. Core concerns of adolescents include body image development and acceptance by the opposite sex or same sex, depending on preference or gender identity.

Relationships with the opposite sex are important (Fig. 33-10). Adolescents engage in sexual activity for pleasure, to satisfy drives and curiosity, as a conquest, for affection and because of peer pressure. Teaching about sexual function, begun during the school years, should expand to cover more in-depth information on the physical, hormonal and emotional changes of puberty. An adolescent needs accurate, complete information on sexuality and cultural and moral values. Information must include how pregnancy occurs; methods of preventing pregnancy—stressing that male and female partners both are responsible for contraception; and transmission of and protection against sexually transmitted infections, especially acquired immunodeficiency syndrome and hepatitis (see Chaps 25 and 26).

A full, confidential sexual or sexuality history should be obtained from adolescents. This history includes questioning previously noted in the reproductive review of systems as well as:

- What is your sexual preference?
- How do you feel about becoming a man/woman?

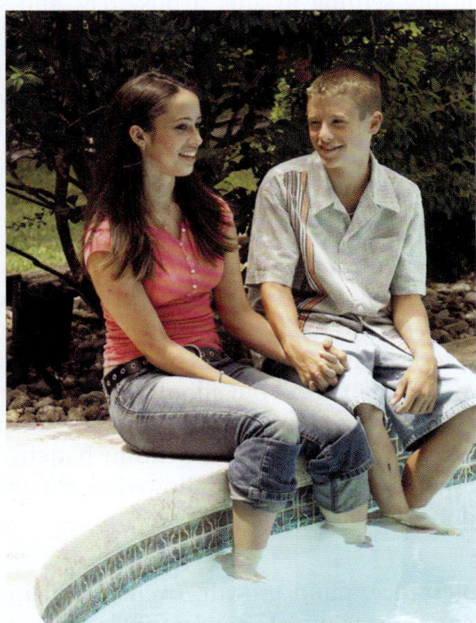

FIGURE 33-10 During adolescence, relationships with the opposite sex are important stepping stones to adulthood. (Klossner, N. J. & Hatfield, N. [2006]. *Introductory maternity and pediatric nursing.* Philadelphia: Lippincott Williams & Wilkins.)

Lifestyle and health practices

Normal nutritional requirements

Proper nutrition is necessary for childhood growth and development. Food and feeding are important parts of growing up, with needs and desires changing as the child grows (Fig. 33-11). General overviews of each phase of nutrition follow.

Toddlers

Growth rate slows dramatically during the toddler years, thus decreasing the need for kilojoules, protein and fluid. Starting at about 12 months, most toddlers are eating the same foods as the rest of the family. At 18 months, many toddlers experience physiological anorexia and become picky eaters. They experience food jags and eat large amounts one day and very little the next. They like to feed themselves and prefer small portions of appetising foods. Frequent, nutritious snacks can replace a meal. Food should not be used as a reward or a punishment. Milk should be limited to no more than 1 L per day to ensure intake and absorption of iron-enriched foods to prevent anaemia. Recommendations for screening for anaemia should be based on age, sex and risk of anaemia.

Preschoolers

Requirements are similar to those of the toddler. Three- and four-year-old children may still be unable to sit with family during meals. Four-year-old children are picky eaters. Five-year-old children are influenced by the food habits of others. A 5-year-old child tends to be focused on the 'social' aspects of eating: table conversation, manners, willingness to try new foods, and help with meal preparation and cleanup.

School-age children

A school-age child's daily kilojoule requirements diminish in relation to body size. Carers should continue to stress the need for a balanced diet from the food pyramid because resources are being stored for the increased growth needs of adolescence. The child is exposed to broader eating experiences in the school lunchroom; he or she may still be a 'picky' eater but

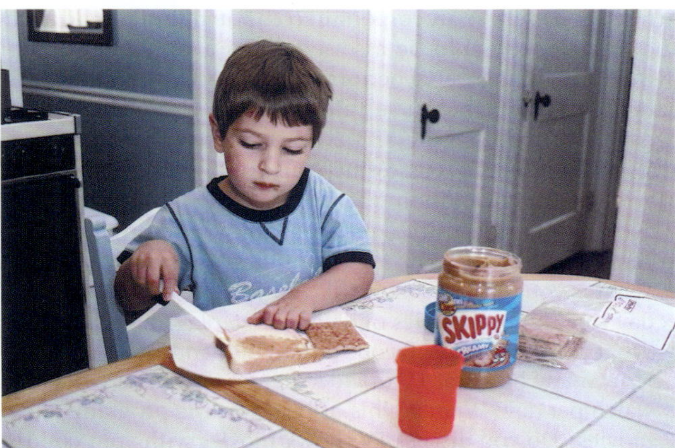

FIGURE 33-11 Many young children enjoy helping to prepare their lunch. (Weber, J.R., & Kelley, J.H. [2018]. *Health Assessment in Nursing* [6th ed.]. © Wolters Kluwer Health.)

should be more willing to try new foods. Children may trade, sell or throw away home-packed school lunches. At home, the child should eat what the family eats; the patterns that develop now stay with the child into adulthood.

Adolescents

An adolescent's daily intake should be balanced among the foods in the pyramid; average daily intake of kilojoules requirements vary with sex and age. Adolescents typically eat whatever they have at break activities; readily available nutritious snacks provide good insurance for a balanced diet. Milk (calcium) and protein are needed in quantity to aid in bone and muscle growth. Maintaining adequate quality and quantity of daily intake may be difficult because of such factors as a busy schedule, the influence of peers and an easy availability of fast foods. Family eating patterns established during the school years continue to influence an adolescent's food selection. Female adolescents are very prone to negative dieting behaviours. Common dietary deficiencies include iron, folate and zinc.

Sample nursing history questions for toddlerhood to adolescence include:

- What does your child eat in a typical day?
- Is your child on any special type of diet? If so, what for?
- What types of food does your child like and dislike most?
- Does your child have any feeding problems?
- Is your child allergic to any foods? If so, how does your child react to those foods?
- Does your child take any vitamin or mineral supplements?
- How much fluid does your child drink per day?
- Is your water fluorinated? If not, does your child take supplements?
- Has your child had any recent weight gain or loss?

These questions should also be asked directly of adolescents when parents are not present:

- Do you have any concerns with body image?
- Have you been on any self-imposed diet?
- How often do you weigh yourself?
- Have you ever used any of the following methods for weight loss: Self-induced vomiting? Laxatives? Diuretics? Excessive exercise? Fasting?

Normal activity and exercise

Activity and exercise are important components of a child's life and, therefore, should be assessed when a complete subjective examination is being performed. Play, activity and exercise patterns can give the nurse valuable clues about the overall health of a child. Display 33-2 describes play characteristics across childhood. This assessment also allows the examiner to provide health-promotion teaching.

Sample nursing history questions for toddlerhood to adolescence include:

- What is your child's activity like during a typical 24-hour day (including activities of daily living, play and school)?
- What are your child's favourite activities and toys?
- How many hours of TV or video games does your child watch per day? What are his or her favourite programs/movies? Do you discuss TV shows/movies with your child?
- Are there any restrictions on TV watching (content, hours, relationship to chores/homework)?
- What chores does your child do at home (school-age child/adolescent)?
- Does the older child/adolescent work outside the home? What does he or she do?
- How many hours does he or she work during the school year?
- Does the work interfere with school or social life?
- Why does the child work?
- Does your child have any problems that restrict physical activity?
- Does your child require any special devices to manage with activities of daily living/play?
- At what age did your child first walk?
- Can your child keep up with his or her peers?
- Does your child have any hobbies/interests (age 6 and older)?
- In what sports does your child participate?

Normal sleep requirements and patterns

Sleep is an integral part of health assessment. Lack of sleep can affect all areas of health, including cognitive, physical and emotional health. Children require varying amounts of sleep based primarily on their age. They also have varying sleep habits that correlate with their developmental status. A safe sleep environment is also important for all young children to reduce the risk of sudden unexpected death in infants. This includes a safe cot, safe mattress and safe bedding.

Toddlers

Total sleep requirements decrease during the second year and average about 12 hours per day. Most toddlers nap once a day until the end of the second or third year. Sleep problems are common and may be due to fears of separation. Bedtime rituals and transitional objects, such as a blanket or stuffed toy, are helpful.

Preschoolers

The average preschooler sleeps 11 to 13 hours per day. Preschoolers typically need an afternoon nap until age 5, when most begin kindergarten. Bedtime rituals persist and sleep problems are common. These include nightmares, night terrors, difficulty settling in after a busy day, and stretching bedtime rituals to delay sleep. Continuing with reassuring bedtime rituals together with some relaxation time before bed should help the child settle in. The daytime nap may be eliminated if it seems to interfere with night-time sleep. For many preschoolers, a security object and night light continue to help relieve anxiety or fear at bedtime (Fig. 33-12).

School-age children

School-age children's individual sleep requirements vary but typically range from 8 to 9.5 hours per night. Because the growth rate has slowed, children actually need less sleep now than during adolescence. The child's bedtime can be later than during the preschool period but should be firmly established and adhered to on school nights. Reading before bedtime may facilitate sleep and set up a positive bedtime pattern. Children may be unaware of fatigue and, if allowed to remain up, they will be tired the next day.

Adolescents

During adolescence, rapid growth, overexertion in activities and a tendency to stay up late commonly interfere with sleep and rest requirements. In an attempt to 'catch up' on missed sleep, many adolescents sleep late at every opportunity. Each adolescent is unique in the number of sleep hours required to stay healthy and rested.

DISPLAY 33-2: CHARACTERISTICS OF PLAY AMONG CHILDREN

Toddlers

Toddlers engage in parallel play—they play alongside, not with, others. Imitation is one of the most common forms of play and locomotion skills can be enhanced with push–pull toys. Toddlers change toys frequently because of short attention spans.

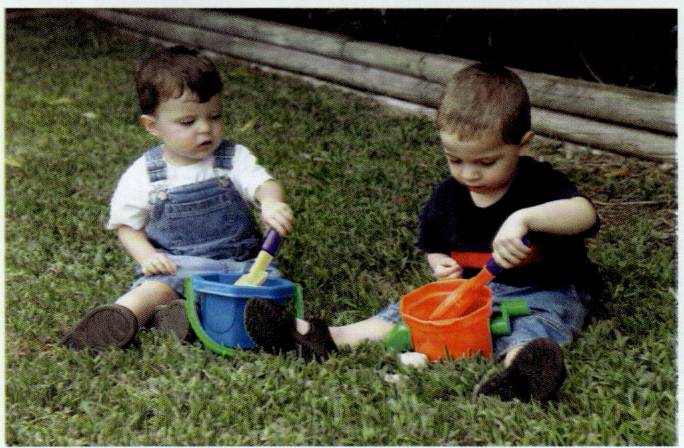

Preschoolers

Typical preschool play is associative—interactive and cooperative with sharing. Preschoolers need contact with age mates. Activities such as jumping, running and climbing promote growth and motor skills. Preschoolers are at a typical age for imaginary playmates. Imitative, imaginative and dramatic play are important. TV and video games should only be a part of the child's play, and parents should monitor content and amount of time spent in use. Associative play materials include dress-up clothes and dolls, housekeeping toys, play tents, puppets, and doctor and nurse kits. Curious and active preschoolers need adult supervision, especially near bodies of water and gym sets.

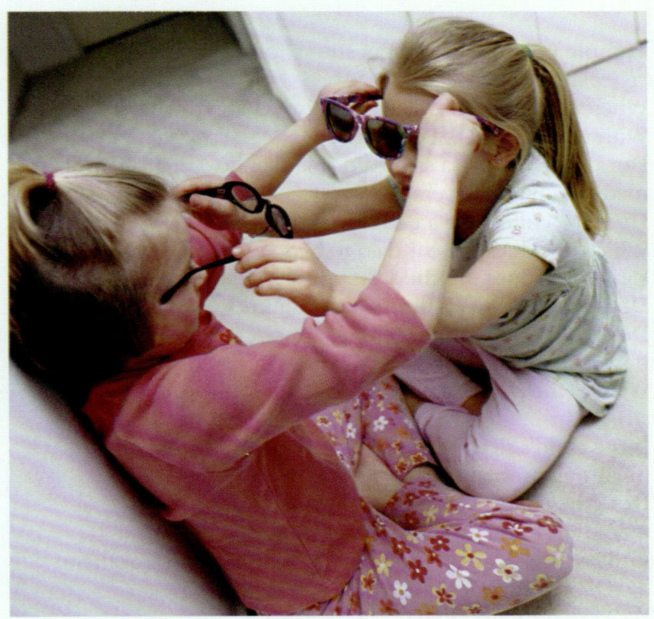

School-age children

Play becomes more competitive and complex during the school-age period. Characteristic activities include joining team sports, secret clubs and 'gangs'; Scouting or like activities; working complex puzzles; collecting; playing quiet board games; reading; and hero worshiping. Rules and rituals are important aspects of play and games.

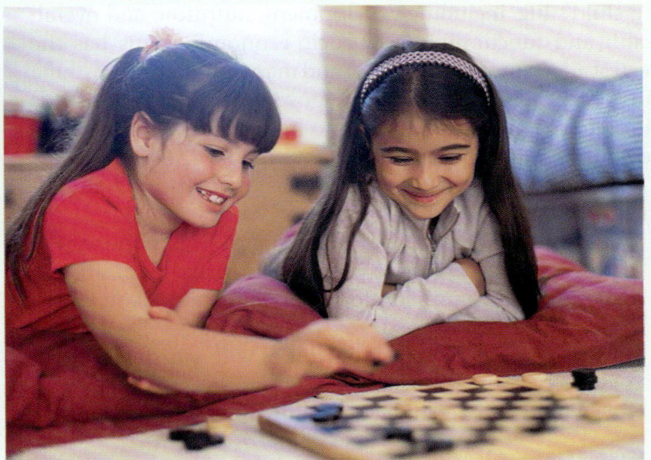

(Weber, J.R., & Kelley, J.H. [2018]. *Health Assessment in Nursing* [6th ed.]. © Wolters Kluwer Health.)

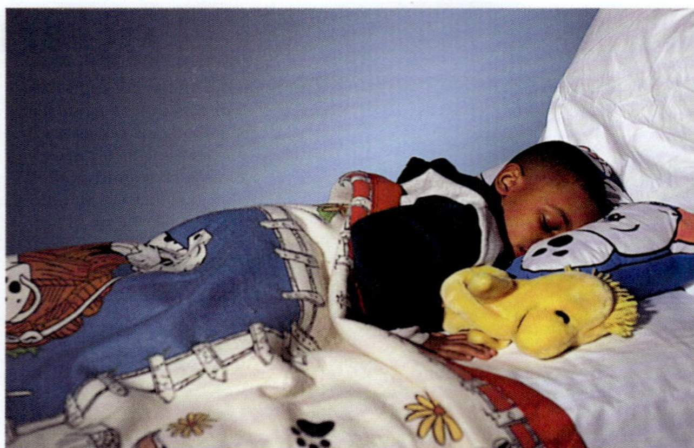

FIGURE 33-12 A security object, such as a favourite toy, can help a preschooler to sleep. (© B. Proud.)

Sample nursing history questions for toddlerhood to adolescence include:

- Where does the child sleep, and on what type of bed?
- With whom does the child sleep?
- Does the child use a sleep aid (blanket, toy, night light, medication and beverage)?
- Does the child have a bedtime ritual?
- What time does the child go to bed at night?
- What time does the child get up in the morning?
- Does the child sleep through the night?
- Does the child require feeding at night and, if so, what and how is it administered (bottle caries)?
- What is the child's nap schedule, and for how long are the sleep naps?
- Is the child's sleep restful or restless; any snoring or breathing problems?
- Does the child sleepwalk or sleep talk?
- Does the child have nightmares or night terrors?
- If the child has sleep problems, what do you do for them?

Socio-economic situation

A family's socio-economic situation greatly affects all aspects of a child's life, including development, nutrition, and overall health and functioning. Low socio-economic status has the greatest adverse effect on health, and many children in Australia and New Zealand live below the poverty level. Therefore, it is critical to obtain this assessment to initiate intervention strategies at the earliest opportunity.

Sample nursing history questions for infancy to adolescence include:

- Would you seek more medical assistance (e.g. in the way of preventive screenings, checkups, sick visits, medication requests, eyeglass prescriptions) for your child if you had the money to do so?
- Do you have any financial difficulties with which you need assistance?
- How would you describe your family's living conditions?

Relationship and role development

The development of relationships and a role within groups is a crucial aspect of childhood. The ability of children to establish high-quality relationships and form specific roles in the early years significantly determines their ability to form high-quality relationships and roles when adulthood is reached.

CULTURAL CONSIDERATIONS

Culture is an important factor in a person's relationship and role development. Things to consider include whether the child's culture or ethnicity is a minority within the major cultural group; the traditional role of children in the particular child's culture; and whether there is male or female dominance in the particular culture.

Another major influence on the child's development of relationships and roles is the structure of the family. Various family structures include two-parent families, single-parent families, blended families, same-sex, transgender and gender diverse parent families, families with an adopted child, or families with a foster child.

Early intervention and early prevention of poor relationships between the child and his or her carers, siblings, peers and influential adults outside the immediate family are vital. Therefore, assessment of this aspect of a child's life is extremely important. It is important to ask questions to the parent or carer as well as the child because they may have differing views concerning the nature of the child's relationships.

Sample nursing history questions for toddlerhood to adolescence specifically geared to the parent or carer include:

- What is your family structure?
- With what culture or ethnic group does your family identify?
- How would you describe your family support system?
- Who is the child's primary carer (especially for smaller children, not in school)?
- What is the child's role in the family?
- What are the family occupations and routines?
- How much time do you spend with your children and what activities do you participate in when you are together?
- Have there been any changes in your family lately—divorce, birth, deaths, moves?
- How does your child get along with parents, siblings, extended family, teachers and peers?
- Discuss your child's circle of friends.
- What disciplinary measures do you use?

Sample nursing history questions for toddlerhood to adolescence specifically geared to the child or adolescent include:

- How do you get along with your parents? Brothers? Sisters?
- What activities do your family do together?
- What chores do you do around the house?
- What would you consider is your role in the family?
- What are the names of your family members and friends?
- Do you have a best friend?
- What do you like best about family and friends?
- What do you dislike about family and friends?
- What do you do or share with your friends?
- Do your parents know your friends? Do they like them?
- Do you get along with the other kids at school?
- Do you get along with your teachers?

Self-esteem and self-concept development

Childhood is the time when an individual develops the self-esteem and self-concept that shapes him or her in adult life

(Table 33-5). Therefore, an assessment of this nature is crucial to providing health-promotion teaching, prevent future problems and intervene with current problems. This is a good time to ask questions regarding the child's values and beliefs because these areas tend greatly to influence a person's self-concept. This assessment requires that the same questions be asked of both the parent and the child because their opinions may be significantly different. Reassure the parent and the child that all answers discussed will be kept confidential.

Sample nursing history questions for toddler to adolescence include (also ask these questions directly to the child; these questions are given in italics):

- How would you describe your child? *How would you describe yourself?*
- What does your child do best? *What do you do best?*
- In what areas does your child need improvement? *In what areas do you think you need improvement?*
- Is your child ever overly concerned about his or her weight? *Do you like your present weight? What would you like to weigh?*
- Are culture and religion important factors in your home? *Are culture and religion important to you?*
- In what religion is the child being reared? *What religion are you?*
- How does your child define right and wrong? *How would you decide if something were right or wrong?*
- What are your family values? *What values are important to you?*
- What are the child's goals in life? *What are your goals in life?*

Coping and stress management

Childhood is full of stressors and fears, including the developmental crises of transition to each life stage and common childhood fears such as the dark and being left alone (Tables 33-6 and 33-7). The ways in which children cope with stress and fear can affect their development and how they will handle subsequent life events. Coping mechanisms vary depending on developmental level, resources, situation, style and previous experience with stressful events (Table 33-8).

The ability of a child to cope is often influenced by individual temperament. Temperament involves the child's style of emotional and behavioural responses across situations. Temperament is biological in origin; however, it is influenced by environmental characteristics and patterned by society. This is significant because short- and long-term psychosocial adjustments are shaped by the goodness of fit between the child's temperament and the social environment.

Sample nursing history questions for infancy to adolescence include (questions asked of the child appear in italic print):

- What does your child do when he or she gets angry or frustrated? *What do you do when you get angry or frustrated?*

Table 33-5 Self-concept development

Toddlers and preschoolers	Greater sense of independence
School-age children	More aware of differences, norms and morals; sensitive to social pressures
Adolescents	Self-concept crystallises in later adolescence when child focuses on physical and emotional changes and peer acceptance

Table 33-6 Stressors in children

Young children	Change in daily structure, new sibling separation
Older children	Starting school, long holidays, moving Change in family structure (remarriage), Christmas
Adolescents	Pregnancy peer loss Breakup with boyfriend or girl friend
All children	Parental loss (divorce, death, jail)

Table 33-7 Common childhood fears

Infants	Loud noises; falling and sudden movements in the environment; stranger anxiety begins around age 6 months
Toddlers	Loss of parents—separation anxiety; stranger anxiety; loud noises; going to sleep; large animals; certain people (doctor, Father Christmas); certain places (doctor's office); large objects or machines
Preschoolers	The dark; being left alone, especially at bedtime; animals (particularly large dogs); ghosts and other supernatural beings; body mutilation; pain; objects and people associated with painful experiences
School-age children	Failure at school; bullies; intimidating teachers; supernatural beings; storms; staying alone; scary things in TV and movies; consequences related to unattractive appearance; death
Adolescents	Relationships with people of the opposite sex; homosexual tendencies; ability to assume adult roles; drugs; acquired immunodeficiency syndrome; divorce; gossip; public speaking; plane and car crashes; death

Table 33-8 Coping mechanisms in children

Infants	Restlessness, rocking, playing with toys, crying, thumb sucking, sleeping
Toddlers/ Preschoolers	Asking questions, wanting order, holding favourite toy, learning by trial and error, tantrums, aggression, thumb sucking, withdrawal, regression
School-age children	Trying problem solving; communicating, fantasising, acting out situations, quiet, denial, regression, reaction formation
Adolescents	Problem solving, philosophical discussions, conforming with peers, asserting control, acting out, using drugs or alcohol, denial, projection, rationalisation, intellectualisation

DISPLAY 33-3: SUICIDE ASSESSMENT: RISKS AND SIGNS

Suicide is a leading killer of young people, particularly teenagers. The nurse can be instrumental in detecting signs of impending suicide and, possibly, intervening to prevent it. During the nursing assessment, several interviewing methods and questions may help uncover a young patient's suicidal thoughts.

- Ask if the child ever thought of hurting or killing self (hurting is different from killing).
- If the answer is 'yes', ask the child when he or she thought of killing self.
- Ask how the child planned to do it.
- Ask if the child ever tried to kill himself or herself before and if any help was received after the incident.
- Ask if the child believes that there are any other options besides suicide to resolve problems.

Children and adolescents who verbalise planned, lethal means to commit suicide, and who feel that they do not have any other options, are at extremely high risk of carrying out their plan—especially if they have attempted suicide in the past. Some risk factors and warning signs of potential suicide include the following:

Risk factors

- Previous attempt
- Suicide of family member or close friend
- History of abuse, neglect or psychiatric hospitalisation
- Persistent depression
- Mental disorder (voices tell child to kill self)
- Substance abuse
- Difficult home situation
- Incarceration
- Few social opportunities; isolated
- Firearms in the home.

Warning signs

- Feeling depressed, irritable or hopeless
- Seems preoccupied with death themes, as in books, music, art, films or TV shows
- Gives away valued possessions
- Talks about death, especially own
- Acts recklessly or adopts antisocial behaviour
- Experiences rapid change in school performance
- Has episode of sudden cheerfulness after being depressed
- Exhibits dramatic change in everyday behaviours, such as sleeping and eating
- Smokes continuously (chain smoking)
- Expresses sense of worthlessness or hopelessness.

- What does your child do when he or she gets tired? *What do you do when you get tired?*
- When your child has a tantrum, how do you handle it?
- What things make your child scared? *What things scare you?*
- What does he or she do when scared? *What do you do when you're scared?*
- What kinds of things does your child worry about? *What kinds of things do you worry about?*
- When your child has a problem, what does he or she do? *When you have a problem, what do you do?*
- Have there been any big problems or changes in your family lately? *Have there been any big problems or changes in your family lately?*
- Is there a problem with alcohol or drugs? *Do you use tobacco, alcohol or drugs?*
- Has your child ever run away from home? *Have you ever run away from home?*
- How does your child react when their needs are not met immediately, and what do you do about it? *What do you do when you are sad? What do you do when you are angry?*
- Is your child 'accident prone', and why do you think that is? *Did you ever think about hurting yourself? Did you ever think about killing yourself?* (See Display 33-3.)

COLLECTING OBJECTIVE DATA: PHYSICAL EXAMINATION

Preparing the patient

In most cases, physical assessment involves a head-to-toe examination that encompasses each body system. When examining children, the sequence should be altered to accommodate the child's developmental needs:

- Less threatening and least intrusive procedures, such as a general inspection and heart and lung auscultation, should be completed first to secure the child's trust.
- Explain what you will be doing and what the child might feel; allow the child to manipulate the equipment before it is used.
- Try to perform an examination in a comfortable, non-threatening area.
- The temperature should be warm, the room well lit and all threatening instruments out of the child's view.
- The room should contain age-appropriate diversions such as toys and cartoons for younger children and posters for adolescents.
- If the child is uncooperative, first assess the reason (usually fear) then intervene appropriately. If still unsuccessful, involve the parents, use a firm approach and complete the examination as quickly but completely as possible.
- Involve the child in the physical examination at all times, unless it is stressful for him or her.

Equipment

- Appropriate assessment tool such as ASQ or PEDS
- Ophthalmoscope (the ophthalmoscope is frequently used in the advanced eye assessment; see Equipment spotlight 17-1)
- Otoscope (the otoscope is frequently used in advanced ear assessment; see Equipment spotlight 18-1)
- Scale or stadiometer
- Snellen Eye Chart
- Stethoscope
- Other relevant equipment and paperwork as per institutional policy

Physical assessment

- Recognise how techniques and demeanour for interviewing and examining children differ among the age groups and from those used for interviewing and examining adults. Display 33-4 gives developmental approaches to the physical examination.

DISPLAY 33-4: DEVELOPMENTAL APPROACHES TO THE PHYSICAL ASSESSMENT

Children in each age group respond differently to the hands-on physical assessment; however, the following guidelines should be kept in mind:

- *Toddlers.* Allow toddler to sit on parent's lap; enlist parent's aid; use play; praise cooperation.
- *Preschoolers.* Use story telling; use doll and puppet play; give choices when able.
- *School-age children.* Maintain privacy; use gown; explain procedures and equipment; teach about their bodies.
- *Adolescents.* Ensure privacy and confidentiality; provide option of having parent present or not; emphasise normality; provide health teaching.

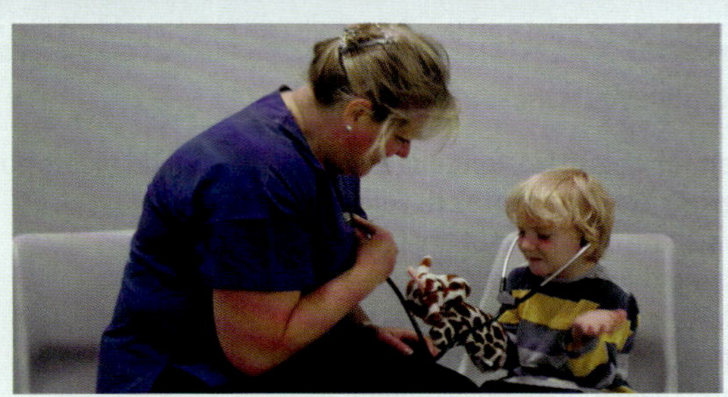

Puppet or doll play is a great way to prepare a preschooler for physical examination.

- Evaluate growth and development patterns according to the different paediatric age groups and across body systems.
- Recognise children who are difficult to examine because of anxiety or fear.
- Develop forms of age-appropriate 'play' to distract less cooperative children so a physical examination can be completed.

CRITICAL THINKING

8. While examining Michael, what techniques would you use to obtain temperature, pulse and respirations accurately?
9. How would you initiate the assessment of Michael without frightening him?

PHYSICAL ASSESSMENT

ASSESSMENT PROCEDURE	NORMAL FINDINGS	ABNORMAL FINDINGS
General appearance and behaviour		
Note overall appearance. Observe hygiene, interaction with parents and yourself (and siblings if present). Note also facial expressions, posture, nutritional status, speech, attention span and level of cooperation. **CLINICAL TIP** **Behavioural observation is one of the most important assessments to make with children because alterations usually signify health problems.**	Child appears stated age, is clean, appears well nourished, and has no unusual body odour. Clothing is in good condition and appropriate for climate. Child is alert, active, responds appropriately to stress of the situation and maintains eye contact. Child is appropriately interactive for age, seeks comfort from parent; appears happy or appropriately anxious because of examination. Child is attentive and speech is appropriate for age, follows age-appropriate commands and is reasonably cooperative. Toddler is lordotic when standing; preschooler is slightly bowlegged; older child demonstrates straight and well-balanced posture.	Lack of eye contact indicates many things including anxiety or significant psychosocial problems. **CULTURAL CONSIDERATIONS** **Lack of eye contact is normal for certain cultural groups such as Asians and Aboriginal and Torres Strait Islander peoples.** Deviations from normal that can be discerned from a child's appearance or behaviour are listed below. Certain faces may indicate fear, anxiety, anger, allergies, acute illness, pain, mental deficiency, or respiratory distress. A child's posture or movement may indicate pain, low self-esteem, rejection, depression, hostility or aggression. Hygiene gives insight into neglect, poverty, mental illness or retardation or knowledge deficit regarding hygiene (e.g. teen parent). Abnormal behaviour may suggest neurological problems (head trauma, cranial lesions), metabolic problems (diabetic ketoacidosis), psychiatric disorders or psychosocial problems. Abnormal development (child does not appear stated age) may indicate mental retardation, abuse, neglect or psychiatric disorders.

Continued on following page

PHYSICAL ASSESSMENT (continued)

ASSESSMENT PROCEDURE	NORMAL FINDINGS	ABNORMAL FINDINGS
Developmental assessment		
Screen for cognitive, language, social, and gross and fine motor developmental delays in the beginning of the physical assessment for preschoolers. Use a standardised assessment tool such as the Ages and Stages Questionnaire and Parents' Evaluation of Developmental Status.	Child meets normal parameters for age.	Child lags in earlier stages.
Vital signs		
Assess temperature. Use axillary, skin or tympanic route when assessing the temperature. The rectal route should only be used in neonates and children age under 3 months. **SAFETY TIP** **Use the rectal route only when absolutely necessary because of increased discomfort in older children. Rectal temperatures are also contraindicated in certain circumstances, such as the immunosuppressed child as well as the child who has diarrhoea, a bleeding disorder, a perforated anus or a history of rectal surgery.** To take a rectal temperature in a toddler, lay the child supine and lift lower legs up into the air, bending the legs at the hips. Insert lubricated rectal thermometer no more than 2 cm into rectum. Temperature registers in 3 to 5 min on a rectal thermometer. Lay a school-age child on the stomach on a table. Maintain firm hold on child's hips so child does not raise buttocks up during the procedure. Separate buttocks with thumb and forefinger of non-dominant hand and insert thermometer. See Chapter 7 for other temperature techniques.	Temperature is 37°C.	Temperature may be altered by exercise, stress, crying, environment, diurnal variation (highest between 4 and 6 p.m.). Both hyperthermic and hypothermic conditions are noted in children. **FIGURE 33-13** Measuring radial pulse in an adolescent.
Assess pulse rate. Count the pulse for a full minute. Children younger than 2 years should have apical pulse measured. Radial pulses may be taken in children over 2 years old (Fig. 33-13).	Awake and resting rates vary with the age of the child: 3 months–2 years: 80–150 2–10 years: 70–110 10 years–adult: 55–90 **CLINICAL TIP** **Athletic adolescents tend to have lower pulse rates.**	Pulse may be altered by apprehension or anxiety, medications, activity and pain, as well as pathological conditions.

PHYSICAL ASSESSMENT (continued)

ASSESSMENT PROCEDURE	NORMAL FINDINGS	ABNORMAL FINDINGS
Assess respiratory rate. Monitor respirations in children older than 1 year the same as for adults.	Normal ranges are as follows: 6 months–2 years: 20–30 3–10 years: 20–28 10–18 years: 12–20	Respiratory rate and character may be altered by medications, positioning, fever, activity and anxiety or fear as well as pathological conditions.
Evaluate blood pressure. Blood pressure should be measured annually in children 3 years and older, and in all ages when conditions warrant it. The appropriate cuff width is 50% to 75% of the upper arm (Fig. 33-14). The length should encircle the circumference without overlapping. A small diaphragm should be used for the stethoscope. If for some reason the arm cannot be used, a measurement can be taken on the thigh. If children younger than 3 years require a blood pressure reading, a Doppler stethoscope should be used.	Normal ranges are as follows: *Systolic:* 1–7 years = age in years + 90 8–18 years = (2 × age in years) + 90 *Diastolic:* 1–5 years = 56 6–18 years = age in years + 52 (see also Table 33-9)	Systolic and diastolic blood pressure above 95th percentiles for age and sex after three readings is considered high blood pressure. **CLINICAL TIP** **If the blood pressure reading is too high for age, the cuff may be too small; it should cover two-thirds of the child's upper arm. If the blood pressure reading is too low for age, the cuff may be too large. Chapter 7 explains how to take a blood pressure reading.**

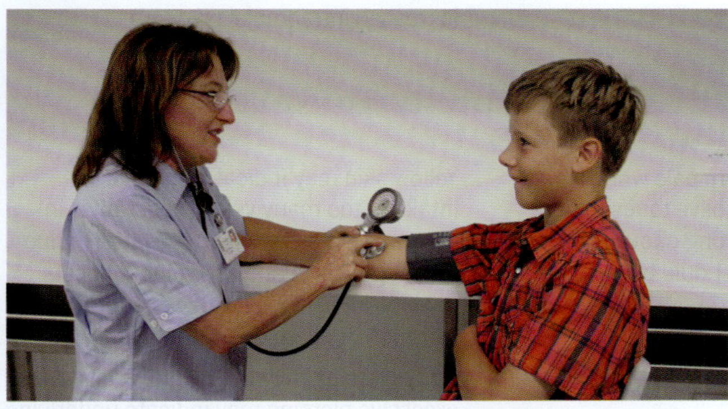

FIGURE 33-14 Measuring a child or an adolescent's blood pressure requires a cuff that is appropriately sized.

Measurements		
Measure height. In a child younger than 2 years, determine height by measuring the recumbent length. Fully extend the body, holding the head in midline and gently grasping the knees and pushing them downwards until the legs are fully extended and touching the table. If using a measuring board, place the head at the top of the board and the heels firmly at the bottom. Without a board, use paper under the child and mark the paper at the top of the head and bottom of the heels. Then measure the distance between the two points. Determine an older child's height by having the shoeless child stand as straight as possible with head midline and vision line parallel between the ceiling and floor (Fig. 33-15). Child's back, buttocks and back of heels should be against the wall; measure height with a stadiometer. Plot height measurement on an age- and gender-appropriate growth chart (birth to 36 months and 2 to 20 years).	See the growth charts in Appendix A for normal findings. **CULTURAL CONSIDERATIONS** **Asian children are smaller at all ages.**	Significant deviation from normal in the growth charts would be considered abnormal.

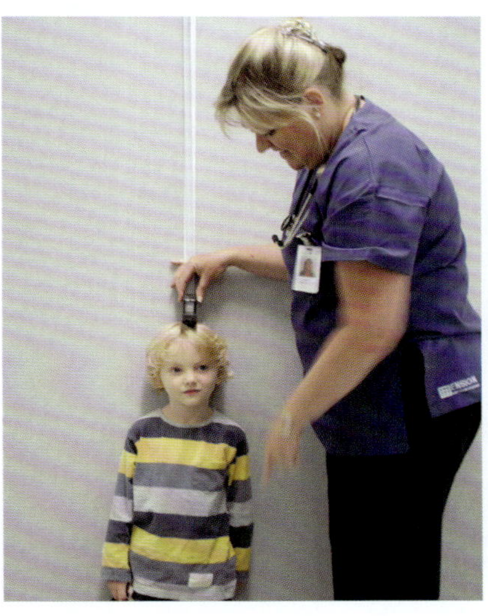

FIGURE 33-15 Measuring the height of a preschooler.

Continued on following page

PHYSICAL ASSESSMENT (continued)

ASSESSMENT PROCEDURE	NORMAL FINDINGS	ABNORMAL FINDINGS
Measure weight on an appropriately sized beam scale with non-detectable weights. Weigh a small child lying or sitting on a scale that measures to the nearest 10 g. Weigh an older child standing on a scale that measures to the nearest 100 g. Weigh an older child in underpants or light gown to respect modesty. Plot weight measurement on age- and gender-appropriate growth chart (birth to 36 months and 2 to 20 years).	See Appendix A for normal findings.	Deviation from the wide range of normal weights is abnormal. See the growth charts in Appendix A and compare differences.
Measure head circumference (HC) or occipital frontal circumference (OFC) at every physical examination for toddlers younger than 2 years and older children when conditions warrant. Plot the measurement on standardised growth charts specific for gender.	HC (OFC) measurement should fall between the 5th and 95th percentiles and should be comparable to the child's height and weight percentiles.	HC (OFC) not within the normal percentiles may indicate pathology. Those greater than 95% may indicate macrocephaly. Those under the 5th percentile may indicate microcephaly. Increased HC (OFC) in children older than 3 years may indicate separation of cranial sutures due to increased intracranial pressure.
Skin, hair and nails		
INSPECTION AND PALPATION		
Observe skin colour, odour and lesions.	Skin colour ranges from pale white with pink, yellow, brown or olive tones to dark brown or black. No strong odour should be evident, and the skin should be lesion free. Normal skin variations (Common variations 33-1) include: • Port wine stains • Haemangiomas • Café-au-lait spots (are normal in small numbers).	Yellow skin may indicate jaundice or intake of too many yellow vegetables in infants (sclera is white in the latter). Blue skin suggests cyanosis, pallor suggests anaemia and redness suggests fever, irritation or allergies. Body piercing may be cultural or a fad, but excessive piercing may indicate underlying self-abusive tendencies. If tattoos appear to be 'homemade', consider the possibility of contamination with hepatitis B virus or human immunodeficiency virus (HIV) from infected needles. Urine odour suggests incontinence, dirty nappy or uraemia. Salty sweat may indicate cystic fibrosis (a parent may report that the child's skin tastes salty when the parent kisses the child). Ecchymoses in various stages or in unusual locations or circular burn areas suggest child abuse. **CULTURAL CONSIDERATIONS** **Bruising or burning may also be from cultural practices such as *cupping* or *coining*. Petechiae, lesions or rashes may indicate serious disorders.** Greater than six café-au-lait spots may indicate neurovascular disease.

Continued on page 723

Table 33-9 Blood pressure levels for the 90th and 95th percentiles of blood pressure for girls and boys, ages 1 to 17

		Systolic BP (mmHg), by height percentile from standard growth curves							Diastolic BP (mmHg), by height percentile from standard growth curves						
Age	BP percentile[a]	5%	10%	25%	50%	75%	90%	95%	5%	10%	25%	50%	75%	90%	95%
Girls															
1	90th	97	98	99	100	102	103	104	53	53	53	54	55	56	56
	95th	101	102	103	104	105	107	107	57	57	57	58	59	60	60
2	90th	99	99	100	102	103	104	105	57	57	58	58	59	60	61
	95th	102	103	104	105	107	108	109	61	61	62	62	63	64	65
3	90th	100	100	102	103	104	105	106	61	61	61	62	63	63	64
	95th	104	104	105	107	108	109	110	65	65	65	66	67	67	68
4	90th	101	102	103	104	106	107	108	63	63	64	65	65	66	67
	95th	105	106	107	108	109	111	111	67	67	68	69	69	70	71
5	90th	103	103	104	106	107	108	109	65	66	66	67	68	68	69
	95th	107	107	108	110	111	112	113	69	70	70	71	72	72	73
6	90th	104	105	106	107	109	110	111	67	67	68	69	69	70	71
	95th	108	109	110	111	112	114	114	71	71	72	73	73	74	75
7	90th	106	107	108	109	110	112	112	69	69	69	70	71	72	72
	95th	110	110	112	113	114	115	116	73	73	73	74	75	76	76
8	90th	108	109	110	111	112	113	114	70	70	71	71	72	73	74
	95th	112	112	113	115	116	117	118	74	74	75	75	76	77	78
9	90th	110	110	112	113	114	115	116	71	72	72	73	74	74	75
	95th	114	114	115	117	118	119	120	75	76	76	77	78	78	79
10	90th	112	112	114	115	116	117	118	73	73	73	74	75	76	76
	95th	116	116	117	119	120	121	122	77	77	77	78	79	80	80
11	90th	114	114	116	117	118	119	120	74	74	75	75	76	77	77
	95th	118	118	119	121	122	123	124	78	78	79	79	80	81	81
12	90th	116	116	118	119	120	121	122	75	75	76	76	77	78	78
	95th	120	120	121	123	124	125	126	79	79	80	80	81	82	82
13	90th	118	118	119	121	122	123	124	76	76	77	78	78	79	80
	95th	121	122	123	125	126	127	128	80	80	81	82	82	83	84
14	90th	119	120	121	122	124	125	126	77	77	78	79	79	80	81
	95th	123	124	125	126	128	129	130	81	81	82	83	83	84	85
15	90th	121	121	122	124	125	126	127	78	78	79	79	80	81	82
	95th	124	125	126	128	129	130	131	82	82	83	83	84	85	86
16	90th	122	122	123	125	126	127	128	79	79	79	80	81	82	82
	95th	125	126	127	128	130	131	132	83	83	83	84	85	86	86
17	90th	122	123	124	125	126	128	128	79	79	79	80	81	82	82
	95th	126	126	127	129	130	131	132	83	83	83	84	85	86	86

Table 33-9 Blood pressure levels for the 90th and 95th percentiles of blood pressure for girls and boys, ages 1 to 17 (continued)

Age	BP percentile[a]	Systolic BP (mmHg), by height percentile from standard growth curves							Diastolic BP (mmHg), by height percentile from standard growth curves						
		5%	10%	25%	50%	75%	90%	95%	5%	10%	25%	50%	75%	90%	95%
Boys															
1	90th	94	95	97	98	100	102	102	50	51	52	53	54	54	55
	95th	98	99	101	102	104	106	106	55	55	56	57	58	59	59
2	90th	98	99	100	102	104	105	106	55	55	56	57	58	59	59
	95th	101	102	104	106	108	109	110	59	59	60	61	62	63	63
3	90th	100	101	103	105	107	108	109	59	59	60	61	62	63	63
	95th	104	105	107	109	111	112	113	63	63	64	65	66	67	67
4	90th	102	103	105	107	109	110	111	62	62	63	64	65	66	66
	95th	106	107	109	111	113	114	115	66	67	67	68	69	70	71
5	90th	104	105	106	108	110	112	112	65	65	66	67	68	69	69
	95th	108	109	110	112	114	115	116	69	70	70	71	72	73	74
6	90th	105	106	108	110	111	113	114	67	68	69	70	70	71	72
	95th	109	110	112	114	115	117	117	72	72	73	74	75	76	76
7	90th	106	107	109	111	113	114	115	69	70	71	72	72	73	74
	95th	110	111	113	115	116	118	119	74	74	75	76	77	78	78
8	90th	107	108	110	112	114	115	116	71	71	72	73	74	75	75
	95th	111	112	114	116	118	119	120	75	76	76	77	78	79	80
9	90th	109	110	112	113	115	117	117	72	73	73	74	75	76	77
	95th	113	114	116	117	119	121	121	76	77	78	79	80	80	81
10	90th	110	112	113	115	117	118	119	73	74	74	75	76	77	78
	95th	114	115	117	119	121	122	123	77	78	79	80	80	81	82
11	90th	112	113	115	117	119	120	121	74	74	75	76	77	78	78
	95th	116	117	119	121	123	124	125	78	79	79	80	81	82	83
12	90th	115	116	117	119	121	123	123	75	75	76	77	78	78	79
	95th	119	120	121	123	125	126	127	79	79	80	81	82	83	83
13	90th	117	118	120	122	124	125	126	75	76	76	77	78	79	80
	95th	121	122	124	126	128	129	130	79	80	81	82	83	83	84
14	90th	120	121	123	125	126	128	128	76	76	77	78	79	80	80
	95th	124	125	127	128	130	132	132	80	81	81	82	83	84	85
15	90th	123	124	125	127	129	131	131	77	77	78	79	80	81	81
	95th	127	128	129	131	133	134	135	81	82	83	83	84	85	86
16	90th	125	126	128	130	132	133	134	79	79	80	81	82	82	83
	95th	129	130	132	134	136	137	138	83	83	84	85	86	87	87
17	90th	128	129	131	133	134	136	136	81	81	82	83	84	85	85
	95th	132	133	135	136	138	140	140	85	85	86	87	88	89	89

Source: Reprinted from National High Blood Pressure Education Program Working Group on Hypertension Control in Children and Adolescents. https://www.nhlbi.nih.gov/files/docs/resources/heart/hbp_ped.pdf

[a]Blood pressure percentile determined by a single measurement.

COMMON VARIATIONS 33-1: COMMON SKIN VARIATIONS IN CHILDREN

Port-wine stain

This birthmark consisting of capillaries is dark red or bluish and darkens with exertion or temperature exposure. It appears as a large, irregular, macular patch on the scalp or face. Unlike a haemangioma, this birthmark does not fade with time.

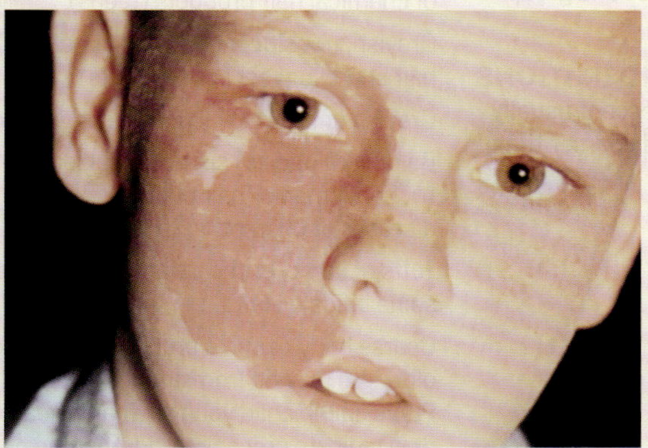

Café-au-lait spot

This birthmark is a light brown, round or oval patch. If there are more than six separate, large (>1.5 cm) patches, an inherited neurocutaneous disease may be present.

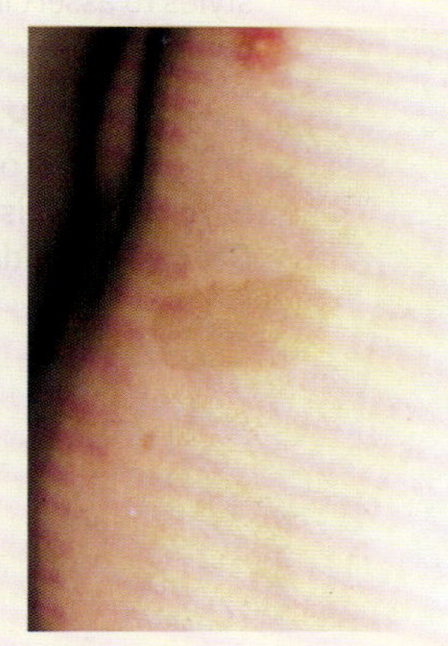

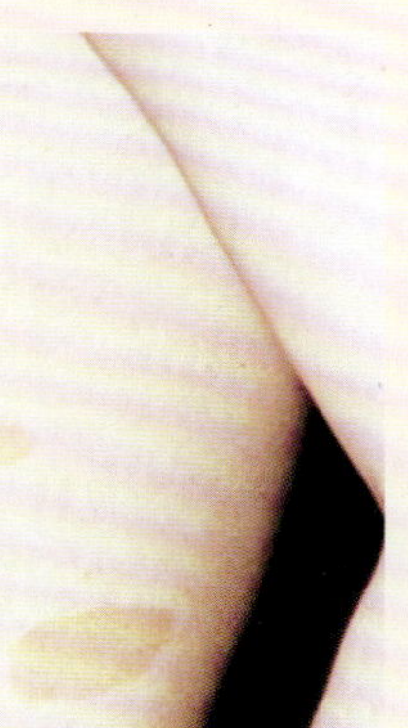

Haemangioma

This skin variation is caused by an increased amount of blood vessels in the dermis.

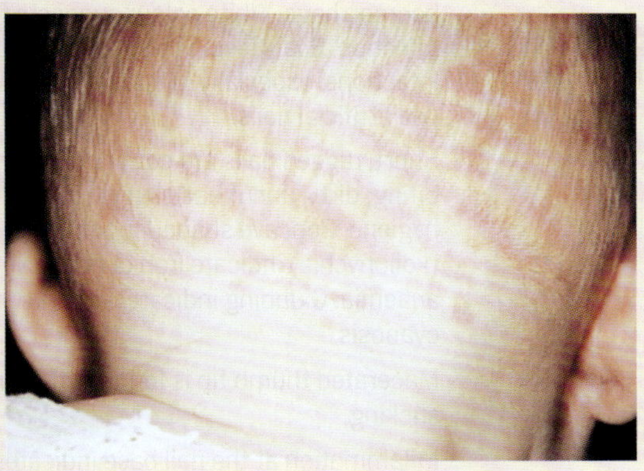

PHYSICAL ASSESSMENT (continued)

ASSESSMENT PROCEDURE	NORMAL FINDINGS	ABNORMAL FINDINGS
Skin, hair and nails (continued)		
Palpate for texture, temperature, moisture, turgor and oedema.	Skin should be soft, warm, slightly moist with good turgor and without oedema. Skin should be soft and elastic, with no tenting when tested for turgor.	Excessive dryness suggests poor nutrition, excessive bathing or an endocrine disorder. Flaking or scaling suggests eczema or fungal infections. Poor skin turgor indicates dehydration or malnutrition; oedema suggests renal or cardiac disorders; periorbital oedema may indicate pathology but may also be due to recent crying, sleeping or allergies. A Russell sign (abrasion or scarring on joints of index and middle fingers) suggests self-induced vomiting. Bite marks may indicate child abuse or self-abusive behaviour (psychiatric disorders, mental retardation).

Continued on following page

PHYSICAL ASSESSMENT (continued)

ASSESSMENT PROCEDURE	NORMAL FINDINGS	ABNORMAL FINDINGS
Inspect and palpate hair. Observe for distribution, characteristics, infestation and presence of any unusual hair on body.	Hair is normally lustrous, silky, strong and elastic. Fine, downy hair covers the body. Adolescents may display a variety of hair styles to assert independence and group conformity. **CULTURAL CONSIDERATIONS** **Children of African descent usually have hair that is curlier and coarser than Caucasian children.**	Dirty, matted hair may indicate neglect. Dull, dry, brittle hair may indicate poor nutrition, hypothyroidism or excessive use of chemical hair products (teens). Greyish, translucent flakes that adhere to hair shaft suggest lice (ova, nits). Greyish or brown oval bodies suggest ticks. Balding (alopecia) suggests neglect, trichotillomania (hair pulling), skin diseases or chemotherapy. Tufts of hair over the spine may indicate spina bifida occulta. Coarse body hair in a prepubertal child or older girl may be from endocrine disorder. Pubic hair in child younger than 8 years may indicate precocious adrenarche or precocious puberty.
Inspect and palpate nails. Note colour, texture, shape and condition of nails.	Nails should be clean and groomed. Adolescents may colour or pierce nails. Pink undertones should be seen. **CULTURAL CONSIDERATIONS** **Dark-skinned children have deeper nail pigment.**	Blue nailbeds indicate cyanosis. Yellow nailbeds suggest jaundice. Blue-black nailbeds are found with nailbed haemorrhage. White colour suggests fungal infection. Scaly lesions also indicate fungal infections, especially in adolescents who use artificial nails. Short, ragged nails are common with nail biting; dirty, uncut nails suggest poor hygiene. Concave shape, 'spoon nails' (koilonychia) indicate iron deficiency anaemia. Clubbing indicates chronic cyanosis. Macerated thumb tip is found with thumb sucking. Inflammation at the nail base indicates paronychia.
Head, neck and cervical lymph nodes		
INSPECTION AND PALPATION		
Inspect and palpate the head. Note shape and symmetry.	Head is normocephalic and symmetrical.	Very large head is hydrocephalus. Oddly shaped head suggests premature closure of sutures (possibly genetic). Third fontanelle located between the anterior and posterior fontanelle indicates Down syndrome. Craniotabes—from osteoporosis of the outer skull bone. Palpating too firmly with the thumb or forefinger over the temporoparietal area will leave an indentation of the bone.
Test head control, head posture and range of motion.	Full range of motion—up, down and sideways—is normal.	Hyperextension suggests opisthotonos or significant meningeal irritation. Limited range of motion suggests torticollis (wryneck).

PHYSICAL ASSESSMENT (continued)

ASSESSMENT PROCEDURE	NORMAL FINDINGS	ABNORMAL FINDINGS
Head, neck and cervical lymph nodes (continued)		
Inspect and palpate the face. Note appearance, symmetry and movement (have child make faces). Palpate the parotid glands for swelling.	Face is normally proportionate and symmetrical. Movements are equal bilaterally. Parotid glands are normal size. **CLINICAL TIP** **Some adolescents may appear to have unusual skin tones or markings from applying makeup as a form of self-expression.**	Unusual proportions (short palpebral fissures, thin lips, and wide and flat philtrum, which is the groove above the upper lip) may be hereditary, or they may indicate specific syndromes, such as Down syndrome (Fig. 33-16) and fetal alcohol syndrome. Other findings may indicate the following: • Unequal movement—facial nerve paralysis • Enlarged parotid gland—mumps or bulimia • Abnormal facial expressions—chromosomal anomaly • Crease across nose, shiners (dark circles under eyes) and mouth agape—allergies (allergic facial expressions).
Inspect and palpate the neck. Palpate the thyroid gland and the trachea. Also inspect and palpate the cervical lymph nodes for swelling, mobility, temperature and tenderness (Fig. 33-17). 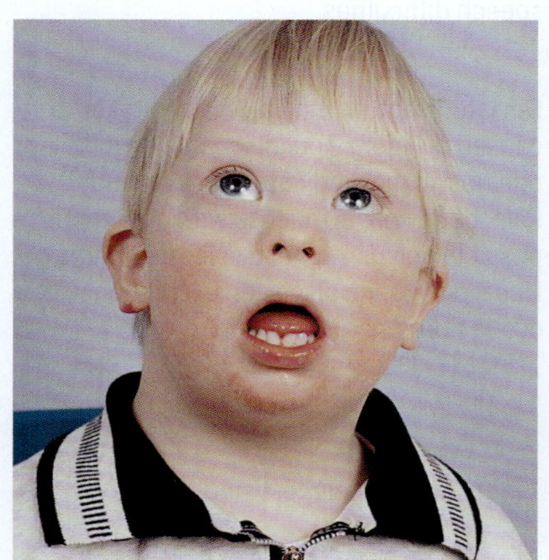 **FIGURE 33-16** Down syndrome results from a genetic abnormality. (© B. Proud.)	The isthmus is the only portion of the thyroid that should be palpable. The trachea is midline. Lymph nodes are usually non-palpable in adolescents. 'Shotty' lymph nodes (small, non-tender, mobile) are commonly palpated in children between the ages of 3 and 12 years. 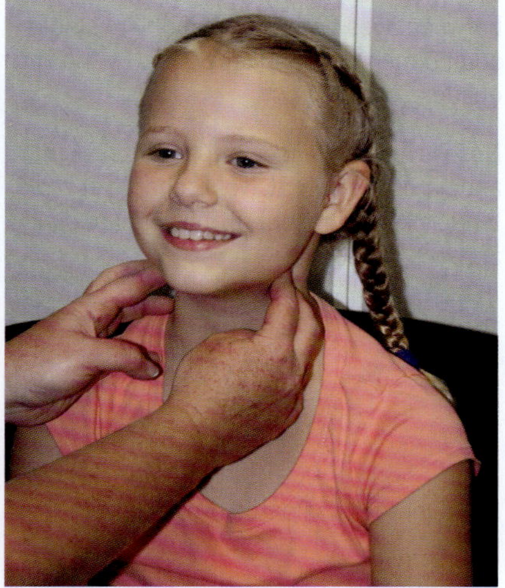 **FIGURE 33-17** Palpating the cervical lymph nodes.	Implications of some abnormal findings include the following: • Short, webbed neck—anomalies or syndromes • Distended neck veins—difficulty breathing • Enlarged thyroid or palpable masses—pathological processes • Shift in tracheal position from midline—serious lung problem (e.g. foreign body or tumour) • Enlarged firm lymph nodes—Hodgkin disease or HIV infection • Enlarged, warm and tender lymph nodes—lymphadenitis or infection in the head and neck area that is drained by the affected node.
Mouth, throat and sinuses		
INSPECTION		
Note the condition of the lips, palates, tongue and buccal mucosa (Fig. 33-18).	Lips, tongue and buccal mucosa appear pink and moist. No lesions are present.	Dry lips may indicate mouth breathing or dehydration. Stomatitis suggests infection or immunodeficiency. Koplik's spots (tiny white spots on red bases) on the buccal mucosa may be a prodromal sign of measles. Cleft lip or palate is a congenital abnormality (Fig. 33-19).

Continued on following page

PHYSICAL ASSESSMENT (continued)

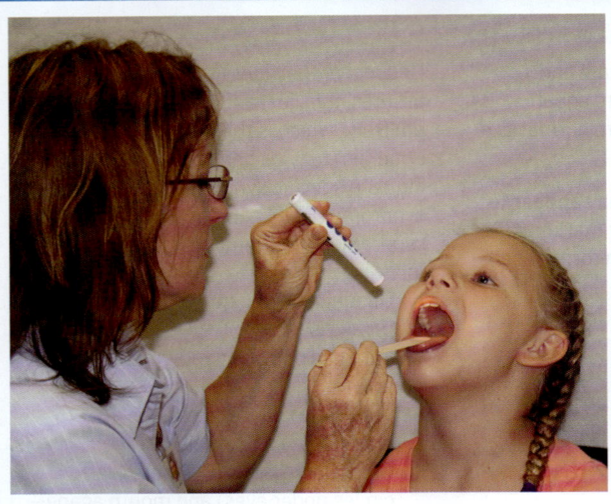

FIGURE 33-18 Inspecting the mouth.

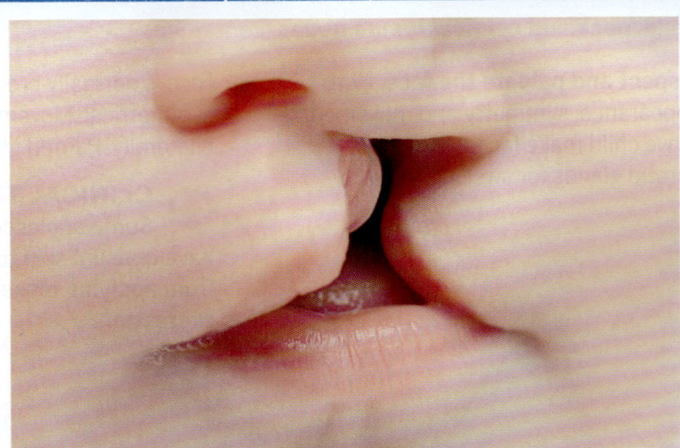

FIGURE 33-19 Cleft lip. (Shutterstock.com/malost.)

ASSESSMENT PROCEDURE	NORMAL FINDINGS	ABNORMAL FINDINGS
Observe the condition of the teeth and gums.	Deciduous teeth begin to develop between 4 and 6 months; all 20 erupt by 36 months; teeth begin to fall out around 6 years, when permanent tooth eruption begins and progresses until all 32 have erupted.	Dental caries may herald 'bottle caries syndrome'. Enamel erosion may indicate bulimia.
Note the condition of the throat and tonsils. Also observe the insertion and ending point of the frenulum.	Tonsils are easily seen by age 6 when they increase to adult dimensions. They reach maximum size (about twice adult size) between ages 10 and 12. Atrophy to stable adult dimensions usually occurs by the end of adolescence.	Tonsillar or pharyngeal inflammation suggests infection. Extension of the frenulum to the tip of tongue may interfere with extension of the tongue, which causes speech difficulties.
Inspect nose and sinuses. To inspect the nose and sinuses, avoid using the nasal speculum in young children. Instead, push up the tip of the nose and shine the light into each nostril. Observe the structure and patency of the nares, discharge, tenderness and any colour or swelling of the turbinates.	Nose is midline in face, septum is straight and nares are patent. No discharge or tenderness is present. Turbinates are pink and free of oedema.	Deviated septum may be congenital or caused by injury. Foul discharge from one nostril may indicate a foreign body. Pale, boggy nasal mucosa with or without possible polyps suggests allergic rhinitis. Nasal polyps are also seen in children with cystic fibrosis.
PALPATION		
Palpate the sinuses in older children if sinusitis is suspected. The sinuses of young children are not palpable.	No tenderness palpated over sinuses.	Tender sinuses suggest sinusitis.
Eyes		
INSPECTION		
Inspect the external eye. Note the position, slant and epicanthal folds of the external eye.	Inner canthus distance approximately 2.5 cm, horizontal slant, no epicanthal folds. Outer canthus aligns with tips of the pinnas (Fig. 33-20).	Wide-set position (hypertelorism), upward slant, and thick epicanthal folds suggest Down syndrome. 'Sun-setting' appearance (upper lid covers part of the iris) suggests hydrocephalus.

PHYSICAL ASSESSMENT (continued)

ASSESSMENT PROCEDURE	NORMAL FINDINGS	ABNORMAL FINDINGS
Eyes (continued)		
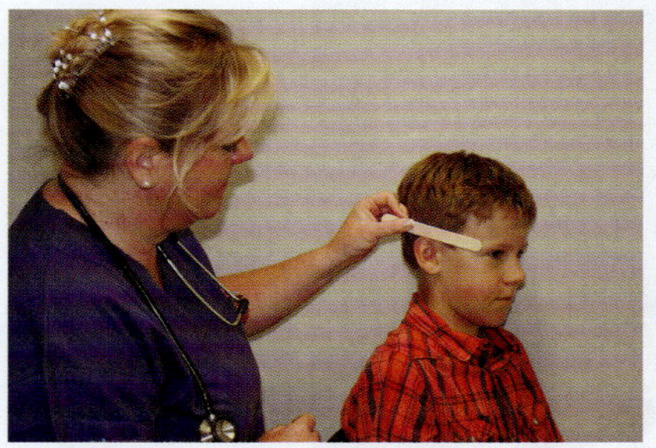 **FIGURE 33-20** Outer canthus is in alignment with the tip of the pinna.	**CULTURAL CONSIDERATIONS** Epicanthal folds (excess of skin extending from roof of nose that partially or completely covers the inner canthus) are normal findings in Asian children, whose eyes also slant upwards.	
Observe eyelid placement, swelling, discharge and lesions.	No swelling, discharge or lesions of eyelids.	Eyelid inflammation may result from blepharitis, hordeolum or dacryocystitis (inflammation or blockage of lacrimal sac or duct). Ptosis (drooping eyelids) suggests oculomotor nerve palsy, congenital syndrome or a familial trait. A painful, oedematous, erythematous area on eyelid may be a hordeolum (stye). A nodular, non-tender lesion on the eyelid may be a chalazion (cyst). Swelling, erythema or purulent discharge may indicate infection or blocked tear ducts. Sunken area around eyelids may indicate dehydration. Periorbital oedema suggests fluid retention.
Inspect the sclera and conjunctiva for colour, discharge, lesions, redness and lacerations.	Sclera and conjunctiva are clear and free of discharge, lesions, redness or lacerations.	Yellow sclera suggests jaundice, blue sclera may indicate osteogenesis imperfecta ('brittle bone disease') and redness may indicate conjunctivitis.
Observe the iris and the pupils.	Pupils are equal, round and reactive to light and accommodation (PERRLA).	Brushfield's spots may indicate Down syndrome. Sluggish pupils indicate a neurological problem. Miosis (constriction) indicates iritis or narcotic use or abuse. Mydriasis (pupillary dilation) indicates emotional factors (fear), trauma or certain drug use.
Finally inspect the eyebrows and eyelashes.	Eyebrows should be symmetrical in shape and movement. They should not meet midline. Eyelashes should be evenly distributed and curled outwards.	Sparseness of eyebrows or lashes could indicate skin disease or deliberate pulling out of hairs (usually due to anxiety or habit). Corneal abrasions are common during childhood and may not be easily visible to the naked eye.
Perform visual acuity tests. Use the following diagnostic tools to perform visual acuity testing: The Sheridan-Gardiner vision screening tool is considered the gold standard for use in children aged 4 years and over. The LEA symbols tool is appropriate for vision surveillance in younger children.	Normal visual acuity measured in metres is as follows: 1 year—6/60 2 years—6/20 5 years—6/9 6 years—6/6 Children should be able to differentiate colours by age 5.	Children with a one-line difference between eyes should be referred. Children should also be referred for abnormal visual acuity or inability to distinguish colours. Visual impairment can indicate congenital defects (cataracts), malignant tumours, chronic disease (diabetes), drugs, trauma, enzyme deficiencies or refractive errors (myopia, hyperopia, astigmatism).

Continued on following page

PHYSICAL ASSESSMENT (continued)

ASSESSMENT PROCEDURE	NORMAL FINDINGS	ABNORMAL FINDINGS
CLINICAL TIP Fatigue, anxiety, hunger and distractions interfere with vision testing. Testing should precede procedures that create discomfort. **Perform extraocular muscle tests.** **CLINICAL TIP** Use a toy, a puppet or the parent to focus the child's eyes. Older children, including adolescents, focus better if they are given something to focus on instead of being told to 'look straight ahead'.	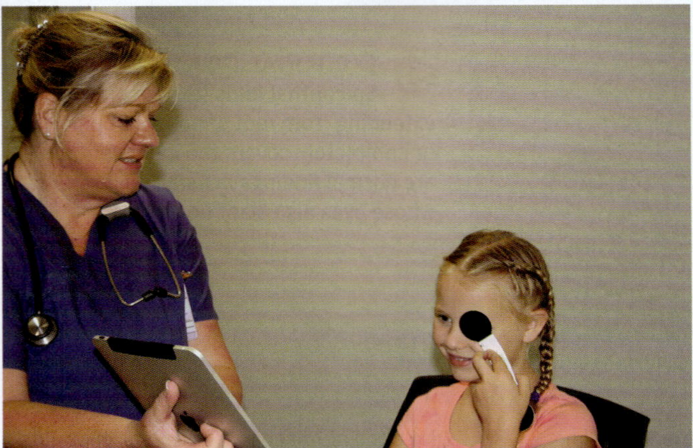 **FIGURE 33-21** Performing the cover test.	
Cover test: Have the child cover one eye and look at an interesting object (Fig. 33-21). Observe the uncovered eye for any movement. When the child is focused on the object, remove the cover and observe that eye for movement.	In the cover test, the eyes remain focused.	Eye movement is present during the cover test; this may indicate strabismus.
Hirschberg test: Shine light directly at the cornea while the child looks straight ahead.	In the Hirschberg test, the light reflects symmetrically in the centre of both pupils.	Unequal alignment of light on the pupils in the Hirschberg test signals strabismus.
Ears		
Inspect external ears. Note placement, discharge or lesions of the ears.	Top of pinna should cross the eye-occiput line and be within a 10-degree angle of a perpendicular line drawn from the eye-occiput line to the lobe. No unusual structure or markings should appear on the pinna.	Low-set ears with an alignment greater than a 10-degree angle suggest mental retardation or congenital syndromes. Abnormal shape may suggest renal disease process, which may be hereditary. Preauricular skin tags or sinuses suggest other anomalies of ears or the renal system.
Inspect internal ear. The internal ear examination requires using an otoscope and, for toddlers, restraint by (1) having a parent hold the seated child in the lap while holding the child's hands with one hand and the child's head sideways against chest or (2) laying the child supine, with the parent holding the child's arms up over head. Then the nurse can gently but firmly hold the child's head to the side. Regardless of technique used, the nurse should always hold the otoscope in a manner that allows for rapid removal if the child moves. Because an infant's external canal is short and straight, pull the pinna down and back. Because an older child's canal shortens and becomes less straight, like the adult's, gently pull the pinna up and back.	No excessive cerumen, discharge, lesions, excoriations or foreign body are in external canal. Tympanic membrane is pearly grey to light pink with normal landmarks. Tympanic membranes redden bilaterally when child is crying or febrile.	Presence of foreign bodies or cerumen impaction. Purulent discharge may indicate otitis externa or presence of foreign body. Purulent, serous discharge suggests otitis media. Bloody discharge suggests trauma, and clear discharge may indicate cerebrospinal fluid leak. Perforated tympanic membrane may also be noted.

PHYSICAL ASSESSMENT (continued)

ASSESSMENT PROCEDURE	NORMAL FINDINGS	ABNORMAL FINDINGS
Eyes (continued)		
Test hearing acuity. Test acuity initially by whispering questions from a distance of approximately 2.5 m. If hearing deficit is suspected, complete audiometric testing should be performed. Audiometry measures the threshold of hearing for frequencies and loudness. In addition, all children should have audiometric testing performed before entering school.	Answers whispered questions. Audiometry results are within normal ranges.	Failure to respond to whispered questions may indicate hearing deficit. Audiometry results outside normal range suggest hearing deficit.
Thorax and lungs		
INSPECTION		
Inspect the shape of the thorax.	By age 5 to 6 years, the thoracic diameter reaches the adult 1:2 or 5:7 ratio (anteroposterior to transverse).	Abnormal shapes of the thorax include pectus excavatum and pectus carinatum.
Children under 7 years old are abdominal breathers.	Respirations should be unlaboured and regular in all ages. Respirations should be: age 2 years to 10 years: 20–28 breaths/minute; 10 years to 18 years: 12–20 breaths/minute.	Retractions (suprasternal, sternal, substernal, intercostal) and grunting suggest increased inspiratory effort, which may be due to asthma, atelectasis, pneumonia or airway obstruction. Periods of apnoea that last longer than 20 seconds and are accompanied by bradycardia may be a sign of a cardiovascular or central nervous system (CNS) disease.
PERCUSSION AND AUSCULTATION		
Percuss and auscultate the lungs. During percussion of the lungs, note tone elicited.	Hyper-resonance is the normal tone elicited in young children because of thinness of the chest wall. This diminishes as the child ages and the chest wall develops.	A dull tone may indicate a mass, fluid or consolidation.
Auscultate for breath sounds and adventitious sounds. If a toddler's lung sounds seem noisy, auscultate the upper nostrils. Toddlers with an upper respiratory infection may transmit noisy breathing from the upper nostrils to the upper lobes of the lungs. Encourage deep breathing in children; try one of the following techniques: blow out light on otoscope (Fig. 33-22), blow cotton ball in air, blow pinwheel, 'race' paper off table.	Breath sounds may seem louder and harsher in young children because of their thin chest wall. No adventitious sounds should be heard, although transmitted upper airway sounds may be heard on auscultation of thorax. 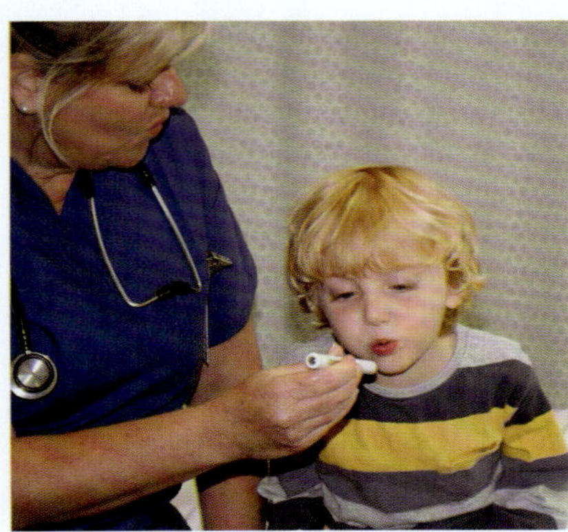 **FIGURE 33-22** To encourage deep breathing, ask a child to blow out the light on an otoscope or a penlight.	Diminished breath sounds suggest respiratory disorders such as pneumonia or atelectasis. Stridor (inspiratory wheeze) is a high-pitched, piercing sound that indicates a narrowing of the upper tracheobronchial tree. Expiratory wheezes indicate narrowing in the lower tracheobronchial tree. Rhonchi and rales (crackles) may indicate a number of respiratory diseases such as pneumonia, bronchitis or bronchiolitis.

Continued on following page

PHYSICAL ASSESSMENT (continued)

ASSESSMENT PROCEDURE	NORMAL FINDINGS	ABNORMAL FINDINGS
Breasts		
Inspect and palpate breasts. Note shape, symmetry, colour, tenderness, discharge, lesions and masses.	Breasts are flat and symmetrical in prepubertal children. Obese children may appear to have breast tissue.	Redness, oedema and tenderness indicate mastitis. Enlargement in adolescent boys suggests gynaecomastia. Masses in the adolescent female breast usually indicate cysts or trauma.
Assess stage of breast and sexual development of girls. Teach breast self-exam to adolescents (see Self-assessment 21-1).	See Tanner sexual maturity rating in Table 33-1.	Breast development before age 8 may indicate precocious puberty or thelarche. Lack of breast development after age 13 may indicate delayed puberty or a pathological process.
Heart		
INSPECTION AND PALPATION		
Inspect and palpate the praecordium. Note lifts and heaves. Palpate apical impulse (Fig. 33-23).	The apical pulse is at the fourth intercostal space until the age of 7 years, when it drops to the fifth. It is to the left of the midclavicular line (MCL) until age 4, at the MCL between ages 4 and 6, and to the right at age 7.	A systolic heave may indicate right ventricular enlargement. Apical impulse that is not in proper location for age may indicate cardiomyopathy, pneumothorax or diaphragmatic hernia.

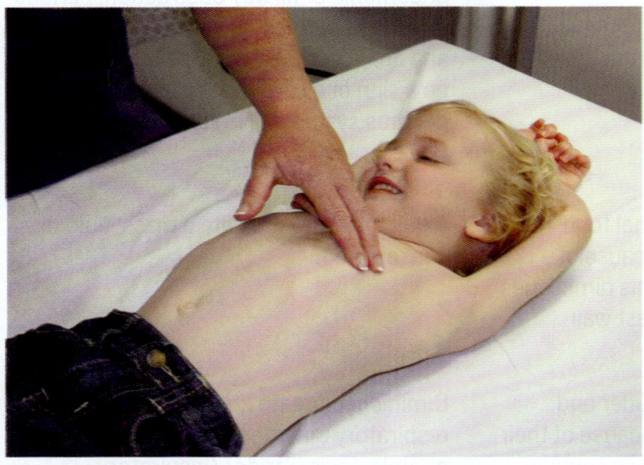

FIGURE 33-23 To palpate a preschooler's apical pulse, place your hand at the fourth intercostal space to the left of the midclavicular line.

ASSESSMENT PROCEDURE	NORMAL FINDINGS	ABNORMAL FINDINGS
AUSCULTATION		
Auscultate heart sounds. Listen to the heart. Note rate and rhythm of apical impulse, S_1, S_2, extra heart sounds and murmurs. **CLINICAL TIP** **Keep in mind that sinus arrhythmia is normal in young children. Heart sounds are louder, higher pitched and of shorter duration in children. A split S_2 at the apex occurs normally in some children, and S_3 is a normal heart sound in some children. A venous hum also may be normally heard in children.**	Normal heart rates are cited in the 'Vital Signs' section above. Innocent murmurs, which are common throughout childhood, are classified as systolic; short duration; no transmission to other areas; grade III or less; loudest in pulmonic area (base of heart); low-pitched, musical or groaning quality that varies in intensity in relation to position, respiration, activity, fever and anaemia. No other associated signs of heart disease.	Murmurs that do not fit the criteria for innocent murmurs may indicate a disease or disorder. Extra heart sounds and variations in pulse rate and rhythm also suggest pathological processes.

PHYSICAL ASSESSMENT (continued)

ASSESSMENT PROCEDURE	NORMAL FINDINGS	ABNORMAL FINDINGS
Abdomen		
INSPECTION		
Inspect the shape of the abdomen.	In children up to age 4 years, the abdomen is prominent in standing and supine positions. After age 4, the abdomen appears slightly prominent when standing, but flat when supine until puberty.	A scaphoid (boat-shaped, i.e. sunken with prominent rib cage) abdomen may result from malnutrition or dehydration.
Inspect umbilicus. Note colour, discharge, evident herniation of the umbilicus.	Umbilicus is pink, no discharge, odour, redness or herniation.	Inflammation, discharge and redness of umbilicus suggest infection. Diastasis recti (separation of the abdominal muscles) is seen as midline protrusion from the xiphoid to the umbilicus or pubis symphysis. This condition is secondary to immature musculature of abdominal muscles and usually has little significance. As the muscles strengthen, the separation resolves on its own. A bulge at the umbilicus suggests an umbilical hernia, which may be seen in newborns; many disappear by the age of 1 year, and most by age 4 or 5 years. **CULTURAL CONSIDERATIONS** **Compared to children of non-African descent, umbilical hernias are seen more frequently in children of African descent.**
AUSCULTATION		
Auscultate bowel sounds. Follow auscultation guidelines for adult patients provided in Chapter 24.	Normal bowel sounds occur every 10 to 30 seconds. They sound like clicks, gurgles or growls.	Marked peristaltic waves almost always indicate a pathological process such as pyloric stenosis.
PALPATION		
Palpate for masses and tenderness. Palpate abdomen for softness or hardness. **CLINICAL TIP** **To decrease ticklishness, have the child help by placing his or her hand under yours, using age-appropriate distraction techniques, and maintaining conversation focused on something other than the examination (Fig. 33-24).**	Abdomen is soft to palpation and without masses or tenderness.	A rigid abdomen is almost always an emergent problem. Masses or tenderness warrants further investigation.

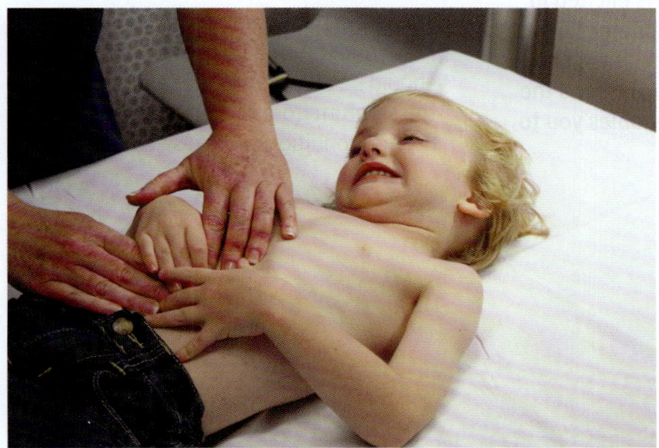

FIGURE 33-24 Let a child help palpate his or her abdomen to decrease ticklishness.

Continued on following page

PHYSICAL ASSESSMENT (continued)

ASSESSMENT PROCEDURE	NORMAL FINDINGS	ABNORMAL FINDINGS
Palpate liver. Palpate the liver the same as you would for adults (see Chap. 24).	Liver is usually palpable 1 to 2 cm below the right costal margin in young children.	An enlarged liver with a firm edge that is palpated more than 2 cm below the right costal margin usually indicates a pathological process.
Palpate spleen. Palpate the spleen the same as you would for adults (see Chap. 24).	Spleen tip may be palpable during inspiration.	Enlarged spleen is usually indicative of a pathological process.
Palpate kidneys. Palpate the kidneys the same as you would for adults (see Chap. 24).	The tip of the right kidney may be palpable during inspiration.	Enlarged kidneys are usually indicative of a pathological process.
Palpate bladder. Palpate the bladder the same as you would for adults (see Chap. 24).	Bladder may be slightly palpable in small children.	An enlarged bladder is usually due to urinary retention but may be due to a mass.
Male genitalia		
Inspect penis and urinary meatus. Inspect the genitalia observing size for age and any lesions. **CLINICAL TIP** **Use distraction or teaching (such as testicular self-examination) when examining the genitalia in older children and adolescents to decrease embarrassment. A chaperone is always recommended.**	Penis is normal size for age and no lesions are seen. The foreskin is retractable in uncircumcised child. Urinary meatus is at tip of glans penis and has no discharge or redness. Penis may appear small in obese boys because of overlapping skin folds.	An unretractable foreskin in a child older than 3 months suggests phimosis. Paraphimosis is indicated when the foreskin is tightened around the glans penis in a retracted position. Hypospadias, urinary meatus on ventral surface of glans, and epispadias, urinary meatus on dorsal surface of glans, are congenital disorders (see Abnormal findings 26-1). Discharge, redness or lacerations may indicate abuse in young children but may occur from infections or foreign body. Discharge in adolescents may be due to sexually transmitted infection, infection or irritation.
Inspect and palpate scrotum and testes. To rule out cryptorchidism, it is important to palpate for testes in the scrotum in infants and young boys. **CLINICAL TIP** **When palpating the testicles in the infant and young boy, you must keep the cremasteric reflex in mind. This reflex pulls the testicles up into the inguinal canal and abdomen and is elicited in response to touch, cold or emotional factors. Have young boys sit with knees flexed and abducted. This lessens the cremasteric reflex and enables you to examine the testicles.**	Scrotum is free of lesions. Testes are palpable in scrotum, with the left testicle usually lower than the right. Testes are equal in size, smooth, mobile and free of masses. If a testicle is missing from the scrotal sac but the scrotal sac appears well developed, suspect physiological cryptorchidism. The testis has originally descended into the scrotum but has moved back up into the inguinal canal because of the cremasteric reflex and the small size of the testis. You should be able to milk the testis down into the scrotum from the inguinal canal. This normal condition subsides at puberty.	Absent testicles and atrophic scrotum suggest true cryptorchidism (undescended testicles; see Chap. 26). This suggests that the testicles never descended. This condition occurs more frequently in preterm than term infants because testes descend at 8 months of gestation. It can lead to testicular atrophy and infertility and increases the risk of testicular cancer. Hydroceles are common in infants. They are fluid-filled masses that can be transilluminated (see Abnormal findings 26-2). They usually resolve spontaneously. A scrotal hernia is usually caused by an indirect inguinal hernia that has descended into the scrotum. It can usually be pushed back into the inguinal canal. This mass will not transilluminate. A painless nodule on the testis may indicate testicular cancer, which appears most frequently in males age 15 to 34 years; therefore, testicular self-examination should be taught to all boys age 14 years and older (see Self-assessment 26-1).

PHYSICAL ASSESSMENT (continued)

ASSESSMENT PROCEDURE	NORMAL FINDINGS	ABNORMAL FINDINGS
Male genitalia (continued)		
Inspect and palpate inguinal area for hernias. Observe for any bulge in the inguinal area. Ask the child to bear down or try to lift something heavy to elicit a possible hernia. Using your little finger, palpate up the inguinal canal to the external inguinal ring if a hernia is suspected.	No inguinal hernias are present.	A bulge in the inguinal area or palpation of a mass in the inguinal canal suggests an inguinal hernia. Indirect inguinal hernias occur most frequently in children (see Abnormal findings 26-3).
Assess sexual development. Note pubic hair pattern, and size and development of penis and scrotum.	See Tanner sexual maturity ratings in Table 33-2.	Pubic hair growth, enlargement of the penis to adolescent or adult size, and enlarged testes in a boy younger than age 8 years suggest precocious puberty.
Female genitalia		
Inspect external genitalia. Note labia majora, labia minora, vaginal orifice, urinary meatus and clitoris. **CLINICAL TIP** **Have female children assist with genitalia examination by using their hands to spread the labia. This helps to decrease any stress and embarrassment. A chaperone is always recommended.**	Labia majora and minora are pink and moist. Young girls have flattened majora, thin minora, small clitoris and thin hymen. Starting at school age, the labia become fuller and the hymen thickens. This progresses until puberty when the genitalia develop adult characteristics. No discharge from vagina or meatus; no redness or oedema present normally.	Partial or complete labia minora adhesions are sometimes seen in girls younger than age 4 years. Referral is necessary to disintegrate the thin, membranous adhesion. An imperforate hymen (no central orifice) is sometimes seen and is not significant unless it persists until puberty and causes problems with menstruation. Discharge from vagina or urinary meatus, redness, oedema or lacerations may suggest abuse in the young child. However, infections or a foreign body in the vagina may cause these symptoms. Discharge in adolescents suggests sexually transmitted infection, infection or irritation.
Inspect internal genitalia. An internal genitalia examination is not routinely performed in the child, although it may be called for if infection, bleeding, a foreign body, disease or sexual abuse is suspected. A paediatric specialist should perform the examination. An internal genital examination consisting of both the speculum and bimanual examinations is recommended for all sexually active adolescents and virgins starting at age 18 years. In addition, an internal examination is indicated in the adolescent who has non-menstrual bleeding or discharge. The procedure is the same as for the adult. Time and care must be taken for adequate teaching and reassurance.	See Chapter 25 for normal findings.	See Chapter 25 for abnormal findings.

Continued on following page

PHYSICAL ASSESSMENT (continued)

ASSESSMENT PROCEDURE	NORMAL FINDINGS	ABNORMAL FINDINGS
Assess sexual development. Note pubic hair pattern.	See Tanner sexual maturity ratings in Table 33-3 for normal findings.	Growth of pubic hair in young girls (age under 8 years) suggests precocious puberty. Unusual pubic hair distribution in pubertal girls may indicate a disorder. For example, a male pattern of hair growth may suggest polycystic ovary disease.
Anus and rectum		
INSPECTION AND PALPATION		
Inspect the anus. The anus should be inspected in children and adolescents. Perform quickly at the end of the genitalia examination to limit embarrassment in the older child and adolescent. Spread the buttocks with gloved hands, and note patency of anal opening, presence of any lesions and fissures, and condition and colour of perianal skin. **CLINICAL TIP** **A chaperone is always recommended.**	The anal opening should be visible, moist and hairless. No haemorrhoids or lesions. Perianal skin should be smooth and free of lesions. A mild nappy rash (red papules) may be seen in infants. Perianal skin tags may be noted.	Haemorrhoids are unusual in children and could be due to chronic constipation, but may be caused by sexual abuse or abdominal pressure from lesion. Bleeding and pain often indicate tears or fissures in the anus, which often cause constipation because of pain of passing stool. Pustules may indicate secondary infection of nappy rash. A dark ring around the anus may indicate heavy metal poisoning. Lacerations, purulent discharge or extreme apprehension during examination may indicate physical or sexual abuse. Nappy rashes with more than mild red or pink papules suggest problems such as seborrhoea, nappy dermatitis and monilial infection.
Palpate rectum. This internal examination is not routinely performed in children or adolescents. However, it should be performed if symptoms suggest a problem. The child should be in a supine position with the legs flexed. Provide reassurance throughout the examination. If the child is old enough, ask him or her to bear down. This helps to relax the sphincter. Slowly insert a gloved, lubricated finger (the little finger may be used for comfort, but the index finger is more sensitive) into the anal opening, aiming the finger towards the umbilicus.	Prostate gland is non-palpable in young boys. Bimanual rectoabdominal exam in girls may reveal small midline mass (cervix).	If other masses are palpated, they are considered abnormal; no other structures are palpable until adolescence.

PHYSICAL ASSESSMENT (continued)

ASSESSMENT PROCEDURE	NORMAL FINDINGS	ABNORMAL FINDINGS
Musculoskeletal		
INSPECTION		
Assess feet and legs. Note symmetry, shape, movement and positioning of the feet and legs. Perform neurovascular assessment. 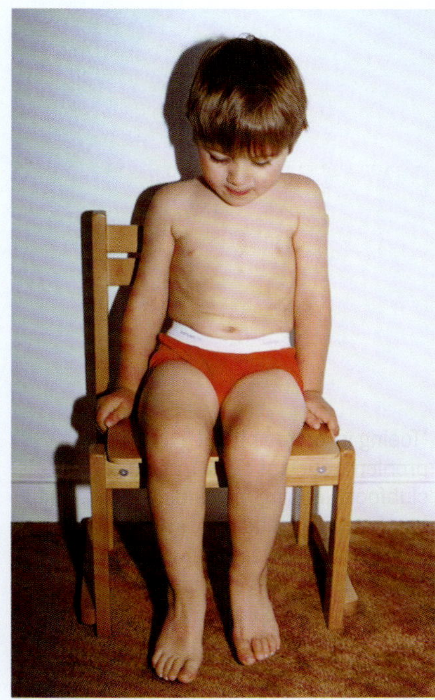 **FIGURE 33-25** Normally positioned feet and legs.	Feet and legs are symmetrical in size, shape, movement and positioning (Fig. 33-25). Extremities should be warm and mobile with adequate capillary refill. All pulses (radial, brachial, femoral, popliteal, pedal) should be strong and equal bilaterally. A common finding in children (up to 2 or 3 years old) is metatarsus adductus deformity. This is an inward positioning of the forefoot with the heel in normal straight position, and it resolves spontaneously. Tibial torsion, also common in infants and toddlers, consists of twisting of the tibia inwards or outwards on its long axis, is usually caused by intrauterine positioning and typically corrects itself by the time the child is 2 years old. 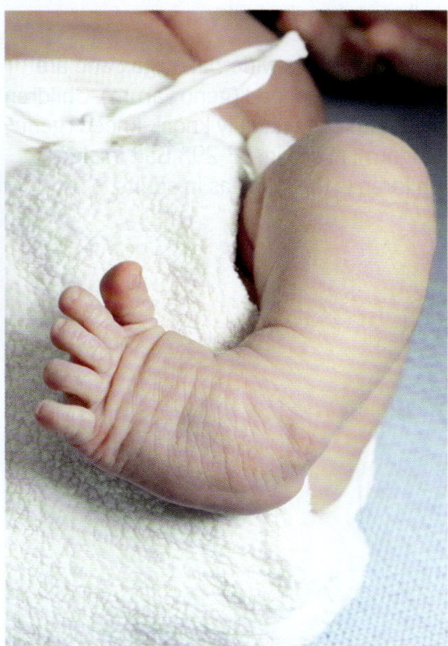 **FIGURE 33-26** Talipes equinovarus, also called clubfoot. (Dreamstime.com/AGLphotoproductions.)	Short, broad extremities, hyperextensible joints and palmar simian crease may indicate Down syndrome. Polydactyly (extra digits) and syndactyly (webbing) are sometimes found in children with mental retardation. Neurovascular deficit in children is usually secondary to trauma (e.g. fracture). Fixed-position (true) deformities do not return to normal position with manipulation. Metatarsus varus is inversion (a turning inwards that elevates the medial margin) and adduction of the forefoot. Talipes varus is adduction of the forefoot and inversion of the entire foot. Talipes equinovarus (clubfoot) is indicated if the foot is fixed in the following position: adduction of forefoot, inversion of entire foot and equinus (pointing downwards) position of entire foot (Fig. 33-26).
Assess spinal alignment. Observe spine and posture. Assess for scoliosis (Fig. 33-27).	By 12 to 18 months, the lumbar curve develops. Toddlers display lordotic posture. Findings in older children and adolescents are similar to those in adults.	Kyphosis may result from poor posture or from pathological conditions. Scoliosis usually is idiopathic and is more common in adolescent girls. Abnormal posture suggests neuromuscular disorders such as cerebral palsy (Fig. 33-28). Extremities that are asymmetrical in size, shape and movement indicate scoliosis or hip disease.

Continued on following page

PHYSICAL ASSESSMENT (continued)

ASSESSMENT PROCEDURE	NORMAL FINDINGS	ABNORMAL FINDINGS
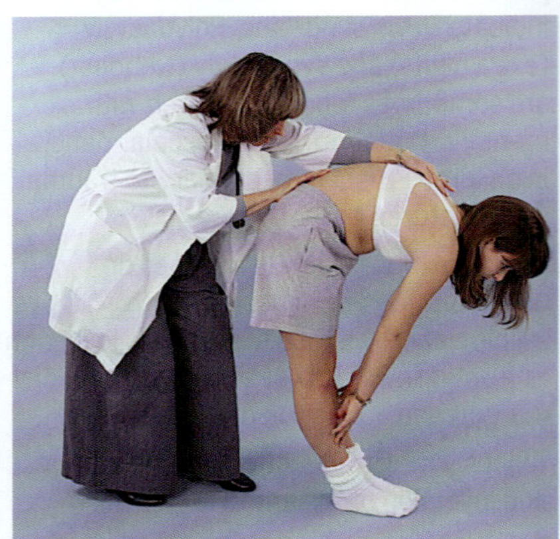 **FIGURE 33-27** Assessing spinal curvature for scoliosis. (© B. Proud.)	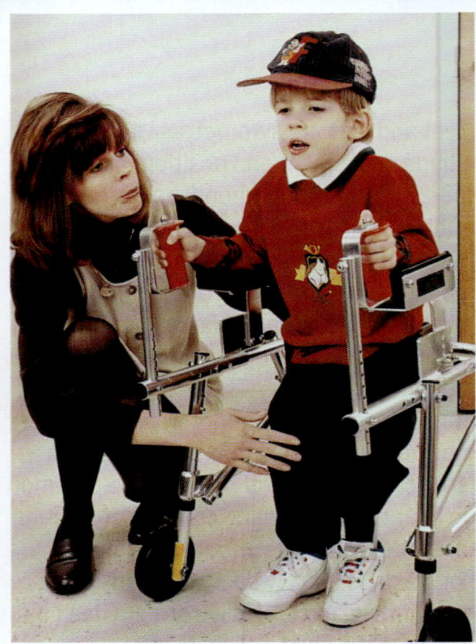 **FIGURE 33-28** Neuromuscular weakness is a hallmark of cerebral palsy.	
Assess gait. Observe gait initially when the child enters the exam room. This enables you to observe the child when he or she is unaware of being observed and gait is most natural. Later have the child walk to and from the parent (the child should be barefoot) and observe gait.	Toddlers have a wide-based gait and are usually bow-legged (genu varum). Children ages 2 to 7 are usually knock-kneed (genu valgum). (See Fig. 33-29.) Gait in older children is the same as in adults.	'Toeing in' or 'toeing out' indicates problems such as tibial torsion or clubfoot. Limping may indicate congenital hip dysplasia (toddlers); synovitis (preschoolers); Legg-Calvé-Perthes disease (school-age children); slipped capital femoral epiphysis, scoliosis (adolescents). When the child is wearing shoes, limping usually suggests poorly fitting shoes or the presence of a pebble. Many abnormal gaits are noted in cerebral palsy.

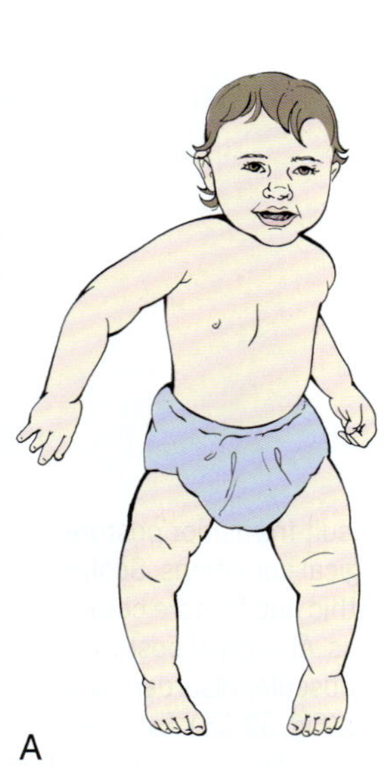

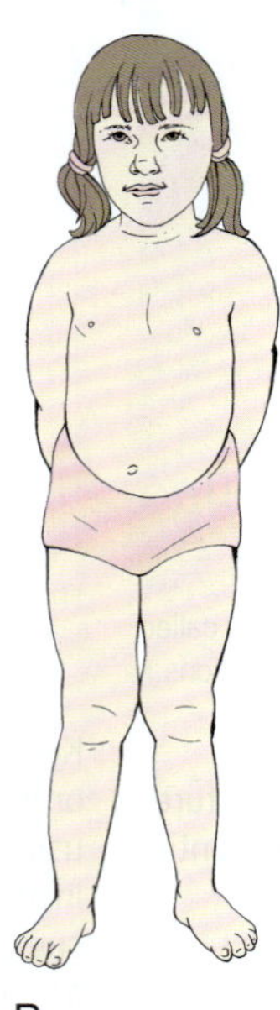

FIGURE 33-29 **(A)** Genu varum (bow legs); **(B)** genu valgum (knock knees).

PHYSICAL ASSESSMENT (continued)

ASSESSMENT PROCEDURE	NORMAL FINDINGS	ABNORMAL FINDINGS
Musculoskeletal (continued)		
Assess joints. Note range of motion, swelling, redness and tenderness.	Full range of motion and no swelling, redness or tenderness.	Limited range of motion, swelling, redness and tenderness indicate problems ranging from mild injuries to serious disorders, such as rheumatoid arthritis.
Assess muscles. Note size and strength.	Muscle size and strength should be adequate for the particular age and should be equal bilaterally.	Inadequate muscle size and strength for the particular age indicate neuromuscular disorders such as muscular dystrophy.
Neurological		
INSPECTION		
Much of the neurological examination of children older than age 2 years is performed in the same way as for adults. **CLINICAL TIP** **As with adults, integrate the neurological assessment into the overall assessment, observing the child first in the natural state, then purposefully. Playing games such as 'Simon says' can help elicit responses from young children.**		
Test cerebral function. Assess level of consciousness, behaviour, adaptation and speech.	The child should be alert and active, respond appropriately and relate well to the parent and the nurse. Increased independence will be demonstrated with age. By age 3 years, speech should be easily understood.	Abnormal findings include altered level of consciousness and inappropriate responses. Maladaptation is displayed by an inability to relate well to parent and nurse, lack of independence with age, inappropriate responses to commands, hyperactivity and poor attention span. Although physiological dysfluency is normal in preschoolers, unintelligible speech by age 3 years, prolonged stuttering, slurring and lisping indicate speech disorders or neurological problems. Slurring may also be indicative of substance abuse, drug toxicity or conditions such as diabetic ketoacidosis.
Test cranial nerve function. Test cranial nerve function in young people the same way as for adults when possible.	Normal findings are the same as for adults.	Alterations in cranial nerve function demonstrate a problem or pathological process.
Test deep tendon and superficial reflexes. Test deep tendon and superficial reflexes in young people the same way as for adults.	Normal findings are the same as for adults, except the Babinski response is normal in children younger than 2 years (this response usually disappears between 2 and 24 months) and triceps reflex is absent until age 6.	Absence or marked intensity of these reflexes, asymmetry and the presence of Babinski response after age 2 years may demonstrate pathology. Sustained (continuous) ankle clonus is abnormal and suggests CNS disease.
Test balance and coordination. Balance and coordination in a child are tested in much the same way as for an adult. Have the child hop, skip and jump, when appropriate for developmental age.	School-age children and adolescents should be able to perform most balance and coordination tests.	Abnormal findings include unstable gait, lack of coordination of movements and positive Romberg. These may indicate a number of problems, including CNS disease and neuromuscular disorders.

Continued on following page

PHYSICAL ASSESSMENT (continued)

ASSESSMENT PROCEDURE	NORMAL FINDINGS	ABNORMAL FINDINGS
Test sensory function. Same as for adults, when possible.	Sensitivity to touch and discrimination should be present. The thresholds of touch, pain and temperature are higher in older children.	Absent or decreased sensitivity to touch and two-point discrimination may indicate paraesthesia.
Test motor function. Tests for motor function in children are similar to tests for adults. Also watch for hand preference.	Gross and fine motor skills should be appropriate for the child's developmental age. Hand preference is developed during the preschool years.	Gross and fine motor skills that are inappropriate for developmental age and lack of head control by age 6 months may indicate cerebral palsy. Hand preference that is not developed during preschool years may indicate paresis on opposite side.
Observe for 'soft sign'. Soft signs of neurological problems are controversial because these signs do not always indicate a pathological process.	Soft signs disappear with age.	Soft signs include but are not limited to: • Short attention span • Poor coordination of position • Hypoactivity • Impulsiveness • Labile emotions • Distractibility • No demonstration of handedness • Language and articulation problems • Learning problems.

VALIDATING AND DOCUMENTING FINDINGS

Documentation for children and adolescents uses the same guiding principles for describing adults, in that documenting findings by describing them as 'good', 'poor' or 'normal' should be avoided. Nurses document what they observe, palpate, percuss and auscultate. Descriptions should be objective, accurate and concise, yet comprehensive. Phrases and standardised abbreviations are preferable to full sentences, and a sequential manner should be followed. Both national and local institutional policies should be adhered to.

Sample of subjective data

Caucasian female, age 13 months. Visiting for well-child health check. Current health and illness status: Has been well since last health care visit at age 9 months; no current problems, health concerns or medications. Past health history: Birth FTNSVD [full-term, normal, spontaneous delivery], BW [birth weight] 3.2 kg; no problems. Otitis media at age 6 months. Allergies (and reaction to same): None. Immunisation status: UTD [up to date].

Growth and developmental milestones: Sat at 6.5 months; walked at 11 months; first word ('dada') at 8 months. Habits: None.

ROS (review of systems [or symptoms]): General: Well child, three 'colds' in first year; Integument: No lesions, bruising; Head: No trauma, headaches; Eyes: Visual acuity, no problems by history; last eye exam (N/A [not applicable]); no drainage, infections; Ears: Hearing acuity, no problems by history; last hearing exam (N/A); no drainage; history of [h/o] otitis media at 6 months treated with amoxicillin); Nose: No bleeding, congestion, discharge; Mouth: No lesions, soreness; no tooth eruption, last dental exam (N/A); Throat: No sore throats, hoarseness, difficulty swallowing; Neck: No stiffness, tenderness; Chest: No pain, cough, wheezing, shortness of breath, asthma, infections; Breasts: No thelarche, lesions, discharge; Cardiovascular: No history of murmurs, exercise intolerance, dizziness, palpitations, congenital defects; Gastrointestinal: Appetite excellent; bowel habits (one soft, brown BM/day); no food intolerances, nausea, vomiting, pain, history of parasites; Genitourinary: No urgency, frequency, discharge, urinary tract infections; Gynaecological: No discharge; Musculoskeletal: No pain, swelling, fractures, mobility problems; Neurological: No tremors, unusual movements, seizures; Lymphatic: No pain, swelling or tenderness, enlargement of spleen or liver; Endocrine/metabolic: Growth patterns follow 50%; no polyuria, polydipsia, polyphagia.

Psychiatric history: No developmental disorder. Family history: Diabetes (maternal grandmother); hypertension (paternal grandfather). Nutritional history: Drinks three 240 mL bottles of whole milk/day; eats three meals consisting of mixture of baby and table foods. Likes finger foods; hates strained meats and string beans. No problems with feeding, feeds self with much assistance, uses spoon and cup. Takes a multivitamin daily.

Determine the quantity and the types of food or formula ingested daily: use 24-hour recall, food diary for 3 days (2 weekdays and 1 weekend day) or food frequency record.

Sleep history: Bedtime is 8 p.m.; awakens at 6 a.m. Takes two brief naps/day. Sleeps with favourite blanket, 'Kermie'.

Psychosocial history: Lives with single mother, age 35 years. Mother is vice president of major company; mother completed university. Cultural background is Italian/Irish; religion: Protestant. Mother has no contact with child's father but does have strong network of friends and family members. No financial difficulties.

Attends day care while mother works. Plays with dolls and push-toys; mother very safety conscious of toys and uses car seat. Discipline: Mother uses distraction and reinforces word 'no'. No history of domestic violence.

Developmental history: Cognitive: Likes to put things in mouth to explore them; likes to feel different textures. Child knows her name and can point to five body parts. Searches for hidden objects. Language: Knows 10 words, including 'no'. Gross motor: Walks without help, starting to climb. Fine motor: Right-handed, builds two-block tower.

Sample of objective data

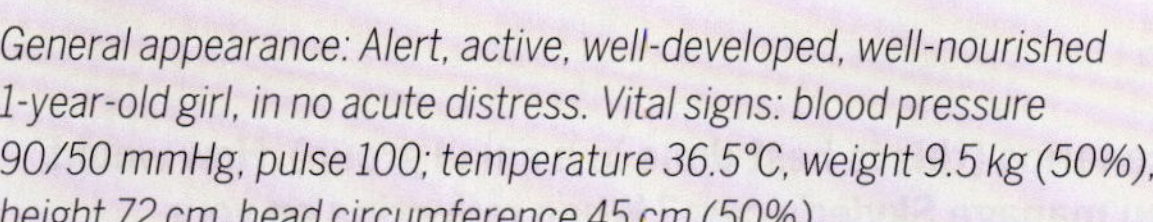

General appearance: Alert, active, well-developed, well-nourished 1-year-old girl, in no acute distress. Vital signs: blood pressure 90/50 mmHg, pulse 100; temperature 36.5°C, weight 9.5 kg (50%), height 72 cm, head circumference 45 cm (50%).

Skin: Pink, moist, appropriate turgor, no lesions; hair curly with normal distribution; nails pink and hard.

Head and neck: Normocephalic, fontanelles not palpable, neck supple, no lymph nodes palpable.

Mouth, throat, nose and sinus: Pharynx clear, no adenopathy, nares patent, turbinates pink with scant clear discharge.

Eyes and ears: Sclera clear, pupils equally round, react to light and accommodation [PERRLA], external ear canal free of cerumen impaction, foreign body, no obvious discharge.

Heart: Normal sinus rhythm, no murmurs auscultated.

Abdomen: Soft, no masses or organomegaly.

Genitalia and rectum: Tanner 1, no discharge or lesions.

Musculoskeletal: Spine straight, no tufts or dimples, full range of movement [FROM], adequate muscle strength and tone.

Neurological: Cranial nerves II to XII intact, deep tendon reflexes 2+, no Babinski, sensitive to touch, coordination, gross and fine motor movement appropriate for age.

Thorax and lungs: Thorax round and symmetrical, hyper-resonance percussed over lung fields.

Heart: 100 beats/minute.

Analysis of data

DIAGNOSTIC REASONING: POSSIBLE CONCLUSIONS

After collecting subjective and objective data pertaining to children and adolescents, identify abnormal findings and patient's strengths. Then cluster the data to reveal any significant patterns or abnormalities. These data may then be used to make clinical judgements about the status of the child or adolescent.

Potential patient risks

- Impaired skin integrity: 'nappy rash' (related to parental knowledge deficit of skin care for a nappy-wearing infant or child)
- Injury (related to open fontanelles)
- Injury to teeth (related to developmental age and play activities)
- Injury to nose (related to insertion of foreign bodies into nasal cavity)
- Injury to ear (related to attempts to insert foreign objects into ear)
- Aspiration (related to improper feeding and small size of stomach in newborns)
- Impaired urinary elimination (related to parental knowledge deficit of toilet-training techniques)
- Injury (related to premature physical developmental level)
- Imbalanced nutrition: less than body requirements

Potential patient problems

- Impaired skin integrity: acne (related to developmental changes)
- Ineffective health maintenance (related to lack of proper mouth care)
- Ineffective airway clearance (related to bronchospasm and increased pulmonary secretions)
- Deficient fluid volume (related to vomiting or diarrhoea)
- Imbalanced nutrition: more than body requirements.

Selected collaborative problems

After grouping the data, it may become apparent that certain collaborative problems emerge. Remember that collaborative problems differ from nursing diagnoses in that they cannot be prevented with nursing interventions alone. However, these physiological complications of medical conditions can be detected and monitored by the nurse. In addition, the nurse can use doctor- and nurse-prescribed interventions to minimise the complications of these problems. The nurse may also have to refer the patient in such situations for further treatment of the problem. The following is a list of collaborative problems seen more frequently in the paediatric patient. However, other collaborative problems seen in the adult are also seen in paediatric patients:

- Severe malnutrition or dehydration
- Delayed growth
- Failure to thrive
- Respiratory distress
- Permanently deformed femoral head
- Hydrocephalus or shunt infections.

Medical problems

After grouping the data, the patient's signs and symptoms may clearly require medical diagnosis and treatment.

ONLINE RESOURCES

An extensive range of additional resources to enhance teaching and learning and to facilitate understanding may be found online at the text's accompanying website, located on thePoint at http://thepoint.lww.com. These include Watch and Learn videos, Concepts in Action animations, journal articles, case studies, discussion topics and quizzes.

Subscribers may also access Lippincott Procedures, an extensive online point-of-care procedure guide that provides reliable step-by-step instructions for more than 1700 procedures, including 450 evidence-based Australian procedures, and skills in a variety of speciality settings, together with a wealth of supporting information.

SIMULATED LEARNING

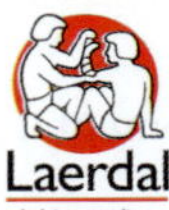

Having completed this chapter, explore the scenarios of Skyler Hansen Part 1 and Part 2. Skyler is an 18-year-old who has been newly diagnosed with type 1 diabetes mellitus. Incorporating the health assessment content in this chapter with your existing theoretical knowledge and clinical experience, progress through the simulation scenarios (this is best done in a small group). How would you manage Skyler's care? When reflecting on your management of Skyler, what do you think you did well and what do you think you can improve? Consider why you think this and also how you might manage a similar problem in the future.

CASE STUDY

The case study demonstrates how to analyse child assessment data for a specific patient. The exercises included in the ancillary product on thePoint that complements this text offer further opportunities to enhance your skills.

Mrs Carter brings 2-year-old Michael to the paediatric emergency department because he has been 'irritable and feverish since last night'. Further history reveals that Michael has also had a runny nose and cough for 2 days and his appetite and fluid intake have decreased since his fever started. Michael is otherwise healthy. You are the assessing nurse.

Michael's physical examination reveals he is a slightly irritable, 2-year-old boy, pulling at his ears, temperature 38.9 °C, and nasal congestion with clear discharge. When the medical officer examined him, he was found to have bilateral red, bulging tympanic membranes; his pharynx was lightly red without exudate; his chest was clear; his abdomen was soft without hepatosplenomegaly; and there were no meningeal signs.

He is diagnosed with an upper respiratory tract infection (URTI) and bilateral otitis media (BOM). Michael's doctor orders amoxicillin 250 mg TDS for 10 days. As Michael's allocated nurse you are to provide Michael's mother with education regarding his home care. During your discussion with Mrs Carter, she tells you that she is concerned that Michael is jealous of his new baby sister because he has occasional tantrums when she holds the baby. She is also concerned about Michael's development because he recently started to refuse using the potty, a newly acquired skill. Mrs Carter is very attentive to both the new baby and Michael throughout the interview, and she asks you for suggestions in how to help Michael cope with the new arrival. While doing so, she points out that her husband has been extra attentive to Michael since his sister was born.

The following concept map illustrates the diagnostic reasoning process.

Applying COLDSPA

Applying COLDSPA for patient symptoms: 'male 2-year-old irritable and feverish'.

Mnemonic	Question	Data provided	Missing data
Character	Describe the sign or symptom (feeling, appearance, sound, smell or taste, if applicable).	'Irritable and feverish'.	Describe the child's irritable behaviours. How high was the temperature? Did the child have chills?
Onset	When did it begin?	'Last night'.	
Location	Where is it? Does it radiate? Does it occur anywhere else?	Nasal congestion with clear discharge; red, bulging bilateral tympanic membranes.	
Duration	How long does it last? Does it recur?	Runny nose and cough for 2 days.	
Severity	How bad is it? or How much does it bother you?	Child pulling at ears and has temperature of 38.9 °C.	
Pattern	What makes it better or worse?	Father gives extra attention to child.	Has the child been given any medications? If so, what type, dose, frequency and affects on fever and irritability? How long has the child's father been giving extra attention to his son? How does the child respond to this?
Associated factors/How it **A**ffects the patient	What other symptoms occur with it? How does it affect you?	Child has had a poor appetite and decreased fluid intake since the onset of the fever; throws temper tantrums when mother holds his new baby sister; refuses to use the potty, a newly acquired skill.	Describe the child's fluid and food intake during the last 2 days as compared to typical intake prior to irritability and fever. Have temper tantrums worsened since runny nose and cough began? How long has the child been introduced to the new potty?

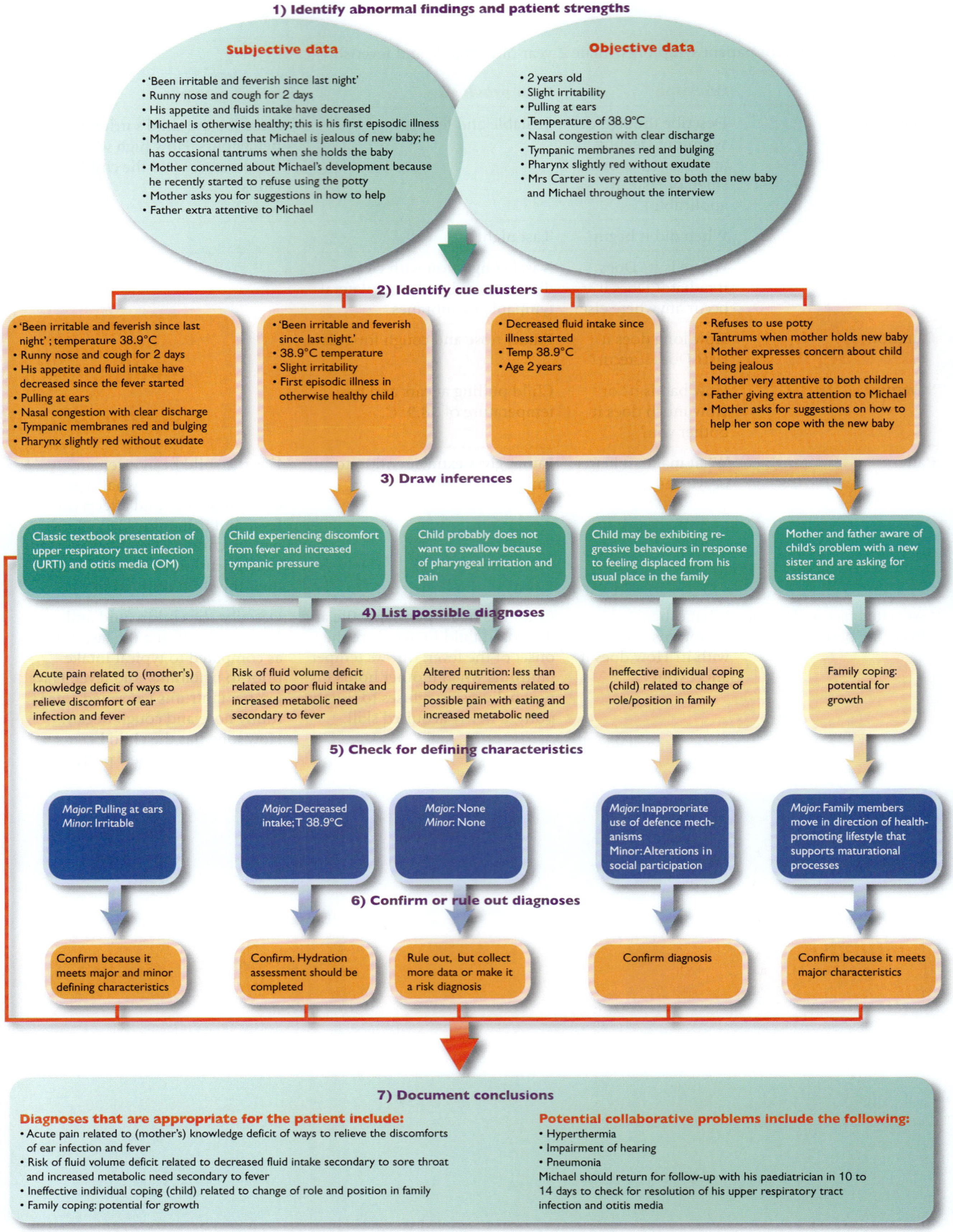

1) Identify abnormal findings and patient strengths

Subjective data

- 'Been irritable and feverish since last night'
- Runny nose and cough for 2 days
- His appetite and fluids intake have decreased
- Michael is otherwise healthy; this is his first episodic illness
- Mother concerned that Michael is jealous of new baby; he has occasional tantrums when she holds the baby
- Mother concerned about Michael's development because he recently started to refuse using the potty
- Mother asks you for suggestions in how to help
- Father extra attentive to Michael

Objective data

- 2 years old
- Slight irritability
- Pulling at ears
- Temperature of 38.9°C
- Nasal congestion with clear discharge
- Tympanic membranes red and bulging
- Pharynx slightly red without exudate
- Mrs Carter is very attentive to both the new baby and Michael throughout the interview

2) Identify cue clusters

- 'Been irritable and feverish since last night'; temperature 38.9°C
- Runny nose and cough for 2 days
- His appetite and fluid intake have decreased since the fever started
- Pulling at ears
- Nasal congestion with clear discharge
- Tympanic membranes red and bulging
- Pharynx slightly red without exudate

- 'Been irritable and feverish since last night.'
- 38.9°C temperature
- Slight irritability
- First episodic illness in otherwise healthy child

- Decreased fluid intake since illness started
- Temp 38.9°C
- Age 2 years

- Refuses to use potty
- Tantrums when mother holds new baby
- Mother expresses concern about child being jealous
- Mother very attentive to both children
- Father giving extra attention to Michael
- Mother asks for suggestions on how to help her son cope with the new baby

3) Draw inferences

- Classic textbook presentation of upper respiratory tract infection (URTI) and otitis media (OM)
- Child experiencing discomfort from fever and increased tympanic pressure
- Child probably does not want to swallow because of pharyngeal irritation and pain
- Child may be exhibiting regressive behaviours in response to feeling displaced from his usual place in the family
- Mother and father aware of child's problem with a new sister and are asking for assistance

4) List possible diagnoses

- Acute pain related to (mother's) knowledge deficit of ways to relieve discomfort of ear infection and fever
- Risk of fluid volume deficit related to poor fluid intake and increased metabolic need secondary to fever
- Altered nutrition: less than body requirements related to possible pain with eating and increased metabolic need
- Ineffective individual coping (child) related to change of role/position in family
- Family coping: potential for growth

5) Check for defining characteristics

- *Major:* Pulling at ears; *Minor:* Irritable
- *Major:* Decreased intake; T 38.9°C
- *Major:* None; *Minor:* None
- *Major:* Inappropriate use of defence mechanisms; Minor: Alterations in social participation
- *Major:* Family members move in direction of health-promoting lifestyle that supports maturational processes

6) Confirm or rule out diagnoses

- Confirm because it meets major and minor defining characteristics
- Confirm. Hydration assessment should be completed
- Rule out, but collect more data or make it a risk diagnosis
- Confirm diagnosis
- Confirm because it meets major characteristics

7) Document conclusions

Diagnoses that are appropriate for the patient include:

- Acute pain related to (mother's) knowledge deficit of ways to relieve the discomforts of ear infection and fever
- Risk of fluid volume deficit related to decreased fluid intake secondary to sore throat and increased metabolic need secondary to fever
- Ineffective individual coping (child) related to change of role and position in family
- Family coping: potential for growth

Potential collaborative problems include the following:

- Hyperthermia
- Impairment of hearing
- Pneumonia

Michael should return for follow-up with his paediatrician in 10 to 14 days to check for resolution of his upper respiratory tract infection and otitis media

References

American College of Obstetricians and Gynecologists. (2014). Primary and preventive health care for female adolescents. In *Tool kit for teen care* (2nd ed.). Washington DC: Author. Viewed July 2019 at https://www.acog.org/Clinical-Guidance-and-Publications/Committee-Opinions/Committee-on-Adolescent-Health-Care/The-Initial-Reproductive-Health-Visit.

Australian Technical Advisory Group on Immunisation (2018). The Australian Immunisation Handbook. Viewed February 2020 at https://immunisationhandbook.health.gov.au/.

Bright Futures and American Academy of Pediatrics. (2019). Recommendations for preventative health care (periodicity schedule). Viewed October 2019 at https://www.aap.org/en-us/Documents/periodicity_schedule.pdf

Erikson, E. H. (1963). *Childhood and society* (2nd ed.). New York: Norton.

Freud, S. (1923/1974). *The ego and the id*. London: Hogarth.

Hockenberry, M. & Wilson, D. (2013). *Wong's essentials of pediatric nursing* (9th ed.). St Louis: Mosby/Elsevier.

Kohlberg, L. (1969). Stage and sequence: The cognitive developmental approach to socialization. In D. Gaslin (Ed). *Handbook of socialization: Theory and research* (pp. 347–380). Chicago: Rand McNally.

Kohlberg, L. (1976). Moral stages and moralization: The cognitive-developmental approach. In T. Lickona (Ed). *Moral development and behaviour*. New York: Holt, Rinehart & Winston.

Kohlberg, L. (1984). *The psychology of moral development: The nature and validity of moral stages* (Vol. 2). New York: Harper & Row.

Piaget, J. (1932). *The moral judgement of the child*. New York: Harcourt Brace Jovanovich.

Piaget, J. (1952). *The origins of intelligence in children*. New York: International Universities Press.

Piaget, J. & Inhelder, B. (1969). *The psychology of the child*. New York: Basic Books.

Tanner, J. (1962). *Growth at adolescence* (2nd ed.). Oxford, England: Blackwell Scientific.

Tanner, J. (1981). Growth and maturation during adolescence. *Nutrition Reviews, 39*(2), 43–55.

The Immunisation Advisory Centre. (2019). Influenza vaccines. Viewed July 2019 at https://www.immune.org.nz/vaccines/available-vaccines/influenza-vaccines.

Selected readings

American Optometric Association. (2019). Infant vision: Birth to 24 months of age. Viewed July 2019 at https://www.aoa.org/patients-and-public/good-vision-throughout-life/childrens-vision/infant-vision-birth-to-24-months-of-age.

Asher, C. & Northington, L. (2017). Society of Pediatric Nurses position statement: Temperature measurement. Viewed October 2019 at .

Australian Breastfeeding Association. (2017). Breastfeeding and co-sleeping. Available at https://www.breastfeeding.asn.au/bfinfo/breastfeeding-and-co-sleeping.

Australian Government Department of Health. (n.d.). National Cervical Screening Program. Viewed July 2019 at http://www.cancerscreening.gov.au/internet/screening/publishing.nsf/Content/cervical-screening-1.

Australian Government Department of Health. (2018a). Australian immunisation handbook. Viewed July 2019 at https://immunisationhandbook.health.gov.au/.

Australian Government Department of Health. (2018b). Human papillomavirus (HPV). Viewed July 2019 at https://immunisationhandbook.health.gov.au/vaccine-preventable-diseases/human-papillomavirus-hpv.

Australian Government Department of Health. (2018c). *Australian National Breastfeeding Strategy 2018 and beyond*. Canberra: Author. Viewed July 2019 at https://consultations.health.gov.au/population-health-and-sport-division/breastfeeding/supporting_documents/Draft%20Australian%20National%20Breastfeeding%20Strategy%20%20%20PDF%20version.pdf.

Australian Government Department of Health. (2018d). Vaccination for migrants, refugees and people seeking asylum in Australia. Viewed July 2019 at https://immunisationhandbook.health.gov.au/vaccination-for-special-risk-groups/vaccination-for-migrants-refugees-and-people-seeking-asylum-in.

Australian Government Department of Health. (2019a). Human papillomavirus (HPV) immunisation Service. Viewed July 2019 at https://www.health.gov.au/health-topics/immunisation/immunisation-services/human-papillomavirus-hpv-immunisation-service.

Australian Government Department of Health. (2019b). National Immunisation Program Schedule. Viewed July 2019 at https://www.health.gov.au/health-topics/immunisation/immunisation-throughout-life/national-immunisation-program-schedule.

Australian Institute of Family Studies (AIFS). (2017). Mandatory reporting of child abuse and neglect. Viewed July 2019 at https://aifs.gov.au/cfca/publications/mandatory-reporting-child-abuse-and-neglect.

Australian Institute of Family Studies (AIFS). (2019). Reporting abuse and neglect: Information for service providers. Viewed July 2019 at www.aifs.gov.au/cfca/pubs/factsheets/a142843/index.html.

Australian Institute of Health & Welfare (AIHW). (2012). A picture of Australia's children. Cat. no. PHE 167. Canberra: Author.

Berger, K. S. (2014). *The developing person through childhood and adolescence* (9th ed.). New York: Worth Publishing.

Better Health Channel. (2018). Sudden unexpected death in infants (SUDI and SIDS). Viewed July 2019 at https://www.betterhealth.vic.gov.au/health/healthyliving/sudden-unexpected-death-in-infants-sudi-and-sids.

Cancer Council. (n.d.). The HPV vaccine. Viewed July 2019 at http://www.hpvvaccine.org.au/the-hpv-vaccine/vaccine-background.aspx.

Coates, D. (2018). Vision screening and assessment in infants and children. Viewed July 2019 at https://www.uptodate.com/contents/vision-screening-and-assessment-in-infants-and-children?search=snellen%20eye%20chart%20scale%20children&source=search_result&selectedTitle=1~150&usage_type=default&display_rank=1.

Iannelli, V. (2019). Dental health guide for children. Viewed July 2019 at https://www.verywellfamily.com/dental-health-guide-for-children-2632281.

Kruger, P., Teague, W., Khanal, R., et al. (2019). Screening for associated anomalies in anorectal malformations: The need for a standardised approach. *ANZ Journal of Surgery*, doi:10.1111/ans.15150.

Ladwig, G. B. & Ackley, B. J. (2014). *Nursing diagnosis handbook* (10th ed.). St Louis: Mosby/Elsevier.

Ministry of Health. (2018). *Immunisation Handbook 2017* (2nd ed.). Wellington: Ministry of Health. Available at https://www.health.govt.nz/publication/immunisation-handbook-2017.

New Zealand Ministry of Health (NZMOH). (2015). Current food and nutrition guidelines. Viewed July 2019 at www.health.govt.nz/our-work/preventative-health-wellness/nutrition/food-and-nutrition-guidelines.

New Zealand Ministry of Health (NZMOH). (2018a). Family violence questions and answers. Viewed July 2019 at https://www.health.govt.nz/our-work/preventative-health-wellness/family-violence/family-violence-questions-and-answers#mandatory.

New Zealand Ministry of Health (NZMOH). (2018b). New Zealand immunisation schedule. Viewed July 2019 at https://www.health.govt.nz/our-work/preventative-health-wellness/immunisation/new-zealand-immunisation-schedule.

New Zealand Ministry of Health (NZMOH). (2018c). Well child Tamariki Ora: My health book. Viewed July 2019 at https://www.healthed.govt.nz/system/files/resource-files/HE7012_Well%20Child%20Tamariki%20Ora%20my%20health%20book_0.pdf.

Peterson, C. (2014). *Looking forward through the lifespan: Developmental psychology* (6th ed.). Sydney: Pearson.

Royal Children's Hospital Melbourne. (2014). Clinical guidelines (nursing): Temperature management. Viewed July 2019 at https://www.rch.org.au/rchcpg/hospital_clinical_guideline_index/Temperature_Management/.

Royal Children's Hospital Melbourne. (2015). *Paediatric handbook* (9th ed.). Melbourne: Wiley Blackwell.

Royal Children's Hospital Melbourne. (2018). Clinical practice guidelines: Family violence. Viewed July 2019 at https://www.rch.org.au/clinicalguide/guideline_index/Family_Violence/.

Royal Children's Hospital Melbourne. (n.d.a). Engaging and assessing the adolescent patient. Available at https://www.rch.org.au/clinicalguide/guideline_index/Engaging_with_and_assessing_the_adolescent_patient/.

Royal Children's Hospital Melbourne. (n.d.b). Clinical guidelines (nursing): Pain assessment and measurement. Viewed July 2019 at https://www.rch.org.au/rchcpg/hospital_clinical_guideline_index/Pain_Assessment_and_Measurement/.

Starship Children's Hospital. (2016). Paediatric pain assessment. Viewed July 2019 at https://www.starship.org.nz/guidelines/paediatric-pain-assessment/.

Sparrow, M. (2014). Pain management. In J. Dempsey, S. Hillege, & R. Hill (Eds). *Fundamentals of nursing: A person-centred approach to care* (2nd ed.). Sydney: Lippincott, Williams & Wilkins.

Online resources

1800 Respect-National Sexual Assault, Domestic Family Violence Counselling Service: https://www.1800respect.org.au/

Ages and Stages Questionnaire: https://agesandstages.com/

Australian Hearing, children: https://www.hearing.com.au/Resources-for-health-professionals/General-Practitioners/How-to-detect-hearing-loss-in-babies-and-children

Australian Institute of Family Studies: www.aifs.gov.au

Beyond Blue: https://www.beyondblue.org.au/

Centre for Adolescent Health, Royal Children's Hospital, Melbourne: www.rch.org.au/cah
Child, Youth & Family, New Zealand: www.cyf.govt.nz
Developmental milestones and the Early Years Learning Framework and the National Quality Standards: https://www.acecqa.gov.au/sites/default/files/2018-02/DevelopmentalMilestonesEYLFandNQS.pdf
Generation Next: www.generationnext.com.au
headspace (Australia's National Youth Mental Health Foundation): www.headspace.org.au
Health*InSite*, child development: www.healthinsite.gov.au/child-development
Human Papilloma Virus: https://immunisationhandbook.health.gov.au/vaccine-preventable-diseases/human-papillomavirus-hpv
Immunisation Advisory Centre New Zealand: www.immune.org.nz
The Australian Immunisation Handbook: https://immunisationhandbook.health.gov.au/
Kids Health New Zealand: www.kidshealth.org.nz
Kids Help Line: https://kidshelpline.com.au/
Kiwi Families, Child Development: https://www.kiwifamilies.co.nz/
Mental Health Foundation New Zealand: https://www.mentalhealth.org.nz/get-help/in-crisis/helplines/
National Health and Medical Research Council, dietary guidelines: https://www.nhmrc.gov.au/about-us/publications/australian-dietary-guidelines#block-views-block-file-attachments-content-block-1
Lifeline: https://www.lifeline.org.au/
New Zealand Immunisation Schedule: https://www.health.govt.nz/your-health/healthy-living/immunisation
Plunkett: https://www.plunket.org.nz/
Teenage Health, Better Health Channel: https://www.betterhealth.vic.gov.au/health/healthyliving/teenage-health
New Zealand Ministry of Health Helping Adolescents: https://www.health.govt.nz/your-health/healthy-living/emergency-management/managing-stress-emergency/helping-adolescents
Red Nose: https://rednose.org.au/
Sydney Children's Hospital at Westmead Adolscent health GP Resource Kit: https://www.schn.health.nsw.gov.au/files/attachments/complete_gp_resource_kit_0.pdf
The Royal Children's Hospital Melbourne-Paediatric Clinical Practice Guidelines: https://www.rch.org.au/clinicalguide/about_rch_cpgs/Welcome_to_the_Clinical_Practice_Guidelines/
Vision Australia: www.visionaustralia.org
White Ribbon: https://www.whiteribbon.org.au

CHAPTER 34

Assessing older people

CASE STUDY

Mrs Janice Kimberley is an 86-year-old lady who has difficulty climbing stairs and maintaining her home of 43 years. However, she receives assistance from her family and the local council, which has a service supporting people at home. She eats two meals a day and has had a gradually improving appetite since receiving extra support. She reports occasional episodes (about once every 2 to 3 weeks) of difficulty swallowing, especially food that is dry or meat that is tough. Mrs Kimberley takes a psyllium-powder bulking-laxative to keep her bowel movements regular and soft. Her current prescription medications are a combined levodopa carbidopa tablet three times a day and sodium hydrochlorothiazide 500 mg each morning.

Challenges and approaches

Common physical findings in older people have been identified in the preceding chapters on body systems. However, it is not just the physiological changes of ageing that warrant a special approach to assessment of the older adult. Many older adults are healthy, active and independent, despite these normal physical changes in their bodies. It is, rather, that advancing age increases the risk of chronic illness and disability. The term 'frail older person' describes the vulnerability of the 'old-old' (generally mid-eighties, nineties and centenarians) to be in poorer health, to have more chronic disabilities and to function less independently (Cesari et al., 2017).

Nearly 20% of people between the ages 64 and 74 years have limitations on activity because of chronic conditions. However, the proportion of older people with disability decreased in the period from 2012 to 2015, and 94.8% older people live in a household rather than residential care. Nevertheless, disability takes a much heavier toll on the very old; almost 9 out of 10 of those age 90 years and over have a disabling physical condition. Over half have one or more severe disabilities, and about 1 in 3 older Australians need assistance with daily activities (Australian Bureau of Statistics [ABS], 2016).

LOSS OF HOMEOSTATIC RESERVE

The loss of homeostatic reserve is the main reason that older people are more likely to be sick and disabled (Cesari et al., 2017). The average 85-year-old person is living with almost 50% less cellular function in their organ systems throughout their bodies. On a daily basis, they may have no ill effects from this loss of reserve. However, if an 85-year-old person is living with a chronic problem such as diabetes and then becomes suddenly ill with what is usually a very treatable problem in a younger person (such as a bladder infection), this loss of reserve can have dramatic consequences.

Presentation of illness

When the physiology of advanced age is combined with comorbidity, their assessment is complicated. Consequently, the signs and symptoms of illness often present differently in the oldest-old. *Adverse events* or *adverse drug effects* in this population often include falls, confusion, incontinence, generalised weakness and lethargy. These complications are also referred to as *geriatric syndromes* and are more commonly signs and symptoms of illness in the very old than are the more common manifestations of illness in younger adults such as fever, pain and abnormal laboratory values.

The population at greatest risk for developing atypical presentations is the very old, who also have cognitive or functional impairment and multiple comorbidities, and who are being treated with multiple medications (Australian Institute of Health and Welfare [AIHW], 2018).

Knowing the older person's usual daily pattern and functional level is the best baseline against which to compare assessment data. For example, a new onset of incontinence for a 92-year-old resident of an assisted living facility who still drives her own car should not be viewed as a normal consequence of ageing. The incontinence could be the result of an infection or worsening heart failure. A more subtle presentation of these same problems could be signalled by complete incontinence in a 92-year-old man with severe cognitive impairment, who until very recently had only occasional incontinence. The key to recognising pathology and illness in the very old is in knowing the person's *baseline functional status* and recognising a deviation from it.

Symptoms of disease and disability in the very old frequently manifest as incontinence, falls, weakness and lethargy, confusion, changes in sleep or level of alertness, and loss of appetite or weight loss. Not only do these syndromes describe the common and most recognisable ways in which disease often presents itself in the frail older person, they also describe the consequences of physiological stress. For example, incontinence and confusion are often signs of infection. The incontinence and confusion can easily lead to a fall when the

DISPLAY 34-1 COMMON PROBLEMS IN THE OLDER PERSON WARRANTING FURTHER INVESTIGATION AS IDENTIFIED BY THE ACRONYM SPICES

- Skin impairment
- Poor nutrition
- Incontinence
- Cognitive impairment
- Evidence of falls or functional decline
- Sleep disturbances (Francis et al., 1998)

older person attempts to walk to the bathroom, but on the way experiences lightheadedness caused by dehydration and postural hypotension. The fall may result in a hip fracture and immobility, which may lead to a pressure ulcer, urinary tract infection and delirium. This cascade of unfortunate events often leads a frail but independent older adult living at home to dependence and disability.

Risk screening tools, such as SPICES (see Display 34-1), may be used to monitor the population of high-risk frail older people for some of the non-specific indicators of disease. Because the oldest-old have the highest prevalence of chronic illness and comorbidity, one disease may mask the symptoms of another. For example, fatigue and dyspnoea of severe congestive heart failure may mask anaemia caused by a duodenal ulcer. A severe illness is more likely to affect multiple organ systems as the body's reserves and ability to respond to physiological stress are impaired. For instance, pneumonia will typically precipitate congestive heart failure.

To complicate the assessment process even more, medications often result in significant adverse effects rather than improve the symptoms in the frail older person. Often a drug is used to treat the adverse drug effect and the problems spiral into a nearly indecipherable collection of symptoms (Holbeach & Yates, 2010). There are medications that should be avoided in people over 65 because their potential risks outweigh potential benefits, regardless of the person's level of frailty (Elliott, 2006).

Thus, collection of subjective data from the frail older person must take into consideration the more common ways in which diseases and disorders present in older people (Nay et al., 2013). Information regarding falls, weakness, incontinence, confusion, sleep difficulties and loss of appetite is essential. Finally, the patient's family, social, economic resources and environment must be assessed to determine any relationship to the patient's symptoms. For example, isolation, physical barriers or neglect may precipitate physiological and functional decline.

The intention of the *National safety and quality health service (NSQHS) Standard 10: Preventing falls and harm from falls* is to reduce the incidence of patient falls and minimise harm from falls. For more information, see www.safetyandquality.gov.au.

CULTURAL CONSIDERATIONS

For older Aboriginal and Torres Strait Islander Australians and New Zealand Indigenous people, there are particular issues that should be considered. Importantly the average lifespan for Aboriginal and Torres Strait Islander and Māori people is less than their Pākehā or European-descended counterparts. Some of the factors that lead to a diminished lifespan in older Aboriginal and Torres Strait Islander Australians are higher rates of smoking, higher body mass index and lower levels of physical activity (Australian Indigenous Health*InfoNet*, 2019). Tuberculosis also has a higher rate of prevalence in older Aboriginal and Torres Strait Islander people and hospitalisation rates are much higher (Department of Health, 2017). Older Aboriginal and Torres Strait Islander people also use residential aged care at higher rates than non-Aboriginal and Torres Strait Islander Australians.

Older Māori compared with Pākehā are four times more likely to live in the most deprived areas (Hunter, 2016). In addition, the health literacy of older Māori is lower than non-Māori, and this may result in a diminished ability to make informed appropriate decisions about their health (Reid & White, 2012). Smoking by older Māori females is significantly higher compared with non-Māori females of the same age, and older Māori are significantly more likely to be overweight or obese (Hunter, 2016). Diabetes mellitus is also a significant issue for both Aboriginal and Torres Strait Islander Australians and Māori. It has a prevalence of 32.1% among Aboriginal and Torres Strait Islander people aged 55 and over (ABS, 2014), and in Māori the rate is reported to be double that of non-Māori in the 65-years-and-over age group (New Zealand Ministry of Health, 2011).

Health assessment

COLLECTING SUBJECTIVE DATA: THE NURSING HEALTH HISTORY

Adapting interview techniques

In today's youth-oriented culture, it is not uncommon to think of physical frailty as a serious problem. If older people experience some degree of declining health, a fear of being increasingly dependent on others may be possible. Many older patients approach clinicians with hesitation because they have known friends and family members who have become sicker or died as a result of intervention. They may also be reluctant to admit health problems because they fear being admitted to a hospital or nursing home. It is essential that the nurse adapt routine interviewing techniques, regardless of the extent of disability and illness being experienced as there is always something positive that the older person is doing. For example, it is important to look for good nutritional habits as well as identify which foods are to be avoided, or to focus on everyday activities that keep an older person ambulatory, just as it is important to identify risk factors for falls. The nurse can acknowledge the older patient's accomplishments that make or have made their lives meaningful.

CASE STUDY

Mrs Kimberley has regular dental examinations and sucks on hard sweets to alleviate her dry mouth. Mrs Kimberley denies any recent falls, fainting or dyspnoea with daily activities. However, she reports that she needs to sit for 5 to 10 minutes before standing to avoid becoming lightheaded. Mrs Kimberley has yearly mammograms and Pap smears. She is a breast cancer survivor and stopped taking supplemental oestrogen when diagnosed and treated 20 years ago. She reports no bleeding or change in moles or skin lesions. She receives vitamin B12 injections once a month and reports she always has more energy for 2 to 3 weeks afterwards. Mrs Kimberley reports she has had to get new eyeglasses twice in the last 4 years and that she sees occasional halos around lights. She can still read the newspaper if she shines a bright light directly on it, and she enjoys knitting. She states she is contented with her life and keeps in touch with family and friends, with frequent phone calls and occasional visits.

Mrs Kimberley has indicated to you she has to take her time standing up and that she may have some diminishing vision. It is possible that she believes these adjustments are part of getting older.

CRITICAL THINKING

1. What further questions about her vision and faintness would you ask?
2. How could you determine how her health problems are affecting her lifestyle?
3. How could you help her to think about these physical frailties so that she is not afraid of seeking help?

Determining functional status

Functional assessment is an evaluation of the person's ability to carry out the basic self-care *activities of daily living* (ADLs) such as bathing, eating, grooming and toileting.

There are many tools available for measuring ability to perform ADLs. One commonly used tool is the Katz Activities of Daily Living (Assessment tool 34-1), which includes those activities necessary for wellbeing as an individual in a society. These activities, known as Instrumental Activities of Daily Living (Assessment tool 34-2), focus primarily on household chores (e.g. cooking, cleaning, laundry), mobility-related activities (e.g. shopping and transportation) and cognitive abilities (e.g. money management, using the telephone and making decisions affecting basic safety and social needs). Functional ability is determined by the dynamic interplay of the frail elder's physiological, emotional and cognitive status, and the physical, interpersonal and social environments. A major purpose of assessing the frail older person is to identify and describe correctly the patient's ability to perform activities of daily living.

CRITICAL THINKING

4. Using the Katz Activities of Daily Living, what problems are you likely to identify in Mrs Kimberley's life at home?
5. If you were to assess Mrs Kimberley's Instrumental Activities of Daily Living, what household chores do you think she would have difficulty with?

ASSESSMENT TOOL 34-1 Katz activities of daily living

Activities	Independence:	Dependence:
Points (1 or 0)	(1 Point) NO supervision, direction or personal assistance.	(0 Points) WITH supervision, direction, personal assistance or total care.
Bathing Points: _______	(1 POINT) Bathes self completely or needs help in bathing only a single part of the body such as the back, genital area or disabled extremity.	(0 POINTS) Needs help with bathing more than one part of the body getting in or out of the bath or shower. Requires total bathing.
Dressing Points: _______	(1 POINT) Gets clothes from cupboards and drawers and puts on clothes and outer garments complete with fasteners. May have help tying shoes.	(0 POINTS) Needs help with dressing self or needs to be completely dressed.
Toileting Points: _______	(1 POINT) Goes to toilet, gets on and off, arranges clothes, cleans genital area without help.	(0 POINTS) Needs help transferring to the toilet, cleaning self or uses bedpan or commode.
Transferring Points: _______	(1 POINT) Moves in and out of bed or chair unassisted. Mechanical transferring aids are acceptable.	(0 POINTS) Needs help in moving from bed to chair or requires a complete transfer.
Continence Points: _______	(1 POINT) Exercises complete self-control over urination and defecation.	(0 POINTS) Is partially or totally incontinent of bowel or bladder.
Feeding Points: _______	(1 POINT) Gets food from plate into mouth without help. Preparation of food may be done by another person.	(0 POINTS) Needs partial or total help with feeding or requires parenteral feeding.
Total points = _______	*6 = High (patient independent)*	*0 = Low (patient very dependent)*

Adapted with permission from Gerontological Society of America. Katz, S., Down, T. D., Cash, H. R. & Grotz, R. C. (1970). Progress in the development of the index of ADL. *Gerontologist, 10,* 20–30.

ASSESSMENT TOOL 34-2 Lawton scale for Instrumental Activities of Daily Living (IADL)

Instructions: Start by asking the patient to describe her/his functioning in each category; then complement the description with specific questions as needed.

Ability to telephone

1. Operates telephone on own initiative: looks up and dials numbers, etc.
2. Answers telephone and dials a few well-known numbers.
3. Answers telephone but does not dial.
4. Does not use telephone at all.

Shopping

1. Takes care of all shopping needs independently.
2. Shops independently for small purchases.
3. Needs to be accompanied on any shopping trip.
4. Completely unable to shop.

Food preparation

1. Plans, prepares and serves adequate meals independently.
2. Prepares adequate meals if supplied with ingredients.
3. Heats and serves prepared meals, or prepares meals but does not maintain adequate diet.
4. Needs to have meals prepared and served.

Housekeeping

1. Maintains house alone or with occasional assistance (e.g. heavy work done by domestic help).
2. Performs light daily tasks such as dishwashing and bedmaking.
3. Performs light daily tasks but cannot maintain acceptable level of cleanliness.
4. Needs help with all home maintenance tasks.
5. Does not participate in any housekeeping tasks.

Laundry

1. Does personal laundry completely.
2. Launders small items; rinses socks, stockings, and so on.
3. All laundry must be done by others.

Mode of transportation

1. Travels independently on public transportation, or drives own car.
2. Arranges own travel via taxi, but does not otherwise use public transportation.
3. Travels on public transportation when assisted or accompanied by another.
4. Travel is limited to taxi or car with assistance.
5. Does not travel at all.

Responsibility for own medication

1. Is responsible for taking medication in correct dosages at correct time.
2. Takes responsibility if medication is prepared in advance, in separated dosages.
3. Is not capable of dispensing own medication.

Ability to handle finances

1. Manages financial matters independently (budgets, writes cheques, pays rent and bills, goes to bank); collects and keeps track of income.
2. Manages day-to-day purchases but needs help with banking, major purchases, controlled spending and so on.
3. Incapable of handling money.

Scoring: Circle one number for each domain. Total the numbers circled. Total score can range from 8 to 28. The lower the score, the more independence. Scores are only good for individual patients. Useful to see score comparison over time.

Lawton, M. P. (1971). Functional assessment of elderly people. *Journal of the American Geriatrics Society, 9*(6), 465–481. Reprinted by permission of Blackwell Science, Inc.

Biographical data

Cultural norms were not always as informal as they are today. Many older people grew up when they were not addressed by their first names except by those very close to them. One should always begin the interview by addressing an older person more formally as 'Mr', 'Mrs' or 'Ms', or with an appropriate title such as 'Reverend' or 'Doctor'. In general, younger people today are more likely to feel comfortable sharing personal information with regard to finances, personal likes and dislikes, and feelings than are older adults. Many older people are also aware of their vulnerability with regard to scams and fraud. Thus, they are reluctant to give out personal information. An important maxim of geriatric care is 'Collect no more information than is essential for optimal care.' If the individual is cognitively impaired, a trusted carer may need to be involved in the history. Being sensitive to the older person's need to be respected and acknowledged is essential.

History of present health concern or current health status

QUESTION	RATIONALE
Mental status	
Have you noticed any changes in your ability to concentrate or think clearly enough to keep up with your daily activities? If so, when did this begin and describe what you have noticed?	A common symptom of acute illness in the frail older person is a about deterioration of cognition. The ageing brain is more easily affected by pathology because it is especially vulnerable to deficits in oxygenation and nutrition. Changes in cognition that have occurred suddenly and recently (e.g. past few days or within past week or two) must ALWAYS be assumed to be the result of a disease or illness and must be thoroughly assessed and appropriately referred for treatment.
CLINICAL TIP **If the older person is too lethargic, agitated or medically unstable to respond, family or professional carers should be queried with regard to how current cognition and behaviour compares with the patient's prior level of function. If the patient appears to be excessively distracted during the interview or has revealed multiple inconsistencies or the inability to describe daily activities or to answer specific questions, it is generally advisable to speak with a family member or carer about noted changes in cognition or behaviour.**	Although intellectual capacity does not diminish with advancing age, the brain as it ages does become more susceptible to injury. Delirium is a change in cognition that develops over a short period of time and is characterised by a change in level of alertness, ranging from extreme lethargy to agitation. People with delirium may continuously shift attention from one stimulus to another. Their speech is often difficult to understand because they shift abruptly and inappropriately from one thought to another. It is usually difficult to hold a conversation with a delirious person. Disorientation is more often to time and place rather than to self and delusions and hallucinations may occur.
Do you believe that you have more problems with memory than most? Do you believe that life is empty? Have you recently had to drop many of your activities and interests?	Depression is not more common in old age. However, symptoms of depression in the older person more commonly manifest as changes in cognition (memory deficits, paranoia and agitation) and physical symptoms (muscle aches, joint pains, gastrointestinal (GI) disturbances, headache and weight loss) than they do in younger adults. Depression in the older person has even been called 'pseudodementia'. It can also be a symptom of certain physical disorders, especially endocrine disorders such as hypothyroidism, pancreatic and adrenal disorders, and cancers of all types. Certain antihypertensives, antianxiety drugs and hormones may also precipitate depressive symptoms.
Open-ended questions usually yield the most beneficial information when screening for depression in the older person. However, when time is limited or whenever warning signs are noted, a screening instrument such as the short version of the Geriatric Depression Scale (Yesavage & Brink, 1983) should be used for further validation. (See Self-assessment 34-1.)	When more than five questions are answered as indicated on the tool, a high probability of depressive symptoms exists. The purpose of a screening tool is not to confirm a diagnosis but rather to point out the need for a more in-depth assessment or referral.
Are you concerned about changes in your memory? Are you bothered by anger or inability to control your frustrations with day-by-day living?	By age 85, nearly half the population will be exhibiting signs of the most common type of dementia, Alzheimer disease (AD). Dementia is a broad diagnostic category that includes multiple physical disorders characterised by alterations in memory, abstract thinking, judgement and perception (Assessment tool 34-3). Unlike delirium, dementias are characterised by gradual decline in cognitive function to the extent that daily functions are affected (activities of daily living [ADLs] or instrumental activities of daily living [IADLs]) usually over months or years. Although memory impairment is generally characterised as the key diagnostic criterion for AD, the earliest signs may more often be behavioural and characterised by irritability, aggression or angry outbursts, suspiciousness or even withdrawal.

Continued on page 753

SELF-ASSESSMENT 34-1 ASSESSING GERIATRIC DEPRESSION

Choose the best answer for how you felt over the past week.

1.	Are you basically satisfied with your life?	yes/no
2.	Have you dropped many of your activities and interests?	yes/no
3.	Do you feel that your life is empty?	yes/no
4.	Do you often get bored?	yes/no
5.	Are you hopeful about the future?	yes/no
6.	Are you bothered by thoughts you can't get out of your head?	yes/no
7.	Are you in good spirits most of the time?	yes/no
8.	Are you afraid that something bad is going to happen to you?	yes/no
9.	Do you feel happy most of the time?	yes/no
10.	Do you often feel helpless?	yes/no
11.	Do you often get restless and fidgety?	yes/no
12.	Do you prefer to stay at home, rather than going out and doing new things?	yes/no
13.	Do you frequently worry about the future?	yes/no
14.	Do you feel you have more problems with memory than most?	yes/no
15.	Do you think it is wonderful to be alive now?	yes/no
16.	Do you often feel downhearted and blue?	yes/no
17.	Do you feel pretty worthless the way you are now?	yes/no
18.	Do you worry a lot about the past?	yes/no
19.	Do you find life very exciting?	yes/no
20.	Is it hard for you to get started on new projects?	yes/no
21.	Do you feel full of energy?	yes/no
22.	Do you feel that your situation is hopeless?	yes/no
23.	Do you think that most people are better off than you are?	yes/no
24.	Do you frequently get upset over little things?	yes/no
25.	Do you frequently feel like crying?	yes/no
26.	Do you have trouble concentrating?	yes/no
27.	Do you enjoy getting up in the morning?	yes/no
28.	Do you prefer to avoid social gatherings?	yes/no
29.	Is it easy for you to make decisions?	yes/no
30.	Is your mind as clear as it used to be?	yes/no

For scoring, reverse the answers for Nos. 1, 5, 7, 9, 15, 19, 21, 27, 29 and 30, then count the total number of 'yes' answers. Scoring: 0–10 = within normal range; 11 or higher = possible indication of depression.

Brink, T. A., et al. (1982). Screening tests for geriatric depression. *Clinical Gerontologist*, 1, 37–44.

ASSESSMENT TOOL 34-3 Short Blessed Test

Patient: ________________ DATE: ________________

Age: ____________

Short Blessed Test (SBT)[1]

'Now I would like to ask you some questions to check your memory and concentration. Some of them may be easy and some of them may be hard.'

1. What year is it now? _______	Correct (0)	Incorrect (1)
2. What month is it now? _______	Correct (0)	Incorrect (1)

Please repeat this name and address after me:

John Brown, 42 Market Street, Sydney or Auckland
John Brown, 42 Market Street, Sydney or Auckland
John Brown, 42 Market Street, Sydney or Auckland
(underline words repeated correctly in each trial)
Trials to learning____________(can't do in 3 trials = C)

Good, now remember that name and address for a few minutes.

ASSESSMENT TOOL 34-3 Short Blessed Test (continued)

3. Without looking at your watch or clock, tell me about what time it is.
   (If response is vague, prompt for specific response) — Correct (0) — Incorrect (1)
   (within 1 hour) ___________
   Actual time: ________________

4. Count aloud backwards from 20 to 1 — 0 1 2 Errors
   (Mark correctly sequenced numerals)
   If subject starts counting forwards or forgets the task, repeat instructions and score one error
   20 19 18 17 16 15 14 13 12 11
   10 9 8 7 6 5 4 3 2 1

5. Say the months of the year in reverse order.
   If the tester needs to prompt with the last name of the month of the year, one error should be scored
   (Mark correctly sequenced months)
   D N O S A JL JN MY AP MR F J — 0 1 2 Errors

6. Repeat the name and address I asked you to remember.
   (The thoroughfare term (Street) is not required)
   (John Brown, 42 Market Street, Sydney or Auckland) — 0 1 2 3 4 5 Errors
   ____, _____, ___, _________, ______________

Check correct items **USE ATTACHED SCORING GRID & NORMS**

Short Blessed Test (SBT) Administration and Scoring Guidelines[2]

A spontaneous self-correction is allowed for all responses without counting as an error.

1. What is the year?
   Acceptable Response: The exact year must be given. An incomplete but correct numerical response is acceptable (e.g. 01 for 2001).
2. What is the month?
   Acceptable Response: The exact month must be given. A correct numerical answer is acceptable (e.g. 12 for December).
3. The clinician should state: 'I will give you a name and address to remember for a few minutes. Listen to me say the entire name and address and then repeat it after me.'

   It is important for the clinician to carefully read the phrase and give emphasis to each item of the phrase. There should be a one second delay between individual items.

   The trial phrase should be re-administered until the subject is able to repeat the entire phrase without assistance or until a maximum of three attempts. If the subject is unable to learn the phrase after three attempts, a 'C' should be recorded. This indicates the subject could not learn the phrase in three tries.

   Whether or not the trial phrase is learned, the clinician should instruct 'Good, now remember that name and address for a few minutes.'
4. Without looking at your watch or clock, tell me about what time it is?
   This is scored as correct if the time given is within plus or minus one hour. If the subject's response is vague (e.g. 'almost 1 o'clock'), they should be prompted to give a more specific response.
5. Counting. The instructions should be read as written. If the subject skips a number after 20, an error should be recorded. If the subject starts counting forwards during the task or forgets the task, the instructions should be repeated and one error should be recorded. The maximum number of errors is two.
6. Months. The instructions should be read as written. To get the subject started, the examiner may state 'Start with the last month of the year. The last month of the year is_______________.' If the subject cannot recall the last month of the year, the examiner may prompt this test with 'December'; however, one error should be recorded. If the subject skips a month, an error should be recorded. If the subject starts saying the months forwards upon initiation of the task, the instructions should be repeated and no error recorded. If the subject starts saying the months forwards during the task or forgets the task, the instructions should be repeated and one error recorded. The maximum number of errors is two.
7. Repeat. The subject should state each item verbatim. The address number must be exact (i.e. '4200' would be considered an error for '42'). For the name of the street (i.e. Market Street), the thoroughfare term is not required to be given (i.e. leaving off 'drive' or 'street') or to be correct (i.e. substituting 'boulevard' or 'lane') for the item to be scored correct.
8. The final score is a weighted sum of individual error scores. Use the table below to calculate each weighted score and sum for the total.

Continued on following page

ASSESSMENT TOOL 34-3 Short Blessed Test (continued)

Final SBT score and interpretation

Item no.	Errors (0–5)	Weighting factor	Final item score
1		×4	
2		×3	
3		×3	
4		×2	
5		×2	
6		×2	
			Sum total = ____________ *(Range 0–28)*

Interpretation

A screening test in itself is insufficient to diagnose a dementing disorder. The SBT is, however, quite sensitive to early cognitive changes associated with Alzheimer disease. Scores in the impaired range (see below) indicate a need for further assessment. Scores in the 'normal' range suggest that a dementing disorder is unlikely, but a very early disease process cannot be ruled out. More advanced assessment may be warranted in cases where other objective evidence of impairment exists.

- In the original SBT (Katzman et al., 1983), 90% of normal scores were 6 points or lower, whereas scores of 7 or higher would indicate a need for further evaluation to rule out a disorder such as Alzheimer disease.
- Based on clinical research findings from the Memory and Ageing Project[3], the following cut-off points may also be considered:
  - 0–4: Normal cognition
  - 5–9: Questionable Impairment (evaluate for early dementing disorder)
  - ≥10: Impairment Consistent with Dementia (evaluate for dementing disorder)

[1]Katzman, R., Brown, T., Fuld, P., Schechter, R. & Schimmel, H. (1983). Validation of a short orientation-memory concentration test of cognitive impairment. *American Journal of Psychiatry*, 140, 734–739.

[2]These guidelines and scoring rules are based on the administration experience of faculty and staff of the Memory and Aging Project, Alzheimer's Disease Research Center, Washington University School of Medicine, St Louis (John C. Morris, MD, Director & PI). For more information about the ADRC, please visit our website at http://alzheimer.wustl.edu.

[3]Morris, J. C., Heyman, A., Mohs, R. C., Hughes, J. P., van Belle, G., Fillenbaum, G., Mellits, E. D. & Clark, C. (1989). The Consortium to Establish a Registry for Alzheimer's Disease (CERAD). Part I. Clinical and neurophysiological assessment of Alzheimer's disease. *Neurology*, 39(9), 1159–1165.

COLDSPA

Example adapted to the older person

Use the COLDSPA mnemonic as a guideline to collect needed information for each symptom the patient shares. In addition, the following questions help elicit important information.

Mnemonic	Question
Character	Describe the sign or symptom. How does it feel, look, sound, smell and so forth?
Onset	When did it begin? Did the onset occur shortly after taking a new medication? Is the onset associated with a certain activity or time of day?
Location	Where is it? Does it radiate?
Duration	How long does it last? Does it recur?
Severity	How bad is it? Does it affect functional ability to perform activities of daily living or instrumental activities of daily living?
Pattern	What makes it better? What makes it worse? Does the pattern fit disease geriatric syndrome?
Associated factors/How it Affects the patient	What other symptoms occur with it? What other data would be useful in solving the answer to the presenting problem?

History of present health concerns (continued)

QUESTION	RATIONALE
Falls	
Do you ever need to grab onto something because you feel like you're going to stumble or fall? Have you ever used anything to steady yourself when you're walking?	Risk factor assessment for falls is important because the fall can be a symptom of another problem needing attention. A fall can be the symptom of a treatable medical condition, the result of an adverse response to a medication or a problem associated with chronic illness and frailty. The nurse must be sensitive to an older person's fears and anxieties. Loved ones are also concerned with the safety threat imposed by falls and the possible guilt associated with not being available at the time that a fall occurs. Although the fear of falling is a realistic and common fear, the need to stay active both before and after a fall is even greater. Falling is not a normal part of ageing. Limitations in activity are not the appropriate response to a positive fall assessment. The risk of falling can be minimised by a comprehensive assessment followed by appropriate medical, exercise and adaptive environmental interventions.
Have you had any recent falls? What were you doing? Where did it occur? What other kinds of feelings or symptoms did you have when you fell (e.g. headache, confusion)? Do you ever feel lightheaded or dizzy when you get up from a chair or a bed?	The history should determine the circumstances surrounding any previous falls of the past 3 months to determine if a pattern exists. The pattern and circumstances surrounding the fall can provide valuable clues to the physical, medication or environmental basis for the fall. For example, falls occurring with standing up and associated with dizziness may point to orthostatic hypotension and an adverse reaction to medication. If the patient reports tripping or slipping in the absence of stiffness or weakness and any symptoms, an environmental basis such as shoes or floors with a slick surface or loose carpeting or rugs may be suspected.
Do you have any difficulty when getting up out of bed or from sitting in a chair? Does stiffness and soreness inhibit your ability to move about? Do you ever feel like your legs are going to 'give way' or that they are weak? If so, describe. What is your usual daily pattern of activity? Exercise routine?	Patients may benefit from exercises to improve flexibility, fitness and endurance and to delay functional decline. Exercises can benefit even those who have led sedentary lifestyles or who already have some functional deficits.
Do you have any discomfort in your legs with activity? Would you describe the discomfort as pain, cramping, aching, fatigue or weakness in the calf? Do your hips, thighs or buttocks hurt with ambulation? If so, how far can you walk before the pain occurs? Does the pain go away with rest?	These symptoms are commonly associated with intermittent claudication, a circulatory disorder affecting the peripheral blood vessels of the leg. Symptoms are usually bilateral and progressive.
Weakness: Fatigue and dyspnoea	
How has your energy level changed in the last few days or weeks? How does it affect your daily activities such as cooking, household chores or activities outside the home (e.g. shopping, social, church)? When is your energy at its lowest level? When does it seem to be at its best? **CLINICAL TIP** **When an older person complains of weakness and fatigue, anaemia must always be ruled out. Anaemia is always a symptom of an underlying pathology. A few common causes in the older person are GI bleeding and nutritional deficiencies (especially B12, folate and iron). Anticoagulants and non-steroidal anti-inflammatory drugs (NSAIDs) increase the risk of GI bleeding.**	Self-reported fatigue and weakness, as well as a decline in physical activity and appetite, are common elements of frailty syndrome. The progression of the weakness and how it relates to ADLs and IADLs provides clues to possible aetiologies. For example, a sudden and severe fatigue that affects self-care activities such as bathing and dressing may be more likely to have an acute cause such as infection, myocardial infarction or arrhythmia such as atrial fibrillation. Diminishing energy over months or weeks is more likely to indicate a more insidious pathology such as a slow gastrointestinal bleed, arthritis and pain, or even depression.

Continued on following page

History of present health concerns (continued)

QUESTION	RATIONALE
Do you ever experience shortness of breath? If so, is it related to activity? (Specific questions about endurance, stair climbing or activities of daily living are necessary for quantifying the extent of the problem.) Does it occur at rest or when lying down? How many pillows do you use? Any pain with breathing?	Dyspnoea is a frequently reported symptom associated with common illnesses among older patients, including chronic obstructive pulmonary disease, asthma, lung cancer and heart failure. Older adults with chronic respiratory or cardiac problems who experience some constant degree of dyspnoea are unlikely to seek care or note dyspnoea unless there is a change in functional capabilities.
Do you seem to be breathing faster? Sweating? Do you experience anorexia (loss of appetite) or fatigue?	In the frail elder, an increase in respirations, sweating or overall malaise may be the only indication of a respiratory problem (American Association of Colleges of Nursing [AACN], 2012).
Do you have a recurrent cough? Does it ever have blood in it? Do you use tobacco or have you in the past?	A recurrent cough, fatigue, weight loss, shortness of breath and productive cough (sometimes blood-tinged) are hallmarks of lung cancer (second most common type of cancer in men over age 75, with incidence rising in women).
Weakness: Nutrition and hydration	
Have you experienced any change in your appetite in the past 6 months? If yes, when did you first notice a decline in appetite? Did you have any other health problem at about this same time? Did you start taking any new medication at this time?	A loss of appetite is a nearly universal co-factor of both physical and mental diseases in older people.
Can you describe what you eat in an average day? Compile a 24-hour food and fluid diary noting food preferences and cravings, vitamin and food supplement intake, and dietary restrictions (e.g. salt). On a day when your appetite is less, how would your eating habits change? A screening tool (e.g. Display 34-2 and Self-assessment 34-2) may be helpful in identifying those at risk of being malnourished.	A sudden loss of appetite is most often a symptom of disease or an adverse medication effect. Because the aged body is housing a 'smaller engine', the minimum kilojoule intake does decrease in old age. Even healthy older adults consume only an estimated 5,000 to 6,700 kJ per day. This has led to the general consensus that older adults need nutrient-dense foods to ingest enough essential nutrients. A 3-day food diary, with 1 day being a weekend day, is the most reliable method of obtaining a diet history.
Do you limit the kind or amount of food you eat because of problems with your teeth or dentures (e.g. biting apples or chewing meat)? An oral health assessment tool (Assessment tool 34-4) may help to detect problems.	Oral health is a vital component of good nutrition, socialisation and a positive self-concept. Untreated oral health problems are a common cause of discomfort that may interfere with chewing and digestion.
Do you ever feel like you're choking when you drink water or feel like food is catching in your throat?	Dysphagia is a frequent problem associated with neurological conditions as well as when food is not sufficiently chewed or there is insufficient saliva to mix with food. Dysphagia increases risk of choking, aspiration, dehydration and malnutrition. Signs and symptoms of dysphagia range from weak or hoarse voice, pocketing of food, coughing after food or fluids to drooling.
How much fluid do you think you drink each day?	Fluid intake of less than 1,500 mL daily (excluding caffeine-containing beverages) is a possible indicator of dehydration. Fluid requirements for older persons without cardiac or renal disease are approximately 30 mL/kg of body weight per day. Loss of appetite almost always coexists with inadequate hydration. Decreased thirst sensation is common with ageing. And decreased mobility makes it less possible for the frail older person to respond to an already diminished sense of thirst. Drug use may contribute to dehydration as well. For example, diuretics are widely used in treating cardiovascular and renal disease as are fluid restrictions.

Continued on page 756

DISPLAY 34-2 MINI–NUTRITIONAL ASSESSMENT (MNA®-SF)

Mini Nutritional Assessment MNA®

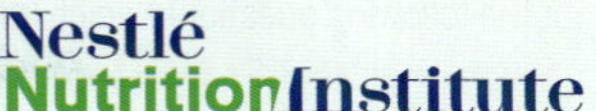

Last name: First name:

Sex: Age: Weight, kg: Height, cm: Date:

Complete the screen by filling in the boxes with the appropriate numbers. Total the numbers for the final screening score.

Screening

A Has food intake declined over the past 3 months due to loss of appetite, digestive problems, chewing or swallowing difficulties?

0 = severe decrease in food intake
1 = moderate decrease in food intake
2 = no decrease in food intake ☐

B Weight loss during the last 3 months

0 = weight loss greater than 3 kg (6.6 lbs)
1 = does not know
2 = weight loss between 1 and 3 kg (2.2 and 6.6 lbs)
3 = no weight loss ☐

C Mobility

0 = bed or chair bound
1 = able to get out of bed / chair but does not go out
2 = goes out ☐

D Has suffered psychological stress or acute disease in the past 3 months?

0 = yes 2 = no ☐

E Neuropsychological problems

0 = severe dementia or depression
1 = mild dementia
2 = no psychological problems ☐

F1 Body Mass Index (BMI) (weight in kg) / (height in m)^2

0 = BMI less than 19
1 = BMI 19 to less than 21
2 = BMI 21 to less than 23
3 = BMI 23 or greater ☐

IF BMI IS NOT AVAILABLE, REPLACE QUESTION F1 WITH QUESTION F2.
DO NOT ANSWER QUESTION F2 IF QUESTION F1 IS ALREADY COMPLETED.

F2 Calf circumference (CC) in cm

0 = CC less than 31
3 = CC 31 or greater ☐

Screening score (max. 14 points)

12 - 14 points: Normal nutritional status
8 - 11 points: At risk of malnutrition
0 - 7 points: Malnourished ☐☐

References

1. Vellas B, Villars H, Abellan G, *et al.* Overview of the MNA® - Its History and Challenges. *J Nutr Health Aging.* 2006;**10**:456-465.
2. Rubenstein LZ, Harker JO, Salva A, Guigoz Y, Vellas B. Screening for Undernutrition in Geriatric Practice: Developing the Short-Form Mini Nutritional Assessment (MNA-SF). *J. Geront.* 2001; **56A**: M366-377
3. Guigoz Y. The Mini-Nutritional Assessment (MNA®) Review of the Literature - What does it tell us? *J Nutr Health Aging.* 2006; **10**:466-487.
4. Kaiser MJ, Bauer JM, Ramsch C, et al. Validation of the Mini Nutritional Assessment Short-Form (MNA®-SF): A practical tool for identification of nutritional status. *J Nutr Health Aging.* 2009; **13**:782-788.

For more information: www.mna-elderly.com

For further information, visit www.mna-elderly.com. Vellas, B., Villars, H., Abellan, G., et al. (2006). Overview of the MNA®—Its history and challenges. *Journal of Nutrition Health and Aging, 10,* 456–465. Rubenstein, L. Z., Harker, J. O., Salva, A., Guigoz, Y., Vellas, B. (2001). Screening for undernutrition in geriatric practice: Developing the Short-Form Mini Nutritional Assessment (MNA-SF). *Journals of Gerontology, 2001;56A,* M366–M377. Guigoz, Y. (2006). The Mini-Nutritional Assessment (MNA®) Review of the literature: What does it tell us? *Journal of Nutrition Health and Aging, 10,* 466–487. Kaiser, M. J., Bauer, J. M., Ramsch, C., et al. (2009). Validation of the Mini Nutritional Assessment Short-Form (MNA®-SF): A practical tool for identification of nutritional status. *Journal of Nutrition Health and Aging, 13,* 782–788. ®Société des Produits Nestlé S.A., Trademark Owners. © Société des Produits Nestlé SA 1994, Revision 2009. N67200 12/99 10M.

SELF-ASSESSMENT 34-2 NUTRITIONAL SCREENING INITIATIVE CHECKLIST TO DETERMINE YOUR NUTRITIONAL HEALTH

The older adult fills out the following questions, which have associated points.

	Yes
I have an illness or condition that made me change the kind or amount of food I eat.	2
I eat fewer than two meals a day.	3
I eat few fruits or vegetables, or milk products.	2
I have three or more drinks of beer, liquor or wine almost every day.	2
I have tooth or mouth problems that make it hard for me to eat.	2
I don't always have enough money to buy the food I need.	4
I eat alone most of the time.	1
I take three or more different prescribed or over-the-counter drugs a day.	1
Without wanting to, I have lost or gained 4.5 kilograms in the last 6 months.	2
I am not always physically able to shop, cook or feed myself.	2
Total nutritional score	______

Scoring:
0–2 indicates good nutrition
3–5 indicates moderate risk
6 or more indicates high nutritional risk

White, J. V., Ham, R. J., Lipschitz, D. A., Dwyer, J. T. & Wellman, N. S. (1991). Consensus of the Nutrition Screening Initiative: Risk factors and indicators of poor nutritional status in older Americans. *Journal of the American Dietetic Society*, 91, 783–787 (used with permission).

History of present health concerns (continued)

QUESTION	RATIONALE
Have you experienced weight loss or changes in your health along with your cough?	Weight loss, night sweats or changes in respiratory status, such as coughing, may be signs of tuberculosis (TB). Debilitated older people are at increased risk of TB. In addition, glucocorticosteroid therapy and nutritional deficiencies depress the immune system, thereby increasing the chances of reactivating a dormant TB infection.
Have you received the pneumococcal vaccine within the past 6 years? Do you get annual flu vaccines?	Pneumonia is the most common cause of infection-related deaths in the older person. The pneumovax is recommended once a lifetime for those over age 65 and every 6 years for high-risk patients. Debilitated and institutionalised elders are particularly at risk for serious influenza-related illness.
Urinary incontinence	
Explain to the patient that many illnesses and medications can cause problems with urine control. This is not normal just because one is getting older, but it is a common problem. Do you ever have any urine leakage or problems controlling your urine flow?	Between 8% and 38% of older adults living at home are incontinent (Anger et al., 2006). The incidence of urinary incontinence is higher for older people who are institutionalised and cognitively impaired. Incidence of new-onset incontinency among hospitalised older adults has been reported at 35% to 42% (Zürcher et al., 2011). Loss of bladder function or control can be an embarrassing and demeaning problem. Unfortunately, many older adults believe that problems with bladder control are a normal and expected part of ageing. Yet this is not an expected part of ageing. Incontinence is often associated with chronic conditions such as stroke, multiple sclerosis, prostatitis and urinary tract infection (UTI). It may also be the result of a faecal impaction or constipation, or an adverse drug effect.

Continued on page 758

ASSESSMENT TOOL 34-4 Oral Health Assessment Tool (OHAT)

Oral Health Assessment Tool

Name ______________ Completed by ______________ Date ______________

- ☐ Is independent
- ☐ Needs reminding
- ☐ Needs supervision
- ☐ Needs full assistance
- ☐ Will not open mouth
- ☐ Grinding or chewing
- ☐ Head faces down
- ☐ Refuses treatment
- ☐ Is aggressive
- ☐ Bites
- ☐ Excessive head movement
- ☐ Cannot swallow well
- ☐ Cannot rinse and spit
- ☐ Will not take dentures out at night

	Healthy	Changes	Unhealthy	Dental Referral
Lips	☐ Smooth, pink, moist	☐ Dry, chapped or red at corners	☐ Swelling or lump, red/white/ulcerated bleeding/ulcerated at corners *	☐ Yes ☐ No
Tongue	☐ Normal moist, roughness, pink	☐ Patchy, fissured, red, coated	☐ Patch that is red and/or white/ulcerated, swollen *	☐ Yes ☐ No
Gums and Oral Tissue	☐ Moist, pink, smooth, no bleeding	☐ Dry, shiny, rough, red, swollen, sore, one ulcer/sore spot, sore under dentures	☐ Swollen, bleeding, ulcers, white/red patches, generalised redness under dentures *	☐ Yes ☐ No
Saliva	☐ Moist tissues watery and free flowing	☐ Dry, sticky tissues, little saliva present, resident thinks they have a dry mouth	☐ Tissues parched and red, very little/no saliva present, saliva is thick, resident thinks they have a dry mouth *	☐ Yes ☐ No

	Healthy	Changes	Unhealthy	Dental Referral
Natural Teeth	☐ No decayed or broken teeth or roots	☐ 1- 3 decayed or broken teeth/roots, or teeth very worn down	☐ 4 or more decayed or broken teeth/roots or fewer than 4 teeth, or very worn down teeth *	☐ Yes ☐ No
Dentures	☐ No broken areas or teeth, worn regularly, and named	☐ 1 broken area or tooth, or worn 1-2 hours per day only or not named	☐ 1 or more broken areas or teeth, denture missing / not worn, need adhesive, or not named *	☐ Yes ☐ No
Oral Cleanliness	☐ Clean and no food particles or tartar in mouth or on dentures	☐ Food, tartar, plaque 1-2 areas of mouth, or on small area of dentures	☐ Food particles, tartar, plaque most areas of mouth, or on most of dentures *	☐ Yes ☐ No
Dental Pain	☐ No behavioural, verbal or physical signs of dental pain	☐ Verbal &/or behavioural signs of pain such as pulling at face, chewing lips, not eating, changed behaviour.	☐ Physical pain signs (swelling of cheek or gum, broken teeth, ulcers), as well as verbal &/or behavioural signs (pulling at face, not eating, changed behaviour) *	☐ Yes ☐ No

* Unhealthy signs usually indicate referral to a dentist is necessary

Assessor Comments

Lewis, A., and Manuel, Eliza. Buiding Better Oral Health Communities: Better Oral Health in Home Care, South Australia Department of Health, Adelaide, © SA Dental Service, Central Adealide Local Health Network.

History of present health concerns (continued)

QUESTION	RATIONALE
(Male) Do you have difficulty starting a stream of urine? Frequency? Night time frequency? Dribbling? If yes, do you ever take any cold or sinus medications or medication to help you sleep?	Benign prostatic hypertrophy occurs in 80% of men over age 70 from exposure to androgen hormones. It may result in urinary frequency, difficulty starting a stream of urine, nocturia and urinary retention with overflow incontinence and an increased risk of UTI. Over-the-counter drugs with anticholinergic side effects (e.g. cold or sinus preparations and sleep medications) may contribute to urinary retention or add to obstructive symptoms.
How long has the leakage (or use patient's descriptive words) been going on? Has it ever suddenly become worse?	Any new onset of incontinence or exacerbation may indicate an infection. In the hospitalised elder, UTI ranks high as a suspected cause for any new onset of incontinence. UTI is the most common hospital-acquired bacterial infection. UTI must also be a concern for elders at home or in long-term care because it is the most frequent source of bacteraemia for these people. A UTI is particularly perplexing in older patients because it presents in such an atypical way (i.e. without fever, or elevation in white blood cell counts, or dysuria, or urinary frequency). Even more common symptoms of a UTI in the frail person may be confusion, lethargy, anorexia and nocturia.
What activities are associated with your loss of urine control?	The patient's activities during an episode of incontinence may help to determine the type of incontinence and, therefore, its treatment. See Display 34-3 for a description of the kinds of urinary incontinence.
Bowel elimination	
Do you have any problems with bowel elimination?	As people age, GI motility decreases because of a loss of muscle tone and atrophy. Dehydration, immobility and poor intake exacerbate the likelihood of constipation. Adequate fluid intake, dietary fibre and moderate exercise are key factors in maintaining efficient elimination.
Have you had a change in bowel habits recently? Have you ever had blood in your stools? Have you had your stools tested for blood? What medications do you take?	The guaiac stool test to detect occult blood is a common test administered to detect abnormalities of the GI tract. Patients with a history of polyps, adenomas and inflammatory bowel disease are at increased risk for colorectal cancer in old age. Warning signs include rectal bleeding, unexplained weight loss and a change in bowel habits. NSAIDs, such as aspirin and naproxen, corticosteroids, and anticoagulants such as warfarin may promote GI bleeding.
Pain assessment	
Do you have pain, discomfort, aching or soreness? If so, is the discomfort worse with activity? Relieved by rest? Do you have problems with grasping, reaching or activities that use your hands, arms, back or legs?	Functional limitations and pain are common consequences of inflammatory joint disease in the frail person. The combination of pain and functional impairment may predispose the patient to social isolation and depression.
Pain scales used with adults are also usually valid in evaluating pain in an older patient except in the more severe stages of dementia. For those with moderate levels of dementia but who are still able to verbalise, short and frequent questioning about pain using words such as 'hurting', 'soreness', 'aching' or 'uncomfortable' may be useful. For non-verbal individuals with dementia, behaviours such as grimacing, striking out and moaning should be routinely evaluated to identify pain and assess the degree to which the pain is being relieved (Display 34-4). Many of the behaviours commonly labelled as 'aggressive' or 'combative' are the result of untreated pain (Douzjian et al., 1998).	As many as 50% of community-dwelling older people suffer from persistent pain and up to 80% of nursing home residents have substantiated pain that is undertreated (British Geriatrics Society/British Pain Society, 2013). Pain can lead quickly to a downward cascade of anxiety, depression, isolation and functional decline. Acute pain frequently manifests as confusion.

DISPLAY 34-3 UNDERSTANDING URINARY INCONTINENCE: ASSESSMENT AND INTERVENTION

Types of incontinence

The signs and symptoms associated with the involuntary loss of urine have been clustered into three categories: urge, stress and overflow incontinence. Any one or a combination of all three types may be present in an individual. Voiding diaries are useful for determining the type of incontinence that is occurring based on the amount, timing and associated symptoms of incontinent episodes.

Urge incontinence

Urge incontinence is the involuntary loss of urine associated with an abrupt and strong desire to void. It is frequently caused by a neurological disorder such as a cerebrovascular accident or multiple sclerosis, which impairs the ability of the bladder or urinary sphincter to contract and relax. However, urge incontinence is commonly associated with bladder overactivity without any underlying neurological disorder.

Stress incontinence

Stress incontinence is the involuntary loss of urine during coughing, sneezing, laughing or other physical activities that increase abdominal pressure. In women, stress incontinence may result from weakened and relaxed muscles from the combined effects of ageing superimposed on the effects of childbirth.

Note: Atrophic vaginitis from oestrogen deficiency usually results in symptoms of urge incontinence as well as stress incontinence (mixed incontinence).

Overflow incontinence

Overflow incontinence is the involuntary loss of urine associated with overdistension of the bladder. Prostatic hypertrophy is a common cause in men, and diabetic neuropathy is a common cause in both sexes.

Functional incontinence

Functional incontinence is the inability to get to the bathroom in time or to understand the cues to void due to problems with mobility or cognition.

Steps of assessment

The nursing assessment varies somewhat depending on the patient's general health status and whether the problem is an acute or chronic one. In general, however, a comprehensive nursing assessment can be described as a five-step process that includes screening for an infection with a urinalysis, obtaining a voiding diary, evaluating functional status, compiling a health history and performing a physical examination. Key features within the five steps follow:

- Record all incontinent and continent episodes for 3 days in a voiding diary.
- Review medication for any newly prescribed drugs that may be triggering incontinence. Follow up with doctor regarding need to discontinue therapy or change medication.
- Rule out constipation or faecal impaction as a source of urinary incontinence. If patient has had no bowel movement within last 3 days or is oozing stool continuously, check for impaction by digital examination or abdominal palpation. Problem should be treated if identified.
- Assess functional status along with signs and symptoms as they relate to incontinence. Contributors to incontinence may include immobility, insufficient fluid intake and confusion. Accompanying signs and symptoms include polyuria, nocturia, dysuria, hesitancy, poor or interrupted urine stream, straining, suprapubic or perineal pain, urgency and characteristics of incontinent episodes (precipitated by walking, coughing, getting in and out of bed and so forth).
- Consult doctor regarding physical examination and need to measure postvoid residual volume using a portable ultrasound device (e.g. bladder scanner). Catheterisation is rarely performed for postvoid residual estimation. Components of the physical examination include direct observation of urine loss using a cough stress test; abdominal, rectal, genital and pelvic examination; and identification of neurological abnormalities. Abdominal and vaginal examinations are performed to detect prolapse or a palpable bladder after micturition.

Interventions

The doctor is responsible for identifying and treating the conditions causing reversible or chronic incontinence. A physiotherapist may play a role in identifying specific activities that are associated with incontinent episodes. Either a nurse or a physiotherapist may be involved in teaching Kegel exercises to help relieve stress incontinence. When functional incontinence and urgency have been identified, the expertise of an occupational therapist in appropriate dressing and undressing and for choosing incontinence aids may be beneficial.

Voiding diary

Time	Drinks		Voiding	
	Kind	How much	How many times	How much
6–7 AM	Coffee	2 cups	I	medium
7–8 AM	orange juice	1 glass	II	lots
8–9 AM	—	—	I	little
9–10 AM	—	—	—	—
10–11 AM	water	1 glass	I	medium

Time	Leaks/accidents	Strength of urge	Activity at the time of leak
6–7 AM		strong	no leak
7–8 AM		strong	
8–9 AM	I		frying eggs
9–10 AM			
10–11 AM			

DISPLAY 34-4 INDICATORS OF PAIN IN THE COGNITIVELY IMPAIRED

- Medical diagnoses known to commonly cause pain such as arthritis, osteoporosis, fractures, cancer and history of back pain
- Pain history and use of analgesics
- Family or professional carer reports of possible pain
- Behavioural patterns of aggressiveness or resisting care
- Rubbing on specific areas of body
- Vocalisations, such as moaning (yelling, or increases in the loudness of existing vocalisations)

COLLECTING OBJECTIVE DATA: PHYSICAL EXAMINATION

CASE STUDY

Until the last 5 to 10 years, Mrs Kimberley was 165 cm and weighed approximately 59 kg. She is now 160 cm tall and weighs 56 kg.

CRITICAL THINKING

6. Make a list of the possible reasons for Mrs Kimberley's loss of height and weight.

There is often a fine line between deterioration of function from ageing and deterioration from disease. For this reason, it is crucial to integrate the subjective, functional and physical assessments. The significance of a physical finding is often determined by the effect it has on the person's level of comfort and ability to function. A medical pathology should be suspected whenever any physical or functional change has occurred suddenly (days to weeks).

An efficient and effective way to determine the significance of physical findings in an older person is to collect subjective data while you are conducting a physical examination. Because medication is often a primary method of treating disease in Australia and New Zealand, and *polypharmacy* is such a common occurrence in the older person, sudden changes or abnormalities noted in the physical examination must always be analysed for the possibility of being the result of an adverse drug effect. Because many diseases have a 'silent' presentation in the older person, an in-depth, comprehensive physical examination is especially important to detect and treat disease in a timely way.

CULTURAL CONSIDERATIONS

For some Aboriginal and Torres Strait Islander Australians, direct eye contact is forbidden, for reasons including gender and seniority. When engaging the older person from this group, position yourself slightly side-on or at arm's length to facilitate communication without the need to make direct eye contact. However, do not avoid contact because you are afraid to cause offense.

Preparing the patient

The nurse needs to examine one's own attitudes or stereotypical assumptions of the older patient. It is essential that the nurse also be sensitive to the patient's need for privacy as well as his or her wishes for a carer to remain in the room during all or parts of the assessment.

The examination of a frail adult usually takes longer than that of a younger adult because of the chronic conditions, disabilities and ensuing discomfort that many frail people experience. It is best to limit the length of the examination. This may mean that a complete assessment may require several sessions over a period of time. The patient may feel less hurried if paperwork, such as a health questionnaire, can be completed at home either by the patient alone or with the help of a carer. Some modifications and techniques appropriate for an examination of the frail person include the following:

- Keep the temperature of the examination room warmer than may be comfortable for younger adults.
- Eliminate background noise as much as possible.
- When interacting with an older patient, remember that it may be more acceptable to be more formal than informal. For example, address the patient by first name only if the patient specifically requests that you do so.
- Keep your voice volume down, even if you anticipate the patient has difficulty hearing. Speaking clearly and at a moderate pace is more beneficial in cases of hearing loss. Remember to face the patient when speaking with him or her.
- Do not assume that the patient cannot answer questions if he or she has a cognitive impairment. However, if the impairment has significantly impaired function or verbal expression, give only one-step directions and avoid questions that require two responses. The cognitively impaired older person with few remaining verbal abilities may have no or only minimal loss of the ability to comprehend non-verbal cues.
- If you need to question carers or collateral sources to validate or clarify information, avoid consulting them in the presence of the patient.
- Older people with physical disabilities may need assistance with dressing and with repositioning themselves during the examination. Allow additional time in deference to the patient's need for independence as well as your need to know how much the patient can do independently.

CLINICAL TIP

When speaking to an older adult who suffers from hearing loss, speak to them face-to-face and use a moderate pace and medium tone rather than raising your voice or speaking too quickly.

Equipment

In addition to the equipment needed for performing a complete adult physical examination, the following items will be needed for assessing the functional capacity of the older adult:

- Newspaper or book and lamp light for vision testing
- Lemon slice or mint for sense of smell test
- Thick fluid or food of pudding consistency and spoon for swallowing examination (a teacup with water to swallow may also be used)
- Food and fluid diary sheets or forms
- Two or three pillows for patient comfort and positioning
- Straight-backed chair for 'Get up and go' test.

PHYSICAL ASSESSMENT

ASSESSMENT PROCEDURE	NORMAL FINDINGS OR VARIATIONS	ABNORMAL FINDINGS
Measure and record the patient's height and weight, noting weight changes and problems with swallowing or chewing. Review laboratory test values (full blood count, and vitamin B12, cholesterol, albumin and prealbumin levels). **CLINICAL TIP** **Suspect drug toxicity in patients taking medications such as digoxin, theophylline, quinidine or antibiotics if patient reports nausea or diarrhoea.**	Antral cells and intestinal villi atrophy, and gastric production of hydrochloric acid decreases with age. Chronic diseases such as cancer and arthritis are associated with increases in inflammatory chemicals that can cause anorexia and fatigue. A certain degree of anorexia also always accompanies pain—especially chronic pain. (See Chap. 8 for a discussion of pain assessment.) Toxic levels of drugs must always be suspected when appetite loss is sudden and severe. The ability to smell and taste decreases with age, which can also diminish appetite. Medications can also decrease sense of smell and taste in older people.	Indicators of malnutrition include: Patient weighs less than 80% ideal body weight. Patient has had 10% loss in body weight over the past 6 months or 5% loss in body weight over the past month. Haemoglobin level is lower than 120 g/L. Haematocrit is lower than 0.37. (*Note:* A value is not given because this is a proportion of the total blood volume, also known as packed cell volume, which can also be expressed as a percentage, i.e. 37%.) Vitamin B12 serum is lower than 120 µmol/L. Indicators of poor nutritional status include: Serum cholesterol level is lower than 4.0 mmol/L. Serum albumin level is lower than 35 g/L. Serum prealbumin levels (used to monitor improvement of nutritional status) do not increase 10 mg/L/day.
Because muscle mass decreases and fatty tissues increase, the older patient is at increased risk for dehydration. Evaluate hydration status as you would nutritional status. Begin with accurate serial measurements of weight, careful review of laboratory test findings (serial serum sodium level, haematocrit, osmolality, blood urea nitrogen [BUN] level, and urine-specific gravity), and a 2- to 3-day diary of fluid intake and output.	Normal findings include stable weight and stable mental status. **CLINICAL TIP** **Increases over time in laboratory values are usually indicators of deteriorating hydration (even though values may be within normal limits).**	Sudden weight loss; fever; dry, warm skin; furrowed, swollen and red tongue; decreased urine output; lethargy and weakness are all signs of dehydration. An acute change in mental status (particularly confusion), tachycardia and hypotension may indicate severe dehydration, which may be precipitated by certain medications such as diuretics, laxatives, tricyclic antidepressants or lithium.

ASSESSMENT PROCEDURE	NORMAL FINDINGS	ABNORMAL FINDINGS
Skin and hair		
INSPECTION AND PALPATION		
Inspect and palpate skin lesions. Wear gloves when palpating lesions. Note whether lesions are flat or raised, palpable or non-palpable. Also note colour, size and exudates, if any. Despite a decrease in the total number of melanocytes, hyperpigmentation occurs in sun-exposed skin (neck, face and arms). Although dermatological lesions are common, many are benign. The combination of environmental exposure and diminished immunity increases the risk of skin cancer and cutaneous infections such as ringworm, *Candida* infections of mouth, vagina and nail beds. This risk is increased by predisposing conditions such as diabetes mellitus, malnutrition, steroid or antibiotic use.	Normal findings include the following: Lentigines: Hyperpigmentation in sun-exposed areas appear as brown, pigmented, round or rectangular patches (Fig. 34-1). Often called liver spots. Venous lakes: Reddish vascular lesions on ears or other facial areas resulting from dilation of small, red blood vessels. Skin tags: Acrochordons, flesh-coloured pedunculated lesions. Seborrhoeic keratoses: Tan, brown or reddish flat lesions commonly found on fair-skinned persons in sun-exposed areas. Cherry angiomas: Small, round, red spots. Senile purpura: Vivid purple patches (lesion should not blanch to touch).	Abnormal findings include: Irregularly shaped lesion or scaly, elevated lesion (squamous cell carcinoma). Actinic keratoses, round or irregularly shaped tan, scaly lesions that may bleed or be inflamed (premalignancy). Waxy or raised lesion, especially on sun-exposed (basal cell carcinoma) areas. Herpes zoster vesicles (shingles) draining clear fluid or pustules atop an erythematous base following a clear linear pattern and accompanied by pain. More than half of older people with shingles will have neuralgia that persists after resolution of the skin lesions. Pinpoint-sized, red-purple, non-blanchable petechiae (a common sign of platelet deficiency).

Continued on following page

PHYSICAL ASSESSMENT (continued)

ASSESSMENT PROCEDURE	NORMAL FINDINGS	ABNORMAL FINDINGS
Skin and hair (continued)		
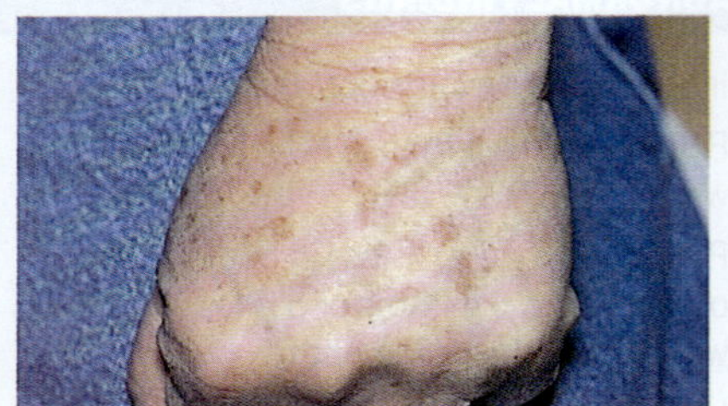 **FIGURE 34-1** Solar lentigines are very common on ageing skin.		Large bruises may result from anticoagulant therapy, a fall, renal or liver failure, or elder abuse.
Note colour, texture, integrity and moisture of skin and sensitivity to heat or cold.	Somewhat transparent, pale, skin with an overall decrease in body hair on lower extremities. Dry skin is common.	Torn skin (possibly the result of abrasive tape used to hold bandages or tubes in place).
Elastic collagen is gradually replaced with more fibrous tissue and loss of subcutaneous tissue. Decreased vascularity and diminished neurological response to temperature changes and atrophy of eccrine sweat glands increases risk of hyperthermia and hypothermia. **CLINICAL TIP** **Room humidifiers, avoidance of harsh deodorants or soaps, and use of lanolin-containing products after bathing (while skin is still moist) may help to relieve the effects of dry skin.**	Skin may wrinkle and tent when pinched. *Note:* Pinching skin is not an accurate test of turgor in the older people.	Extremely thin, fragile skin (friable skin) with excessive purpura (possibly from corticosteroid use). Dry, warm skin, furrowed tongue and sunken eyes from dehydration (especially when the patient has decreased urinary output, increased serum sodium, BUN and creatinine levels, increased osmolality and haematocrit values, tachycardia; and mental confusion). Sudden heat or cold intolerance could be signs of thyroid dysfunction.
Inspect and palpate hair and scalp.	Loss of pigmentation causes greying of scalp, axillary and pubic hair. Mild hair growth on the upper lip of women may appear as result of decreased oestrogen to testosterone ratio. Toenails usually thicken whereas fingernails often become thinner. Both usually become yellowish and dull.	Patchy or asymmetric hair loss is abnormal.
Head and neck		
INSPECTION		
Inspect head and neck for symmetry and movement. Observe facial expression (Fig. 34-2). 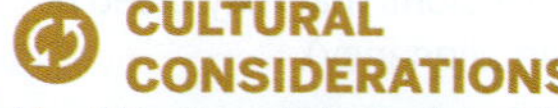 **CULTURAL CONSIDERATIONS** **For Māori, certain parts of the body are regarded as *tapu* or sacred, for example, the head, the heart and the genitalia. If you need to touch a person's head, show respect by asking for his or her consent and explaining what needs to be done.**	Atrophy of face and neck muscles. Reduced range of motion of head and neck. Shortening of neck due to vertebral degeneration and development of 'buffalo hump' at the top of the cervical vertebrae. 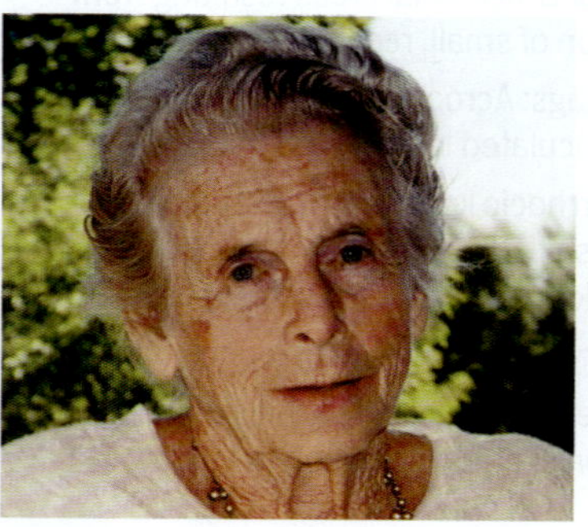 **FIGURE 34-2** Observe facial expression.	Abnormalities include: Asymmetry of mouth or eyes possibly from Bell palsy or cerebrovascular accident (CVA). Marked limitation of movement or crepitation in back of the neck from cervical arthritis. Involuntary facial or head movements from an extrapyramidal disorder such as Parkinson disease or some medications. Reported episodic, unilateral, shocklike or burning pain of the face or continuous pain, which may be postherpetic or caused by a dental caries or abscess. *Note:* In cognitively impaired elders, sleep disturbances or agitation may be the only sign of neuropathic pain.

PHYSICAL ASSESSMENT (continued)

ASSESSMENT PROCEDURE	NORMAL FINDINGS	ABNORMAL FINDINGS
Mouth and throat		
INSPECTION		
Inspect the gums and buccal mucosa for colour and consistency.	Slight decrease in saliva production.	Saliva-depressing medications include antihistamines, antipsychotics, antihypertensives and any drug with anticholinergic side effects may promote dental caries and increase risk of pneumonia.
If the patient is wearing dentures, inspect them for fit. Then ask the patient to remove them for the rest of the oral examination.	Resorption of gum ridge commonly results in poorly fitting dentures. Tooth surfaces may be worn from prolonged use.	Loose-fitting dentures or inability to close mouth completely may also be the result of a significant weight gain or loss. Foul-smelling breath may indicate periodontal disease. Whitish or yellow-tinged patches in mouth or throat may be candidiasis from use of steroid inhalers or antibiotics.
Examine the tongue. Observe symmetry and size.	Tongue pink and moist.	A swollen, red and painful tongue may indicate vitamin B or riboflavin deficiency.
Observe the patient swallowing food or fluids (Fig. 34-3). **SAFETY TIP** **Help the patient who reports dysphagia to lean slightly forwards with the chin tucked in towards the neck when swallowing and offer food of pudding consistency to minimise the risk of aspiration.**	Mild decrease in swallowing ability.	Coughing, drooling, pocketing or spitting out food after intake are all possible signs of dysphagia. A drooping mouth, chronic congestion or a weak or hoarse voice (especially after eating or drinking) also suggests dysphagia. Observed swallowing difficulties in which case a nutritional assessment should be completed and the patient referred for a barium swallow examination.

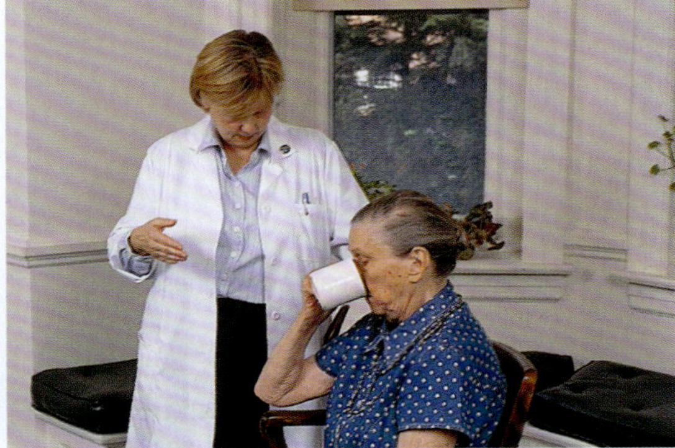

FIGURE 34-3 Assessing for swallowing problems. (© B. Proud.)

ASSESSMENT PROCEDURE	NORMAL FINDINGS	ABNORMAL FINDINGS
Nose and sinuses		
INSPECTION		
Inspect the nose for colour and consistency.	Nose and nasal passages are not inflamed, and skin and mucous membranes are intact. Nose may seem more prominent on face because of loss of subcutaneous fat. Nasal hairs are coarser.	Oedema, redness, swelling or clear drainage, which may indicate allergies or rhinitis.

Continued on following page

PHYSICAL ASSESSMENT (continued)

ASSESSMENT PROCEDURE	NORMAL FINDINGS	ABNORMAL FINDINGS
Nose and sinuses (continued)		
		CLINICAL TIP **Relocation into a newly constructed residential or long-term care facility should be investigated further as a possible cause of allergic or non-allergic rhinitis. New carpet, chipboard cupboards and paint fumes can elicit a non-allergic vasomotor response as well as an allergic one.**
Evaluate the sense of smell. Have the patient close his or her eyes and smell a common substance, such as mint, lemon or soap (Fig. 34-4). **SAFETY TIP** **Alert patients with diminished smell to the importance of smoke alarms and routine inspections of stoves and furnaces.**	Slightly diminished sense of smell and ability to detect odours.	Patient cannot identify strong odour. This may cause a decrease in appetite and may be a safety concern.
Test nasal patency by asking the patient to breathe while blocking one nostril at a time (Fig. 34-5).	Breathes with reasonable ease.	Patient reports feeling of inadequate breath intake, which may result from nasal polyps, a deviated septum, or allergic or infectious rhinitis or sinusitis.

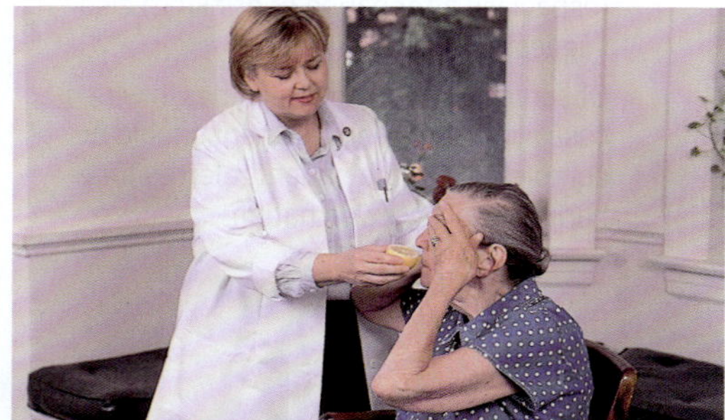
FIGURE 34-4 Assessing sense of smell. (© B. Proud.)

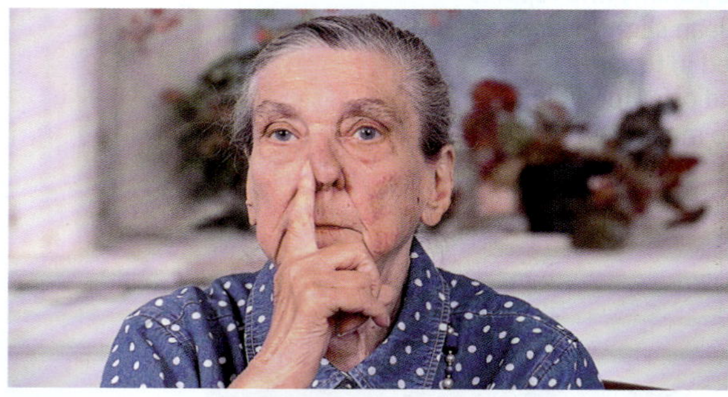
FIGURE 34-5 Testing nasal patency. (© B. Proud.)

ASSESSMENT PROCEDURE	NORMAL FINDINGS	ABNORMAL FINDINGS
PALPATION		
Palpate the frontal and maxillary sinuses for consistency and to elicit possible pain. **SAFETY TIP** **Older patients with nasogastric feeding tubes are at increased risk for sinusitis related to the obstruction.**	No lesions or pain.	Patient reports pain and dryness; inflammation is evident. **CLINICAL TIP** **Older patients may self-treat sinus pain or nasal congestion with decongestants and antihistamines, which may further dry the nasal passages and prevent normal sinus drainage. These drugs may also aggravate hypertension (in patients taking antihypertensive drugs) and exacerbate cardiac arrhythmias. In patients taking antibiotics for sinusitis, watch for adverse effects on renal function. Because antibiotics also may kill normal bacteria, watch for signs of candidal or *Clostridium difficile* infection in the gastrointestinal (GI) tract, mouth or vagina.**

PHYSICAL ASSESSMENT (continued)

ASSESSMENT PROCEDURE	NORMAL FINDINGS	ABNORMAL FINDINGS
Eyes and vision		
INSPECTION		
Inspect eyes, eyelids, eyelashes and conjunctiva. Also observe eye and conjunctiva for dryness, redness, tearing or increased sensitivity to light and wind.	Skin around the eyes becomes thin, and wrinkles appear normally with age. Stretched skin in eyelid may produce feeling of heaviness and a tired feeling. In the lower eyelid, 'bags' form. Excessive stretching of the lower eyelid may cause it to droop downwards, which keeps it from shutting completely and can cause dryness, redness or sensitivity to light and wind. Eyes are described as irritated or having a 'scratchy sensation'.	A turning in of the lower eyelid (entropion) is more common and causes the eyelashes to touch the conjunctiva and cornea. Severe entropion may result in an ulcerous corneal infection. Abnormalities in blinking may result from Parkinson disease; dull or blank staring may be a sign of hypothyroidism.
Inspect the cornea and lens. Also ask the patient when he or she last had an eye and vision examination. **CLINICAL TIP** **To detect glaucoma, tonometry should be performed every 1 to 2 years on everyone older than 35. Elevated intraocular pressure indicates the need for referral to an ophthalmologist and confirmation with applanation tonometry.**	An arcus senilis, a cloudy or greyish ring around the iris, and decreased pigment in iris are age-related changes. The lens loses elasticity, which results in decreased ability to change shape (presbyopia). A loss of transparency in the crystalline lens of the eyes is a natural part of the ageing process. Exposure to sunlight, smoking and inherited tendencies increase risk.	Cataracts most commonly affect people after age 55 and result in a yellowish or brownish discolouration of the lens. Common symptoms include painless blurring of vision, glare and halos around lights, poor night vision, and colours that look dull or brownish. Location and extent of cloudiness determine degree to which a person's vision is affected. A thickening of the bulbar conjunctiva that grows over the cornea (called pterygium) may interfere with vision.
Inspect the pupils. With a penlight or similar device, test pupillary reaction to light (Fig. 34-6).	Overall decrease in pupil size and ability to dilate in dark and constrict in light may occur with advanced age; this results in poorer night vision and decreased tolerance to glare.	An irregularly shaped pupil may indicate removal of a cataract. Asymmetrical response may be due to a neurological condition.
Test vision. Ask the patient to read from a newspaper or magazine. Use only room lighting for the initial reading. Use task lighting for a second reading (Fig. 34-7). Ask about changes in vision, trouble with night vision or differences in vision with left versus right eye.	Impaired near vision is indicative of presbyopia (farsightedness), a common finding in older adults. Also common are slight decreases in peripheral vision and difficulty in differentiating blues from greens. **CLINICAL TIP** **Older adults generally require two to three times more diffuse and task lighting.**	A significant decrease in central vision, to the extent needed for activities of daily living, may signal a cataract in one or both eyes. *Macular degeneration* (thin membrane in the centre of the retina) is suspected if the patient has difficulty in seeing with one eye (see Abnormal findings 34-1). The disorder almost always becomes bilateral. Related abnormal findings include blurry words in the centre of the page or door frames that don't appear straight. This condition should be referred and evaluated.

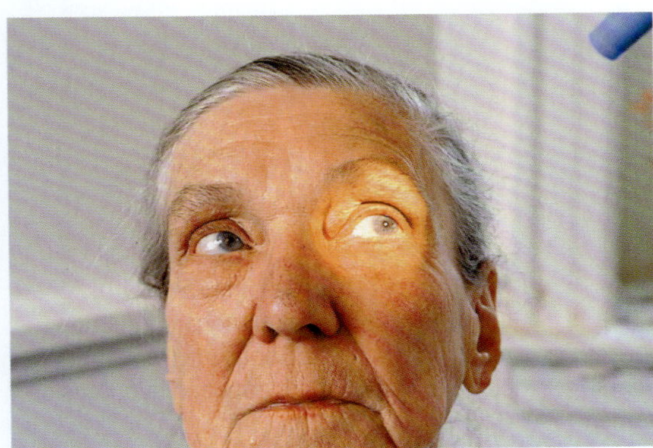

FIGURE 34-6 Testing pupillary reaction. (© B. Proud.)

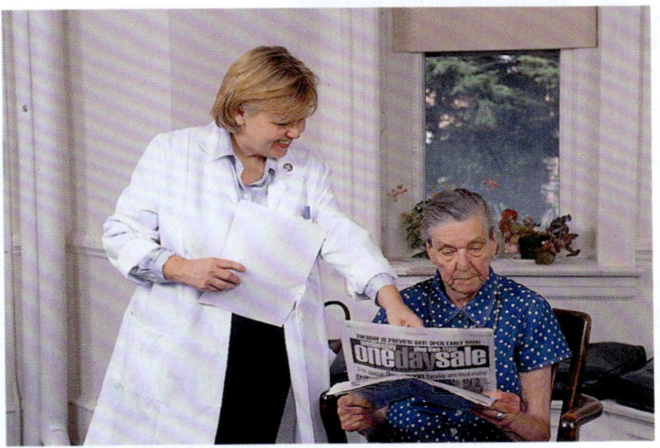

FIGURE 34-7 Reading with room lighting. (© B. Proud.)

Continued on following page

PHYSICAL ASSESSMENT (continued)

ASSESSMENT PROCEDURE	NORMAL FINDINGS	ABNORMAL FINDINGS
Eyes and vision (continued)		
Also ask patient about small specks or 'clouds' that move across the field of vision.	With ageing, tiny clumps of gel may develop within the eye. These are referred to as 'floaters'. They should occur occasionally and not increase significantly in frequency.	A noticeable loss of vision—including cloudiness, distortion of familiar objects and occasionally blind spots or floaters—is a common symptom of diabetic retinopathy. New floaters, an increase in frequency of floaters associated with flashes of light may be a sign of retinal detachment. This requires immediate referral to prevent blindness (see Abnormal findings 34-1).
Ears and hearing		
INSPECTION		
Inspect the external ear. Observe shape, colour and hair growth. Also look for lesions or drainage.	Hairs may become coarser and thicker in the external ear, especially in men. Earlobes may elongate and penna increases in length and width.	Inflammation, drainage or swelling may be from infection.
Perform an otoscopic examination to determine quantity, colour and consistency of cerumen.	Cerumen production decreases, leading to dryness and tendency towards accumulation.	Hard, dark brown cerumen signals impaction of the auditory canal, which commonly causes a conductive hearing loss. A darkened hole in the tympanic membrane or patches indicates perforation or scarring of the tympanic membrane.
Perform the *voice–whisper test*, a functional examination to detect obvious (conversational) hearing loss. Instruct the patient to put a hand over one ear and to repeat the sentence you say. Stand approximately 60 cm away from the patient and whisper a sentence (Fig. 34-8). 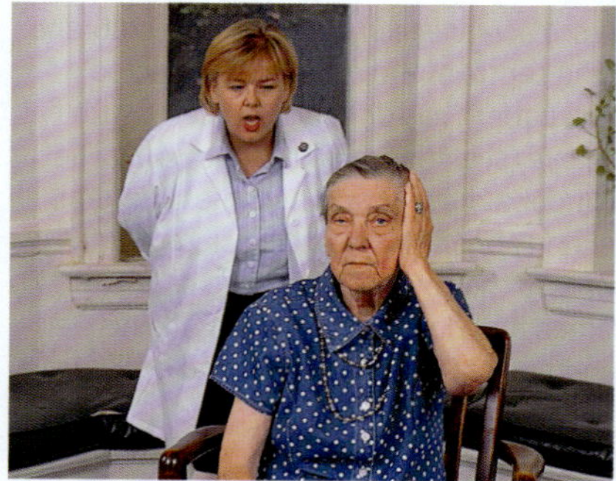 **FIGURE 34-8** Assessing hearing with the voice-whisper test. (© B. Proud.)	The inability to hear high-frequency sounds (presbycusis) or to discriminate a variety of simultaneous sounds and soft consonant sounds or background noises is due to degeneration of hair cells of inner ear. **CLINICAL TIP** **Assess hearing acuity before as well as after the otoscopic examination, if cerumen is removed during the examination. If you are facing the patient, hold your hand close to your mouth so the patient cannot read your lips.**	Inability to hear the whispered sentence indicates a hearing deficiency and the need to refer the patient to an audiologist for testing. **CLINICAL TIP** **Raising one's voice to someone with presbycusis usually only makes it more difficult for them to hear. Speaking more slowly will usually lower the frequency and be more therapeutic.**
Thorax and lungs		
INSPECTION		
Inspect shape of thorax. Note respiratory rate, rhythm and quality of breathing.	Decreased elasticity of alveoli causes lungs to recoil less during expiration and loss of resilience that holds thorax in a contracted position, loss of skeletal muscle strength in thorax and abdomen, decreased vital capacity, increased residual volume and slight barrel chest.	Respiratory rate exceeding 25 breaths/minute may signal a pulmonary infection along with increased sputum production, confusion, loss of appetite and hypotension (McGann, 2000). Respiratory rate of less than 16 breaths/minute may be a sign of neurological

PHYSICAL ASSESSMENT (continued)

ASSESSMENT PROCEDURE	NORMAL FINDINGS	ABNORMAL FINDINGS
	Increased reliance on diaphragmatic breathing and increased work of breathing.	impairment, which may lead to aspiration pneumonia. Significant loss of aerobic capacity and dyspnoea with exertion is usually due to disease, exposure over a lifetime to pollutants, smoke, or severe or prolonged lack of exercise.
PERCUSSION		
Percuss lung tones as you would in a younger adult.	Resonant, except in the presence of structural changes such as kyphosis or a slight barrel chest, when hyperresonance may occur.	Consolidation of infection will cause dullness to percussion; alveolar retention of air, as occurs in emphysema, results in hyperresonance. **SAFETY TIP** **Supine positioning, shallow breathing and poor dental hygiene increase the risk of pulmonary infection. Pneumonia is the most common cause of infection-related deaths in the older person and is called the 'silent killer'. It seldom presents as the classic triad of cough, fever and pleuritic pain. Instead, subtle changes such as an increase in respiratory rate and sputum production, confusion, loss of appetite and hypotension are more likely to be the presenting symptoms (Fitzpatrick et al., 2000).**
AUSCULTATION		
Auscultate lung sounds as you would in a younger adult.	Vesicular sounds should be heard over all areas of air exchange. However, because lung expansion may be diminished, it may be necessary to emphasise taking deep breaths with the mouth open during the exam. Following an instruction to take a deep breath may be very difficult for those with dementia.	Breath sounds may be distant over areas affected by kyphosis or the barrel chest of ageing. Wheezes and crackles are heard only with diseases, such as pulmonary oedema, pneumonia or restrictive disorders. Diminished breath sounds, wheezes, crackles, rhonchi that do not clear with cough and egophony are common signs of consolidation caused by pneumonia.
Heart and blood vessels		
BLOOD PRESSURE		
Take blood pressure to detect actual or potential orthostatic hypotension and, therefore, the risk for falling. Measure pressure with the patient in lying, sitting and standing positions. Also measure pulse rate. Have the patient lie down for 5 minutes; take the pulse and blood pressure; at 1 minute, take blood pressure and pulse after patient is sitting and again at 1 minute after patient stands (Fig. 34-9).	An older person's baroreceptor response to positional changes is slightly less efficient. A slight decrease in blood pressure may occur. Blood pressure increases as elasticity decreases in arteries with proportionately greater increase in systolic pressure, resulting in a widening of pulse pressure.	A greater than 10 mmHg drop in systolic or diastolic pressure and an increase in heart rate of 20 beats or more per minute indicate orthostatic hypotension. A serious consequence is the potential for lightheadedness and dizziness, which may precipitate hip fracture or head trauma from a fall.

Continued on following page

PHYSICAL ASSESSMENT (continued)

ASSESSMENT PROCEDURE	NORMAL FINDINGS	ABNORMAL FINDINGS
Heart and blood vessels (continued)		
SAFETY TIP If dizziness occurs, instruct patient to sit a few minutes before attempting to stand up from a supine or reclining position.	**CLINICAL TIP** Any patient with blood pressure exceeding 160/90 mmHg should be referred to the health care provider for follow-up.	**CLINICAL TIP** Some sources of orthostatic hypotension include medications, such as antihypertensives, diuretics and drugs with anticholinergic side effects (anxiolytics, antipsychotics, hypnotics, tricyclic antidepressants and antihistamines). A sudden and increasingly widened pulse pressure, especially in combination with other neurological abnormalities and a change in mental status, is a classic sign of increased intracranial pressure (which in older patients may be due to a haemorrhagic stroke or haematoma).

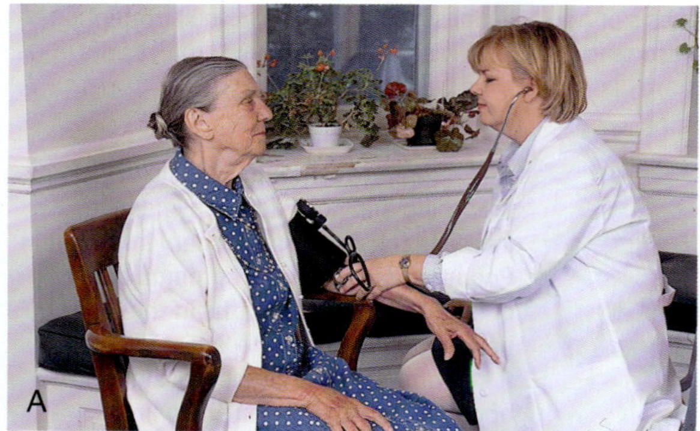

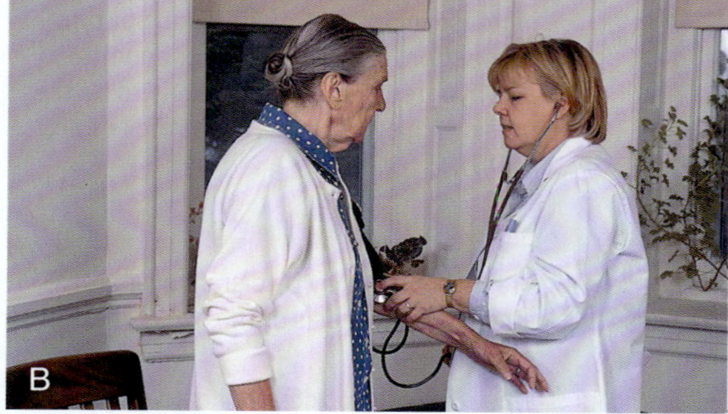

FIGURE 34-9 (A) Assessing blood pressure when sitting. **(B)** Assessing blood pressure when standing. (© B. Proud.)

ASSESSMENT PROCEDURE	NORMAL FINDINGS	ABNORMAL FINDINGS
EXERCISE TOLERANCE		
Measure activity tolerance. Evaluate, either by reviewing results of stress testing or by observing the patient's ability to move from a sitting to a standing position (Fig. 34-10) or to flex and extend fingers rapidly. **CLINICAL TIP** Poor lower body strength, especially in the ankles, may impair the ability of the frail person to rise from a chair to a standing position. Poor upper body strength, especially in the shoulders, may impede the ability to push up from a bed or chair or to extend and flex fingers.	The maximal heart rate with exercise is less than in a younger person. The heart rate will also take longer to return to its pre-exercise rate. Rise in pulse rate should be no greater than 10 to 20 beats/minute. The pulse rate should return to the baseline rate within 2 minutes.	A rise in pulse rate greater than 20 beats/minute and a rate that does not return to baseline within 2 minutes is an indicator of exercise intolerance. Cardiac arrhythmias as determined by stress testing are also indicative of exercise intolerance.

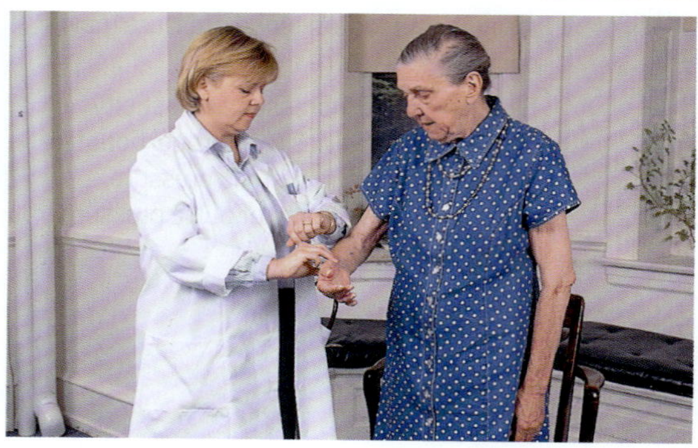

FIGURE 34-10 Assessing heart rate after the patient rises from a sitting position provides clues to his or her tolerance of physical exertion. (© B. Proud.)

PHYSICAL ASSESSMENT (continued)

ASSESSMENT PROCEDURE	NORMAL FINDINGS	ABNORMAL FINDINGS
Determine adequacy of blood flow by palpating the arterial pulses in all locations (carotid, brachial, radial, femoral, popliteal, posterior tibial and dorsalis pedis) for strength and quality (Fig. 34-11). **SAFETY TIP** Palpate carotid arteries gently and one side at a time to avoid stimulating vagal receptors in the neck, dislodging existing plaque or causing syncope or a stroke.	Proximal pulses may be easier to palpate because of loss of supporting surrounding tissue. However, distal lower extremity pulses may be more difficult to feel or even non-palpable. The dorsalis pedis pulse is absent in approximately 20% of older people (Mezey et al., 1993).	Insufficient or absent pulses are likely to be an indication of arterial insufficiency. Partially obstructed blood flow increases the risk of ulcers and infection; completely obstructed blood flow is a medical emergency requiring immediate intervention to prevent gangrene and possible amputation.

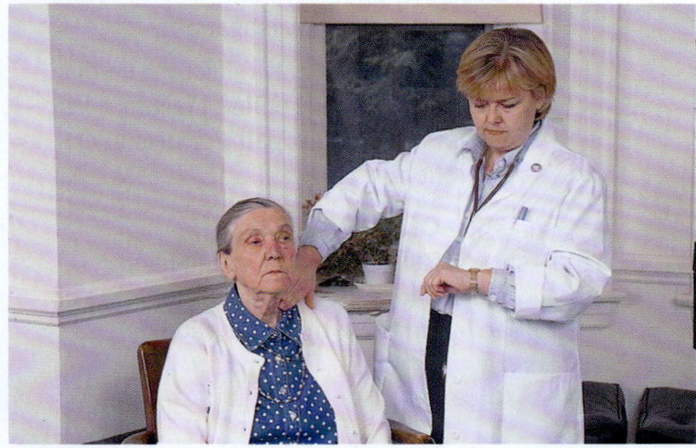

FIGURE 34-11 Palpating the carotid artery to assess blood flow. (© B. Proud.)

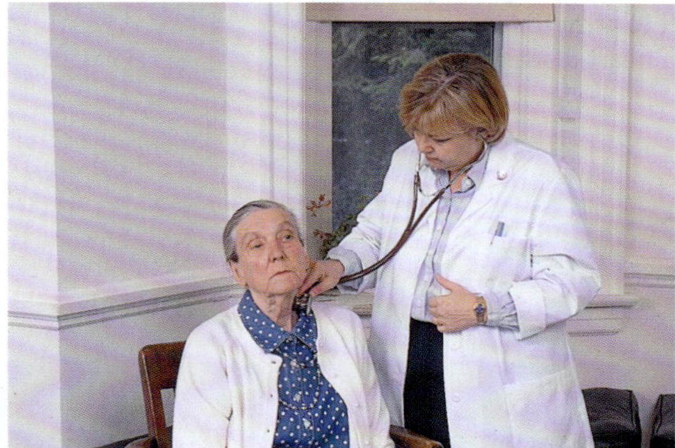

FIGURE 34-12 Use the bell of the stethoscope to listen for bruits. (© B. Proud.)

ASSESSMENT PROCEDURE	NORMAL FINDINGS	ABNORMAL FINDINGS
ARTERIES AND VEINS		
Auscultate the carotid, abdominal and femoral arteries (Fig. 34-12).	No unusual sounds should be heard.	A bruit is abnormal, and the patient needs a prompt referral for further care because of the high risk of CVA from a carotid embolism or an abdominal or femoral aneurysm.
Evaluate arterial and venous sufficiency of extremities. Elevate the legs above the level of the heart and observe colour, temperature, size of the legs and skin integrity.	Hair loss with advanced age (cannot be used singly as an indicator of arterial insufficiency).	Leg pain associated with walking, burning or cramping, duskiness or mottling when the leg is in a dependent position; paleness with elevation; cool, thin, shiny skin; thickened, brittle nails; and diminished pulses are signs of arterial insufficiency.
Inspect and palpate veins while patient is standing.	Prominent, bulging veins are common. Varicosities are considered a problem only if ulcerations, signs of thrombophlebitis or cords are present. Cords are non-tender, palpable veins having a rubber tubing consistency.	Unilateral warmth, tenderness and swelling may be indications of thrombophlebitis.
Heart		
Inspect and palpate the praecordium.	The praecordium is still, not visible and without thrills, heaves, palpable pulsations (noted exception may be the apex of the heart if close to the surface).	Heaves are felt with an enlarged right or left ventricular aneurysm.

Continued on following page

PHYSICAL ASSESSMENT (continued)

ASSESSMENT PROCEDURE	NORMAL FINDINGS	ABNORMAL FINDINGS
Heart (continued)		
		Thrills indicate aortic, mitral or pulmonic stenosis and regurgitation that may originate from rheumatic fever. Pulsations suggest an aortic or ventricular aneurysm, right ventricular enlargement or mitral regurgitation.
Auscultate heart sounds. **The accumulation of lipofuscin, amyloid, collagen and fats in the pacemaker cells of the heart and loss of pacemaker cells in the sinus node predispose the older adult to arrhythmias, even in the absence of heart disease.**	A soft systolic murmur heard best at the base of the heart may result from calcification, stiffening and dilation of the aortic and mitral valve.	Abnormal heart sounds are generally considered to be disease-related only if there is additional evidence of compromised cardiovascular function. However, any previously undetected extra heart sound warrants further investigation. S_3 and S_4 sounds may reflect the cardiac and fluid overloads of heart failure, aortic stenosis, cardiomyopathy or myocardial infarction. **CLINICAL TIP** **Falls, dyspnoea, fatigue and palpitations are common symptoms of arrhythmias in the older people.**
Breasts		
INSPECTION AND PALPATION		
Inspect and palpate breast and axillae. When viewing axillae and contour of breasts, assist a patient with arthritis to raise the arms over the head. Do this gently and without force and only if it is not painful for the patient. If the breasts are pendulous, assist the patient to lean slightly so the breasts hang away from the chest wall, enabling you to best observe symmetry and form. **CLINICAL TIP** **A greater percentage of older women have had radical mastectomies. If so, inquiring about pain and swelling from lymphoedema is important.**	The breasts of older women are often described as pendulous because of the atrophy of breast tissue and supporting tissues and the forward thrust of the patient brought about by kyphosis. Decreases in fat composition and increase in fibrotic tissue may make the terminal ducts feel more fibrotic and palpable as linear, spokelike strands. Nipples may retract because of loss in musculature. Unlike nipple retraction due to a mass, nipples retracted because of ageing can be everted with gentle pressure (Mezey et al., 1993).	Pain upon palpation may indicate an infectious process or cancer. Breast tenderness, pain or swelling may be side effects of hormone replacement therapy and an indication that a lower dosage is needed. Male breast enlargement (gynaecomastia) may result from a decrease in testosterone. Macerated skin under the breasts may result from perspiration or fungal infection (usually seen in an immunocompromised patient).
Inspect skin under breasts.	Skin intact without lesions or rashes.	
Abdomen		
MOTILITY		
Assess GI motility and auscultate bowel sounds. Review fibre intake and laxative use.	5 to 30 sounds/minute are heard. A decrease in gastric emptying time occurs with ageing and may cause early satiety. Intestinal motility is generally reduced from a general loss of muscle tone. Risk of constipation is increased by diminished physical activity, fluid intake, fibre in diet and by certain medications such as iron or narcotics.	Absence of bowel sounds and vomiting of undigested food is abnormal. Decreased motility is exacerbated by common pathologies such as Parkinson, stroke and diabetes mellitus that results in propensity for chronic constipation and diverticula.

PHYSICAL ASSESSMENT (continued)

ASSESSMENT PROCEDURE	NORMAL FINDINGS	ABNORMAL FINDINGS
		SAFETY TIP **If diverticula become infected, emergency treatment may be required to prevent perforation and sepsis.** Hiatal hernia that manifests by postprandial chest fullness, heartburn or nausea.
Determine absorption or retention problems in older patients receiving enteral feedings. *Note:* An abdominal radiograph, flat plate, should be taken to check for correct placement of newly inserted nasogastric tubes.	Less than 100 mL residual is a normal finding for intermittent feedings.	More than 100 mL residual measured before a scheduled feeding is a sign of insufficient absorption and excessive retention. Abdominal distension, diarrhoea, fluid overload, aspiration pneumonia, or fluid or electrolyte imbalances may indicate excessive retention, although mental status changes may be the first or only sign.
Inspect and percuss abdomen in same manner as for younger adults. **CLINICAL TIP** **The loss of abdominal musculature that occurs with ageing may make it easier to palpate abdominal organs.** Atrophy of intestinal villi is a common ageing change.	Liver, pancreas and kidneys normally decrease in size, but the decrease is not generally appreciable upon physical examination.	Anorexia, abdominal pain and distension, impaired protein digestion and vitamin B12 malabsorption suggest inflammatory gastritis or a peptic ulcer. Abdominal distension, cramping, diarrhoea and increased flatus are signs of lactose intolerance, which may occur for the first time in old age. Bruits over aorta suggest an aneurysm. If present, do not palpate because this could rupture the aneurysm. Guarding upon palpation, rebound tenderness or a friction rub (sounds like pieces of sandpaper rubbing together) often suggests peritonitis, which could be secondary to ruptured diverticuli, tumour or infarct.
Palpate the bladder. (Ask patient to empty bladder before the examination.) If the bladder is palpable, percuss from symphysis pubis to umbilicus. If the patient is incontinent, postvoid residual content may also need to be measured.	Empty bladder is not palpable or percussible.	Full bladder sounds dull. More than 100 mL drained from bladder is considered abnormal for a postvoid residual. A distended bladder with an associated small-volume urine loss may indicate overflow incontinence. (See Display 34-3.)
Genitalia		
Note: It is not common practice for nurses to assess an older person's genitalia, but if assessment is required, proceed as follows.		
FEMALE		
Inspect external genitalia. Assist the patient into the lithotomy position. Inspect the urethral meatus and vaginal opening. **CLINICAL TIP** **Arthritis may make the lithotomy position particularly uncomfortable for the older woman, necessitating changes. If the patient has breathing difficulties, elevating the head to a semi-Fowler position may help.**	Many atrophic changes begin in women at menopause. Pubic hair is usually sparse, and labia are flattened. Clitoris is decreased in size. The size of ovaries, uterus and cervix also decreases.	White, glistening particles attached to pubic hair may be a sign of lice. Redness or swelling from the urethral meatus indicates a possible urinary tract infection.

Continued on following page

PHYSICAL ASSESSMENT (continued)

ASSESSMENT PROCEDURE	NORMAL FINDINGS	ABNORMAL FINDINGS
Genitalia (continued)		
Ask the patient to cough while in the lithotomy position. **CLINICAL TIP** **Incontinence is not a normal part of ageing. If embarrassment or acceptance is preventing the patient from acknowledging the problem, the genital examination may be a more acceptable time to introduce the topic.**	No leakage of urine occurs.	Leakage of urine that occurs with coughing is a sign of stress incontinence and may be due to lax pelvic muscles from childbirth, surgery, obesity, cystocoele, rectocele or a prolapsed uterus. *Note:* In non-communicative patients, an excoriated perineum may be the result of incontinence, which warrants further investigation.
Test for prolapse. Ask the patient to bear down while you observe the vaginal opening.	No prolapse is evident.	A protrusion into the vaginal opening may be a cystocele, rectocele or uterine prolapse, which is a common sequela of relaxed pelvic musculature in older women.
Perform a pelvic examination. Put on disposable gloves and use a small speculum if the vaginal opening has narrowed with age. Use lubrication on speculum and hand because natural lubrication is decreased.	Vagina narrows and shortens. A loss of elastic tissue and vascularity in vagina results in a thin, pale epithelium. Atrophic changes are intensified by infrequent intercourse. Loss of elasticity and reduced vaginal lubrication from diminishing levels of oestrogen can cause dyspareunia (painful intercourse). Sexual desire, pleasure are not necessarily diminished by these structural changes, nor do women lose capacity for orgasm with age. Because the ovaries, uterus and cervix shrink with age, the ovaries may not be palpable.	Malignancy, vulvar dystrophies, urinary tract infections and other infections, such as *Candida albicans,* bacterial vaginosis, gonorrhoea or *Chlamydia,* can mimic atrophic vaginitis (Kennedy-Malone et al., 2000).
Test pelvic muscle tone. Ask the woman to squeeze muscles while the examiner's finger is in the vagina. Assess perineal strength by turning fingers posterior to the perineum while the woman squeezes muscles in the vaginal area.	The vaginal wall should constrict around the examiner's finger, and the perineum should feel smooth.	If the patient has a cystocele, the examiner's finger in the vagina will feel pressure from the anterior surface of the vagina. In patients with uterine prolapse, protrusion of the cervix is felt down through the vagina. A bulging of the posterior vaginal wall and part of the rectum may be felt with a rectocele.
MALE		
Inspect the male genital area with the patient in standing position if possible.	The decline in testosterone brings about atrophic changes. Pubic hair is thinner. Scrotal skin is slightly darker than surrounding skin and is smooth and flaccid in the older man. Penis and testicular size decreases, scrotum hangs lower.	Scrotal oedema may be present with portal vein obstruction or heart failure. Lesions on the penis may be a sign of infection. Associated symptoms frequently include discharge, scrotal pain and difficulty with urination.
Observe and palpate for inguinal swelling or bulges suggestive of hernia in the same manner as for a younger male.	No swelling or bulges are present.	Masses or bulges are abnormal, and pain may be a sign of testicular torsion. A mass may be due to a hydrocoele, spermatocele or cancer.
Auscultate the scrotum if a mass is detected; otherwise, palpate the right and left testicle using the thumb and first two fingers.	No detectable sounds or masses are present.	Bowel sounds heard over the scrotum may suggest an indirect inguinal hernia. Masses are abnormal, and the patient should be referred to a specialist for follow-up examination.

PHYSICAL ASSESSMENT (continued)

ASSESSMENT PROCEDURE	NORMAL FINDINGS	ABNORMAL FINDINGS
Anus, rectum and prostate		
Note: It is not common practice for nurses to assess an older person's prostate, but if assessment is required, proceed as follows.		
INSPECTION AND PALPATION		
Inspect the anus and rectum.	The anus is darker than the surrounding skin. Bluish, grapelike lumps at the anus are indicators of haemorrhoids.	Lesions, swelling, inflammation and bleeding are abnormalities. If haemorrhoids account for discomfort, the degree to which bleeding, swelling or inflammation interferes with bowel activity generally determines if treatment is warranted.
Put on gloves to palpate the anus and rectum. Also palpate the prostate in the male patient. **CLINICAL TIP** **The left side-lying position with knees tucked up towards the chest is the preferred one for comfort. Pillows may be needed for positioning and patient comfort.**	The prostate is normally soft or rubbery-firm and smooth, and the median sulcus is palpable. Some degree of enlargement (BPH) almost always occurs by age 85 as does a decrease in amount and viscosity of seminal fluid. Sperm count may decrease by as much as 50%. Orgasm may be briefer and time to obtain an erection may increase. These changes alone, however, do not usually result in any loss of libido or satisfaction.	Palpation of internal masses could indicate polyps, internal haemorrhoids, rectal prolapse, cancer or faecal impaction. Obliteration of the median sulcus is felt with prostatic hyperplasia. A hard, asymmetrically enlarged and nodular prostate is suggestive of malignancy (Mezey et al., 1993). A tender and softer prostate is more common with prostatitis. Fever and painful urination are common with acute prostatitis. Obstructive symptoms are seen with both malignancy and infection of prostate.
Musculoskeletal system		
INSPECTION AND PALPATION		
Observe the patient's posture and balance when standing, especially the first 3 to 5 seconds. **CLINICAL TIP** **The ability to reach for everyday items without losing balance can be assessed by asking the patient to remove an object from a shelf that is high enough to require stretching or standing on the toes and to bend down to pick up a small object, such as a pen, from the floor.**	Patient stands reasonably straight with feet positioned fairly widely apart to form a firm base of support. This stance compensates for diminished sense of proprioception in lower extremities. Body usually bends forwards as well.	A 'humpback' curvature of the spine, called kyphosis, usually results from osteoporosis. The combination of osteoporosis, calcification of tendons and joints, and muscle atrophy makes it difficult for the frail older person to extend the hips and knees fully when walking. This impairs the ability to maintain balance early enough to prevent a fall. Patient cannot maintain balance without holding onto something or someone. Postural instability increases the risk of falling and immobility from the fear of falling.
Observe the patient's gait by performing the timed 'Get up and go' test (Fig. 34-13): 1. Have the patient rise from a straight-backed armchair, stand momentarily and walk about 3 m towards a wall. 2. Ask the patient to turn without touching the wall and walk back to the chair, then turn around and sit down. 3. Using a watch or clock with a second hand, time how long it takes the patient to complete the test.	Widening of pelvis and narrowing of shoulders. Patient walks steadily without swaying, stumbling or hesitating during the walk. The patient does not appear to be at risk of falling. Older patients without impairments in gait or balance can complete the test within 10 seconds.	Shuffling gait, characterised by smaller steps and minimal lifting of the feet, increases the risk of tripping when walking on uneven or unsteady surfaces. Abnormal findings from the timed 'Get up and go' test include hesitancy, staggering, stumbling and abnormal movements of the trunk and arms. People who take more than 30 seconds to complete the test tend to be dependent in some activities of daily living such as bathing, getting in and out of bed, and climbing stairs.

Continued on following page

PHYSICAL ASSESSMENT (continued)

ASSESSMENT PROCEDURE	NORMAL FINDINGS	ABNORMAL FINDINGS
Musculoskeletal system (continued)		
4. Score performance on a 1 to 5 scale: 1 = normal 2 = very slightly abnormal 3 = mildly abnormal 4 = moderately abnormal 5 = severely abnormal.		
Inspect the general contour of limbs, trunk and joints. Palpate wrist and hand joints.	Enlargement of the distal, interphalangeal joints of the fingers, called Heberden nodes, are indicators of *degenerative joint disease* (DJD), a common age-related condition involving joints in the hips, knees and spine as well as the fingers (Fig. 34-14).	With accumulated damage and loss of cartilage, bony overgrowths protrude from the bone into the joint capsule, causing deformities, limited mobility and pain. Hand deformities such as ulnar deviation, swan-neck deformity and boutonnière deformity are of concern because of the limitations they impose on activities of daily living and related pain.

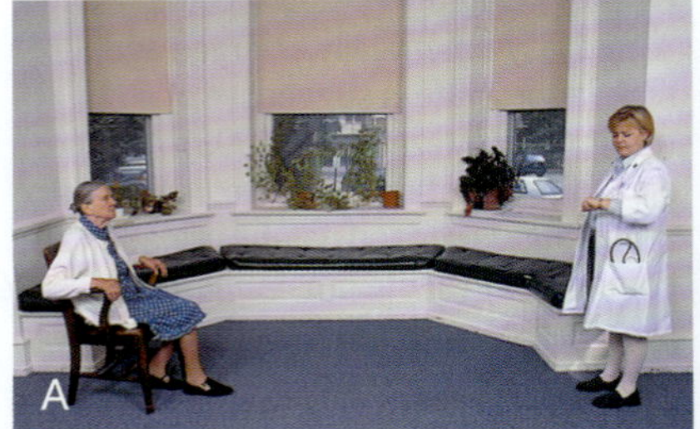

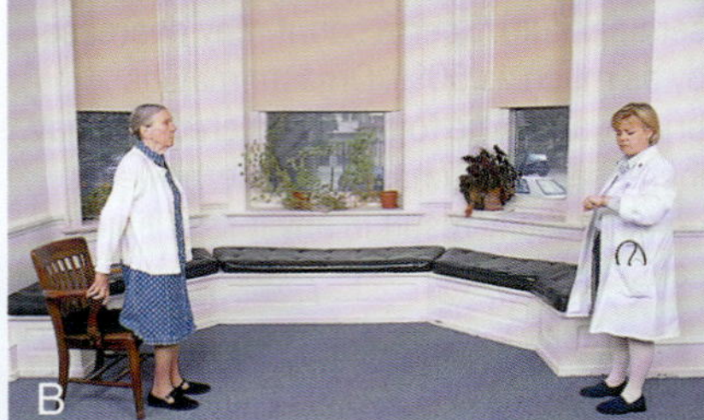

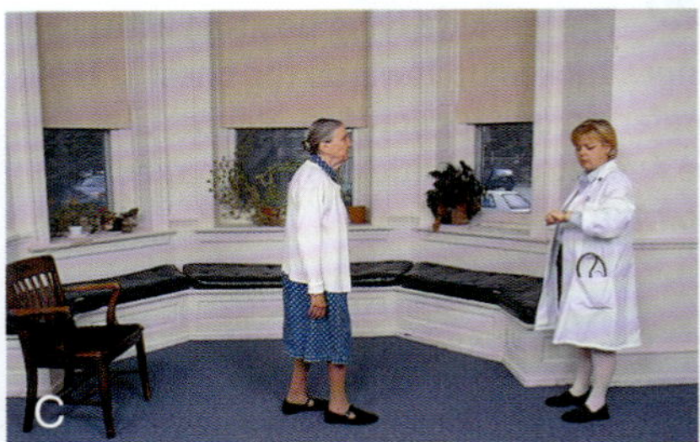

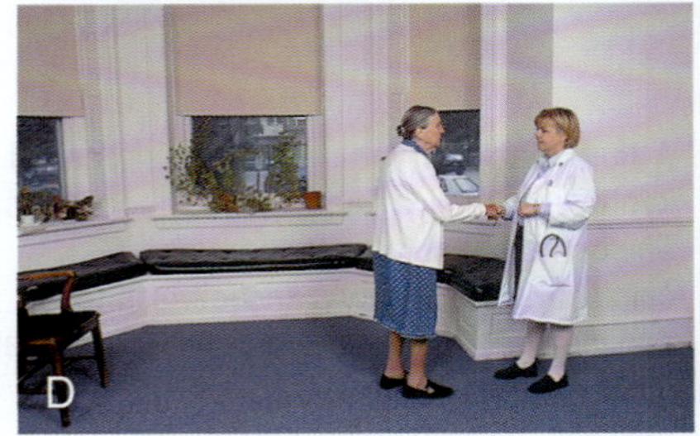

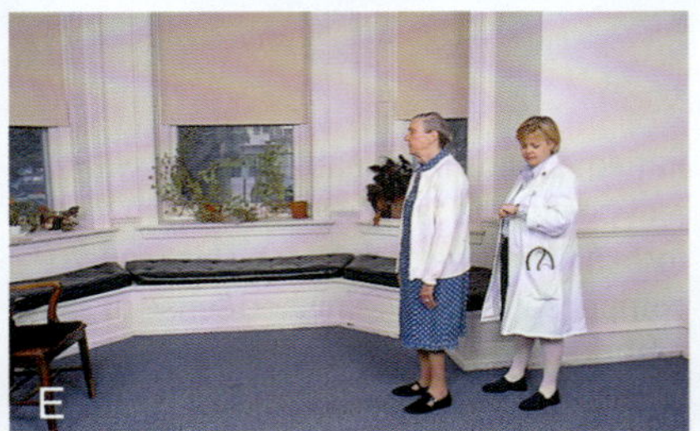

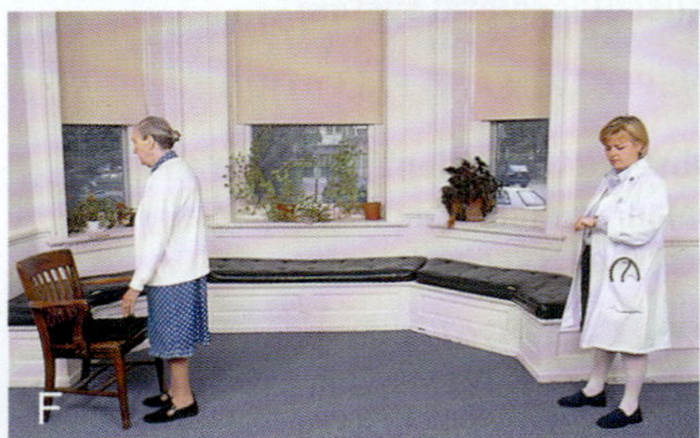

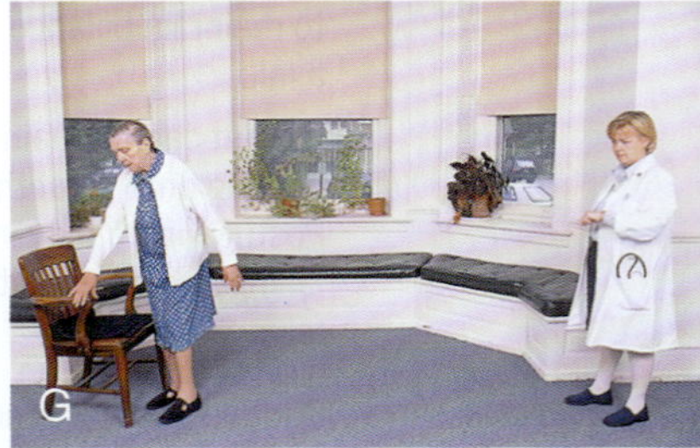

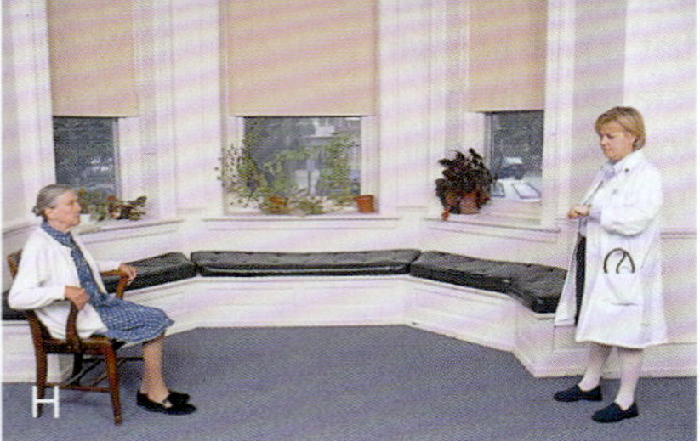

FIGURE 34-13 'Get up and go' test. (© B. Proud.)

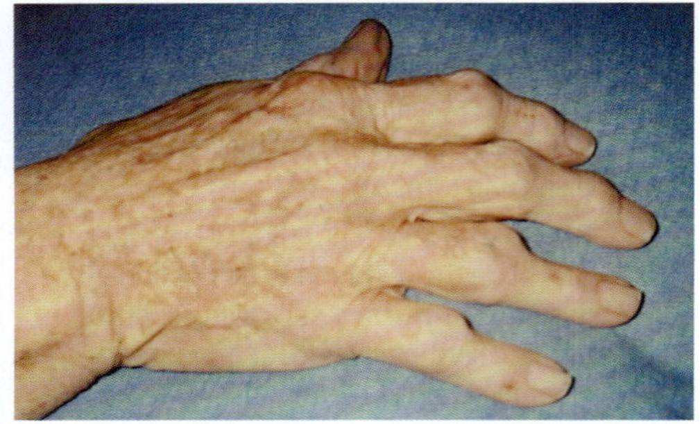

FIGURE 34-14 Degenerative joint disease.

PHYSICAL ASSESSMENT (continued)

ASSESSMENT PROCEDURE	NORMAL FINDINGS	ABNORMAL FINDINGS
Test range of motion (ROM). Ask patient to touch each finger with the thumb of the same hand, to turn wrists up towards the ceiling and down towards the floor, to push each finger against yours while you apply resistance and to make a fist and release it (Fig. 34-15).	There is full ROM of each joint and equal bilateral resistance.	Limitations in ROM or strength may be due to DJD, rheumatoid arthritis or a neurological disorder, which, if unilateral, suggests CVA. Signs of pain such as grimacing, pulling back or verbal messages are indicators of the need to do a pain assessment. Grating, popping, crepitus and palpation of fluid are also abnormalities. Crepitus and joint pain that is worse with activity and relieved by rest in the absence of systemic symptoms are often associated with DJD.

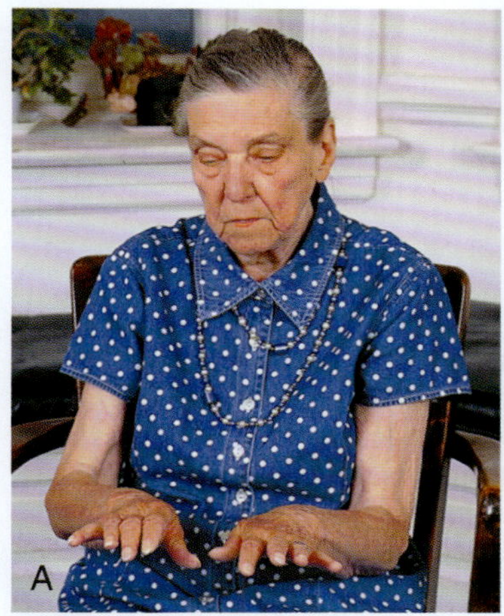
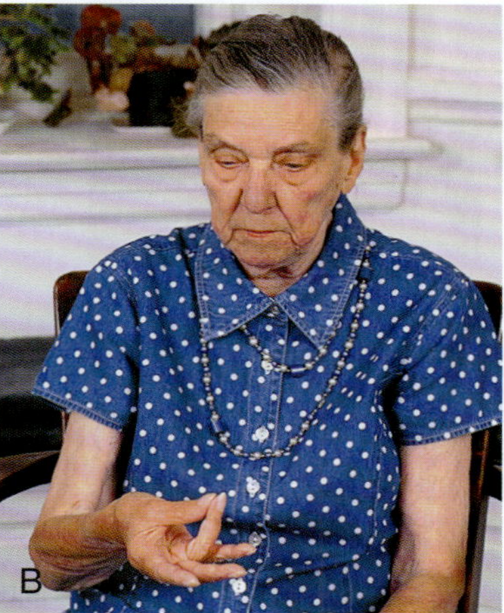
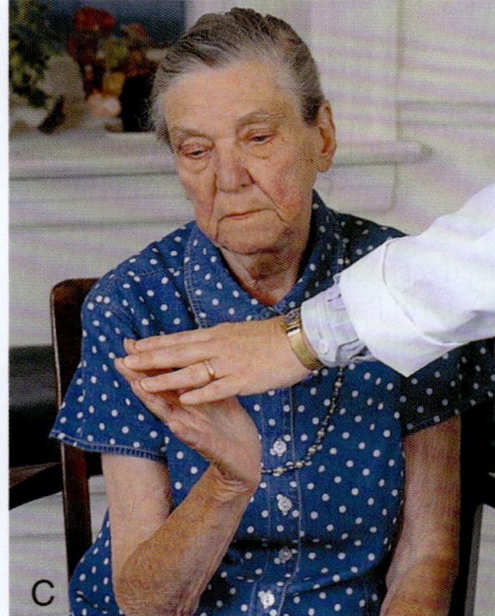
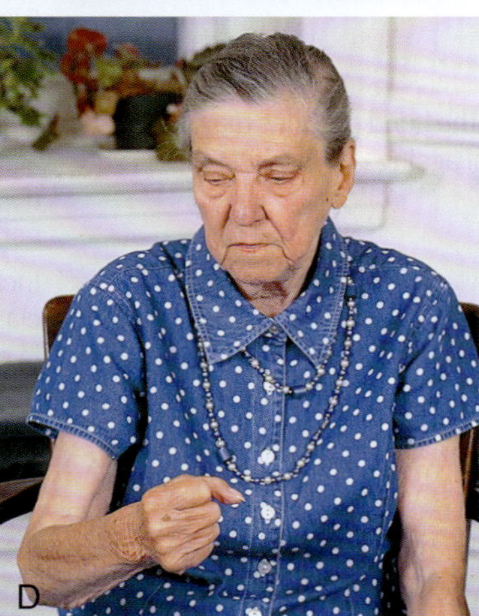

FIGURE 34-15 Testing range of motion. (© B. Proud.)

ASSESSMENT PROCEDURE	NORMAL FINDINGS	ABNORMAL FINDINGS
Similarly assess ROM and strength of shoulders (left) and elbows (right) (Fig. 34-16).	There is full ROM of each joint and equal strength.	Tenderness, stiffness and pain in the shoulders and elbows (and hips), which is aggravated by movement, are common signs associated with *polymyalgia rheumatica*.
Assess hip joint for strength and ROM in the same manner as for a younger adult.	Intact flexion, extension, and internal and external rotation.	Hip pain that is worse with weight bearing and relieved with rest may indicate DJD. There is usually also an associated crepitation and decrease in ROM. Complaints of hip or thigh pain, external rotation and adduction of the affected leg,

Continued on following page

PHYSICAL ASSESSMENT (continued)

ASSESSMENT PROCEDURE	NORMAL FINDINGS	ABNORMAL FINDINGS
Musculoskeletal system (continued)		
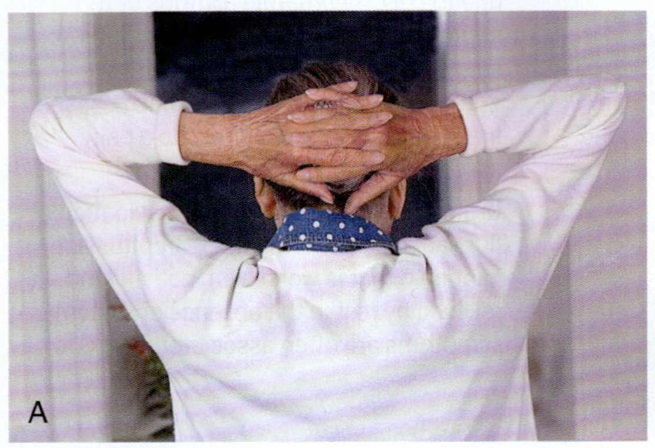 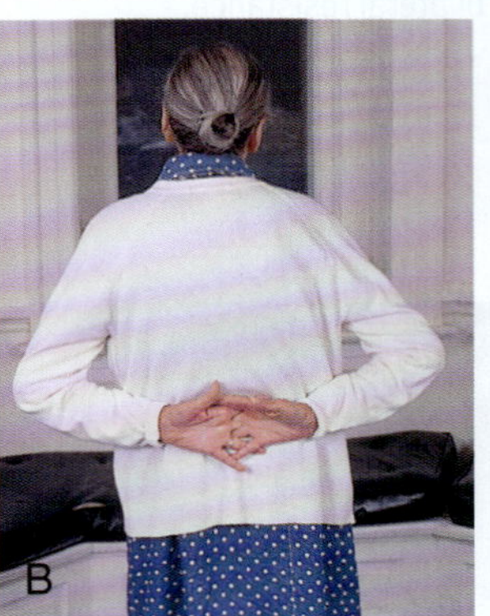 **FIGURE 34-16** Testing range of motion. (© B. Proud.)		and an inability to bear weight are the most common signs of a hip fracture. Much less common signs may be mild discomfort and minimal shortening of the leg (Burke & Walsh, 1997).
Inspect and palpate knees, ankles and feet. Also assess comfort level particularly with movement (flexion, extension, rotation).	The common problems associated with the aged foot, such as soreness and aching, are most frequently due to improperly fitting footwear.	A great toe overriding or underlying the second toe may be hallux valgus (bunion). Other abnormal findings may be enlargement of the medial portion of the first metatarsal head and inflammation of the bursae over the medial aspect of the joint. Bunions are associated with pain and difficulty walking.
Inspect patient's muscle bulk and tone.	Atrophy of the hand muscles may occur with normal ageing.	Muscle atrophy can result from rheumatoid arthritis, muscle disuse, malnutrition, motor neuron disease or diseases of the peripheral nervous system. Increased resistance to passive ROM is a classic sign of Parkinson disease, especially in patients with bradykinesia. Decreased resistance may also suggest peripheral nervous system disease, cerebellar disease or acute spinal cord injury.
Neurological system		
Observe for tremors and involuntary movements.	Resting tremors increase in the aged. In the absence of an identifiable disease process, they are not considered pathological.	The tremors of Parkinson disease may occur when the patient is at rest. They usually diminish with voluntary movement. They usually begin in the hand and may affect only one side of the body (especially early in the disease). The tremors are accompanied by muscle rigidity.
Sensory system		
Test sensation to pain, temperature, touch position and vibration as you would for a younger adult.	Touch and vibratory sensations may diminish normally with ageing.	Unilateral sensory loss suggests a lesion in the spinal cord or higher pathways; a symmetrical sensory loss suggests a neuropathy that may be associated with a condition such as diabetes.
Assess positional sense by using the Romberg test as presented in Chapter 29**.** The exceptions to the test are patients who must use assistive devices such as a walker.	There is minimal swaying without loss of balance.	Significant swaying with appearance of a potential fall.

ABNORMAL FINDINGS 34-1 Age-related abnormalities of the eye

Common age-related abnormalities of the eye include glaucoma, macular degeneration, retinal detachment and diabetic retinopathy.

GLAUCOMA

The patient with glaucoma is usually symptom-free. In older people, diabetes and atherosclerosis are conditions that increase the risk of glaucoma. The disorder is caused by increased pressure that can destroy the optic nerve and cause blindness if not treated properly. An acute form of glaucoma can occur at any age and is a true medical emergency because blindness can result in a day or two without treatment. Rainbowlike halos or circles around lights, severe pain in the eyes or forehead, nausea and blurred vision may occur with the acute form of glaucoma.

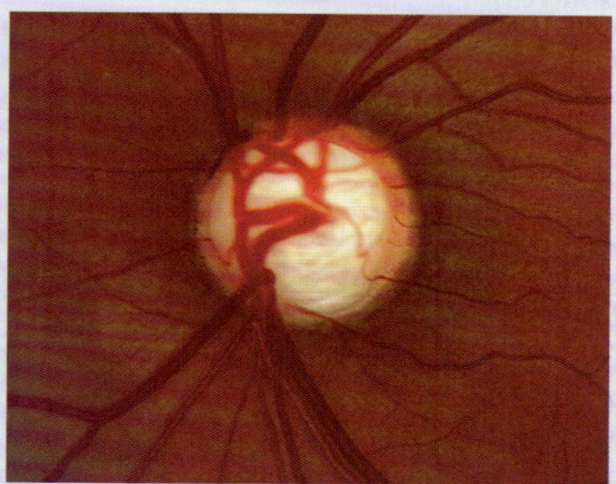

Glaucomatous cupping. (Shutterstock.com/memorisz.)

MACULAR DEGENERATION

Macular degeneration, a gradual loss of central vision, is caused by ageing and thinning of the micro-thin membrane in the centre of the retina called the macula. Additional risk factors include sunlight exposure, family history and fair skin. Most cases begin to develop after age 50, but damage may be occurring for months to years before symptoms occur. Peripheral vision is not affected, and the condition may occur initially in only one eye. Only about 10% of all age-related macular degeneration leaks occur in the small blood vessels in the retinal pigment epithelium. This type accounts for the most serious loss of vision.

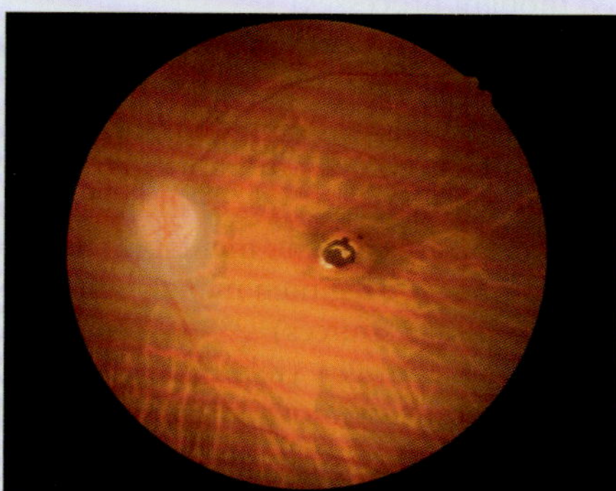

Funduscopic view of intermediate-age–related macular degeneration. (Used with permission from the National Eye Institute, National Institutes of Health, Baltimore, MD.)

RETINA DETACHMENT

Retinal detachment occurs at a greater frequency with ageing as the vitreous pulls away from its attachment to the retina at the back of the eye, causing the retina to tear in one or more places. A retinal detachment is always a serious problem. Blindness will result if the detachment is not treated.

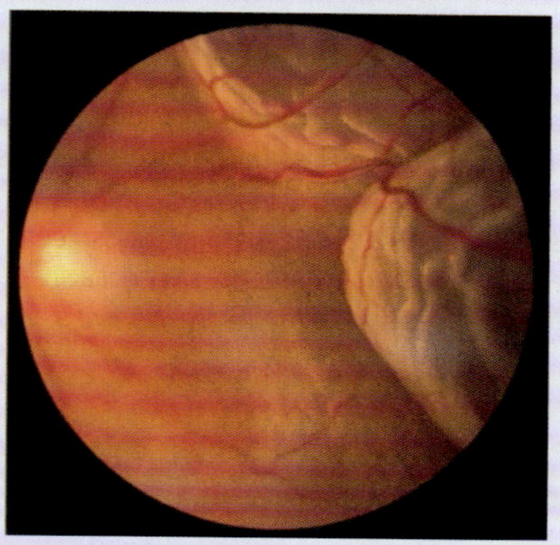

Ophthalmoscopic photograph of retinal detachment. (Used with permission from Moore, K. L. & Dailey, A. F. [2006]. *Clinically oriented anatomy* [5th ed., p. 967]. Philadelphia: Lippincott Williams & Wilkins.)

DIABETIC RETINOPATHY

Many older adults have diabetes, which can lead to cataracts, glaucoma and diabetic retinopathy. Of those with diabetes mellitus, about 90% will develop diabetic retinopathy to some degree. The more serious of the two forms of the disease, proliferative diabetic retinopathy, occurs most often among those who have had diabetes for more than 25 years. People with the advanced form of the disease usually experience a noticeable loss of vision, including cloudiness, distortion of familiar objects and, occasionally, blind spots or floaters. If not treated, diabetic retinopathy will lead to connective scar tissue, which over time can shrink, pulling on the retina and resulting in a retinal detachment. In the early stages of the milder form of the disease, background diabetic retinopathy, the person may be unaware of problems because the loss of sight is usually gradual and mainly affects peripheral vision.

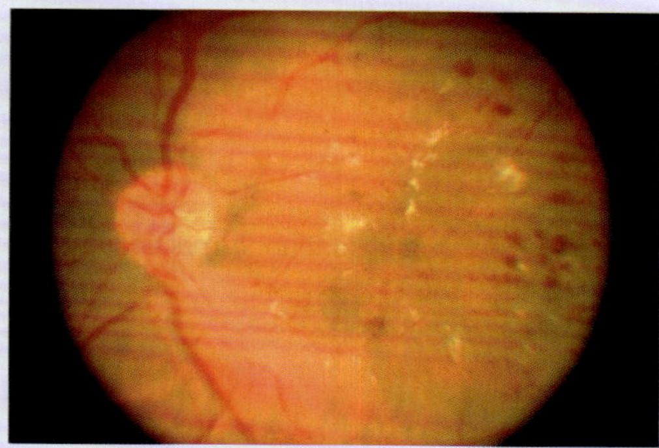

Ocular fundus of a patient with background diabetic retinopathy. (Used with permission from Klintworth, G. K. [2008]. The eye. In R. Rubin & D. E. Strayer [Eds]. *Rubin's pathology: Clinicopathologic foundations of medicine* [5th ed., p. 1257]. Philadelphia: Lippincott Williams & Wilkins.)

VALIDATING AND DOCUMENTING FINDINGS

The prevalence of chronic conditions in the older person redefines the meaning of wellness. The ability of the older person to function in everyday activities, albeit with environmental and pharmacological interventions, is a more meaningful measure of wellness than are physical findings alone. Thus, the objective and subjective data must reflect a functional and physical assessment.

Sample of subjective data

Health complaints or abnormalities are as likely to be the result of an adverse reaction to drug therapy as they are to a disease process. Compiling a profile of prescription and over-the-counter medications is an essential component of any assessment of the frail older person—whether it is being performed to treat a specific health complaint or for compiling baseline data of the patient's health status.

Objective data for Mrs Kimberley

Mrs Kimberley has no significant blood pressure difference between lying and standing (lying 150/85 mmHg, heart rate 88 beats/minute sitting 148/84 mmHg, heart rate 90 beats/minute; standing 148/84 mmHg, heart rate 90 beats/minute); respiratory rate 22 breaths/minute.

Mrs Kimberley is independent in transfers and uses a walker. She has a pill-rolling tremor at rest. She completes the timed 'Get up and go' test within the expected time. Physical examination reveals a soft systolic murmur, absent pedal pulses, and soft and non-distended abdomen. She has no pedal oedema; toenails are thick and yellowish; no ulcerations or discolouration of skin on legs. No abdominal or carotid bruits noted on auscultation; lungs are clear on auscultation. The patient's tongue is pink and moist. Her skin is thin and transparent. Numerous moles and brown, pigmented flat lesions (lentigines) are noted on her hands, lower arms and neck. Her fingernails are yellowish and brittle. A yellowish discolouration is noted in the lenses of both eyes. Slight accumulation of dry earwax in outer ear; tympanic membrane is pink and intact. Mini–Mental Status exam is normal. Mrs Kimberley has no noted difficulties in conversation to do with memory, judgement, comprehension or word recall.

CRITICAL THINKING

7. What are the most significant abnormal findings for Mrs Kimberley?
8. What is she managing well?

Analysis of data

DIAGNOSTIC REASONING: POSSIBLE CONCLUSIONS

After collecting subjective and objective data pertaining to the frail older person assessment, identify abnormal findings and patient strengths. Then cluster the data to reveal any significant patterns or abnormalities. These data may then be used to make clinical judgements about the status of the patient's health.

Potential patient risks

- Carer role strain (related to complexity of illness and lack of resources)
- Ineffective family coping (related to emotional conflicts secondary to chronic illness of parent)
- Social isolation (related to inability to communicate effectively, decreased mobility, effects of chronic illness or pain)
- Imbalanced nutrition: less than body requirements (related to dysphagia or decreased desire to eat secondary to altered level of consciousness)
- Constipation (related to decreased physical mobility, decreased intestinal motility, lower fluid intake, reduced fibre and bulk in diet and effects of medications)
- Impaired skin integrity (related to loss of subcutaneous tissue, immobility and malnutrition)
- Ineffective thermoregulation (related to loss of subcutaneous tissue, atrophy of eccrine sweat glands, decreased functioning of sebaceous glands)
- Disturbed sensory perception (related to dry eyes, loss of lens transparency, slow pupil constriction; or presbycusis)
- Impaired gas exchange (related to diminished recoil of lungs, less elastic alveoli and loss of skeletal muscle strength)
- Loneliness (related to changing role and decreasing functional status)
- Diversional activity deficit (related to impaired mobility or impaired thought processes)
- Fatigue (related to compromised circulatory or respiratory system or effects of medications)
- Grieving (related to debilitating effects of chronic illness)
- Hopelessness (related to deteriorating physical condition)
- Chronic sorrow of partner, carer or individual patient (related to chronic physical or mental disability of patient)
- Ineffective therapeutic regimen management (related to lack of community resources)
- Impaired physical mobility (related to pain, age, pathological changes in joints or neuromuscular impairment)
- Powerlessness (related to unpredictability of complex disease processes and complex treatments)
- Ineffective protection (related to decreased immunity)
- Activity intolerance (related to weakness, fatigue or pain related to joint and muscle deterioration and subsequent disuse of joints)
- Ineffective role performance (related to chronic illness)
- Functional urinary incontinence (related to immobility or dementia)

- Wandering (related to cognitive impairment, disorientation and sedation)
- Bathing, hygiene, grooming self-care deficit (related to impaired physical or cognitive functioning)
- Acute confusion (related to adverse effects of medication, infection or dehydration).

Selected collaborative problems

Often, abnormalities identified in the nursing assessment (including functional) will require a collaborative approach. Since *geriatric syndromes* are usually caused by acute pathology, they almost always require referral and collaboration with medical staff and the multidisciplinary team.

After grouping the data, certain collaborative problems may become apparent. Remember that collaborative problems differ from nursing diagnoses in that nursing interventions cannot prevent them. However, these physiological complications of medical conditions can be detected and monitored by the nurse. In addition, the nurse can use doctor- and nurse-prescribed interventions to minimise the complications of the problems. The following is a list of collaborative problems that may be identified when assessing the frail patient. It is important to remember, however, that any complication in the very old is likely to manifest as any one of the geriatric syndromes.

Geriatric syndromes: Falls

- Cardiac—syncope, orthostasis, arrhythmias
- Musculoskeletal—loss of strength, osteoporosis, osteoarthritis
- Neurological—dizziness, poor balance and gait, intracranial haemorrhage
- Sensory—loss of vision
- Infection

Geriatric syndromes: Urinary incontinence

- Urinary obstruction—prostatic hypertrophy
- Infection
- Constipation, faecal impaction
- Adverse medication effect

Geriatric syndromes: Acute mental status decline

- Infection—pneumonia, urinary tract, sepsis
- Adverse medication effect
- Dehydration
- Cardiovascular—heart failure, cerebrovascular accident (CVA)
- Metabolic—hypothyroidism or hyperthyroidism, hypoglycaemia
- Depression

Geriatric syndromes: Weakness, fatigue, anorexia and dyspnoea

- Cancer
- Pain
- Dysphagia
- Adverse medication effect
- Renal failure
- Infection

ONLINE RESOURCES

An extensive range of additional resources to enhance teaching and learning and to facilitate understanding may be found online at the text's accompanying website, located on thePoint at http://thepoint.lww.com. These include Watch and Learn videos, Concepts in Action animations, journal articles, case studies, discussion topics and quizzes.

Subscribers may also access Lippincott Procedures, an extensive online point-of-care procedure guide that provides reliable step-by-step instructions for more than 1700 procedures, including 450 evidence-based Australian procedures, and skills in a variety of speciality settings, together with a wealth of supporting information.

SIMULATED LEARNING

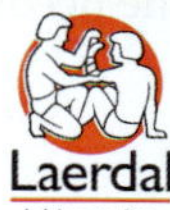

Having completed this chapter, explore the scenarios of Vincent Brody Part 1 and Part 2. Vincent is a 67-year-old male with long-standing chronic obstructive pulmonary disease. Incorporating the health assessment content in this chapter with your existing theoretical knowledge and clinical experience, progress through the simulation scenarios (this is best done in a small group). How would you manage Vincent's care? When reflecting on your management of Vincent, what do you think you did well and what do you think you can improve? Consider why you think this and also how you might manage a similar problem in the future.

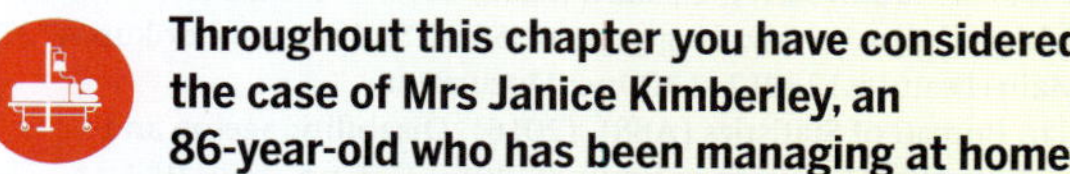

Throughout this chapter you have considered the case of Mrs Janice Kimberley, an 86-year-old who has been managing at home but is now having some difficulties. In the simulation scenario based on Mrs Kimberley and available to your lecturer online, you will continue to assess Mrs Kimberley's activities of daily living, instrumental activities of daily living, present health concern and nutritional status as well as assessing her for any evidence of:

- **Delirium or dementia**
- **Depression**
- **Frailty.**

In this simulation you will be using the assessment tools described in this chapter.

CASE STUDY

The case study demonstrates how to analyse assessment data for an older person. The exercises included in the ancillary product on thePoint that complements this text offer further opportunities to enhance your skills.

Mrs Janice Kimberley is an 86-year-old lady who has difficulty climbing stairs and maintaining her home of 43 years. However, she receives assistance from her family and the local council, which has a service supporting people at home. She eats two meals a day and has had a gradually improving appetite since receiving extra support. She reports occasional episodes (about once every 2 to 3 weeks) of some difficulty swallowing, especially food that is dry or meat that is tough. Mrs Kimberley takes a psyllium-powder bulking-laxative to keep her bowel movements regular and soft. Her current prescription medications are a combined levodopa carbidopa tablet three times a day and sodium hydrochlorothiazide 500 mg each morning.

Mrs Kimberley has regular dental examinations and sucks on hard sweets to alleviate her dry mouth. Mrs Kimberley denies any recent falls, fainting or dyspnoea with daily activities. However, she reports that she needs to sit for 5 to 10 minutes before standing to avoid becoming lightheaded. Mrs Kimberley has yearly mammograms and Pap smears. She is a breast cancer survivor and stopped taking supplemental oestrogen when diagnosed and treated 20 years ago. She reports no bleeding or change in moles or skin lesions. She receives vitamin B12 injections once a month and reports she always has more energy for 2 to 3 weeks afterwards. Mrs Kimberley reports she has had to get new eyeglasses twice in the last 4 years and that she sees occasional halos around lights. She can still read the newspaper if she shines a bright light directly on it, and she enjoys knitting. She states she is contented with her life and keeps in touch with family and friends, with frequent phone calls and occasional visits.

Mrs Kimberley has indicated to you she has to take her time standing up and that she may have some diminishing vision. It is possible that she believes these adjustments are part of getting older.

References

American Association of Colleges of Nursing (AACN). (2012). Competencies to improve care of older adults. Available at www.aacn.nche.edu/education-resources/competencies-older-adults.

Anger, J. T., Saigal, C. S. & Litwin, M. S. (2006). The prevalence of urinary incontinence among community-dwelling adult women: Results from the National Health and Nutrition Examination Survey. Urologic Diseases in America Project. *Journal of Urology, 175*(2), 601–604.

Australian Bureau of Statistics (ABS). (2014). *Australian Aboriginal and Torres Strait Islander health survey: Updated results, 2012–13*. Canberra: Author. Available at https://www.abs.gov.au/AUSSTATS/abs@.nsf/Lookup/4727.0.55.006Main+Features122012–13?OpenDocument.

Australian Bureau of Statistics (ABS). (2016). Disability, ageing and carers, Australia: Summary of findings, 2015. Cat. no. 4430.0. Canberra. Available at https://www.abs.gov.au/ausstats/abs@.nsf/Lookup/4430.0main+features302015.

Australian Indigenous Health*InfoNet*. (2019). *Overview of Aboriginal and Torres Strait Islander health status 2018*. Perth: Australian Indigenous Health*InfoNet*. Available at https://healthinfonet.ecu.edu.au/healthinfonet/getContent.php?linkid=617557&title=Overview+of+Aboriginal+and+Torres+Strait+Islander+health+status+2018.

Australian Institute of Health and Welfare (AIHW). (2018). *Older Australia at a glance*. Cat. no. AGE 87. Canberra. Available at https://www.aihw.gov.au/reports/older-people/older-australia-at-a-glance/contents/summary.

British Geriatrics Society and British Pain Society. (2013). *Guidance on the management of pain in older people*. London: Author. A special edition of *Age and Ageing, 42* (Supp. 1).

Burke, M. & Walsh, M. (1997). Gerontologic nursing: Holistic care of the older adult (2nd ed.). St Louis: Mosby.

Cesari, M., Calvani, R. & Marzetti, E. (2017). Frailty in older persons. *Clinics in Geriatric Medicine, 33*(8), 293–303.

Department of Health. (2017). Tuberculosis notifications in Australia, 2014. *Communicable Diseases Intelligence, 41*(3). Available at https://www1.health.gov.au/internet/main/publishing.nsf/Content/cdi4103-k.

Douzjian, M., Wilson, C., Shultz, M., et al. (1998). A program to use pain control medication to reduce psychotropic drug use in residents with difficult behavior. *Annals of Long-Term Care, 6*(5), 174–178.

Elliott, R. A. (2006). Problems with medication use in the elderly: An Australian perspective. *Journal of Pharmacy Practice and Research, 36*(1), 58–66.

Fitzpatrick, J., Fulmer, T., Wallace, M., et al. (Eds). (2000). *Geriatric nursing research digest* (pp. 80–84). New York: Springer.

Francis, D., Fletcher, K. & Simon, L. (1998). The geriatric resource model of care. *The Nursing Clinics of North America, 33*(3), 482–496.

Holbeach, E. & Yates, P. (2010). Prescribing in the elderly. *Australian Family Physician, 39*(10), 728–733.

Hunter, S. (2016). Addressing diversity of older adults. In S. Hunter & C. Miller (Eds). *Miller's nursing for wellness in older adults* (2nd Australian & New Zealend ed.). Sydney: Lippincott Williams & Wilkins.

Katz, S., Down, T. D., Cash, H. R., et al. (1970). Progress in the development of the index of ADL. *The Gerontologist, 10*, 20–30.

Katzman, R., Brown, T., Fuld, P., et al. (1983). Validation of a short orientation-memory concentration test of cognitive impairment. *American Journal of Psychiatry, 140*, 734–739.

Kennedy-Malone, L., Fletcher, K. R. & Plank, L. M. (2000). *Management guidelines for gerontological nurse practitioners*. Philadelphia: F.A. Davis.

Klintworth, G. K. (2008). The eye. In R. Rubin & D. E. Strayer (Eds). *Rubin's pathology: Clinicopathologic foundations of medicine* (5th ed., p. 1257). Philadelphia: Lippincott Williams & Wilkins.

Lawton, M. P. (1971). Functional assessment of elderly people. *Journal of the American Geriatrics Society, 9*(6), 465–481.

McGann, E. (2000). Pulmonary changes in elders. In J. Fitzpatrick, T. Fulmer, M. Wallace, et al. (Eds). *Geriatric nursing research digest* (pp. 80–84). New York: Springer.

Mezey, M., Rauckhorst, L. & Stokes, S. (1993). *Health assessment of the older individual* (2nd ed.). New York: Springer.

Moore, K. L. & Dailey, A. F. (2006). *Clinically oriented anatomy* (5th ed., p. 967). Philadelphia: Lippincott Williams & Wilkins.

Morris, J. C., Heyman, A., Mohs, R. C., et al. (1989). The Consortium to Establish a Registry for Alzheimer's Disease (CERAD). Part I. Clinicial and neurophysiological assessment of Alzheimer's disease. *Neurology, 39*(9), 1159–1165.

Nay, R., Garratt, S. & Fetherstonhaugh, D. (2013). *Older people: Issues and innovations in care* (4th ed.). Sydney: Churchill Livingstone.

New Zealand Ministry of Health. (2011). *Tatau kura tangata: Health of older Māori chart book 2011*. Wellington: Author.

Reid, S., Te Rarawa & White, C., Ngāti Tama. (2012). Understanding health literacy. *Best Practice Journal, 45*, 4–7.

Tasman, W. & Jaeger, E. (Eds). (2001). *The Wills Eye Hospital atlas of clinical ophthalmology* (2nd ed.). Philadelphia: Lippincott Williams & Wilkins.

White, J. V., Ham, R. J., Lipschitz, D. A., et al. (1991). Consensus of the nutrition screening initiative. Risk factors and indicators of poor nutritional status in older Americans. *Journal of the American Dietetics Society, 91*, 783–787.

Williams, M. (2009). The basic geriatric respiratory examination. Available at www.medscape.com/viewarticle/712242.

Yesavage, J. A. & Brink, T. L. (1983). Development and validation of a geriatric depression screening scale: A preliminary report. *Journal of Psychiatric Research*, *17*, 37–49.

Zürcher, S., Saxer, S. & Schwendimann, R. (2011). Urinary incontinence in hospitalised elderly patients: Do nurses recognise and manage the problem? *Nursing Research & Practice (online)*, *11*, 1–5. Available at www.hindawi.com/journals/nrp. Art. ID 671302.

Selected readings

Australian Government Department of Health and Ageing. (2014). National Bowel Cancer Screening Program. Available at www.cancerscreening.gov.au.

Peterson, C. (2014). *Looking forward through the lifespan: Developmental psychology* (6th ed.). Sydney: Pearson.

Online resources

Aged and Community Services, Australia (ACSA): www.agedcare.org.au
Alzheimer's Australia: www.fightdementia.org.au
Alzheimer's New Zealand: www.alzheimers.org.nz
Australian Association of Gerontology (AAG): www.aag.asn.au
Australian Bureau of Statistics, ageing: www.abs.gov.au
Australian Indigenous Health*InfoNet*: www.healthinfonet.ecu.edu.au
Cancer Council Australia: www.cancer.org.au
Cancer Society of New Zealand: www.cancernz.org.nz
Centre for Diversity in Aged Care: www.culturaldiversity.com.au
Centre for Independent Living New Zealand: www.independentliving.org.nz
Australian Government: https://www.myagedcare.gov.au/
Dietitians Association of Australia: www.daa.asn.au
Eldernet: www.eldernet.co.nz
Health*Insite*, health information service: www.healthinsite.gov.au/seniors
Independent Living Centres Australia: www.ilcaustralia.org.au
International Research Centre for Healthy Ageing & Longevity: www.irchal.org
National Ageing Research Institute (NARI): https://www.nari.net.au/
New Zealand Association of Gerontology: www.gerontology.org.nz
New Zealand Institute for Research on Ageing: www.victoria.ac.nz/nzira
New Zealand Ministry of Health, health of older people: www.health.govt.nz/our-work/life-stages/health-older-people
Statistics New Zealand, older people in New Zealand: www.stats.govt.nz
Tatau kura tangata: Health of older Māori chart book 2011: www.health.govt.nz/publication/tatau-kura-tangata-health-older-maori-chart-book-2011

CHAPTER 35

Assessing families

CASE STUDY

You are talking with the Ross family, who have returned to the clinic for help dealing with Dan's recent diagnosis and treatment for type 1 diabetes mellitus. Dan is a 17-year-old school student who is scheduled to leave for university in 6 months. He was diagnosed with type 1 diabetes mellitus 4 months ago. Since then he has been seen in the emergency department five times for complications resulting from not following his diet–exercise–insulin protocol.

The doctor refers the Ross family to the nurse to help the family address the identified problem of Dan's refusal to follow the protocol. Because the diet and food preparation affect the whole family, Dan's sister Jenna attends the family session as well. Dan's file includes a genogram (Fig. 35-6).

Conceptual background

Nurses are well aware of the need for establishing a relationship with all patients, but Wright and Bell (2009) assert that the relationship between the nurse and the family is at a deeper level than the average nurse–patient relationship. Illness reverberates within and outside relationships, especially as a result of serious illness. As these authors argue, serious illness can strengthen and reinforce relationships or cause relationships to become difficult and divided. It is for this reason that Wright and Bell recommend focusing family assessment on relationships, and beliefs about the illness that the patient and family members hold which may influence these relationships. The nurse family assessment processes can be used to help identify family strengths and support development of the nurse–family relationship based on common understanding and respect (Smith & Ford, 2013).

FOCUS OF FAMILY ASSESSMENT

Family assessment varies with the nurse's level of education in family nursing and with the type of family nursing care to be provided. The usual approach to family assessment taken by nurses who are not specialists in family nursing is to focus on the individual as patient and the family as context for the patient's illness and care. This type of family assessment focuses on determining strengths and problem areas within the family's structure and function that influence the family's ability to support the patient.

A more advanced knowledge of family nursing is required to care for the family as patient. Using this approach, the nurse views the family unit as a system and does not focus on any one family member. Instead, the nurse works at all times simultaneously with a mental picture of the family system and the individuals in the system, which is particularly the case for Aboriginal and Torres Strait Islander peoples and New Zealand Māori patients and their families (see, for example, Chaps 11 and 12). The nurse caring for the family system can still provide care to the individual when necessary, but the primary assessment and interventions are directed towards the family as a dynamic system. The information provided in this chapter is relevant to either approach but omits expert family systems nursing concepts. The ability to ascertain use of cultural health care beliefs and practices is also important when assessing families. See Chapter 10 for information on providing culturally competent care and specific health practices.

Terms related to family assessment

To assess a family, the nurse must first determine who constitutes a family. The traditional definition of family was based on relationships of blood, marriage or adoption. This definition has evolved over the years, and a number of different groups of people living together are now considered to be families (e.g. single-parent families, extended families, communes, gay and lesbian couples, multigenerational families; Fig. 35-1). Therefore, at the turn of the 21st century, those involved in family nursing incorporated a broader definition of family, thought to be more relevant to the times. This definition is as follows: 'The family is a social system composed of two or more persons who coexist within the context of some expectations of reciprocal affection, mutual responsibility, and temporal duration. The family is characterized by commitment, mutual decision making and shared goals' (Department of Family Nursing, Oregon Health Sciences University, 1985, quoted in Hanson & Boyd, 1996, p. 6).

Based on this definition, it is relatively simple for the nurse to determine who constitutes a family for the purpose of a family assessment: the family is whoever they say they are. Other definitions of family may be used for other purposes. For example, for statistical reporting purposes, the Australian Bureau of Statistics (ABS) defines a family as a group two or more persons related by blood, marriage (registered or de facto), adoption, step or fostering, and who are usually resident in the same household (ABS, 2017). The New Zealand definition is similar: 'A couple, with or without children, or one

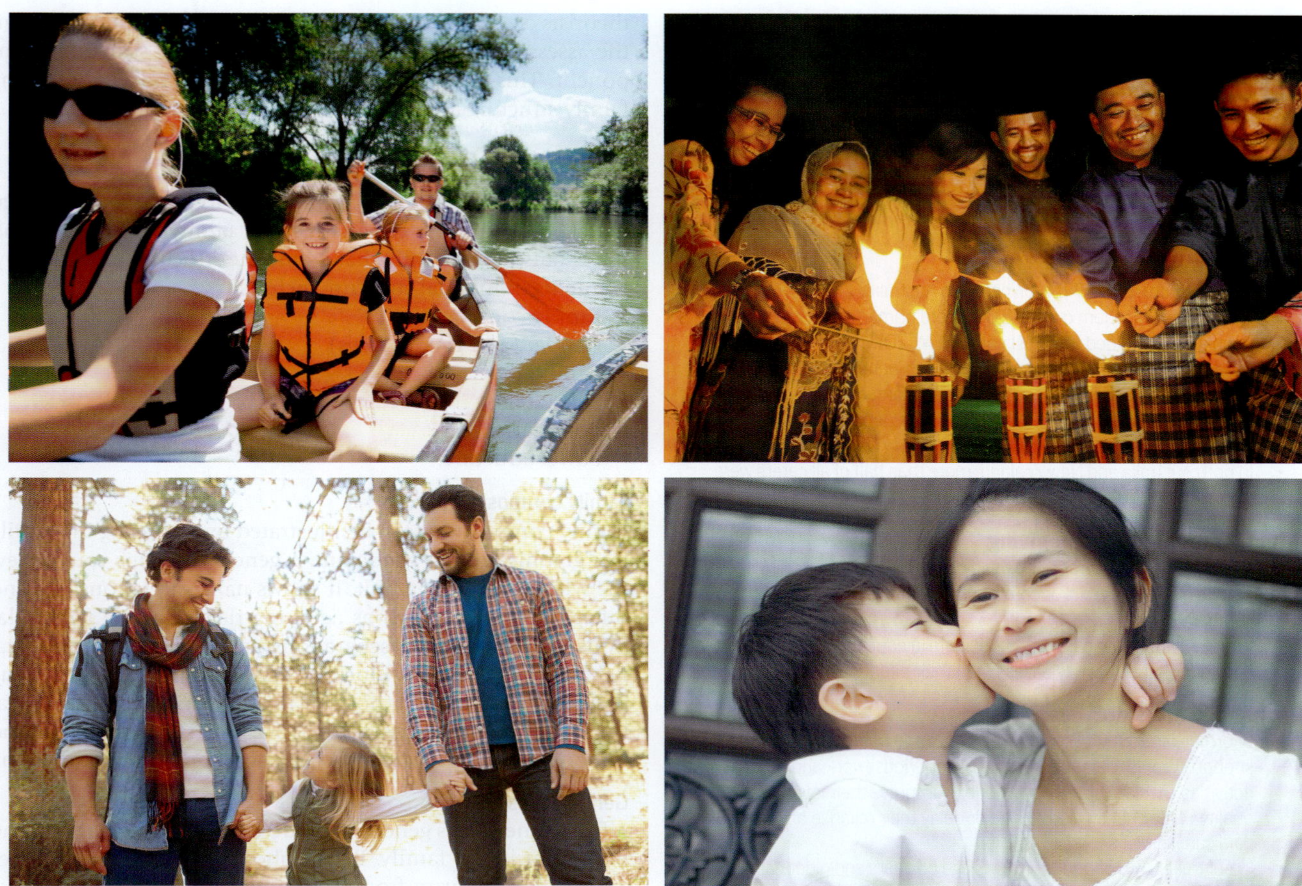

FIGURE 35-1 Some examples of many family compositions. (**A,** Shutterstock.com/nullplus; **B,** Shutterstock.com/Abdul Razak Latif; **C,** Shutterstock.com/Monkey Business Images; **D,** Shutterstock.com/wong sze yuen.)

parent with children, usually living together in a household' (Stats NZ Tatauranga Aotearoa, 2017). Chapter 2 provides examples of approaches towards different types of families. However, although definitions have evolved over time and in response to different purposes, it is important to remember that the functions of a 'family' retain commonalities, that is, in providing individual members an environment within which all can meet their health, wellness and developmental needs (Conway & Dempsey, 2014).

CLINICAL TIP

If there is disagreement within a family about who is a part of the family and who is not, the nurse should note this difference of opinion and determine that the family for the assessment consists of those people who interact the most frequently.

Relationship between families and illness

Among the many reasons for nurses to understand the concepts of family assessment, three stand out as important to a nursing assessment text:

- An ill person's family is an essential part of the context in which the illness occurs.
- The family members, the ill person and even the illness itself interact in such a way that no single component can be separated from the rest.
- The statistics on family caregiving show that families are very much involved in providing care for an ill family member. (For an overview of the many people involved in caring for family members who are ill, chronically ill or have disabilities in Australia and New Zealand, see Display 35-1.)

The dynamic interactions of the ill family member, the illness and other family members will become clear as the elements of family assessment are described throughout this chapter.

FRAMEWORK OF FAMILY ASSESSMENT

A variety of nursing models or frameworks have been developed as tools for assessing the family. Nurses have developed these models on the basis of family theories because none of the non-nursing fields has captured the necessary elements of the nursing of families. The framework used in this chapter for assessing the family is a modified combination of the Calgary Family Assessment Model (Wright & Leahey, 2005) and the Friedman (2002) Family Assessment Model. Regardless of which model or framework you use to assess the family, there are three essential components of family assessment especially prominent in all family assessment models:

- Structure
- Development
- Function.

Environmental components, cultural–ethnic variations and areas of family coping, family stress and family communication are usually incorporated into these three essential

DISPLAY 35-1 WHAT IS A CARER?

An informal carer is someone who provides care to others who need help or support due to disability, health conditions or ageing, outside the formal care sector (where paid care is provided by trained professionals) (AIHW, 2017). Carers are a diverse group and form an important part of the Australian and New Zealand aged and community health care systems.

Carer statistics

- In 2015, there were 2.7 million carers in Australia (1 in 9 Australians), of whom over 850,000 were primary carers, i.e. the people who provided the most care (AIHW, 2017).
- In New Zealand, data from the 2013 census identified 431,649 carers, which include those who look after someone who does not live in their household (i.e. 12.8% of the total population are carers) (Statistics New Zealand Census, 2013, cited in Grimmond, 2014).
- In both Australia and New Zealand, more than half of all carers were women (56% for Australia; 63% for New Zealand).

Impact of informal caregiving

- Access of primary carers (the main carers) to education, employment and social or community life may be affected by their caring role.
- The ability of young carers to participate in education, employment and social activities may be less than their peers.

What do carers do?

- Informal carers such as family members and friends may provide support through personal care, transport, housework and other activities. This assistance may not only improve their loved ones' quality of life but can also reduce or delay their reliance on formal, paid care services.
- In Australia, 76% of primary carers age 65 years and older care for their spouse or partner (AIHW, 2017).

Effect of caring on carers

There can be both positive and negative effects from being a carer, and there is evidence that many carers have unmet needs (AIHW, 2017).

- 40% of older carers report that the caring role contributed to a closer relationship with the person concerned.
- 2 in 5 carers (41%) report there is no backup carer.
- Nearly 1 in 5 (19%) report they often feel worried or depressed.

In New Zealand, a Carers' Strategy Action Plan (2019–2023) is being developed to improve the wellbeing of carers and to support those who provide care. Strategies proposed include more accurately identifying carers, their needs and their work, and supporting carers through information, navigation and respite care provision (Ministry of Social Development, 2019).

What does the future hold?

The future supply of carers in Australia and New Zealand may be at risk because of demographic factors.

The increase in the ageing population will increase the level of demand for carers. With proportionally fewer numbers of people of working age, there will be increased pressure for potential carers in this group to remain in the workforce for longer.

components. However, some models of family assessment may address them separately.

Family structure

Family structure has three elements: internal structure, external structure and context. Some theorists focus on a structural–functional framework that, when applied to family assessment, examines the interaction between the family and its internal and external environment (Friedman, 2002). Other theorists separate the assessment of family structure from the assessment of family function within the structural component. This chapter focuses on the interaction between the family structure and its internal and external environments.

Internal structure

The internal structure of a family refers to the ordering of relationships within the confines of that family. It consists of all the details in the family that define the structure of the family. Elements of internal structure include:

- Family composition
- Gender (and gender roles)
- Rank order
- Subsystems
- Boundaries
- Power structure.

Family composition

Family composition can be illustrated by recording the family tree graphically as a genogram. A genogram helps you to view the whole family as a unit. It shows names, relationships and other information such as ages, marriages and de facto relationships, divorces and separations, adoptions and health data. Behaviour and health–illness patterns can be examined using the genogram because both of these patterns tend to repeat through the generations. Figure 35-2 illustrates the format and symbols used for a simple three-generation family genogram.

Gender roles

A family member's gender often determines his or her role and behaviour in the family. Beliefs about male and female roles and behaviours vary from one family to another. Also there may be female or male subsystems that share common interests or activities.

Rank order

Rank order refers to the sibling rank of each family member. For instance, families treat the oldest child differently from the way they treat the youngest child. The rank order and gender of each family member in relation to other siblings' rank order and gender make a difference in how the person will eventually relate to a spouse or de facto partner and children. For example, an older sister of a younger brother may bring certain expectations of how women relate to men into a relationship. If the older sister marries a man who is an older brother to a younger sister, there may be conflict or competition because each may expect to be the responsible leader.

Subsystems

Each member of a family may belong to several subsystems. Subsystems may be related to gender, generational position (parents, grandparents, children), shared interests or activities (e.g. music, sports, hobbies) or function (work at home, work away from home). Examples of subsystems are: parent–child, spousal, sibling, grandmother–granddaughter, mother–daughter and father–son. Subsystems in a family relate to one another according to rules and patterns, which often are not perceived by the family until pointed out by an outsider.

Boundaries

Boundaries keep subsystems separate and distinct from other subsystems. They are maintained by rules that differentiate the particular subsystem's tasks from those of other subsystems. The most functional families have subsystems with clear

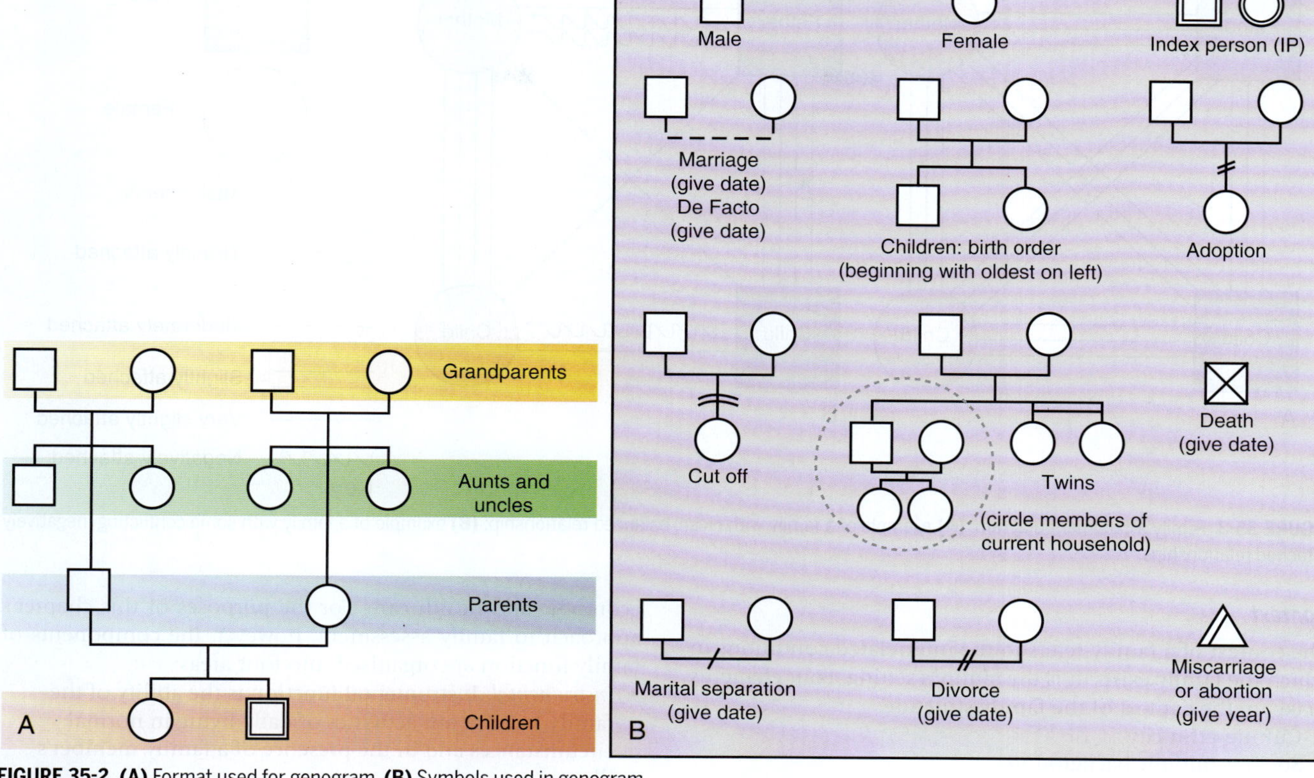

FIGURE 35-2 **(A)** Format used for genogram. **(B)** Symbols used in genogram.

boundaries; however, some connection between subsystems is maintained along with the boundaries. According to a theory by the family therapist Salvador Minuchin, the family and its subsystems may have problems with connectedness, so that boundaries are either too rigid or too diffuse (Miller, 2011). Disengaged families have rigid boundaries, which lead to low levels of effective communication and support among family members. Enmeshed families have diffuse boundaries, which make it difficult for individuals to achieve individuation from the family.

Power structure

Power structure has to do with the influences each member has on the family processes and function. Some distribution of power is necessary to maintain order so the family can function. There is usually a power hierarchy, with the parents having more authority than the children. In the most functional families, parents have a sense of shared power and children gain increasing power as they mature and become more responsible.

A tool to help the nurse and family examine family structure and function is the Family Attachment Diagram. This is a diagram of the family members' interactions. It represents the reciprocal nature and quality of the interactions. Figure 35-3 represents both a family with close and balanced relationships and a family with some conflicting, negatively attached relationships.

External structure

External structure refers to those outside groups or things to which the family is connected. External structures may influence aspects of the internal structure of the family. Two elements of external structure include extended family and external systems.

Extended family

Extended family may consist of family members not residing in the home but with whom the family interacts frequently, such as grandparents or an aunt and uncle who live only 5 minutes away. It also may include family members with whom the family interacts infrequently such as a first cousin who lives across the country and with whom the family communicates only through Christmas cards and a visit once every few years. However, the family feels confident that this cousin would be supportive in times of need. Another type of extended family is the 'cut off' family member. An example would be a brother who left home 10 years ago and with whom there is no contact at all. This brother may still be considered extended family.

External systems

External systems are those systems that are larger than the family and with which the family interacts. These systems include institutions, agencies and significant people outside the family. Some specific examples of external systems include a family's local health centre, school, jobs, church, recreational organisations, friends, neighbours, work colleagues and extended family (only those with whom interaction is frequent).

An ecomap can be used to assess the family members' interactions with the systems outside the family. The diagram, illustrated in Figure 35-4, is similar to the attachment diagram and shows the positive or conflicting nature of the family's relationships with outside groups or organisations.

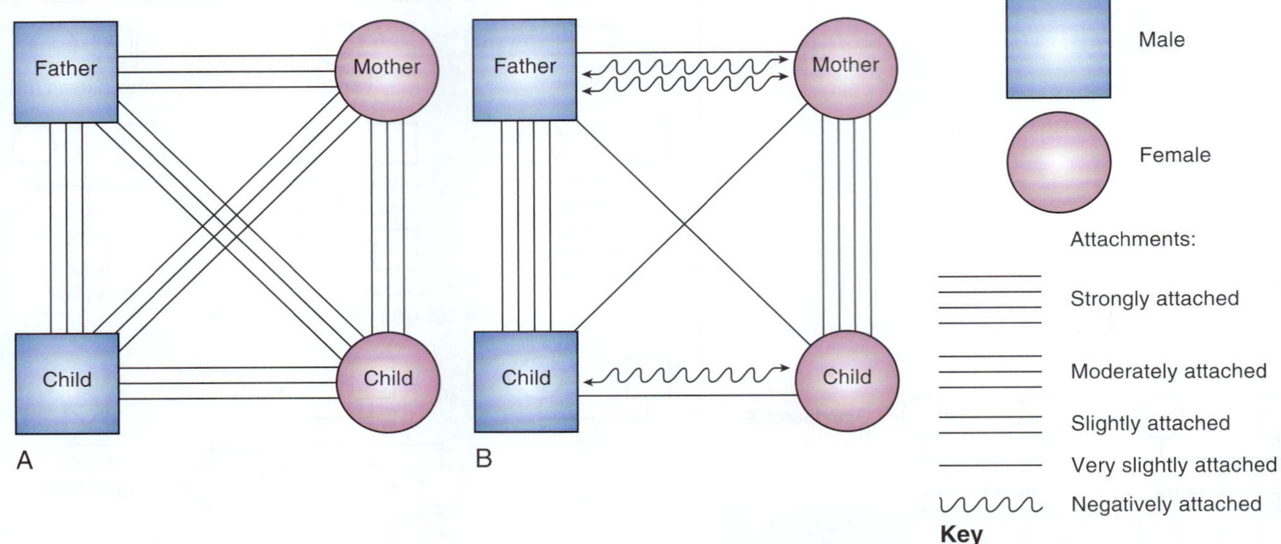

FIGURE 35-3 Family attachment diagram: **(A)** example of a family with close, balanced relationship; **(B)** example of a family with some conflicting, negatively attached relationships.

Context

The context of a family refers to the interrelated conditions in which the family exists: it is the family's setting. Four elements make up the context of the family structure:

- Culture-ethnicity
- Socio-economic background
- Religion
- Environment.

Culture or ethnicity may influence family structure and interactions. Assessment should include how much the family identifies with and adheres to traditional practices of a particular culture, whether the family's practices are similar to those of the neighbourhood of residence and whether the family has more than one ethnic or cultural makeup.

The effects of socio-economic background and religion provide context for the family structure and lifestyle. A couple from different social classes or different religions may bring different expectations into the family system.

Environmental characteristics of the residence and neighbourhood, and family and neighbourhood interactions clarify the context for the family structure and interactions.

Family development

Like individuals, families go through stages of growth and development. These stages of development are as important to the health and wellbeing of the family as they are to the individual. In fact, a static family structure is dysfunctional. Friedman (2002) developed theories about family lifecycle stages and their associated tasks. Although largely traditional family types are not necessarily reflective of the diversity currently present in Australia and New Zealand, they are still useful to consider. The stages and tasks of three of these cycles—the traditional nuclear family, divorced family and remarried family—are described by Wright and Leahey (2005) and are presented in Display 35-2.

Family function

Friedman (1998, 2002) defined five basic family functions: affective, socialisation and social placement, reproductive, economic and health care. For the purposes of this chapter's approach to family assessment, however, the components of family function are organised into four areas:

- *Instrumental:* Instrumental function is the ability of the family to carry out activities of daily living in normal circumstances and in the presence of a family member's illness.
- *Affective and socialisation:* Affective function refers to the family's response to all members' needs for support, caring, closeness and intimacy, and the balance of needs for separateness and connectedness. Socialisation function refers to the family's ability to bring about healthy socialisation of children.
- *Expressive:* Expressive function refers to communication patterns used within the family. Members of well-functioning families are able to: express a broad range of emotions; clearly express feelings and needs; encourage feedback; listen attentively to one another; treat one another with respect; avoid displacing, distorting or masking verbal messages; avoid negative circular communication patterns; and use encouraging versus punishment methods to influence behaviour.
- *Health care:* Assessment of health care function is useful for the nurse. It refers to family members' beliefs about a health problem; its aetiology, treatment and prognosis; and the role of professionals. Whether all family members agree or some members disagree with the beliefs helps the nurse to understand the family. The family's health promotion practices are also assessed.

THEORETICAL CONCEPTS OF FAMILY FUNCTION

Some components of family function are based on theoretical concepts found in systems theory, Bowen family system theory and communication theory. It is important for the nurse to have a good understanding of these concepts before performing an assessment of family function.

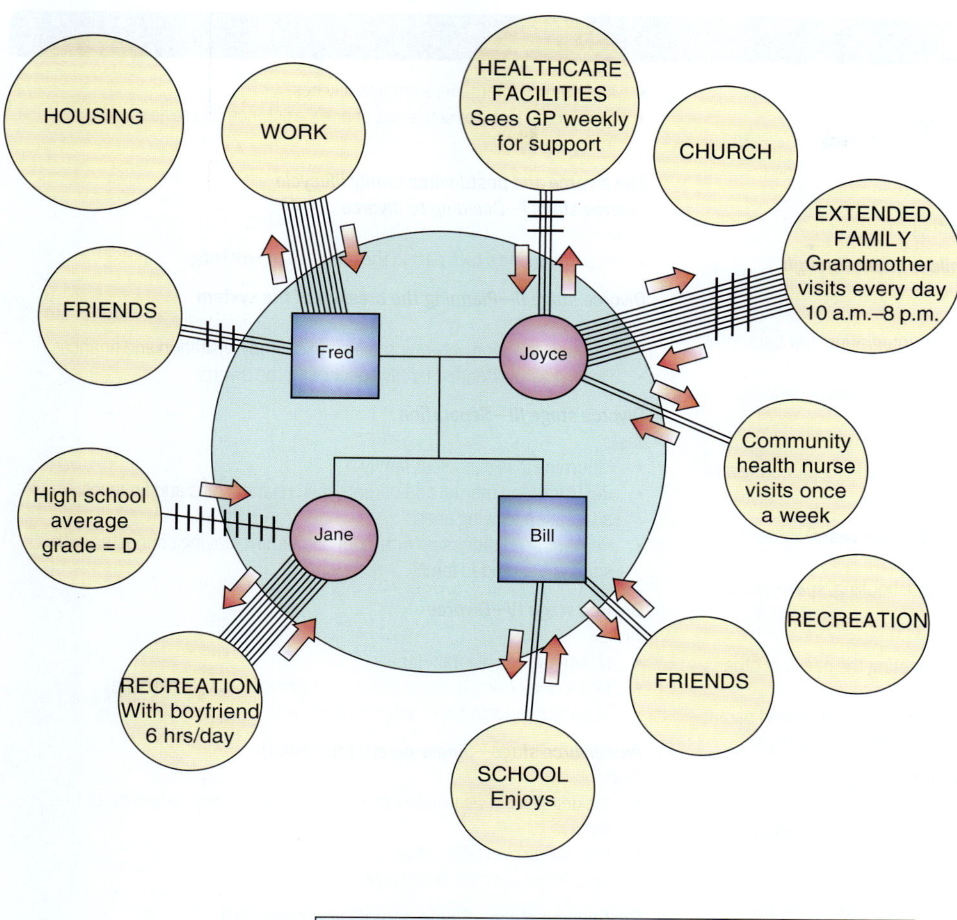

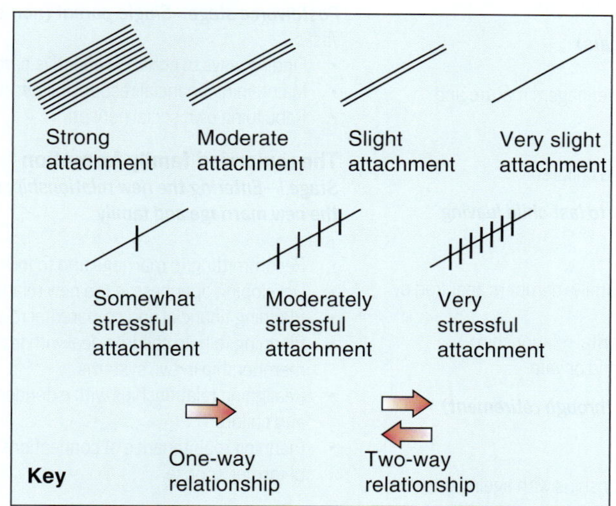

FIGURE 35-4 An ecomap is used to assess family members' interactions with systems outside the family.

Systems theory

Systems theory holds that a system is composed of subsystems interconnected to the whole system and to each other by means of an integrated and dynamic self-regulating feedback mechanism. Systems theory can be applied to any group with reciprocal dynamic interaction.

Wright and Leahey (2005) list the major concepts of systems theory that apply to families: A family is part of a larger suprasystem and is also composed of many subsystems (e.g. parent–child, sibling, spouse); the family as a whole is greater than the sum of its parts; a change in one family member affects all family members; the family is able to create a balance between change and stability; and family members' behaviours are best understood from a view of circular rather than linear causality. For example, any behaviour of family member A affects family member B, and B's behaviour then affects A. Therefore, rather than an individual causing a family problem, the behaviour pattern or system causes another behaviour.

Bowen family system theory

The family therapist Bowen (Bowen Center, n.d.; Titelman, 2008) developed several concepts that are widely used to

DISPLAY 35-2 FAMILY LIFECYCLES

Two-parent nuclear family lifecycle

Stage I—Beginning families (stage of marriage)

Tasks

- Establishing a mutually satisfying marriage
- Relating harmoniously to the kin network
- Planning a family (decisions about parenthood)

Stage II—Childbearing families (oldest child is infant through 30 months)

Tasks

- Setting up the young family as a stable unit (integrating new baby into family)
- Reconciling conflicting developmental tasks and needs of various family members
- Maintaining a satisfying marital relationship
- Expanding relationships with extended family by adding parenting and grandparenting roles

Stage III—Families with preschool children (2.5 to 6 years)

Tasks

- Meeting family members' needs for adequate housing, space, privacy and safety
- Socialising the children
- Integrating new child members while still meeting the needs of other children
- Maintaining healthy relationships within the family (marital and parent–child) and outside the family (extended family and community)

Stage IV—Families with schoolchildren (6 to 13 years)

Tasks

- Socialising the children, including promoting school achievement and fostering of healthy peer relations of children
- Maintaining a satisfying marital relationship
- Meeting the physical health needs of family members

Stage V—Families with teenagers (13 to 20 years)

Tasks

- Balancing of freedom with responsibility as teenagers mature and become increasingly autonomous
- Refocusing the marital relationship
- Communicating openly between parents and children

Stage VI—Launching young adults (from first to last child leaving home)

Tasks

- Expanding the family circle to include new family members acquired by marriage of children
- Continuing to renew and re-adjust in the marital relationship
- Assisting ageing and ill parents of the husband or wife

Stage VII—Middle-aged parents (empty nest through retirement)

Tasks

- Providing a health-promoting environment
- Sustaining satisfying and meaningful relationships with ageing parents and adult children
- Strengthening the marital relationship

Stage VIII—Family in retirement and old age (retirement to death of both spouses)

Tasks

- Maintaining a satisfying living arrangement
- Adjusting to a reduced income
- Maintaining marital relationships
- Adjusting to loss of spouse
- Maintaining intergenerational family ties
- Continuing to make sense out of one's existence (life review and integration)

The divorce and postdivorce family lifecycle

Divorce stage I—Deciding to divorce

Tasks

- Accepting one's own part in the failure of the marriage

Divorce stage II—Planning the breakup of the system

Tasks

- Working cooperatively on problems of custody, visitation and finances
- Dealing with extended family concerning the divorce

Divorce stage III—Separation

Tasks

- Mourning loss of nuclear family
- Restructuring marital and parent–child relationships and finances; adaptation to living apart
- Realigning relationships with extended family; staying connected with spouse's extended family

Divorce stage IV—Divorce

Tasks

- Mourning loss of intact family
- Retrieving hopes, dreams and expectations from the marriage
- Staying connected with extended families

Postdivorce stage—Single-parent (custodial)

Tasks

- Making flexible visitation arrangements with ex-spouse and his or her family
- Rebuilding own financial resources
- Rebuilding own social network

Postdivorce stage—Single-parent (non-custodial)

Tasks

- Finding ways to continue effective parenting relationship with children
- Maintaining financial responsibilities to ex-spouse and children
- Rebuilding own social network

The remarried family formation

Stage I—Entering the new relationship; conceptualising and planning the new marriage and family

Tasks

- Recommitting to marriage and to forming a family
- Developing openness in the new relationship
- Planning financial and co-parental relationships with ex-spouse
- Planning to help children deal with fears, loyalty conflicts and membership in two systems
- Realigning relationships with extended family to include new spouse and children
- Planning maintenance of connections for children with extended family of former spouse

Stage II—Remarriage and family reconstitution

Tasks

- Restructuring family boundaries to allow for inclusion of new spouse or stepparent
- Realigning relationships and financial arrangements throughout subsystems
- Making room for relationships of all children with custodial and non-custodial parents and grandparents

Adapted from Friedman, M. (1998). *Family nursing: Theory and practice* (4th ed., p. 141). Norwalk, CT: Appleton & Lange.

assess family function. Bowen views the nuclear family as part of a multigenerational extended family with patterns of relating that tend to repeat over generations. When the pattern of projecting anxiety onto a child continues across generations, it is called the *multigenerational transmission process.* Bowen theorises that familial emotional and interaction patterns are reflected in eight interwoven concepts. Two of these concepts—differentiation of self and triangles—are especially important to grasp for assessment of family function.

Differentiation of self

Differentiation of self is assessed in relation to the boundaries of the subsystems in the structure of the family. This concept is based on a balance of emotional and intellectual levels of function. The emotional level, associated with lower brain centres, relates to feelings. The intellectual level, associated with the cerebral cortex, relates to cognition. How connected these levels, or systems, are affects the person's social functioning. The greater the balance between thinking and feeling, the higher the differentiation of self and the better the person is at managing anxiety.

The Bowen Center (n.d.) provides a summary of key elements of the concept of differentiation of self. The family with highly differentiated adult members is flexible in its interactions, seeks to support all members, understands each member as unique and encourages members to develop differently from one another. Family roles are assigned on the basis of knowledge, skill and interest.

The family with low levels of differentiation has adult members who demonstrate impulsive actions, who have difficulty delaying gratification, who cannot analyse a situation before reacting and who cannot maintain intimate interpersonal relationships (similar to the developmental level of a 2-year-old child). Intense, short-term relationships are the norm, and emotionally based reactions can escalate into violence. Family roles are assigned on the basis of family tradition.

A moderately differentiated person is less dominated by emotions, but personal relationships are often emotion-dominated. Life is rule-bound and thinking is usually dualistic (things and people are black and white, good or bad, smart or stupid). A situation cannot be perceived from any but a personal perspective. The person tends to 'fuse' or become enmeshed with another in emotional relationships, losing themselves in the efforts to please the other. Families with moderately differentiated members exhibit rigid patterns of interactions that are rule-bound and have defined roles and acceptable behaviours.

Triangles

Triangles are discussed in relation to subsystems of family structure. Titelman (2008) describes the Bowen triangle as a relational pattern or emotional configuration that exists among one or two family members and another person, object or issue. Triangles exist in all families; who makes up a triangle can change depending on the situation. However, when two people avoid dealing with emotional closeness or an issue that produces anxiety, they may use a third person to evade the stress. For instance, a wife may pull in a child as a third person in the couple's relationship; the husband may distance himself from the conflict by deeper involvement in work. As the intensity of the relationship changes, the amount of interaction is usually balanced, so that as two members move closer, the third withdraws.

Communication theory

Communication theory concerns the sending and receiving of both verbal and non-verbal messages. The focus is on how individuals interact with one another. According to Wright and Leahey (1994), the major concepts of communication theory applied to families are:

- All non-verbal communication is meaningful.
- All communication has two major channels for transmission (verbal and non-verbal including body language, facial expression, voice tone, music, poetry, painting and so forth).
- A dyadic (two-person) relationship has varying degrees of symmetry and complementarity (both of which may be healthy depending on context).
- All communication consists of two levels: content (what is said) and relationship (of those interacting).

It is important to remember that what is functional for one family or culture may not be helpful in another. During the assessment process the nurse can role model clear communication patterns and acknowledge effective communication within the family.

Circular communication

Circular communication is a reciprocal form of communication between two people. Another way of looking at this concept is to consider the pattern of communication that develops when two or more people communicate regularly. Wright and Leahey (1994) note that most relationship issues have a pattern of circular communication. One person speaks and another interprets what is heard, then reacts and speaks on the basis of that interpretation, creating a circular feedback loop based on each individual's perceptions and reactions.

Circular communication can be positive or negative. An example of negative circular communication is as follows: An angry wife or husband criticises her or his spouse; the spouse feels angry and withdraws; the wife or husband becomes even angrier and criticises more; the spouse becomes angrier and withdraws further. Each person sees the problem as the other's and each person's communication influences the other person's behaviour. Positive and negative circular communication patterns are illustrated in Figure 35-5.

Family assessment

Wright and Leahey (2005) assert that family knowledge can be obtained and applied even in very brief meetings with a family. They provide a guide to a 15-minute (or shorter) family interview. Key elements of the interview, which occurs only in the context of a therapeutic relationship, are communicating in a respectful manner, therapeutic conversation, family genogram (and ecomap as appropriate), therapeutic questions and acknowledgement of the family's strengths. See Display 35-3 for a summary of the interview technique.

FAMILY INTERVIEW TECHNIQUES

The brief interview consists of several elements, which are described by Wright and Leahey in the context of the Calgary

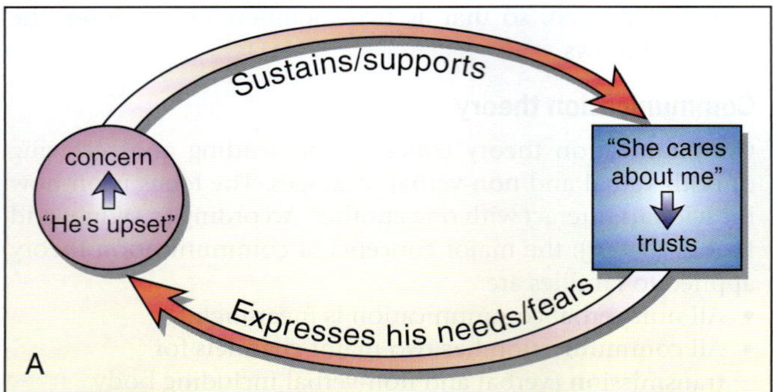

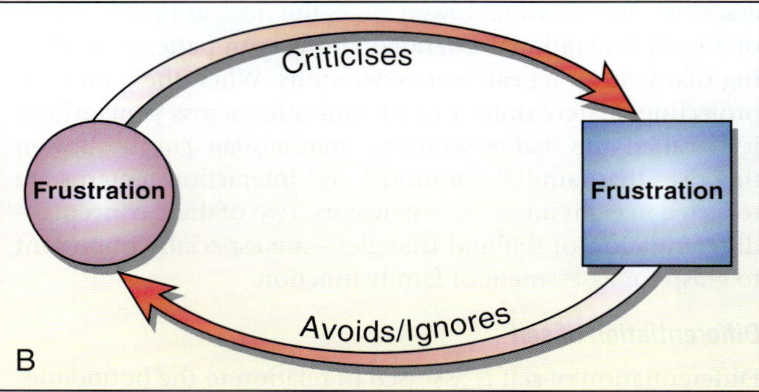

FIGURE 35-5 (A) Positive circular communication. **(B)** Negative circular communication.

CASE STUDY

Mr and Mrs Ross express concern and caring for Dan's wellbeing and request assistance with dealing with Dan's diagnosis and treatment. You ask how everyone feels about Dan's disease and treatment. Both the parents and Jenna appear tense when describing the effect of trying to deal with Dan's disease and his refusal to follow the protocol. Mr and Mrs Ross express frustration with their inability to get Dan to follow the doctor's orders. Dan expresses frustration at having a disease and at being asked to follow a protocol that makes him different from his friends and unable to do the things that they do (e.g. diet, exercise, partying). Dan expresses frustration at having his parents tell him what to do. Jenna expresses frustration at Dan for upsetting the family, especially at mealtimes, and particularly in regard to what family members eat and how they interact. When you ask the family to tell you about Dan's disease and treatment, Dan and his parents describe a good understanding of the disease and reasons for the protocol.

CRITICAL THINKING

1. You decide to explore the impact of Dan's diagnosis on the whole family. What importance could family rank order have on the impact of Dan's diagnosis on family functioning? How would you incorporate this aspect into your assessment?
2. Would you ask the family members about their communication styles and patterns? Why or why not?

Family Assessment Model and the Calgary Family Intervention Model. Essential points follow.

Communicating with respect

The simple acts of communicating with respect that invite a trusting relationship are:

- Always call the patient by name.
- Introduce yourself by name.
- Examine your attitude and adjust responses to convey interest and acceptance.

DISPLAY 35-3 TIPS FOR CONDUCTING THE 15-MINUTE FAMILY INTERVIEW

- Introduce yourself and use respect in interactions.
- Seek opportunities to involve family in care delivery and decision making.
- Use active listening, create family genograms (ecomaps) and ask therapeutic questions to help family members (and the nurse) better understand the family's needs and beliefs about themselves and the illness.
- Seek opportunities to acknowledge the strengths of individuals and the family.

- Explain your role for the time you will spend with the patient or family.
- Explain any procedure before entering the room with equipment to perform the procedure.
- Keep appointments and promises to return.
- Be honest.

Therapeutic conversation

Therapeutic conversation is purposeful and time-limited. The arts of listening and empathising are paramount. You should not only make information giving and patient involvement in decision making an integral part of the care delivery process but also seek opportunities to engage in purposeful conversations with families. Nurse–family therapeutic conversations can include basic ideas such as:

- Offering to accompany the patient to the clinic or hospital
- Including family members in health care facility admission procedures
- Encouraging family members to ask questions during patient orientation to a health care facility
- Acknowledging the patient's and family's expertise in managing health problems by asking about routines at home
- Presenting opportunities to practise how the patient will handle different interactions in the future, such as telling family members and others that they cannot eat certain foods
- Consulting with families and patients about their ideas for treatment and discharge (Wright & Leahey, 2000, p. 280).

The principles above can also be used to support communication with children and young people in the family; however, the communication approach used by the nurse needs to be tailored to the child or young person concerned and his or age and developmental stage (Smith & Ford, 2013). The nurse also needs to have a sound understanding of the child's or young person's situation and communication preferences, particularly if he or she is the family member affected by illness.

Family genograms and ecomaps

The genogram (see Fig. 35-1) acts as a continuous visual reminder to carers to 'think family' In addition, the ecomap (see Fig. 35-4) illustrates the family's interactions with outside systems.

Acknowledgement of strengths

Acknowledge the family's strengths at least once or twice during each meeting with the family. The individual or family can be commended on strengths, resources or competencies observed or reported to the nurse. With these observations of behaviour look for patterns, not one-time occurrences, to commend. Examples include 'Your family shows much courage in living with your wife's cancer for 5 years' and 'Your son is so gentle despite feeling so ill' (Wright & Leahey, 2000, p. 282). This positive feedback offers family members a new view of themselves. Wright and Leahey propose that many families experiencing illness, disability or trauma have a 'commendation-deficit disorder' (p. 282). Offering a different view of themselves helps the family members to look differently at the health problem and more towards solutions. Some assessment tools such as the Australian Family Strengths Nursing Assessment Guide can be used to support solutions-focused conversations with any family member, which can help to identify and build on family strengths (Smith & Ford, 2013).

CRITICAL THINKING

3. Family assessment in the context of a health care problem requires the gathering of relevant clinical information as well as assessment of the family's verbal and non-verbal communication patterns. Review the earlier sections on family structure, development and function and determine why it is important that Dan and his family should be assessed together rather than assessing Dan alone.
4. Before reading the following section on family assessment, consider how communication patterns and styles could influence the impact of a diagnosis of diabetes on a younger family member. How could the diagnosis have a positive impact? How could it have a negative impact?
5. Consider what impact the diagnosis could have on Dan as the only male child in the family with regard to his self-image and self-esteem. Is it important to assess the other family members' understanding of this aspect, as well as their understanding of the disease and treatment? Why or why not?

Assessment procedure

To complete a family assessment of structure, function and development, the following outline provides a pattern and suggested questions. As appropriate, incorporate some of the following interview components and techniques in your practice.

FAMILY ASSESSMENT

ASSESSMENT PROCEDURE	NORMAL FINDINGS	ABNORMAL FINDINGS
Family structure		
INTERNAL FAMILY STRUCTURE		
Assess family composition. Use a genogram and fill in as much information as possible. Ask the following questions: • What is the family type (two-parent, three-generation, single-parent)? • Who does the family consider to be family? • Has anyone recently moved in or out? Has anyone recently died?	Family identifies family type and members of the family. A new baby born into family or young adult moving out reflects normal lifecycle tasks. Death is also a normal part of life, but it is not often viewed as a family strength.	A new baby or a young adult moving out may cause excessive stress for family. Death of a family member often causes a variety of different reactions including extreme grief, depression, anger and even relief. Serious family problems may result when family members react to, and deal with, the death differently.
Determine gender roles in the family. Gender often determines an expected family role. Ask each family member the following question: What are the expected behaviours for men in your family? For women? **CLINICAL TIP** **It is important to ask both the men and the women what they perceive to be the roles of men and the woman in the family because they may perceive the roles differently.**	Family members understand and agree on expected gender-related behaviours; expected behaviours are flexible.	Rigid, gender-related behaviours reduce the family's flexibility for meeting family needs. One or more family members have different beliefs about expected behaviours for men and women, which can lead to family conflict.

Continued on following page

FAMILY ASSESSMENT (continued)

ASSESSMENT PROCEDURE	NORMAL FINDINGS	ABNORMAL FINDINGS
Evaluate rank order. Spousal rank order often plays a significant role in family harmony. Ask spouses: What rank order did you have in your childhood family (e.g. older sister, youngest brother)? Using the family's answers and information you know concerning birth order, ask yourself: Are spouses' birth rank orders likely to be complementary or competitive?	Complementary birth order of spouses can support each spouse's interaction with the other based on past experiences with siblings (e.g. older brother in one family marries younger sister in another).	Competitive birth order of spouses may result in problems. For example, if an older brother in one family marries an older sister in another, both may be used to being the responsible leader.
Assess subsystems. Ask the family questions about attachments within the family. For example, is there a mother–daughter relationship? How strong is it? Use a family attachment diagram to determine family subgroups. Assessment of the function of family subgroups is covered under assessment of family function.	Family subgroups are present and appear healthy.	Family subgroups are absent or appear excessively strong, excluding other family members. For instance, a strong female subgroup of mother and daughters may work to exclude the father or husband from important family activities or decision making. Or an overly strong spousal subsystem may impose an emotional distance between parents and children.
Assess family boundaries. Boundaries separate family subsystems. Ask the family questions about how the subsystems are fixed within the family. For example, is the mother–daughter subsystem totally separated from the father–son subsystem? Based on the family's answers, ask yourself the following questions: Are there boundaries between subsystems? What types of boundaries are present? *Note:* Assessment of the function of family boundaries is covered under 'Family function'.	Permeable boundaries are present.	Rigid or diffuse boundaries are present.
Evaluate the family power structure. Ask the family to rate the structure of the family on a scale with chaos (no leader) at one end, equality in the middle and domination by one individual at the other end. If the family is dominated by one individual, ask the patients who that person is.	A power hierarchy with parents equally in control, but tending towards egalitarian and flexible power shifts, is considered normal. This type of structure demonstrates respect for all family members and encourages family development and effective functioning.	Chaotic or authoritarian power structures tend to prevent effective family functioning and individual development.
EXTERNAL STRUCTURE		
Assess the extended family. Ask 'Are extended family members available to help support your immediate family?'	Extended family can provide emotional and other support to the family.	Lack of extended family or no contact with extended family results in no support for immediate family.
Assess external systems. Ask the family questions about relationships with external systems (e.g. agencies and people outside immediate family). Use an ecomap to record and view these relationships. Then ask yourself the following questions based on the ecomap: What relationship is there between the family and external systems? Are external systems overinvolved or underinvolved with the family?	Positive relationships with external systems are beneficial to the family. Balanced involvement with external systems adds to the health of the family.	Conflictual relationships with external systems add stress to the family. Too little or too much involvement with external systems can prevent the family from effectively using resources to meet its needs. In addition, either overinvolvement or underinvolvement with external systems can add great stress to the immediate family.

FAMILY ASSESSMENT (continued)

ASSESSMENT PROCEDURE	NORMAL FINDINGS	ABNORMAL FINDINGS
Family structure (continued)		
Assess context. Ask questions that relate to ethnicity, socio-economic background, religion and environment. How does the family's culture or ethnicity affect the family structure and function? How does the family's culture or ethnicity affect interactions with neighbours? How does the family's culture or ethnicity affect interactions with external systems?	The family has strong and mutually supportive connections with others of like ethnicity or culture.	Cultural or ethnic difference from the neighbourhood or larger society can produce misunderstanding and negatively affect communications and interactions.
What socio-economic background is most representative of the family? Do socio-economic background factors affect the family's ability to meet its needs?	Cultural, social and economic factors of the family's socio-economic background support the family's ability to meet its needs.	Cultural, social and economic resources associated with social class may be inadequate to meet family needs.
Is religion important to the family?	Religion provides the family with supportive spiritual beliefs.	Religious controversies among family members may produce family conflict.
Are environmental characteristics of the residence and neighbourhood adequate to meet family needs?	The residence and neighbourhood are safe, and necessary resources are available.	The residence or neighbourhood is not safe. Resources are not readily available.
Family development: Lifecycle stages and tasks		
Ask the family questions about the family's lifecycle stage. Can the family meet the tasks of the current lifecycle stage with which it is dealing?	The family has successfully met the tasks of previous lifecycle stages and can meet the tasks of its current lifecycle stage.	The family has not adequately met tasks of previous lifecycle stages and may be unable to meet tasks of the current stage.
Family function		
Assess instrumental function. Evaluate if the family can carry out routine activities of daily living.	The family has successfully met routine daily living needs of all family members.	The family cannot carry out one or more activities of daily living.
Does a family member's illness affect the family's ability to carry out activities of daily living?	The family can continue to carry out activities of daily living even with the added stress of an ill family member.	The added stress of caring for an ill family member prevents the family from adequately carrying out one or more activities of daily living.
Note affective and socialisation function. Observe family interactions and ask questions to determine if family members provide mutual support and nurturance to one another.	Families that can meet psychological needs for support and nurturance of family members provide an opportunity for each individual to self-differentiate and reach emotional maturity.	Families that cannot provide for psychological needs for support and nurturance make self-differentiation and emotional health of the members unlikely.
Are parenting practices appropriate for healthy socialisation of the children?	Parenting practices based on respect, guidance and encouragement (rather than punishment) encourage socialisation.	Parenting practices based on control, coercion and punishment discourage socialisation. Chapter 9 discusses nursing assessment of families that use violence.
What function do subgroups serve within the family?	Subgroups are flexible and assist the family in meeting changing needs.	Rigid subgroups do not easily change to meet individual needs.

Continued on following page

FAMILY ASSESSMENT (continued)

ASSESSMENT PROCEDURE	NORMAL FINDINGS	ABNORMAL FINDINGS
Are there alliances that produce triangles?	Flexible alliances and triangles form to maintain family functioning.	Rigid alliances and triangles are formed to balance negative forces and stress. They are a coping mechanism.
What function do boundaries serve within the family?	Permeable boundaries encourage emotional development and self-differentiation of family members.	Rigid or diffuse boundaries discourage emotional development and self-differentiation.
Are family members enmeshed (overly involved with each other)? Disengaged (underinvolved with each other)?	Adequate involvement of family members without enmeshment or disengagement serves as support for family function and individual development.	Enmeshed or disengaged family members cannot adequately self-differentiate.
Evaluate expressive function. Ask the family and observe interactions to *assess emotional communication:* Do all family members express a broad range of both negative and positive emotion?	Open expression and acceptance of feelings and emotions within a family encourages positive family functioning.	Lack of acceptance of emotional expression or acceptance of emotional expression by only some family members tends to prevent effective family development and functioning.
Assess *verbal communication:* Are verbal messages clearly stated?	Clear verbal messages increase open communication.	Displaced, masked or distorted messages obstruct open communication and may reflect underlying problems in family functioning.
Assess *non-verbal communication:* Do non-verbal communications match verbal content?	Clear and open communications have verbal and non-verbal elements that match.	Non-verbal communications that do not match verbal content suggest a lack of honesty or openness in the communication.
Assess *circular communication:* Is there an evident pattern of circular communication? If so, is it negative or positive?	Positive circular communication helps to build up the family members.	Negative circular communication reinforces interpersonal conflict and prevents an understanding of the intended message.
Assess the family's health care function. Ask the following questions: What do family members believe about the aetiology, treatment, prognosis of the health problem? What do family members believe about the role of professionals, the role of the family and the level of control the family has relative to the health problem? Are family members' beliefs in agreement or discord?	Agreement among family members reduces conflict.	Disagreement among family members produces conflict and draws on energy and emotional resources needed to handle the health problem.
What strengths does the family believe it has for coping with the health problem?	If the family perceives strengths, it will be more likely to cope effectively.	If the family does not perceive strengths, it will have difficulty coping with the health problem.
Are the family's health promotion practices supportive of family health?	A pattern of health promotion practices provides a basis for building in health care for a particular health problem.	A family that has little practice of health promotion behaviours will have difficulty incorporating health care practices for a particular problem into its routines.
Assess for multigenerational patterns. Look back over the assessment and determine if there are any multigenerational patterns evident in any categories.	Multigenerational patterns of positive behaviours are often seen in effectively functioning families.	Multigenerational patterns of ineffective or destructive behaviours make change more difficult.

VALIDATING AND DOCUMENTING FINDINGS

After establishing a therapeutic relationship with the Ross family, the nurse interviews the family, using therapeutic questions. The family reports family stress and conflict about Dan's recent diagnosis of type 1 diabetes mellitus. The nurse explores this health concern using the COLDSPA mnemonic.

Sample of subjective and objective data

The nurse interviews the family about structure. The family is composed of two parents and two adolescent children (son Dan, 17 years old, and daughter Jenna, 12 years old)—a two-generation family. Family members agree on expected gender-related behaviours, which are flexible. The wife is the youngest daughter of her family, and the husband is the oldest son of his family. Subgroups and triangles between family members are flexible. The boundaries between subgroups are permeable.

The nurse explores power. The two parents report that they are equally in control, but the children are consulted for decisions that affect the family. The nurse asks about extended family and support systems. Mr Ross's mother lives in a nearby town but is not able to provide physical support to the family, although she is emotionally supportive. The family is positively involved in local sporting clubs, Dan has a group of supportive friends, and the parents enjoy being involved with the local garden club. Time spent with groups outside the family is balanced evenly with time spent with the immediate family.

The nurse asks about the environment. The family lives in a safe home and in a neighbourhood with people of similar ethnicity. The family's cultural, social and economic factors support their ability to live well. The family is currently able to meet the tasks of its lifecycle stage, although the family is facing Dan's departure for university in 6 months' time. The family has met routine activities of daily living needs of its members.

Family provides the psychological needs for support and nurturance of all family members, although Dan does not feel supported and the family is conflicted on how best to support him with the new diagnosis and treatment protocol. Family members feel free to express and accept feelings and emotions openly, although Dan's increasingly rebellious attitude and anger are new and are increasing family stress. Completing the Ross family assessment, the nurse asks questions about diabetes within the family and how the family has handled stressful situations in the past.

The nurse asks how everyone feels about Dan's disease and treatment. Both the parents and Jenna appear tense when describing the effect of trying to deal with Dan's disease and his refusal to follow the protocol. Mr and Mrs Ross express frustration with inability to get Dan to follow the doctor's orders. Dan expresses frustration at having a disease and at being asked to follow a protocol that makes him different from his friends and unable to do the things they do

Continued on following page

COLDSPA

Mnemonic	Question	Patient response example
Character	Describe the sign or symptom (feeling, appearance, sound, smell or taste, if applicable). In this case, describe the family members' reactions to the diagnosis and treatment of Dan's diabetes.	Family conflict has developed over Dan not following the prescribed diet–exercise–insulin protocol. Repeated visits to the emergency department (ED) and the threats to his long-term health have exacerbated the family stress.
Onset	When did it begin?	Four months ago at diagnosis.
Location	Where is it? Does it radiate? Does it occur anywhere else?	The conflicts between Dan and his parents and his sister have escalated.
Duration	How long does it last? Does it recur?	The conflicted interactions have become more frequent as the time nears for Dan to go away to university.
Severity	How bad is it? How much does it bother you?	All family members describe the conflict and its effect as very stressful, both to their interactions as a family and to Dan's interactions with his peers.
Pattern	What makes it better or worse?	Mealtimes make it worse, and there is increasing family stress with repeated visits to the ED.
Associated factors/How it **A**ffects the patient	What other symptoms occur with it? How does it affect you?	Dan's age of 17 brings up the issue of family development states beginning to change, anticipating family exit when he leaves for university, as well as his developmental tasks being threatened by his inability to 'be like his friends'.

(e.g. diet, exercise, partying). Dan expresses frustration at having his parents tell him what to do. Jenna expresses frustration at Dan for upsetting the family, especially at mealtime, particularly in regard to what family members eat and how they interact. When the nurse asks the family about Dan's disease and treatment, Dan and his parents describe a good understanding of the disease and reasons for the protocol.

Multigenerational patterns of positive behaviours are described by this family. The nurse observes family interactions during the assessment. Negative circular communication is seen between Dan and his parents and sister.

Analysis of data

DIAGNOSTIC REASONING: POSSIBLE CONCLUSIONS

After collecting subjective and objective data pertaining to the family, identify abnormal data and patient strengths. Then cluster the data to reveal any significant patterns or abnormalities. These data may be used to make clinical judgements about the status of the family.

Potential patient risks

- Risk of carer role strain
- Risk of impaired parent, infant or child attachment
- Risk of impaired parenting
- Risk of compromised family coping
- Risk of dysfunctional family processes
- Risk of impaired home maintenance

Potential patient problems

- Carer role strain
- Compromised family coping
- Ineffective family coping: disabling
- Dysfunctional family processes: alcoholism
- Interrupted family processes
- Impaired home maintenance
- Ineffective family therapeutic regimen management
- Parental role conflict
- Impaired parenting
- Impaired social interaction
- Social isolation
- Spiritual distress
- Ineffective role performance

Selected collaborative problems

After grouping the data, certain collaborative problems may emerge. Remember that collaborative problems cannot be prevented by nursing interventions. However, these physiological complications of medical conditions can be detected and monitored by the nurse. In addition, the nurse can use doctor- and nurse-prescribed interventions to minimise the complications of these problems. The nurse may also have to refer the patient in such situations for further treatment of the problem. The following is a list of collaborative problems that may be identified when assessing the family:

- Spousal conflict
- Child abuse
- Domestic violence.

Medical problems

After grouping the data, it may become apparent that the family has signs and symptoms that may require medical or mental health professional diagnosis and treatment. Referral to a primary care provider is necessary.

ONLINE RESOURCES

An extensive range of additional resources to enhance teaching and learning and to facilitate understanding may be found online at the text's accompanying website, located on thePoint at http://thepoint.lww.com. These include Watch and Learn videos, Concepts in Action animations, journal articles, case studies, discussion topics and quizzes.

Subscribers may also access Lippincott Procedures, an extensive online point-of-care procedure guide that provides reliable step-by-step instructions for more than 1700 procedures, including 450 evidence-based Australian procedures, and skills in a variety of speciality settings, together with a wealth of supporting information.

CASE STUDY

The case study demonstrates how to analyse assessment data for a family. The exercises included in the ancillary product on thePoint that complements this text offer further opportunities to enhance your skills.

You are talking with the Ross family, who have returned to the clinic for help dealing with Dan's recent diagnosis and treatment for type 1 diabetes mellitus. Dan is a 17-year-old school student who is scheduled to leave for university in 6 months. He was diagnosed with type 1 diabetes mellitus 4 months ago. Since then he has been seen in the emergency department five times for complications resulting from not following his diet–exercise–insulin protocol.

The doctor refers the Ross family to the nurse to help the family address the identified problem of Dan's refusal to follow the protocol. Because the diet and food preparation affect the whole family, Dan's sister Jenna attends the family session as well. Dan's file includes a genogram (Fig. 35-6).

Mr and Mrs Ross express concern and caring for Dan's wellbeing and request assistance with dealing with Dan's diagnosis and treatment. You ask how everyone feels about Dan's disease and treatment. Both the parents and Jenna appear tense when describing the effect of trying to deal with Dan's disease and his refusal to follow the protocol. Mr and Mrs Ross express frustration with their inability to get Dan to follow the doctor's orders. Dan expresses frustration at having a disease and at being asked to follow a protocol that makes him different from his friends and unable to do the things that they do (e.g. diet, exercise, partying). Dan expresses frustration at having his parents tell him what to do. Jenna expresses frustration at Dan for upsetting the family, especially at mealtimes, and particularly in regard to what family members eat and how they interact. When you ask the family to tell you about Dan's disease and treatment, Dan and his parents describe a good understanding of the disease and reasons for the protocol.

The following concept map illustrates the diagnostic reasoning process.

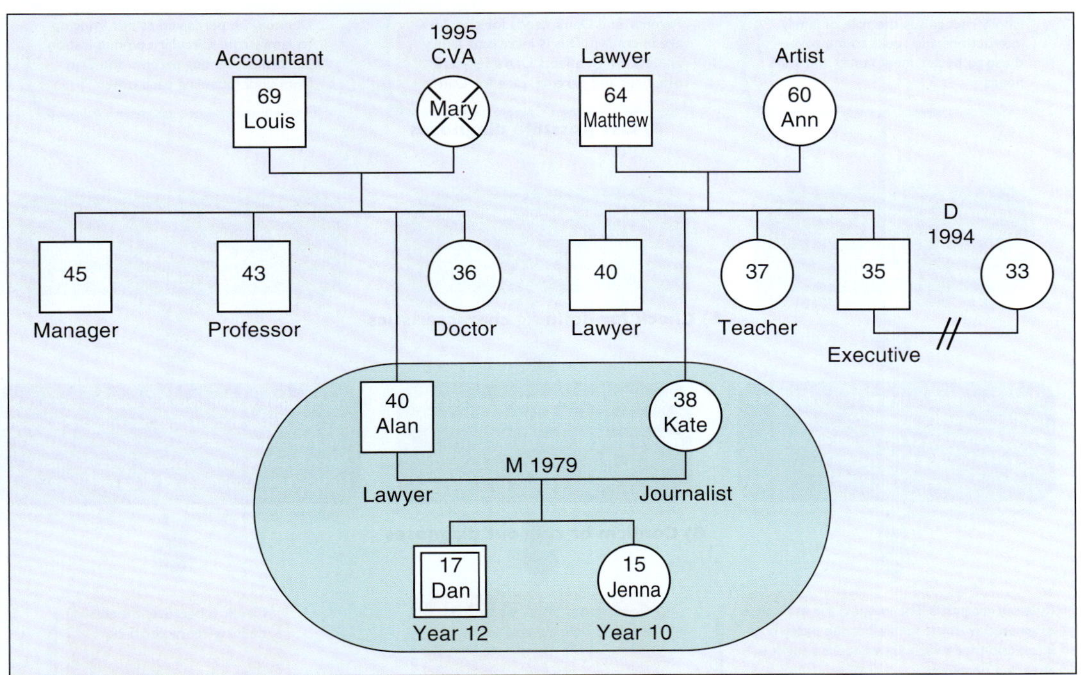

FIGURE 35-6 Genogram of the Ross family.

1) Identify abnormal findings and patient strengths

Subjective data

- Dan refuses to follow prescribed diabetes protocol
- Parents express concern and caring for Dan's well-being and request assistance with dealing with Dan's diagnosis and treatment
- Parents express frustration with inability to get Dan to follow the doctor's orders
- Dan expresses frustration at having a disease and at a protocol that makes him different from his friends
- Dan expresses frustration at having his parents tell him what to do
- Jenna expresses frustration at Dan for upsetting the family, especially at mealtimes

Objective data

- Family members appear tense when describing the effect of trying to deal with Dan's disease and his refusal to follow the protocol
- Dan is a 17-year-old school student who is scheduled to leave for university in 6 months. He was diagnosed with type I diabetes mellitus 4 months ago
- Dan has been seen by the doctor and in the emergency department five times in the past 4 months for complications resulting from not following the protocol
- Dan and his parents describe a good understanding of the disease and reasons for the protocol
- A circular pattern of communication has developed: Between the parents and between the father and Dan. Dan is not following the protocol, which increases the parents' anxiety and frustration. In addition, the parents' expressions of displeasure cause Dan's sense of loss of control, anxiety, and frustration to increase

2) Identify cue clusters

- Family asks for assistance with dealing with Dan's diagnosis and treatment

- Dan has returned to doctor and ED five times in 4 months
- Parents express frustration at inability to get Dan to follow treatment protocol
- Family members appear tense
- Circular communication pattern increasing anxiety

- Circular communication pattern increasing parents' and Dan's anxiety
- Dan is not following diabetes treatment protocol

3) Draw inferences

Family recognises the role of family interactions and seeks to improve these to better meet family and son's needs

Parents' and Dan's needs for control are in conflict. This is increasing family anxiety, which affects Dan's self-care practices and parents' care for Dan

Dan may be perceived as not living up to family role. Circular communication pattern preventing parents and Dan from understanding each other

4) List possible diagnoses

(Family) Health-seeking behaviours: request for assistance to improve the ability to deal with son's diagnosis and treatment

Risk of impaired home maintenance related to interaction of disease protocol, family lifecycle stage and family communication patterns

Interrupted family processes related to interaction of disease, treatment protocol, family lifecycle stage, multigenerational gender roles and family communication process

5) Check for defining characteristics

Major: Expressed desire to seek information for (family) health promotion
Minor: Expression of desire for increased control of health practice (family)

Major: Outward expression of difficulty by family in caring for a family member
Minor: Impaired carers: anxious

Major: Family system does not adapt constructively to crisis. Family system does not support open and effective communication.
Minor: Family system cannot or does not meet physical/emotional needs of all its members

6) Confirm or rule out diagnoses

Rule out diagnosis. The request for assistance originated with the family, but the pattern of interaction for which assistance is sought is already a problem

Confirm the diagnosis because it meets defining characteristics

Confirm because it meets defining characteristics

7) Document conclusions

Diagnoses that are appropriate for this patient include:
- Risk of impaired home maintenance
- Interrupted family processes

Possible collaborative problems include the following:
- Depression
- Marital conflict

References

Australian Bureau of Statistics (ABS). (2017). Labour force, Australia: Labour force status and other characteristics of families, June 2016. ABS cat. no. 6224.0.55.001. Canberra: Author.

Australian Institute of Health and Welfare (AIHW) (2017). Australia's welfare 2017. Australia's welfare series no. 13. AUS 214. Canberra: Author. Available at https://www.aihw.gov.au/getmedia/088848dc-906d-4a8b-aa09-79df0f943984/aihw-aus-214-aw17.pdf.

Bowen Center. (n.d.). Bowen theory. Available at www.thebowencenter.org/pages/theory.html.

Conway, J. & Dempsey, J. (2014). Health of the individual, family and community. Chap. 3. In J. Dempsey, S. Hillege, & R. Hill (Eds). *Fundamentals of nursing: A person-centred approach to care* (2nd ed.). Sydney: Lippincott Williams & Wilkins.

Friedman, M. (1998). *Family nursing: Theory and practice* (4th ed.). Norwalk, CT: Appleton & Lange.

Friedman, M. (2002). *Family nursing: Theory and practice* (5th ed.). Norwalk, CT: Appleton & Lange.

Grimmond, D. (2014, June). The economic value and impacts of informal care in New Zealand. Report prepared for Carers New Zealand and the NZ Carers Alliance. Infometrics. Viewed August 2019 at https://cdn.auckland.ac.nz/assets/auckland/about-us/equity-at-the-university/equity-information-staff/information-for-carers/The%20economic%20value%20of%20informal%20care%20in%20New%20Zealand%20Final%20copy.pdf.

Hanson, S. & Boyd, S. (Eds). (1996). *Family health care nursing*. Philadelphia: F.A. Davis.

Miller, A. (2011). Instructor's manual for Salvador Minuchin on family therapy with Minucin, S and Lappin, J. psychotherapy.net. Available at https://www.psychotherapy.net/data/uploads/5113e45715ce5.pdf

Ministry of Social Development. (2019). Mahi Aroha Caring for the Carers: Discussion document on the proposed Carers' Strategy Action Plan 2019-2023. New Zealand Government.

Smith, L. M. & Ford, K. (2013). Family strengths and the Australian Family Strengths Nursing Assessment Guide. In M. Barnes & J. Rowe (Eds). *Child, youth and family health: Strengthening communities* (pp. 98–105). Australia: Elsevier.

Stats NZ Tatauranga Aotearoa. (2017) Family. Viewed August 2019 at http://datainfoplus.stats.govt.nz/Item/nz.govt.stats/728b04b1-c460-4729-a311-b02f1117795b?_ga=2.256884747.1020476086.1565502084-67535932.1560148735#/nz.govt.stats/f0d2a392-c52d-4107-875b-29b581d49d7c/5.

Titelman, P. (Ed). (2008). *Triangles: Bowen family systems theory perspectives*. New York: The Haworth Press.

Wright, L. & Leahey, M. (2000). *Nurses and families: A guide to family assessment and intervention*. Philadelphia: F.A. Davis.

Wright, L. & Leahey, M. (2005). *Nurse and families: A guide to family assessment and intervention* (4th ed.). Philadelphia: F.A. Davis.

Wright, L. M. & Bell, J. M. (2009). *Beliefs and illness: A model for healing*. Calgary, Alberta: 4th Floor Press.

Wright, L. M. & Leahey, M. (1994). *Nurses and families: A guide to family assessment and intervention* (2nd ed.). Philadelphia: F.A. Davis.

Selected readings

Coyne, E., Grafton, E., El Reid, A., et al. (2017). Understanding family assessment in the Australian context: What are adult oncology nursing practices? *Collegian (Royal College of Nursing, Australia)*, *24*, 175–182.

Dempsey, J., Hillege, S. & Hill, R. (2014). *Fundamentals of nursing: A person-centred approach to care* (2nd ed.). Sydney: Lippincott Williams & Wilkins.

Kaakinen, J. R., Coehlo, D. P., Steele, R., et al. (2014). *Family health care nursing: Theory, practice, and research* (5th ed.). Philadelphia: F.A. Davis.

Online resources

Australian Bureau of Statistics: www.abs.gov.au
Australian Government Department of Human Services: www.humanservices.gov.au
Australian Government Department of Social Services: www.dss.gov.au
Australian Institute for Patient- and Family-Centered Care: www.aipfcc.org.au
Australian Institute of Family Studies: www.aifs.gov.au
Australian Institute of Health & Welfare: www.aihw.gov.au
Carers Australia: www.carersaustralia.com.au
Carers New Zealand: www.carers.net.nz
Centre for Cultural Competence Australia: http://ccca.com.au
Centre for Cultural Diversity in Ageing: www.culturaldiversity.com.au
Centre for Culture, Ethnicity and Health: www.ceh.org.au
Journal of Transcultural Nursing: http://tcn.sagepub.com/
Kiwi Families: www.kiwifamilies.co.nz
Mental Health in Multicultural Australia: www.mhima.org.au
Ministry of Social Development (New Zealand): www.msd.govt.nz
Stats NZ Tatauranga Aotearoa: www.stats.govt.nz
Strengthening Families/Whakapiripiri Nga Whānau: www.strengtheningfamilies.govt.nz
Transcultural Nursing and Health Care Consulting: http://transculturalnursingandhcc.com.au
Transcultural Nursing Society: www.tcns.org

CHAPTER 36

Assessing alcohol, tobacco and other drug-related issues

CASE STUDY

John Williams is a 46-year-old builder. He is married with two teenage sons. He is fit and active and very involved with the local rugby league club: he attends rugby training twice per week and games on the weekends and helps organise social functions for the club.

John was admitted to the hospital after falling from a roof at his worksite. He sustained a fracture of his pelvis and right humerus, multiple abrasions and contusions. On arrival at the hospital, he was taken to surgery for internal fixation of the right humerus and internal fixation of his pelvis. He is now an inpatient for postsurgical observation and recovery. He has morphine patient-controlled analgesia for pain relief, additional analgesia for breakthrough pain as required and regular antiemetics (ondansetron) ordered on his medication chart.

Conceptual foundations

Use of alcohol, tobacco and other drugs (ATODs) can be seen as a beneficial way of relaxing, and exciting when mixing with friends and having some fun. At the same time, ATOD use can present direct and indirect risks and dangers to the individual user and to the community. Problems caused by ATOD use can have an impact on all areas of health care. Some problems are easily identified, such as respiratory disease caused by smoking, liver disease caused by harmful levels of alcohol consumption and overdose from heroin injection. However, other problems can be more subtle and often missed by health care professionals as an underlying cause of a wide range of physical, psychological and psychosocial harm. Personal and social problems caused by ATOD use can be substantial and affect many aspects of a person's life, including relationships, family life, employment, and physical and psychological health. Additionally, various cultural groups may be affected differently by ATOD use.

ATOD use is common in our community and nurses are frequently required to assess and provide care for people who have been affected by alcohol, tobacco and other drugs. ATOD use includes both legal (readily available–but with some states and territories imposing certain restrictions) and illegal substances. Legal substances such as alcohol, tobacco and over-the-counter and prescribed medications may be misused or used illicitly, for example, selling diazepam or quetiapine to another person once the prescription has been dispensed. In many cases, presentation or admission to a hospital can be affected by ATOD use, which may be:

- The cause for presentation or admission (e.g. alcohol intoxication or acute withdrawal)
- A causal factor in the primary diagnosis (e.g. smoking and respiratory disease)
- Affecting different aspects of the patient's treatment during admission (e.g. pain management for a patient with opiate dependency).

This chapter introduces concepts around ATOD assessment in the hospital setting. Many people using ATODs are stigmatised and discriminated against in our society. This can have an impact on the decision of patients to honestly report their ATOD use and the quality of care that is provided to them. The care of patients experiencing issues related to ATOD use can be complex and, where available, referral to professional ATOD clinicians for specialist advice and treatment is appropriate.

The terms 'substances' and 'psychoactive drugs' are sometimes used collectively to refer to alcohol, tobacco and other drugs, but this chapter uses the term ATODs.

EPIDEMIOLOGY OF ATOD USE

The media and popular culture portray many stereotypical images of drug users. In reality, however, ATOD use and misuse is present at all socio-economic levels and affects people of all ages. A high proportion of the Australian and New Zealand populations drink alcohol. Recent national surveys show similar rates of use in the two counties: 12.2% of Australians and 15% of adult New Zealanders smoke tobacco daily, and 77% of Australians above age 14 and 79% of adult New Zealanders have consumed alcohol in the last 12 months (Australian Institute of Health and Welfare [AIHW], 2016a; New Zealand Ministry of Health [NZMOH], 2018a).

It was reported that 17.1% of Australians (2016 data), and 20% of New Zealanders (2017–2018 data) drink alcohol at risky or hazardous levels, and both countries report that males are twice as likely as females to drink alcohol in quantities that put them at risk of incurring an alcohol-related chronic disease, accident or injury over their lifetime. The consequences of these patterns of ATOD consumption are reflected in the chronic health conditions and the acute episodes of harm that are seen in Australian and New Zealand hospitals, creating a significant cost to health care systems.

Patterns of drug use differ by certain population characteristics depending on the drug type of interest. Harm caused by ATOD among Aboriginal and Torres Strait Islander Australians and New Zealand Indigenous peoples is at a much higher rate than the rest of the population. Smoking rates among Aboriginal and Torres Strait Islander Australians remains high, but recent data show the commencement of a decline. In 2018, 52% of Aboriginal and Torres Strait Islander adults were current smokers, more than double the rate of non-Aboriginal and Torres Strait Islander peoples who smoked (AIHW, 2018a).

Compared with non-Aboriginal and Torres Strait Islander Australians, a higher proportion of Aboriginal and Torres Strait Islander peoples abstain from both alcohol use and binge drinking. Around 27% of Aboriginal and Torres Strait Islander Australians have recorded not drinking over a 12-month period (AIHW, 2011), which is double the rate of non-Aboriginal and Torres Strait Islander Australians. However, of those who did drink, Aboriginal and Torres Strait Islander peoples (15% 2014–2015 data [AIHW, 2018b]) were almost twice as likely as non-Aboriginal and Torres Strait Islander Australians (8%) to binge, and there is almost twice the rate of alcohol-attributed deaths in the Aboriginal and Torres Strait Islander population (National Health and Medical Research Council [NHMRC], 2011). The proportion of Aboriginal and Torres Strait Islander peoples and non-Aboriginal and Torres Strait Islander Australians who drank at long-term (chronic), risky or high-risk levels is similar, at 15% and 14%, respectively (AIHW, 2018b).

Comparative statistics are available for Māori and Pacific people. Higher smoking rates persist among Māori and Pacific adults, at 31% and 20%, respectively although these figures have dropped significantly since the last survey conducted in 2012. Māori have similar alcohol consumption rates to the total New Zealand population, but have higher rates of drinking at hazardous levels. One in three (40%) Māori aged 15 years or more who drank alcohol in the previous year (2017–2018) had a potentially hazardous drinking pattern, with Māori men (48%) more likely to drink hazardously than Māori women (32%) (New Zealand Ministry of Health, 2018a). Similarly, Pacific people have been reported as drinking at potentially hazardous levels. One in three (36%) Pacific people aged 15 years or more who drank alcohol in the past year has a potentially hazardous drinking pattern, with Pacific men (46%) much more likely to drink hazardously than Pacific women (25%) (New Zealand Ministry of Health, 2018b). In Australia, recent illicit drug use (over 12 months) was recorded at 16% of the population aged 14 and over (AIHW, 2018c). This demonstrates an increasing trend from previous years mainly due to an increase in the proportion of people who had used cannabis, ecstasy, cocaine and methamphetamines (AIHW, 2018c). Approximately a quarter (23%) of Aboriginal and Torres Strait Islander Australians had recently used an illicit substance, whereas 43% reported they had used at least one illicit substance in their lifetime (AIHW, 2018b). In New Zealand, 11% of adults aged 15 years and over reported using cannabis in the last 12 months. Cannabis was used by 15% of men and 8.0% of women. Male cannabis users were more likely to report using cannabis at least weekly in the last 12 months (NZMOH, 2015). In another survey, 16.6% of adults reported that they had used 'any drugs' for recreational purposes. Cannabis, benzodiazepines and 'party pills', ecstasy, amphetamines, LSD and other synthetic hallucinogens were reported to be the most common drugs used in New Zealand for recreational purposes from 2007 to 2008 (NZMOH, 2010).

CRITICAL THINKING

1. Reflect on your recent clinical practice. Given the statistics outlined above, how many patients do you think you have cared for who may have had an undiagnosed drug use problem? Alternatively, reflect on your personal experiences. How many people do you know, or have you witnessed, who may have been affected by ATOD use?
2. Think about the case study above. For what signs and symptoms would you monitor Mr Williams post surgery?

Rationale for conducting an ATOD assessment

AOTD use may cause or exacerbate many health problems. Table 36-1 lists examples of health problems caused by

Table 36-1 Examples of common health problems related to alcohol, tobacco and other drug use

Substance	Associated health problems
Tobacco	Coronary heart disease, cerebrovascular disease, peripheral vascular disease, chronic obstructive airways disease, acute and chronic rhinitis, exacerbation of hay fever and asthma, cancer, peptic ulcer disease, Crohn disease, gastro-oesophageal reflux disease, complications related to pregnancy and reproduction, osteoporosis, dependence
Alcohol	Depression, anxiety, altered sleep patterns, hypertension, weight gain, gastritis, impotence, fatty liver, memory loss, cirrhosis of the liver, pancreatitis, oesophageal varices, peripheral neuritis, cancer (oesophagus, head, neck and lung), heart failure, impaired blood clotting, vitamin deficiency, poor nutrition, complications related to pregnancy and reproduction, memory loss, dementias, Wernicke encephalopathy or Korsakoff psychosis, dependence
Opioids	Harm related to injecting, overdose, dependence, constipation, hyperalgesia, dry mouth
Benzodiazepines	Anxiety, altered sleep patterns, impaired memory, impaired cognition, dependence, emotional blunting
Cannabis	Dependence, subtle cognitive impairment, exacerbation of respiratory conditions, reduced sperm count, strong association with comorbid mental health conditions

commonly used substances. Because the effects of ATOD use are far-reaching, it is relevant to consider an ATOD assessment to determine whether substance use could be a cause or a contributing factor to a patient's health problems and recovery.

REVIEW OF ALCOHOL, TOBACCO AND OTHER DRUGS

ATODs are described as chemical substances that affect the way users think, feel or act because of their effects on the central nervous system (CNS). ATODs interact in the brain to alter perception, mood, consciousness and behaviour for varying periods, depending on the type and combinations of drugs used, as well as the personality and physical characteristics of the person taking the substances. (Review Chap. 29 to understand how the CNS works.) ATODs can be categorised according to their effect on the CNS. Three broad categories are CNS depressants, CNS stimulants and other drugs such as party drugs methylenedioxymethamphetamine (MDMA, Ecstasy), gamma-hydroxybutyrate (GHB), mephedrone ('meow meow') and benzylpiperazine (BPZ). Examples of ATODs in each of these categories are listed in Table 36-2.

CASE STUDY

Twenty-four hours post surgery, John Williams complains of poor sleep, which he blames on constant interruptions by the staff and the noisy environment of the hospital. During the morning shift you notice he is gradually becoming more agitated, and by the afternoon you notice he also has a significant tremor in his extremities. Recent observations show an increase in his blood pressure and temperature. He is also complaining of feeling nauseous.

CRITICAL THINKING

3. What are the possible causes of some of the objective and subjective signs and symptoms that Mr Williams is exhibiting?

An understanding of the way each category affects the CNS will provide a framework for recognising and assessing potential ATOD-related issues in patients. Generally, similar effects would be expected from substances belonging to the same category, but some specific differences are evident between each substance. In addition, these categories are not rigid, as some drugs have attributes that can place them into more than one category. For example, cannabis is primarily a CNS depressant, but it may also have some hallucinogenic effects. Table 36-3 outlines general expectations for effects, intoxication and withdrawal symptoms for substances in each of the three categories.

PATTERNS OF DRUG USE

Patterns of ATOD use can be described by a continuum ranging from non-use to the dependent use of one or more substances (see Fig. 36-1). Five patterns of drug use have been identified. The pattern of use can move along the continuum in either direction and may remain at any point. Although some people steadily increase their ATOD use, there is no evidence confirming that gradual progression is inevitable for all users. Adopting a specific style of substance use may be a conscious decision or an unconscious decision resulting from a range of factors. Drug use patterns describe the style in which a person uses a particular substance; for example, a person may be a dependent user of one substance and an experimental user with other substances.

Table 36-2 Alcohol, tobacco and other drug categories

CNS depressants	CNS stimulants	Other drugs (hallucinogens and party drugs)
Alcohol	Nicotine	3,4-methylenedioxymethamphetamine (MDMA, ecstasy)
Opioids	Caffeine	Gamma-hydroxybutyrate (GHB)
Benzodiazepines	Amphetamines	Ketamine
Cannabis sativa (delta-9-tetrahydrocannabinol, THC)	Cocaine	Psilocybin (mushrooms) Lysergic acid diethylamide (LSD)
Volatile substances (inhalants)		Phencyclidine hydrochloride (PCP)

Table 36-3 The effects of alcohol, tobacco and other drugs

Substance	Effects	Intoxication symptoms	Withdrawal symptoms
CNS depressants			
Alcohol	Initial relaxation, sense of wellbeing, decreased inhibitions, impaired judgement, impaired coordination, ataxia, slurred speech, hypotension, bradycardia, bradypnoea, constricted pupils, labile mood, potential for aggression, unpredictable behaviour	Nausea, vomiting, memory loss, sleepiness, poor response to external stimuli, respiratory failure, coma, possible death	**Mild** Anxiety, agitation, tremor, nausea, tachycardia, hypertension, disturbed sleep, raised temperature **Severe** Vomiting, extreme agitation, disorientation, confusion, paranoia, hyperventilation, delirium tremens

Table 36-3 The effects of alcohol, tobacco and other drugs (continued)

Substance	Effects	Intoxication symptoms	Withdrawal symptoms
Opioids	Analgesia, euphoria, hypotension, bradypnoea, drowsiness, pupillary constriction, nausea, vomiting, constipation, itching, sweating, flushed skin, dry mouth, dry skin and eyes, decreased libido	Slow shallow respirations, constricted pupils, sedation, coma, possible death	Lacrimation, rhinorrhoea, sweating, yawning, agitation, irritability, piloerection, hot and cold flushes, appetite loss, strong cravings, stomach cramps, diarrhoea, nausea, vomiting, pain in joints, legs and arms, headache, poor sleep, lethargy, poor concentration
Benzodiazepines	Sedation, reduced anxiety, potentiation of other CNS depressants, paradoxical euphoria	Drowsiness, lethargy, motor incoordination, ataxia, decreased reaction time, impaired cognition, impaired memory, confusion, muscle weakness, depression, nystagmus, vertigo, dysarthria, slurred speech, blurred vision, dry mouth, headaches	**Mild** Anxiety, insomnia, irritability, restlessness, agitation, depression, tremor, dizziness, muscle twitching, anorexia, nausea, metallic taste, fatigue, tinnitus, hyperacusis, photophobia, perceptual disturbances, blurred vision **Severe** Seizures, delirium
Cannabis	Relaxation, sense of wellbeing, disinhibition, heightened visual and auditory perceptions, increased appetite, altered perception of time, alterations in concentration (difficulty in focusing or over-focusing)	Anxiety, paranoia, hallucinations, impaired coordination, short-term memory loss, tachycardia, supraventricular arrhythmias, not associated with fatal overdose	Anxiety, restlessness, irritability, anorexia, disturbed sleep, increase in vivid dreams, gastrointestinal disturbances, night sweats, tremor
Volatile substances (inhalants)	Euphoria, excitation, exhilaration, sense of invulnerability, nausea, vomiting, headaches, diarrhoea, abdominal pain	Slurred speech, disorientation, confusion, delusions, weakness, tremor, headaches, visual distortions, visual hallucinations, ataxia, stupor, seizures, coma, cardiopulmonary arrest, death	None
CNS stimulants			
Nicotine	Increased arousal, alertness, performance enhancement, tachycardia, increased cardiac output, hypertension, headache, decreased appetite, insomnia, dreams, nausea, vomiting, heartburn, diarrhoea, myalgias, arthralgias	Nausea	Cravings, irritability, restlessness, mood swings, increased appetite, hunger, insomnia, fatigue, dizziness, anxiety, depression, difficulty concentrating
Caffeine	Mild mood elevation, increased alertness, anxiety, irritability, jitteriness, insomnia, increased gastrointestinal motility, diuresis, psychomotor agitation	Delirium, nausea	Headaches, irritability, drowsiness, fatigue
Amphetamines	Tachycardia, hypertension, palpations, arrhythmia, tachypnoea, insomnia, overstimulation, euphoria, restlessness, talkativeness, increased confidence, increased self-awareness, appetite suppression, pupillary dilation, mild confusion, panic, increased energy, increased stamina, heightened alertness, improved performance and concentration, headache, teeth grinding, increased libido, nausea,	Unpredictable behaviour, violent or irrational behaviour, mood swings including hostility and aggression, pressured or slurred speech, paranoid thinking, confusion, perceptual disorders, headache, blurred vision, dizziness, psychosis, cerebrovascular accident, seizures, coma, teeth grinding, gross body image distortions, cardiac stimulation (tachycardia, angina, arrhythmia, myocardial infarction), vasoconstriction,	Fatigue, exhaustion, hunger, irritableness, agitation, depression, overwhelming desire to sleep, disrupted sleeping patterns, cravings, headaches, generalised aches and pains, possible paranoia, possible misinterpretation of surroundings

Continued on following page

Table 36-3 The effects of alcohol, tobacco and other drugs (continued)

Substance	Effects	Intoxication symptoms	Withdrawal symptoms
	vomiting, constipation, diarrhoea, abdominal cramps, pale sweaty skin, hyperpyrexia, increased deep tendon reflexes	hypertension, cardiovascular collapse, respiratory difficulties or failure, dry mouth, nausea, vomiting, abdominal cramps, flushing, pallor, hyperpyrexia, diaphoresis	
Cocaine	Euphoria, sociability, gregariousness, talkativeness, increased confidence, increased feelings of control, energy, decreased need for sleep, improved task performance, improved concentration, suppressed appetite, local anaesthesia, pupillary dilation, vasoconstriction, tachypnoea, tachycardia, hypertension, pyrexia	Repetitive behaviour, anxiety, severe agitation, panic, aggression, hostility, muscle twitches, tremors, loss of coordination, heightened reflexes, respiratory failure, hypertension, angina, pulmonary oedema, acute renal failure, convulsions, blurred vision, cerebrovascular accident, pallor, confusion, delirium, hallucinations (auditory and tactile), dizziness, muscle rigidity, weak rapid pulse, cardiac arrhythmias, myocardial ischaemia and infarction, diaphoresis, hyperpyrexia, headache, stomach pain, nausea, vomiting	Dysphoric mood, fatigue, insomnia or hypersomnia, psychomotor agitation or retardation, cravings, increased appetite, vivid unpleasant dreams
Other drugs (hallucinogens and party drugs)			
Ecstasy	Heightened sensory perception, euphoria, talkativeness, increased energy, reduced anxiety, feelings of comfort, feeling of belonging, feeling of love, empathic feelings, pupillary dilation, increased jaw tension, teeth grinding, loss of appetite, hyperpyrexia, dry mouth, tachycardia, sweaty palms, hot and cold flushes	Nausea, vomiting, insomnia, hyperthermia, impaired cognition, headaches, dizziness	None
GHB	Mild euphoria, disinhibition, feeling of calmness	Drowsiness, dizziness, nausea, vomiting, respiratory depression, coma	None
Ketamine	Thought disorders, out-of-body experiences, aphrodisiac effects, hallucinations, perceptual distortion, stimulant effects, analgesia	Anxiety, agitation, nausea, vomiting, tachycardia, angina, hypertension, temporary paralysis, analgesia, sensory dissociation, coma	None
Psilocybin (mushrooms)	Euphoria, giggling, laughter, creativeness, philosophical, feeling of wonder, emotionally sensitive, altered time perception, lethargy	Headache, nausea, vomiting, mild to severe anxiety, confusion	None
LSD	Energy, creative thinking, euphoria, increased awareness of senses, pupillary dilation, poor concentration, mood changes, unusual thoughts, altered time perception	Anxiety, tension, diaphoresis, nausea, dizziness, confusion, insomnia, paranoia, fear, panic, unwanted and overwhelming feelings, difficulty in regulating body temperature	None
PCP	Energy, euphoria, disconnected thoughts, sense of calm, disinhibition, shifts in perception of reality, tachycardia, altered time perception, analgesia, feelings of invulnerability, dissociation, confusion, disorientation, hallucinations	Severe anxiety, nausea, vomiting, physical aggression, disturbing hallucinations, temporary amnesia, severe confusion, disorganised thinking, bradycardia, hypotension, bradypnoea, seizures, ataxia, coma	None

Source: National Centre for Education and Training on Addiction (NCETA) Consortium (2004). Alcohol and other drugs: A handbook for health professionals. Canberra: Department of Health and Ageing. Available at http://nceta.flinders.edu.au/files/3012/5548/2429/EN199.pdf.

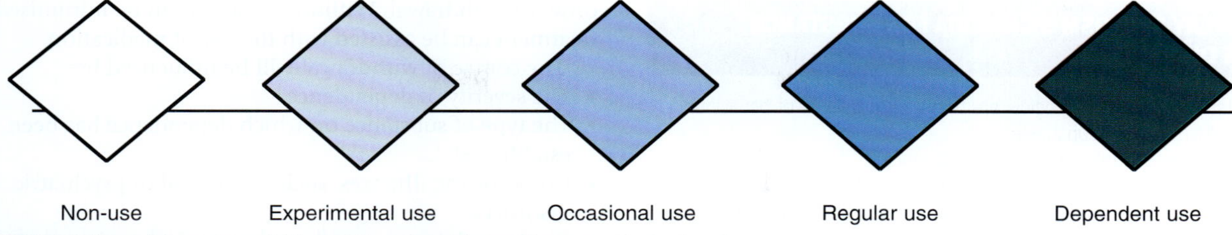

FIGURE 36-1 Pattern of drug use model (a variation of models used by many other authors).

Non-use

Factors supporting the non-use of ATODs may include cultural, religious, health or personal reasons, for example, choosing not to smoke tobacco because of the risks of developing respiratory conditions or lung cancer (health reasons). Some people have never used ATODs and have no plans to use them in the future, particularly if ATOD use does not feature in their family environment. Non-users also include people with a history of substance dependence who are now abstinent from that substance for whatever reason.

Experimental use

Experimental use can be defined as a person 'trying' a particular substance. It refers to once-only or short-term ATOD use. The decision to try ATODs and experience their effects is part of the process of determining whether to abstain or continue their use. Experimentation is a common feature of adolescence across a range of lifestyle behaviours. In this context, exploration of ATOD use can be considered part of the developmental process. As a result, many people may have experimented with ATOD use as an adolescent, often in the company of their peers. This pattern of use may be safe or risky depending on the substance and the context in which it is used.

Occasional use

Occasional use tends to be irregular and indicates that the individual does not have an established pattern of use, for example, an occasional joint of cannabis, a couple of alcoholic drinks with friends or the rare use of amphetamines. This pattern may have little impact on the individual's lifestyle, but it can potentially lead to harm (e.g. if binging or when intoxicated) even though the person is not using in an established pattern.

Regular use

Regular use occurs when a person uses ATODs on a regular basis and often with an established pattern. It occurs at both safe and risky levels. Some individuals may be able to use regularly and continue managing other activities such as school, work and study. Others may be at greater risk if they use large quantities of ATODs on a regular basis; for example, binge drinking of alcohol increases the risks of intoxication, accidents, poor decision making, memory loss and alcohol-related violence.

Dependent use

Individuals may become physiologically and psychologically dependent on ATODs. Dependence occurs with regular and repeated exposure to the substance. At this stage, the individual has little or no control over their ATOD use and is compelled to use in order to feel normal or to cope with everyday tasks. ATOD use often dominates the individual's life, leading to difficulties in many areas such as relationships, finances, legal matters, housing, school and work, as well as physical and psychological wellbeing. Individuals are likely to experience significant physical withdrawal symptoms upon ceasing use of the substance and to experience problems associated with psychological dependence, such as anxiety and depression.

CASE STUDY

You start to investigate the reasons behind John Williams's symptoms. You recall from a discussion with him yesterday that he enjoys drinking beer with his mates after work and at the footy. When you ask him about the amount of beer he normally drinks, he replies he probably buys two cartons of beer per week, as well as drinking beer at the football club after training and games, and at social events. He says he has drunk these amounts for years, can hold his grog fine and rarely gets 'drunk'. When his wife visits him later, she confirms his alcohol intake. She says he drinks daily and she often worries about the impact of his drinking on his health.

CRITICAL THINKING

4. Based on this information, are you concerned about Mr Williams's alcohol intake? Do you think the information provided is an accurate description of his actual alcohol intake? What other information might you like to obtain, if any?

DEFINITIONS RELATED TO SUBSTANCE USE

The DSM-5 (American Psychiatric Association, updated in 2017) is an internationally established diagnostic manual for mental disorders. The diagnoses detailed include substance use disorders and substance-induced disorders such as intoxication, withdrawal and other substance- or medication-induced mental disorders. These diagnostic criteria can be used routinely as part of the initial assessment, or to assess the patient's suitability to enter ATOD treatment. It is useful as a guide and should be used in conjunction with the patient's clinical presentation and symptoms and other assessment such as psychological and social assessments.

Substance use disorder

The DSM-5 describes the essential features of *substance use disorder* as a 'cluster of cognitive, behavioral, and physiological symptoms indicating that the individual continues using the substance despite significant substance-related problems' (APA, 2017). The DSM-5 criteria for substance use disorder are

DISPLAY 36-1 DSM-5 CRITERIA FOR SUBSTANCE USE DISORDER

The summarised points below are based on a pattern of behaviours related to use of the substance:

- Impaired control over use of the substance
- Persistent desire to cut down on use of the substance
- A great deal of time spent obtaining and using the substance
- Cravings to use the substance
- Failure to fulfil life obligations (e.g. work or school) because of use of the substance
- Social, occupational or recreational activities are interrupted because of use of the substance
- Substance use in situations that are physically hazardous
- Continues to use the substance despite recurrent physical and psychological problems caused by use
- Increased tolerance
- Withdrawal symptoms evident following use of the substance.

Detailed descriptions of each point can be obtained from the DSM-5 (APA, 2017).

divided into the following main groupings: *impaired control, social impairment, risky use* and *pharmacological* criteria. Display 36-1 lists the criteria for substance use disorder.

Substance-induced disorder

The DSM-5 describes substance-induced disorder as the overall category of substance-induced disorders as including intoxication, withdrawal and other substance- or medication-induced mental disorders (e.g. substance-induced psychotic disorder and substance-induced depressive disorder [APA, 2017]).

Intoxication

Acute intoxication results from the pharmacological effects of the substance being used. For intoxication to occur, the amount of substance taken must exceed the individual's tolerance level. The amount required to produce a state of intoxication differs considerably across individuals because of varying levels of tolerance, and any user can experience intoxication whether he or she is a naive, experienced or dependent user. Intoxication may become life-threatening if it causes the following: significant alteration of CNS function, such as respiratory depression and sedation; physiological stressors such as hypertension, tachycardia and hyperthermia; and alteration in mental functioning (e.g. panic, paranoia or psychosis) resulting in accidental injuries or self-harm and self-destructive behaviour.

Withdrawal

Withdrawal is one of the clinical indicators of dependence. Withdrawal can occur following a cessation or reduction in the use of a substance that was previously used repeatedly over a long time or at high doses and on which the individual is typically dependent. The onset and course of withdrawal is time-limited and is related to the type of substance and dose being used prior to abstinence. Withdrawal symptoms are often the opposite of the effects produced by the presence of the substance in the body (refer to Table 36-3 for information on specific substance withdrawal symptoms). In addition to the physiological symptoms experienced in withdrawal, psychological cravings or a strong desire to use drugs will be present. The substance's half-life represents the time taken for the body to eliminate half of the drug: this is used as an indicator for the onset of withdrawal. Withdrawal states can be minimised and treatment can be assisted with the use of medication.

The course of withdrawal will be influenced by:

- The severity of dependence
- The type of substance on which dependence has been established
- Co-occurring illnesses, such as physical or psychiatric disorders
- Psychosocial factors such as the physical environment, fears and expectations
- Medical, psychological and social support available.

Alcohol withdrawal can be complex and, in some cases, life-threatening. The following may predict a more severe withdrawal: a history of seizures, hallucinations or delirium; a long period of use or a high amount of use; the presence of other illnesses or injury; and the use of other psychotropic medication. Withdrawal from benzodiazepines—although the drug is rarely life-threatening when used alone—can also be severe and involve seizures and delirium, particularly when the benzodiazepine is used in high doses or with alcohol. A thorough assessment assists in identifying patients at risk of severe or complex withdrawal, and medical management is required for a safe withdrawal from alcohol and benzodiazepines.

Substance- or medication-induced mental disorders

The DSM-5 states that 'the substance/medication-induced mental disorders are potentially severe, usually temporary, but sometimes persisting CNS syndromes that develop in the context of the effects of substances of abuse, medications, or several toxins'. All substance- or medication-induced disorders share common characteristics and they are described as follows:

- The disorder represents a clinically significant symptomatic presentation of a relevant mental disorder.
- There is evidence from the clinical history, physical examination or laboratory findings of both of the following:
  - The disorder developed during or within 1 month of a substance intoxication or withdrawal or taking a medication; and
  - The involved substance or medication can produce the mental disorder.
- The disorder is not better explained by an independent mental disorder. Such evidence of an independent mental disorder could include the following:
  - The disorder preceded the onset of severe intoxication or withdrawal or exposure to the medication; or
  - The full mental disorder persisted for a substantial period (e.g. at least 1 month) after the cessation of acute withdrawal or severe intoxication or taking the medication. This criterion does not apply to substance-induced neurocognitive disorders or hallucinogen persisting perception disorder, which persists beyond the cessation of acute intoxication or withdrawal.
- The disorder does not occur exclusively during a delirium.
- The disorder causes clinically significant distress or impairment in judgement, social, occupational or other important areas of functioning (APA, 2017).

NATIONAL DRUG POLICIES

The national drug policies of Australia and New Zealand are outlined in Display 36-2.

DISPLAY 36-2 NATIONAL DRUG POLICIES OF AUSTRALIA AND NEW ZEALAND

The national drug policies of Australia and New Zealand are based on the principle of harm minimisation, which encompasses the three areas of supply reduction, demand reduction and harm reduction. Harm minimisation policies and programs are aimed at reducing the harmful effects of drug use for individuals and the community, and improving social, economic and health outcomes. Harm minimisation does not condone drug use but rather recognises the actual harm associated with use, whether the substances are legal or illegal. The goal of harm minimisation is to reduce this harm.

- *Supply reduction* is managed primarily by customs and law enforcement systems. This is achieved by monitoring the trafficking of drugs across national borders, as well as reducing the supply of illegal drugs in the community.
- *Demand-reduction activities* range from campaigns to prevent an increase in the number of new users to helping regular users to access treatment programs such as detoxification, substitution programs, and rehabilitation and counselling services.
- *Harm-reduction interventions* are used in society for a range of situations where there is inherent risk, such as wearing seat belts in cars and swimming between the flags at the beach. For ATOD use, harm-reduction interventions aim to educate people on how to minimise harm if they choose to continue using ATODs. The implementation of needle and syringe programs in Australia has been a very cost-effective harm-reduction strategy. These programs have produced a positive impact on the health outcomes of the injecting population (averting more than 32,000 new HIV infections and 96,000 new HCV infections) and provide health care cost savings for the community. For every $1 invested in needle and syringe programs, more than $4 are returned, with greater returns expected over longer time frames (National Centre in HIV Epidemiology and Clinical Research, 2009).

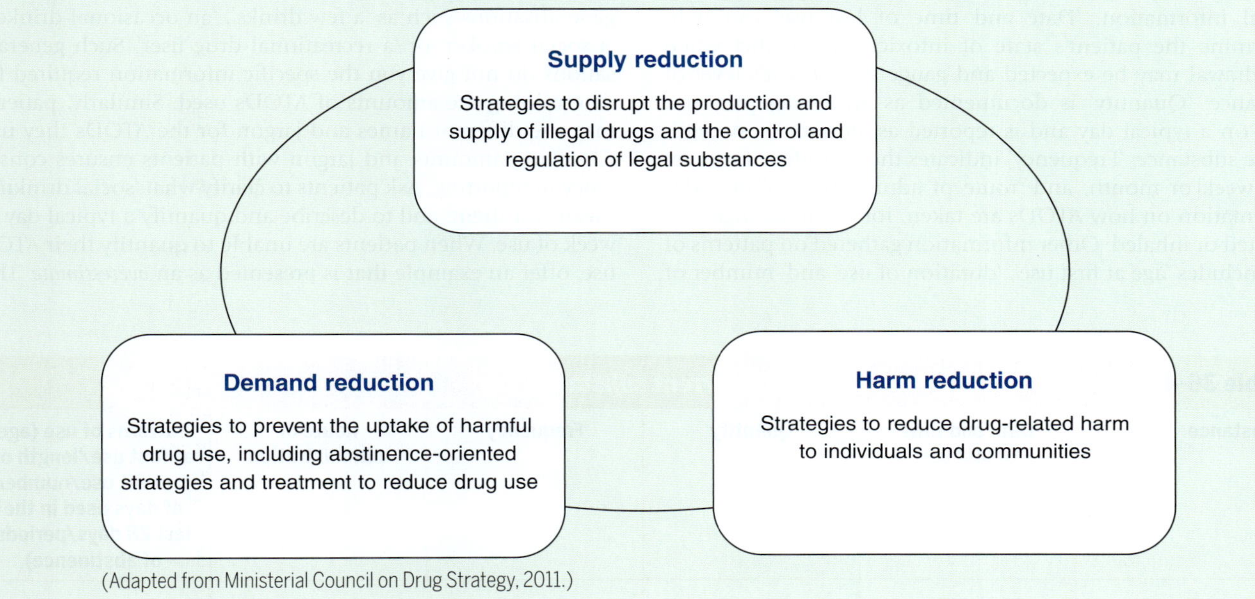

(Adapted from Ministerial Council on Drug Strategy, 2011.)

The ATOD assessment

COLLECTING SUBJECTIVE DATA: THE NURSING HEALTH HISTORY

As a nurse you may find it difficult to raise the topic of ATOD use with your patients for fear of being offensive. Asking about ATOD use is a skill that you can develop with practice and weave into the conversation gently, so that it seems natural to ask such questions. During the interview, you need to strike a balance between being inquisitive and remaining non-confrontational so that the patient does not become defensive and then not provide you with an accurate history. Seek the patient's permission to ask questions about ATOD use. This can help to create a therapeutic relationship where the patient and nurse work collaboratively. The goal is to be friendly and factual while avoiding subjective statements. Below are examples of questions that you can use to start a discussion about ATOD use:

- 'You mentioned before that you enjoy an alcoholic drink; can you tell me how many drinks you have in an average week?'
- 'A lot of us like a drink or a cigarette to relax. How about you: what do you like to use?'

CLINICAL TIP

When dealing with an intoxicated patient, assess the level of intoxication and any associated risks, and place importance on collecting objective data (see below).

The information you gather from an ATOD assessment may include:

- The principal drug of concern and any other secondary drug of concern
- The quantity, frequency and patterns of use:
  - Baseline for current drug use
  - Level of dependence on ATODs
- The effects of intoxication, including the assessment of any life-threatening potential

- The possibility of current or impending withdrawal
- Potential drug interactions
- A correct diagnosis as a differential or comorbid diagnosis may exist
- Any problems related to drug use
- Drug use triggers
- Life events and trauma that may contribute to drug use
- Special needs due to factors such as culture, religion, sexuality and gender.

Assessing current and past ATOD use

A useful tool that you can use to obtain information about a patient's ATOD use is shown in Table 36-4. Ask patients about their use of all substances, as they may not recognise the relevance of some ATOD use. For example, a patient may identify cannabis as their primary drug of concern but may not recognise tobacco as a drug or consider its effect on their health.

Using the framework in Table 36-4 enables you to gather useful information. 'Date and time of last use' can help determine the patient's state of intoxication, predict when withdrawal may be expected and gauge the patient's level of tolerance. 'Quantity' is documented as an average amount used on a typical day and is reported as amount or strength of the substance. 'Frequency' indicates the episodes of use per day, week or month, and 'route of administration' provides information on how ATODs are taken, for example, ingested, injected or inhaled. Other information gathered on patterns of use includes 'age at first use', 'duration of use' and 'number of days used in the last 28 days'. All this information can help to identify the patient's level of or risk of dependence, the priority of substance use in the patient's life and other risks associated with ATOD use. 'Periods of abstinence' may prompt questioning around previous episodes of withdrawal, symptoms experienced and the subsequent risk of severe withdrawal (e.g. seizure activity), as well as whether the patient was engaged in any treatment at this time.

There are many mixed messages about safe and unsafe levels of alcohol consumption, and suggested levels vary between countries (see Display 36-3). Alcohol consumption can provide many risks to the health and wellbeing of individuals, and this is heavily supported by research internationally. Note that there is a significant amount of research indicating that no level of tobacco smoking can be considered safe.

Clarifying patient information

Patients will report ATOD use in different ways and often use generalisations such as 'a few drinks', 'an occasional drinker', 'a social smoker' or 'a recreational drug user'. Such generalisations do not give you the specific information required for determining the amounts of ATODs used. Similarly, patients may use different names and jargon for the ATODs they use. Clarifying amounts and jargon with patients ensures consistency in reporting. Ask patients to clarify what 'social drinking' means for them, and to describe and quantify a typical day or week of use. When patients are unable to quantify their ATOD use, offer an example that is presented as an *overestimate.* This

Table 36-4 Sample table to record patient's current substance use

Substance	Date and time of last use	Quantity	Frequency	Route of administration	Patterns of use (age at first use/length of current use/number of days used in the last 28 days/periods of abstinence)
Tobacco					
Alcohol					
Benzodiazepines					
Opiates					
Cannabis					
Amphetamines					
Ecstasy					
Inhalants					
Hallucinogens					
Other (e.g. steroids)					

Note: This table is not prescriptive and may be modified for different working environments. Most hospitals have their own system for assessing ATOD use.

DISPLAY 36-3 SAFE AND UNSAFE LEVELS OF ALCOHOL USE

In Australia and New Zealand, 10 g of alcohol is considered to equal one standard drink. Both countries provide guidelines indicating recommended levels of alcohol intake described as 'standards drinks'. These guidelines for safe drinking can be found at:

- https://www.nhmrc.gov.au/health-advice/alcohol (Australia)
- https://www.alcohol.org.nz/help-advice/advice-on-alcohol/low-risk-alcohol-drinking-advice (New Zealand)

The websites also provide diagrammatic representation of the number of standard drinks for commonly purchased beverages in Australia and New Zealand.

allows patients to give a more accurate response without fear of being judged. Sample questions are given below:

- 'Would it be easy for you to drink a carton of beer when watching the footy?'
- 'Do you drink in rounds at the pub? How many people are in the round and how many turns do you take to go to the bar?'
- 'On days when everything just goes wrong, how many tablets do you take to get you through?'

Determining accurate amounts of use can be difficult, but there are some instances where accuracy is extremely important. For example, a patient dependent on alcohol or benzodiazepines or both may be at risk of severe withdrawal, which may be life-threatening, and an opioid-dependent patient may require analgesia outside of what would be considered the normal parameters. Display 36-4 shows examples of some commonly used substances in doses or amounts.

Attitudes play a vital role in influencing patient behaviour and willingness to access treatment for ATOD use. Attitudes towards ATOD use are influenced by several different sources, including the media, family, friends, education, religion, culture, personal experiences and defence mechanisms. The nurse's attitudes and feelings about ATOD use and misuse can affect the quality of patient care. Acceptance and a non-judgemental attitude towards patients, and knowledge about ATOD use issues, will increase referral rates for treatment. Cultural differences can influence nurse and patient behaviours that could be misinterpreted. For further information on cultural issues in healthcare, refer to Chapters 10 to 13.

DISPLAY 36-4 COMMONLY USED SUBSTANCES IN DOSES OR AMOUNTS

Alcohol—number of standard drinks per day (10 g alcohol = 1 standard drink)
Amphetamines—points or grams per day
Benzodiazepines—milligrams or tablets per day
Cannabis—grams, cones, joints or foils per day or week
Ecstasy—tablets per day
Hallucinogens—number of trips
Heroin—grams or dollars per day
Methadone—milligrams per day
Prescription opiates (e.g. morphine)—milligrams or tablets per day
Subutex or suboxone—milligrams per day
Tobacco—number of cigarettes per day
Volatile substances—number of episodes or days of substance use, or sniffing time

COLLECTING OBJECTIVE DATA: THE PHYSICAL EXAMINATION

Assessing the health of patients with ATOD use issues

ATOD use can be identified through changes in the biological, psychological and social (or biopsychosocial) components of the health assessment. Some of the factors you need to assess include:

- Physical changes due to impaired functioning of major organs
- Increased or decreased energy levels
- Any experience of hangovers, their regularity and impact on the patient's lifestyle
- Accidents due to intoxication or withdrawal symptoms due to substance use
- Changes in mental health
- Impact on social circumstances.

ATOD use can affect the patient's presentation and have an impact on the patient's biological health status. For example, people who consume large amounts of alcohol may have impaired liver function or liver disease. Note that the patient's presentation may be difficult to diagnose if they have taken multiple substances from different categories.

Considerations for the biological assessment

Patients who misuse ATODs may show some variations in their biological assessment. Taking core observations such as temperature, blood pressure, pulse rate, respiratory rate, pupil size and reactivity can provide you with important information on the patient's state of intoxication or withdrawal. (Refer to Table 36-3 for information on the physiological effects of different substances.) You can obtain collateral information about the patient from the patient's family and friends, doctor or community case manager.

CLINICAL TIP

For a patient who is compromised from overdose of a CNS depressant, maintenance of the airway, breathing and circulation becomes a priority.

By observing the patient's integumentary system, you may be able to detect previous or current ATOD use. For example, one of the side effects of smoking tobacco is premature ageing of the skin, and injecting drug use may leave significant scarring on the body. People inject substances in a range of different sites over the body. Common sites include the anterior cubital fossa; peripheries such as the arms, hands, legs and feet; and the groin and neck. When assessing for evidence of injecting drug use look for fresh and healing injection sites, scarred surface veins (fresh or old sites), multiple injection sites, track marks, abscesses, redness and signs of skin infections. Injection marks are easily concealed by clothing and tattooed areas of the skin and may not be obvious. Use of amphetamine-based substances can cause changes in behaviour that may lead to repetition of some activities. An example is continual picking of the skin, particularly in amphetamine users, which leads to significant scarring on the backs of hands arms and even the face. If any signs are present, try to gather more information on the patient's use of injectable substances.

The patient's medical and surgical history may indicate past problems that are affected by ATOD use. Additional data that can contribute information to the state of the patient's health include tests such as analysis of liver function and electrolyte level, urine drug screening and examination of blood alcohol level. Obtaining a list of the patient's current medications (both prescribed and non-prescribed) may assist you in identifying other health issues.

Measuring the patient's bloodborne virus status is also informative, as injecting drug users are at a significantly higher risk of contracting infections such as hepatitis B virus (HBV), hepatitis C virus (HCV) and human immunodeficiency virus (HIV). These viruses can have an impact on the patient's health and the effectiveness of treatments. Patients in this high-risk group may be advantaged by being offered an HBV immunisation regimen.

A patient's menstrual cycle can be altered for many reasons, including significant use of ATODs and nutritional and metabolic changes brought about by ATOD use. This may be further compounded by a chaotic lifestyle and associated risk-taking behaviours. Special considerations are needed if a woman is pregnant and using ATODs. Some substances can have teratogenic effects on the fetus, and many complications can arise during the pregnancy if the mother uses ATODs. Where a pregnant woman is using ATODs, referral to and treatment by specialist antenatal and ATOD services will improve the outcome for both the mother and the baby. Further information is available in Chapter 31.

Considerations for the psychological assessment

Patients using ATODs commonly experience co-existing mental health problems, such as anxiety and depression. Mental health symptoms are more likely to be substance induced if the symptoms subside when the intoxicating effects of ATODs subside. Depending on the substance and the level of use, substance-induced mental health symptoms may continue for 1 month after the patient ceases ATOD use. If the mental health symptoms continue after this period, or they were prominent prior to ATOD use, or there is a family history of a mental health problem, consider that the patient may have a mental disorder. With a high prevalence of co-existing ATOD use and mental health disorders, it is best practice to address both issues at the same time, and collaboration with mental health services is an important aspect of the treatment plan. Mental health symptoms need to be monitored and treatment commenced where indicated.

ATOD misuse can have an impact on cognitive function. In particular, alcohol consistently targets and injures specific parts of the brain in patients, who then exhibit signs of alcohol-related brain injury. Wernicke encephalopathy and Korsakoff psychosis are serious conditions that are precipitated by heavy alcohol consumption and inadequate nutrition, particularly thiamine intake. Furthermore, non-fatal opioid or benzodiazepine overdose can result in significant permanent brain injury, primarily due to long periods of respiratory depression. Conditions such as these may cause changes in memory capacity, ability to adapt to new situations and impaired retention of new learning.

The use of ATODs has the potential to increase the risk of suicidal tendencies, and it is possible that some substances may increase the risk of suicidal acts. The disinhibiting effects of alcohol can lead patients to express ideas of suicide while intoxicated, particularly if there is a co-existing diagnosis of depression or a history of suicidal intent. For further information on assessment of the patient's mental status, refer to Chapter 6.

Considerations for the social assessment

ATOD misuse can have a significant impact on patients' social circumstances. Use and misuse of ATODs are present at all socio-economic levels and affect people of all cultures and ages. Parts of the substance use disorder criteria (outlined above) identify how ATOD use can become a priority for those who are dependent such that the patient's social circumstances may deteriorate; for example, the patient's personal relationships may suffer as the priority for maintaining these relationships reduces.

There are many ways in which ATOD use is interwoven with social factors. Some examples are provided below (but note that this list is not exhaustive):

1. Social factors may predict ATOD use—for example, adolescents may socialise with friends using ATODs and feel pressured to use with them.
2. ATOD use may have an impact on social factors—for example, a relationship may break down because a person cannot tolerate his or her partner's drinking or the behaviour associated with drinking.
3. Social factors may play a role in a patient presenting for treatment—for example, the individual's medical condition may worsen because he or she is homeless.

Patients may express concerns about the effects of their ATOD use on certain social aspects of their lives; some examples of these are provided in Table 36-5. You should acknowledge these concerns and refer the patient to a social worker where appropriate. The way that social circumstances are affected by ATOD use can provide information on the patient's ability to form and access social support, take on information about his or her health condition, manage his or her finances and manage life stressors. Good social support can enhance a patient's prognosis, and you should identify whether the patient has such support during the assessment.

Table 36-5 Social circumstances affected by ATOD use

- Life view
- Relationships with family, friends and social supports
- Family history of substance use
- Responsibilities for children and/or contact with children
- Education
- Employment
- Living circumstances
- Legal issues
- Finances
- Involvement with other agencies
- Strengths including interests, hobbies and leisure activities

CRITICAL THINKING

5. Based on the information supplied, do you think Mr Williams's presentation could be caused by alcohol use? In what ways could his alcohol intake be affecting his hospital admission and the biopsychosocial elements of his health?
6. What patient education could you provide to Mr Williams in the form of harm reduction?

Analysis of data

DIAGNOSTIC REASONING: POSSIBLE CONCLUSIONS

After collecting subjective and objective data and, if possible, collateral data pertaining to the patient's ATOD use, identify abnormal findings and patient strengths. Then cluster the data to reveal any significant patterns or abnormalities. These data may be used to make clinical judgements about the possible implications of the patient's ATOD use.

Potential patient risks

- Risk of injury (related to ATOD intoxication)
- Risk of hyperthermia (related to ATOD pharmacodynamics)
- Risk of ineffective breathing pattern (related to ATOD pharmacodynamics)
- Risk of infection (related to injecting drug use)
- Risk of violence (related to ATOD intoxication)

Potential patient problems

- Potential for impaired cardiovascular efficiency (related to infection from non-sterile injecting practices)
- Potential for dysfunctional family processes (related to domestic violence)
- Potential for impaired memory (related to impaired gas exchange during ATOD overdose)
- Potential for disturbed body image (related to dental cavities caused by impaired oral mucous membranes)

Selected collaborative problems

After grouping the data, it may become apparent that certain collaborative problems emerge. Remember that collaborative problems cannot be prevented by nursing interventions. However, these physiological complications of medical conditions can be detected and monitored by the nurse. In addition, the nurse can use doctor- and nurse-prescribed interventions to minimise the complications of these problems. The nurse may also have to refer the patient in such situations for further treatment of the problem. The following is a non-exhaustive list of collaborative problems that may be identified when assessing ATOD-related issues:

- Endocarditis
- Lung cancer
- Oesophageal varices
- Gastro-oesophageal reflux disease
- Dental cavities and chipping of teeth
- Acquired communicable diseases
- Anxiety
- Depression
- Associated history of trauma and abuse
- Potential ATOD and medication interaction
- Cognitive impairment
- Poor decision making.

Medical problems

If, after grouping the data, it becomes apparent that the patient has signs and symptoms that may require medical diagnosis and treatment, referral to a primary care provider is necessary.

ONLINE RESOURCES

An extensive range of additional resources to enhance teaching and learning and to facilitate understanding may be found online at the text's accompanying website, located on thePoint at http://thepoint.lww.com. These include Watch and Learn videos, Concepts in Action animations, journal articles, case studies, discussion topics and quizzes.

Subscribers may also access Lippincott Procedures, an extensive online point-of-care procedure guide that provides reliable step-by-step instructions for more than 1700 procedures, including 450 evidence-based Australian procedures, and skills in a variety of speciality settings, together with a wealth of supporting information.

CASE STUDY

The case study demonstrates how to analyse ATOD assessment data for a specific patient. The exercises included in the ancillary product on thePoint that complements this text offer further opportunities to enhance your skills.

John Williams is a 46-year-old builder. He is married with two teenage sons. He is fit and active and very involved with the local rugby league club: he attends rugby training twice per week and games on the weekends and helps organise social functions for the club.

John was admitted to the hospital after falling from a roof at his worksite. He sustained a fracture of his pelvis and right humerus, multiple abrasions and contusions. On arrival at the hospital, he was taken to surgery for internal fixation of the right humerus and internal fixation of his pelvis. He is now an inpatient for postsurgical observation and recovery. He has morphine patient-controlled analgesia for pain relief, additional analgesia for breakthrough pain as required and regular antiemetics ordered on his medication chart.

Twenty-four hours post surgery, John complains of poor sleep, which he blames on constant interruptions by the staff and the noisy environment of the hospital. During the morning shift you notice that he is gradually becoming more agitated, and by the afternoon you notice

Continued on following page

that he also has a significant tremor in his extremities. Recent observations show an increase in his blood pressure and temperature. He is also complaining of feeling nauseous.

You start to investigate the reasons behind John's symptoms. You recall from a discussion with him yesterday that he enjoys drinking beer with his mates after work and at the footy. When you ask him about the amount of beer that he normally drinks, he replies that he probably buys two cartons of beer per week, as well as drinking beer at the football club after training and games, and at social events. He says that he has drunk these amounts for years, can hold his grog fine and rarely gets 'drunk'. When his wife visits him later, she confirms his alcohol intake. She says that he drinks daily and she often worries about the impact of his drinking on his health.

The following concept map illustrates the diagnostic reasoning process.

Applying COLDSPA

Applying COLDSPA can be used to explore the patient's symptoms of ATOD use as illustrated below.

Mnemonic	Question	Data provided	Missing data
Character	Describe the sign or symptom (feeling, appearance, sound, smell or taste, if applicable).	Complains of poor sleep, agitation, tremor, increased blood pressure, increased temperature, nausea	How did you get to the clinic today?
Onset	When did it begin?	Day 1 post surgery	
Location	Where is it? Does it radiate? Does it occur anywhere else?	Tremors in extremities (hands and feet); nausea; generally unsettled from poor sleep and agitation	
Duration	How long does it last? Does it recur?		Have you ever had these symptoms before? If so, how long did they last? How did they resolve?
Severity	How bad is it? or How much does it bother you?	Increasing agitation and tremors over time; worsening observations (blood pressure, temperature); nausea and poor sleep reducing comfort levels	
Pattern	What makes it better or worse?	Symptoms are getting worse as time passes	Do you normally sleep well? Have you suffered from tremors in the past? What has improved these symptoms in the past?
Associated factors/How it Affects the patient	What other symptoms occur with it? How does it affect you?	Poor appetite; communication difficult with agitation; problems with fine motor skills due to tremor	

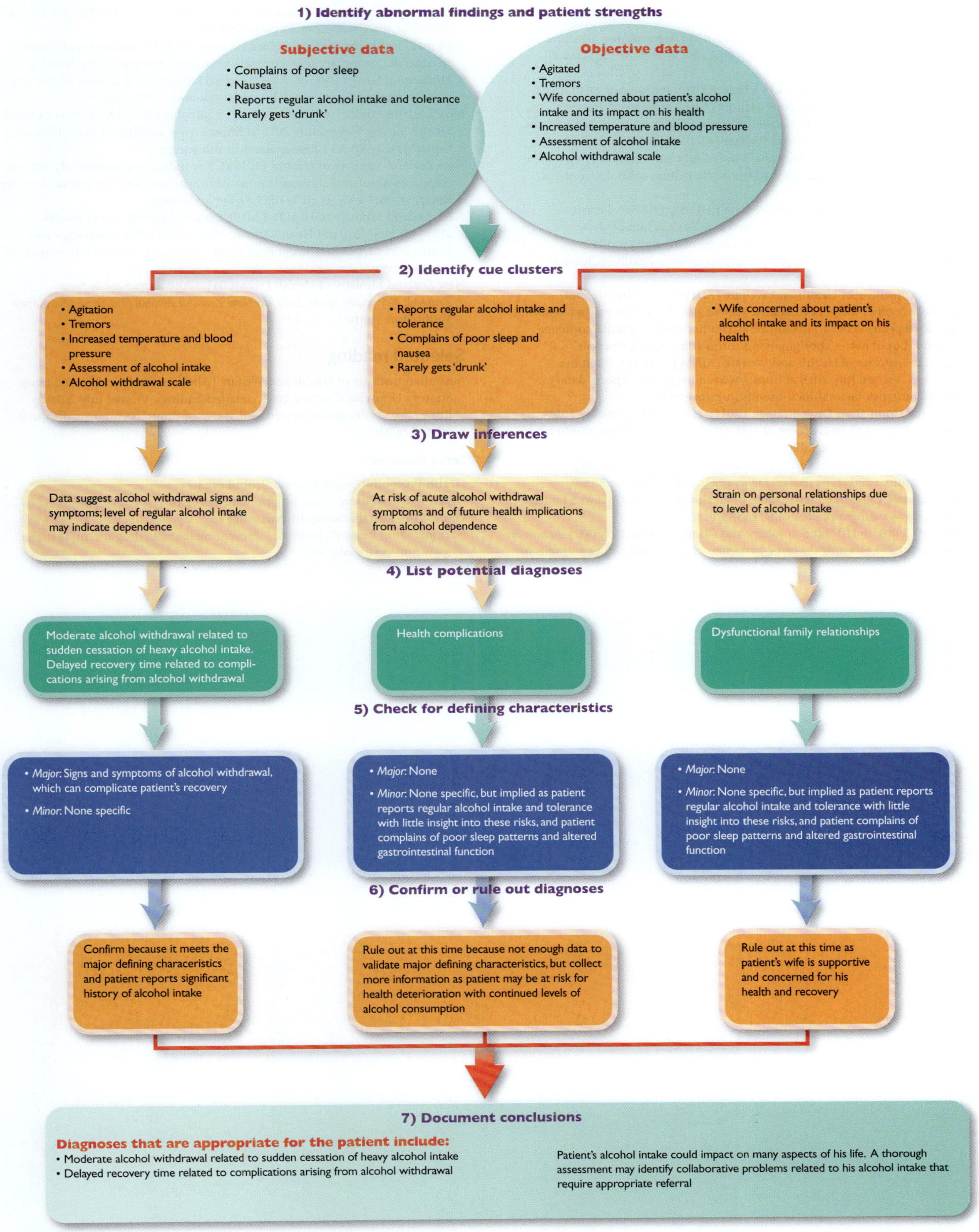

1) Identify abnormal findings and patient strengths

Subjective data
- Complains of poor sleep
- Nausea
- Reports regular alcohol intake and tolerance
- Rarely gets 'drunk'

Objective data
- Agitated
- Tremors
- Wife concerned about patient's alcohol intake and its impact on his health
- Increased temperature and blood pressure
- Assessment of alcohol intake
- Alcohol withdrawal scale

2) Identify cue clusters

- Agitation
- Tremors
- Increased temperature and blood pressure
- Assessment of alcohol intake
- Alcohol withdrawal scale

- Reports regular alcohol intake and tolerance
- Complains of poor sleep and nausea
- Rarely gets 'drunk'

- Wife concerned about patient's alcohol intake and its impact on his health

3) Draw inferences

Data suggest alcohol withdrawal signs and symptoms; level of regular alcohol intake may indicate dependence

At risk of acute alcohol withdrawal symptoms and of future health implications from alcohol dependence

Strain on personal relationships due to level of alcohol intake

4) List potential diagnoses

Moderate alcohol withdrawal related to sudden cessation of heavy alcohol intake. Delayed recovery time related to complications arising from alcohol withdrawal

Health complications

Dysfunctional family relationships

5) Check for defining characteristics

- *Major:* Signs and symptoms of alcohol withdrawal, which can complicate patient's recovery
- *Minor:* None specific

- *Major:* None
- *Minor:* None specific, but implied as patient reports regular alcohol intake and tolerance with little insight into these risks, and patient complains of poor sleep patterns and altered gastrointestinal function

---

- *Major:* None
- *Minor:* None specific, but implied as patient reports regular alcohol intake and tolerance with little insight into these risks, and patient complains of poor sleep patterns and altered gastrointestinal function

6) Confirm or rule out diagnoses

Confirm because it meets the major defining characerisctics and patient reports significant history of alcohol intake

Rule out at this time because not enough data to validate major defining characteristics, but collect more information as patient may be at risk for health deterioration with continued levels of alcohol consumption

Rule out at this time as patient's wife is supportive and concerned for his health and recovery

7) Document conclusions

Diagnoses that are appropriate for the patient include:
- Moderate alcohol withdrawal related to sudden cessation of heavy alcohol intake
- Delayed recovery time related to complications arising from alcohol withdrawal

Patient's alcohol intake could impact on many aspects of his life. A thorough assessment may identify collaborative problems related to his alcohol intake that require appropriate referral

References

American Psychiatric Association (APA). (2017) *Diagnostic and Statistical Manual of Mental Disorders*, (5th ed.). Update October 2017. (DSM 5) Arlington, VA.

Australian Institute of Health and Welfare. (2011). Indigenous Australians substance use. Viewed July 2019 at https://www.aihw.gov.au/reports/indigenous-australians/substance-use-among-indigenous-people/formats.

Australian Institute of Health and Welfare (AIHW). (2016a). Alcohol, tobacco & other drugs in Australia. Viewed July 2019 at https://www.aihw.gov.au/reports/alcohol/alcohol-tobacco-other-drugs-australia/contents/introduction.

Australian Institute of Health and Welfare (AIHW). (2018a). Report on Indigenous smoking status. Viewed July 2019 at https://www.aihw.gov.au/reports/indigenous-australians/nkpis-indigenous-australians-health-care-2018/contents/preventative-health-indicators/smoking-status-results.

Australian Institute of Health and Welfare (AIHW). (2018b). Alcohol, tobacco & other drugs in Australia. Viewed July 2019 at https://www.aihw.gov.au/reports/alcohol/alcohol-tobacco-other-drugs-australia/contents/priority-populations/aboriginal-and-torres-strait-islander-people.

Australian Institute of Health and Welfare (AIHW). (2018c). Illicit use of drugs. Viewed July 2018 at https://www.aihw.gov.au/reports-data/behaviours-risk-factors/illicit-use-of-drugs/overview.

Ministerial Council on Drug Strategy. (2011). *National drug strategy 2010–2015: A framework for action on alcohol, tobacco and other drugs*. Canberra: Commonwealth of Australia.

National Centre for Education and Training on Addiction (NCETA) Consortium. (2004). *Alcohol and other drugs: A handbook for health professionals*. Canberra: Department of Health and Ageing. Viewed January 2014 at www.drugsandalcohol.ie/13585/#.

National Centre in HIV Epidemiology and Clinical Research. (2009). *Return on investment 2: Evaluating the cost-effectiveness of needle and syringe programs in Australia*. University of New South Wales Department of Health and Ageing. Available at www.apo.org.au/node/19432.

National Health and Medical Research Council. (2011). Alcohol and health in Australia. Summary based on data from 2007 National Drug Strategy Household Survey (AIHW, 2008). Viewed January 2014 at www.nhmrc.gov.au/your-health/alcohol-guidelines/alcohol-and-health-australia.

New Zealand Ministry of Health. (2015). Cannabis use 2012/13: New Zealand Health Survey. Viewed July 2019 at https://www.health.govt.nz/publication/cannabis-use-2012-13-new-zealand-health-survey.

New Zealand Ministry of Health. (2018a). Key indicators. Viewed July 2019 at https://minhealthnz.shinyapps.io/nz-health-survey-2017-18-annual-data-explorer/_w_0811ceee/_w_5c3a7ba5/#!/key-indicators.

New Zealand Ministry of Health. (2018b). Annual update of key results 2016/17: New Zealand Health Survey. Viewed July 2019 at https://www.health.govt.nz/publication/annual-update-key-results-2016-17-new-zealand-health-survey.

New Zealand Ministry of Health (NZMOH). (2010). *Drug use in New Zealand: Key results of the 2007/08 New Zealand Alcohol and Drug Use Survey*. Wellington: Author.

Selected reading

Australian Institute of Health and Welfare (AIHW). (2016b). National Drug Strategy Household Survey 2016: detailed findings. Viewed July 2019 at https://www.aihw.gov.au/reports/illicit-use-of-drugs/2016-ndshs-detailed/related-material.

Online resources

Health Promotion Agency: www.alcohol.org.nz
NZ Drug Foundation: www.drugfoundation.org.nz
DrinkWise Australia: www.drinkwise.org.au
National Drug Research Institute—Preventing harmful drug use in Australia: www.ndri.curtin.edu.au

CHAPTER **37**

Assessing people with intellectual disabilities

CASE STUDY

James is a 37-year-old man with moderate to severe intellectual disability. He will say 'yes' or 'no' and is able to ask for particular types of food that he really likes, such as chocolate biscuits: 'chocky bikkies'. He also uses expletives when angry or wishing to exclaim. Today he is brought to your health centre because for two days he has been intermittently hitting his head against the wall and now there is a laceration on his temple that is bleeding and needs to be sutured.

Definitions and explanations of challenges

DEFINITION

In Australia *intellectual disability* (ID) is described as occurring when a person has significant limitations in their cognitive function, measured as IQ. This is usually below 70. The person with ID will also have impairments in at least two of the following areas: communication, self-care and social skills. Intellectual disability is therefore a combination of reduced IQ and diminished adaptive functions; it is not just a result of below-average IQ. This means that the person requires assistance to manage these limitations. To fit the definition of ID these impairments need to have occurred before the age of 18 (Centre for Disability Studies [CDS], 2006). New Zealand disability experts suggest that a similar definition be used, with the exception that IQ is said to be below 75 for someone with ID (Bray, 2003); however, the New Zealand Intellectual Disability (Compulsory Care and Rehabilitation) Act 2003 sets IQ for a person with ID also at lower than 70.

HEALTH OF PEOPLE WITH INTELLECTUAL DISABILITY

People with ID often have more health problems than the general population because the cause of their ID may contribute to other health problems; for example, Down syndrome is associated with thyroid disease. These problems tend to be chronic and complex (Banks, 2016). In addition to genetically associated health problems, lifestyle-associated health problems are more likely in people with ID, and these lead to obesity and reduced aerobic fitness. For example, reduced muscle tone and diminished coordination associated with several forms of ID will discourage people with ID from being more active. Unfortunately, despite having an increase in morbidity, people with ID have more barriers to accessing health care and are less likely to be screened for hypertension and cancer. They are also less likely to be immunised (CDS, 2006).

CASE STUDY

James is quite active around the residential facility where he has lived for 20 years. However, although he is physically active, he eats excessively, particularly high-kilojoule, high-fat foods. As a consequence, he is obese. Being 37 years old, obese and living in an institutional setting will increase James's chances of having several preventable health problems.

CRITICAL THINKING

1. List the health problems you think James might be at risk of.

FACTORS COMPLICATING HEALTH ASSESSMENT

Communication

Communication impairments often include problems with expressive language that make it difficult for people with ID to tell other people about their symptoms of pain, and they frequently find it hard to describe their illness. Many people with ID have very limited or no expressive language and so they rely on family or support workers to recognise and describe the symptoms of their illness. However, these carers may not know what symptoms the person has, even when they have known the person for many years. This can be made even more difficult because support workers may not have worked in the role for very long and may not know the person they are accompanying very well.

CASE STUDY

James is accompanied by a personal support worker (PSW) on this visit to your health facility.

CRITICAL THINKING

2. What questions will you ask the PSW?
3. Will you direct your questions to the PSW, or will you ask James?
4. How will you involve James in the collection of subjective data?
5. How will you determine the accuracy of the subjective data you collect?

Health assessment

COLLECTING SUBJECTIVE DATA

Adapting interview techniques and communication

Begin communicating with the person with ID rather than with their carer, but check to see if the person wants their carer to stay or if they agree for this person to speak on their behalf. If they struggle to answer questions, then ask their carer; however, the person with ID and their carer may not agree with each other.

Although people with ID may have difficulty expressing themselves, they may still understand what is said to them. To check this, first find out how they indicate 'yes' or 'no'. Then ask them questions requiring 'yes' or 'no' responses, and confirm the accuracy of these responses with the person who is accompanying them.

The person with ID may use augmentative and alternative communication (AAC), and their use of an AAC needs to be determined early and made use of (see Display 37-1). AAC can include the use of communication books, sign language, voice output communication aids or a picture exchange communication system. Whatever AAC the patient uses, ask them to show you how they use it.

Before you begin collecting the subjective data, explain what you are going to do and why you are going to do it. Then check that the patient has understood this. Use models and pictures to assist you. You should also point to the relevant body parts as necessary. Remember that hearing may be a problem and the person may have trouble understanding what is being said. You should speak clearly and carefully, using short, simple sentences. Each sentence should contain only one concept (Hardy et al., 2006).

Begin by asking the person questions you are certain they can answer. This will build confidence, increase their trust in you and reduce their anxiety. Don't ask questions that include or suggest an answer because people with ID are more likely to agree, particularly with a positive response such as 'yes'. Check their answers by asking the same question using different words.

When interviewing patients with ID, you will need to take more time than with patients without an ID. In particular, you should allow for some time for patients with ID to respond. It is generally regarded that waiting 10 seconds for a response is reasonable, and this can seem like a long time (CDS, 2006).

Text with pictures and symbols can help with explanations and assist the person to remember what you have described. However, you will need to assess their literacy first. Some people with ID can have a wide, expressive language vocabulary but are illiterate, whereas others appear to have quite limited speech capabilities but are functionally literate.

Expressive language is not always an accurate indicator of a person's literacy abilities. Abstract concepts, particularly those associated with numeracy, are more likely to be difficult for the person with ID to understand. This can also mean they may have trouble understanding or describing time. Therefore, it is important to use daily routines such as meals, rather than numerical time references, to describe or ask about occurrences. For example, if asking about when a period of pain might have occurred, don't ask if it occurred twice a day. Rather, ask if it occurred near a particular daily event. Wherever possible, be concrete in your questions and descriptions (Hardy et al., 2006).

DISPLAY 37-1 AUGMENTATIVE AND ALTERNATIVE COMMUNICATION

Augmentative and alternative communication (AAC) is the term used to describe additional or other ways that people with difficulty using spoken language communicate. Using sign language or an electronic device that translates typed phrases into spoken words is an example of AAC.

Cultural considerations

The same cultural considerations that are described in Chapters 10, 11 and 12 need to be included when assessing the person with ID. In addition, there needs to be an emphasis on including the family/*whānau* in any assessment. Although this is always important for both Māori and Aboriginal and Torres Strait Islander peoples, it is also important for all people with ID. This is because many people with ID live with their family and usually rely on them for their care.

In New Zealand, health assessors should refer to the 'Guidelines for cultural assessment under the Intellectual Disability (Compulsory Care and Rehabilitation) Act 2003' for further direction on how to provide care competently. This document is available from the New Zealand Ministry of Health's website via www.health.govt.nz.

Health records

Wherever possible, a continuous record of the person's health should be kept. Intellectual disability is life long, so a record of the person's health history that accompanies them to any health assessment is valuable and should be encouraged. This record needs to include a list of diagnoses and treatments, as well as immunisations, allergies and drug reactions, of the patient with ID. It should also indicate what screening tests and preventative health measures have been instigated (CDS, 2006).

To ensure you address the most relevant details, Lennox et al. (2005b) have created a checklist for common presentations and a guide for collecting details about the patient (see Assessment tool 37-1).

ASSESSMENT TOOL 37-1 Checklist of patient details

Patient details of primary importance:

- Past and current medications
- Allergies
- Diet
- History of illnesses and operations
- Family history
- Person responsible for medical decisions

And if bowel problems, seizures or challenging behaviour exists:

- A bowel care plan
- Seizure charts
- Behavioural records

And also a personal history, including:

- Family involvement
- Favourite activities
- Past residential information

Lennox, N., et al. (2005b). Common presentations. Boxes 1 and 2. *Management guidelines: Developmental disability* (p. 8). Melbourne: Therapeutic Guidelines Inc.

CASE STUDY

Unfortunately, James does not have a health record with him, and his personal support worker did not bring one, either. You decide to phone his residential facility to learn more about his past history and treatments.

CRITICAL THINKING

6. What questions would be appropriate to ask James's carers at his residential facility?
7. Would any privacy or confidentiality matters apply if you ring about James's past history? How can you ensure that his privacy is adequately protected?

An example of recording a 'Health assessment for people with an intellectual disability' is available online at www.health.gov.au.

CASE STUDY

The problem with a health record is that it could contain information only about James's health and might not document what he likes, what he eats, how he behaves and what upsets him. You are concerned he might injure himself or the property of other people if he is upset.

You decide to ask James's personal support worker what she knows about James. She tells you that James hates having his blood pressure measured and does not like to be touched by people he doesn't know.

CRITICAL THINKING

8. How will you measure James's blood pressure?
9. How will you conduct a physical examination if he is unlikely to let you touch him?
10. What record-keeping would you recommend?

A good resource to help you answer these questions has been produced by MOIRA: Disability and Youth Service, Melbourne, via www.moira.org.au.

Atypical presentations and 'diagnostic overshadowing'

Even people with ID who are able to communicate their needs may still have difficulty recognising the symptoms of their illness, so they may not tell anyone about their discomfort. For example, those with otitis media may become bad tempered with earache and their speech may deteriorate, but they cannot describe what is wrong. At the same time, their carers may not recognise the subtle decline in their speech until the symptoms become more obvious or the illness becomes more severe, such as a rupture of the tympanic membrane.

The distress endured by the person with ID may manifest as concerning behaviours that their family or support workers might describe as self-injuring, unexplained irritability, aggression and excessive or unusual vocalisations (Charlot et al., 2011). The person may also regress in their behaviour so that they act in a more immature way.

When assessing people with ID who have difficulties expressing their experience of symptoms, a health professional may misinterpret clinical manifestations of their illness as a usual feature of their disability. Called 'diagnostic overshadowing', this health assessment problem is particularly likely for behavioural problems, which can be seen as a characteristic of intellectual disability rather than a mental health issue (Cheetham & McMillan, 2017). It also occurs with physical illness; for example, a change in motor activity in someone with cerebral palsy is attributed to the cerebral palsy rather than to a spinal injury or brain injury. Diagnostic overshadowing is more likely when the health care provider is not familiar with the care of people with ID (Cheetham & McMillan, 2017). People with cerebral palsy often do not have an ID; however, communication difficulties can impede assessment, so that diagnostic overshadowing is still possible.

Common problems

As many of the health problems endured by people with ID have not been detected and are therefore not treated (Zeldin & Bazzano, 2016), it is important that health professionals are particularly vigilant and begin by considering common problems. These problems include respiratory illness, sensory impairments, dental problems, eating disorders (including malnutrition and obesity), gastrointestinal problems, epilepsy and mental health problems.

Respiratory illness

A predominant cause of death in people with ID is respiratory disease (Tyrer & McGrother, 2009). This is because of aspiration associated with reflux and swallowing problems.

Aspiration is also increased in people with epilepsy, which is also more prevalent.

Immunisation against respiratory diseases such as influenza is also less likely because of poorer preventative health measures for people with ID.

Having Down syndrome also increases the risk of respiratory disease because of abnormalities of the lungs, diminished immunity and mouth breathing, which bypasses some of the protective effects of nasal breathing.

Vision and hearing impairments

Problems with hearing and vision are common in people with ID, with up to 40% having hearing problems, and a similar proportion being affected by diminished vision (Beange et al., 1995). Hearing and vision problems are exacerbated by frequent infections of the ears and eyes.

Vision impairment

Assessing vision is more complex in people with ID because they may not have enough literacy to identify letters used in a Snellen chart. If the nurse using the eye chart does not recognise this inability, an incorrect measurement of visual acuity may occur.

People with ID are also less likely to visit an optician who is able to perform accurate visual acuity tests (Beange et al., 1995). Furthermore, several causes of ID are associated with sight problems, in particular Down syndrome, cerebral palsy, fragile X syndrome and fetal rubella syndrome.

Although there is a very high incidence of visual problems in people with ID, they are less likely to have these conditions assessed and treated. Consequently, when people with ID present for assessment, visual acuity needs to be a part of their comprehensive physical assessment.

Hearing impairment

Many people with ID have diminished hearing either as a result of the syndrome they have or because of recurrent ear infections. In particular, Down syndrome, which is associated with decreased immunity, predisposes the person to recurrent ear infections (Manickam et al., 2016). It is therefore important to check for a history of repeated ear infections, especially in people with Down syndrome. This is also important for similar reasons in people with fragile X syndrome and cerebral palsy. In people who have fetal rubella syndrome there is frequently hearing impairment as a result of neural damage. Consequently, many people with ID need hearing aids but do not use them. This is usually because the person has not been diagnosed with a hearing impairment rather than as a result of not complying with instructions to wear hearing aids. The uncorrected hearing impairment consequently exacerbates communication problems.

Problems with hearing may also be compounded by impacted cerumen, a common problem in people with ID. Therefore, a careful inspection of the ears is warranted and hearing must be assessed.

Dental health

People with ID have more dental caries, loose teeth and gingivitis that are often unrecognised and untreated (Anders & Davis, 2010). Poor diet and ineffective dental hygiene causes many of these ailments (Hardy et al., 2006).

Despite subsidised dental care in Australia, people with ID are less likely to visit a dentist. Health assessment of the person with ID must therefore include an inspection of the mouth. Problems with this part of the body, particularly painful problems, may explain behavioural changes.

Nutritional problems

Swallowing

According to Cheetham and McMillan (2017), the more profound the cognitive impairment of a person, the more likely his or her swallowing will be affected. Dysphagia is also associated with anatomical abnormalities of the mouth associated with several syndromes and impaired neuromuscular control. Aspiration or choking is therefore more likely. Nurses should therefore ensure that a patient's swallowing ability is carefully assessed, preferably by a speech therapist. This is particularly important in people with cerebral palsy and in people with neuromuscular disorders.

Weight problems

The assessment of body mass index and waist circumference are important indicators of overnutrition and obesity, which is more prevalent in people with milder cognitive impairment. These measurements should be regularly collected as part of a preventative health program. Resultant obesity from overeating is more likely in the person with ID because of an overconsumption of high-kilojoule foods, inactivity, medication (antipsychotics and anticonvulsants) and genetic conditions such as Prader-Willi syndrome and Down syndrome. Conversely, some people with ID are at risk of being malnourished through insufficient food intake and some metabolic disorders such as phenylketonuria (Cheetham & McMillan, 2017).

Gastrointestinal problems

Helicobacter pylori

Infection with *Helicobacter pylori* is more prevalent in people with ID, particularly if they live in (or have lived in) institutional care. Therefore, people with ID should be assessed for *H. pylori* infection, although the ability to do the urea breath test may be compromised, making tests for *H. pylori* using other methods necessary. Hardy et al. (2006) believe *H. pylori* tests and subsequent treatment will need to occur for much of the rest of the patient's lives. Infection with *H. pylori* may be the cause of unexplained abdominal discomfort.

Gastro-oesophageal reflux disease

People with ID need to be assessed for gastro-oesophageal reflux disease (GORD) because GORD can affect up to 50% of this patient population (Cheetham & McMillan, 2017). Gastro-oesophageal reflux disease is more prevalent in people with fragile X syndrome and when their impairment is more profound.

Constipation

For people with more profound ID and for those who have reduced mobility, constipation is likely. Coleman and Spurling (2010) found that up to 70% of people with ID who are in institutional care have constipation. This problem is associated with medication, reduced fluid intake, low-fibre diet and inactivity. Constipation can be a significant threat to the health of people with ID and has been related to several deaths. To assess for constipation, it is recommended to ask the patient or carer about bowel motion, particularly faecal overflow. Also ask about abdominal pain. Abdominal palpation may enable the detection of faeces.

Epilepsy

People with ID need to be assessed for a history of seizures because these could be an explanation for unusual behaviour such as vacant staring or stereotypical movement. Assessing people with ID for previous occurrences of seizures is important and more likely because about one-third (25% to 35%) of all people with ID have epilepsy, compared with a prevalence of about 2% in the wider population (Lennox et al., 2005c). Kerr et al. (2009) report that epilepsy is often more difficult to control in people with ID. With more profound ID, the frequency of epilepsy increases, an important consideration when assessing people whose ID is severe.

As a result of using multiple medications to control more complex, more frequent and more prevalent seizures, the likelihood of *polypharmacy* increases, so the side effects of anticonvulsant medication need to be looked for in the health assessment of people with ID (Lennox et al., 2005c).

Mental health

The assessment of mental health is important because people with ID are twice as likely to have mental health problems because of their syndrome, their medications, their physical health problems or the restrictions on their lives (Einfeld et al., 2011). Particular mental health problems that are more likely in this population include anxiety disorders, depression, bipolar disorders and schizophrenia. In addition, they are also more likely to act in ways that can be difficult for or confronting to the people around them. There are also syndromes within autism spectrum disorders that are associated with very specific mental health issues.

Anxiety disorders

When assessing the health of the person with ID, physical signs of anxiety such as rapid breathing, tense muscles and agitated movements might be observed. In addition, aggression, screaming and repetitive actions could also indicate an anxiety disorder.

These signs could indicate general anxiety, phobias or panic disorders, which are more likely in people with ID (Lennox et al., 2005a); however, confirming anxiety by asking about the patient's thoughts is difficult to assess. Anxiety is often seen in people with autistic spectrum disorders, and these patients are likely to exhibit signs of aggression, repetitive acts or verbal outbursts when their routines are interrupted or their daily structure is changed.

Mood

Evidence of mood disorders and depression in people with ID is similar to that of the rest of the population who may be depressed; however, there are signs and behaviours that are characteristic of people with ID. Signs of depression in the person with ID can manifest as changes in mood, a loss of interest in usual activities, increased activity and other changes in behaviour. Irritability, a sign of depression, can be exhibited by increasing verbal and physical aggression, with resultant damage to property.

A mood disturbance that might indicate depression is a depressed mood, with tearfulness, a sad appearance and less laughter. People with ID may also lose interest in things that usually bring them pleasure such as their favourite television programs. Other signs might include spending more time alone, losing physical skills, having new sleep patterns, losing or gaining weight, becoming agitated or moving less (Lennox et al., 2005a). Self-injury, aggression, uncharacteristic incontinence and screaming are also associated with depression in people with ID (Hardy et al., 2006).

Psychosis and schizophrenia

Hardy et al. (2006) report that the occurrence of schizophrenia is three times more likely in people with ID. The symptoms of psychosis in people with ID tend to be less complicated and not as obvious as in people who do not have an ID. However, the range of psychotic manifestations is still the same. The signs to look for include delusions, but these can be hard to distinguish from fantasies associated with cognitive impairment. The continual and unexplained targeting of another person may be an indication of paranoid delusions (Lennox et al., 2005a). Other signs to look for include bizarre and disorganised behaviour. Schizophrenia is difficult to diagnose in people with profound ID because diagnosis relies on the person being able to communicate his or her thoughts. Because of the increasing prevalence of mental health issues, the difficulty of identifying these issues and the significant impact of mental illness on a person's life, it is important that health professionals are aware of the significance of psychosis and other psychiatric disorders. Where psychotic symptoms are suspected in a person with ID, he or she will need psychiatric referral.

Challenging behaviour

Behaviour that is confronting, aggressive, destructive or self-injuring is the most common reason for performing a health assessment (Lennox et al., 2005d). A challenging behaviour has many possible causes and is often the primary means of communicating distress by the person with ID; however, it may also be part of the intellectual disability without any other cause. This creates a difficulty for the health professional assessing the person with ID because the challenging behaviour may be usual for the patient, or it could indicate a serious illness and significant pain. To assume that a challenging behaviour is simply part of the impairment of a person with ID risks a serious problem being overlooked. This is termed 'diagnostic overshadowing' (Lennox et al., 2005a, p. 124). By being aware that diagnostic overshadowing is possible, health professionals are more likely to uncover health problems that might otherwise be missed.

Musculoskeletal problems

Some people with ID are prone to fractures, usually because of problems with osteoporosis. Bone density is reduced because of inactivity, insufficient dietary calcium, vitamin D deficiency and anticonvulsant medication. Several mechanisms also increase the chance of a fracture, including ataxia contributing to falls, and trauma as a result of challenging behaviour (Cheetham & McMillan, 2017). It is therefore important to assess for fractures if there is a history of falls or traumatic injury. Skeletal injuries should also be checked in the presence of an unexplained behavioural change.

People with ID who have cerebral palsy or have severe cognitive impairment are more likely to endure spasticity and contractures. These abnormalities can be a source of pain and discomfort and so should be assessed as part of the comprehensive health assessment.

Medications

Medications to treat seizures (anti-epileptics) and those that affect perception and behaviour (psychotropics) are frequently prescribed to people with ID. It is possible that these patients have been taking such medications for many years without a change in dosage or frequency. However, as ageing occurs, it is increasingly likely that these medications may interact or cause side effects because of ageing-related changes to drug metabolism and excretion.

Therefore, when assessing the health of people with ID it is important to list carefully the medications they are taking and consider the possibility that one or more of these drugs is contributing to their symptoms or behavioural changes (Lennox et al., 2005d). As a consequence of these many issues, it is recommended that people with ID should be regularly screened for more prevalent health problems. See Table 37-1 for a health care checklist and screening frequency.

Table 37-1 Health care checklist for an adult with developmental disability

Health concern	Review frequency	Practitioner
General health		
blood pressure	yearly	GP
oral health (teeth, gums and oral cavity)	every 6 months	dentist
hearing		
• assessment	• Down syndrome—every 2 to 3 years • non-Down syndrome—every 3 to 5 years	audiologist
• correct use of hearing aids	regularly	GP or audiologist
• otoscopy	opportunistically	GP
vision		
• assessment	• Down syndrome—every 2 to 3 years • non-Down syndrome—every 3 to 5 years	optometrist/ophthalmologist
• correct use of glasses	regularly	GP or optometrist/ ophthalmologist
medication review	at least every 6 to 12 months	medication review pharmacist
thyroid function	• Down syndrome—yearly • non-Down syndrome—yearly or less frequently (depending on cause of disability)	GP
dyslipidaemia	regularly*	GP
diabetes	fasting plasma glucose • Down syndrome—yearly • non-Down syndrome—at least every 3 years (more frequently if taking antipsychotic drugs)	GP
skin check	yearly	GP
Lifestyle		
alcohol	yearly	GP
smoking	yearly	GP
nutrition	yearly	GP
weight	yearly	GP
physical activity	yearly	GP
Women's health		
breast cancer		
• breast examination	regular review (frequency not clear)	GP
• mammography	every 2 years from ages of 50 to 69 years	radiographer
cervical cancer (Papanicolaou [Pap] smear)	every 2 years from ages of 18 to 69 years, if patient has ever been sexually active	GP
Men's health		
testicular examination	on first presentation and yearly after that	GP
prostate cancer screen	according to clinical assessment (routine screening is not recommended at the time of writing)	GP

Table 37-1 Health care checklist for an adult with developmental disability (continued)

Health concern	Review frequency	Practitioner
Immunisation		
	according to the schedule in *The Australian Immunisation Handbook*	GP
Other		
epilepsy	continually aware of risk; if taking antiepileptic drugs, consider vitamin D supplementation	GP
urinary incontinence	continually	GP
mobility	continually	GP/allied health professionals
problem behaviour (physical/ psychological/social)	opportunistically, if indicated	GP/psychologist
depression (especially in high-risk patients [e.g. previous diagnosis of psychiatric disorder])	maintain high level of clinical awareness of people at high risk of depression screen opportunistically	GP
dementia (Down syndrome patients from age of 35 years)	heightened clinical awareness enquire opportunistically about memory and functioning	GP/psychologist/psychiatrist
sexual health (advice on contraception, safe sex and sexually transmitted infections)	opportunistically, if indicated	GP
bone health	• Down syndrome—measure bone mineral density: – in early adulthood – at menopause in women – at approximately 40 years of age in hypogonadal men	GP
	• non-Down syndrome—enquire opportunistically about risk factors	GP

Reproduced with permission from Adult health care. In: *Management guidelines: developmental disability. Version 3*. Melbourne: Therapeutic Guidelines Limited; 2012. The Management Guidelines: Developmental Disability are currently being revised, with publication scheduled for December 2020. Please see https://www.tg.org.au for more information.

* Much of this advice is the same as for the general population. Royal Australian College of General Practitioners. (2009). *Guidelines for preventive activities in general practice* [The red book] [7th ed.]. Melbourne: Author.

Indicators of distress

People with ID may not present with typical behaviours or symptoms that are usually associated with illness or pain. It is therefore important to discover from the carer how the person behaves when he or she is distressed. A tool that can formalise this process, particularly for individuals with very limited communication, is the Disability Distress Assessment Tool, or 'DisDAT' (see Assessment tool 37-2). This tools relies on the carer's abilities to discern when the person is content and when he or she is distressed, and to describe the difference between these two states. The current tool can be downloaded from www.disdat.co.uk. (There are no restrictions on making copies, but it cannot be altered in any way without the author's permission.)

COLLECTING OBJECTIVE DATA: PHYSICAL EXAMINATION

Before beginning a physical examination of a person with ID, first explain what you are planning to do and why you are doing it. Use pictures, gestures and equipment to help you explain.

Any equipment to be used should be demonstrated first. For example, show how you are going to measure the patient's

CASE STUDY

James has a laceration on his scalp from hitting his head against the wall. Some of your colleagues thought James's actions were part of his usual behaviour and associated with his intellectual disability. However, you are concerned that James's behaviour has been an indication that he's experiencing distress and discomfort.

James's personal support worker thinks that he is protecting his abdomen. You would like to examine him, but his obesity and unwillingness to let you touch him are going to make assessment difficult.

CRITICAL THINKING

11. How will you assess James's abdomen to check for signs of peritonitis and other indicators of abdominal discomfort?

ASSESSMENT TOOL 37-2 DisDAT: Disability distress assessment tool

v21

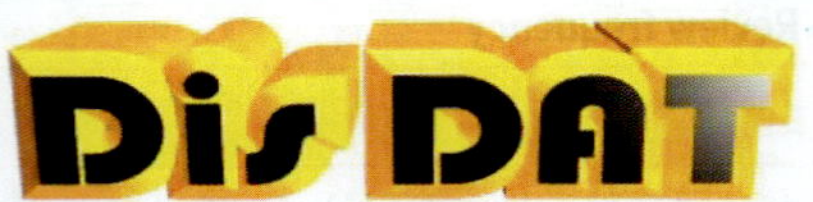

Distress and Discomfort Assessment Tool

Individual's name:

DoB: Gender:

NHS No:

Your name:

Date completed:

Names of others who helped complete this form:

THE DISTRESS PASSPORT

Summary of signs and behaviours when content and when distressed

	When CONTENT	When DISTRESSED
Face Jaw & tongue Eyes		
Vocal sounds Speech		
Habits & mannerisms Comfortable distance		
Body posture Body observations		

Known triggers of distress (write here any actions or situations that usually cause or worsen distress)

ASSESSMENT TOOL 37-2 DisDAT: Disability distress assessment tool (continued)

Distress and Discomfort Assessment Tool

v21

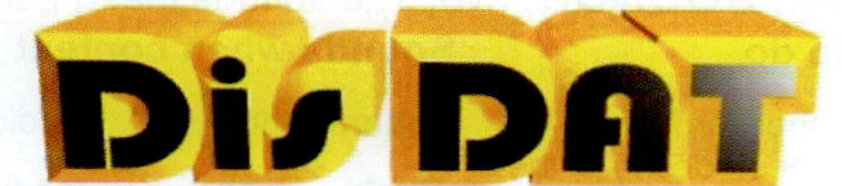

Please take some time to think about and observe the individual under your care, especially their appearance and behaviours when they are both content and distressed. Use these pages to document these.

We have listed words in each section to help you to describe the signs and behaviours. You can circle the word or words that best describe the signs and behaviours when they are content and when they are distressed.

Your descriptions will provide you with a clearer picture of their 'language' of distress.

COMMUNICATION LEVEL *

This individual is unable to show likes or dislikes		Level 0
This individual is able to show that they like or don't like something		Level 1
This individual is able to show that they want more, or have had enough of something		Level 2
This individual is able to show anticipation for their like or dislike of something		Level 3
This individual is able to communicate detail, qualify, specify and/or indicate opinions		Level 4

* This is adapted from the Kidderminster Curriculum for Children and Adults with Profound Multiple Learning Difficulty (Jones, 1994, National Portage Association).

FACIAL SIGNS

Appearance

What to do	Appearance when content	Appearance when distressed
Ring the words that best fit the facial appearance. Add your words if you want.	Passive Laugh Smile Frown Grimace Startled **In your own words:**	Passive Laugh Smile Frown Grimace Startled **In your own words:**

Jaw or tongue movement

What to do	Movement when content	Movement when distressed
Ring the words that best fit the jaw or tongue movement. Add your words if you want.	Relaxed Drooping Grinding Biting Rigid Shaking **In your own words:**	Relaxed Drooping Grinding Biting Rigid Shaking **In your own words:**

Appearance of eyes

What to do	Appearance when content	Appearance when distressed
Ring the words that best fit the appearance of the eyes. Add your words if you want.	Good eye contact Little eye contact Avoiding eye contact Closed eyes Staring Sleepy eyes 'Smiling' Winking Vacant Tears Dilated pupils **In your own words:**	Good eye contact Little eye contact Avoiding eye contact Closed eyes Staring Sleepy eyes 'Smiling' Winking Vacant Tears Dilated pupils **In your own words:**

BODY OBSERVATIONS: SKIN APPEARANCE

What to do	Appearance when content	Appearance when distressed
Ring the words that best fit the describe the appearance of the skin. Add your words if you want.	Normal Pale Flushed Sweaty Clammy **In your own words:**	Normal Pale Flushed Sweaty Clammy **In your own words:**

Continued on following page

ASSESSMENT TOOL 37-2 DisDAT: Disability distress assessment tool (continued)

VOCAL SOUNDS (NB. The sounds that a person makes are not always linked to their feelings)

What to do	Sounds when content	Sounds when distressed
Ring the words that best describe the sounds *Write down* commonly used sounds (write it as it sounds; 'tizz', 'eeiow', 'tetetetete'):	**Volume:** high medium low **Pitch:** high medium low **Duration:** short intermittent long **Description of sound / vocalisation:** Cry out Wail Scream laugh Groan / moan shout Gurgle **In your own words:**	**Volume:** high medium low **Pitch:** high medium low **Duration:** short intermittent long **Description of sound / vocalisation:** Cry out Wail Scream laugh Groan / moan shout Gurgle **In your own words:**

SPEECH

What to do	Words when content	Words when distressed
Write down commonly used words and phrases. If no words are spoken, write NONE		
Ring the words which best describe the speech	Clear Stutters Slurred Unclear Muttering Fast Slow Loud Soft Whisper Other, eg. swearing:	Clear Stutters Slurred Unclear Muttering Fast Slow Loud Soft Whisper Other, eg.swearing:

HABITS & MANNERISMS

What to do	Habits and mannerisms when content	Habits and mannerisms when distressed
Write down the habits or mannerisms, eg. "Rocks when sitting"		
Write down any special comforters, possessions or toys this person prefers.		
Please Ring the statements which best describe how comfortable this person is with other people being physically close by	Close with strangers Close only if known No one allowed close Withdraws if touched	Close with strangers Close only if known No one allowed close Withdraws if touched

BODY POSTURE

What to do	Posture when content	Posture when distressed
Ring the words that best describe how this person sits and stands.	Normal Rigid Floppy Jerky Slumped Restless Tense Still Able to adjust position Leans to side Poor head control Way of walking: Normal / Abnormal Other:	Normal Rigid Floppy Jerky Slumped Restless Tense Still Able to adjust position Leans to side Poor head control Way of walking: Normal / Abnormal Other:

BODY OBSERVATIONS: OTHER

What to do	Observations when content	Observations when distressed
Describe the pulse, breathing, sleep, appetite and usual eating pattern, eg. eats very quickly, takes a long time with main course, eats puddings quickly, "picky".	Pulse: Breathing: Sleep: Appetite: Eating pattern:	Pulse: Breathing: Sleep: Appetite Eating pattern:

ASSESSMENT TOOL 37-2 DisDAT: Disability distress assessment tool (continued)

Information and Instructions

DisDAT is

Intended to help identify distress cues in individuals who have severely limited communication.

Designed to describe an individual's usual content cues, thus enabling distress cues to be identified more clearly.

NOT a scoring tool. It documents what many carers have done instinctively for many years thus providing a record against which subtle changes can be compared.

Only the first step. Once distress has been identified the usual clinical decisions have to be made by professionals.

Meant to help you and the individual in your care. It gives you more confidence in the observation skills you already have, which in turn will give you more confidence when meeting other carers.

When to use DisDAT

When the carer believes the individual is NOT distressed

The use of DisDAT is optional, but it can be used as a
- baseline assessment document
- transfer document for other carers.

When the carer believes the individual IS distressed

If DisDAT has already been completed it can be used to compare the present signs and behaviours with previous observations documented on DisDAT. It then serves as a baseline to monitor change.

If DisDAT has not been completed:

a) When the person is well known DisDAT can be used to document previous content signs and behaviours and compare these with the current observations

b) When the person is new to a carer, or the distress is new, DisDAT can be used document the present signs and behaviours to act a baseline to monitor change.

How to use DisDAT

1. **Observe the individual** when content and when distressed- document this on the inside pages. *Anyone* who cares for them can do this.
2. **Observe the context** in which distress is occurring.
3. **Use the clinical decision distress checklist** on this page to assess the possible cause.
4. **Treat or manage** the likeliest cause of the distress.
5. **The monitoring sheet** is a separate sheet, which will help if you want to observe a pattern of distress or see how the distress changes over time. It's use is optional. There are three types to choose from the website- use whichever suits you best.
6. **The goal** is a reduction the number or severity of distress signs and behaviours.

Remember

- Most information comes from several carers together.
- The assessment form need not be completed all at once and may take a period of time.
- Reassessment is essential as the needs may change due to improvement or deterioration.
- Distress can be emotional, physical or psychological. What is a minor issue for one person can be major to another.
- If signs are recognised early then suitable interventions can be put in place to avoid a crisis.

Clinical decision distress checklist

Use this to help decide the cause of the distress

Is the new sign or behaviour?

- Repeated rapidly?

Consider pleuritic pain (in time with breathing)
Consider colic (comes and goes every few minutes)
Consider: repetitive movement due to boredom or fear.

- Associated with breathing?

Consider: infection, COPD, pleural effusion, tumour

- Worsened or precipitated by movement?

Consider: movement-related pains

- Related to eating?

Consider: food refusal through illness, fear or depression
Consider: food refusal because of swallowing problems
Consider: upper GI problems (oral hygiene, peptic ulcer, dyspepsia) or abdominal problems.

- Related to a specific situation?

Consider: frightening or painful situations.

- Associated with vomiting?

Consider: causes of nausea and vomiting.

- Associated with elimination (urine or faecal)?

Consider: urinary problems (infection, retention)
Consider: GI problems (diarrhoea, constipation)

- Present in a normally comfortable position or situation?

Consider: anxiety, depression, pains at rest (eg. colic, neuralgia), infection, nausea.

If you require any help or further information regarding DisDAT please contact:
Lynn Gibson 01670 394 260
Dorothy Matthews 01670 394 808
Dr. Claud Regnard 0191 285 0063 or e-mail on claudregnard@stoswaldsuk.org

For more information see
www.disdat.co.uk

Further reading

Regnard C, Matthews D, Gibson L, Clarke C, Watson B. Difficulties in identifying distress and its causes in people with severe communication problems. *International Journal of Palliative Nursing,* 2003, 9(3): 173-6.

Regnard C, Reynolds J, Watson B, Matthews D, Gibson L, Clarke C. Understanding distress in people with severe communication difficulties: developing and assessing the Disability Distress Assessment Tool (DisDAT). J Intellect Disability Res. 2007; **51(4)**: 277-292.

Distress may be hidden, but it is never silent

ASSESSMENT TOOL 37-3 The 6 A's of assessment

Assess communication skills
Allow sufficient time and develop rapport
Arrange adequate follow-up and collect information from multiple sources
Adopt a biopsychosocial approach
Be **Aware** of syndrome-specific conditions and the 'occults'
Assume there is a cause of the health problem beyond the developmental disability

Lennox, N., et al. (2005b). Box 1: Common presentations. *Management guidelines: Developmental disability* (p. 7). Melbourne, Vic.: Therapeutic Guidelines.

blood pressure by first performing the procedure on the carer or on yourself. Then check that the patient has understood what you are going to do and ask if they will allow you to perform the procedure on them. A useful mnemonic that can help is the '6 A's of assessment' (see Assessment tool 37-3).

CASE STUDY

After carefully demonstrating and explaining what you are going to do using the help of the PSW (who knows James well and whom he trusts), you are able to inspect and palpate James's abdomen. However, because of his obesity you cannot determine anything much by palpation, except that he is obviously tender. Consequently, an abdominal radiograph is organised, and it reveals extensive constipation.

James will require admission to hospital for a general anaesthetic and disimpaction.

CRITICAL THINKING

12. What information could you have gathered to help you determine constipation as a problem earlier?
13. Do you think a bowel chart will be appropriate for James in his residential setting?

CONCLUSION

Many health problems are more common in people with ID, and these conditions are often not diagnosed. They may be associated with the cause of the person's disability, or continue because they have not been identified and treated.

The identification of illness and chronic health in people with ID is less straightforward because of the difficulties patients often have in communicating their symptoms. The detection of pain is also not easy because of their communication difficulties; however, any change in behaviour should be investigated as a sign of discomfort.

Effective health care for people with ID can be undermined by the negative attitudes of health professionals and poor health support systems. Therefore, health professionals must treat people with ID with dignity and carefully assess for infirmity.

When assessing the health of people who have ID, it is important to consider what problems are more likely because of their intellectual impairment. It is also necessary to involve them in all aspects of assessment and to avoid touching them until you have their permission.

Where possible, the family must be included for cultural and practical reasons. In most circumstances the family will be able to provide details of the presenting problem and past health. However, before talking with the family, first ask the person with ID.

ONLINE RESOURCES

An extensive range of additional resources to enhance teaching and learning and to facilitate understanding may be found online at the text's accompanying website, located on thePoint at http://thepoint.lww.com. These include Watch and Learn videos, Concepts in Action animations, journal articles, case studies, discussion topics and quizzes.

Subscribers may also access Lippincott Procedures, an extensive online point-of-care procedure guide that provides reliable step-by-step instructions for more than 1700 procedures, including 450 evidence-based Australian procedures, and skills in a variety of speciality settings, together with a wealth of supporting information.

SIMULATED LEARNING

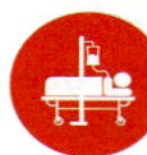

Throughout this chapter you have considered the case of James, who has an intellectual disability. In the simulation scenario based on James and available to your lecturer online, you will continue to assess James and the issues that have been complicated by his difficulty communicating. In this simulation you will be using the assessment tools described in this chapter.

CASE STUDY

This case study illustrates how to analyse assessment data for a specific patient. The exercises included in the ancillary product on thePoint that complements this text offer further opportunities to enhance your skills.

James is a 37-year-old man with moderate to severe intellectual disability. He will say 'yes' or 'no' and is able to ask for particular types of food that he really likes, such as chocolate biscuits: 'chocky bikkies'. He also uses expletives when angry or wishing to exclaim. Today he is brought to your health centre because for two days he has been intermittently hitting his head against the wall. Now there is a laceration on his temple that is bleeding and needs to be sutured.

James is quite active around the residential facility where he has lived for 20 years. However, although he is physically active, he eats excessively, particularly high-kilojoule, high-fat foods. As a consequence, he is obese. Being 37 years of age, obese and living in an institutional setting will increase James's chances of having several preventable health problems.

James is accompanied by a personal support worker (PSW) on this visit to your health facility. Unfortunately, James does not have a health record with him, and his PSW did not bring one, either. You decide to phone his residential facility to learn more about his past history and treatments.

The problem with a health record is that it could contain information only about James's health and might not document what he likes, what he eats, how he behaves and what upsets him. You are concerned James might injure himself or the property of other people if he is upset.

You decide to ask James's PSW what she knows about James. She tells you James hates having his blood pressure measured and does not like to be touched by people he doesn't know.

James has a laceration on his scalp from hitting his head against the wall. Some of your colleagues thought James's actions were part of his usual behaviour and associated with his intellectual disability. However, you are concerned that James's behaviour has been an indication that he's been experiencing distress and discomfort.

His PSW thinks that he is protecting his abdomen. You would like to examine him, but his obesity and unwillingness to let you touch him are going to make assessment difficult.

After carefully demonstrating and explaining what you are going to do using the help of the PSW (who knows James well and whom he trusts), you are able to inspect and palpate James's abdomen. However, because of his obesity you cannot determine anything much by palpation, except that he is obviously tender. Consequently, an abdominal radiograph is organised, and it reveals extensive constipation.

James will require admission to hospital for a general anaesthetic and disimpaction.

References

Anders, P. L. & Davis, E. L. (2010). Oral health of patients with intellectual disabilities: A systematic review. *Special Care in Dentistry, 30*(3), 110–117.

Banks, S. (2016). Chronic illness and people with intellectual disability: Prevalence, prevention and management. National Disability Services. Department of Education and Training, Australian Governement. Available at https://www.nds.org.au/images/LearnNDevelop/Chronic-Illness-and-People-with-Intellectual-Disability.PDF.

Beange, H., et al. (1995). Medical disorders of adults with mental retardation: A population study. *American Journal of Mental Retardation, 99*(6), 595–604.

Bray, A. (2003). Definitions of intellectual disability: Review of the literature prepared for the National Advisory Committee on Health and Disability to inform its project on services for adults with an intellectual disability. National Advisory Committee on Health and Disability. Wellington: National Health Committee and Donald Beasley Institute. Available at http://www.moh.govt.nz/notebook/nbbooks.nsf/0/E9228E058EC737A6CC257D6900751918/$file/definition%20of%20intellectual%20disability.pdf.

Centre for Disability Studies (CDS [previously CDDS]). (2006). *Health care in people with intellectual disability: Guidelines for general practitioners*. Sydney: NSW Health. Available at https://www.aci.health.nsw.gov.au/__data/assets/pdf_file/0016/231514/Health_Care_in_People_with_Intellectual_Disability_Guidelines.pdf.

Charlot, L., Abend, S., Ravin, P., et al. (2011). Non-psychiatric health problems among psychiatric inpatients with intellectual disabilities. *Journal of Mental Deficiency Research, 55*(2), 199–209.

Cheetham, T. & McMillan, S. (2017). Physical Health. In M. L. Wehmeyer, I. Brown, M. Percy, et al. (Eds). *A comprehensive guide to intellectual and developmental disabilities* (2nd ed., pp. 665–678). Baltimore: Paul H Brookes.

Coleman, J. & Spurling, G. (2010). Constipation in people with learning disability. *British Medical Journal, 340*, c222.

Einfeld, S. L., Ellis, L. A. & Emerson, E. (2011). Comorbidity of intellectual disability and mental disorder in children and adolescents: A systematic review. *Journal of Intellectual and Developmental Disability, 36*(2), 137–143.

Hardy, S., Woodward, P., et al. (2006). *Meeting the health needs of people with learning disabilities: Guidance for nursing staff*. London: Royal College of Nursing.

Kerr, M., Scheepers, M., Arvio, M., et al. (2009). Consensus guidelines into the management of epilepsy in adults with an intellectual disability. *Journal of Intellectual Disability Research, 53*(8), 687–694.

Lennox, N., et al. (2005a). Assessment of psychiatric disorders. In *Management guidelines: Developmental disability* (pp. 123–134). Melbourne: Therapeutic Guidelines Ltd.

Lennox, N., et al. (2005b). Common presentations. Boxes 1 and 2. In *Management guidelines: Developmental disability* (pp. 7–8). Melbourne: Therapeutic Guidelines.

Lennox, N., et al. (2005c). Epilepsy. In *Management guidelines: Developmental disability* (pp. 151–162). Melbourne: Therapeutic Guidelines Ltd.

Lennox, N., et al. (2005d). Preventative health care and health promotion. In *Management guidelines: Developmental disability* (pp. 95–99). Melbourne: Therapeutic Guidelines Ltd.

Manickam, V., Shott, G. S., Heithaus, D., et al. (2016). Hearing loss in Down syndrome revisited—15 Years later. *International Journal of Pediatric Otorhinolaryngology, 88*, 203–207.

New Zealand Ministry of Health. (2004). Guidelines for cultural assessment—Māori. Under the Intellectual Disability (Compulsory Care and Rehabilitation) Act 2003. Viewed January 2014 at www.health.govt.nz/system/files/documents/publications/idccrguidelines-culturalassessment.pdf.

Royal Australian College of General Practitioners. (2009). *Guidelines for preventive activities in general practice* (7th ed.). Melbourne: Author.

Tyrer, F. & McGrother, C. (2009). Cause-specific mortality and death certificate reporting in adults with moderate to profound intellectual disability. *Journal of Intellectual Disability Research, 53*(11), 898–904.

Zeldin, A. S. & Bazzano, A. T. F. (2016). Intellectual disability. *eMedicine*. Available at https://emedicine.medscape.com/article/1180709-overview.

Selected readings

Australian Government Department of Health and Ageing. (2014). *Australian immunisation handbook* (10th ed.). Canberra: Author.

Tracy, J., Burbridge, M., Butler, J., et al. (2016). Working with people with intellectual disabilities in healthcare settings. Centre for Developmental Disability Health, Monash Health, Victoria. Available at https://www.cddh.monashhealth.org/wp-content/uploads/2016/11/2016-working-with-people-with-intellectual-disabilities.pdf.

Online resources

Australasian Society for Intellectual Disability: www.asid.asn.au

Centre for Developmental Disability Health Victoria (CDDH), Monash University: www.cddh.monash.org

Centre for Disability Studies (CDS [previously CDDS]), Sydney University: https://cds.org.au/

IHC New Zealand: https://ihc.org.nz/

MOIRA: Disability and Youth Service: https://moira.org.au/

Council for Intellectual Disability: https://cid.org.au/

New Zealand Ministry of Health, Disability services: https://www.health.govt.nz/your-health/services-and-support/disability-services

National Institute for Health and Care Excellence (NICE)—People with learning disabilities: https://www.nice.org.uk/guidance/population-groups/people-with-learning-disabilities

Queensland Centre for Intellectual and Developmental Disability (QCIDD): www.qcidd.com.au

Therapeutic Guidelines Limited *(Management Guidelines: Developmental Disability)*: https://tgldcdp.tg.org.au/fulltext/quicklinks/management_guideline.pdf

CHAPTER **38**

Assessing communities

CASE STUDY

As part of a state-wide public health initiative and assessment of resources, a nurse evaluates the town of Pine Tree Valley. This small town is in a semi-rural area around 50 km from a regional centre. It was originally settled in the 1850s and over the years has strengthened its focus on farming and forestry. In recent decades, the economic basis has deteriorated, and over the last 10 years the population has decreased to fewer than 2,500 people. Median household and median personal income are below the national averages, and the unemployment rate is higher than the national average. Ethnic composition is predominantly Caucasian of European descent and the predominant religion is Lutheran. Health care resources are available in the region, but only a few are located in the community itself. Primary health care and social services are available in the community, but specialist services are accessed in the tertiary level hospital in the larger regional centre. The nurse's assessment of Pine Tree Valley will be discussed throughout the chapter. It is an abbreviated case study of an assessment of a small town. In actual practice, a thorough assessment of a community would require more in-depth data collection than is described in this vignette. Such assessments may be quite lengthy and beyond the scope of this book.

Conceptual foundations

The purpose of community assessment is to determine the health-related concerns of its members, regardless of the type of the community. The nurse learns about the community, its people, its history and its culture through the assessment process. A thorough and accurate assessment provides the foundation for diagnosis and for planning appropriate nursing interventions.

DEFINITION OF COMMUNITY

A thorough assessment of a community first requires an understanding of the concept of community. *Community* may be defined in several ways, depending on the conceptual view of the term, but two common ways of understanding it are as a community of place and as a community of interest. A combination of place and interest are reflected in the sociological perspective. Three definitions are offered from the field of sociology (Sociology Guide, 2014):

1. Collections of people with a 'particular social structure'
2. A group with a 'sense of belonging or community spirit'
3. A group for which 'all the daily activities of a community, work and non-work, take place within the geographical area, which is self contained'.

Another definition of *community* that is broad enough to encompass place and interest is an 'open social system characterised by people in a place over time who have common goals' (Maurer & Smith, 2012, p. 341). Communities are also created through collaboration, interaction with other people and the environment and through people depending on one another for various purposes (McMurray & Clendon, 2011).

From these definitions, it can be seen that people can belong to several different communities at varying and overlapping times. The context in which a community exists is also important as there are significant differences in the sociopolitical contexts of individual countries, such as Australia and New Zealand. The classification of a specific community, then, depends on the definition. For purposes of assessment, communities are classified according to either location or social relationship. The first classification is a geopolitical community in which people have a time and space relationship. Geopolitical communities may be determined by natural boundaries such as rivers, lakes or mountain ranges For example, the Murray River separates a length of the states of Victoria and New South Wales in Australia. Geopolitical boundaries also may be physical constructions: cities, towns, voting districts or councils. Another example of a geopolitical community is a census area, which is determined by the government to organise demographic data collection.

As noted previously, communities also may be classified by relationships among a group of people. These communities are usually centred on a specific goal or function. For example, Parent to Parent Inc. in New Zealand provides training, information and support to parents of children with special needs, or a group such as the Parent's Jury in Australia may collectively advocate for legislation to improve children's food and physical activity environments. Communities can also be organised to address a common interest or problem, such as a nurses' association or a consumer-led support group for family and friends of people with diabetes. Similarly, women who have experienced domestic violence may link in with a shelter or support group to gain peer support. Another example of this type of community is a group of people with similar religious or political beliefs. There are also cultural-specific communities (see Chap. 10 for cultural assessment, and Chaps 11 and 12 for detailed discussion on assessment of Aboriginal and Torres Strait Islander peoples and Māori, respectively). Any number of social communities may exist within the boundaries of a geopolitical community.

MODELS OF COMMUNITY ASSESSMENT

A number of different models or frameworks have been used to provide the structure for assessing both geopolitical and social communities. Assessment of a community is a two-way, collaborative process. Engaging community members in the assessment process and the use of a framework of assessment result in a comprehensive picture of the health of the community concerned. Community engagement in this process assists the identification of health questions or concerns that are relevant, and can also lead to improved health and health behaviours in disadvantaged groups (Cyril et al., 2015). It is also understood that the potential impact on community health should be considered in all government policy development (World Health Organization & Government of South Australia, 2010; New Zealand Ministry of Health [NZMOH], 2013) and based on evidence including research data (Makkar et al., 2016).

A concept also explored in the Australian and New Zealand setting is that of a community's *degree of resilience.* This is seen as the ability of the community to adapt to changes outside its control, for example, a natural disaster (e.g. earthquake, fire, flood), or a change in the economic context within which the community is operating. The capacity of the community to learn and adapt to a changing situation can demonstrate its ability to grow and evolve to cope successfully with the change (Maguire & Cartwright, 2008). Public health systems have a crucial part to play in community resilience, and assessment of the community's health care capacity in both conventional circumstances and crisis situations can help to strengthen disaster preparedness (Nunes-Vaz et al., 2019).

It is useful to also understand that public health care provision in community settings usually incorporates primary health care models. Primary health care is defined by the World Health Organization (WHO) as a 'whole-of-society approach to health and well-being centred on the needs and preferences of individuals, families and communities' (WHO, 2019). It includes broader and interrelated aspects of health including physical, mental and social health. Nurses working in primary health care settings contribute through support of patient engagement, decision making and health system navigation, as well as nursing care provision (McKittrick & McKenzie, 2018).

The Community as Partner model provides a comprehensive guide for data collection (Francis et al., 2013a, 2013b). Central to the model are the people, or core, of the community. This component includes demographic information as well as information about the history, culture, and values and beliefs of the people. Also identified are eight subsystems that are affected by the people of the community and that directly contribute to the health status of the community. These include housing, fire and safety, health, education, economics, politics and government, communication and recreation. The community as partner model has been adapted for use in this chapter.

Community assessment

Community assessment involves both subjective and objective data collection using a variety of methods. Subjective data collection includes perceptions of the community by the nurse as well as by members of the community. The nurse should spend time in the community to 'get to know' the people and get a sense of their values and beliefs. Through the process of participant observation, the nurse hopes to become accepted as a member of the community. This method of data collection allows the nurse to participate in the daily life of the community, make observations and obtain information about the structures and influences that affect the community. The nurse should ask key members or leaders of the community as well as 'typical' residents to provide further information and insight about the community. Assessing the needs of the marginalised members of the community and their ability to access services is also important because, although social services may be supporting the majority of community members, they may not be accessible to those with multiple or pre-existing needs. For example, a sole parent with health care needs may find it difficult to access health care during working hours if appropriate child care is not available. The cost of public transport (or the lack of public transport) may also be a barrier to accessing health care.

Objective methods of data collection include using surveys and analysing existing data such as census information, health records and other public documents. The assessment section outlines a step-by-step assessment of the community. Within each assessment topic, three aspects of community should be considered: people, environment and health. The nursing component is inherent throughout each topic considered.

CASE STUDY

You decide to assess the health of the Pine Tree Valley community to determine any actual and potential health risks to community groups.

CRITICAL THINKING

1. What types of community groups could there be in a small country town, and how may this be different from a more urban community setting?
2. Before reading the following section, consider how you might approach assessing this community; for example, could more than one method of assessment be used, and how?

COMMUNITY ASSESSMENT

ASSESSMENT PROCEDURE	NORMAL FINDINGS	ABNORMAL FINDINGS
Community history		
Study the history of the community. Look for this information at the local library or ask local residents. Use this information to gain insights into the health practices and belief systems of community members.	The community history should include initial development, any specific ethnic groups that may have settled there, past economic trends and past population trends.	The history of some communities may include episodes that have had a disruptive influence on the people of the community such as relocation because of repeated flooding, a history of racial or ethnic problems or the closing of a factory.
Demographic information		
Obtain age and gender information from census data. Age is the most important risk factor for health-related problems. Gender may be another important risk factor.	A healthy or typical community has a distribution of individuals in various age ranges: younger than 5, 5 to 19, 20 to 34, 35 to 54, 55 to 64, and 65 and older, as well as no significant difference between percentages of males and females.	Communities with a large percentage of elderly people or very young children generally have more health-related problems. Communities with a preponderance of women of childbearing age may need to improve access to or expand family planning and antenatal services as well as postnatal programs.
Study census figures and state and territory population reports. Use this information to learn about racial and ethnic groups that reside in the community.	Programs and special screenings are congruent with the needs of the racial and ethnic groups in the community.	Special programs and screenings are not available in proportion to the racial and ethnic population. For example, Aboriginal and Torres Strait Islander peoples, Māori and Pacific Islander people often have a higher incidence of diabetes or alcohol-related health problems, and thalassaemia is prevalent among people from Mediterranean countries. Therefore, special screenings and programs to meet the needs of particular racial or ethnic groups become more important to these communities.
Obtain vital statistics data. These data can be obtained from the Australian Institute of Health and Welfare (AIHW, 2019a), Statistics New Zealand (2013) and government health departments. These include birth and death records as well as crude death rates (age and cause), specific death rates and infant–maternal mortality. Morbidity (disease) data also are important indicators of the health status of the community.	Expected birth, death and morbidity data should generally reflect overall rates for Australia and New Zealand. See Displays 38-1 to 38-8 for age-related causes of mortality and life expectancy.	Higher-than-expected birth, death and morbidity rates, especially age- and cause-specific rates, may indicate a lack of services or programs in critical areas. For example, higher-than-expected teen birth rates may be related to a lack of family planning services or education; high mortality rates associated with motor vehicles, especially when alcohol is involved, indicate that alcohol awareness programs should be instituted; and greater than expected rates of tuberculosis or sexually transmitted infections indicate that primary and secondary prevention efforts should be increased.

Continued on page 833

DISPLAY 38-1 CAUSES OF PERINATAL* MORTALITY, AUSTRALIA

Congenital abnormalities
Unexplained antepartum death
Spontaneous preterm
Specific perinatal conditions

* Perinatal in this instance means a fetal or neonatal death of at least 20 weeks' gestation or at least 400 g birth weight.
Source: Australian Institute of Health and Welfare. (2018). *Australia's mothers and babies 2016–In brief* (p. 90). Perinatal Statistics series no. 34. Cat. no. PER 97. Canberra: Author. CC BY 3.0 license.

DISPLAY 38-2 CAUSES OF INFANT MORTALITY (LESS THAN 1 YEAR), AUSTRALIA

Male
Fetus and newborn affected by maternal factors and by complications of pregnancy, labour and delivery
Other disorders originating in the perinatal period
Disorders related to length of gestation and fetal growth
Ill-defined and unknown causes of mortality (includes sudden infant death syndrome)

Female
Fetus and newborn affected by maternal factors and by complications of pregnancy, labour and delivery
Ill-defined and unknown causes of mortality
Congenital malformations of the circulatory system
Other disorders originating in the perinatal period

Australian Bureau of Statistics. (2018). *Causes of death, Australia, 2017*. Cat. no. 3303.0. Viewed September 2019 at https://www.abs.gov.au/AUSSTATS/abs@.nsf/Lookup/3303.0Explanatory%20Notes12017?OpenDocument. CC BY 4.0 International License.

DISPLAY 38-3 CAUSES OF CHILD AND TEENAGE MORTALITY (1 TO 14 YEARS), AUSTRALIA

Male
Malignant neoplasms of eye, brain and other parts of the central nervous system
Pedestrian injured in transport accident
Accidental drowning and submersion
Intentional self-harm

Female
Malignant neoplasms of eye, brain and other parts of the central nervous system
Accidental drowning and submersion
Intentional self-harm
Car occupant injured in transport accident
Episodic and paroxysmal disorders

Australian Bureau of Statistics. (2018). *Causes of death, Australia, 2017*. Cat. no. 3303.0. Viewed September 2019 at https://www.abs.gov.au/AUSSTATS/abs@.nsf/Lookup/3303.0Explanatory%20Notes12017?OpenDocument. CC BY 4.0 International License.

DISPLAY 38-4 CAUSES OF TEENAGE AND ADULT MORTALITY, AUSTRALIA

Ages 15 to 24
Male
Intentional self-harm
Car occupant injured in transport accident
Motorcycle rider injured in transport accident
Accidental poisoning by and exposure to noxious substances

Female
Intentional self-harm
Car occupant injured in transport accident
Accidental poisoning by and exposure to noxious substances
Malignant neoplasms of lymphoid, haematopoietic and related tissue

Ages 25 to 44
Male
Intentional self-harm
Accidental poisoning by and exposure to noxious substances
Ischaemic heart disease
Car occupant injured in transport accident

Female
Intentional self-harm
Accidental poisoning by and exposure to noxious substances
Malignant neoplasm of breast
Malignant neoplasms of digestive organs

Ages 45 to 64
Male
Malignant neoplasms of digestive organs
Ischaemic heart disease
Malignant neoplasms of respiratory and intrathoracic organs
Intentional self-harm

Female
Malignant neoplasms of digestive organs
Malignant neoplasm of breast
Malignant neoplasms of respiratory and intrathoracic organs
Ischaemic heart disease

Ages 65 to 84
Male
Malignant neoplasms of digestive organs
Ischaemic heart disease
Malignant neoplasms of respiratory and intrathoracic organs
Chronic lower respiratory diseases

Female
Malignant neoplasms of digestive organs
Ischaemic heart disease
Chronic lower respiratory diseases
Malignant neoplasms of respiratory and intrathoracic organs

Australian Bureau of Statistics. (2018). *Causes of death, Australia, 2017*. Cat. no. 3303.0. Viewed September 2019 at https://www.abs.gov.au/AUSSTATS/abs@.nsf/Lookup/3303.0Explanatory%20Notes12017?OpenDocument. CC BY 4.0 International License.

DISPLAY 38-5 CAUSES OF INFANT MORTALITY (LESS THAN 1 YEAR), NEW ZEALAND

Certain conditions originating in the perinatal period
Congenital malformations, deformations and chromosomal abnormalities
Symptoms, signs, and abnormal clinical and laboratory findings, not elsewhere classified
External causes of morbidity and mortality

New Zealand Ministry of Health. (2019). *Mortality 2016 data tables.* Viewed September 2019 at https://www.health.govt.nz/publication/mortality-2016-data-tables.

DISPLAY 38-6 CAUSES OF CHILD AND TEENAGE MORTALITY (1 TO 14 YEARS), NEW ZEALAND

External causes of morbidity and mortality
Neoplasms
Diseases of the respiratory system
Diseases of the nervous system

New Zealand Ministry of Health. (2019). *Mortality 2016 data tables.* Viewed September 2019 at https://www.health.govt.nz/publication/mortality-2016-data-tables.

DISPLAY 38-7 CAUSES OF TEENAGE AND ADULT MORTALITY, NEW ZEALAND

Ages 15 to 24
External causes of morbidity and mortality
Neoplasms
Diseases of the nervous system
Diseases of the circulatory system

Ages 25 to 44
External causes of morbidity and mortality
Neoplasms
Diseases of the circulatory system
Diseases of the nervous system

Ages 45 to 64
Neoplasms
Diseases of the circulatory system
External causes of morbidity and mortality
Diseases of the respiratory system

Ages 65 to 84
Neoplasms
Diseases of the circulatory system
Diseases of the respiratory system
Diseases of the nervous system

New Zealand Ministry of Health. (2019). *Mortality 2016 data tables.* Viewed September 2019 at https://www.health.govt.nz/publication/mortality-2016-data-tables.

DISPLAY 38-8 LIFE EXPECTANCY AT BIRTH, AUSTRALIA AND NEW ZEALAND

In Australia, based on the latest mortality rates, a boy born between 2015 and 2017 can expect to live 80.5 years, whereas a girl can expect to live 84.6 years. In comparison, Aboriginal and Torres Strait Islander life expectancy for the same period for boys was estimated to be 71.6 years and for girls, 75.6 years (AIHW, 2019a).

In 2013, life expectancy at birth was 73.0 years for Māori males and 77.1 years for Māori females, compared with 80.3 years for non-Māori males and 83.9 years for non-Māori females (Statistics New Zealand, 2018).

Overall, Australia and New Zealand compare well internationally in terms of life expectancy, with Australia ranking ninth (82.6 years) and New Zealand eleventh (81.9 years) for both males and females (Organisation for Economic Cooperation and Development, 2019).

COMMUNITY ASSESSMENT (continued)

ASSESSMENT PROCEDURE	NORMAL FINDINGS	ABNORMAL FINDINGS
Demographic information (continued)		
Refer to the Australian Bureau of Statistics or Statistics New Zealand for the following information: Number of people per household, their marital status and the mobility of the population. 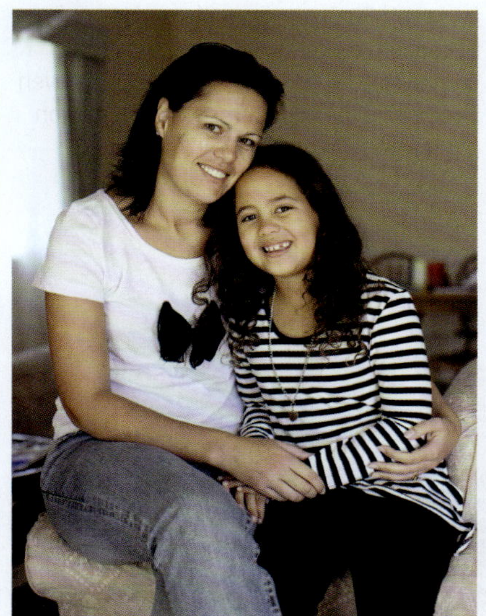 **FIGURE 38-1** In Australia and New Zealand there are various types of family households. (iStockphoto.com/pamspix.)	The Australian Bureau of Statistics identifies three types of households: family household, lone household and group household. In 2016, 71.3% of the 8.2 million households in Australia contained one or more families. A family is defined as two or more persons, one of whom is at least age 15 years, who are related by blood, marriage (registered or de facto), adoption, step- or fostering, and who are usually resident in the same dwelling (Fig. 38-1). Lone person households constituted 24% of Australian households, and group households accounted for the remaining 4%. Couple families with or without children made up 83% of all families in Australia, whereas sole parent families made up the remaining 16%. The proportion of lone person households has not changed significantly over the last 13 years; however, the number of lone women households has risen consistently overall (Australian Bureau of Statistics [ABS], 2019). For Statistics New Zealand, a family is identified as a couple with or without children or one parent and their children. A household is one person who usually lives alone or two or more people who usually live together and share facilities. New Zealand census data show that there has been a decline in the average household size from 3.7 people per household in 1951 to 2.7 people per household in 2013 (Statistics New Zealand, 2014). Australians and New Zealanders are a mobile population, moving for education, jobs or retirement. A healthy community adjusts to these changes and organises to meet the needs of the population.	Sole parents (teenage parents in particular) are at greater risk for health problems, especially those related to role overload. This occurs because sole parents often have to assume the role of the missing parent in addition to their own roles. Sole parents report a higher incidence of children's academic and behavioural problems than parents in two-parent families. Single people have a higher mortality rate than do partnered people. Elderly people living alone also are at higher risk for health problems. In addition, some immigrant groups, such as migrant farm families, are at higher risk. Communities that do not adapt to meet the needs of the mobile population compromise the continuity and quality of care for these people.

Continued on following page

COMMUNITY ASSESSMENT (continued)

ASSESSMENT PROCEDURE	NORMAL FINDINGS	ABNORMAL FINDINGS
Obtain data to determine religious beliefs of the community. These data can be obtained from the Australian Bureau of Statistics, Statistics New Zealand, and personal observation and interviews. Each community's values are unique, rooted in tradition and exist to meet the needs of the population. Religious beliefs and culture are closely related to the community's values (Fig. 38.2).	Healthy communities demonstrate an awareness and respect for different values and religions. There is a deliberate effort among various subgroups to communicate and to work together. Many communities form ministerial alliances, in which various denominations collaborate to meet the needs of the community. They may provide emergency shelters, operate soup kitchens or food banks and provide help for special populations. Certain religious beliefs directly affect health practices such as use of family planning services.	Some communities exhibit conflict among subgroups. Different values, beliefs and practices are seen as a threat to one group's own values and beliefs. An unhealthy community may fail to recognise the existence of cultural or religious differences and believe that all members of the community should conform to one set of values. In such communities, anyone who does not fit the accepted norm is 'suspect'. Such an atmosphere does not enhance the overall health status of the community, which makes it difficult or even impossible for members to collaborate on problem solving.

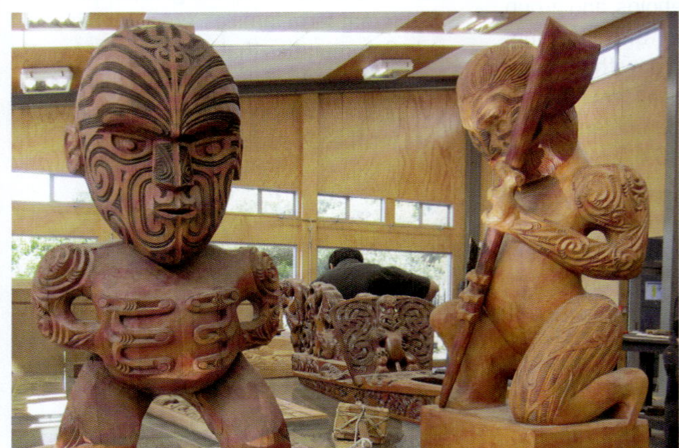

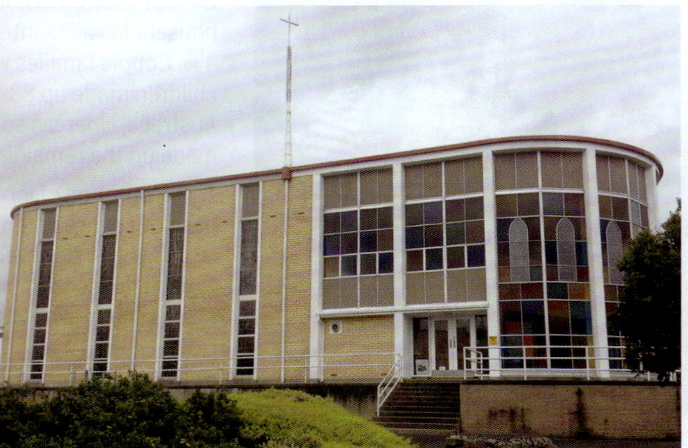

FIGURE 38-2 Information about the history, culture, and values and beliefs of the people in a community are included in a community as partner assessment model. (**Left,** iStockphoto.com; **Right,** © Kate Cameron)

Physical environment		
Identify geographic boundaries of the community. This information may be obtained from the local council or Australian Bureau of Statistics or Statistics New Zealand.	Boundaries of a community should be clear, uncontested and accepted by all members.	Boundaries may not always be clearly identified, and communities may not be able to resolve disputes without legal action. One community may seek to annex part of another because of access to certain resources, or a group or neighbourhood may attempt to separate legally from the larger community because of ideological differences, zoning regulations or other issues. Disagreement about such issues may disrupt delivery of services.
Identify the neighbourhoods that make up the area. Note characteristics. Neighbourhoods have specific populations and boundaries and may vary a great deal in culture, leadership and ties to the larger community. They may be composed of certain ethnic groups, socio-economic backgrounds or age groups.	Neighbourhoods should be cohesive with a sense of identity while having strong ties to the larger community.	Some neighbourhoods may seek to isolate themselves from the larger community or may be resistant to others who wish to move into the neighbourhood. In such situations, conflicts often arise and mistrust may be widespread.

COMMUNITY ASSESSMENT (continued)

ASSESSMENT PROCEDURE	NORMAL FINDINGS	ABNORMAL FINDINGS
Physical environment (continued)		
Obtain housing information from census reports and local council information. A community should provide a variety of housing options.	A healthy community can provide enough safe, affordable housing to meet the needs of its members. Of the almost 288,800 Australians who accessed specialist homelessness services from 2017 to 2018, more than 83,000 were under age 18 years (AIHW, 2019b). Although currently there is no precise measure of homelessness in New Zealand, there are 12,311 on the Housing New Zealand waiting list in categories A and B; that is, they are assessed as being at risk or having serious need (New Zealand Ministry of Social Development, 2019).	A lack of adequate housing may be a serious problem in some communities. A shortage of safe, low-income housing contributes directly to the growing number of homeless individuals and families. Other communities may have a serious shortage of adequate rental property or special housing for the elderly or disabled. Inadequate housing contributes to various health problems related to safety and communicable diseases.
Determine climate and geographic terrain of the area. This information may be obtained from the Bureau of Meteorology, government agencies and direct observation. Climate varies from region to region as does geographic terrain. Both have a direct effect on the health of the community.	Healthy communities have the resources to deal with whatever problems climate and terrain present. Such problems include extreme cold or heat, floods, fires, blizzards, cyclones and earthquakes. Certain health problems may be more prevalent in particular geographic areas (e.g. dengue fever in North Queensland). Government and district council safety programs and disaster plans, and health education programs should be in place.	Communities inadequately prepared to deal with disasters or health problems related to climate or terrain do not adequately meet the needs of their members. This may result in a higher incidence of the following problems: heat exhaustion, deaths due to overexposure to cold, skin cancers, infectious diseases, and deaths and injuries related to other natural disasters.
Health and social services		
Determine the number of health care facilities and providers available to the community. Information about health services can be obtained from the government health departments, local professional organisations, telephone directories, and personal interviews and observations.	A healthy community provides adequate primary health care services. These services include private and non-profit facilities staffed with doctors, nurse practitioners and nurses who provide medical, surgical, obstetric, gynaecological, paediatric, emergency (Fig. 38-3), and various diagnostic and preventive services. Specialty services, such as neonatal intensive care, should be easily accessible to the community (Fig. 38-4). In addition to doctors and nurses, the health care delivery system should include dentists, physiotherapists and dietitians, among others.	Many communities (particularly rural ones) cannot provide needed services, especially in obstetric care. It is not unusual for a person to be 100 km or more away from the nearest services. In addition, funding problems have caused many small rural hospitals to close, leaving residents a significant distance from health care services. Access to ambulance services also may be of concern for rural and remote communities. Accessibility may be limited because fewer health care providers are willing to accept some types of third-party reimbursement.

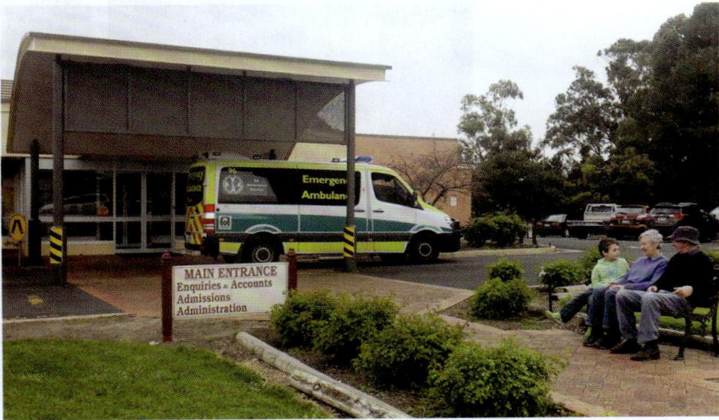

FIGURE 38-3 Access to emergency health care is important for residents in rural and remote communities. (© Kate Cameron.)

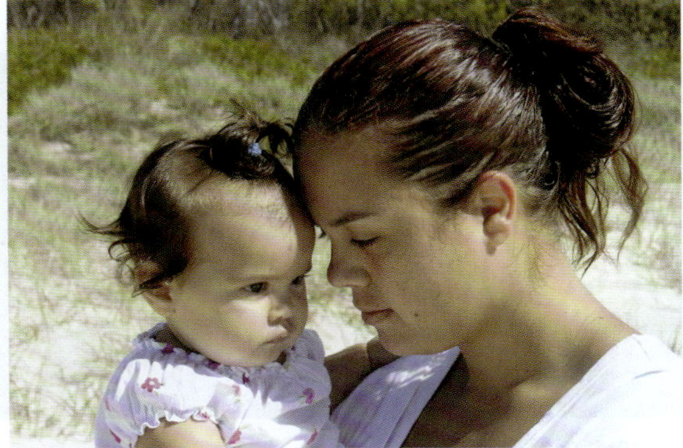

FIGURE 38-4 Healthy communities provide access to adequate primary health care services for people of all ages. (iStockphoto.com/chemc.)

Continued on following page

COMMUNITY ASSESSMENT (continued)

ASSESSMENT PROCEDURE	NORMAL FINDINGS	ABNORMAL FINDINGS
Obtain data concerning public health and home health services. This information can be obtained from local directories, the government health departments and personal interviews. Local public health agencies have the responsibility of protecting and promoting the health of the general population. Program objectives are related to primary prevention and early diagnosis, and are supported by current national policy both in Australia (Australian Government Department of Health and Ageing, 2010) and in New Zealand (NZMOH, 2011). Home health care is a fast growing component of the health care system as hospital stays become shorter, whereas the need for skilled care remains.	Local public health services are usually delivered through state or territory government health departments. Home health services may be provided through a number of different agencies such as a government-funded community or visiting nursing services and private agencies. Services provided include skilled nursing care, home health aides, medical social services, nutritional consultation and rehabilitation services (Fig. 38-5).	Areas of rapidly increasing density of population may outstrip the population's health care infrastructure and services. Changes in population groups such as the ageing population may also mean that services are inadequate for the growing community's needs.
Determine what level of social services is available in the community. Information may be obtained through local directories, the government health departments or personal interviews.	A community should provide social services—both public and through non-government organisations—for people of all ages. Official agencies include mental health facilities and government departments of children and family services. Other agencies may be drug and alcohol treatment facilities, centres for victims of domestic violence, hospices and shelters for the homeless. Charities and non-government agencies (such as OzHarvest and The Wayside Chapel, Sydney; see Fig. 38-6) also offer community services. Additional social programs may come from groups such as the YMCA and Parents Without Partners. Accredited child care facilities for children and the elderly should also be available.	Access to social service agencies may be an obstacle in urban areas. In addition, funding may limit the number of programs and people these agencies serve. Availability of programs may be limited in rural areas. For example, homeless shelters and shelters for victims of domestic violence are non-existent in many rural areas. Lack of transportation in rural areas may also make programs inaccessible. The cost of treatments not covered by government subsidies can limit accessibility for those without private health insurance.

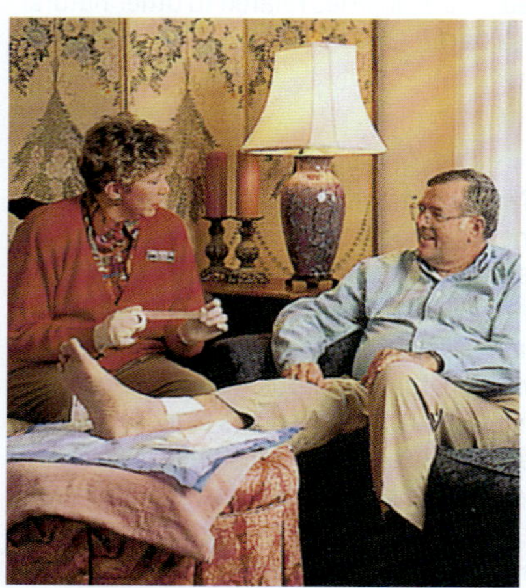

FIGURE 38-5 Healthy communities have adequate and available home health and skilled nursing care, among other services.

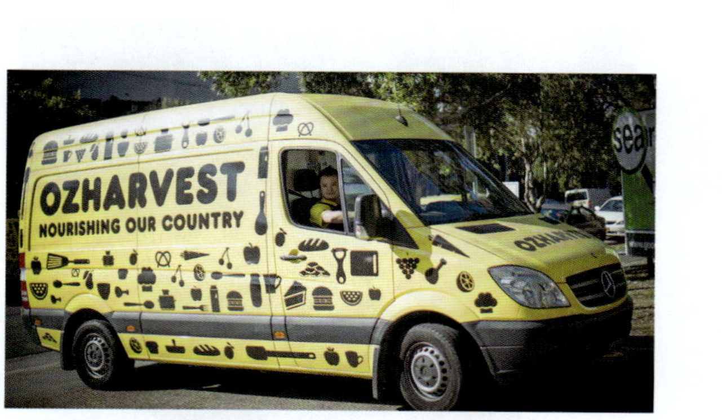

A

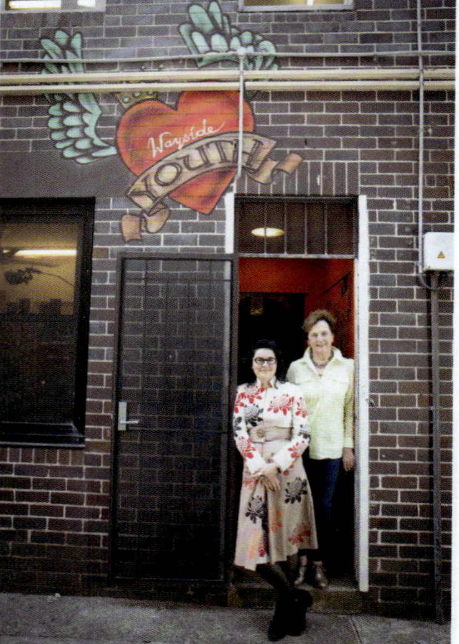

B

FIGURE 38-6 Charities and non-government agencies provide a range of community services, including health promotion. (**A,** Image supplied with kind permission of OzHarvest Sydney; **B,** Fairfax Syndication/Renee Nowytarger.)

COMMUNITY ASSESSMENT (continued)

ASSESSMENT PROCEDURE	NORMAL FINDINGS	ABNORMAL FINDINGS
Health and social services (continued)		
Determine if long-term care services are available in the community. Long-term care services are those that meet the needs of elderly members, those with a chronic disabling illness and those who have suffered disabilities due to accidents. Information can be obtained from local directories and the government health departments.	A community should provide services for long-term care assistance in the home as well as extended care for those who can no longer function in their homes. For example, personal care assistance or a visiting nurse and skilled nursing and intermediate care facilities for those needing certain levels of nursing care should be available. Rehabilitation centres, boarding homes, continuing care and retirement or assisted living centres are other types of long-term care facilities.	The capacity of available agencies may not meet the needs of a given community. Facilities that provide care for special concerns (e.g. Alzheimer disease) may not be available in all communities. Facilities in urban areas may be inaccessible because of cost. Rural areas, in general, are likely to have inadequate long-term care resources. This is especially true in areas such as respite care and personal care assistance in the home.
Gather community economic data. These data should include median household income, per capita income, percentage of households or individuals below the poverty level, percentage of people on public assistance and unemployment statistics. In addition, collect data about local business and industry, types of occupations or jobs in which people are employed and occupational health risks associated with certain occupations. Data can be collected from census records, government reports (such as Australia's Health from AIHW and QuickStats from Statistics New Zealand) and community employment agencies.	Income has a direct relationship to the health of the residents of the community. For example, the income of community members determines their ability to access appropriate housing and a nutritious diet. Businesses and other local employment opportunities are key factors in economic wellbeing. Businesses provide not only jobs but also goods and services such as groceries, pharmaceuticals and clothing.	Economic instability in a community can lead to a number of health-related concerns. Poverty is associated with higher morbidity and mortality rates. High unemployment creates a stressful environment and a threat to the psychological wellbeing of the community. Occupationally related death and injuries cost the nation millions of dollars a year, with lung diseases and musculoskeletal injuries being the most frequent causes.
Gather information regarding fire, police and environmental services in the community. This information can be obtained from local and regional police departments, fire departments, environmental agencies and government health departments. Fire, police and environmental services also are given the responsibility to protect the community from direct and indirect threats to its health and safety (Fig. 38-7). These services have both a direct and an indirect relationship to a community's wellbeing in knowing that it is safe from a variety of threats.	Police should be equipped with personnel, equipment and facilities to protect the community. Property and personal identification programs and support programs such as Neighbourhood Watch may also be run by the police department. The number of firefighters, equipment, response time and education programs contribute to adequate fire protection services. Environmental protection includes a wide range of programs such as water and air quality, solid and hazardous waste disposal, sewage treatment, food and restaurant inspection, and monitoring of public swimming pools, motels and other public facilities.	Violent crimes, such as murder, rape, robbery and assault or increases in loss of life and property due to fires, may indicate that police and fire protection services are inadequate. This also contributes to a general sense of fear or uneasiness throughout the community and can lead to increased levels of stress and a loss of a sense of wellbeing. Poor environmental protection can result in repeated cases of illnesses, injuries and even death. A number of health problems can be linked to the environment (e.g. waterborne illnesses and lead poisonings).

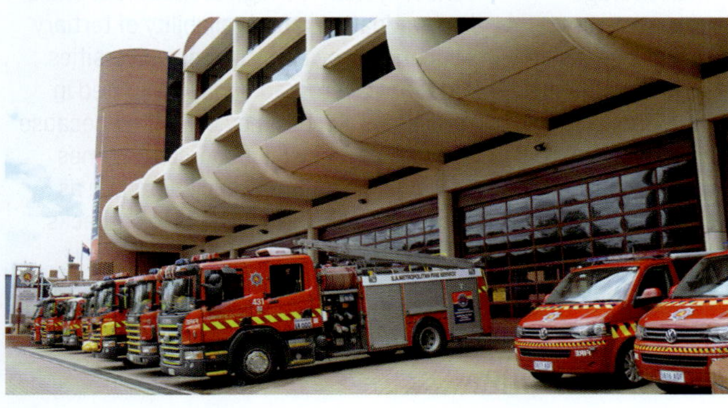

FIGURE 38-7 Adequate fire and police department protection are hallmarks of health communities. (SA Metropolitan Fire Service.)

Continued on following page

COMMUNITY ASSESSMENT (continued)

ASSESSMENT PROCEDURE	NORMAL FINDINGS	ABNORMAL FINDINGS
Determine transportation options available in the community. Obtain information from local businesses through interviews, government transport departments and direct observation.	The most common means of transportation in most communities is the private car. Other sources of transportation locally, in addition to walking, are taxis, buses, trams and trains. Long-distance transportation, in addition to the car, includes air, rail and bus service. Roads, freeways and footpaths should be kept in good repair, and communities should have adequate programs for maintenance. Special transportation needs to include school transportation and transportation for the elderly or disabled people.	Lack of a private car is a particular problem in rural areas, where public means of transportation are often non-existent. Personal safety or cost may make public transportation inaccessible for many in urban areas. Inability to access health care services because of transportation difficulties is a particular problem for the elderly and for parents with young children (Fig. 38-8).

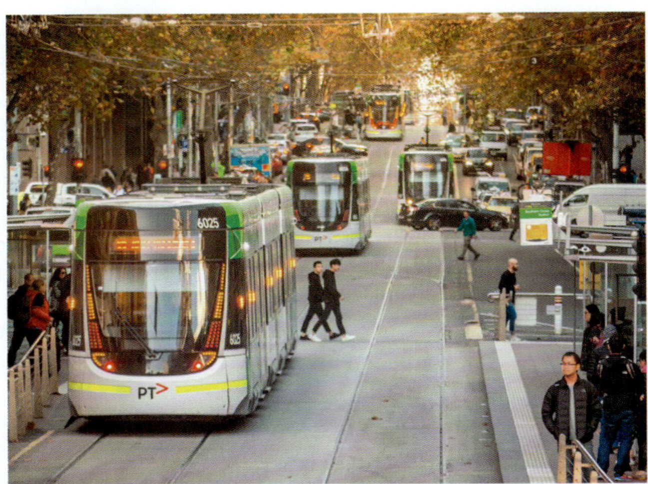

FIGURE 38-8 Access to transportation has a direct relationship to access to health care and other essential services. (Shutterstock.com/ Shuang Li.)

ASSESSMENT PROCEDURE	NORMAL FINDINGS	ABNORMAL FINDINGS
Review levels of education, current school enrolment and education resources in the community. Information may be obtained from census reports, local schools and government education departments.	In general, the higher the community's education level, the healthier the community. Resources needed to meet community educational needs include preschool and early intervention programs, public or private primary and secondary schools, and access to advanced education. Adequate supply of qualified educators, up-to-date facilities and equipment (Fig. 38-9), and programs that meet the needs of those with special needs are keys to a successful education system. Low absenteeism and higher-than-average scores on standardised achievement tests are indicators of effectiveness. Adult education should be available. Additionally, comprehensive school health programs directed by nurses, healthy school canteen food and after-school programs contribute to the health of a community. Public libraries are an important community supplement to the school system.	Adequate funding for schools in rural areas and in areas with dwindling populations of young families is a growing problem for many communities, especially where the economy is weak. Where there are low numbers of students, schools may need to cut back spending in areas such as equipment purchases, special programs and extracurricular activities such as music and athletics. School violence is a growing problem for many communities. Another indication of problems in the school system is a high dropout rate and a low graduation rate. Availability of tertiary education providers such as universities or technical programs may be limited in rural areas. Access may be limited because of a lack of financial resources. In times of economic difficulty, facilities such as community libraries often face cutbacks.

COMMUNITY ASSESSMENT (continued)

ASSESSMENT PROCEDURE	NORMAL FINDINGS	ABNORMAL FINDINGS
Health and social services (continued)		

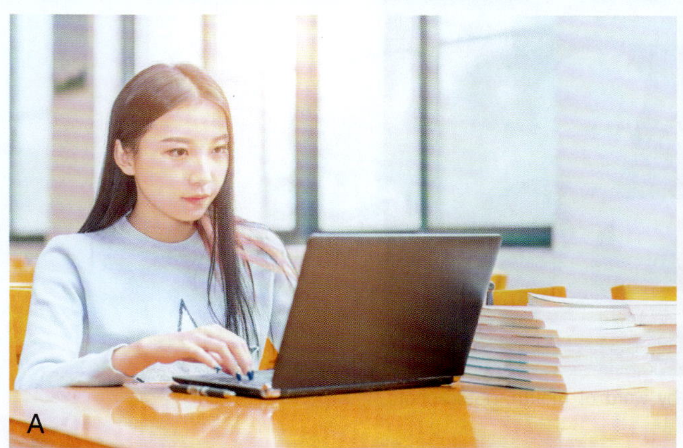

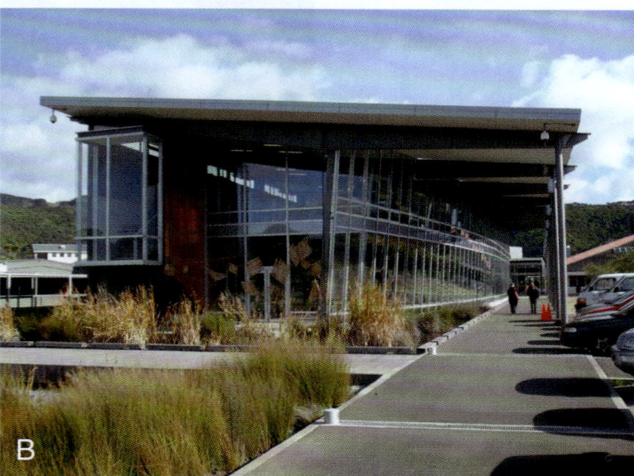

FIGURE 38-9 **(A)** Secondary school students need access to up-to-date equipment and facilities. **(B)** Whitireia New Zealand's library building. (**A,** Shutterstock.com/xiao yu; **B,** Wikimedia Commons/WCPWM. CC by-SA 3.0. https://commons.wikimedia.org/wiki/File:TeKeteWananga_WhitireiaCommunityPolytechnic.jpg.)

ASSESSMENT PROCEDURE	NORMAL FINDINGS	ABNORMAL FINDINGS
Review the government and political structures of the community. Information may be obtained from local government agencies, local political organisations and local directories. Government departments are often directly involved in planning and implementing programs that affect the health of the community. In addition, the political system is responsible for health-related legislation. It is important to assess both the formal and the informal power structures in the community.	The government of a community and its leaders should be responsible and accessible to the community. Members should participate in the governance of the community as evidenced by voter registration and percentage of registered voters who actually vote in elections. Open community meetings should be held to allow citizens a forum in which they may express their views. Political organisations should represent the differing views of the citizens; there should be an atmosphere of tolerance among the different groups.	If the government is not responsive to the views of the citizens, members of the community will become increasingly apathetic. As a result, the formal power structure becomes ineffective in meeting the needs of the community. Low voter turnout and little representation of groups with different views and interests may be indicative of an unresponsive or unrepresentative government.
Determine both the formal and the informal means of communication in the community. Sources of information include the census data, telephone book and personal interviews and observations.	Open channels of communication are an important factor in maintaining the health of a community. Larger communities usually have many types of formal communication sources including local free-to-air television and radio stations, paid satellite television channel access and one or more daily newspapers. Smaller communities usually have access to fewer television and radio stations, and newspapers are typically published weekly. Mail delivery may also be limited. However, online services are usually available in all but more remote communities. Informal communications include word of mouth (Fig. 38-10); newsletters; bulletin board notices at community centres, stores, businesses and churches; and fliers distributed by mail or door-to-door.	Traditional means of communication may not be sufficient for some people in the community. Those who do not speak or understand English may not be able to obtain necessary information through either formal or informal means. Some people may not have access to telephone or other means of communication. Elderly people and others who are isolated also may be at a disadvantage.

Continued on following page

COMMUNITY ASSESSMENT (continued)

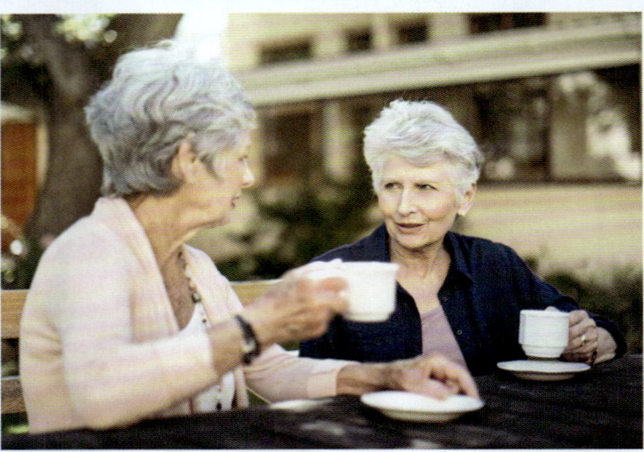

FIGURE 38-10 News may travel by word of mouth. (iStockphoto.com/shapecharge.)

ASSESSMENT PROCEDURE	NORMAL FINDINGS	ABNORMAL FINDINGS
Determine availability of community recreation and leisure programs for individuals and groups in all age ranges in the community. Information may be obtained from the census data, park and recreation departments, churches, schools, businesses and personal interviews.	Schools in the area should have a regular program of physical education in which all students participate. In addition, schools should provide equipment and programs for extracurricular activities, including both team and individual sports (e.g. tennis, football), art, music, and other types of recreational programs. Churches and non-government organisations may provide recreational programs, senior citizen dinners and outings, youth programs, church festivals, and special holiday activities. A comprehensive, community-based program is essential. Indoor or outdoor facilities (e.g. swimming pools, playing fields) should be available to all citizens, easily accessible and kept in good repair. Organised activities for individuals and groups of all ages, genders, social status and physical abilities should be available at minimal or no cost (Fig. 38-11).	Communities with a poor economic base or those with a large percentage of rural residents may not be able to provide adequate programs for recreation. Finding funds for building and maintaining recreational facilities is difficult: Lack of transportation may seriously limit access. Social isolation may become a problem for these people. In a community where there are no programs available for young people, gang activity and alcohol or drug abuse may develop. In communities where activities such as water sports or beach sports are common, lack of programs related to safety issues could result in serious injury or even death.

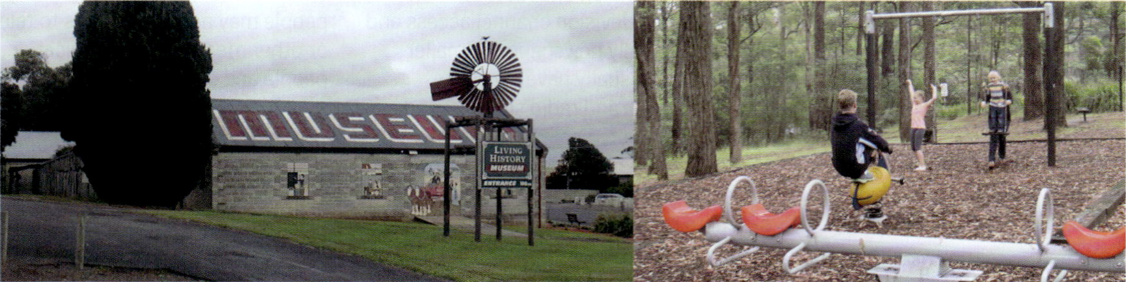

FIGURE 38-11 Recreational and leisure activities are directly related to a community's health status in that they connect people in the community and provide opportunities to socialise. (© Dr Kate Cameron.)

CASE STUDY

Your initial assessment shows there are areas of potential risk such as a lower-than-average median income and a lack of public transport; however, the overall availability and quality of health care seems adequate. Review the information presented in the previous section about community engagement and assessment and consider the following questions.

CRITICAL THINKING

3. Whom should you speak to, to find out more about these concerns and their impact; for example, would it help to talk with policy makers or health care professionals?
4. Has the community responded successfully to other challenges related to resource limitations in the past? If so, how was this outcome achieved?

CASE STUDY

Assessment of the community reveals limited health resources available to the community. Several residents have expressed their concern about this to the nurse. The nurse explores this health concern using the COLDSPA mnemonic.

The nurse further assesses the community, starting with the history. Aboriginal and Torres Strait Islander peoples first inhabited the area in and around Pine Tree Valley. Later, German immigrants settled in the region and the timber or logging industry became the economic base of the community. The town derived its name from the large numbers of pine trees that grew in the area.

The nurse then explores the demographics. The total population for the town of Pine Tree Valley as of 2016 was 2,352, a decrease of 13.6% from the 2001 census. Of the total number of residents, 56% are female and 26.3% are age 65 years or older. Racial distribution includes 94.5% Caucasian, 3% Aboriginal, 1.3% Italian and 1.2% other. Of residents age15 years and older, 65.4% are married; 10.1% are either separated or divorced; 12.3% are single; and 12.2% are widowed. The leading cause of death in Pine Tree Valley is cardiovascular disease. The German immigrants who originally settled the area brought with them their Lutheran faith; over 80% still practise that religion. There is also a small Baptist congregation as well as small Methodist and Catholic churches.

The nurse notes that Pine Tree Valley is situated in a very rural area and is bordered on the north by national park land. The Cache River runs along its western border and an interstate highway lies 4 km from the city limits on the east. The southern edge of the town is surrounded by farmland. The average temperature in January is 31.2 °C and in June, 14.3 °C.

The nurse assesses the health and social services. Pine Tree Valley has no hospital; the nearest is 50 km away and is an 85-bed, full-service facility. It is the only hospital in the district. A family practice doctor and a nurse practitioner have an office in Pine Tree Valley. The office is open 4 days a week. There is also a government-funded community health centre and services include immunisations, advice on health diet and lifestyle, sexually transmitted infection screening, family planning, and environmental services. A local district nurse office offers home health services as well as hospice care. The nearest mental health centre is approximately 50 km away, as are many other services including regional council government offices. There is a 50-bed aged care facility in Pine Tree Valley operating at full capacity. Several residents have expressed their concern about this to the nurse and commented that a committee has been formed to examine ways in which the capacity of the facility could be increased.

The median household income for Pine Tree Valley is $33,845, which is lower than the national average. Of the nearly 2,400 residents, 15.1% live below the poverty level (the national average is 13.3%). The single largest employer in the community is a minimum-security state correctional facility. Other areas of employment include forestry-related occupations, farming, and local businesses such as car sales, farm implement sales and supermarkets. The unemployment rate is 7.8%, which is higher than the state average.

Pine Tree Valley maintains a small local police force of five full-time officers, two part-time officers and one office worker. There is also a fire department with seven part-time firemen and a small group of volunteer firemen. There are no trained emergency medical personnel working with the fire department. The equipment is slightly outdated but still functional. Environmental services are provided through the shire health department. The crime rate is relatively low, with the incidence of violent crime below the state average.

There is no public transportation in Pine Tree Valley, except for a small taxi service (one taxicab) and a community minibus supported by the regional council, which provides transportation for senior citizens. There is an interstate bus service available on a limited basis. The nearest airport is 140 km away.

Pine Tree Valley supports a primary school and a high school, with a total of approximately 450 students in kindergarten through Year 12. There is no school nurse

Continued on following page

available. School administrators expressed some concern about this. Although health-related problems are referred to the local health department, schools have difficulty getting the required screenings completed and school immunisation records are not up to date. The school principals also are concerned there is no one available to care for illness or injuries when they occur. The high school provides a limited number of extracurricular activities including boys' and girls' basketball, football and athletics. The nearest university is 220 km from Pine Tree Valley. There is a small library open in the afternoons and on Saturday. The community residents are proud of their library because it is entirely funded through contributions; they often hold quiz nights, raffles and other fundraising events to support it.

Pine Tree Valley has a mayor or shire council form of government. The mayor was more than willing to meet with the nurse and invited her to attend the council meeting on the first Monday of the month. Those members of the community with whom the nurse talked indicated they felt comfortable with their elected officials and they were free to voice concerns and opinions at any time. There are two major political parties and both are active in the town. The number of registered voters who voted in the last election was higher than the state average.

A radio station is located approximately 50 km away, and the nearest television station is 100 km from Pine Tree Valley. The town has satellite television service and a post office. A small local newspaper is published weekly. Dial-up and broadband Internet access is available.

Pine Tree Valley has a small town park equipped with playground equipment, three playing fields and a picnic shelter. There are netball and football leagues for children ages 7 to 18, along with Scout and Guide troops. Other organised recreational activities, such as senior citizen programs, are offered through the churches.

Applying COLDSPA

A COLDSPA can be used to explore the community's position, as illustrated below.

Mnemonic	Question	Data provided
Character	Describe the sign or symptom (feeling, appearance, sound, smell or taste, if applicable).	'Our 50-bed skilled nursing facility is always full, and the nearest alternative is 40 km away.'
Onset	When did it begin?	'The facility was built 10 years ago and quickly filled up.'
Location	Where is it? Does it radiate? Does it occur anywhere else?	Not applicable
Duration	How long does it last? Does it recur?	'This has put a strain on so many people and families over several years now.'
Severity	How bad is it? or How much does it bother you?	'This puts many families under long-term stress if they have a family member who may need skilled care. They worry and then if the person has to go to another town, there is the worry about travel and travel expenses to see their loved one.'
Pattern	What makes it better or worse?	'There is no change in pattern of worry, except that a committee has been formed that gives some hope for the future. But a few years ago, another committee did not make a difference.'
Associated factors/How it Affects the patient	What other symptoms occur with it? How does it affect you?	'Family members often have to stay home from work or give up work to care for an ageing and sick relative. This puts an economic burden on the family and the whole community.'

CRITICAL THINKING

5. Would it be useful for community members to make contact with representatives from the health care providers in the town to discuss the lack of resources, or has this step been done already?
6. Is there other information you could seek in relation to the health care resources issue that residents have identified, and how could you obtain this?

VALIDATING AND DOCUMENTING FINDINGS

Validate the community assessment data you have collected. This step is necessary to verify that the data are reliable and accurate. Document the assessment data following the health care facility or organisation policy.

Analysis of data

DIAGNOSTIC REASONING: POSSIBLE CONCLUSIONS

After collecting subjective and objective data pertaining to a community assessment, identify abnormal findings and the community's strengths. Then cluster the data to reveal any significant patterns or abnormalities. These data may then be used to make clinical judgements about the status of the community's health. The following sections provide possible conclusions the nurse may make after assessing a community.

CRITICAL THINKING

7. How could you find out if there are communities in other areas who have dealt with this type of situation in innovative ways? Can these strategies be adopted by the community of Pine Tree Valley?
8. What is likely to be the future demand and potential issues for health care resources in this community?

Potential community problems, complications or risks

- Risk of ineffective community coping (related to low income and high unemployment)
- Risk of ineffective community protection (related to lack of a school nurse and resulting inadequate vaccination and screening programs)

Selected collaborative problems

After grouping the data, certain collaborative problems may emerge. Remember that collaborative problems differ from nursing diagnoses in that they cannot be prevented or treated by nursing interventions alone. However, these physiological complications of medical conditions can be detected and monitored by the nurse. In addition, the nurse can use doctor- and nurse-prescribed interventions to minimise the complications of these problems. The nurse may also have to refer the patient in such situations for further treatment of the problem. The following is a list of collaborative problems that may be identified when assessing a community:

- Post-traumatic stress disorder, community
- Lack of access to routine screening programs (e.g. mammography, Pap tests, bowel screening) and vaccinations for infectious diseases.

ONLINE RESOURCES

An extensive range of additional resources to enhance teaching and learning and to facilitate understanding may be found online at the text's accompanying website, located on thePoint at http://thepoint.lww.com. These include Watch and Learn videos, Concepts in Action animations, journal articles, case studies, discussion topics and quizzes.

Subscribers may also access Lippincott Procedures, an extensive online point-of-care procedure guide that provides reliable step-by-step instructions for more than 1700 procedures, including 450 evidence-based Australian procedures, and skills in a variety of speciality settings, together with a wealth of supporting information.

CASE STUDY

The case study demonstrates how to analyse community assessment data. The exercises included in the ancillary product on thePoint that complements this text offer further opportunities to enhance your skills.

The following is an abbreviated case study of an assessment of a small town. In actual practice, a thorough assessment of a community would require more in-depth data collection than is described in this vignette. Such assessments may be quite lengthy and beyond the scope of this book.

The following concept map illustrates the diagnostic reasoning process.

History

Pine Tree Valley (PTV) was first inhabited by Aboriginal and Torres Strait Islander peoples. Then German immigrants settled in the region and the timber or logging industry became the economic base.

Demographics

Total population as of 2016 was 2,352, a decrease of 13.6% from the 2001 census. Residents: 56% are female and 26.3% are age 65 years or older. Racial distribution: 94.5% Caucasian, 3% Aboriginal, 1.3% Italian and 1.2% other. Of the population, 65.4% of those over 15 are married; 10.1% are either separated or divorced; 12.3% are single; and 12.2% are widowed. The leading cause of death is cardiovascular disease. Over 80% of residents practise Lutheran faith. PTV also has small Baptist, Methodist and Catholic churches.

Physical environment

Pine Tree Valley is in a very rural area, bordered on the north by national park land. The Cache River is on the western border; an interstate highway lies 4 km from the city limits on the east. The south is surrounded by farmland. The average temperature in January is 31.2°C and in June, 14.3°C.

Health and social services

Pine Tree Valley has no hospital; the nearest is 50 km away and is an 85-bed, full-service facility. It is the only hospital in the district. A family practice doctor and nurse practitioner have an office in PTV that is open 4 days a week. A government-funded community health centre offers immunisations, advice on healthy diet and lifestyle, sexually transmitted infection screening, family planning, and environmental services. Local district nurse office offers home health and hospice care. Mental health centre is 50 km away. PTV has a 50-bed aged care facility that operates at full capacity. A committee has been formed to examine ways in which the capacity of the facility can be increased.

Economics

Median household income is $33,845 (below national average). Of the PTV population, 15.1% live below the poverty level. The largest employer in the community is a minimum-security state correctional facility. Other jobs include forestry-related occupations, farming and local businesses such as car sales, farm implement sales and supermarkets. The unemployment rate is 7.8% (higher than the state average).

Safety

Pine Tree Valley has a small local police force of five full-time officers, two part-time officers and one dispatcher or office worker. There is a fire department with seven part-time firefighters and a small group of volunteer firefighters. There are no trained emergency medical personnel working. The equipment is outdated but functional. Environmental services are provided through the shire health department. The crime rate is low, with the incidence of violent crime below the state average.

Transportation

There is no public transportation, except for one taxicab and a community minibus, which provides transportation for senior citizens. Interstate bus service is available on a limited basis. The nearest airport is 140 km away.

Education

Pine Tree Valley has a primary school and a high school, with a total of approximately 450 students. There is no school nurse available (school administrators expressed concern). Schools have difficulty getting the required screenings completed and school immunisation records are not up to date. High school provides a limited number of extracurricular activities. University is 220 km away. A small library funded by contributions is open part time.

Government

Pine Tree Valley has a mayor or shire council form of government. The mayor is cooperative. Community members indicate they are comfortable with their elected officials and free to voice concerns. There are two major parties and both are active in the town. The number of registered voters who voted in the last election was higher than the state average.

Communication

A radio station is 50 km away, and a television station is 100 km away. Satellite television service and a post office are available. A small local newspaper is published weekly. Dial-up and broadband Internet access are available.

Recreation

Pine Tree Valley has a small town park with playground equipment, playing fields and a picnic shelter. There are netball and football leagues for children ages 7 to 18 along with Scout and Guide troops. Other organised recreational activities, such as senior citizen programs, are offered through the churches.

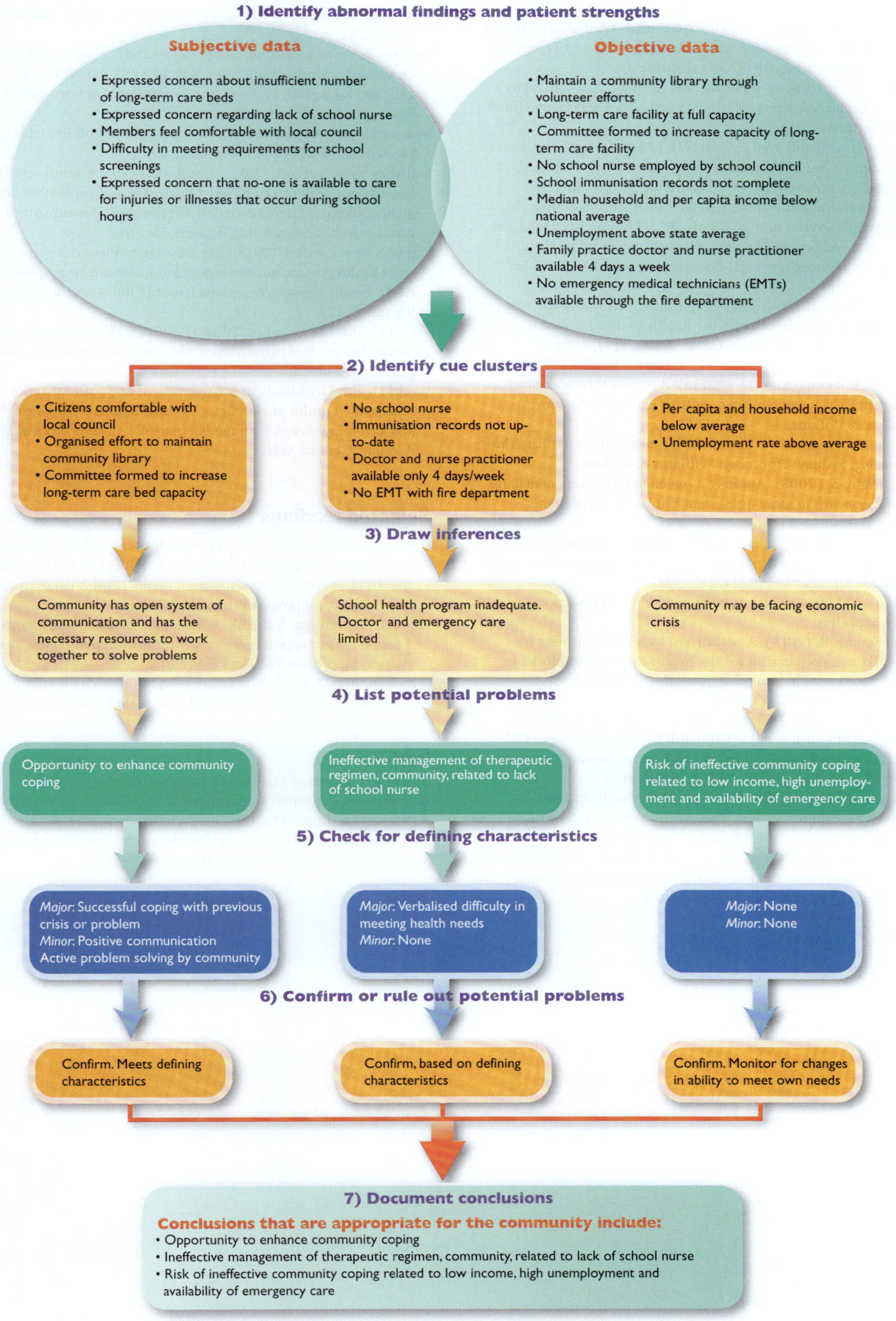

1) Identify abnormal findings and patient strengths

Subjective data

- Expressed concern about insufficient number of long-term care beds
- Expressed concern regarding lack of school nurse
- Members feel comfortable with local council
- Difficulty in meeting requirements for school screenings
- Expressed concern that no-one is available to care for injuries or illnesses that occur during school hours

Objective data

- Maintain a community library through volunteer efforts
- Long-term care facility at full capacity
- Committee formed to increase capacity of long-term care facility
- No school nurse employed by school council
- School immunisation records not complete
- Median household and per capita income below national average
- Unemployment above state average
- Family practice doctor and nurse practitioner available 4 days a week
- No emergency medical technicians (EMTs) available through the fire department

2) Identify cue clusters

- Citizens comfortable with local council
- Organised effort to maintain community library
- Committee formed to increase long-term care bed capacity

- No school nurse
- Immunisation records not up-to-date
- Doctor and nurse practitioner available only 4 days/week
- No EMT with fire department

- Per capita and household income below average
- Unemployment rate above average

3) Draw inferences

Community has open system of communication and has the necessary resources to work together to solve problems

School health program inadequate. Doctor and emergency care limited

Community may be facing economic crisis

4) List potential problems

Opportunity to enhance community coping

Ineffective management of therapeutic regimen, community, related to lack of school nurse

Risk of ineffective community coping related to low income, high unemployment and availability of emergency care

5) Check for defining characteristics

Major: Successful coping with previous crisis or problem
Minor: Positive communication
Active problem solving by community

Major: Verbalised difficulty in meeting health needs
Minor: None

Major: None
Minor: None

6) Confirm or rule out potential problems

Confirm. Meets defining characteristics

Confirm, based on defining characteristics

Confirm. Monitor for changes in ability to meet own needs

7) Document conclusions

Conclusions that are appropriate for the community include:

- Opportunity to enhance community coping
- Ineffective management of therapeutic regimen, community, related to lack of school nurse
- Risk of ineffective community coping related to low income, high unemployment and availability of emergency care

References

Australian Bureau of Statistics (ABS). (2019). 2016 Census QuickStats. Viewed September 2019 at https://quickstats.censusdata.abs.gov.au/census_services/getproduct/census/2016/quickstat/036?opendocument.

Australian Government Department of Health and Ageing. (2010). *Building a 21st century primary health care system: Australia's first National Primary Health Care Strategy*. Canberra: Author.

Australian Institute of Health and Welfare (AIHW). (2019a). Deaths in Australia. Viewed September 2019 at https://www.aihw.gov.au/reports/life-expectancy-death/deaths-in-australia/contents/life-expectancy.

Australian Institute of Health and Welfare (AIHW). (2019b). Australia's specialist homelessness services annual report 2017–18. Cat. no. HOU 299. Canberra: Author. Viewed September 2019 at https://www.aihw.gov.au/reports/homelessness-services/specialist-homelessness-services-2017-18/contents/contents.

Cyril, S., Smith, B. J., Possamai-Inesedy, A., et al. (2015). Exploring the role of community engagement in improving the health of disadvantaged populations: A systematic review. *Global Health Action, 8*(1), 29842. doi:10.3402/gha.v8.29842.

Francis, K., Chapman, Y., Hoare, K., et al. (2013a). *Australia & New Zealand community as partner: Theory and practice in nursing* (2nd ed.). Sydney: Lippincott Williams & Wilkins.

Francis, K., Chapman, Y., Hoare, K., et al. (2013b). *Community as partner: Theory and practice in nursing*. Sydney: Lippincott Williams & Wilkins.

Maguire, B. & Cartwright, S. (2008). *Assessing a community's capacity to manage change: A resilience approach to social assessment*. Canberra: Australian Government Bureau of Rural Sciences.

Makkar, S. R., Brennan, S., Turner, T., et al. (2016). The development of SAGE: A tool to evaluate how policymakers' engage with and use research in health policymaking. *Research Evaluation, 25*(3), 315–328.

Maurer, F. & Smith, C. (2012). *Community/public health nursing practice* (5th ed.). St Louis: Elsevier/Saunders.

McKittrick, R. & McKenzie, R. (2018). A narrative review and synthesis to inform health workforce preparation for the health care homes model in primary healthcare in Australia. *Australian Journal of Primary Health, 24*, 317–329. https://doi.org/10.1071/PY18045.

McMurray, A. & Clendon, J. (2011). *Community health and wellness: Primary health care in practice* (4th ed.). Sydney: Churchill Livingstone/Elsevier.

New Zealand Ministry of Health (NZMOH). (2011). *Better, sooner, more convenient health care in the community*. Wellington: Author.

New Zealand Ministry of Health (NZMOH). (2013). About health impact assessment. Viewed September 2013 at www.health.govt.nz/our-work/health-impact-assessment/about-health-impact-assessment.

New Zealand Ministry of Social Development. (2019). Housing register. Viewed September 2019 at https://www.msd.govt.nz/about-msd-and-our-work/publications-resources/statistics/housing/index.html.

Nunes-Vaz, R., Arbon, P. & Steenkamp, M. (2019). Imperatives for health sector decision-support modelling. *International Journal of Disaster Risk Reduction, 38*, 101234.

Organisation for Economic Cooperation and Development. (2019). Life expectancy at birth (indicator). doi: 10.1787/27e0fc9d-en.

Sociology Guide. (2014). Community. Available at www.sociologyguide.com/basic-concepts/Community.php.

Statistics New Zealand. (2013). New Zealand period life tables, 2010–2012. Viewed January 2014 at www.stats.govt.nz.

Statistics New Zealand. (2014). Census QuickStats about families and households: 2006 (base)-2031 update. Viewed September 2019 at http://archive.stats.govt.nz/Census/2013-census/profile-and-summary-reports/qstats-families-households/households.aspx.

Statistics New Zealand. (2018). Life expectancy. Viewed September 2019 at https://www.health.govt.nz/our-work/populations/maori-health/tatau-kahukura-maori-health-statistics/nga-mana-hauora-tutohu-health-status-indicators/life-expectancy.

World Health Organization (WHO). (2019). Primary health care. Viewed November 2019 at https://www.who.int/news-room/fact-sheets/detail/primary-health-care.

World Health Organization & Government of South Australia. (2010). *Adelaide statement on health in all policies: Moving towards a shared governance for health and well-being. Report from the International Meeting on Health in All Policies, Adelaide*. Geneva: WHO.

Selected readings

Conway, J. & Dempsey, J. (2014). Health of the individual, family and community. Chap. 3. In J. Dempsey, S. Hillege, & R. Hill (Eds). *Fundamentals of nursing: A person-centred approach to care* (2nd Australian and New Zealand ed.). Sydney: Lippincott Williams & Wilkins.

Dempsey, J., Hillege, S. & Hill, R. (2014). *Fundamentals of nursing and midwifery: A person-centred approach to care* (2nd Australian and New Zealand ed.). Sydney: Lippincott Williams & Wilkins.

Johnston, K. A. & Lane, A. B. (2019). An authenticity matrix for community engagement. Public Relations Review. Available at https://doi.org/10.1016/j.pubrev.2019.101811.

Online resources

Australian Bureau of Statistics: www.abs.gov.au
Australian Government Department of Social Services: www.dss.gov.au
Australian Institute of Health and Welfare: www.aihw.gov.au
New Zealand Ministry of Social Development: www.msd.govt.nz
Statistics New Zealand: www.stats.govt.nz

UNIT 5 HEALTH ASSESSMENT AND SIMULATION-BASED LEARNING

CHAPTER 39

The value of simulation-based learning

INTRODUCTION

Health care simulation is a technique used to engage students in an environment that resembles authentic clinical practice. *Fidelity* describes the extent to which students perceive the simulation to mimic reality, whereas *immersion* is the ability to have students so entranced in the simulation environment that disbelief is suspended, enabling students to exhibit natural behaviours and responses during the simulation activity.

A simulated learning environment reflects the clinical setting. It offers the ability to facilitate a wide range of clinical experiences or events that nurses may encounter in practice. Simulation scenarios are developed to represent patients with ill health or deteriorating health so that students may apply clinical reasoning and nursing care processes. These scenarios are usually standardised and repeatable and have predetermined learning outcomes that students explore in self-reflection, feedback or debriefing.

Simulation in nursing is a methodology that promotes a safe, non-judgemental environment where students learn from their errors and identify knowledge and performance gaps with no risk of harm to patients. It encourages critical thinking, problem-based learning, skill development, clinical decision making, interdisciplinary teamwork, communication skills and behaviour modification. This consolidates nursing competency and confidence for clinical practice, contributing to the quality of health care delivery, improved patient safety and the professional expertise of the nurse.

LEARNING IN A SIMULATED ENVIRONMENT

Learner benefits

Learning in a simulated learning environment offers several benefits for the student, particularly when compared with learning that occurs in a passive way through lectures or other didactic techniques. This is because the simulated learning environment offers students the opportunity to actively participate and practise their skills in a way that is relevant (Murray & Boulet, 2012). When combined with effective debriefing using evidence-based tools by expert facilitators, simulated learning improves students' critical thinking (Goodstone et al., 2013).

A measurable outcome of using realistic simulation learning activities that enhance critical thinking is that deteriorating patients are recognised more promptly (Theilen et al., 2013). This form of learning is not just appropriate for the management of acutely unwell patients; it is also effective for health assessment, as the process enables students to improve their physical assessment skills (Pacsi, 2008). Health assessments are a vital part of nursing practice, and simulation facilitates the opportunity to experience and explore numerous assessment techniques. The scope of potential simulation scenarios is unlimited, and so simulation may offer opportunities for clinical encounters and responsibilities that may not be available to students on clinical placements.

Apart from offering a safe environment to put theory into practice, the benefits of learning through simulation include:

- Newly graduated nurses are better prepared for clinical practice.
- Students can improve their competence in targeted areas.
- Students can practise team-based activities such as detecting and managing deteriorating patients.
- Using scenarios involving team communication, students can improve their collaboration skills and the resultant patient care.
- It is an effective method to prepare nurses for new procedures, communication processes and skills-based techniques.
- It is an effective method to evaluate a student's performance and competence.
- It is a suitable activity for purposefully performing skills required to be a competent clinically based nurse (Aebersold & Tschannen, 2013).

Regardless of the simulation approach and level of education, students report increased self-confidence as a result of participating in simulation scenarios. Simulation should therefore be used throughout all phases of nurse education (Tosterud et al., 2013).

A safe learning environment

The measurable outcomes and practical benefits of learning in a simulated environment are not just a function of the scenarios used; they are also dependent on the participants' feelings of safety. Exposure to a broad array of experiences in a safe environment helps enhance student confidence while also improving their clinical competence (Fisher & King, 2013). It is therefore important that throughout the simulated learning experience students feel safe and able to explore their practice. This does not mean that challenging scenarios should be avoided; however, if students feel threatened or if facilitators are too critical, students may withdraw and subsequently gain less from the experience.

Simulation is also safe for patients because students practise on mannequins or use actors. However, simulation also improves patient safety by giving students the opportunity to practise and develop their skills and communication techniques before they use them on actual patients. Additionally, student procedural competence can be assessed before students move into clinical practice. For example, use of an otoscope on a squirming child can be simulated and potential for damage to the auditory canal demonstrated, so that the student understands the risks and acquires safe practice habits.

Simulated learning is consequently able to connect safe knowledge with safe action. Without a simulated experience there is a risk that students will learn techniques in the clinical setting with no supporting explanation—or, if they learn the theory of a technique, they may not learn the corresponding psychomotor skills. An endorsed simulated learning experience connects theory to practice and helps prevent dangerous practice (McAllister et al., 2013).

In addition, simulation activities can be used to apply legal and ethical principles (Smith et al., 2013). For example, using a scenario with an actor about to have an invasive procedure can reinforce for students the legal practice of gaining consent, and a simulated patient refusing to eat can illustrate the ethics of freedom versus control.

Authenticity and immersion

For students to fully participate in a simulation environment they need to suspend their expectations that the situation is not real and become immersed in the activity. To assist this process, the simulated activity is set as close to reality as possible and students receive a briefing beforehand from a simulation facilitator. With increasing exposure and simulation fidelity students can learn to enter a simulation and treat it as real. Being authentic in the simulation scenario helps students to realise the activity's relevance to practice and subsequently assists the transfer of learning and application skills to the clinical area (Handley & Dodge, 2013).

SIMULATION TECHNOLOGIES AND TECHNIQUES

There are different types of simulation technologies and techniques.

- **Human patient simulators.** Simulators resembling adults, children and babies can be highly complex or simple in design (Fig. 39-1).

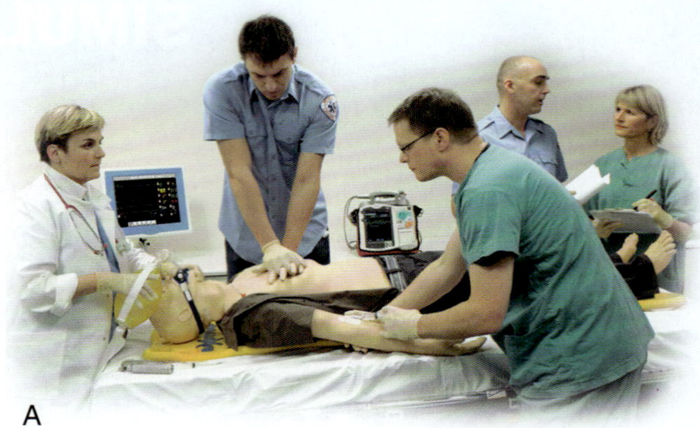
A

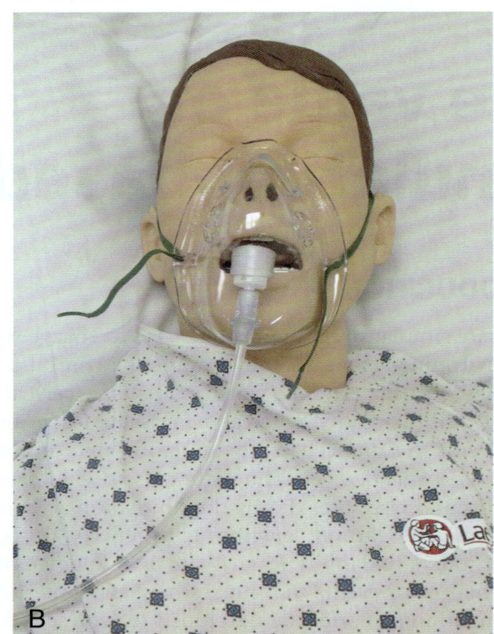
B

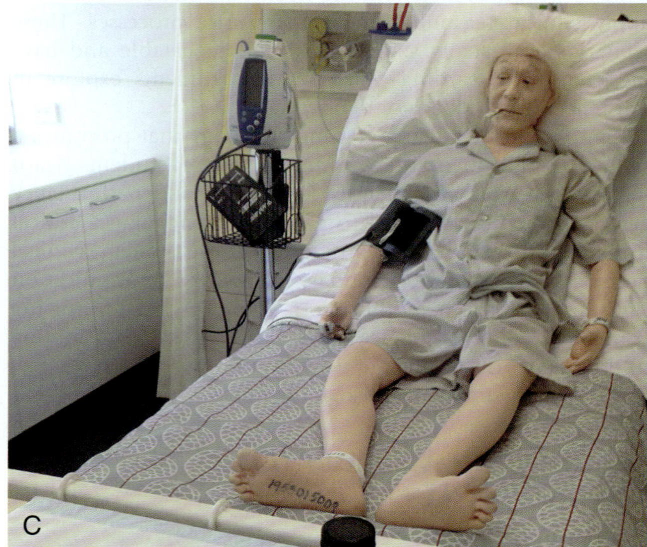
C

FIGURE 39-1 Human patient simulators: **(A)** Laerdal's SimMan 3G; **(B)** and **(C)** patient simulators in QUT's Clinical Simulation Centre. (Image (A) courtesy of Laerdal; images (B) and (C) courtesy of QUT Clinical Simulation Centre.)

- High-technology human patient simulators have sophisticated computer software and hardware to mimic many human physiological and pathological conditions. They respond to clinical interventions, procedures and virtual pharmacology.
- Advanced-technology human patient simulators are operated by a person who controls the physiological and pathological responses to clinical interventions. They are used for basic clinical conditions, vital signs and auscultation interpretation.
- Low-technology human patient simulators are usually simple mannequins with no electronics. They are used for manual handling, hygiene and bathing skills.

- **Part task trainers.** Generally considered to be low technology, these static models or parts of anatomy are used for developing and assessing skills related to techniques or procedures (Fig. 39-2). They range from arms for venipuncture, to pelvic torsos for urinary catheterisation, torsos with heads for nasogastric care or tracheostomy care and body part models for wound management.
- **Hybrid virtual reality (VR) simulators.** High-technology, computer-generated 2D or 3D images associated with a model, a body part or a simulated patient are used to develop competency in procedures that need highly skilled nurses (Fig. 39-3). An example is an ultrasound simulator that has a male or female torso for scanning cardiac, abdominal or fetal images in real time. As these systems are software-driven, a variety of pathologies mimicking real ultrasound scanning can be created.
- **VR simulators with haptic feedback.** This high-technology simulation equipment usually replicates a medical or surgical procedure and is responsive to the user's actions (Fig. 39-4). This type of simulator provides tactile feedback for skills training. It is usually linked to a computer for 2D or 3D virtual anatomy and pathologies to enhance the fidelity of the experience. These systems use imitations of real instruments and associated tools for biopsies and excisions. Examples of skills that can be practised include bronchoscopy, colonoscopy, endoscopy, laparoscopy and vascular catheterisation.
- **VR simulation or worlds.** Avatars or character roles in a 2D or 3D environment can be created to simulate reality through computer software programs (Fig 39-5). The usual clinical scenario is a branching pathway that unfolds as decision making and actions are undertaken.
- **Simulated patients.** Actors or staff may play the role of a patient in a simulation scenario (Fig. 39-6). They

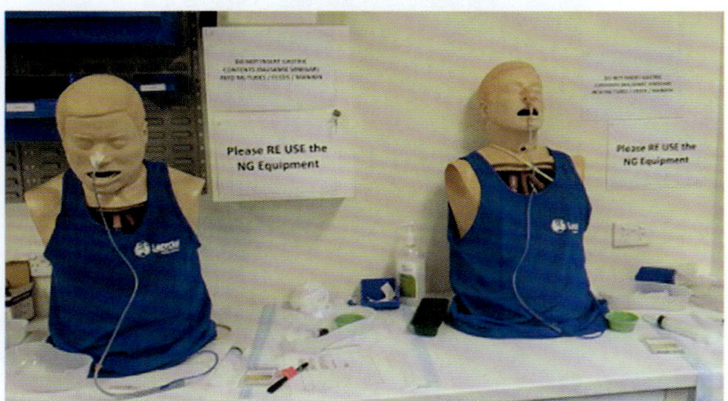

FIGURE 39-2 Part task trainers. (Image courtesy of QUT Clinical Simulation Centre.)

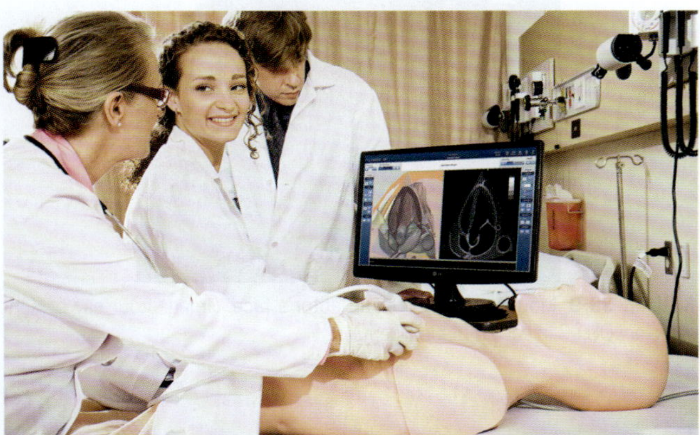

FIGURE 39-3 VIMEDIX ultrasound simulator. (Image courtesy of CAE Healthcare. © CAE healthcare.)

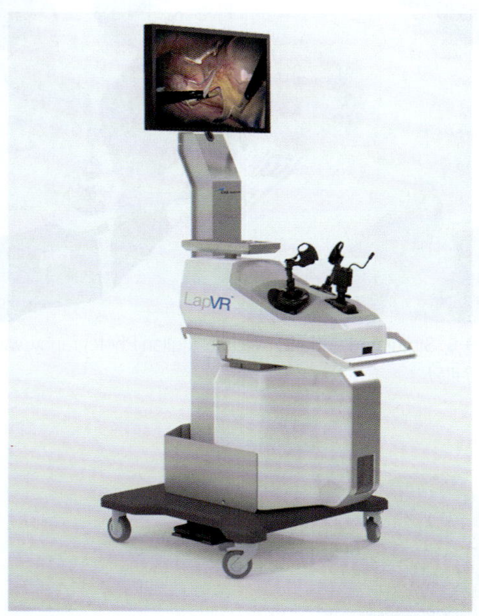

FIGURE 39-4 LapVR surgical simulator. (Image courtesy of CAE Healthcare. © CAE Healthcare.)

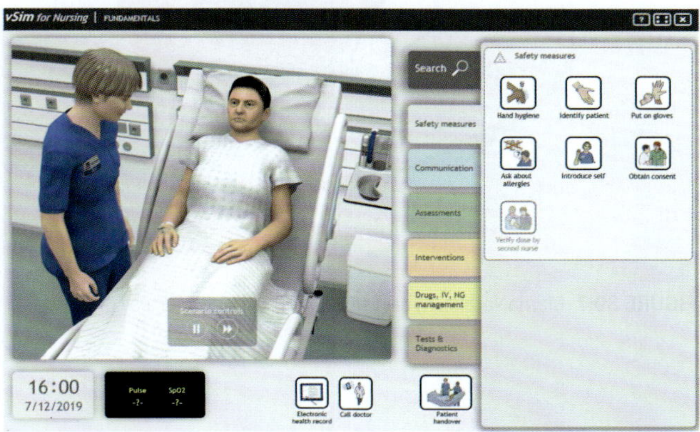

FIGURE 39-5 Virtual reality simulation. (© Laerdal.)

will be trained in the role they are portraying, including signs, symptoms, emotions and behaviours. Simulated patients can be trained to give feedback to participants to add to the quality of the debriefing process. In some situations individuals with illnesses or conditions may act as simulated patients, providing even greater realism to the scenario.

- **Hybrid simulation.** A hybrid simulation is a combination of a simulated patient or an actor with a part task trainer. Examples include a scenario where an injection pad is placed onto the arm of a simulated patient, and a birthing simulator used for procedural, technique and communication skills training (Fig. 39-7).
- **Video case studies and role playing.** These techniques involve exploration of clinical situations through video or in class acting with analysis including self-reflection, peer group or facilitated learning activities, debriefing or feedback (Fig. 39-8).
- **Moulage.** Moulage is the art of enhancing simulation through makeup, artificial secretions, smells or sounds that increase the fidelity of the simulation scenario and evoke the senses of the participants. Examples of moulage include trauma wounds, injuries, scars, ulcers, blood, pus, vomit and faeces (Fig. 39-9). It can be applied to simulators or actors.

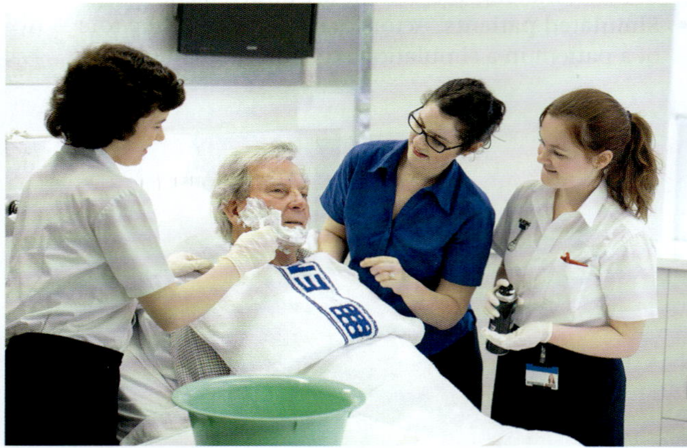

FIGURE 39-6 Simulated patient. (Michael Mullan Photography, www.michaelmullan.com.au.)

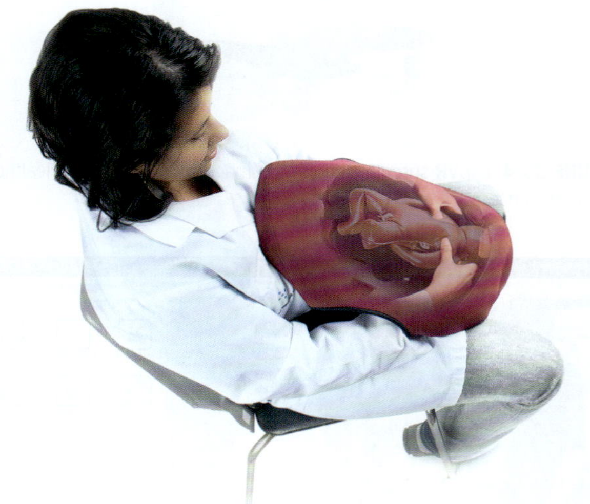

FIGURE 39-7 MamaNatalie, hybrid simulation. (Image courtesy of Laerdal.)

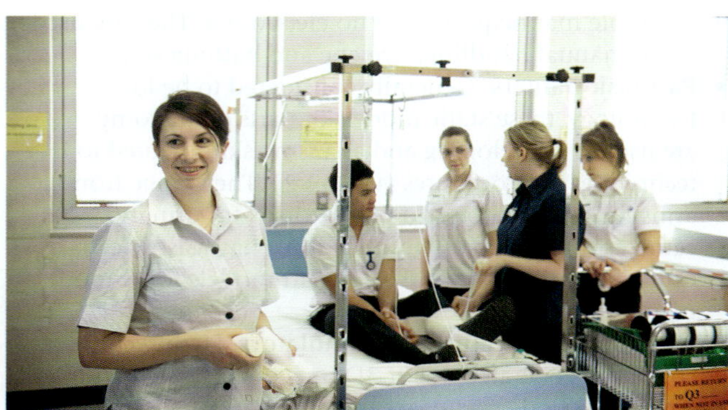

FIGURE 39-8 Role playing. (Michael Mullan Photography, www.michaelmullan.com.au.)

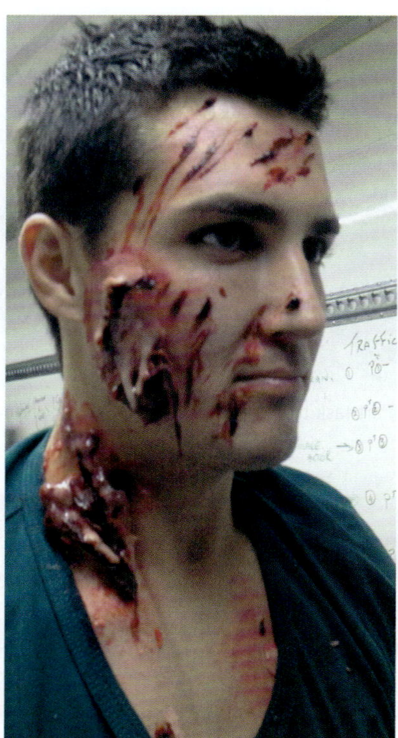

FIGURE 39-9 Moulage applied to an actor's face. (Image courtesy of Kent Jackson, QUT Clinical Simulation Centre.)

EMERGING TECHNOLOGIES: VIRTUAL REALITY SOFTWARE FOR NURSING ASSESSMENTS

The novice nurse requires assistance to develop clinical competencies associated with judgement, prioritisation and safe patient care (Borg Sapiano et al., 2018; Meakim et al., 2013). To develop these competencies teachers can use interactive virtual reality (VR) with virtual patients portrayed in virtual environments. This virtual nursing can integrate theory and evidence-based practice to develop clinical reasoning and instil confidence in learners in a low stakes environment (Cant & Copper, 2017; Foronda & Bauman, 2014; Jenson & Forsyth, 2012). The learning is immersed into the virtual clinical environment to manage unlimited clinical scenarios, matched to individual student learning by incorporating guidance and assessment in the software (Smith & Hamilton, 2015). Assessment in the software can be tailored to the competency level of the learners. When the students first enter the virtual clinical environment they are prompted and assisted, but as they progress, prompting is reduced and eventually removed so that the learners act independently. This reinforces learning, leading to assessment demonstrating the learners' newly developed knowledge, skills and behaviours (Georg & Zary, 2014).

Nursing assessment can be conducted on virtual patients from fundamental nursing and then advanced to complex scenarios of patient care. Practising fundamental activities such as handwashing techniques, medication administration and basic dressings can be undertaken in an augmented, clinical VR. In augmented VR, digital elements are overlaid on to existing physical reality. This could mean visible virtual microbes appear on the students' hands, which can then be 'washed' away with real water. By using augmented VR, more detailed immersive scenarios can be created with patients with deteriorating conditions, patients with complex conditions and patients with mental health issues.

The reproducibility of VR reinforces learning, which is then developed in skills classes, simulation scenarios and ultimately the clinical environment (Zhu et al., 2014). The adoption of this pedagogy by nursing appears to be gradual with new software technologies evolving to enhance learner's experiences (Foronda & Bauman, 2014; Padilha et al., 2018). Nursing VR software offers a safe and readily available environment for learning that students can repeat, access at any time and is free from peer or facilitator pressure (Butt et al., 2016; Verkuyl et al., 2017).

REVIEWING NURSING ASSESSMENTS WITH AUDIO-VISUAL MANAGEMENT SYSTEMS

If you participate in a simulation scenario you may have an audio-visual (AV) recording made of your performance along with incorporated assessments for enhancing the review of your developing nursing competencies (Fig. 39-10) (Bensfield et al., 2012). Utilisation of AV systems in the nursing curriculum creates an assessment record of the acquired learning outcomes throughout a nurse's training (Kothari et al., 2017). Assessment using nursing simulations can be formative or summative and aims to evaluate knowledge, skills and behaviours of learners with an AV system, enhancing the learning and assessment process (Oermann, 2016; Tavares et al., 2014; Wright et al., 2018).

Audio visual recording systems with integrated assessment have the facility to store recordings of participants for faculty to observe and critique student performance that is assessed against predetermined learning outcomes (Ali & Miller, 2018; Noureldin et al., 2018; So et al., 2019) (Fig. 39-11). Institutions may also make the recording available for students and their peers to reflect on their actions, decisions and behaviours when performing patient assessments. The recordings with incorporated assessments also enable self- or peer evaluation, enhancing the development of nursing competence.

Simulation scenario video recordings can be annotated for debriefing and feedback. This can be enhanced with assessment checklists designed for each scenario and linked to each recording in the system (Fig. 39-12). Teachers use the assessment templates to feedback and critique the learner's performance, then learners use this with the video recording as evidence of their learning (Noveanu et al., 2017). Consequently, learners can be critiqued through feedback or debriefing that can be in real time or later through the recording. Narrative observations can also be included and associated with the video recordings to enhance patient assessment skills (Lockeman et al., 2017; Paige et al., 2018). Audio-visual recording of student performance is a powerful tool for developing nursing competence; however, students find it threatening, and the technique should be used with sensitivity.

MAXIMISING THE SIMULATION EXPERIENCE

In order to maximise the simulation experience, simulation activities should follow a standardised format that includes:

- Objectives
- A plan of the activity with resources described
- A period of debriefing
- Formative or summative assessment.

Objectives

Clear objectives available before students undertake the activity will guide what occurs during the simulation. Objectives are necessary to define successful achievement of the learning experience. They also help determine whether mannequins or actors are needed and the technology that is required (Lioce et al., 2013). In other words, the required learning outcomes direct the selection of simulation style used (Tosterud et al., 2013). However, some objectives may not be available to students until after the scenario has been concluded. For example, in a scenario about a deteriorating patient, students may be given an objective regarding managing the patient, but they may not be given an objective that provides answers or gives clues that enable them to easily recognise the problem. These 'hidden' objectives are available to facilitators.

Facilitation style

There are many ways in which the simulation experience can be facilitated; the specific facilitation style is determined by the learning requirements of students and the objectives. The facilitation style should be adjusted according to individual and cultural differences that determine comprehension, abilities and behaviours (Franklin et al., 2013). This is

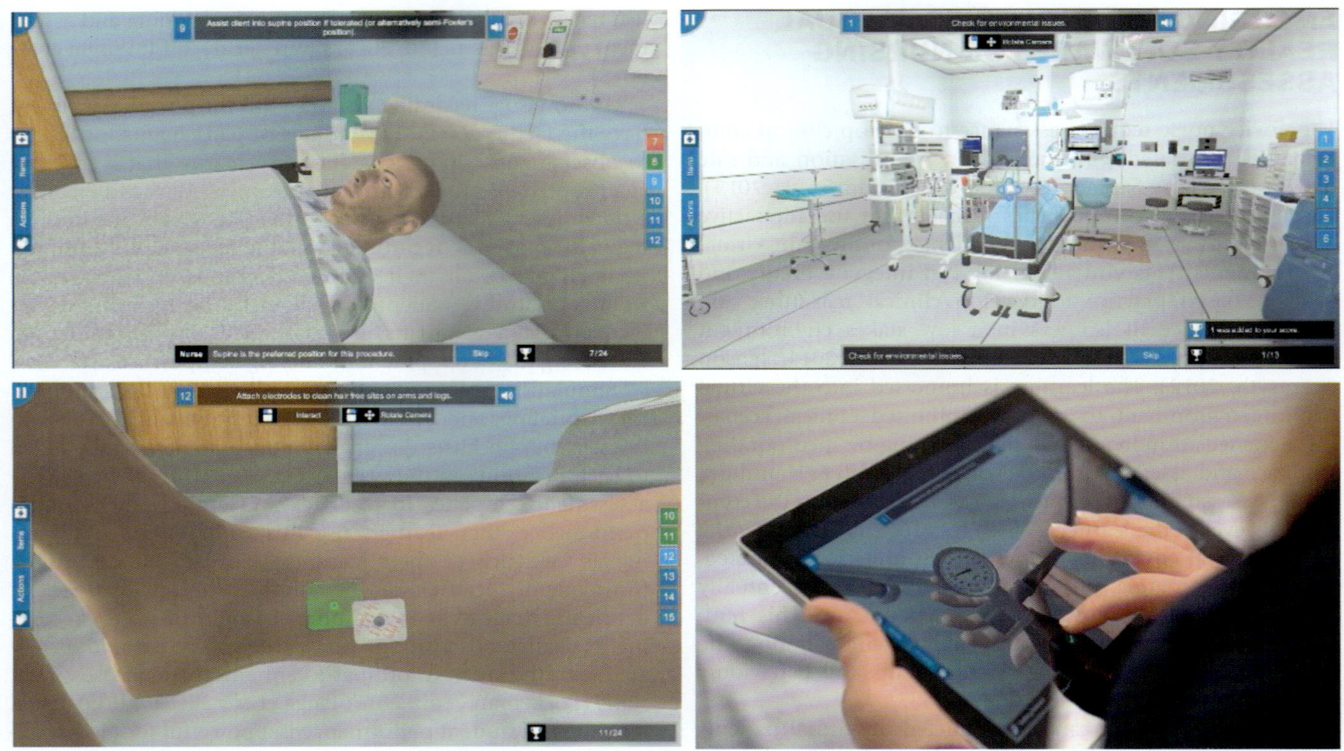

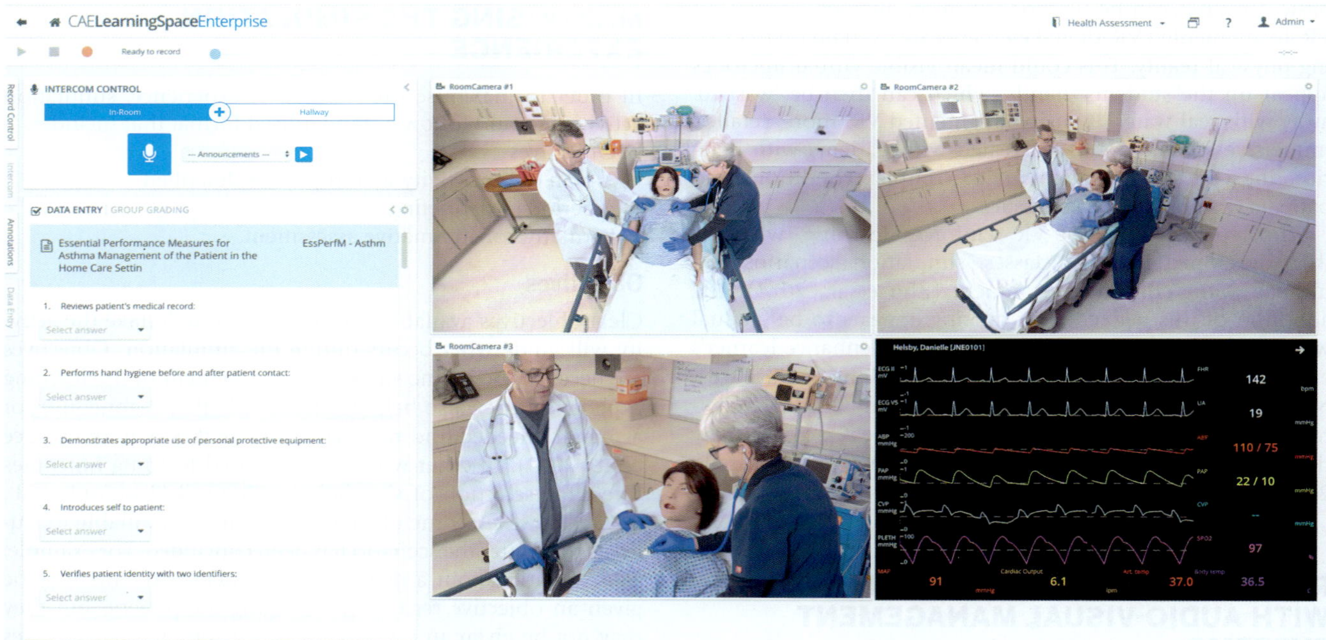

FIGURE 39-10 Simulation technologies and techniques. (Images courtesy of ETRAIN Interactive. Provided by QUT Clinical Simulation Centre.)

particularly valuable for students for whom English is a second language or who come from a culture different from the facilitator.

Debriefing

Debriefing is one of the most important parts of simulation learning (Dufrene & Young, 2014; Levett-Jones & Lapkin, 2014) because of its ability to promote student learning (Decker et al., 2013) and to give students feedback about their communication style (Yoder-Wise, 2013). Learning depends on the process of reflection to lead to new understanding, so all simulated learning experiences should incorporate a debriefing period that stimulates reflection. Debriefing is guided by the facilitator, who supports students to transfer their simulation

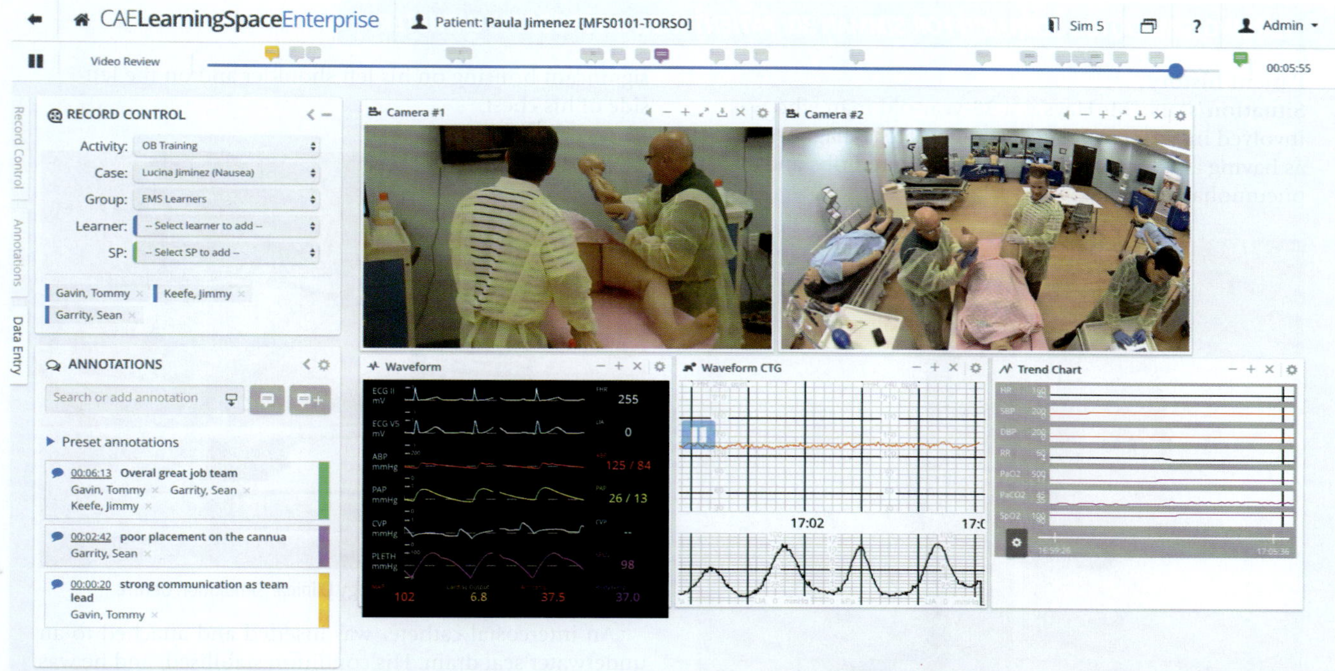

FIGURE 39-11 Simulation technologies and techniques. (Image courtesy of QUT – Clinical Simulation Centre and CAE Healthcare, CAE Learning Space Enterprise.)

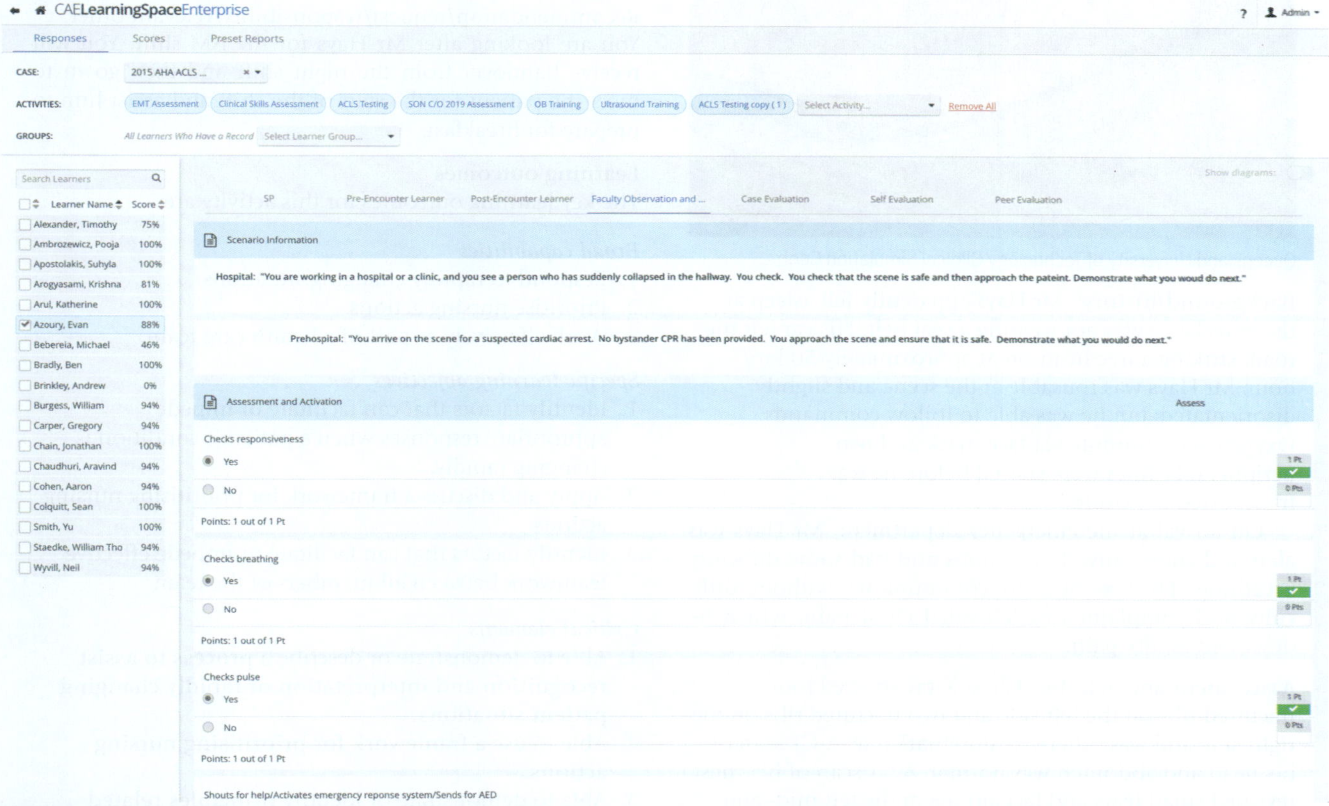

FIGURE 39-12 Simulation technologies and techniques. (Image courtesy of QUT – Clinical Simulation Centre and CAE Healthcare, CAE Learning Space Enterprise.)

experiences into concrete behaviours (McAllister et al., 2013). Facilitators will also point out any errors that occurred during the scenario and guide students to learn from them.

The following scenario is an example of what students can expect to experience in a high-fidelity simulation. The scenario for Mr Hays is planned so that the simulator is programmed with physiological or pathological conditions. The nurse educator can alter the simulator in response to students' clinical decisions and behaviours; consequently, Mr Hays's condition will improve or deteriorate based on students' actions.

NURSING SIMULATION SCENARIO FOR SIMMAN 3G: PATIENT WITH INTERCOSTAL CATHETER

Patient history

Situation/stats: Mr Hays is a 33-year-old man who was involved in a car crash late last night. He is diagnosed as having a pulmonary contusion, fractured ribs and a pneumohaemothorax.

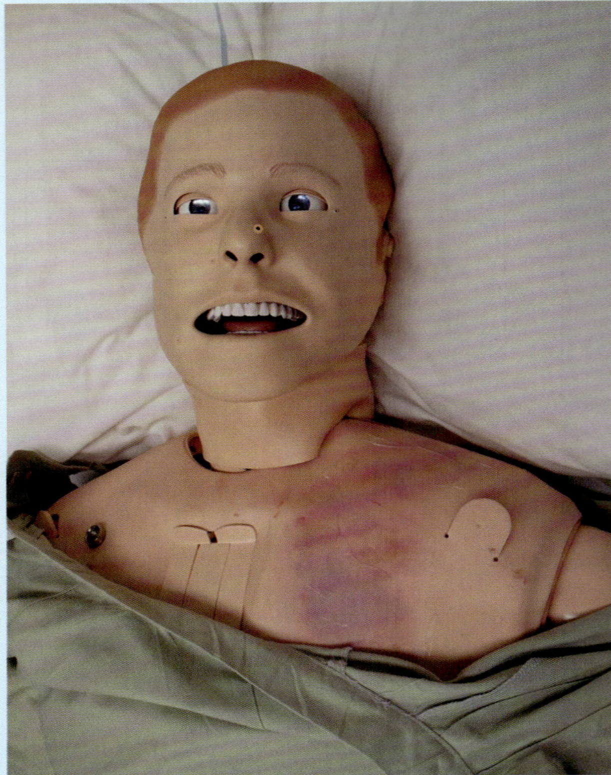

Queensland University of Technology Clinical Simulation Centre.

Background/history: Mr Hays apparently fell asleep at the wheel and was not wearing a seat belt. His car left the road, striking a tree head-on at approximately 50 km/hour. Mr Hays was rousable at the scene and slightly disorientated, but he was able to follow commands. Oxygen at 6 L/minute via face mask and two peripheral IV lines were started before he was transported to hospital.

On arrival at the emergency department, Mr Hays was alert and cooperative but anxious and had some difficulty breathing. He was able to communicate without difficulty and complained of left-sided chest pain, which he described as 'rib' pain.

Assessment and actions: Chest X-ray showed four fractured ribs on the left side and two fractured ribs on the right side and was otherwise unremarkable. A CT scan of his head and abdomen was normal. A CT scan of his chest revealed small tears and lacerations in the left mid- and lower lobes and a left-sided pneumothorax. ECG revealed sinus tachycardia and no other abnormalities. He has significant bruising on his left shoulder and on the left side of his chest.

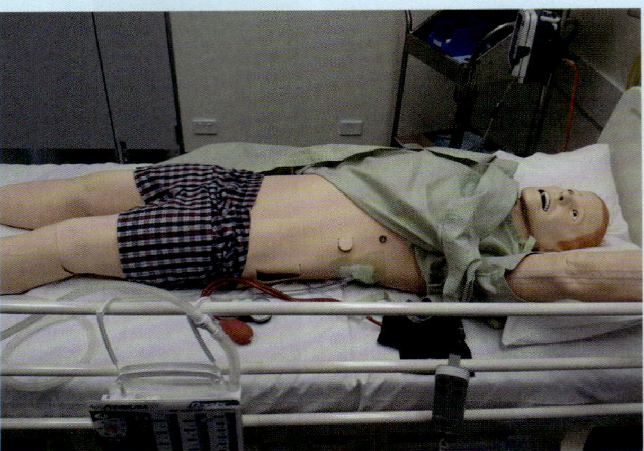

Queensland University of Technology Clinical Simulation Centre.

An intercostal catheter was inserted and attached to an underwater seal drain. His condition stabilised, and he was transferred to our surgical ward. Mr Hays has no previous medical history. He is a smoker and his previous injuries include several broken bones due to motorcycle accidents.

Recommendation/request/responsibility/relevant other: You are looking after Mr Hays for the AM shift. You will receive handover from the night shift and then go in to meet the patient for the start of the shift and assist him to prepare for breakfast.

Learning outcomes

The key learning outcomes for this activity are:

Broad capabilities

1. Respond to rapidly changing situations.
2. Prioritise nursing actions.
3. Work effectively as part of a health care team.

Specific learning objectives

1. Identify factors that can facilitate or impede appropriate responses when a patient's condition is changing rapidly.
2. Apply and discuss a framework for prioritising nursing actions.
3. Identify factors that can facilitate or impede effective teamwork between all members of the team.

Critical elements

1. Able to demonstrate or describe a **process to assist recognition and interpretation of rapidly changing patient situations.**
2. Able to use a **framework for prioritising nursing actions.**
3. Able to demonstrate or identify **principles related to effective teamwork in rapidly changing patient situations.**

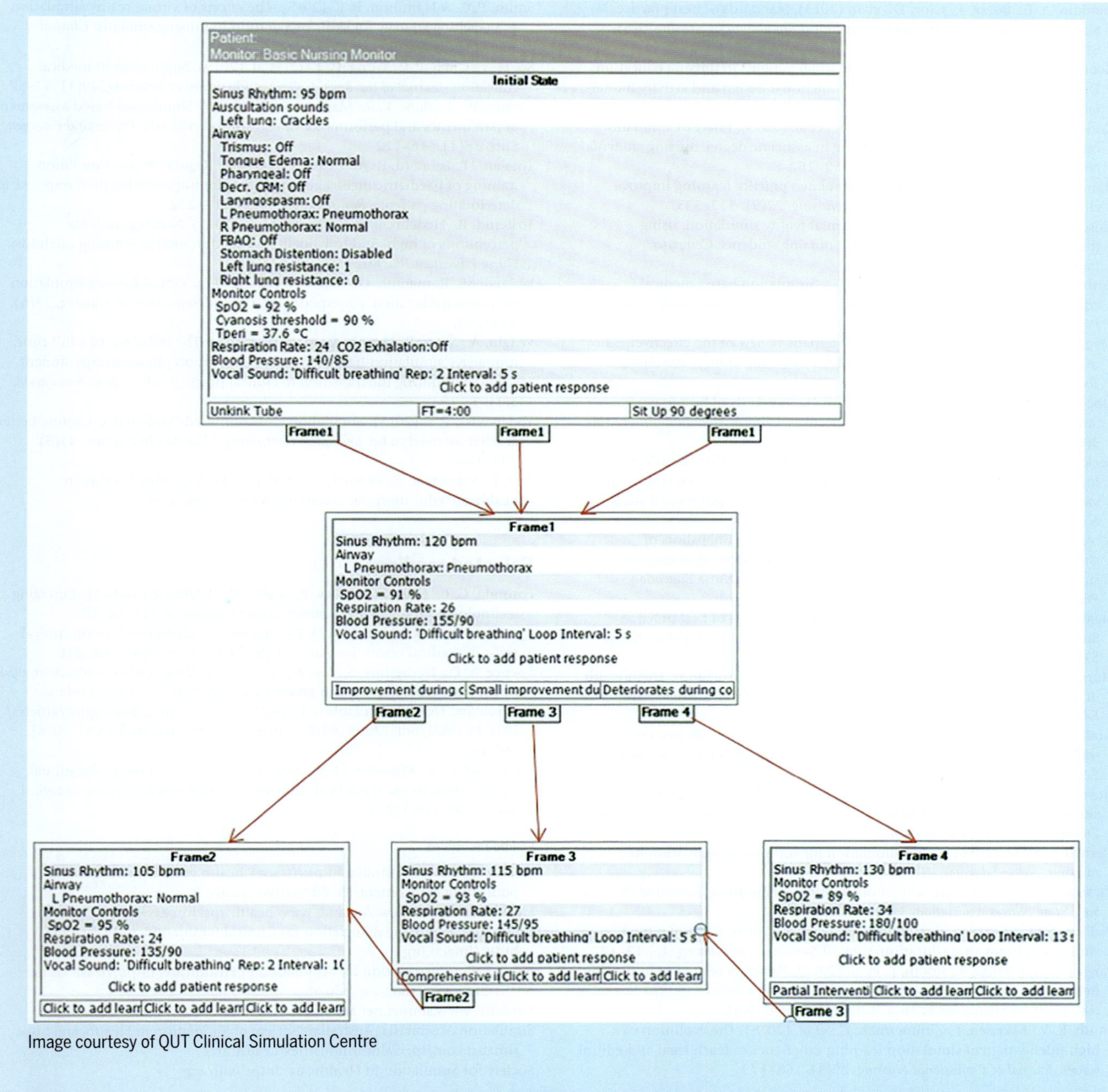

Image courtesy of QUT Clinical Simulation Centre

References

Aebersold, M. & Tschannen, D. (2013). Simulation in nursing practice: The impact on patient care. *Online Journal of Issues in Nursing, 18*(2), 6.

Ali, A. A. & Miller, E. T. (2018). Effectiveness of video-assisted debriefing in health education. *An Integrative Review Journal of Nursing Education, 57*(1), 14–20.

Bensfield, L. A., Olech, M. J. & Horsley, T. L. (2012). Simulation for high-stakes evaluation in nursing. *Nurse Educator, 37*(2), 71–74.

Borg Sapiano, A., Sammut, R. & Trapanib, J. (2018). The effectiveness of virtual simulation in improving student nurses' knowledge and performance during patient deterioration: A pre and post test design. *Nurse Education Today, 62*, 128–133.

Butt, A. L., Kardong-Edgren, S. & Ellertson, A. (2016). Using game-based virtual reality with haptics for skill acquisition. *Clinical Simulation in Nursing, 16*, 25–32.

Cant, R. P. & Cooper, S. J. (2017). Use of simulation-based learning in undergraduate nurse education: An umbrella systematic review. *Nurse Education Today, 49*, 63–71.

Decker, S., Fey, M., Sideras, S., et al. (2013). Standards of best practice: Simulation standard VI: The debriefing process. *Clinical Simulation in Nursing, 9*(6), S26–S29.

Dufrene, C. & Young, A. (2014). Successful debriefing—Best methods to achieve positive learning outcomes: A literature review. *Nurse Education Today, 34*(3), 372–376.

Fisher, D. & King, L. (2013). An integrative literature review on preparing nursing students through simulation to recognise and respond to the deteriorating patient. *Journal of Advanced Nursing, 69*(11), 2375–2388.

Foronda, C. L. & Bauman, E. B. (2014). Strategies to incorporate virtual simulation in nurse education. *Clinical Simulation in Nursing, 10*(1), 412–418.

Franklin, A. E., Boese, T., Gloe, D., et al. (2013). Standards of best practice: Simulation standard IV: Facilitation. *Clinical Simulation in Nursing, 9*(6), S19–S21.

Georg, C. & Zary, N. (2014). Web-based virtual patients in nursing education: Development and validation of theory-anchored design and activity models. *Journal of Medical Internet Research, 16*(4), e105.

Goodstone, L., Goodstone, M. S., Cino, K., et al. (2013). Effect of simulation on the development of critical thinking in associate degree nursing students. *Nursing Education Perspectives, 34*(3), 159–162.

Handley, R. & Dodge, N. (2013). Can simulated practice learning improve clinical competence? *British Journal of Nursing, 22*(9), 529–535.

Jenson, C. E. & Forsyth, D. M. (2012). Virtual reality simulation: using three-dimensional technology to teach nursing students. *Computer, Informatics, Nursing, 30*(6), 312–318.

Kothari, L. G., Shah, K. & Barach, P. (2017). Simulation based medical education in graduate medical education training and assessment programs. *Progress in Pediatric Cardiology, 44*, 33–42.

Levett-Jones, T. & Lapkin, S. (2014). A systematic review of the effectiveness of simulation debriefing in health professional education. *Nurse Education Today, 34*(6), e58–e63.

Lioce, L., Reed, C. C., Lemon, D., et al. (2013). Standards of best practice: Simulation standard III: Participant objectives. *Clinical Simulation in Nursing, 9*(6), S15–S18.

Lockeman, K. S., Appelbaum, N. P., Dow, A. W., et al. (2017). The effect of an interprofessional simulation-based education program on perceptions and stereotypes of nursing and medical students: A quasi-experimental study. *Nurse Education Today, 58*, 32–37.

McAllister, M., Levett-Jones, T., Downer, T., et al. (2013). Snapshots of simulation: Creative strategies used by Australian educators to enhance simulation learning experiences for nursing students. *Nurse Education Practice, 13*(6), 567–572.

Meakim, C., Boese, T., Decker, S., et al. (2013). Standards of best practice: Simulation standard I: Terminology. *Clinical Simulation in Nursing, 9*(6S), S3–S11.

Murray, D. J. & Boulet, J. R. (2012). Simulation-based curriculum: The breadth of applications in graduate medical education. *Journal of Graduate Medical Education, 4*(4), 549–550.

Noureldin, Y. A., Lee, J. Y., McDougall, E. M., et al. (2018). Competency-based training and simulation: Making a 'Valid' argument. *Journal of Endourology, 32*(2), 84–93.

Noveanu, J., Amsler, F., Ummenhofer, W., et al. (2017). Assessments of simulated emergency scenarios: Are trained observers necessary? *Prehospital Emergency Care, 21*(4), 511–524.

Oermann, M. H. (2016). Using simulation for summative evaluation in nursing. *Nurse Educator, 41*(3), 133.

Pacsi, A. L. (2008). Human simulators in nursing education. *Journal of the New York State Nurses Association, 39*(2), 8–11.

Padilha, J. M., Machado, P. P., Ribeiro, A. L., et al. (2018). Clinical virtual simulation in nursing education. *Clinical Simulation in Nursing, 15*, 13–18.

Paige, J. T., Fairbanks, T., Rollin, J., et al. (2018). Priorities related to improving healthcare safety through simulation. Simulation in healthcare. *The Journal of the Society for Simulation in Healthcare, 13*(3S), S41–S50.

Smith, K. V., Klaassen, J., Zimmerman, C., et al. (2013). The evolution of a high-fidelity patient simulation learning experience to teach legal and ethical issues. *Journal of Professional Nursing, 29*(3), 168–173.

Smith, P. C. & Hamilton, B. K. (2015). The effects of virtual reality simulation as a teaching strategy for skills preparation in nursing students. *Clinical Simulation in Nursing, 11*(1), 52–58.

So, H. Y., Chen, P. P., Wong, G. K. C., et al. (2019). Simulation in medical education. *Journal of the Royal College of Physicians of Edinburg, 49*(1), 52–57.

Tavares, W., LeBlanc, V. R., Mausz, J., et al. (2014). Simulation-based assessment of paramedics and performance in real clinical contexts. *Prehospital Emergency Care, 18*(1), 116–122.

Theilen, U., Leonard, P., Jones, P., et al. (2013). Regular in situ simulation training of paediatric medical emergency team improves hospital response to deteriorating patients. *Resuscitation, 84*(2), 218–222.

Tosterud, R., Hedelin, B. & Hall-Lord, M. L. (2013). Nursing students' perceptions of high- and low-fidelity simulation used as learning methods. *Nurse Education Practice, 13*(4), 262–270.

Verkuyl, M., Romaniuk, D., Atack, L., et al. (2017). Virtual gaming simulation for nursing education: An experiment. *Clinical Simulation in Nursing, 13*(5), 238–244.

Wright, A., Moss, P., Dennis, D. M., et al. (2018). The influence of a full-time, immersive simulation-based clinical placement on physiotherapy student confidence during the transition to clinical practice. *Advances in Simulation, 3*(1), 3.

Yoder-Wise, P. S. (2013). Simulation and continued competence: Getting better at what we need to be. *Journal of Continuing Education in Nursing, 44*(5), 195–196.

Zhu, E., Hadadgar, A., Masiello, I., et al. (2014). Augmented reality in healthcare education: An integrative review. *PeerJ, 2*, e469.

Selected readings

Foronda, C. L., Alfes, C. M., Dev, P., et al. (2017). Virtually nursing: Emerging technologies in nursing education. *Nurse Educator, 42*(1), 14–17.

Mete, I. & Brannick, M. T. (2017). Estimating the reliability of, nontechnical skills in medical teams. *Journal of Surgical Education, 74*(4), 596–611.

Spence, A. D., Derbyshire, S., Ian, K., et al. (2016). Does video feedback analysis improve CPR performance in phase 5 medical students? *BMC Medical Education, 16*, 203. Available at https://www.ncbi.nlm.nih.gov/pmc/articles/PMC4983021/pdf/12909_2016_Article_726.pdf. (Accessed 3 Oct. 2018). online.

Umscheid, C. A., Maenner, M. J., Mull, N., et al. (2016). Using educational prescriptions to teach medical students evidence-based medicine. *Medical Teacher, 38*(11), 112–1117.

Online resources

Health Workforce Australia: https://www1.health.gov.au/internet/main/publishing.nsf/Content/Health%20Workforce-2

Health Workforce New Zealand: www.healthworkforce.govt.nz

International Nursing Association for Clinical Simulation and Learning: https://inacsl.org

New Zealand Association for Simulation in Healthcare: http://nzash.co.nz

NHET-Sim: www.nhet-sim.edu.au

SimNET: www.simnet.net.au

Simulation Australasia, Australian Society of Simulation in Healthcare: https://simaust.com/specialties/industries/healthcare/

Society for Simulation in Healthcare: http://ssih.org

APPENDIX A

Growth charts

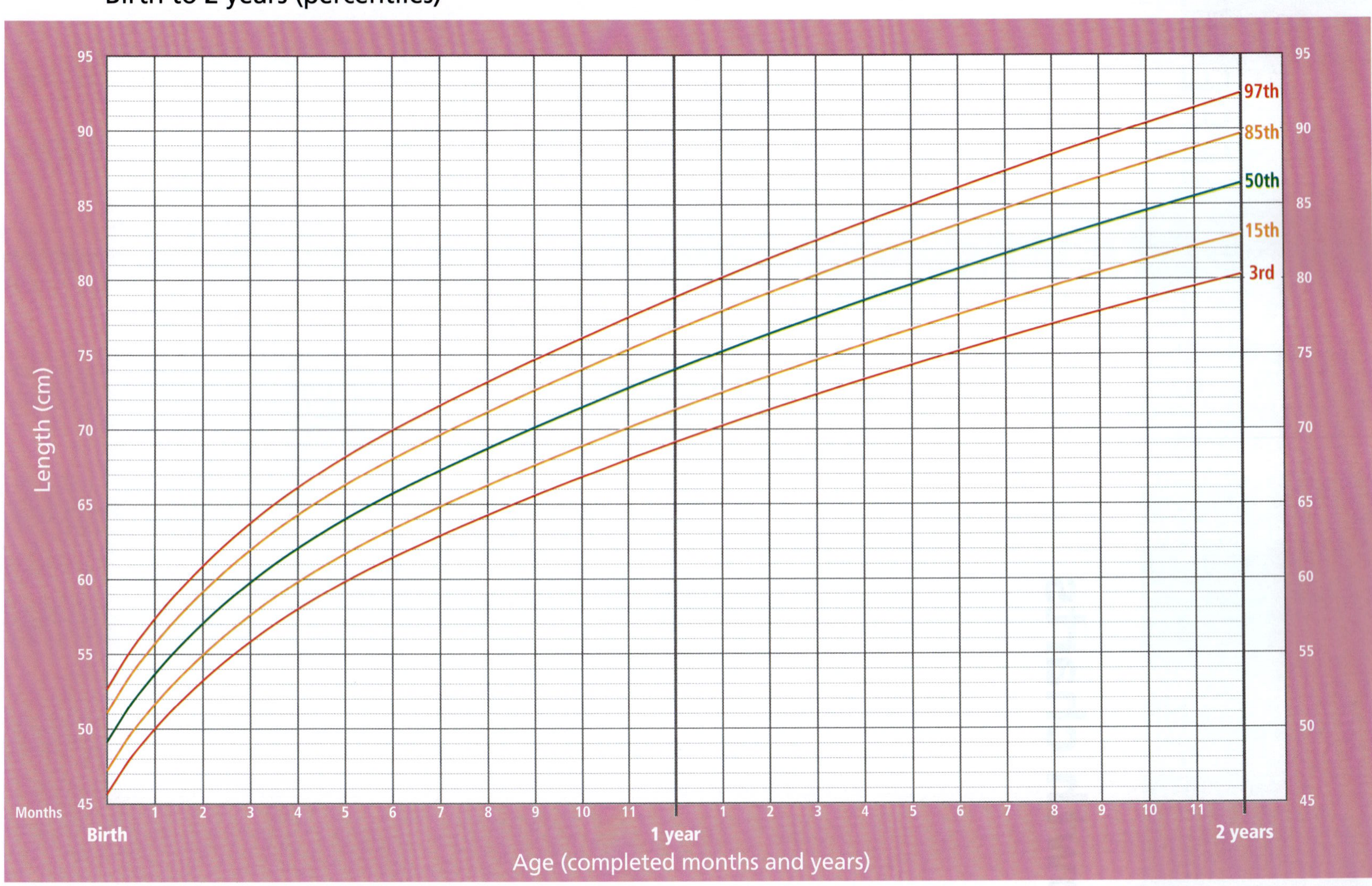

(World Health Organisation Child Growth Standards. © 2019 WHO. Available at https://www.who.int/childgrowth/standards/en/ Accessed 22 Oct. 2019.)

Weight-for-age GIRLS

Birth to 2 years (percentiles)

World Health Organization

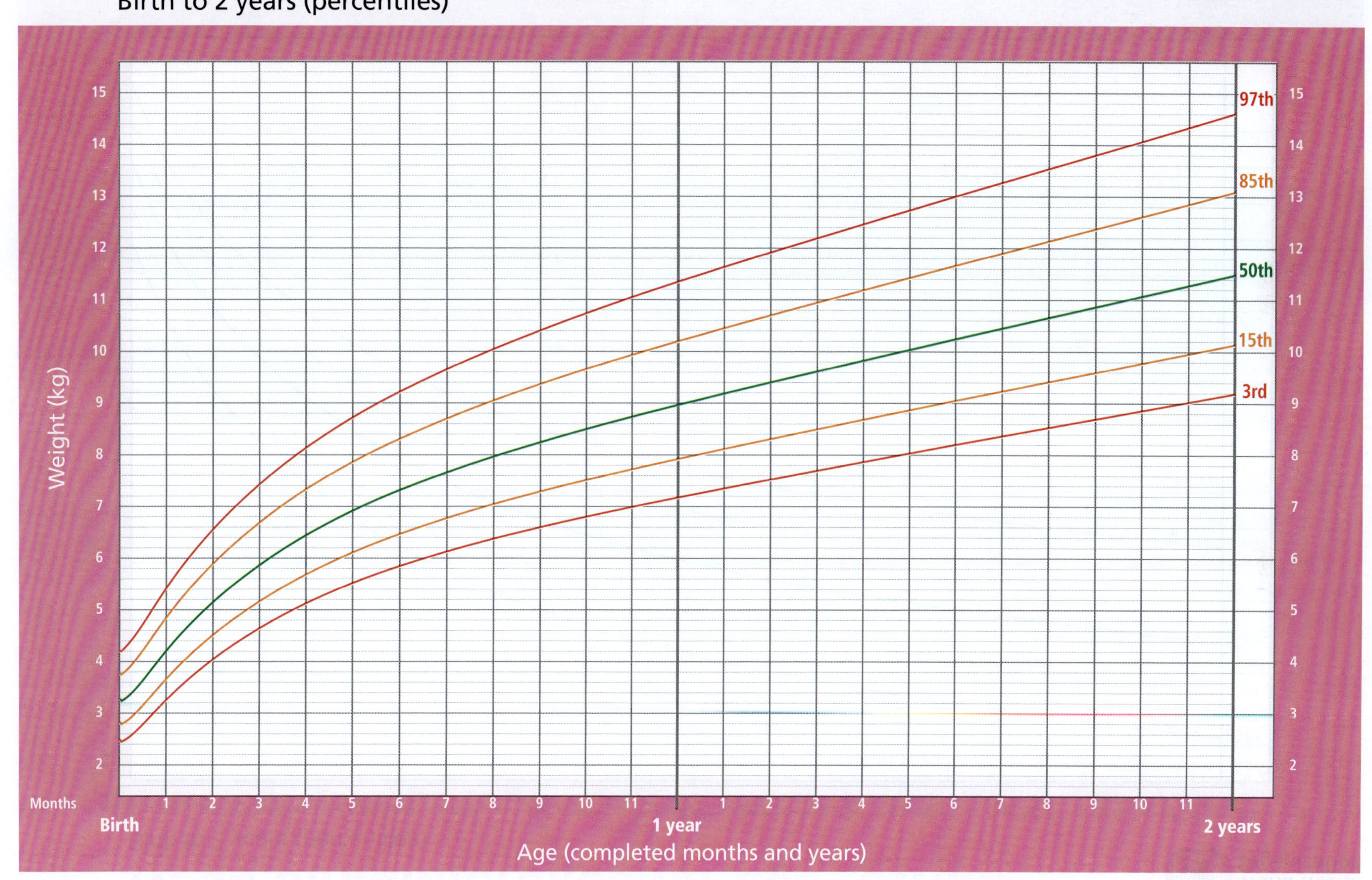

WHO Child Growth Standards

Head circumference-for-age GIRLS

Birth to 2 years (percentiles)

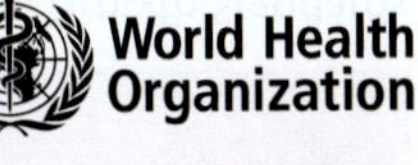
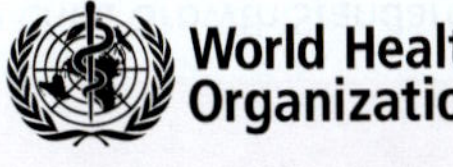

Head circumference (cm)

51 50 49 48 47 46 45 44 43 42 41 40 39 38 37 36 35 34 33 32 31

97th
85th
50th
15th
3rd

Months
Birth 2 4 6 8 10 1 year 2 4 6 8 10 2 years

Age (completed months and years)

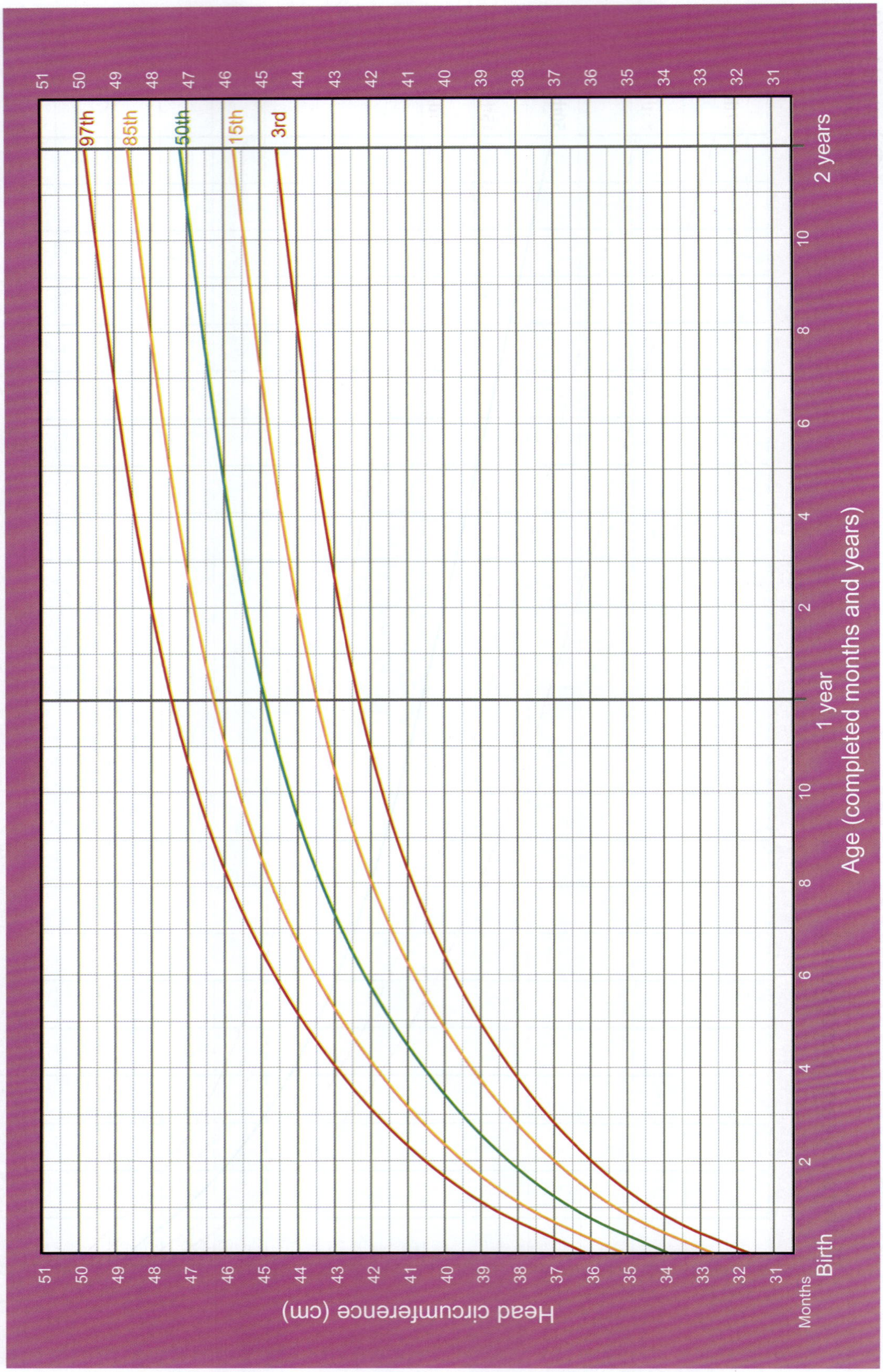

WHO Child Growth Standards

Length-for-age BOYS

Birth to 2 years (percentiles)

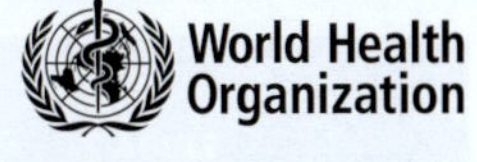

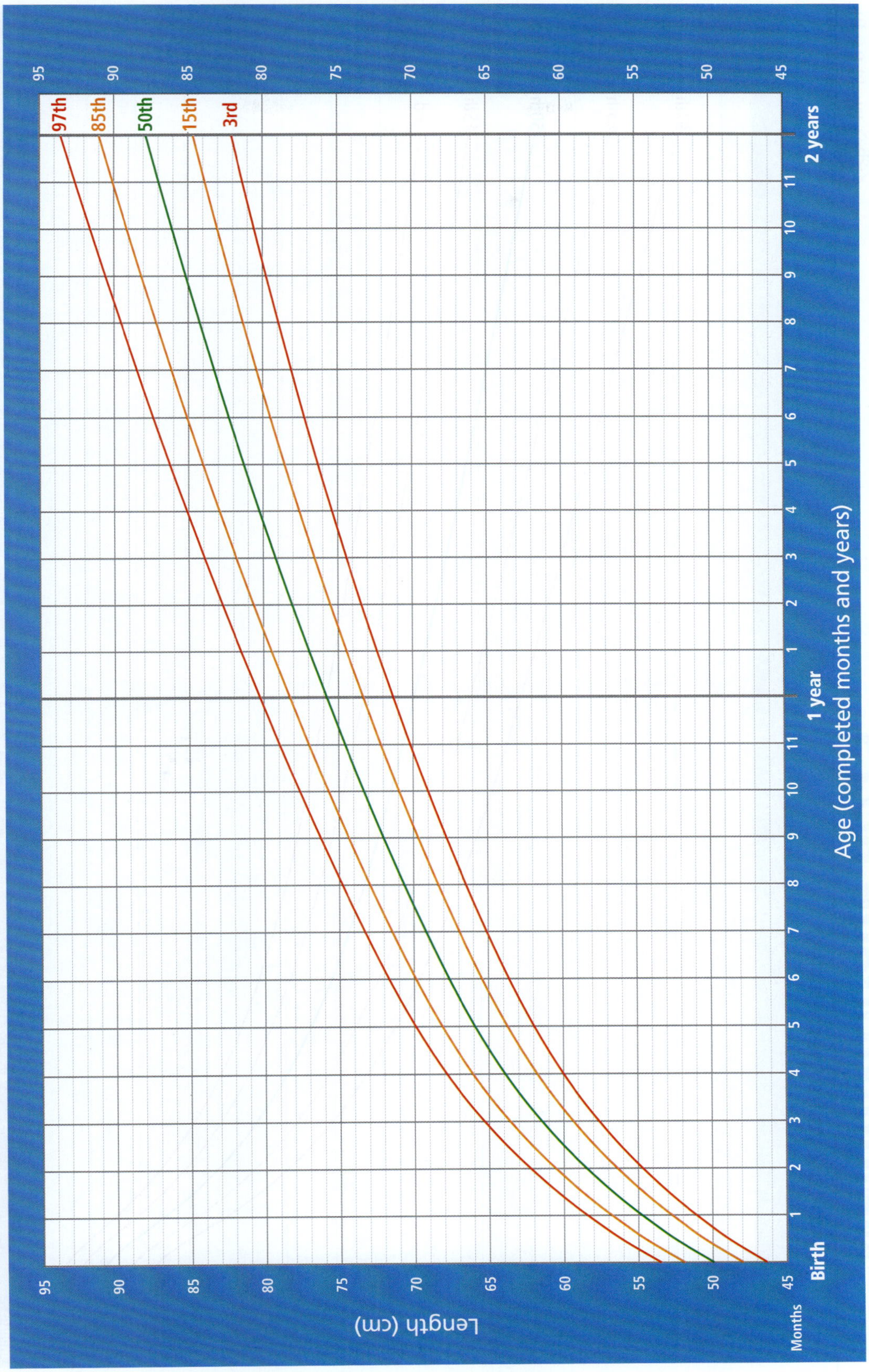

Length (cm)

95
90
85
80
75
70
65
60
55
50
45

97th
85th
50th
15th
3rd

Months
Birth 1 2 3 4 5 6 7 8 9 10 11 1 year 1 2 3 4 5 6 7 8 9 10 11 2 years

Age (completed months and years)

WHO Child Growth Standards

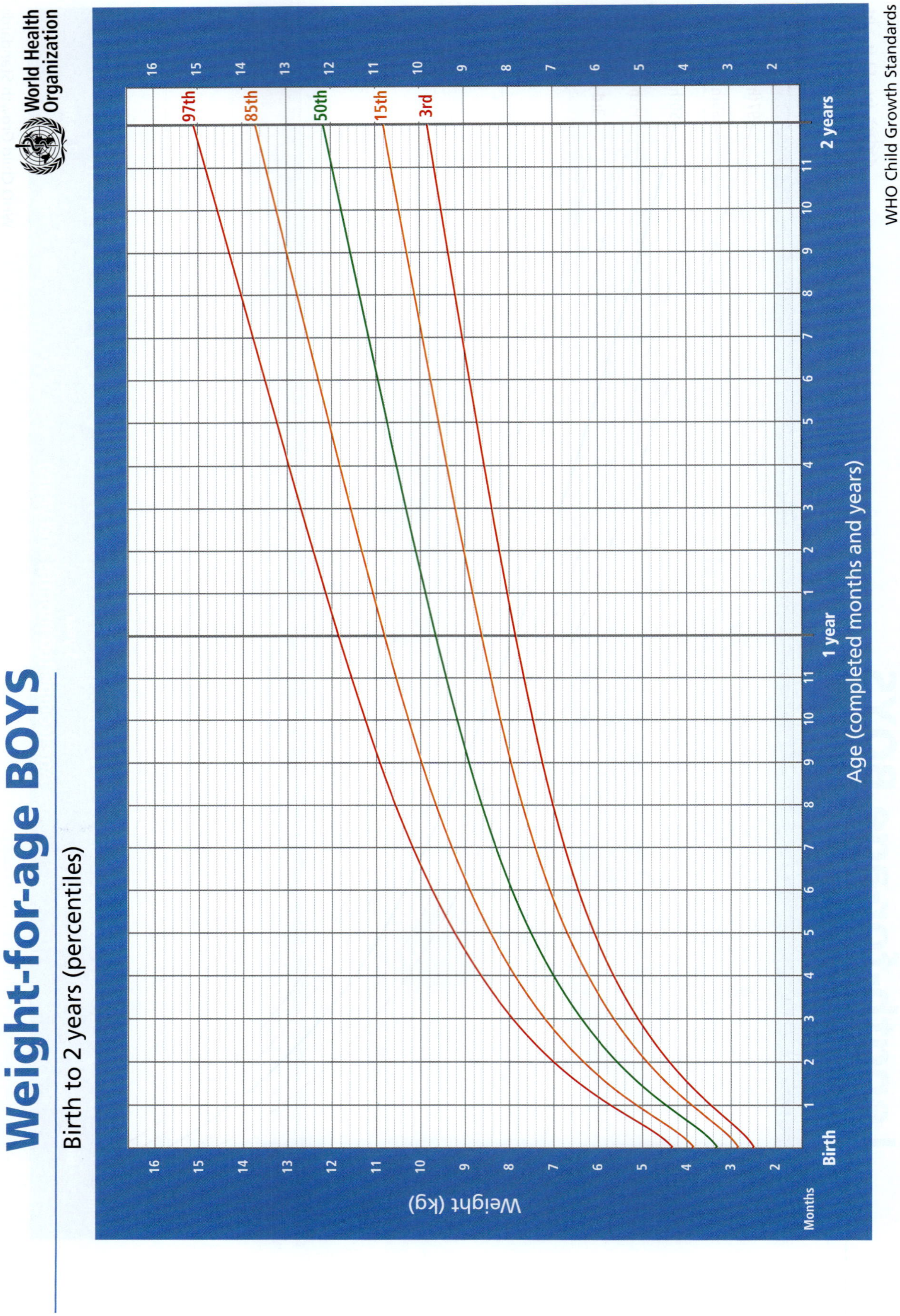

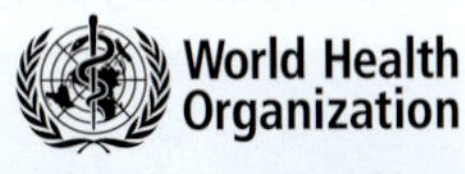

Weight-for-age BOYS

Birth to 2 years (percentiles)

Weight (kg)

16 15 14 13 12 11 10 9 8 7 6 5 4 3 2

97th
85th
50th
15th
3rd

Months
1 2 3 4 5 6 7 8 9 10 11 1 2 3 4 5 6 7 8 9 10 11

Birth
1 year
2 years

Age (completed months and years)

WHO Child Growth Standards

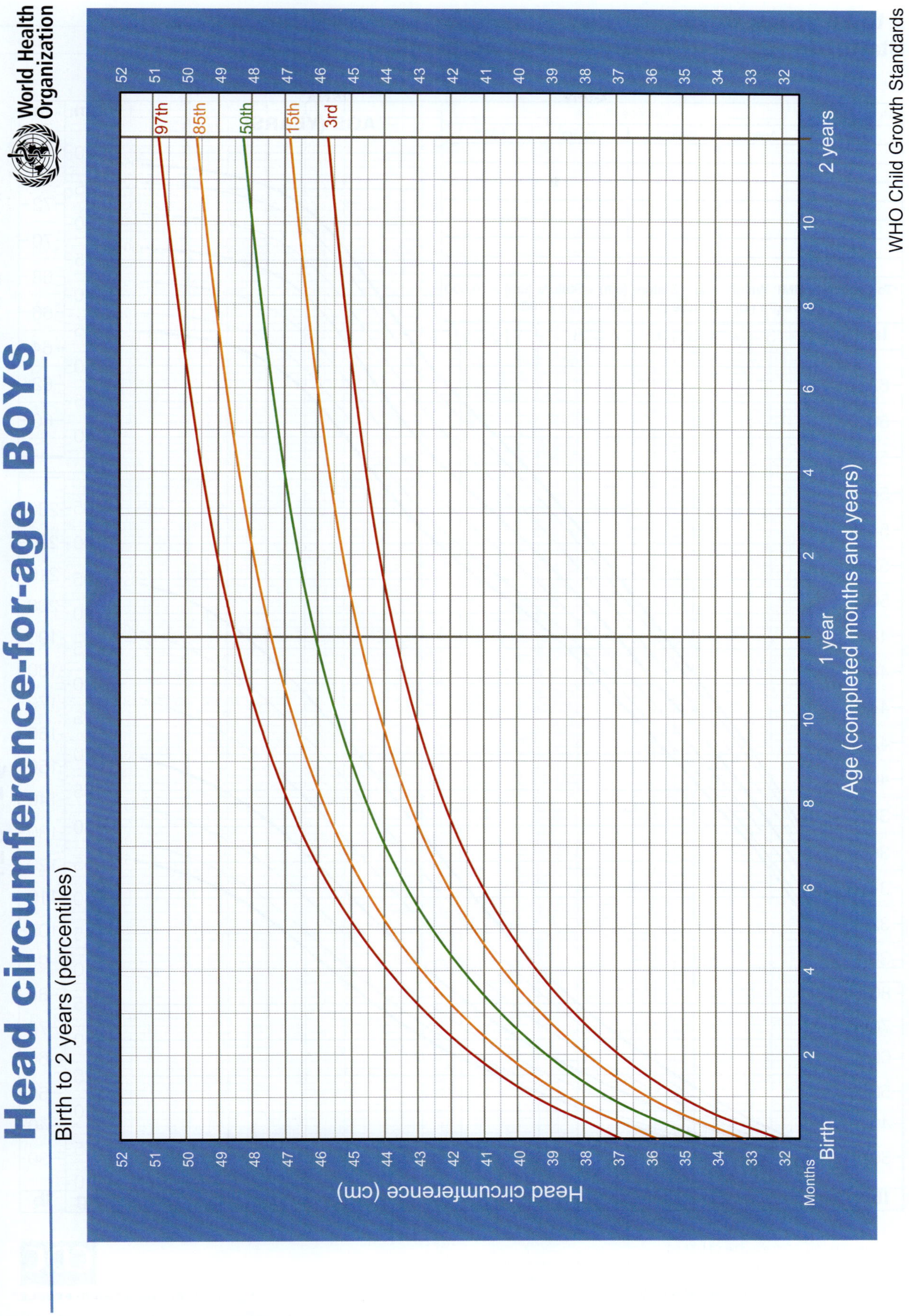

Head circumference-for-age BOYS

Birth to 2 years (percentiles)

World Health Organization

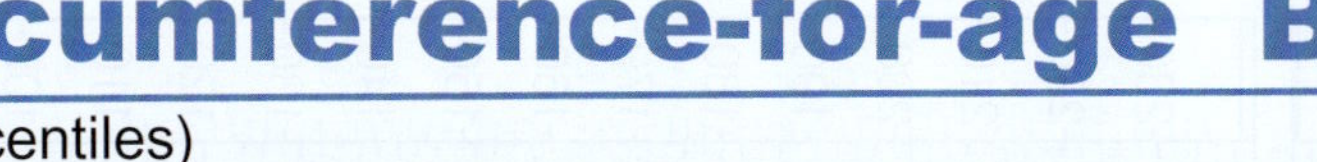

WHO Child Growth Standards

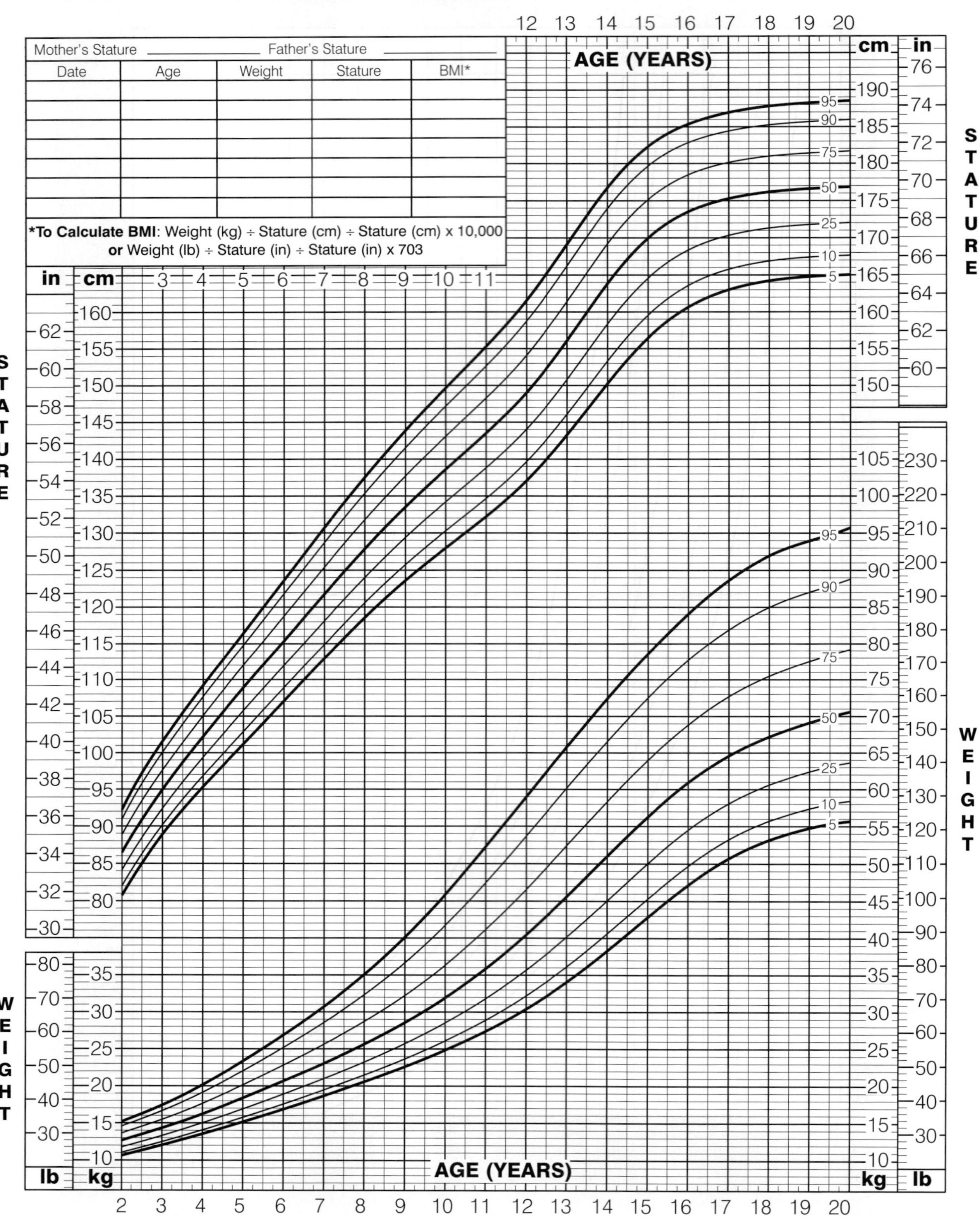

(Developed by the National Center for Health Statistics in collaboration with the National Center for Chronic Disease Prevention and Health Promotion (2000). http://www.cdc.gov/growthcharts Published May 30, 2000 (modified 11/21/00).)

2 to 20 years: Girls
Stature-for-age and Weight-for-age percentiles

NAME ______________________

RECORD # ______________

Mother's Stature ____________ Father's Stature ____________

Date	Age	Weight	Stature	BMI*

***To Calculate BMI**: Weight (kg) ÷ Stature (cm) ÷ Stature (cm) x 10,000
or Weight (lb) ÷ Stature (in) ÷ Stature (in) x 703

AGE (YEARS)

STATURE

WEIGHT

Published May 30, 2000 (modified 11/21/00).
SOURCE: Developed b y the National Center for Health Statistics in collaboration with the National Center for Chronic Disease Prevention and Health Promotion (2000).
http://www.cdc.gov/growthcharts

CDC
SAFER • HEALTHIER • PEOPLE™

(Developed by the National Center for Health Statistics in collaboration with the National Center for Chronic Disease Prevention and Health Promotion (2000). http://www.cdc.gov/growthcharts Published May 30, 2000 (modified 11/21/00).)

2 to 20 years: Boys
Body mass index-for-age percentiles

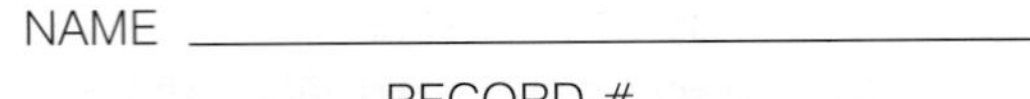

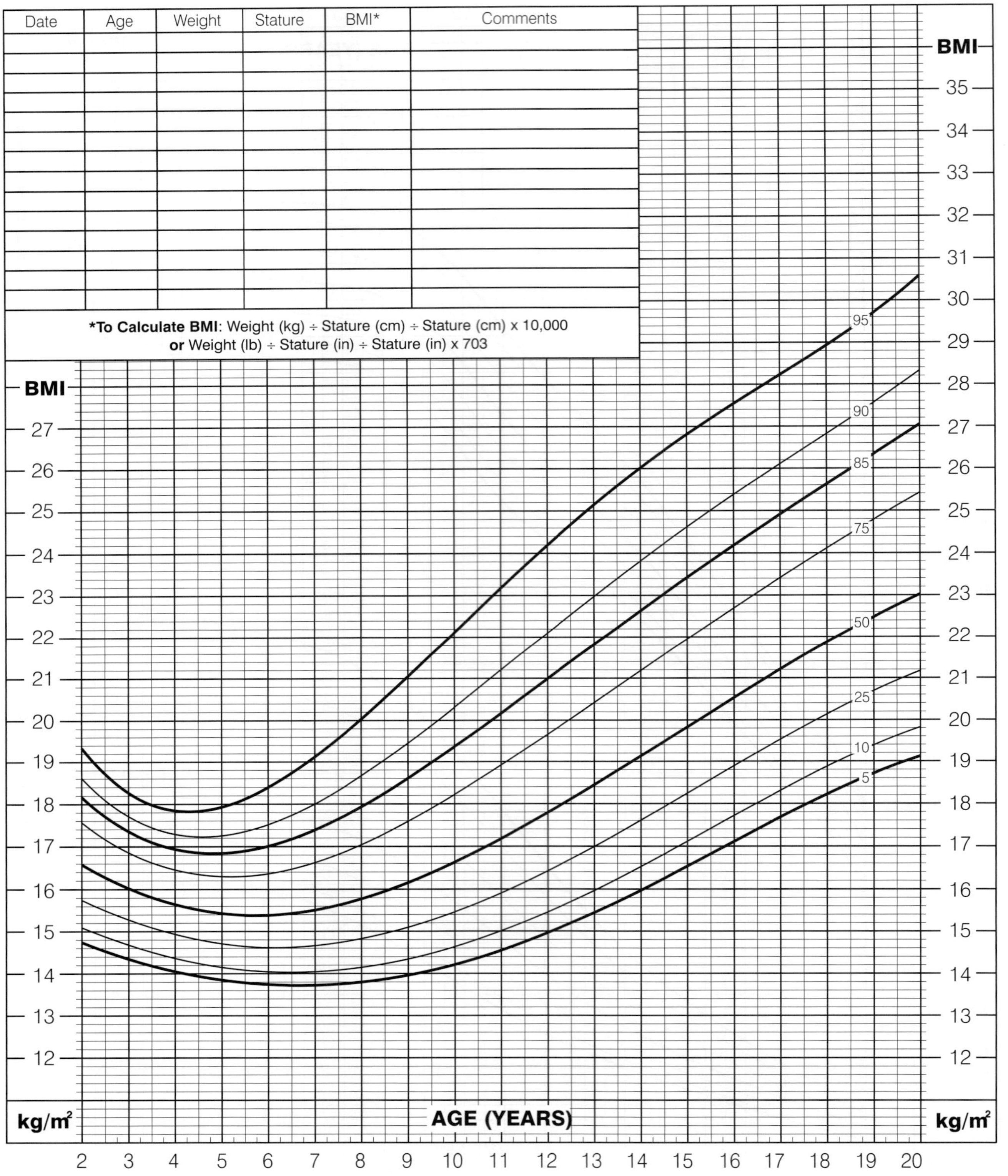

Date	Age	Weight	Stature	BMI*	Comments

***To Calculate BMI**: Weight (kg) ÷ Stature (cm) ÷ Stature (cm) x 10,000
or Weight (lb) ÷ Stature (in) ÷ Stature (in) x 703

BMI

35 34 33 32 31 30 29 28 27 26 25 24 23 22 21 20 19 18 17 16 15 14 13 12

95 90 85 75 50 25 10 5

kg/m²

AGE (YEARS)

2 3 4 5 6 7 8 9 10 11 12 13 14 15 16 17 18 19 20

Published May 30, 2000 (modified 10/16/00).
SOURCE: Developed b y the National Center for Health Statistics in collaboration with the National Center for Chronic Disease Prevention and Health Promotion (2000).
http://www.cdc.gov/growthcharts

CDC
SAFER • HEALTHIER • PEOPLE™

(Developed by the National Center for Health Statistics in collaboration with the National Center for Chronic Disease Prevention and Health Promotion (2000). http://www.cdc.gov/growthcharts Published May 30, 2000 (modified 11/21/00).)

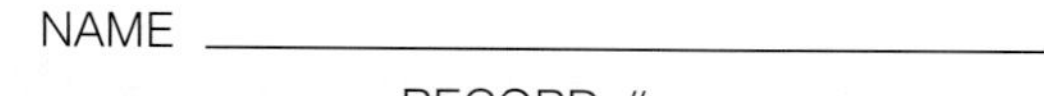

2 to 20 years: Girls
Body mass index-for-age percentiles

NAME ______________________

RECORD # ____________

Date	Age	Weight	Stature	BMI*	Comments

***To Calculate BMI**: Weight (kg) ÷ Stature (cm) ÷ Stature (cm) x 10,000
or Weight (lb) ÷ Stature (in) ÷ Stature (in) x 703

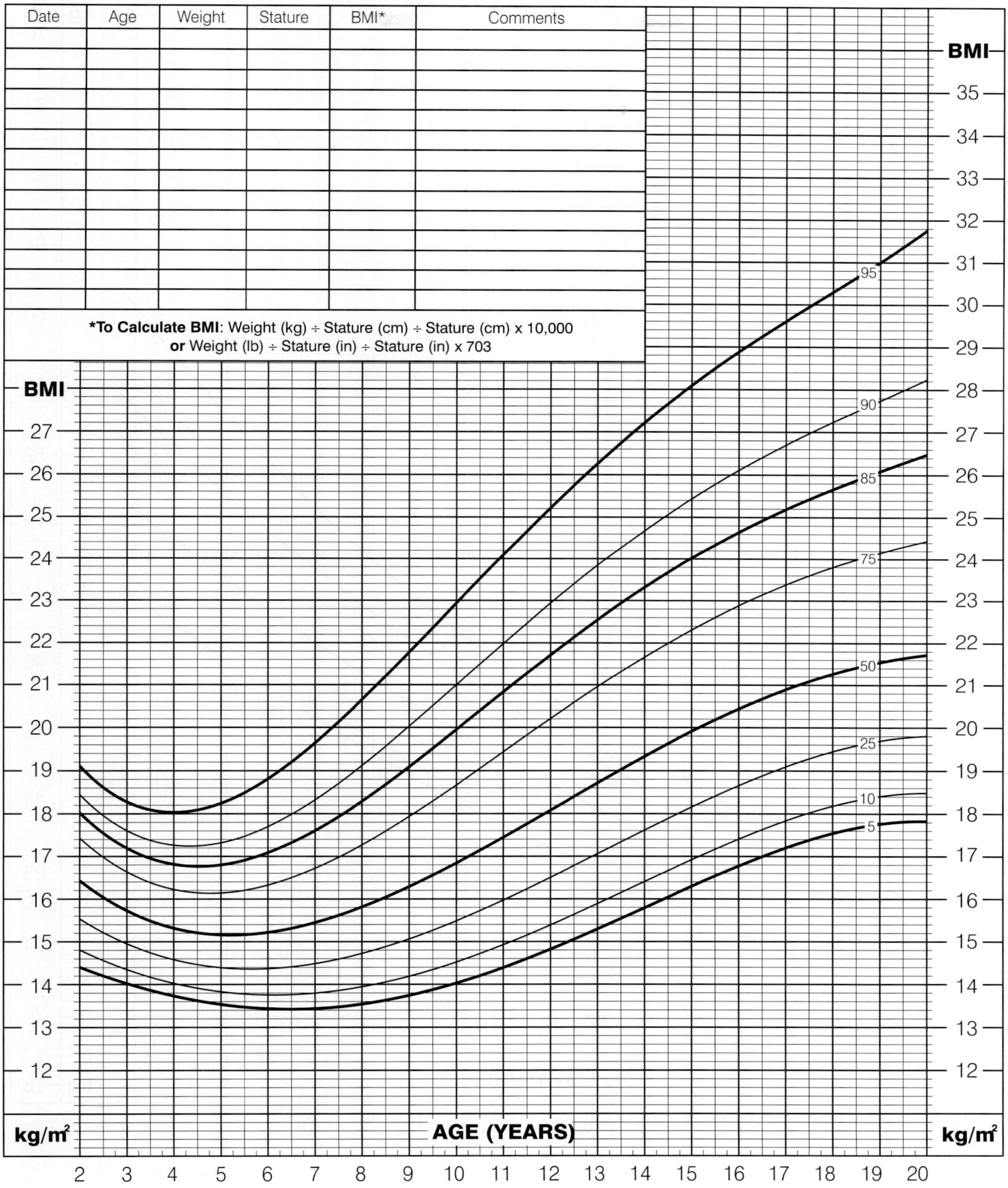

BMI

95
90
85
75
50
25
10
5

35 34 33 32 31 30 29 28 27 26 25 24 23 22 21 20 19 18 17 16 15 14 13 12

kg/m²

AGE (YEARS)

2 3 4 5 6 7 8 9 10 11 12 13 14 15 16 17 18 19 20

Published May 30, 2000 (modified 10/16/00).
SOURCE: Developed b y the National Center for Health Statistics in collaboration with
the National Center for Chronic Disease Prevention and Health Promotion (2000).
http://www.cdc.gov/growthcharts

CDC
SAFER • HEALTHIER • PEOPLE™

(Developed by the National Center for Health Statistics in collaboration with the National Center for Chronic Disease Prevention and Health Promotion (2000). http://www.cdc.gov/growthcharts Published May 30, 2000 (modified 11/21/00).)

NAME ______________

Weight-for-stature percentiles: Boys

RECORD # ______________

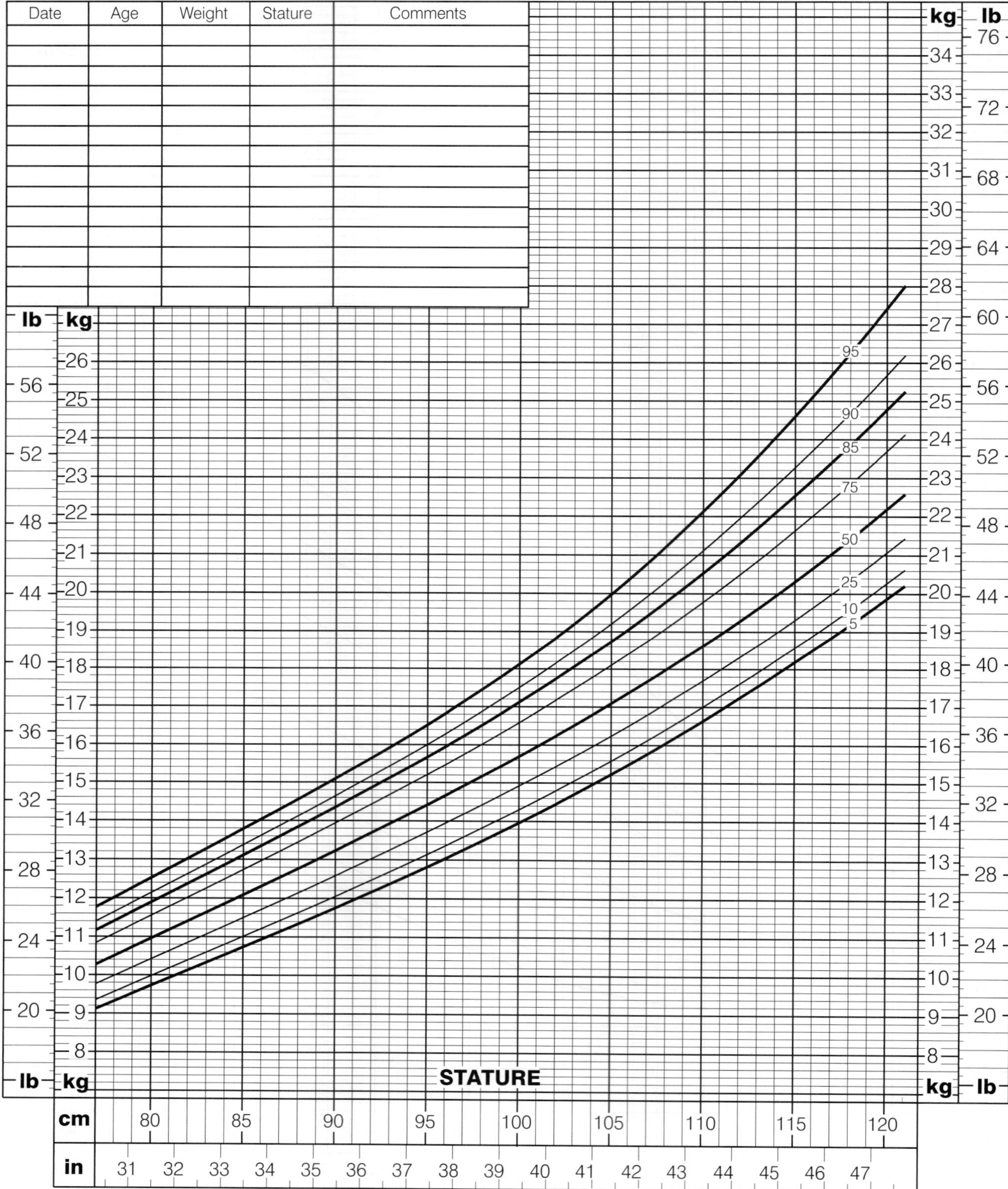

Published May 30, 2000 (modified 10/16/00).
SOURCE: Developed b y the National Center for Health Statistics in collaboration with the National Center for Chronic Disease Prevention and Health Promotion (2000).
http://www.cdc.gov/growthcharts

CDC
SAFER • HEALTHIER • PEOPLE™

(Developed by the National Center for Health Statistics in collaboration with the National Center for Chronic Disease Prevention and Health Promotion (2000). http://www.cdc.gov/growthcharts Published May 30, 2000 (modified 11/21/00).)

NAME ______________________

Weight-for-stature percentiles: Girls

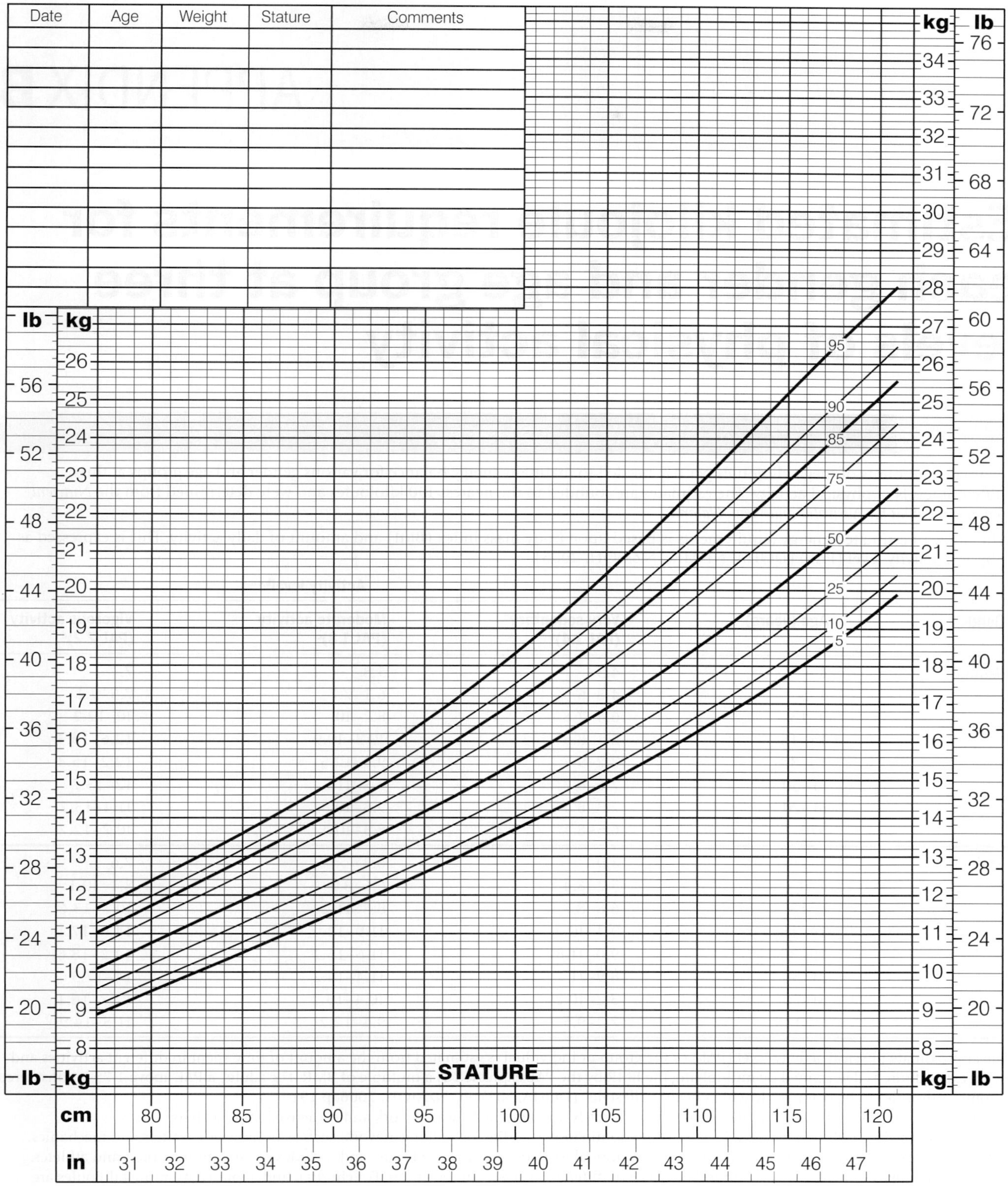

RECORD # ______________

Date	Age	Weight	Stature	Comments

STATURE

Published May 30, 2000 (modified 10/16/00).
SOURCE: Developed by the National Center for Health Statistics in collaboration with the National Center for Chronic Disease Prevention and Health Promotion (2000).
http://www.cdc.gov/growthcharts

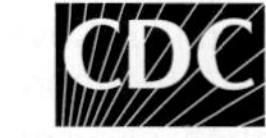

SAFER • HEALTHIER • PEOPLE™

(Developed by the National Center for Health Statistics in collaboration with the National Center for Chronic Disease Prevention and Health Promotion (2000). http://www.cdc.gov/growthcharts Published May 30, 2000 (modified 11/21/00).)

APPENDIX **B**

Estimated kilojoule requirements for each gender and age group at three levels of physical activity

Estimated amounts of mega kilojoules per day needed to maintain energy balance for various gender and age groups at three different levels of physical activity. The estimates are rounded to the nearest 100 kilojoules and were determined from the *Nutrient Reference Values for Australia and New Zealand.*

The range of estimated energy requirements is based upon body mass index (BMI) and amount of daily activity. This is expressed as physical activity level (PAL) (DOHA, NHMRC NZMOH, 2006).

		Activity level[b,c,d]		
Gender	**Age (years)**	**Very sedentary (PAL 1.4)[b]**	**Moderate activity (PAL 1.8)[c]**	**Vigorous activity (PAL 2.2)[d]**
Female	3	4.5	5.8	7.1
	4–8	4.8–6	6.1–7.7	7.5–9.4
	9–13	6.4–7.8	8.2–10	10–12.2
	14–18	8.1–8.5	10.3–10.9	12.6–13.3
	19–30	7.7–9.7	9.9–12.5	12.2–15.3
	31–50	7.6–8.7	9.8–11.2	12–13.7
	51–70	7.3–8.4	9.3–10.8	11.4–13.2
	>70	6.5–8.1	8.3–10.4	10.2–12.7
Male	3	4.9	6.3	7.6
	4–8	5.2–6.4	6.6–8.2	8.1–10.1
	9–13	6.8–8.7	8.8–11.2	10.7–13.6
	14–18	9.3–10.9	11.9–14	14.6–17.1
	19–30	9.0–11.8	11.6–15.2	14.2–18.6
	31–50	8.9–11	11.4–14.2	14–17.3
	51–70	8.2–10.2	10.4–13.2	12.7–16.1
	> 70	7.3–9.5	9.4–12.2	11.5–14.9

"The approximate physical activity level (PAL) of the group or individual is estimated from the amount of time spent in different activities and energy expenditure is determined by multiplying the BMR by the PAL expressed as a multiple of BMR. For adults, a PAL above 1.75 is considered by some authorities to be compatible with a healthy lifestyle" (DOHA, NHMRC NZMOH, 2006, p 19)

b Very sedentary (PAL 1.4) means a lifestyle that is exclusively sedentary with seated work and no active leisure activity.

c Moderately active (PAL 1.8) means a lifestyle of predominantly standing or walking at work, such as housewives, waiters and mechanics.

d Vigorously active means a lifestyle with heavy occupational work or highly active leisure and includes construction workers and athletes.

The kilojoule ranges shown are to accommodate needs of different ages within the group. For children and adolescents, more kilojoules are needed at older ages. For adults, fewer kilojoules are needed at older ages.

Australian Government, Department of Health and Ageing, National Health and Medical Research Council New Zealand Government, Ministry of Health 2006, *Nutrient Reference Values for Australia and New Zealand including Recommended Dietary Intakes*, NHMRC publications. Available online: www.nhmrc.gov.au/_files_nhmrc/file/publications/synopses/n35.pdf. Version 1.2, updated September 2017. CC BY 4.0 International license.

GLOSSARY

A

ADLs—activities of daily living

adrenarche—adrenocortical maturation, which occurs during puberty

adventitious breath sounds—abnormal breath sounds heard during auscultation of the lung fields; may include rales (crackles), rhonchi (wheezes) or pleural friction rubs

alopecia—hair loss

AMB—as manifested by

anorexia—loss of appetite for food

anthropometer—a type of caliper used for measuring elbow breadth and other body parts

anthropometric measurements—measurements of the human body (e.g. height and weight, head circumference, waistline, percentage of body fat, and so forth)

anticholinergic effects—responses to anticholinergic medications, which inhibit the parasympathetic nervous system; in older adults, symptoms are associated with increased or decreased heart rate (depending on dosage), constipation, urinary retention, dilated pupils and vision problems, dry mouth and drowsiness

anxiety—apprehensiveness related to an unknown source; occurs in different degrees

apical impulse—a normal visible pulsation in the area of the midclavicular line in the left fifth intercostal space; impulse can be seen in about half of the adult population

apnoea—cessation of breathing

Argyll Robertson pupils—small, irregular pupils unresponsive to light

arthritis—inflammation of a joint

articulation—place of union or junction between two or more bones of the skeleton

atelectasis—collapse of a lung

atopic—allergic

atrial gallop—low-frequency heart sound known as S_4; occurs at the end of diastole when the atria contract and produced by vibrations from blood flowing rapidly into the ventricles after atrial contraction; S_4 has the rhythm of the word 'Ten-nes-see' and may increase during inspiration

auscultation—assessment technique that uses a stethoscope to hear body sounds inaudible to the naked ear (e.g. heart sounds, movement of blood through the vessels, bowel sounds and air moving through the respiratory tract)

AV—atrioventricular

B

BCP—birth control pills

benign breast disease—non-malignant disease of the breast, such as fibrocystic breast disease

biological variation—changes in physical status as a result of genetics and/or environment and/or the interaction of genetics and environment; human variation of a biological and physiological nature

Biot's respiration—breathing pattern marked by several short breaths followed by long irregular periods of apnoea; may be seen with increased intracranial pressure or head trauma

bipolar disorder—mood disorder categorised as a psychosis and characterised by emotional ups and downs ranging from extreme depression to extreme elation

BP—blood pressure

bradycardia—heart rate less than 60 beats per minute

bradypnoea—slow breathing pattern less than 10 breaths per minute

Braxton Hicks contractions—painless, irregular contractions of the uterus

Brudzinski's sign—flexion of the hips and knees in response to neck flexion; a sign of meningeal inflammation

bruit—abnormal sound; blowing, swishing or murmuring sound caused by turbulent blood flow; heard during auscultation

bruxism—grinding the teeth

Buerger disease—obliterative vascular disease marked by inflammation in small and medium-sized blood vessels

bursa—small sac filled with synovial fluid that lubricates and cushions a joint

C

calcium—chemical element (Ca^{2+}) that is a major component of bone structure and a necessary element for muscle contractions

capillary refill time—time it takes for reperfusion to occur after circulation has been stopped; test for capillary refill involves pressing on a fingernail firmly enough to stop circulation to the digit (signalled by blanching of the underlying tissue), releasing the pressure and measuring the time it takes for colour to return to the tissue; test is used to assess cardiac output

cardiac conduction—process of excitation initiated in the SA node, resulting in contraction of the heart muscle

cardiac cycle—cyclic filling and emptying of the heart
carotid artery—major coronary vessel that transports blood from the heart to the rest of the body
cataract—loss of transparency or presence of cloudiness in the crystalline lens of the eye
Cheyne-Stokes respirations—breathing pattern characterised by a period of apnoea of 10 to 60 seconds, followed by increasing then decreasing rate, followed by another period of apnoea
chloasma—darkening of the skin on the face, known as the 'mask of pregnancy'
chorionic villi sampling (CVS)—test to detect birth defects
closed-ended question—question that can be answered with a yes, no, maybe or other one- or two-word answers; typically used to clarify or specify information contributed in answers to open-ended questions; often begins with the words Are? Do? Did? Is? or Can?
clubbing—enlargement of fingertips and flattening of the angle between the fingernail and nailbed, as a result of heart and/or lung disease
CO—cardiac output
collaborative problems—physiological complications that nurses monitor to detect their onset or changes in status
colonoscopy—internal examination and visualisation of the colon performed by a doctor with a colonoscope—fibre-optic endoscope with a miniature camera attachment
compulsion—repetitive act that the patient must perform and over which he or she has no control
crepitus—a crackling sound/tactile sensation due to air under the skin; may also be heard in joints
critical thinking—complex thought process that has many definitions; in this textbook, critical thinking is best described as a thinking process used to arrive at a conclusion about information that is available; necessary when trying to reason or analyse what a patient's diagnosis is or is not; investigational process or inquiry used to examine data in order to arrive at a conclusion
culture—all verbal and behavioural systems that transmit meaning
culture-bound syndrome—condition or state defined as an illness by a specific cultural group but not interpreted or perceived as an illness by other groups; may have a mental illness component or a spiritual cause
CVA—cerebrovascular accident, stroke
CVS—*see* chorionic villi sampling
cyanosis—bluish or grey colouring of the skin due to decreased amounts of haemoglobin in the blood suggesting reduced oxygenation
cystocoele—herniation of the urinary bladder through the vaginal wall

D

delirium—potentially reversible alteration in mental status that has developed over a short time and is characterised by a change in level of alertness
delusion—false feelings of self that are unreal; may be symptoms of psychotic disorders, delirium or dementia
dementia—diagnostic category that includes multiple physical disorders characterised by slowly deteriorating memory and alterations in abstract thinking, judgement and perception to the degree that the person's ability to perform everyday activities is affected
diastole—period when the heart relaxes and the ventricles fill with blood; in blood pressure measurements, the 'bottom' value represents diastole
diastolic blood pressure—pressure between heartbeats (the pressure when the last sound is heard)
dimpling—indentation or retraction of subcutaneous tissue
direct percussion—direct tapping of a body part with one or two fingertips to elicit tenderness
documentation—committing findings in writing to the patient's record
DRE—digital rectal examination
drug resistance—phenomenon that occurs when microorganisms develop a resistance to the effects of drug therapy, particularly antibiotic therapy
dyskinesia—incoordination marked by darting movements of the tongue and jerking movement of the arms and legs
dysphagia—difficulty swallowing solids or liquids
dystonia—abnormal muscle tone

E

ectopic pregnancy—pregnancy outside of the uterus; also called tubal pregnancy
ectropion—eversion of the lower eyelid
ejection click—high-frequency heart sound auscultated just after S_1; produced by a diseased valve in mid-to-late systole
embryonic milk line—line formed during embryonic development; line starts in the axillary area, runs through the nipple and extends down the abdomen on the outer side of the umbilicus down onto the upper, inner thigh; supernumerary breasts may occur along this line
entropion—inversion of the lower eyelid
epistaxis—nasal bleeding
erythema—redness due to capillary dilation
ethnicity—identification with a socially, culturally and politically constructed group of people with common characteristics not shared by others with whom the group member comes in contact
ethnocentrism—perception that our worldview is the only acceptable truth and that our beliefs, values and sanctioned behaviours are superior to all others
exophthalmos—protruding eyes
extrapyramidal tract—descending pathway of the nervous system outside of the pyramidal tract and responsible for conducting impulses to the muscles for maintaining muscle tone and body control
exudate—any fluid that has exuded out of tissues (e.g. pus)

F

fasciculations—fine tremors
fibroid adenoma—abnormal formation of tissue or tumour of the glandular epithelium-forming fibrous tissue
FOBT—faecal occult blood test; examination of a stool specimen to detect bleeding of unknown origin
fremitus—tactile vibration felt in neck and over the upper thorax from the transmission of vocal sounds from the airways to the surface of the chest wall
friction rub—auscultatory sound resulting from inflammation of the pericardial sac, as with pericarditis
fundus—top of the uterus

G

GCS—Glasgow Coma Scale, an instrument for evaluating level of consciousness

geriatric syndrome—symptoms that are common harbingers of disease and disability in an elderly person

graphaesthesia—ability to identify letters and numbers and drawing by touch and without sight

H

haemorrhoids—varicose veins in the rectum

heart murmur—sounds made by turbulent blood flow through the valves of the heart

hepatomegaly—enlargement of the liver

Homan's sign—aching or cramping pain in the calf felt with passive dorsiflexion of the foot; sign of thrombosis of deep veins in the calf

HR—heart rate

hyperemesis gravidarum—severe and lengthy nausea with pregnancy

I

ICS—intercostal space

illusion—false interpretation of actual stimuli

indirect percussion—also known as mediate percussion; most common percussion method in which tapping elicits a tone that varies with the density of underlying structures (e.g. as density increases, the tone decreases)

induration—hardening

inframammary transverse ridge—firm compressed tissue that may be palpated below the mammary gland in the lower edges of the breasts, especially in large breasts; normal variation and not a tumour

inspection—physical examination technique using the senses (vision, smell and hearing) to observe the condition of various body parts, including normal and abnormal findings

intercostal spaces—spaces between the ribs; the first intercostal space is directly below the first rib, the second intercostal space is below the second rib, and so forth

J

jaundice—yellowness of the skin, eye whites or mucous membranes due to a deposit of bile pigments related to excess bilirubin in the blood; often seen in patients with liver or gallbladder disease, haemolysis and some anaemias

joint—place where two or more bones meet, providing a variety of ranges of motion; a joint may be classified as fibrous, cartilaginous or synovial

jugular veins—major neck vessels that transport blood from the head and neck to the heart

K

keratin—protein that is the chief component of skin, hair and nails

Kernig sign—pain and resistance to extension of the knee in response to flexion of the leg at the hip and the knee; bilateral pain and resistance are signs of meningeal irritation

Korsakoff syndrome—psychosis induced by excessive alcohol use and characterised by disorientation, amnesia, hallucinations and confabulation

kyphosis—abnormally increased forward curvature of the upper spine

L

lanugo—fine, downy hairs that cover newborn's body

leading statement—statement made to elicit more information from the patient; statements may begins with Explain, Describe, Tell or Elaborate

lentigines—benign, spotty, brown skin discolourations, known as age spots or liver spots

lesion—abnormal change of tissue usually from injury or disease

leucoplakia—thick white patches of cells that adhere to oral tissues; condition is precancerous

ligament—strong dense band of fibrous connective tissue that joins the bones in synovial joints

linea nigra—dark line associated with pregnancy that extends from the umbilicus to the mons pubis

lordosis—exaggerated lumbar concavity often seen in pregnancy or obesity

M

macular degeneration (age-related)—thinning or torn membrane in the centre of the retina

mania—hyperexcitation; 'manic' stage of manic–depressive disorder currently known as bipolar disorder

MCL—midclavicular line

melanin—pigment responsible for hair and skin colour

menarche—first menstrual period

mucous plug—clump of mucus that seals the endocervical canal and prevents bacteria from ascending into the uterus

N

nonverbal communication—communication through body language including stance or posture, demeanour, facial expressions and so forth

norms—learned behaviours that are perceived to be appropriate or inappropriate

NSR—normal sinus rhythm

nursing diagnosis—clinical judgement about individuals, family or community responses to actual and potential health problems and life processes; provides the basis for selecting nursing interventions to achieve outcomes for which the nurse is accountable

nystagmus—rhythmic oscillation of the eyes

O

objective data—findings that are directly or indirectly observed through measurements; data can be physical characteristics (e.g. skin colour, rashes, posture), body functions (e.g. heart rate, respiratory rate), appearance (e.g. dress, hygiene), behaviour (e.g. mood, affect), measurements (e.g. blood pressure, temperature, height, weight) or the results of laboratory testing (e.g. platelet count, X-ray findings)

obsession—uncontrollable thought or thoughts that are unacceptable to the patient; characteristic of some neurotic disorders

OD—right eye (from the Latin *oculus dexter*)

oedema—accumulation of fluid in body tissues, which may cause swelling

open-ended question—question that cannot be answered with a yes, no or maybe; usually requires a descriptive or explanatory answer; often begins with the words What? How? When? Where? or Who?
opening snap—extra heart sound occurring in early diastole and resulting from the opening of a stenotic or stiff mitral valve; often mistaken for a split S_2 or an S_3
orthopnoea—difficulty breathing unless in a sitting or standing position; not uncommon in severe cardiac and pulmonary disease
orthostatic hypotension—drop in blood pressure when client arises from a sitting or lying position
OS—left eye (from the Latin *oculus sinister*)
osteoporosis—low bone density that occurs when bone-forming cells cannot keep pace with bone-destroying cells
OU—each eye (from the Latin *oculus uterque*)

P

PAD—peripheral artery disease
pallor—paleness, lack of colour
palpation—examination technique in which the examiner uses the hands to touch and feel certain body characteristics, such as texture, temperature, mobility, shape, moisture and motion
PAOD—peripheral arterial occlusive disease
paralytic strabismus—condition in which eyes deviate from normal position depending on the direction of gaze
parkinsonism—symptoms of Parkinson disease that are secondary to another condition such as cerebral trauma, brain tumour, infection or an adverse drug reaction
Parkinson disease—chronic progressive degeneration of the brain's dopamine neuronal systems that is characterised by muscle rigidity, tremor and slowed movements
percussion—tapping a body chamber with fingers to elicit the sounds from underlying organs and structures
perforator vein—vein that connects a superficial vein with a deep vein; also called communicator vein
pica—a craving for non-nutritional substances such as dirt or clay
pneumothorax—accumulation of air in the pleural space
point localisation—ability to identify points touched on the body without seeing the points touched
polyhydramnios—excessive amniotic fluid associated with multiple gestation or fetal abnormalities
postural hypotension—orthostatic hypotension characterised by dizziness or light-headedness upon rising from a lying or sitting position
praecordium—anterior surface of the body overlying the heart and great vessels
presbycusis—inability to hear high-frequency sounds or to discriminate a variety of simultaneous sounds caused by degeneration of the hair cells in the inner ear
presbyopia—farsightedness; person can see print and objects from further away than considered normal
primary pain—original source of pain
proctosigmoidoscopy—internal examination and visualisation of the sigmoid colon performed by a doctor with a sigmoidoscope—fibre-optic endoscope with miniature camera attachment
prodromal—precursor or early warning symptom of disease (e.g. aura before a migraine headache or seizure)
proprioception—sensory faculties mediated by sensory nerves located in tissues such as the muscles and tendons
prostatic hyperplasia—enlargement of the prostate gland
pruritus—itching
PSA—prostate-specific antigen
pseudodementia—depressive symptoms that are commonly mistaken in the elderly for a dementia
pterygium—thickening of the bulbar conjunctiva that grows over the cornea and may interfere with vision
ptosis—drooping eyelids
ptyalism—excessive salivation
pulse amplitude—strength of the pulse
pyramidal tract—descending pathway of the nervous system; carries impulses that produce voluntary movements requiring skill and purpose

R

range of motion (ROM)—natural distance and direction of movement of a joint
referral problem—problem that requires the attention or assistance of other healthcare professionals besides nurses
referred pain—pain perceived in an area that is not related to its original source (e.g. gallbladder pain may radiate to the right shoulder and pancreatic pain may radiate to the back)
reinforcement technique—presentation of a stimulus so as to modify a response; increasing of a reflex response by causing the person to perform a physical or mental task while the reflex is being tested
retraction—indentation
ruga—wrinkle, or fold of skin or mucous membrane

S

SA—sinoatrial
satiety—fullness, satisfaction commonly associated with meals
scleroderma—degenerative disease characterised by fibrosis and vascular abnormalities in the skin and internal organs
scoliosis—lateral curvature of the spine with an increase in convexity on the side that is curved
splenomegaly—enlargement of the spleen
stereognosis—ability to identify an object by touch rather than sight
sternal retraction—pulling in of sternum during respiration in a physiological attempt to take in more oxygen; seen in hypoxia or air hunger
STI—sexually transmitted infection; previously termed sexually transmitted disease
subjective data—descriptive rather than measurable information; symptoms, sensations, feelings, perceptions, desires, preferences, beliefs, ideas, values and personal information contributed by a patient or other person and verifiable only by the patient or other person
supernumerary nipple—more than two nipples
SV—stroke volume; the volume of blood pumped with each contraction of the heart
synovitis—inflammation of the synovial membrane; synovial membrane surrounds the joint space and contains synovial fluid that lubricates the joint and enhances movement; characterised by painful movement of the joint
system—interacting whole formed of many parts

systole—cardiac phase during which the ventricles contract and eject blood into the pulmonary and circulatory systems

systolic blood pressure—pressure of the blood flow when the heart beats (the pressure when the first sound is heard)

T

tachycardia—heart rate exceeding 100 beats per minute

tachypnoea—rapid, shallow breathing pattern exceeding 20 breaths per minute

temporal event—relating to a particular time of day or activity

tendon—strong fibrous cord of connective tissue continuous with the fibres of a muscle; tendon attaches muscle to bone or cartilage

TENS—transcutaneous electrical nerve stimulation; treatment modality associated with muscle pain, particularly low back pain

thelarche—time during puberty when breasts develop in females

thrill—palpable vibration over the praecordium or an artery; usually the result of stenosis or partial occlusion

TIA—transient ischaemic attack; minor stroke, sometimes called mini-stroke

TMJ syndrome—temporomandibular joint problems; limited range of motion, swelling, tenderness, pain or crepitation in the jaw area

torus palatinus—bony protuberance on the hard palate where the intermaxillary transverse palatine sutures join

trigger factors—factors (e.g. touch, pressure and/or chemical substances) that initiate or stimulate a response such as pain

turgor—normal skin tone, tension and elasticity

U

uterine prolapse—protrusion of the cervix down through the vagina

UTI—urinary tract infection

V

validation—verification

values—learned beliefs about what is held to be good or bad

varicocoele—varicose veins of the scrotum, which feels like a bag of worms upon palpation

venous hum—benign chest sound like roaring water caused by turbulence of blood in the jugular veins; common in children

ventricular gallop—another term for S_3, the third heart sound, which has low frequency and is often accentuated during inspiration; sound has rhythm of the word 'Kentucky' and results from vibrations produced as blood hits the ventricular wall during filling

verbal communication—conversation with words, either spoken or written

viscera (solid, hollow)—internal organs; may consist of solid tissue (e.g. liver) or be hollow to fill with fluids or other substances (e.g. stomach or bladder)

visual field—what a person sees with one eye; field has four parts of quadrants—upper temporal, lower temporal, upper nasal and lower nasal

vital signs—measurable signs of cardiopulmonary and thermoregulatory health status; signs include pulse rate, respiratory rate and character, blood pressure and temperature. (*Note:* Some experts do not consider temperature a vital sign.)

voluntary guarding—person's wilful attempt to protect the body against pain by holding the breath or tightening muscles

INDEX

B

F

I

J

K

N

T

W